Disorders of Voluntary Muscle

Disorders of Voluntary Muscle

Eighth edition

Edited by

George Karpati

David Hilton-Jones

Kate Bushby

Robert C. Griggs

CAMBRIDGE
UNIVERSITY PRESS

CAMBRIDGE UNIVERSITY PRESS
Cambridge, New York, Melbourne, Madrid, Cape Town, Singapore,
São Paulo, Delhi, Dubai, Tokyo

Cambridge University Press
The Edinburgh Building, Cambridge CB2 8RU, UK

Published in the United States of America by
Cambridge University Press, New York

www.cambridge.org
Information on this title: www.cambridge.org/9780521876292

First published 1964, J & A Churchill Ltd
Second edition 1969
Third edition 1974
Fourth edition 1981, Longman Group Ltd
Fifth edition 1988
Sixth edition 1994, Longman Group Ltd
Seventh edition 2001, Cambridge University Press
Eighth edition 2010

Printed in the United Kingdom at the University Press, Cambridge

A catalog record for this publication is available from the British Library

Library of Congress Cataloging-in-Publication Data

Disorders of voluntary muscle / edited by George Karpati … [et al.]. – 8th ed.
p. ; cm.
Includes bibliographical references and index.
ISBN 978-0-521-87629-2 (hardback)
1. Muscles–Diseases. I. Karpati, George. II. Title.
[DNLM: 1. Muscular Diseases. 2. Muscle, Skeletal–physiopathology.
3. Neuromuscular Diseases. WE 550 D612 2010]
RC925.D535 2010
616.7′4–dc22

2009034843

ISBN 978-0-521-87629-2 Hardback

Contents

Contributors

Amelia Evoli
Neuroscience Department, Catholic University,
Rome, Italy

Ami K. Mankodi
Department of Neurology,
Johns Hopkins University,
Baltimore, MD, USA

Ana Ferreiro
INSERM U523,
Institut de Myologie,
Institut Fédératif de Recherche,
Paris, France

Anders Oldfors
Institute of Biomedicine, Sahlgrenska Academy,
University of Gothenburg, Gothenburg, Sweden

Anne K. Lampe

Anneke J. van der Kooi
Department of Neurology,
Academic Medical Centre, University of Amsterdam,
Amsterdam, The Netherlands

Bernard Brais
CHUM Research Centre – Hôpital Notre-Dame,
Laboratoire de neurogénétique de la motricité,
Montreal, Quebec, Canada

Bertrand Fontaine
Assistance Publique-Hôpitaux de Paris,
Reference Center for Muscle Ion Channelopathies,
Groupe Hôpitalier, Pitié-Salpêtrière, Paris, France

Bjarne Udd
Neuromuscular Center,
Tampere University and Hospital,
Tampere, Finland

Carina Wallgren-Pettersson
The Folkhälsan Department of Medical Genetics,
Helsinki, Finland

Caroline A. Sewry
Department of Musculoskeletal Pathology
and Wolfson Centre for Inherited Neuromuscular
Diseases, Robert Jones and Agnes Hunt Orthopaedic
Hospital
NHS Trust, Oswestry, UK
Dubowitz Neuromuscular Centre,
Great Ormond Street Hospital
and Institute of Child Health,
London, UK

Carsten G. Bönnemann
Division of Neurology,
The Children's Hospital of Philadelphia,
University of Pennsylvania School of Medicine,
Philadelphia, PA, USA

Cecilia Jimenez-Mallebera
Neuromuscular Unit,
Department of Clinical Neuroscience,
Charing Cross Hospital,
Imperial College Healthcare NHS Trust,
London, UK
Unitat Patologia Muscular,
Hospital Sant Joan de Deu,
Barcelona, Spain

Chad Heatwole
Department of Neurology,
University of Rochester,
Rochester, NY, USA

Charles A. Thornton
Department of Neurology,
University of Rochester Medical Center,
Rochester, NY, USA

Corrado Angelini
Neurosciences Department,
University of Padova, Italy

David Hilton-Jones
Department of Clinical Neurology,
University of Oxford, Oxford, UK

Doreen Fialho
Department of Neurology,
King's College Hospital NHS Foundation Trust,
London, UK

Duygu Selcen
Mayo Clinic, Department of Neurology,
Rochester, MN, USA

Edward J. Cupler
Neuromuscular Disease Center,
Oregon Health and Sciences University,
Portland, OR, USA

Emma Ciafaloni
University of Rochester,
Rochester, NY, USA

Enrico Bertini
Department of Laboratory Medicine,
Unit of Molecular Medicine,
Bambino Gesù Children's Research Hospital,
Rome, Italy

Eric A. Shoubridge
Montreal Neurological Institute,
Montreal,
Quebec, Canada

Eric Logigian
University of Rochester,
Rochester, NY, USA

Erin O'Ferrall
Neuromuscular Research Department,
Montreal Neurological Institute,
Montreal, Quebec, Canada

Eugenio Mercuri
Academic Medical Centre,
Department of Neurology,
Amsterdam, The Netherlands

Franco Taroni
Department of Diagnostics and Applied Technology,
Fondazione IRCCS Istituto Neurologico "Carlo Besta",
Milan, Italy

Frank L. Mastaglia
Australian Neuromuscular Research Institute,
The University of Western Australia,
Crawley, WA, Australia

Frederic Relaix
Avenir team Mouse Molecular Genetics,
UMR-S 787, INSERM, Institut de Myologie,
Faculté de Médecine Pitié-Salpétrière,
Paris, France

George Karpati
Department of Neurology and Neurosurgery,
McGill University and the Montreal Neurological Institute,
Montreal, Quebec, Canada

Giovanni Meola
Full Professor and Chairman of Neurology
at Department of Neurology,
University of Milan,
IRCCS Policlinico San Donato,
San Donato Milanese-Milan, Italy
Visiting Professor of Neurology,
Department of Neurology,
University of Rochester,
NY, USA
University of Belgrade, Serbia

Gisèle Bonne
Inserm U582, Institut de Myologie,
Groupe Hôpitalier, Pitié- Salpêtrière,
Paris, France

Hannah R. Briemberg
University of British Columbia,
Vancouver, Canada

Hanns Lochmüller
Institute of Human Genetics,
University of Newcastle upon Tyne,
International Centre for Life,
Newcastle upon Tyne, UK

Heinz Jungbluth
Evelina Children's Hospital,
St Thomas' Hospital,
London, UK

Ichizo Nishino
Department of Neuromuscular Research,
National Institute of Neuroscience,
Tokyo, Japan

Jenny E. Morgan
The Dubowitz Neuromuscular Centre,
UCL Institute of Child Health,
London, UK

John Day
University of Minnesota Medical Center,
Minneapolis, MN, USA

John Vissing
Neuromuscular Clinic,
Department of Neurology,
Rigshospitalet, University of Copenhagen,
Copenhagen, Denmark

John T. Kissel
Department of Neurology,
Division of Neuromuscular Disease,
The Ohio State University,
Columbus, OH, USA

Kate Bushby
Institute of Human Genetics,
International Centre for Life,
Newcastle upon Tyne, UK

Leslie Morrison
Department of Neurology,
University of New Mexico,
Albuquerque, NM, USA

Maria J. Molnar
Centre for Molecular Neurology,
Department of Neurology,
Semmelweis University, Budapest

Marianne de Visser
Academic Medical Center,
Department of Neurology,
Amsterdam,
The Netherlands

Marinos C. Dalakas
Neuromuscular Diseases Section, Imperial College,
London Hammersmith Hospital, London, UK

Mary Kay Floeter
Chief, Electromyography Section,
National Institute of Neurological Disorders and Stroke,
National Institutes of Health, 10 Center Drive,
Bethesda, MD, USA

Mariz Vainzof
Human Genome Research Center,
Biosciences Institute,
University of Sao Paulo,
Cidade Universitária,
São Paulo, Brazil

Maxwell S. Damian
Department of Neurology,
University Hospitals of Leicester,
Leicester, UK

Michael G. Hanna
The National Hospital for Neurology and Neurosurgery,
London, UK
MRC Centre for Translational Research
in Neuromuscular Diseases, Institute of Neurology,
University College London,
London, UK

Michael Rose
Department of Neurology,
King's College Hospital,
London, UK

Michael Sinnreich
Department of Neurology and Neurosurgery,
McGill University,
Montreal Neurological Institute and Hospital,
Montreal, Quebec, Canada

Michael Swash
Department of Neurology,
Royal London Hospital,
London, UK
Emeritus Professor of Neurology
at Barts and the London School of Medicine,
Queen Mary University of London,
London, UK
Honorary Professor of Neurology,
Department of Neuroscience,
University of Lisbon, Lisbon, Portugal

Miranda D. Grounds
School of Anatomy and Human Biology,
University of Western Australia, Australia

Mohammed Kian Salajegheh
Department of Neurology,
Brigham & Women's Hospital and Harvard Medical School,
Boston, MA, USA

Nigel G. Laing
Centre for Medical Research,
University of Western Australia,
Western Australian Institute for Medical Research,
QEII Medical Centre,
Western Australia, Australia

Patrick F. Chinnery
Mitochondrial Research Group,
The Medical School, Framlington Place,
Newcastle upon Tyne, UK

Rabi Tawil
Department of Neurology,
University of Rochester School of Medicine,
Rochester, NY, USA

Rénald Gilbert

Richard Orrell
MRC Centre for Neuromuscular Diseases,
Department of Clinical Neurosciences,
University College London,
London, UK

Robert C. Griggs
Department of Neurology,
University of Rochester School of Medicine
and Dentistry and Strong Memorial Hospital,
Rochester, New York, USA

Roberto Massa
Department of Neurology,
University of Rome "Tor Vergata",
Rome, Italy

Saiju Jacob
Queen Elizabeth Neuroscience Centre,
University Hospitals of Birmingham,
Birmingham, UK

Shannon L. Venance
London Health Sciences Centre,
University Hospital,
London ON, Canada

Stefano Di Donato
Fondazione IRCCS Istituto Neurologico "Carlo Besta",
Milan, Italy

Stella Mitrani-Rosenbaum
Goldyne Savad Institute of Gene Therapy,
Hadassah Hebrew University Medical Center,
Hadassah Hospital, Mount Scopus,
Jerusalem, Israel

Stephen Gee
Faculty of Medicine,
University of Ottawa.
Ottawa, Ontario, Canada

Stuart Viegas
Department of Clinical Neurology,
John Radcliffe Hospital, Oxford, UK

Susan C. Brown
Department of Cellular and Molecular Neuroscience,
Imperial College, London, UK

Tahseen Mozaffar
UC Irvine-MDA, ALS and Neuromuscular Centre,
University of California,
Irvine, CA, USA

Tanja Taivassalo
Department of Neurology & Neurosurgery,
Montreal Neurological Institute,
Montreal, Quebec, Canada

Valeria A. Sansone
University of Milan,
IRCCS Policlinico San Donato

Violeta Mihaylova
Department of Neurology,
University Hospital "Alexandrovska",
Sofia, Bulgaria

Yaacov Anziska
Muscular Dystrophy Association (MDA) Clinic,
SUNY-Downstate Medical Center,
Brooklyn, NY, USA

Zohar Argov
Department of Neurology,
Hadassah Hebrew University Medical Center,
Hadassah Hospital, Mount Scopus,
Jerusalem, Israel

On-line Updates

As part of the modernization of this leading textbook, regular update bulletins on each chapter will be published on the website: www.cambridge.org/Karpati

On-line Updates will be authored by a team of outstanding neuromuscular disease specialists who do not currently contribute to the book. The updates will be published every six months, starting in June 2010 and will include selected new references. All content will be peer-reviewed by the Editorial team prior to release on the website.

We hope that this service will be of value to readers. The Editors and Publisher would welcome your feedback.

Foreword by John Walton (Lord Walton of Detchant)

I can hardly believe that this book is now entering its eighth edition. As I said in my foreword to the seventh, it was about 57 years ago when I first began to work on diseases of muscle at the request of the late Professor F.J. Nattrass of Newcastle upon Tyne. During the first few years I endeavoured to identify all of the patients with neuromuscular disease in its many varieties in the northeast of England, and this work led eventually to the introduction of a new classification of the muscular dystrophies, published by Nattrass and myself in *Brain* in 1954. I was fortunate to be able to spend a year learning neuropathology and the pathology of muscle from Raymond Adams at the Massachusetts General Hospital in Boston between 1953 and 1954, before spending a year in the Neurological Research Unit at the National Hospital Queen Square in London, where I continued with my clinical research. Our paper in *Brain* resulted in my receiving a substantial research grant from the Muscular Dystrophy Association of America, which enabled me to expand my research programme when I eventually returned to Newcastle in 1955. Later, with further grants from the Muscular Dystrophy Association of Canada and the embryo Muscular Dystrophy Group of Great Britain and Northern Ireland (which Nattrass and I founded in the early 1950s), I was able to embark upon a much expanded programme, for the first time involving basic research into neuropathology, histochemistry, electrophysiology and the biochemical aspects of neuromuscular disease, among other techniques of investigation. I had also developed the first service in electromyography and related techniques in Newcastle. Later still, with the aid of a programme grant from the Medical Research Council and support from the Wellcome Trust, among other charitable organizations, we were able to build a major research unit in the privately funded laboratories adjacent to the Regional Neurological Centre in Newcastle.

I presume that it was because of these developments that I was invited in 1962, by Mr. J.A. Rivers, of J&A Churchill Ltd, to edit a comprehensive volume on disorders of voluntary muscle, embracing basic science, clinical investigative techniques, clinical diagnosis and genetics, among other disciplines. Thus was *Disorders of Voluntary Muscle* born, and I was delighted to be able, as knowledge expanded at a remarkable rate, to see the book through five subsequent editions. In 1994, however, I recognized that, as I had passed my 72nd birthday and was not involved directly in clinical and laboratory research, or indeed in clinical practice, it was no longer appropriate for me to edit this volume, and was delighted when George Karpati of Montreal, David Hilton-Jones of Oxford and Robert C. Griggs of Rochester, New York, agreed to take it on. It was under their skilled and innovative editorship that the seventh edition appeared in 2001 and proved, in my opinion and in that of many others, to be the most outstanding textbook on diseases of muscle then available. But even since 2001, the virtual explosion of knowledge in molecular biology and other related techniques, and indeed in methods of investigation and management of muscle disease, has meant that a new edition was essential if readers were to be able to consult an authoritative source on such recent developments.

I am delighted that the editors have chosen Professor Kate Bushby of Newcastle to join their team, in view of her outstanding contributions to the field and her distinguished membership of the team of investigators and clinical collaborators now working in Newcastle, partly in a joint Medical Research Council unit, created jointly between the University of Newcastle and University College, London.

This new volume has been remarkably well designed and constructed, the first section dealing with the scientific basis of muscle disease, and the second with methods of investigation. The editors themselves present in Section 3A outstanding descriptions of clinical assessment and a guide to classification, and the principles of prevention, management and treatment, while the extensive Section 3B deals with individual muscle diseases in comprehensive detail. Naturally, because of my involvement in the birth and subsequent lusty development of this volume, I look upon the emergence of a fascinating and comprehensive eighth edition with a mixture of avuncular, even paternal, pride and pleasure. The editors have done a magnificent job in providing a volume which will stand as an outstandingly comprehensive guide to anyone interested in muscle in health or disease, whether basic scientist, clinical scientist, caring doctor or other healthcare professional: it will be read with pleasure and profit, to the ultimate benefit of patients whose future, because of massive developments in the last few years, is so much brighter than it was when the book originally appeared all those years ago.

Addendum

After I had completed this Foreword I learnt the devastating news of the sudden, untimely, and unexpected death of the principal editor of this volume, my good friend George Karpati. Without question, every doctor or scientist working in the field of neuromuscular disease in all parts of the world will be familiar with and will have admired the outstanding contributions which George has made to our understanding of the clinical and scientific aspects of neuromuscular disease throughout his distinguished professional lifetime. Hungarian by birth, George nevertheless became a proud and adopted Canadian, and his department in Montreal acted as a magnet to researchers and interested clinicians from across the world. So much more could be said, and no doubt will be in obituary notices, but speaking for myself I can only say that I have lost a dear and valued friend, whose wise counsel and comment at innumerable scientific meetings has always been to me a source of continuing edification and admiration. He has left a mark upon the field of neuromuscular disease which can never be erased, and will be deeply mourned throughout the scientific world. I shall remember him with pleasure and affection, and hope that this edition of *Disorders of Voluntary Muscle* will stand as an appropriate tribute to his contributions and to his memory.

John Walton (Lord Walton of Detchant)
Belford, Northumberland
June 2009

Preface

Myology as a discipline has continued to expand and increase in complexity since the previous edition of this book appeared in 2001. This growth has been due, mainly, to the application of molecular science to the field, which has led to the discoveries of new entities, a better understanding of the pathogenesis of the relevant diseases, improved diagnostic approaches, and a surge of advanced treatments. The editors have made every effort to ensure that the eighth edition of *Disorders of Voluntary Muscle* reflects these advances. This has been achieved by adding new chapters and by expanding the authorship; however, maintaining a manageable size necessitated condensing and combining chapters. Our ultimate aim is to provide the reader with an up-to-date, authoritative text that will facilitate patient care. Therefore, the authors have concentrated on practical aspects of muscle diseases supported by the use of first class illustrations. While the scientific basis of muscle disease has been addressed, we believe that for more detailed scientific aspects of muscle biology, the reader can consult appropriate reference books and journal articles.

In order to keep abreast of new developments in the future, we have introduced an on-line supplementary section [www.cambridge.org/Karpati] in which additional information and illustrations will be periodically generated, mainly by rising stars of myology.

The editors and the publisher welcome Dr. Kate Bushby of Newcastle upon Tyne, UK as a new editor. She brings vast experience and wisdom to the editorial process. Lord Walton's contribution of a new Foreword remains a valuable nostalgic feature of the book

The editors wish to thank the contributing authors for their expert contributions and the publisher for expediting timely publication.

Ever since the *Disorders of Voluntary Muscle* was first published by John Walton in 1964, it has been considered as the leading comprehensive clinical resource in myology. The editors are confident that this preeminent role will continue with the publication of the eighth edition.

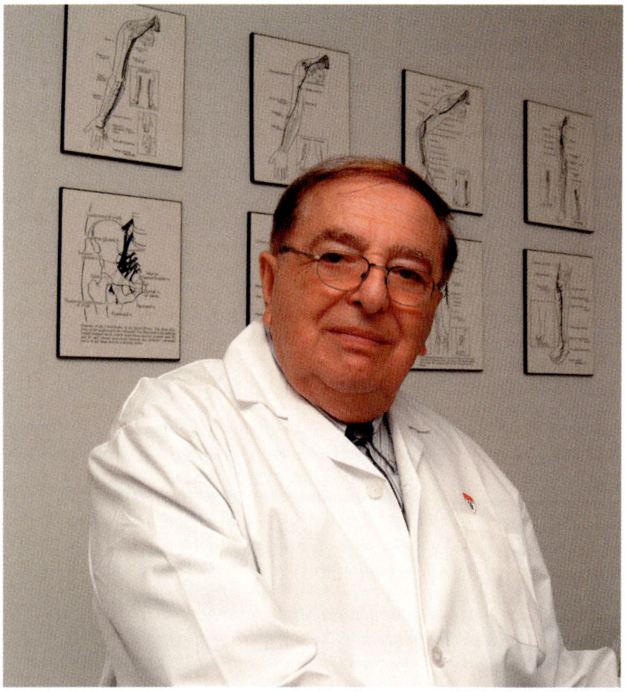

George Karpati (1934–2009)

George Karpati, senior editor of this textbook and leading molecular myologist and experimental neuropathologist of our generation, died suddenly February 7, 2009. George possessed the outstanding skills of a clinical neurologist, an experimental neuropathologist, and a molecular biologist. George's monumental contributions to neuromuscular disease include his seminal studies of inclusion body myositis, critical illness myopathy, Duchenne muscular dystrophy, and carnitine deficiency. He first showed the localization of dystrophin to the muscle fiber surface in Duchenne dystrophy and demonstrated success with dystrophin gene replacement. Over the past two decades Dr. Karpati has been on the forefront of research on the molecular pathogenesis of muscle disease and he has become a dominant figure in approaches to the gene and cellular treatments of first animal models and then on to developing human trials of gene therapy for muscular dystrophy. He has received the highest level of recognition in Canada and abroad. He trained 30 research fellows now in leadership positions in Canada, the USA and around the world. His many awards included the Distinguished Scientist Award, Canadian Society of Clinical Investigation, 1997; Fellow of the Royal Society of Canada, 1999; Officer of the Order of Canada, 2001; Chevalier of the Order of Quebec, 2005; Member of the Canadian Academy of Health Sciences, 2005; Recipient of Prix du Québec, 2006; and Lifetime Achievement Award, World Federation of Neurology Congress, 2006.

George had finished coordinating and overseeing the editing of virtually this entire text at the time of his death. All three remaining editors knew George personally as well as professionally. We all had immense admiration for George's creativity, energy, intensity, tenacity, and enthusiasm. We had all experienced first-hand his relentless pursuit of answers to the pathogenesis of the diseases that are his and our lives' work. George is survived by his wife, Shira, and his two sons. George's family, friends, and all of clinical neuroscience have suffered a great loss. We dedicate this book to our friend: George Karpati.

Kate Bushby
David Hilton-Jones
Robert C. Griggs

Section 1 Chapter 1

The scientific basis of muscle disease

Structure and function of muscle fibers and motor units

Mary Kay Floeter

Introduction

The term "motor unit" was introduced by Sir Charles Sherrington, a founder of modern neurophysiology, who observed that force occurred in discrete steps when a muscle contracted in the stretch reflex [1]. He postulated that each step was produced by the all-or-none action of a single motor neuron upon the muscle fibers it innervated. Sherrington's concept of the motor unit assumed that each muscle fiber receives innervation from only one motor neuron, and that the muscle fiber faithfully responds to every impulse of the motor neuron. These assumptions have subsequently been shown to be true in healthy adult skeletal muscles. The motor unit has become a fundamental concept in understanding the physiology of muscle and the control of movement.

A motor unit consists of one motor neuron and all the muscle fibers it innervates. The term muscle unit has been introduced to refer to the group of muscle fibers innervated by a given motor neuron [2]. The motor neuron and its muscle unit are inseparable in function because each action potential in the neuron activates all fibers of the muscle unit. Thus motor units are the indivisible quantal elements in all movements. The electrophysiological, metabolic, mechanical, and anatomical properties of the motor neuron and its muscle unit are coordinated in a manner that allows efficient muscle contraction over a wide range of motor behaviors. The coordinated expression of the proteins that govern these properties reflects the interplay between the trophic control that motor neurons exert over their muscle fibers through activity patterns and chemical trophic factors, as well as trophic feedback from the muscle fiber to the motor neuron. Although most of the properties of a given motor unit become specified during the early postnatal period of development, physical activity and disease processes can modify certain properties to a limited extent. In this chapter, the basic structural and physiological properties of motor units and muscle fibers will be introduced, with a particular emphasis on humans and other mammals.

Anatomy of motor units

Motor neurons

Motor neurons are the only central neurons with axons that leave the central nervous system (CNS) to innervate non-neuronal tissue. Their cell bodies are located in the anterior horn of the gray matter of the spinal cord (Figure 1.1). The motor neurons that innervate the same muscle cluster together in motor nuclei that form elongated columns that generally extend over several spinal cord segments [3]. The number of motor neurons innervating each muscles varies, ranging from the estimates of 30–40 motor neurons innervating the delicate tenuissimus muscle in the cat [4] to estimates of 100–200 motor neurons innervating human thenar muscles [5, 6]. In the lumbar and cervical enlargements of the spinal cord, the motor neurons that innervate distal limb muscles are located most laterally within the anterior horn, and motor neurons innervating proximal muscles lie more medially [7, 8]. The axons of motor neurons exit the spinal cord through the adjacent anterior roots. When motor axons innervating the same muscle exit from roots of several segments, they rejoin in a muscle nerve after traversing peripheral plexuses and nerve trunks. The muscle nerve contains motor axons innervating the muscle and the sensory axons arising from receptors within the muscle, such as the muscle spindles and tendon organs.

In mammals, there are three kinds of motor neurons in the motor nucleus. Alpha motor neurons are large cells [9, 10] that innervate the striated muscle fibers that make up the bulk of skeletal muscle tissue (extrafusal fibers). Gamma, or fusimotor, neurons are considerably smaller [11] and exclusively innervate one or more of the three types of specialized muscle fibers within the muscle spindle – stretch receptor organs that are present in virtually all somatic muscles [12, 13]. A third class of motor neuron, called skeleto-fusimotor or beta motor neurons, innervates both intra- and extrafusal muscle fibers [14]. Beta motor neurons have been found in higher primates [15] and probably also occur in humans. Because beta motor

Disorders of Voluntary Muscle, 8th edn., eds. George Karpati, David Hilton-Jones, Kate Bushby and Robert C. Griggs. Published by Cambridge University Press.

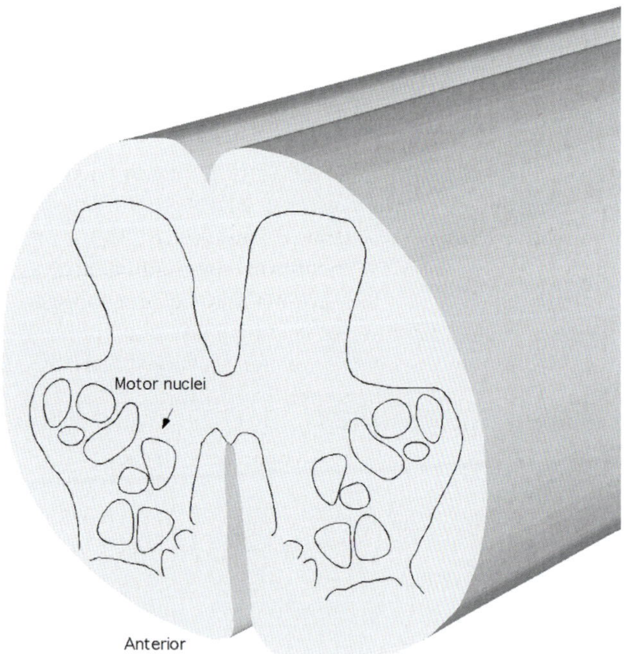

Figure 1.1. Cross-section of the lumbar spinal cord, showing the location of the motor neuron pools.

neurons are difficult to identify in physiological experiments, there is little direct evidence about their properties. What little is known indicates that the properties of beta motor neurons and their extrafusal muscle fibers are essentially the same as those of alpha motor neurons [16]. For this reason, alpha and beta motor neurons will not be distinguished in this chapter.

Alpha motor neurons have extensive dendritic trees that receive synaptic input over their entire extent [17, 18, 19]. Their myelinated axons have large diameters with correspondingly fast conducting velocities, ranging from 40 to 60 m/s in human motor nerves [20]. Faster conduction velocities, 50–120 m/s, have been reported in cats and smaller mammals [21]. The axons of motor neurons can be extremely long, up to a meter in length for those motor neurons innervating the distal foot muscles of a tall adult. The length and diameter of the motor axons mean that the volume of axoplasm may exceed the volume in the cell body and dendrites by tenfold or more (Figure 1.2). The large metabolic demands of maintaining the peripheral axon presumably account for the large size of the motor neuron cell body.

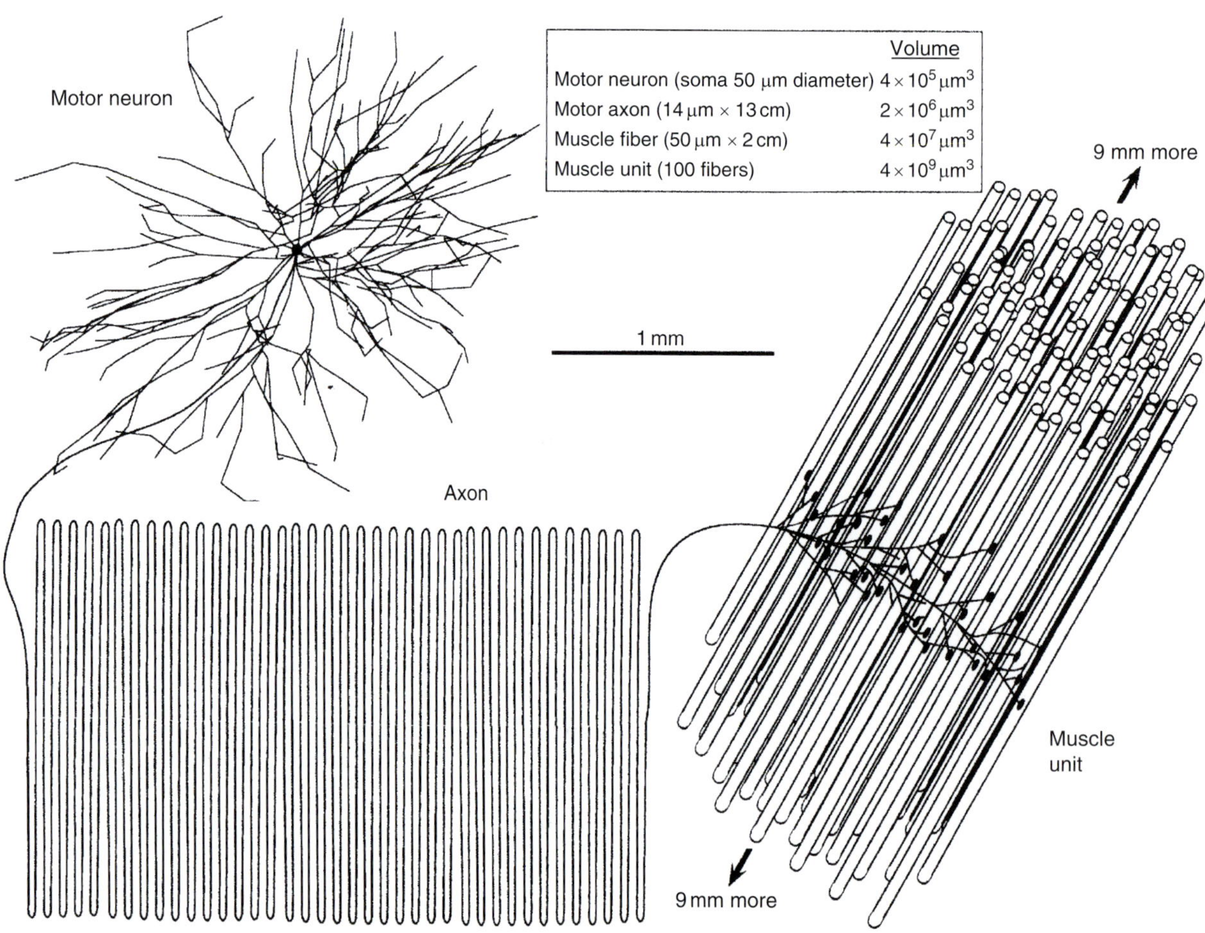

Figure 1.2. Diagram of a motor unit with its components drawn to scale. Note the smaller size of the motor neuron cell body compared with its extensive dendritic tree and very long motor axon. The volume of a single muscle fiber is more than tenfold greater than the volume of cytoplasm in the motor neuron plus its axon. Contributed by R. E. Burke.

Neuromuscular junctions

As the myelinated motor axons near their target muscle, they begin to divide into tens or hundreds of terminal branches, which lose their myelin sheaths as they near the neuromuscular junctions (NMJs). The NMJ is a large, highly specialized synapse between the motor nerve terminal and the muscle fiber [22]. In somatic muscles there is only one NMJ per muscle fiber [23], but exceptions are found in some cranial muscles, such as the laryngeal [24] and extraocular muscles [25]. On a given muscle fiber, the NMJ is located approximately equidistant from its ends, allowing action potential depolarization to spread equally to both ends from the center of the muscle fiber. The NMJ is a complex structure that undergoes remodeling during development and aging and in response to denervation. At the NMJ, the motor nerve terminal is separated from the postsynaptic muscle membrane by a synaptic space containing basal lamina with synapse-specific glycoproteins. On the postsynaptic side, the muscle membrane is highly folded. Acetylcholine receptors are found on the crests of the junctional folds apposing the vesicle release sites on the presynaptic terminal, whereas the voltage-gated sodium channels responsible for action potential generation are densest in the depths of the folds [26]. NMJs exhibit structural specializations related to the size and type of muscle fiber [27]. The structure and function of NMJs will be covered more fully in Chapter 23.

Muscle fibers

The skeletal muscle fiber is a cylindrical, multinucleated cell that is formed by the fusion of myoblast cells during development. The muscle fiber has a highly organized structure, with several distinct spatial domains. Nuclei are positioned along the periphery of the fiber beneath the plasma membrane, or sarcolemma. The center of the muscle fiber is packed with the contractile apparatus, which consists of longitudinally oriented myofibrils and scaffolding proteins. The contractile apparatus is encircled by a network of sarcoplasmic reticulum (SR), a form of endoplasmic reticulum specialized for calcium release and reuptake. The sarcolemma has numerous narrow infoldings, called T-tubules, that penetrate deep into the muscle fiber, where they become closely apposed to regions of the SR at specialized junctions called triads or "calcium release junctions." The T-tubule membrane is continuous with the sarcolemma membrane, but it is specifically enriched in certain membrane proteins, such as voltage-gated calcium channels, chloride channels, and transporters (Figure 1.3) [28, 29]. The T-tubule "interior" is in continuity with the extracellular space, although diffusion occurs more slowly from this narrow space than at the surface membrane. The triads, where T-tubules meet the SR, are the sites where action potential depolarization is coupled to the mechanical contraction. Excitation–contraction coupling occurs through protein–protein interactions between the sarcoplasmic domains of the voltage-gated calcium channels on T-tubule membranes and the calcium release proteins, known as ryanodine receptors, on the SR membrane [30].

The contractile apparatus of the muscle is organized into a series of repeated units a few microns long called sarcomeres [31]. The sarcomere is the smallest unit of contraction. It consists of highly organized protein assemblies that give the muscle fiber a characteristic striated appearance (Figure 1.4b). The sarcomere contains the myofibrils, longitudinal arrays of thick and thin filaments that are maintained in a hexagonal lattice by a scaffolding network (Figure 1.4a). Proteins in the scaffolding network condense at the ends and middle of the sarcomere to form transverse bands called Z-disks and M-bands [32]. The thin filaments consist of filamentous actin entwined by tropomyosin and troponin, a calcium-binding protein. Thick filaments consist of myosin, a large molecule with heavy and light chains. The myosin heavy chains have a tail region and a globular head. Thick filaments are formed by the assembly of myosin monomers with their tails centrally and heads protruding outwards, with an antiparallel orientation on opposite ends of the filament. Z-disks, which mark the border between sarcomeres, serve to anchor the thin filaments. The Z-disks are formed by an ensemble of several proteins, including alpha-actinin. Titin, a large elastic protein spanning from the Z-disk to the M-band, binds to the myofibrils, keeping them centered in the sarcomere, and transmitting tension to the Z-disk during sarcomere shortening [33]. Titin and proteins that comprise the M-band essentially form an intra-sarcomeric cytoskeleton that maintains the regular spacing of the thick and thin filaments [32, 34].

The myosin heads on the thick filament contain an ATPase activity and binding sites for actin. When contraction is initiated by a muscle fiber action potential, calcium released from the SR binds troponin, uncovering binding sites on actin. This leads to the formation of cross-bridges between actin and myosin. The ATPase activity of myosin is enhanced by formation of cross-bridges, and as ATP is hydrolyzed the cross-bridge is broken, freeing the myosin head to swivel to the next actin-binding site. The repeated formation and cleavage of actomyosin cross-bridges produces the sliding action of thin and thick filaments that causes shortening of the sarcomere and muscle contraction [35, 36]. The actomyosin cross-bridges serve as the mechanical linkage between thick and thin filaments for transmitting tension to the insertions of the muscle fiber. The amount of tension is proportional to the number of cross-bridges, reaching a maximum at sarcomere lengths when thick and thin filaments have the greatest overlap [37, 38].

The muscle fiber has a rich cytoskeletal network underlying the membrane and surrounding the myofibrils. In subsarcolemmal regions, protein complexes of dystrophin, syntrophins, and other molecules bind to F-actin and other cytoskeletal proteins. By binding as well to intracellular domains of membrane proteins such as sarcoglycans these effect a linkage between the muscle interior and the extracellular matrix. Beneath the subsarcolemmal cytoskeleton, networks of

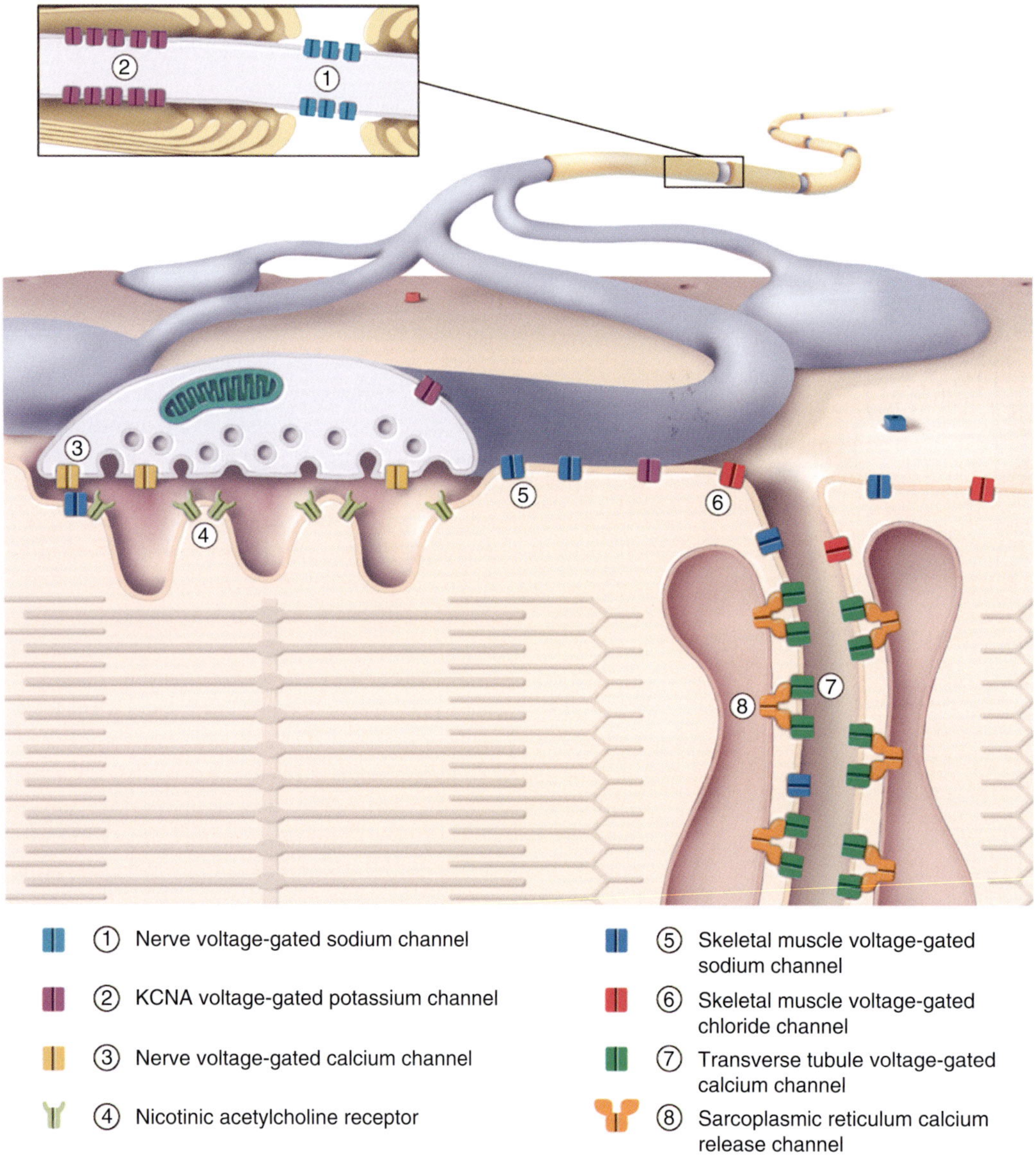

Figure 1.3. Spatial organization of ion channels of the motor nerve, neuromuscular junction (NMJ) and skeletal muscle. The drawing shows a myelinated axon branching to form synaptic contacts with a muscle fiber. The upper inset shows the location of the channels at the node of Ranvier and internodal regions of the motor axon. The lower portion of the drawing depicts the outer surface of a presynaptic terminal and muscle fiber in cut section. Note the location of acetylcholine receptors at the crests of the junctional folds at the NMJ, and the location of channels on the T-tubules and sarcoplasmic reticulum (SR). Used with permission from Cooper and Jan (1999) [175].

intermediate filaments, of which desmin is the most prominent, play a role in the positioning and morphology of organelles within the muscle (reviewed in [39, 40]). Desmin connects Z-disks, SR, myofibrils, and other organelles to the subsarcolemmal cytoskeleton. Mitochondria are usually found in two locations within the muscle fiber, beneath the sarcolemma and among the myofibrils, mostly near the Z-disks. Subsarcolemmal and interfibrillar mitochondria appear to be functionally distinct, with differing cytochrome content, capacity for ADP-stimulated respiration, and susceptibility to apoptotic stimuli [41, 42]. Deficiencies of desmin lead to subsarcolemmal accumulation of mitochondria in mice, supporting a key role for desmin in mitochondrial positioning [43]. Intermediate filaments also bind to proteins on the surface of lysosomes, which are relatively sparse in normal muscle, but become prominent in some myopathies. Glycogen particles, sometimes termed glycosomes, are found in myofibrillar and subsarcolemmal locations.

Extracellular matrix

The muscle fiber is surrounded by an extracellular matrix which consists of several distinct layers [44]. The innermost layer, the basal lamina, contains the carbohydrate-rich extracellular domains of membrane proteins, such as dystroglycan and integrins, that interact with the muscle cytoskeleton; secreted glycoproteins such as members of the laminin family;

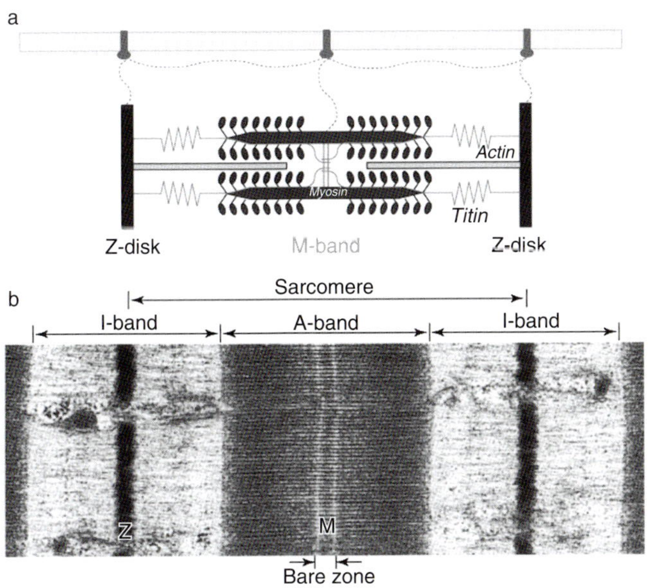

Figure 1.4. Sarcomere structure. The upper drawing shows the myofibrillar proteins, actin and myosin, in longitudinal orientation with titin in the sarcomere. The Z-disk and M-band are transversely oriented. Intermediate filaments (dotted lines) anchor to the cytoskeletal proteins. The lower figure shows the appearance of a complete sarcomere, bordered by two partial sarcomeres, in an electron microscope picture. The A-band is formed by the overlap of actin and myosin filaments. The I-band is formed by thin filaments anchored to the Z-disk, which forms the border between adjacent sarcomeres. (From Agarkova and Perriard (2005) [34], with permission).

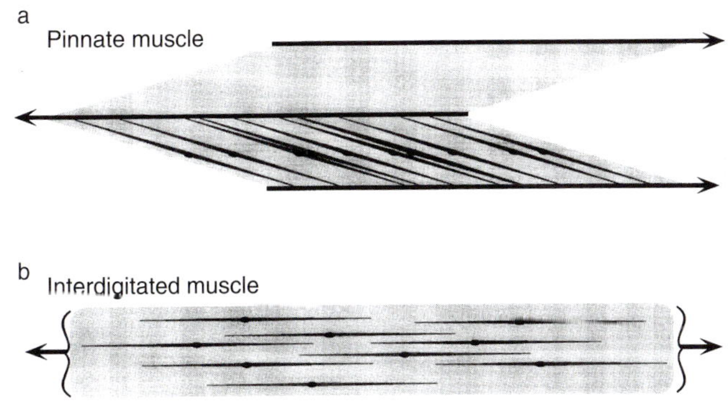

Figure 1.5. The two basic designs of muscle architecture. (a) Pinnate arrangements of muscle fibers in parallel arrays that run at an angle between the aponeuroses of origin and insertion. The fibers of an individual muscle are depicted in the lower half, with central neuromuscular junctions aligned along the axis of the muscle belly. All of the muscle unit fibers contribute to the effective cross-sectional areas of the muscle unit in force generation. (b) An interdigitated muscle, showing tapered muscle unit fibers and their neuromuscular junctions scattered along the length of the muscle belly in irregular arrays. Forces produced by individual fibers are transmitted to the tendons of origin and insertion by internal connective tissue stroma. The effective cross-sectional area of the muscle unit is less than its total cross-sectional area. Contributed by R. E. Burke.

and a variety of ligands and proteoglycans that bind to the extracellular matrix proteins. The outermost layer is rich in collagen fibers, forming a connective tissue layer, the endomysium. The extracellular matrix is specialized at the NMJ, containing synaptic laminins, ligands such as agrin, and the enzyme acetylcholinesterase. The basal lamina and the extracellular matrix molecules play a key role in supporting muscle fiber development and regeneration after injury. Lying beneath the basal lamina are satellite cells, myogenic precursors that are able to proliferate and differentiate into myoblasts [45].

Muscles

Most mammalian muscle fibers are only a few centimeters long, much shorter than the length of most muscles. The length of a muscle fiber is thought to be limited by the need for sarcomeres to be activated nearly simultaneously to produce an effective contraction, which in turn is limited by the time needed for an action potential to travel the length of the muscle fiber. The conduction velocity of muscle fibers is relatively slow, in the range of 2–10 m/s [46, 47]. To achieve an effective mechanical action over a larger length, groups of muscle fibers, called fascicles, are bound together by perimysial connective tissue to form a muscle. Muscle fascicles are arranged in various ways that allow a common direction of force to be delivered to the muscle's points of origin and insertion [48]. There are two general schemes [49]: pinnate, in which the muscle fibers are oriented at an angle to the muscle's primary direction of force; and parallel, in which the orientation of muscle fibers is the same as the force vector. In pinnate muscles, the fascicles are arranged in parallel bundles, often in a feather-like pattern along one or more tendinous aponeuroses (Figure 1.5a). Muscles with pinnate architecture have relatively limited distensibility, but can deliver large output forces. Pinnation is commonly seen in muscles with relatively short lever arms that operate over a limited range of physiological lengths, for example the gastrocnemius muscles of the leg. At the other extreme are muscles with parallel arrangements of interdigitated muscle fascicles, staggered at different longitudinal locations along a web-like intramuscular stroma (Figure 1.5b; [47, 50]). This arrangement allows a small amount of slippage of fascicles past each other, and is commonly seen in muscles that span multiple joints or undergo large changes in length during movement. As might be expected, some muscles exhibit mixtures of these designs (e.g., tibialis anterior in the cat; [51]). A few long, strap-like muscles, such as the biceps femoris, have two or more bellies arranged in series separated by tendinous inscriptions that create distinct anatomical compartments [52].

Most muscles have an optimal range of working lengths. When muscles are stretched during natural movements, they offer some resistance. Most of the tension is related to the number of cross-bridges between overlapping thick and thin filaments [37, 38]. Additional contributions from tendons and internal connective tissue enter into consideration primarily when a muscle is stretched beyond its optimal working range. Because connective tissue is less elastic than muscle fibers, tension rises quickly at these lengths. Contributions from connective tissue to muscle length–tension curves are referred to as passive, in contrast to the active contributions from the myofibrillar cross-bridges. Passive contributions to muscle tension differ between healthy and diseased muscle.

Degenerative muscle diseases, or even the prolonged disuse of muscles, such as after a stroke, may result in markedly increased connective tissue within the muscle with stiffness and increased resistance to stretch [53].

Functional organization of motor units

Distribution of motor unit fibers

The spatial distribution of muscle fibers belonging to an individual motor unit has been studied experimentally with the glycogen depletion technique [54]. In this method, prolonged stimulation of a motor axon is used to deplete muscle fibers of endogenous glycogen stores, enabling the depleted fibers to be identified histochemically. The glycogen depletion method showed that muscle fibers belonging to the same motor unit were arranged in a mosaic fashion among muscle fibers belonging to other motor units [54, 55]. Relatively few muscle fibers from the same unit occurred immediately adjacent to one another [56, 57]. Statistical studies suggest that the distribution of fibers in single units is basically random [58]. Nevertheless, the arrangement of the muscle unit's fibers must accommodate to the internal architecture of the parent muscle to produce a meaningful pattern of force. In pinnate muscles, fibers from one motor unit were found to be scattered more or less evenly through territories that were relatively large, but smaller than the total cross-section of the muscle (Figure 1.6). In multicompartment muscles, motor unit fibers were usually distributed only within one compartment [59]. However, there are examples, such as the extensor digitorum muscle of the monkey forelimb, in which fibers of one motor unit are distributed among several compartments to exert a common force on multiple tendons [60].

Electromyographic (EMG) studies of single motor units in humans suggest a similar spatial organization of muscle unit fibers. Using a technique called scanning EMG, in which a motor unit action potential is recorded as an electrode is advanced in successive steps of 50 μm through the muscle, Stalberg and colleagues [61, 62] recorded territories with cross-sectional areas of 2–10 mm for single motor units in the biceps and tibialis anterior muscles. Within the same region of muscle, they found that several dozen motor units had overlapping territories. For an individual motor unit, at some places the muscle fiber action potentials were grouped, and separated from other regions, suggestive of fractions of the muscle unit innervated by different branches of the motor axon (arrows, Figure 1.7).

One way to describe the size of a motor unit is according to its innervation ratio: the number of muscle fibers innervated by a given motor neuron. The number of muscle fibers

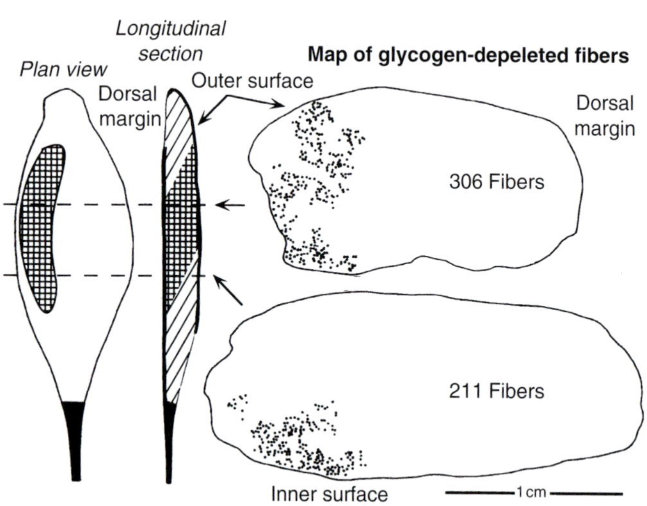

Figure 1.6. The distribution of glycogen-depleted fibers in a Type FR motor unit (fast twitch, fatigue resistant) in the medial gastrocnemius muscle of the cat. The cross-hatched areas in the whole muscle diagrams on the left indicate the extent of the motor unit territory, which occupies only a fraction of the muscle volume. The diagonal hatching on the longitudinal section denotes the angulation of the fibers in this unipinnate muscle. Maps of the spatial distribution of depleted fibers at two levels along the muscle belly are shown on the right. Note the irregular boundaries of the unit territory but relatively even distribution of fibers within it. Adapted from Burke and Tsairis (1973) [56], (with permission from Wiley-Blackwell Publishing Ltd and the authors).

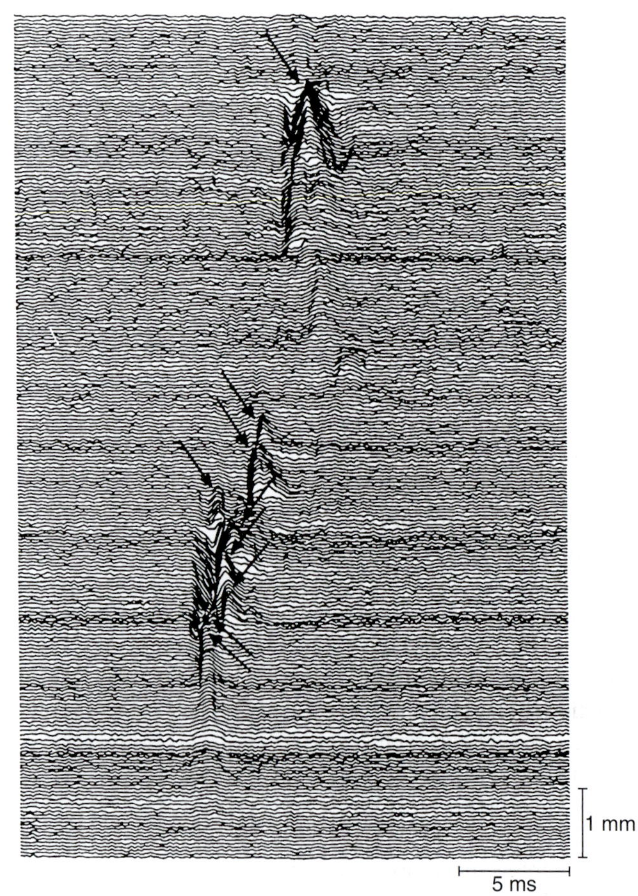

Figure 1.7. Topographical territory of a motor unit from human biceps, as measured by scanning EMG. Each line represents successive steps of 50 μm through the muscle and the motor unit action potential is recorded at each step. For the biceps, the mean cross-sectional length of a motor unit territory was approximately 5 mm. In patients with nerve injury and reinnervation, the territories were of similar size. From Stalberg and Trontelji (1994) [62] with permission.

Table 1.1. Estimates of innervation ratios of motor units in human muscles

Muscle	Number of motor axons	Number of muscle fibers	Innervation ratio	Reference
Biceps	774	580 000	750	Buchthal, 1961 [64]
Brachioradialis	315	129 000	410	Feinstein *et al.*, 1955 [63]
First dorsal interosseous	119	40 500	340	Feinstein *et al.*, 1955 [63]
Medial gastrocnemius	579	1 120 000	1934	Feinstein *et al.*, 1955 [63]
Tibialis anterior	445	250 200	562	Feinstein *et al.*, 1955 [63]

innervated by one motor neuron varies widely between different muscles. In humans, innervation ratios have been estimated by dividing an estimate of the total number of muscle fibers in a muscle by counts of the number of large axons in cross-sections of the muscle nerve. Such calculations have produced estimates of innervation ratios ranging from less than a dozen for the extraocular muscles to over a thousand for motor units of large limb muscles (Table 1.1) [63, 64]. Physiological methods have also been used to estimate the number of motor units innervating certain muscles, and these studies have also shown similar ranges [6]. However, using the glycogen depletion method to identify the fibers of individual motor units in animals, Burke and Tsairis [56] found considerable variation in the innervation ratios for different units within a given muscle. The innervation ratio of the motor unit is a major factor governing its force output. Variation in innervation ratios is likely to provide much of the variability in force output produced by different motor units within a muscle [65, 66].

Muscle fiber types

For more than a century, it has been recognized that mammalian muscles fall into two general groups: dark "red" muscles with slow contraction times and lighter "white" muscles with fast contraction times. Histological and physiological studies have shown that most muscles contain a mixture of muscle fibers with differing contraction speeds and force outputs; muscles composed of purely fast or slow muscle fibers are exceptional (for reviews see [67, 68]). The isoform of the myosin heavy chain (MHC) expressed in the muscle fiber is one of the most important factors influencing the speed of contraction, because the rate of ATP hydrolysis determines the speed of cross-bridge cycling and sarcomere shortening [69, 70]. Other factors affecting the contractile speed of muscle fibers include the isoforms of the calcium reuptake and release proteins expressed and the density of the SR [71, 72, 73, 74]. There are three major isoforms of MHC expressed in adult human limb muscles: MHC I, also called slow myosin; and the two fast isoforms, MHC IIA and MHC IIX (also called MHC IID). Subtypes of these isoforms, as well as embryonic and neonatal forms of MHCs, generate further diversity. The fast and slow isoforms of myosin were first able to be distinguished histochemically because of their differing amounts of ATPase activity at acid and alkaline pH [75]. This histochemical difference allowed fast and slow muscle fibers to be classified into two types. Fast and slow muscle fiber types are further subdivided by their dependence on aerobic or anaerobic metabolic pathways. Muscle fibers that utilize oxidative metabolism for energy needs have abundant mitochondria and lipid droplets. In contrast, muscle fibers using anaerobic pathways for energy tend to be richer in glycolytic enzymes with more abundant glycogen stores. Histochemical methods for demonstrating mitochondrial enzymes combined with myosin ATPase activity have traditionally been used to define three major types of muscle fiber in adult human limb muscles, described below. The histochemical properties of different fiber types correspond fairly well to their contractile properties, allowing muscle fibers to be grouped into a small number of types by either histochemical or physiological measures. It should be recognized, however, that qualitative and quantitative differences in expression of fiber-type-specific proteins generate a continuous range of physiological properties.

Type 1 muscle fibers have a slow twitch and use oxidative metabolism. Type 1 fibers express MHC I, the slow isoform of myosin, and contain many mitochondria. These muscle fibers can be visualized histochemically by strong myosin ATPase activity at low pH and by dense staining for mitochondrial enzymes such as NADH dehydrogenase (i.e., nicotinamide adenine dinucleotide, reduced) and SDH (i.e., succinate dehydrogenase) (Table 1.2). Compared to Type 2 fibers, their SR is less abundant, and it contains a slower isoform of the SR calcium ATPase. Type 1 fibers contain myoglobin, a protein that binds oxygen and confers a red color, and have a rich capillary blood supply [76]. The metabolic profile and vascularization render Type 1 muscle fibers highly resistant to fatigue, and thus suitable for sustained contraction under aerobic conditions. The acronym "SO," slow oxidative, is used by some to denote these fibers.

Type 2 muscle fibers are fast-twitch fibers, expressing fast isoforms of myosin which exhibit strong ATPase activity at alkaline pH. There are several subtypes of Type 2 fibers, but two major subtypes occur in human limb muscles. Type 2A fibers express the MHC IIA isoform of myosin. Compared to Type 1 fibers, their SR is denser, and expresses isoforms of calcium handling proteins that allow a more rapid cycling of calcium ions from SR [71, 72, 73]. Mitochondria are relatively abundant in Type 2A fibers. In addition Type 2A fibers

Table 1.2. Features of muscle fiber and motor unit types. Cox, Cyclo-oxygenase; EPSPs, excitatory postsynaptic potentials; FF, fast twitch, fatigable; FR, fatigue resistant; IPSPs, inhibitory postsynaptic potentials; NADH dehydrogenase, nicotinamide adenine dinucleotide, reduced; PAS, periodic acid Schiff; S, slow twitch, fatigue resistant; SDH, succinate dehydrogenase

Histochemical properties	**Muscle fiber types**		
	1	**2A**	**2B**
Myosin ATPase (pH 9.4)	Low	High	High
Myosin ATPase (pH 4.6)	High	Low	Medium
Oxidative enzymes (SDH, NADH dehydrogenase, Cox)	High	Medium	Low
Phosphorylase	Very low	High	High
Glycogen (PAS)	Low	High	Medium
	Motor unit types		
Mechanical properties	**S**	**FR**	**FF**
Twitch contraction time	Slow	Fast	Fast
Maximum tetanic force	Small	Moderate	High
Fatigue resistance	Very high	Moderate/ high	Low
"Sag"	No	Yes	Yes
Motor neuron properties			
Axon conduction velocity	Slower	Fast	Fast
Soma diameter, membrane area	Smallest	Large	Largest
Input resistance	Highest	Low	Lower
Rheobase (excitability)	Low	Higher	Highest
AHP duration	Longer	Short	Short
Properties of synaptic organization			
Monosynaptic Ia EPSPs	Largest	Large	Small
Disynaptic Ia IPSPs	Largest	Large	Small
Recurrent (Renshaw) IPSPs	Largest	Large	Small
Cutaneous inputs from distal limbs	Mainly IPSPs	Mainly EPSPs	Mainly EPSPs

Notes: Adapted from Burke, R. E., The structure and function of motor units. In *Disorders of Voluntary Muscle*, 7th edn., ed. G. Karpati, D. Hilton-Jones, R. C. Griggs. (Cambridge: Cambridge University Press, 2001), pp. 3–25.

contain glycolytic enzymes, such as phosphorylase, and have abundant glycogen stores. These metabolic properties allow Type 2A to function under aerobic and anaerobic conditions, and provide them with a fairly high resistance to fatigue. Type 2A fibers have been denoted by the acronym "FOG" because they are fast twitch with oxidative and glycolytic metabolic capabilities. The third major muscle fiber type that occurs in human limb muscles is the Type 2B fiber. Type 2B fibers express the fastest isoform of myosin, MHC IIX (also known as IID). Their SR is dense and contains a fast isoform of SR calcium ATPase. Type 2B fibers have relatively sparse mitochondria, but contain glycolytic enzymes and stores of glycogen. Type 2B muscle fibers fatigue easily, but are suitable for short bursts of anaerobic exercise. The acronym "FG," fast, glycolytic, is sometimes used.

Other isoforms of myosin are found in specialized muscle or at different developmental stages. In a number of animal species, Type 2B fibers express a very fast form of myosin, the MHC IIB isoform, particularly in muscles with very fast speeds of contraction [77, 78, 79, 80]. In humans, MHC IIB expression has been reported in some cranial muscles [81] but it is not expressed to a significant extent in limb muscles. Immature forms of myosin are expressed by muscle fibers prior to completing their differentiation during development [82, 83]. Fibers expressing immature forms of myosin that stain for ATPase activity at acid and alkaline pH, Type 2C fibers, are found in small numbers in normal adult limb muscles. The Type 2C profile occurs in regenerating fibers, which can be common in several muscular dystrophies. Muscle spindles also express a mixture of immature and slow isoforms of myosin [84].

The classification of the major muscle fiber types by their pattern of MHC expression agrees relatively well with the histochemical classification of fiber Types 1, 2A, and 2B that is based on myosin ATPase activity at differing pH. However, histochemical methods are relatively insensitive to hybrid muscle fibers expressing more than one MHC isoform. Hybrid muscle fibers can be demonstrated with immunocytochemical methods or *in-situ* hybridization for different isoforms of MHCs [80, 85]. Combinations of MHC IIA with IIx expression are relatively common in Type 2 fibers, for example [85, 86]. In some muscles hybrid fibers make up a sizeable fraction of the muscle fibers [78, 79, 85]. Hybrid fibers may play a role in the ability of muscle fibers to undergo rapid adaptations in response to training and use [87, 88, 89, 90].

Association of motor unit types with muscle fiber types

All muscle fibers belonging to the same motor unit have the same type, as judged from their staining for ATPase activity [54, 91, 92] and MHC isoforms [93, 94, 95]. Within a muscle unit the fibers also appear to have similar metabolic enzyme capacities [94, 96]. It is, therefore, assumed that muscle fibers within the motor unit also have essentially identical mechanical properties. Edström and Kugelberg [54] were the first to use the glycogen depletion method to examine the association between the mechanical properties and histochemical characteristics of the muscle fibers of individual motor units for two types of fast-twitch motor unit in rats. Burke and coworkers [55, 56] later used the same approach to examine the histochemistry of muscle fibers within the full range of physiologically identified motor units in the cat gastrocnemius muscle. In these studies, motor neurons were characterized physiologically with intracellular recordings, including stimulation with short stimulus trains while measuring force output and

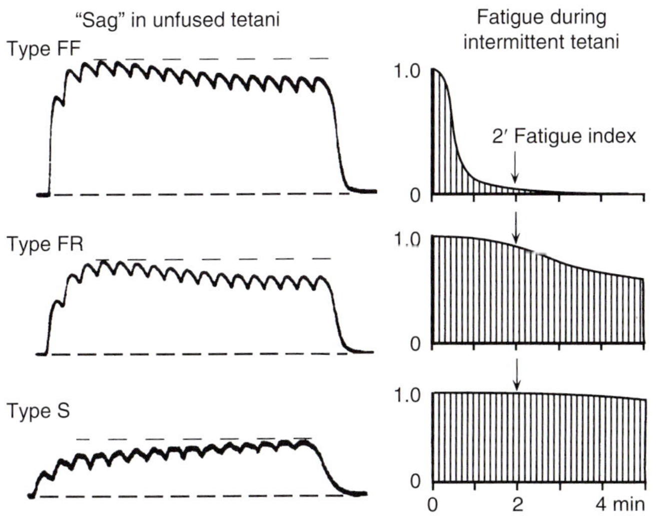

Figure 1.8. Mechanical responses from three muscle units to illustrate the properties used to identify motor unit types physiologically: FF, fast twitch, fatigable; FR, fast twitch, fatigue resistant; and S, slow twitch, fatigue resistant. The records in the left column are unfused tetani produced by repetitive stimulation at intervals near 1.25 times the respective twitch contraction times. The FF and FR unit responses show an early maximum force and subsequent "sag." The graphs on the right show the peak force produced by a sequence of short, unfused tetani produced by 13 stimulus pulses at 40 Hz, delivered every second for 5 min (duty cycle 0.33). The fatigue index is calculated as the ratio of the peak tetanic force after 2 min of repetitive stimulation (arrows) divided by the force produced by the first tetanus. The fatigue index of Type FF units was less than 0.25 while values for the FR and S units were greater than 0.75. The two properties taken together serve to distinguish three groups, with a fourth group, F(int), having a fatigue index between 0.25 and 0.75 and "sag" in unfused tetani. Contributed by R. E. Burke.

prolonged stimulation to deplete glycogen stores in active muscle fibers. Burke and coworkers found that motor units differed in several mechanical properties, not just the speed of contraction. These properties included the magnitudes of force produced by individual twitches (twitch force) and the maximal force produced by repetitive stimulation (tetanic force), resistance to fatigue during sustained activation, and the ratio of the twitch to the tetanic force [67]. These properties each exhibited continuous distributions that initially made it problematic to define distinct groups of motor units. However, two criteria were found that permitted relatively clear clustering of motor units into fast and slow groups in the cat: a "fatigue index" based on the decline in force output during a defined sequence of intermittent tetanization and a "sag property" based on the shape of unfused isometric tetanic contractions (Figure 1.8) [55, 91, 92, 97, 98]. Using these criteria, Burke and colleagues were able to define three main types of motor units: Type FF (fast twitch, fatigable), Type FR (fast twitch, fatigue resistant) and Type S (slow twitch, fatigue resistant). Some fast-twitch units exhibited fatigue resistance intermediate between those of FF and FR units and were, therefore, referred to as F(int) or FI [56, 92, 99]. Physiologically, there was a perfect match between S, FR and FF motor units with the histochemically defined muscle fiber Types 1, 2A, and 2B, respectively (Table 1.2; see also [97, 98, 100]). They also found some evidence that fibers in the minority F(int) unit type were histochemically distinct from the three main types [56, 98]. These same physiological criteria have been used with somewhat more variable success in classifying motor units in rat muscles (e.g., [101, 102]). It is possible that some of the variation in properties such as contraction time within a given motor unit type are associated with hybrid combinations of myosin isoforms, but this remains to be investigated systematically.

Motor units in human muscles

There is a wealth of information available from EMG studies in humans about the behavior of motor units in normal and diseased muscle, and it has been known for some time that fast- and slow-twitch muscle fibers coexist in human muscle [103]. However, for obvious technical reasons, it is difficult to examine the mechanical responses of individual motor units under the controlled conditions possible in animal experiments. Denny-Brown and Pennybacker [104] were the first to record individual twitches from the fasciculations of motor units in patients with motor neuron disease, using an indirect pneumatic transducer. Buchthal and Schmalbruch [105] used a mechanical transducer attached to a needle inserted into tendons, plus intramuscular stimulation of small nerve branches, to demonstrate that small groups of human motor units in normal muscles generate a wide range of twitch speeds, which varied in relation to the predominant local fiber type (see also [106]). The introduction of spike-triggered computer averaging into clinical neurophysiology made it possible to record the responses of individual motor units with greater assurance [107]. In this technique, discharges of single motor units during steady voluntary contractions are used to trigger an averaging computer while measuring the force produced by an appendage (e.g., a finger) attached to a force transducer. There are two limitations of this technique. First, the recorded twitch responses are not isolated twitches but rather components of unfused tetani, leading to errors in estimating the twitch forces and contraction times [108, 109]. Intra-neural stimulation of single motor axons to produce twitches has been used in an attempt to overcome this problem [110, 111, 112]. Secondly, the mechanical responses measured can be significantly degraded by the compliance of components between the active muscle fibers and the force transducer, including tendons of various lengths. Despite these technical limitations, most of the contractile properties measured from human motor units are generally similar to those from animals [113, 114]. There is disagreement about whether fatigability and "sag" can be used to classify human motor unit types in the same manner as in animals, and whether force measurements relate to the fatigability in the same way [110, 112, 115]. However, when motor units have been identified by glycogen depletion in muscle biopsy samples, these properties were consistent with histochemical identification [116]. Overall, the available physiological evidence and correspondence with the histochemical classification strongly suggest that the basic characteristics of Types S, FF, and FR human motor units are similar to those described for the cat and rat.

Functional correlates of fiber properties and motor unit types

It is clear that many factors contribute to mechanical properties of the different motor unit types: in addition to the expression of MHC isoforms, there are fiber-type-specific differences in myosin light chains, troponin and tropomyosin proteins, proteins involved in calcium release and reuptake, and sarcotubular structures [72, 73, 74, 117]. It seems likely that the "sag" property, which differs sharply in fast and slow units, is produced by interactions among these factors [67, 68, 118]. Resistance to fatigue is directly related to the oxidative capacity of the different fiber types (Table 1.2; [91, 119]), as well as to their mitochondrial content [72] and local capillary supply [120]. These correlations are certainly causally related. The forces produced by individual motor units can vary by over two orders of magnitude during tetanization, and this variation is correlated with motor unit type (Figure 1.8 and Table 1.2). The force produced by a motor unit is a function of the effective cross-sectional area of its muscle fibers and the specific force output of that fiber type per unit area. Estimation of the effective cross-sectional area must take into account the effective innervation ratio [121], which may approximate the actual innervation ratio in pinnate muscles [91] but would be less in interdigitated muscles which have unit fibers in serial arrays (Figure 1.5). In general, Type 1 and 2A fibers have smaller diameters than Type 2B, making fiber area an important component of the equation. In humans, Type 2 fibers exhibit the greatest variability in diameter; in general fiber diameters tend to be larger in men than women [122]. There is some controversy about whether specific force output, which cannot be measured directly, differs between units with Type 1 and 2 muscle fibers [65, 69, 91, 92].

Motor neurons and synaptic specializations

In view of the differences between muscle fiber types, it is not surprising that the motor neurons that innervate them exhibit corresponding physiological differences (Table 1.3; reviewed by [67]). In general, motor neurons of Type S motor units have slower axonal conduction velocities, longer durations of post-spike hyperpolarized after-potentials (AHPs), and higher whole-cell input resistance values than the cells that innervate either FR or FF motor units. The AHP duration is particularly important because it is a key factor that controls the rate of motor neuron firing; motor neurons of Type S units have the longest AHPs and generally fire more slowly than those of FR or FF units. When examined with intracellular labeling methods, the motor neurons of Type S units tend to be smaller in membrane area than Type FF cells; Type FR motor neurons are intermediate in size [9, 10]. There is no systematic difference between axonal conduction velocities of FF and FR unit groups [123]. Although the distributions of motor neuron properties are continuous and exhibit large overlaps when sorted according to muscle unit type, the relative excitability of the motor neurons to depolarizing currents injected directly, measured as the rheobase (the amount of current required to produce action potentials reliably), is more closely related to unit type than other measures [124, 125]. The rheobase data imply that intrinsic motor neuron excitability varies according to the sequence S > FR > FF, which has important implications for the recruitment order of motor units (Figure 1.9).

Table 1.3. Functional specialization of motor unit types

Functions	Motor unit type		
	S	FR	FF
Recruitment threshold	Low	Intermediate	High
Duty cycle	Long/ continuous	Intermediate	Short/ intermittent
Fatigue resistance	High	Medium/ high	Low
Metabolic cost at rest	High	Medium/ high	Low
Metabolic optimum action	Isometric	Shortening	Shortening
Force gradation with recruitment	Fine	Intermediate	Coarse

The strength of several synaptic inputs to motor neurons shows type-related differences that are undoubtedly related to the way in which the various types of motor units are used during activity. For example, the average amplitudes of monosynaptic excitatory postsynaptic potentials (EPSPs) produced in motor neurons by group Ia muscle spindle afferents, which are largely responsible for the stretch reflex, are ordered as S > FR > FF (Table 1.2) [126, 127]. The same ordering is evident with the disynaptic inhibition produced by stimulation of group Ia afferents from antagonist muscles [126] and with disynaptic recurrent inhibition produced by Renshaw interneurons activated from motor axon collaterals [128]. The organization of synaptic efficacy is a key factor that controls the function of motor unit populations [129], and for most inputs to motor neurons, the ordering of synaptic efficacy follows the size principle. However, there is evidence that certain cutaneous inputs and supraspinal systems, notably the rubrospinal tract, tend to excite relatively high-threshold motor neurons while inhibiting low-threshold cells [130, 131, 132], a pattern opposite to that found in group Ia excitation. Although there would be potential advantages to competing control systems that could bypass low-threshold, slow-twitch motor units that are slow to relax, the idea that large,

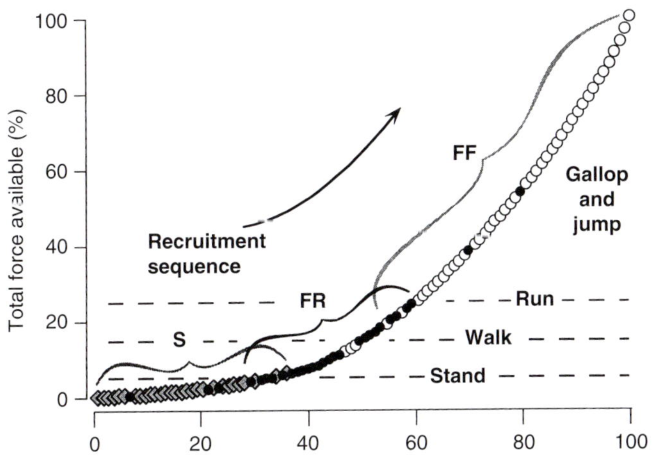

Figure 1.9. The nonlinear increase in force output (ordinate) from the cat medial gastrocnemius (MG) muscle if its motor unit population were recruited (abscissa) strictly in order of the force produced by each motor unit. The initial stage of recruitment is dominated by Type S motor units (gray diamonds) up to approximately 30% of the motor neuron pool, which produces in aggregate about 5% of the total force that the muscle is capable of producing. As indicated by the dashed line, the MG muscle produces this force range in the Achilles tendon during quiet stance in cats. The next region, between 30% and 60% of the motor neuron pool, is dominated by Type FR units (filled circles). Recruitment of Types FR and S together account for about 25% of the total force output available, which is in the range found during walking and running on a treadmill. The final region, above 60% recruitment of the motor pool, is dominated by Type FF units. Forces in this range are seen in the MG muscle only during galloping and jumping. Although the data for this diagram were pooled from different animals and studies [126, 139], the motor unit types exhibit relatively little overlap when arranged in this way.

fast-twitch motor units might be selectively recruited before, or even without, recruitment of normally lower-threshold smaller units is controversial.

Motor units and the control of muscle force

Recruitment

The force produced by a muscle during voluntary contraction is controlled by the recruitment and derecruitment of active motor units and regulation of their firing rates. Much of our knowledge about motor unit recruitment comes from observations in human muscles (e.g., [133, 134]). Under most conditions of isotonic and isometric contraction, small force units are the first to be recruited [104], followed by larger and larger units as force demand increases [67, 135]. The term "size principle" has come into wide use to encapsulate this orderly recruitment sequence [136]. When directly tested by studying recruitment order in pairs of motor units, the smaller force unit exhibits the lower functional threshold in a high proportion of trials [21]. In fact several of the interrelated properties of motor units (Table 1.2) can predict relative excitability equally well [137], so size-ordered recruitment is more-or-less equivalent to type-ordered recruitment. For example, if recruitment were to occur strictly in order of increasing force output, most of the early recruited units would be fatigue-resistant Type S, followed by Type FR, and finally by Type FF (Figure 1.9). The diagram would change little if recruitment were ordered by motor unit type alone. The same basic sequence, although with greater overlaps, would occur if units were recruited strictly in order of decreasing amplitude of monosynaptic group Ia EPSPs. Similarly, gradations of intrinsic motor neuron excitability (i.e., rheobase; Table 1.2) would give the same general pattern. There is abundant evidence that organization of synaptic inputs and intrinsic motor neuron properties are both critical to recruitment control, and in the case of group Ia excitation and many other inputs, both factors cooperate to produce size-ordered recruitment.

There are mechanical as well as metabolic advantages to size-ordered recruitment (Table 1.3). In Type S motor units, slow contraction, small unit force, and fatigue resistance are all advantageous properties for motor units active during sustained, precisely graded actions at modest total force, such as are needed for postural maintenance. There is also evidence that Type 1 muscle fibers are metabolically more efficient during isometric force production than when shortening [138]. At the other extreme, the large-force, fatigable Type FF motor units are clearly best suited for rapid, large force contractions that are intermittent and occur relatively infrequently, to be paid for metabolically by subsequent re-formation of stored glycogen. The Type FR units occupy a middle ground, combining relatively rapid contraction and moderate force increments with considerable resistance to fatigue and the ability to use either aerobic or anaerobic metabolic pathways.

The composition of the motor unit population in the cat medial gastrocnemius can be matched against the forces actually produced by that muscle during unrestrained activity (Figure 1.9) [139]. Given size-ordered recruitment, this comparison suggests that the Type S population is sufficient to generate the relatively small forces needed to maintain quiet standing, while walking and running require additional participation of the Type FR population. Activation of the Type FF population is required only during infrequent actions such as gallop and jumping. The motor unit pools of other hind limb muscles in the cat exhibit differences in composition that fit the mechanical demands as well as the life style of these sedentary predators that must gallop and jump only occasionally [92, 123, 140, 141].

Muscles vary in the proportion of different motor unit types that they contain (Table 1.4; [142]). In many muscles, Type 2B fibers make up 50%–70% of muscle bulk but probably are seldom called into use. It seems likely that the size and proportion of Type FF motor units that are represented by this bulk represent an evolutionary compromise between occasional demand for large output forces and the need to minimize the metabolic cost of muscle maintenance. Muscle fibers of high oxidative activity have a higher resting blood flow [76] and, by inference, higher rates of oxygen and substrate extraction than fibers with low oxidative capacity. Therefore, the

Table 1.4. Proportions of Type I fibers in selected human muscles (from Johnson *et al.*, 1973 [142])

Muscle	Percent Type 1 fibers
Triceps	33
Biceps	42
First dorsal interosseous	57
Lateral gastrocnemius	49
Tibialis anterior	73

energetic cost of Type S and FR motor units is probably considerably higher than that of Type FF units even at rest, making the latter relatively cheap to maintain (Table 1.3).

Control of muscle unit force by motor neuron firing rates and patterns

During most movements, motor neurons fire repetitively with fairly regular frequencies that depend on the strength of contraction and the particular muscle. As a general rule, in humans, motor unit firing frequency ranges from minimum rates of approximately 5–10 Hz to maximum frequencies of 25–40 Hz [143]. Motor neuron firing frequencies are constrained by the AHPs that follow each action potential [135], but motor units also tend to exhibit preferred firing frequencies. Preferred firing frequencies are influenced in part by voltage-sensitive channels on motor neuron dendrites that produce depolarization with a very slow time course of inactivation [144, 145]. The activation of these channels is influenced by neuromodulation, particularly through catecholaminergic systems. Once activated these channels generate persistent inward currents (PICs) that can maintain a relatively steady level of depolarization. Evidence is emerging that PICs may be activated at lower voltage ranges and decay more slowly in low-threshold Type S motor neurons than in high-threshold motor neurons (reviewed in [146]). Such firing behavior fits the motor neuron's functional role in activating muscle fibers that are inherently slow and nonlinear. The maximum tension that can be produced by an individual muscle unit at different motor neuron firing frequencies varies in a sigmoidal fashion, with low force produced by isolated twitches to a maximal force, typically five to ten times higher, when motor neurons fire at high frequencies. This tetanic force reaches 75%–80% of the maximum possible when motor neuron firing intervals equal the twitch contraction time, at which individual twitch responses reach their maximum force.

It is instructive to estimate motor unit output as the force–time integral under a sequence of responses during isometric tetani at different stimulation frequencies, which would be roughly equivalent to the work that the unit would generate if the muscle were free to contract. The force–time curve also reaches a fairly sharp peak at interstimulus intervals near the twitch contraction time in both fast- and slow-twitch units [118]. Therefore, if a muscle unit twitch contraction time is 33 ms (fairly typical of Type FF or FR units in cats; Figure 1.8), its optimum frequency for work output would be about 30 Hz, while for a Type S unit with a twitch contraction time of 80 ms, the optimum would be 12.5 Hz. These frequencies are well within the range actually observed for animal and human motor units. The highly nonlinear behavior of individual muscle units during constant frequency activation illustrates the dependence of muscle unit force output on its short-term activation history. Enhancement as well as reduction (i.e., fatigue) of force output reflect longer-term activation history. For example, repeated bursts of stimulation at relatively high frequency induce increases in force output and changes in the shape of mechanical responses, called post-tetanic potentiation (PTP), that can last for many seconds to minutes (Figure 1.10). Twitch responses are very sensitive to PTP, as can be seen by comparing the first components (dotted falling phases) in unfused tetani in Figure 1.10a, b.

Motor units are remarkably sensitive to the pattern of stimulus intervals as well as to their rate. For example, a single short interval, or doublet, inserted into an otherwise low-frequency stimulus train can produce sustained enhancement of isometric force production, referred to as a "catch property," in both fast- and slow-twitch muscle units [118, 147]. The effect of an initial doublet in Type FF or FR muscle units enhances force output for a few hundred milliseconds but the force profile returns to the baseline level because the "sag" property curtails the duration of catch in these units (Figure 1.10). However, the ability of motor neurons to sustain FF unit force for even brief periods by modulation of their firing patterns may be functionally relevant [148]. Figure 1.10b shows, in the same unit, that catch enhancement is markedly reduced when the unit responses are enhanced through PTP, an effect also observed in Type S units. Catch enhancement can be quite prolonged in Type S units because they have little or no "sag" to curtail it. In Figure 1.10c, different levels of sustained force were produced by changing only one or two intervals within otherwise constant (low) frequency tetani, showing that catch enhancement does not require closely spaced doublet firing. Nevertheless, doublet firing is found in normal human motor units particularly at the onset of rapid, forceful contractions [134, 149] and presumably can cause similar force enhancements. Clearly, the pattern as well as the rate of motor neuron firing can provide significant modulation of the force output from individual motor units.

Plasticity of muscle fiber and motor unit types

Muscle displays a remarkable ability to adapt to altered conditions of use. Adaptation to exercise has been studied intensively in humans and animals because of the wide interest in optimizing fitness and athletic performance. Endurance exercise training increases oxidative enzyme capacity and capillary perfusion in muscle fibers of all fiber types, but produces little

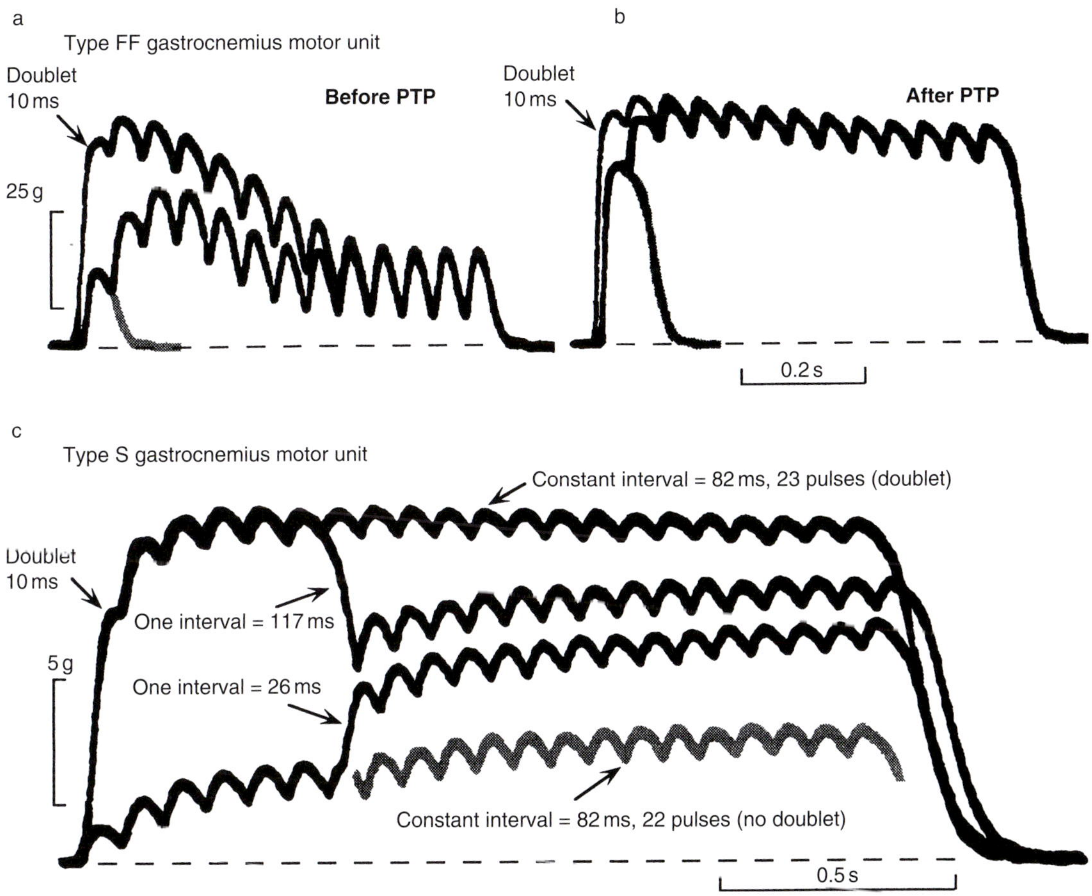

Figure 1.10. Force enhancement, or "catch," produced by changing one or two stimulus intervals in unfused tetanic responses produced by fast and slow- twitch motor units when stimulated by otherwise constant low-frequency stimulus trains. (a) Photographically superimposed isometric unfused tetanic responses produced by a fast-twitch motor unit in a cat gastrocnemius muscle unit by a low-frequency train with (larger response) and without a single extra pulse (doublet) at the onset. The enhanced force produced by the doublet decayed to the baseline force with the same time course as the "sag" evident in the basic response. (b) Responses with and without an initial doublet after repeated tetanization of the muscle unit to produce post-tetanic potentiation (PTP). The responses with and without the doublet are larger than before PTP and the force enhancement produced by the doublet is correspondingly reduced. Note also the marked difference produced by PTP in the first "twitch" responses in each tetanic sequence (gray traces show twitch falling phases.) (c) Superimposed responses from a Type S motor unit in cat gastrocnemius muscle showing persistent catch enhancement produced by an initial doublet in otherwise constant low-frequency trains (interval 82 ms – 11.5 Hz; compare with gray trace that denotes the output in the absence of a doublet). The traces with intermediate forces were produced by altering one interval in the first third of the responses with and without an initial doublet, showing that sustained force was modulated over a threefold range by small changes in stimulation pattern. (Adapted from [118, 147]). Contributed by R. E. Burke.

interconversion between histochemically defined Type 1 and Type 2 fiber types (reviewed in [150, 151]. There is, however, evidence that MHC isoforms can undergo changes in response to different forms of activity and exercise training, with a characteristic sequential transition from MHC I to MHC IIa to MHC IIx [45, 150, 152] as well as changes in the proportions of hybrid fibers [86, 87, 88, 89, 153]. With disuse, e.g., unloading or spinal injury, similar transitions in MHC expression tend to occur in the direction toward fast fiber types. However, the motor unit types S, FF, and FR appear to remain stable with altered conditions of usage within the physiological range (i.e., when innervation remains intact and muscles are not artificially stimulated). In animal studies, the interrelations between muscle unit properties that are used to recognize motor unit types are robust in the face of altered conditions that produce muscle atrophy [154, 155] or compensatory hypertrophy [156, 157].

Denervation and reinnervation

When a muscle nerve is partially injured, the distal portions of surviving axons sprout new collaterals that innervate nearby denervated muscle fibers. The magnitude of sprouting is correlated, in part, with the size of the distal motor axon. Because axonal caliber is correlated with the motor unit type, innervation ratios will tend to be re-established according to the motor unit type [158]. The reinnervated muscle fibers undergo changes in many, but not all, of their metabolic and contractile characteristics to conform to the new motor unit type, a process that involves interactions between the motor neuron and muscle. A classic example is cross-reinnervation of a predominately fast muscle (e.g., the flexor digitorum longus (FDL) of the cat) by the motor axons that originally innervated a predominately slow muscle (soleus). This slow-to-fast reinnervation causes the FDL to become markedly slower [159] and its motor unit population switches quite completely to Type S [160]. However, the effect is not symmetrical. Fast-to-slow cross-reinnervation of the soleus by FDL motor axons produces some speeding of the soleus contraction, but the cross-reinnervated soleus muscle fibers remain histochemically Type 1, even though they are hybrid fibers, coexpressing a form of fast-twitch myosin as well as slow myosin [161]. Cross-reinnervated soleus motor units, like the whole muscle, exhibit shorter than normal twitch contraction times but otherwise retain Type S characteristics [162]. The muscle fibers in the histochemically mixed FDL and homogeneous soleus clearly display different degrees of plasticity when reinnervated by foreign motor neurons. The interpretation of such cross-reinnervation experiments is complicated because the foreign motor neurons do not change their activity patterns, which forces the cross-reinnervated muscle units to function under very different conditions of loading than their normal patterns [163].

Self-reinnervation of a denervated muscle is a simpler situation, and more comparable to the clinical situation of partial nerve injury. To a large but variable extent, the normal muscle fiber and motor unit types re-form in self-reinnervated muscles [158, 164, 165], although wider ranges of tetanic force output and innervation ratios are evident. However, the normal spatial distribution of fibers is disorganized, with more grouping of fibers from the same motor unit than in normal muscle [57, 160, 162, 165]. Some studies have found histochemical uniformity within a given muscle unit after reinnervation ([57, 160] see also [161]), but more recent studies report some degree of nonuniformity of myosin isoforms in some fibers of the same glycogen-depleted muscle units after self-reinnervation [95, 164]. Such observations, like those after cross-reinnervation, suggest that some muscle fibers are more resistant than others to re-specification when innervated by a foreign motor neuron, for reasons that remain unclear.

Electrical activity

Prolonged repetitive electrical stimulation produces slowed contraction times and increased resistance to fatigue of normally innervated as well as denervated muscles. These changes are associated with increases in oxidative capacity and capillarity, and loss of total force output (for review see [86]). These adaptations begin shortly after the onset of chronic stimulation and before evident transformations in myosin isoforms, though the latter eventually occur [166]. The transformation of fast fibers into slow occurs irrespective of the frequency of chronic stimulation [167, 168, 169], and the effect is completely reversible on cessation of imposed stimulation [170]. The reverse transformation (i.e., slow to fast) occurs only under a more limited set of conditions (very short bursts of high-frequency stimulation in denervated muscle [171]). The effect of chronic electrical stimulation, either indirectly through the nerve or directly in the muscle, on individual motor units has been studied in cat medial gastrocnemius muscle [172]. This work showed essentially complete conversion of all tested motor units to physiological Type S and of muscle fibers to Type 1, although the histochemical characteristics were not identical to those of Type 1 fibers in the control muscles. The Type S units in stimulated muscles contracted more slowly than the original population of Type S units. Chronic stimulation also produced changes in the innervating motor neurons in the direction expected of cells that innervate Type S muscle units [173].

The dramatic muscle fiber conversions produced by self- and cross-reinnervation are good evidence that the innervating motor neuron exerts powerful, albeit less than total, control over the expression of the features that make up muscle fiber type [95, 158]. From the changes that occur with electrical stimulation and athletic training, it is also clear that usage is an important component in the control exerted by the motor neuron [87, 88, 89, 90]. Nevertheless, the classic notion of trophic substances acting between motor neuron and its muscle unit remains as a viable adjunct mechanism. There is growing evidence that differentiation of fiber types is partly specified early in development before fibers are singly innervated by a motor neuron [174]. The initial specification of muscle fibers, counterbalancing the neural-based influences on fiber-type-specific expression of muscle proteins [45,150], may account for the incomplete transformation of muscle fibers.

References

1. E. Liddell, C. Sherrington, Recruitment and some other features of reflex inhibition. *Proc. R. Soc. Lond.* **97B** (1925), 488–518.
2. R. E. Burke, Motor unit types of cat triceps surae muscle. *J. Physiol. (Lond.)* **193**:1 (1967), 141–160.
3. R. E. Burke, P. L. Strick, K. Kanda, C. C. Kim, B. Walmsley, Anatomy of medial gastrocnemius and soleus motor nuclei in cat spinal cord. *J. Neurophysiol.* **40**:3 (1977), 667–680.
4. A. Lev-Tov, C. A. Pratt, R. E. Burke, The motor-unit population of the cat tenuissimus muscle. *J. Neurophysiol.* **59**:4 (1988), 1128–1142.
5. T. J. Doherty, W. F. Brown, The estimated numbers and relative sizes of thenar motor units as selected by multiple point stimulation in young and older adults. *Muscle Nerve* **16**:4 (1993), 355–366.
6. A. J. McComas, Invited review: motor unit estimation: methods, results, and present status. *Muscle Nerve* **14**:7 (1991), 585–597.
7. B. Rexed, The cytoarchitectonic organization of the spinal cord in the cat. *J. Comp. Neurol.* **96**:3 (1952), 414–495.
8. J. R. Fetcho, A review of the organization and evolution of motoneurons innervating the axial musculature of vertebrates. *Brain Res.* **434**:3 (1987), 243–280.
9. R. E. Burke, R. P. Dum, J. W. Fleshman, L. L. Glenn, A. Lev-Tov, M. J. O'Donovan, *et al.*, A HRP study of the relation between cell size and motor unit type in cat ankle extensor motoneurons. *J. Comp. Neurol.* **209**:1 (1982), 17–28.

10. S. Cullheim, J. W. Fleshman, L. L. Glenn, R. E. Burke, Membrane area and dendritic structure in type-identified triceps surae alpha motoneurons. *J. Comp. Neurol.* **255**:1 (1987), 68–81.

11. A. K. Moschovakis, R. E. Burke, R. E. Fyffe, The size and dendritic structure of HRP-labeled gamma motoneurons in the cat spinal cord. *J. Comp. Neurol.* **311**:4 (1991), 531–545.

12. R. Granit, The functional role of the muscle spindles – facts and hypotheses. *Brain* **98**:4 (1975), 531–556.

13. P. B. Matthews, Recent advances in the understanding of the muscle spindle. *Sci. Basis Med. Annu. Rev.* (1971), 99–128.

14. P. Bessou, F. Emonet-Denand, Y. Laporte, Motor fibres innervating extrafusal and intrafusal muscle fibres in the cat. *J. Physiol. (Lond.)* **180**:3 (1965), 649–672.

15. K. S. Murthy, W. D. Letbetter, E. Eidelberg, W. E. Cameron, J. Petit, Histochemical evidence for the existence of skeletofusimotor (beta) innervation in the primate. *Exp. Brain Res.* **46**:2 (1982), 186–190.

16. R. E. Burke, P. Tsairis, Histochemical and physiological profile of a skeletofusimotor (beta) unit in cat soleus muscle. *Brain Res.* **129**:2 (1977), 341–345.

17. T. Brannstrom, Quantitative synaptology of functionally different types of cat medial gastrocnemius alpha-motoneurons. *J. Comp. Neurol.* **330**:3 (1993), 439–454.

18. R. M. Ichiyama, J. Broman, V. R. Edgerton, L. A. Havton, Ultrastructural synaptic features differ between alpha- and gamma-motoneurons innervating the tibialis anterior muscle in the rat. *J. Comp. Neurol.* **499**:2 (2006), 306–315.

19. K. A. Starr, J. R. Wolpaw, Synaptic terminal coverage of primate triceps surae motoneurons. *J. Comp. Neurol.* **345**:3 (1994), 345–358.

20. L. J. Dorfman, The distribution of conduction velocities (DCV) in peripheral nerves: a review. *Muscle Nerve* **7**:1 (1984), 2–11.

21. F. E. Zajac, J. S. Faden, Relationship among recruitment order, axonal conduction velocity, and muscle-unit properties of type-identified motor units in cat plantaris muscle. *J. Neurophysiol.* **53**:5 (1985), 1303–1322.

22. B. W. Hughes, L. L. Kusner, H. J. Kaminski, Molecular architecture of the neuromuscular junction. *Muscle Nerve* **33**:4 (2006), 445–461.

23. M. C. Brown, P. B. Matthews, An investigation into the possible existence of polyneuronal innervation of individual skeletal muscle fibres in certain hind-limb muscles of the cat. *J. Physiol. (Lond.)* **151** (1960), 436–457.

24. G. Rossi, G. Cortesina, Multi-motor endplate muscle fibers in the human vocalis muscle. *Nature* **206** (1965), 629–630.

25. J. A. Buttner-Ennever, Anatomy of the oculomotor system. *Dev. Ophthalmol.* **40** (2007), 1–14.

26. B. E. Flucher, M. P. Daniels, Distribution of Na^+ channels and ankyrin in neuromuscular junctions is complementary to that of acetylcholine receptors and the 43 kd protein. *Neuron* **3**:2 (1989), 163–175.

27. G. C. Sieck, Y. S. Prakash, Morphological adaptations of neuromuscular junctions depend on fiber type. *Can. J. Appl. Physiol.* **22**:3 (1997), 197–230.

28. G. L. Dohm, R. W. Dudek, Role of transverse tubules (T-tubules) in muscle glucose transport. *Adv. Exp. Med. Biol.* **441** (1998), 27–34.

29. K. Jurkat-Rott, M. Fauler, F. Lehmann-Horn, Ion channels and ion transporters of the transverse tubular system of skeletal muscle. *J. Muscle Res. Cell Motil.* **27**:5–7 (2006), 275–290.

30. B. E. Flucher, C. Franzini-Armstrong, Formation of junctions involved in excitation-contraction coupling in skeletal and cardiac muscle. *Proc. Natl. Acad. Sci. U. S. A.* **93**:15 (1996), 8101–8106.

31. K. A. Clark, A. S. McElhinny, M. C. Beckerle, C. C. Gregorio, Striated muscle cytoarchitecture: an intricate web of form and function. *Annu. Rev. Cell Dev. Biol.* **18** (2002), 637–706.

32. S. Lange, E. Ehler, M. Gautel, From A to Z and back? Multicompartment proteins in the sarcomere. *Trends Cell Biol.* **16**:1 (2006), 11–18.

33. H. L. Granzier, S. Labeit, Titin and its associated proteins: the third myofilament system of the sarcomere. *Adv. Protein Chem.* **71** (2005), 89–119.

34. I. Agarkova, J. C. Perriard, The M-band: an elastic web that crosslinks thick filaments in the center of the sarcomere. *Trends Cell Biol.* **15**:9 (2005), 477–485.

35. R. Cooke, The sliding filament model: 1972–2004. *J. Gen. Physiol.* **123**:6 (2004), 643–656.

36. A. F. Huxley, Cross-bridge action: present views, prospects, and unknowns. *J. Biomech.* **33**:10 (2000), 1189–1195.

37. T. L. Hill, G. M. White, On the sliding-filament model of muscular contraction, IV. Calculation of force-velocity curves. *Proc. Natl. Acad. Sci. U. S. A.* **61**:3 (1968), 889–896.

38. A. M. Gordon, A. F. Huxley, F. J. Julian, The variation in isometric tension with sarcomere length in vertebrate muscle fibres. *J. Physiol. (Lond.)* **184**:1 (1966), 170–192.

39. Y. Capetanaki, R. J. Bloch, A. Kouloumenta, M. Mavroidis, S. Psarras, Muscle intermediate filaments and their links to membranes and membranous organelles. *Exp. Cell Res.* **313**:10 (2007), 2063–2076.

40. D. Paulin, Z. Li, Desmin: a major intermediate filament protein essential for the structural integrity and function of muscle. *Exp. Cell Res.* **301**:1 (2004), 1–7.

41. P. J. Adhihetty, V. Ljubicic, K. J. Menzies, D. A. Hood, Differential susceptibility of subsarcolemmal and intermyofibrillar mitochondria to apoptotic stimuli. *Am. J. Physiol. Cell Physiol.* **289**:4 (2005), C994–C1001.

42. A. M. Cogswell, R. J. Stevens, D. A. Hood, Properties of skeletal muscle mitochondria isolated from subsarcolemmal and intermyofibrillar regions. *Am. J. Physiol.* **264**:2 Pt 1 (1993), C383–C389.

43. Y. Capetanaki, Desmin cytoskeleton: a potential regulator of muscle mitochondrial behavior and function. *Trends Cardiovasc. Med.* **12**:8 (2002), 339–348.

44. J. R. Sanes, The basement membrane/basal lamina of skeletal muscle. *J. Biol. Chem.* **278**:15 (2003), 12601–12604.

45. S. D. Harridge, Plasticity of human skeletal muscle: gene expression to in vivo function. *Exp. Physiol.* **92**:5 (2007), 783–797.

46. L. Arendt-Nielsen, K. R. Mills, The relationship between mean power frequency of the EMG spectrum and muscle fibre conduction velocity. *Electroencephalogr. Clin. Neurophysiol.* **60**:2 (1985), 130–134.

47. G. E. Loeb, C. A. Pratt, C. M. Chanaud, F. J. Richmond, Distribution and innervation of short, interdigitated muscle fibers in parallel-fibered muscles of the cat hindlimb. *J. Morphol.* **191**:1 (1987), 1–15.
48. J. A. Trotter, Structure-function considerations of muscle-tendon junctions. *Comp. Biochem. Physiol. A. Mol. Integr. Physiol.* **133**:4 (2002), 1127–1133.
49. C. Gans, A. S. Gaunt, Muscle architecture in relation to function. *J. Biomech.* **24** Suppl 1 (1991), 53–65.
50. J. A. Trotter, Functional morphology of force transmission in skeletal muscle. A brief review. *Acta Anat. (Basel)* **146**:4 (1993), 205–222.
51. R. R. Roy, A. Garfinkel, M. Ounjian, J. Payne, A. Hirahara, E. Hsu, *et al.*, Three-dimensional structure of cat tibialis anterior motor units. *Muscle Nerve* **18**:10 (1995), 1187–1195.
52. C. M. Chanaud, C. A. Pratt, G. E. Loeb, Functionally complex muscles of the cat hindlimb. II. Mechanical and architectural heterogeneity within the biceps femoris. *Exp. Brain Res.* **85**:2 (1991), 257–270.
53. R. L. Lieber, S. Steinman, I. A. Barash, H. Chambers, Structural and functional changes in spastic skeletal muscle. *Muscle Nerve* **29**:5 (2004), 615–627.
54. L. Edström, E. Kugelberg, Histochemical composition, distribution of fibres and fatiguability of single motor units. Anterior tibial muscle of the rat. *J. Neurol. Neurosurg. Psychiatry* **31**:5 (1968), 424–433.
55. R. E. Burke, D. N. Levine, F. E. Zajac, 3rd., Mammalian motor units: physiological-histochemical correlation in three types in cat gastrocnemius. *Science* **174**:10 (1971), 709–712.
56. R. E. Burke, P. Tsairis, Anatomy and innervation ratios in motor units of cat gastrocnemius. *J. Physiol. (Lond.)* **234**:3 (1973), 749–765.
57. E. Kugelberg, L. Edstrom, M. Abbruzzese, Mapping of motor units in experimentally reinnervated rat muscle. Interpretation of histochemical and atrophic fibre patterns in neurogenic lesions. *J. Neurol. Neurosurg. Psychiatry* **33**:3 (1970), 319–329.
58. S. C. Bodine, A. Garfinkel, R. R. Roy, V. R. Edgerton, Spatial distribution of motor unit fibers in the cat soleus and tibialis anterior muscles: local interactions. *J. Neurosci.* **8**:6 (1988), 2142–2152.
59. A. W. English, O. I. Weeks, Compartmentalization of single muscle units in cat lateral gastrocnemius. *Exp. Brain Res.* **56**:2 (1984), 361–368.
60. M. H. Schieber, M. Chua, J. Petit, C. C. Hunt, Tension distribution of single motor units in multitendoned muscles: comparison of a homologous digit muscle in cats and monkeys. *J. Neurosci.* **17**:5 (1997), 1734–1747.
61. E. Stalberg, L. Antoni, Electrophysiological cross section of the motor unit. *J. Neurol. Neurosurg. Psychiatry* **43**:6 (1980), 469–474.
62. E. Stalberg, J. V. Trontelji, *Single Fiber Electromyography. Studies in Healthy and Diseased Muscle* (New York: Raven Press, 1994).
63. B. Feinstein, B. Lindegard, E. Nyman, G. Wohlfart, Morphologic studies of motor units in normal human muscles. *Acta Anat. (Basel)* **23**:2 (1955), 127–142.
64. F. Buchthal, The general concept of the motor unit. *Res. Publ. Assoc. Res. Nerv. Ment. Dis.* **38** (1961), 3–30.
65. S. C. Bodine, R. R. Roy, E. Eldred, V. R. Edgerton, Maximal force as a function of anatomical features of motor units in the cat tibialis anterior. *J. Neurophysiol.* **57**:6 (1987), 1730–1745.
66. V. F. Rafuse, M. C. Pattullo, T. Gordon, Innervation ratio and motor unit force in large muscles: a study of chronically stimulated cat medial gastrocnemius. *J. Physiol. (Lond.)* **499**: Pt 3 (1997), 809–823.
67. R. E. Burke, Motor units: anatomy, physiology, and functional organization. In *Handbook of Physiology, Sect. 1: The Nervous System*, Vol. II, Ed. V. B. Brooks. (Washington, DC: American Physiological Society, 1981), pp. 345–522.
68. R. M. Enoka, Morphological features and activation patterns of motor units. *J. Clin. Neurophysiol.* **12**:6 (1995), 538–559.
69. R. Bottinelli, M. Canepari, M. A. Pellegrino, C. Reggiani, Force-velocity properties of human skeletal muscle fibres: myosin heavy chain isoform and temperature dependence. *J. Physiol. (Lond.)* **495**:Pt 2 (1996), 573–586.
70. S. D. Harridge, R. Bottinelli, M. Canepari, M. A. Pellegrino, C. Reggiani, M. Esbjornsson, *et al.*, Whole-muscle and single-fibre contractile properties and myosin heavy chain isoforms in humans. *Pflügers Arch.* **432**:5 (1996), 913–920.
71. A. E. Rossi, R. T. Dirksen, Sarcoplasmic reticulum: the dynamic calcium governor of muscle. *Muscle Nerve* **33**:6 (2006), 715–731.
72. B. R. Eisenberg, D. J. Dix, Z. W. Lin, M. P. Wenderoth, Relationship of membrane systems in muscle to isomyosin content. *Can. J. Physiol. Pharmacol.* **65**:4 (1987), 598–605.
73. H. H. Trinh, G. D. Lamb, Matching of sarcoplasmic reticulum and contractile properties in rat fast- and slow-twitch muscle fibres. *Clin. Exp. Pharmacol. Physiol.* **33**:7 (2006), 591–600.
74. W. Fiehn, J. B. Peter, Properties of the fragmented sarcoplasmic reticulum from fast twitch and slow twitch muscles. *J. Clin. Invest.* **50**:3 (1971), 570–573.
75. L. Guth, F. J. Samaha, Qualitative differences between actomyosin ATPase of slow and fast mammalian muscle. *Exp. Neurol.* **25**:1 (1969), 138–152.
76. T. C. Ong, D. A. Hayes, R. B. Armstrong, Distribution of microspheres in plantaris muscles of resting and exercising rats as a function of fiber type. *Am. J. Anat.* **182**:4 (1988), 318–324.
77. L. C. Rome, Design and function of superfast muscles: new insights into the physiology of skeletal muscle. *Annu. Rev. Physiol.* **68** (2006), 193–221.
78. L. M. Acevedo, J. L. Rivero, New insights into skeletal muscle fibre types in the dog with particular focus towards hybrid myosin phenotypes. *Cell Tissue Res.* **323**:2 (2006), 283–303.
79. J. L. Rivero, R. J. Talmadge, V. R. Edgerton, Fibre size and metabolic properties of myosin heavy chain-based fibre types in rat skeletal muscle. *J. Muscle Res. Cell Motil.* **19**:7 (1998), 733–742.
80. J. L. Rivero, R. J. Talmadge, V. R. Edgerton, A sensitive electrophoretic method for the quantification of myosin heavy chain isoforms in horse skeletal muscle: histochemical and immunocytochemical verifications. *Electrophoresis* **18**:11 (1997), 1967–1972.
81. M. J. Horton, C. A. Brandon, T. J. Morris, T. W. Braun, K. M. Yaw, J. J. Sciote, Abundant expression of myosin heavy-chain IIB RNA in a subset of human masseter muscle fibres. *Arch. Oral Biol.* **46**:11 (2001), 1039–1050.

82. G. A. Unguez, R. J. Talmadge, R. R. Roy, D. Dalponte, V. R. Edgerton, Distinct myosin heavy chain isoform transitions in developing slow and fast cat hindlimb muscles. *Cells Tissues Organs* **167**:2–3 (2000), 138–152.

83. R. S. Staron, Human skeletal muscle fiber types: delineation, development, and distribution. *Can. J. Appl. Physiol.* **22**:4 (1997), 307–327.

84. J. M. Walro, J. Kucera, Why adult mammalian intrafusal and extrafusal fibers contain different myosin heavy-chain isoforms. *Trends Neurosci.* **22**:4 (1999), 180–184.

85. G. M. Stephenson, Hybrid skeletal muscle fibres: a rare or common phenomenon? *Clin. Exp. Pharmacol. Physiol.* **28**:8 (2001), 692–702.

86. D. Pette, The adaptive potential of skeletal muscle fibers. *Can. J. Appl. Physiol.* **27**:4 (2002), 423–448.

87. T. A. Kohn, B. Essen-Gustavsson, K. H. Myburgh, Exercise pattern influences skeletal muscle hybrid fibers of runners and nonrunners. *Med. Sci. Sports Exerc.* **39**:11 (2007), 1977–1984.

88. A. C. Parcell, R. D. Sawyer, R. Craig Poole, Single muscle fiber myosin heavy chain distribution in elite female track athletes. *Med. Sci. Sports Exerc.* **35**:3 (2003), 434–438.

89. D. L. Williamson, P. M. Gallagher, C. C. Carroll, U. Raue, S. W. Trappe, Reduction in hybrid single muscle fiber proportions with resistance training in humans. *J. Appl. Physiol.* **91**:5 (2001), 1955–1961.

90. R. J. Talmadge, R. R. Roy, V. R. Edgerton, Myosin heavy chain profile of cat soleus following chronic reduced activity or inactivity. *Muscle Nerve* **19**:8 (1996), 980–988.

91. R. E. Burke, D. N. Levine, P. Tsairis, F. E. Zajac, 3rd, Physiological types and histochemical profiles in motor units of the cat gastrocnemius. *J. Physiol. (Lond.)* **234**:3 (1973), 723–748.

92. J. C. McDonagh, M. D. Binder, R. M. Reinking, D. G. Stuart, A commentary on muscle unit properties in cat hindlimb muscles. *J. Morphol.* **166**:2 (1980), 217–230.

93. L. Larsson, Is the motor unit uniform? *Acta Physiol. Scand.* **144**:2 (1992), 143–154.

94. G. C. Sieck, M. Fournier, Y. S. Prakash, C. E. Blanco, Myosin phenotype and SDH enzyme variability among motor unit fibers. *J. Appl. Physiol.* **80**:6 (1996), 2179–2189.

95. G. A. Unguez, R. R. Roy, D. J. Pierotti, S. Bodine-Fowler, V. R. Edgerton, Further evidence of incomplete neural control of muscle properties in cat tibialis anterior motor units. *Am. J. Physiol.* **268**:2 Pt 1 (1995), C527–C534.

96. P. M. Nemeth, L. Solanki, D. A. Gordon, T. M. Hamm, R. M. Reinking, D. G. Stuart, Uniformity of metabolic enzymes within individual motor units. *J. Neurosci.* **6**:3 (1986), 892–898.

97. R. P. Dum, T. T. Kennedy, Physiological and histochemical characteristics of motor units in cat tibialis anterior and extensor digitorum longus muscles. *J. Neurophysiol.* **43**:6 (1980), 1615–1630.

98. J. C. McDonagh, M. D. Binder, R. M. Reinking, D. G. Stuart, Tetrapartite classification of motor units of cat tibialis posterior. *J. Neurophysiol.* **44**:4 (1980), 696–712.

99. B. R. Botterman, G. A. Iwamoto, W. J. Gonyea, Classification of motor units in flexor carpi radialis muscle of the cat. *J. Neurophysiol.* **54**:3 (1985), 676–690.

100. T. M. Hamm, P. M. Nemeth, L. Solanki, D. A. Gordon, R. M. Reinking, D. G. Stuart, Association between biochemical and physiological properties in single motor units. *Muscle Nerve* **11**:3 (1988), 245–254.

101. K. Kanda, K. Hashizume, Factors causing difference in force output among motor units in the rat medial gastrocnemius muscle. *J. Physiol. (Lond.)* **448** (1992), 677–695.

102. J. E. Totosy de Zepetnek, H. V. Zung, S. Erdebil, T. Gordon, Motor-unit categorization based on contractile and histochemical properties: a glycogen depletion analysis of normal and reinnervated rat tibialis anterior muscle. *J. Neurophysiol.* **67**:5 (1992), 1404–1415.

103. A. Eberstein, J. Goodgold, Slow and fast twitch fibers in human skeletal muscle. *Am. J. Physiol.* **215**:3 (1968), 535–541.

104. D. Denny-Brown, J. B. Pennnybacker, Fibrillation and fasciculation in voluntary muscle. *Proc. R. Soc. Lond., Series B. Biol. Sci.* **104** (1939), 131–252.

105. F. Buchthal, H. Schmalbruch, Contraction times and fibre types in intact human muscle. *Acta Physiol. Scand.* **79**:4 (1970), 435–452.

106. R. E. Sica, A. J. McComas, Fast and slow twitch units in a human muscle. *J. Neurol. Neurosurg. Psychiatry* **34**:2 (1971), 113–120.

107. H. S. Milner-Brown, R. B. Stein, R. Yemm, The contractile properties of human motor units during voluntary isometric contractions. *J. Physiol. (Lond.)* **228**:2 (1973), 285–306.

108. B. Calancie, P. Bawa, Limitations of the spike-triggered averaging technique. *Muscle Nerve* **9**:1 (1986), 78–83.

109. J. M. Elek, R. Dengler, Human motor units studied by intramuscular microstimulation. *Adv. Exp. Med. Biol.* **384** (1995), 161–171.

110. V. G. Macefield, A. J. Fuglevand, B. Bigland-Ritchie, Contractile properties of single motor units in human toe extensors assessed by intraneural motor axon stimulation. *J. Neurophysiol.* **75**:6 (1996), 2509–2519.

111. C. K. Thomas, B. Bigland-Ritchie, G. Westling, R. S. Johansson, A comparison of human thenar motor-unit properties studied by intraneural motor-axon stimulation and spike-triggered averaging. *J. Neurophysiol.* **64**:4 (1990), 1347–1351.

112. C. K. Thomas, R. S. Johansson, B. Bigland-Ritchie, Attempts to physiologically classify human thenar motor units. *J. Neurophysiol.* **65**:6 (1991), 1501–1508.

113. P. Romaiguere, J. P. Vedel, S. Pagni, A. Zenatti, Physiological properties of the motor units of the wrist extensor muscles in man. *Exp. Brain Res.* **78**:1 (1989), 51–61.

114. J. A. Stephens, T. P. Usherwood, The mechanical properties of human motor units with special reference to their fatiguability and recruitment threshold. *Brain Res.* **125**:1 (1977), 91–97.

115. J. M. Elek, A. Kossev, R. Dengler, M. Schubert, K. Wohlfahrt, W. Wolf, Parameters of human motor unit twitches obtained by intramuscular microstimulation. *Neuromuscul. Disord.* **2**:4 (1992), 261–267.

116. R. A. Garnett, M. J. O'Donovan, J. A. Stephens, A. Taylor, Motor unit organization of human medial gastrocnemius. *J. Physiol. (Lond.)* **287** (1979), 33–43.

117. D. Pette, R. S. Staron, Cellular and molecular diversities of mammalian skeletal muscle fibers. *Rev. Physiol. Biochem. Pharmacol.* **116** (1990), 1–76.

118. R. E. Burke, P. Rudomin, F. E. Zajac 3rd., The effect of activation history on tension production by individual muscle units. *Brain Res.* **109**:3 (1976), 515–529.

119. E. Kugelberg, B. Lindegren, Transmission and contraction fatigue of rat motor units in relation to succinate dehydrogenase activity of motor unit fibres. *J. Physiol. (Lond.)* **288** (1979), 285–300.

120. F. C. Romanul, Capillary supply and metabolism of muscle fibers. *Arch. Neurol.* **12** (1965), 497–509.

121. D. L. Morgan, U. Proske, On the branching of motoneurons. *Muscle Nerve* **24**:3 (2001), 372–379.

122. M. H. Brooke, W. K. Engel, The histographic analysis of human muscle biopsies with regard to fiber types. 1. Adult male and female. *Neurology* **19**:3 (1969), 221–233.

123. F. Emonet-Denand, C. C. Hunt, J. Petit, B. Pollin, Proportion of fatigue-resistant motor units in hindlimb muscles of cat and their relation to axonal conduction velocity. *J. Physiol. (Lond.)* **400** (1988), 135–158.

124. J. W. Fleshman, J. B. Munson, G. W. Sypert, W. A. Friedman, Rheobase, input resistance, and motor-unit type in medial gastrocnemius motoneurons in the cat. *J. Neurophysiol.* **46**:6 (1981), 1326–1338.

125. J. E. Zengel, S. A. Reid, G. W. Sypert, J. B. Munson, Membrane electrical properties and prediction of motor-unit type of medial gastrocnemius motoneurons in the cat. *J. Neurophysiol.* **53**:5 (1985), 1323–1344.

126. R. E. Burke, W. Z. Rymer, Relative strength of synaptic input from short-latency pathways to motor units of defined type in cat medial gastrocnemius. *J. Neurophysiol.* **39**:3 (1976), 447–458.

127. R. P. Dum, T. T. Kennedy, Synaptic organization of defined motor-unit types in cat tibialis anterior. *J. Neurophysiol.* **43**:6 (1980), 1631–1644.

128. W. A. Friedman, G. W. Sypert, J. B. Munson, J. W. Fleshman, Recurrent inhibition in type-identified motoneurons. *J. Neurophysiol.* **46**:6 (1981), 1349–1359.

129. M. D. Binder, C. J. Heckman, R. K. Powers, Relative strengths and distributions of different sources of synaptic input to the motoneurone pool: implications for motor unit recruitment. *Adv. Exp. Med. Biol.* **508** (2002), 207–212.

130. R. E. Burke, E. Jankowska, G. ten Bruggencate, A comparison of peripheral and rubrospinal synaptic input to slow and fast twitch motor units of triceps surae. *J. Physiol. (Lond.)* **207**:3 (1970), 709–732.

131. J. P. Gossard, M. K. Floeter, Y. Kawai, R. E. Burke, T. Chang, S. J. Schiff, Fluctuations of excitability in the monosynaptic reflex pathway to lumbar motoneurons in the cat. *J. Neurophysiol.* **72**:3 (1994), 1227–1239.

132. K. Kanda, R. E. Burke, B. Walmsley, Differential control of fast and slow twitch motor units in the decerebrate cat. *Exp. Brain Res.* **29**:1 (1977), 57–74.

133. H. S. Milner-Brown, R. B. Stein, R. Yemm, The orderly recruitment of human motor units during voluntary isometric contractions. *J. Physiol. (Lond.)* **230**:2 (1973), 359–370.

134. J. E. Desmedt, E. Godaux, Fast motor units are not preferentially activated in rapid voluntary contractions in man. *Nature* **267**:5613 (1977), 717–719.

135. D. Kernell, Organized variability in the neuromuscular system: a survey of task-related adaptations. *Arch. Ital. Biol.* **130**:1 (1992), 19–66.

136. E. Henneman, Relation between size of neurons and their susceptibility to discharge. *Science* **126**:3287 (1957), 1345–1347.

137. T. C. Cope, B. D. Clark, Motor-unit recruitment in the decerebrate cat: several unit properties are equally good predictors of order. *J. Neurophysiol.* **66**:4 (1991), 1127–1138.

138. C. J. Barclay, J. K. Constable, C. L. Gibbs, Energetics of fast- and slow-twitch muscles of the mouse. *J. Physiol. (Lond.)* **472** (1993), 61–80.

139. B. Walmsley, J. A. Hodgson, R. E. Burke, Forces produced by medial gastrocnemius and soleus muscles during locomotion in freely moving cats. *J. Neurophysiol.* **41**:5 (1978), 1203–1216.

140. D. Kernell, E. Hensbergen, Use and fibre type composition in limb muscles of cats. *Eur. J. Morphol.* **36**:4–5 (1998), 288–292.

141. R. P. Dum, R. E. Burke, M. J. O'Donovan, J. Toop, J. A. Hodgson, Motor-unit organization in flexor digitorum longus muscle of the cat. *J. Neurophysiol.* **47**:6 (1982), 1108–1125.

142. M. A. Johnson, J. Polgar, D. Weightman, D. Appleton, Data on the distribution of fibre types in thirty-six human muscles. An autopsy study. *J. Neurol. Sci.* **18**:1 (1973), 111–129.

143. J. H. Petajan, AAEM minimonograph #3: motor unit recruitment. *Muscle Nerve* **14**:6 (1991), 489–502.

144. R. H. Lee, J. J. Kuo, M. C. Jiang, C. J. Heckman, Influence of active dendritic currents on input-output processing in spinal motoneurons in vivo. *J. Neurophysiol.* **89**:1 (2003), 27–39.

145. H. Hultborn, M. E. Denton, J. Wienecke, J. B. Nielsen, Variable amplification of synaptic input to cat spinal motoneurones by dendritic persistent inward current. *J. Physiol. (Lond.)* **552**:Pt 3 (2003), 945–952.

146. C. J. Heckmann, M. A. Gorassini, D. J. Bennett, Persistent inward currents in motoneuron dendrites: implications for motor output. *Muscle Nerve* **31**:2 (2005), 135–156.

147. R. E. Burke, P. Rudomin, F. E. Zajac 3rd., Catch property in single mammalian motor units. *Science* **168**:927 (1970), 122–124.

148. Y. Laouris, L. Bevan, R. M. Reinking, D. G. Stuart, Associations between force and fatigue in fast-twitch motor units of a cat hindlimb muscle. *Can. J. Physiol. Pharmacol.* **82**:8–9 (2004), 577–588.

149. A. Christie, G. Kamen, Doublet discharges in motoneurons of young and older adults. *J. Neurophysiol.* **95**:5 (2006), 2787–2795.

150. D. A. Hood, I. Irrcher, V. Ljubicic, A. M. Joseph, Coordination of metabolic plasticity in skeletal muscle. *J. Exp. Biol.* **209**:Pt 12 (2006), 2265–2275.

151. D. Freyssenet, Energy sensing and regulation of gene expression in skeletal muscle. *J. Appl. Physiol.* **102**:2 (2007), 529–540.

152. D. Pette, Historical perspectives: plasticity of mammalian skeletal muscle. *J. Appl. Physiol.* **90**:3 (2001), 1119–1124.

153. D. Pette, R. S. Staron, Myosin isoforms, muscle fiber types, and transitions. *Microsc. Res. Tech.* **50**:6 (2000), 500–509.

154. R. F. Mayer, R. E. Burke, J. Toop, J. A. Hodgson, K. Kanda, B. W. Walmsley, The effect of long-term immobilization on the motor unit population of the cat medial gastrocnemius muscle. *Neuroscience* **6**:4 (1981), 725–739.

155. R. F. Mayer, R. E. Burke, J. Toop, B. Walmsley, J. A. Hodgson, The effect of spinal cord transection on motor units in cat medial gastrocnemius muscles. *Muscle Nerve* 7:1 (1984), 23–31.

156. J. V. Walsh, Jr., R. E. Burke, W. Z. Rymer, P. Tsairis, Effect of compensatory hypertrophy studied in individual motor units in medial gastrocnemius muscle of the cat. *J. Neurophysiol.* **41**:2 (1978), 496–508.

157. A. E. Olha, B. J. Jasmin, R. N. Michel, P. F. Gardiner, Physiological responses of rat plantaris motor units to overload induced by surgical removal of its synergists. *J. Neurophysiol.* **60**:6 (1988), 2138–2151.

158. T. Gordon, C. K. Thomas, J. B. Munson, R. B. Stein, The resilience of the size principle in the organization of motor unit properties in normal and reinnervated adult skeletal muscles. *Can. J. Physiol. Pharmacol.* **82**:8–9 (2004), 645–661.

159. A. J. Buller, J. C. Eccles, R. M. Eccles, Interactions between motoneurones and muscles in respect of the characteristic speeds of their responses. *J. Physiol. (Lond.)* **150** (1960), 417–439.

160. R. P. Dum, M. J. O'Donovan, J. Toop, R. E. Burke, Cross-reinnervated motor units in cat muscle. I. Flexor digitorum longus muscle units reinnervated by soleus motoneurons. *J. Neurophysiol.* **54**:4 (1985), 818–836.

161. G. F. Gauthier, R. E. Burke, S. Lowey, A. W. Hobbs, Myosin isozymes in normal and cross-reinnervated cat skeletal muscle fibers. *J. Cell Biol.* **97**:3 (1983), 756–771.

162. R. P. Dum, M. J. O'Donovan, J. Toop, P. Tsairis, M. J. Pinter, R. E. Burke, Cross-reinnervated motor units in cat muscle. II. Soleus muscle reinnervated by flexor digitorum longus motoneurons. *J. Neurophysiol.* **54**:4 (1985), 837–851.

163. M. J. O'Donovan, M. J. Pinter, R. P. Dum, R. E. Burke, Kinesiological studies of self- and cross-reinnervated FDL and soleus muscles in freely moving cats. *J. Neurophysiol.* **54**:4 (1985), 852–866.

164. V. F. Rafuse, T. Gordon, Incomplete rematching of nerve and muscle properties in motor units after extensive nerve injuries in cat hindlimb muscle. *J. Physiol. (Lond.)* **509**:Pt 3 (1998), 909–926.

165. V. F. Rafuse, T. Gordon, Self-reinnervated cat medial gastrocnemius muscles. I. Comparisons of the capacity for regenerating nerves to form enlarged motor units after extensive peripheral nerve injuries. *J. Neurophysiol.* **75**:1 (1996), 268–281.

166. H. J. Green, D. Pette, Early metabolic adaptations of rabbit fast-twitch muscle to chronic low-frequency stimulation. *Eur. J. Appl. Physiol. Occup. Physiol.* **75**:5 (1997), 418–424.

167. O. Eerbeek, D. Kernell, B. A. Verhey, Effects of fast and slow patterns of tonic long-term stimulation on contractile properties of fast muscle in the cat. *J. Physiol. (Lond.)* **352** (1984), 73–90.

168. D. Kernell, O. Eerbeek, B. A. Verhey, Y. Donselaar, Effects of physiological amounts of high- and low-rate chronic stimulation on fast-twitch muscle of the cat hindlimb. I. Speed- and force-related properties. *J. Neurophysiol.* **58**:3 (1987), 598–613.

169. C. Brownson, H. Isenberg, W. Brown, S. Salmons, Y. Edwards, Changes in skeletal muscle gene transcription induced by chronic stimulation. *Muscle Nerve* **11**:11 (1988), 1183–1189.

170. J. M. Brown, J. Henriksson, S. Salmons, Restoration of fast muscle characteristics following cessation of chronic stimulation: physiological, histochemical and metabolic changes during slow-to-fast transformation. *Proc. R. Soc. Lond. B. Biol. Sci.* **235**:1281 (1989), 321–346.

171. D. Pette, G. Vrbova, Adaptation of mammalian skeletal muscle fibers to chronic electrical stimulation. *Rev. Physiol. Biochem. Pharmacol.* **120** (1992), 115–202.

172. T. Gordon, N. Tyreman, V. F. Rafuse, J. B. Munson, Fast-to-slow conversion following chronic low-frequency activation of medial gastrocnemius muscle in cats. I. Muscle and motor unit properties. *J. Neurophysiol.* **77**:5 (1997), 2585–2604.

173. J. B. Munson, R. C. Foehring, L. M. Mendell, T. Gordon, Fast-to-slow conversion following chronic low-frequency activation of medial gastrocnemius muscle in cats. II. Motoneuron properties. *J. Neurophysiol.* **77**:5 (1997), 2605–2615.

174. W. J. Thompson, L. C. Soileau, R. J. Balice-Gordon, L. A. Sutton, Selective innervation of types of fibres in developing rat muscle. *J. Exp. Biol.* **132** (1987), 249–263.

175. E. C. Cooper, L. Y. Jan, Ion channel genes and human neurological disease: recent progress, prospects, and challenges. *Proc. Natl. Acad. Sci. U. S. A.* **96**:9 (1999), 4759–4766.

Chapter 2

Myogenic precursor cells

Miranda D. Grounds and Frederic Relaix

Introduction

Formation of skeletal muscle

Skeletal muscle fibers (myofibers) are long syncytial cells with thousands of nuclei. Careful histological observation in the late 1800s clearly demonstrated a great capacity for new muscle formation in many species and it is now widely accepted that during development and in regenerating muscle new myonuclei result from proliferation of mononucleated muscle precursor cells (myoblasts) that fuse together to form multinucleated cells (myotubes) and these mature into myofibers (Figure 2.1).

Origin of myogenic precursor cells and different muscles during development

A detailed discussion of the origin and formation of skeletal muscle during embryogenesis (for reviews see [1, 2, 3]) falls beyond the scope of this chapter, which is focused largely on postnatal muscle. Skeletal muscle is distributed throughout the whole organism, and, when one considers spatial regulation, it is striking that different muscle groups are subjected during development to distinct signaling environments. Highlighting the complexity of understanding muscle formation, little is known about how muscle patterning is regulated. However, it is now widely accepted that all the skeletal muscle of the vertebrate trunk and limbs is derived from progenitor cells located in the somites, pairs of transient epithelial segments derived from paraxial mesoderm that form following an anterior–posterior progression on either side of the neural tube in birds and mouse embryos. Somites arise from the mesenchymal paraxial mesoderm in a regular sequence in an anteroposterior direction as pairs of epithelial spheres budding off on each side of the neural tube. This process is controlled by a segmentation clock involving the *Notch*, *Fgf* and *Wnt* signaling pathways [4]. The peripheral nervous system, which is the other component of the nerve–muscle motor unit, is formed at the same time from neural crest cells that migrate from the dorsal neural tube [5]. In response to environment cues, the somites differentiate into a ventral mesenchymal domain, the sclerotome, and a dorsal epithelium, the dermomyotome. While the sclerotome provides the tendons, cartilage, and bones of the axis (vertebral column and ribs), the latter gives rise to the dermis and the skeletal muscle of the trunk, limbs, pharynx and tongue, in addition to some blood vessels.

In brief, there are three major sources of different groups of skeletal muscles (reviewed in [1, 2, 3]). The somitic **myotome** gives rise to cells that develop into the epaxial trunk and back muscles whereas others in the lateral/ventral domain develop into hypaxial muscles, including body wall, intercostal, and abdominal muscles. While the embryological development of epaxial muscles has been well described, less is known about postnatal satellite cells and molecular signaling in these muscles, compared with limb muscles that have been the focus of much research using animal models. Yet disturbed function of the back muscles has many medical consequences, e.g., related to kyphosis and lower back problems. Some of the **hypaxial somites** (the cervical somites and somites facing the limbs) do not contribute to the myotome and body muscle masses but instead undergo long-range migration to form distant muscles, such as those of the limb, tongue, and diaphragm. The **paraxial head and prechordal mesoderm** give rise to craniofacial muscles including extraocular, branchial and laryngoglossal, and esophageal muscles. Strikingly little is currently known about the distinct genetic networks at work in the formation of facial and head muscles [1]. However, because certain diseases (e.g., oculopharyngeal muscular dystrophy) appear to target or spare specifically all, or groups of, head muscles (e.g., extraocular muscles are generally not affected in patients with Duchenne muscular dystrophy, DMD), understanding the developmental and molecular specificity of these muscles is of much interest.

The populations of muscle precursor cells that give rise to these disparate types of muscles will eventually contribute to the satellite cell pool (Figure 2.1) of postnatal myogenic precursors [6]. From embryonic day 16.5 in the mouse, satellite cells are formed from the Pax7-expressing fetal muscle progenitor cells that progressively become embedded under the basal lamina, in close contact with the myofibers [7]. Satellite

Disorders of Voluntary Muscle, 8th edn., eds. George Karpati, David Hilton-Jones, Kate Bushby and Robert C. Griggs. Published by Cambridge University Press.

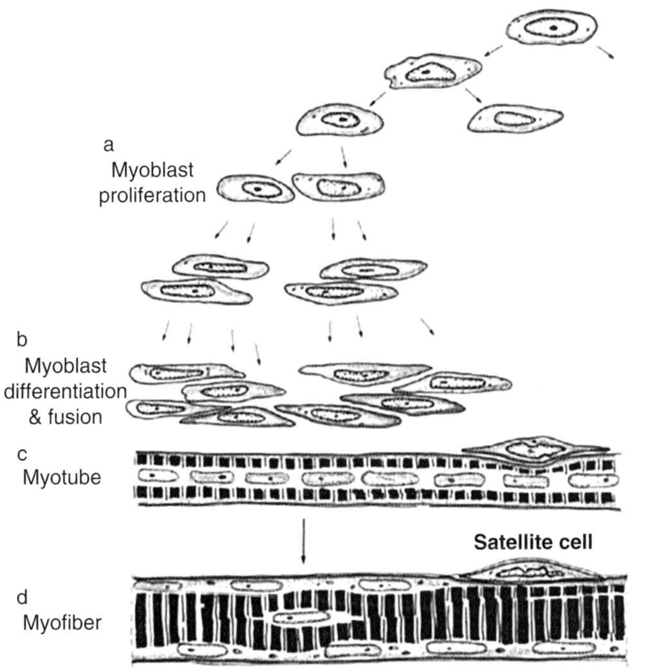

Figure 2.1. Formation of skeletal myofibers and satellite cells. Diagram of myogenesis. This simple diagram illustrates (a) the proliferation of mononucleated myogenic precursor cells called myoblasts; followed by (b) myoblast alignment associated with cessation of proliferation and onset of differentiation; (c) fusion of many myoblasts to form multinucleated young muscle fibers (myotubes) that (d) differentiate further to mature into functional myofibers (under the influence of innervation – not shown). A similar sequence of myogenic events occurs during both embryogenesis and regeneration of damaged adult muscles. The satellite cell is a resident quiescent mononucleated myogenic precursor cell located on the surface of the myofiber beneath the basal lamina.

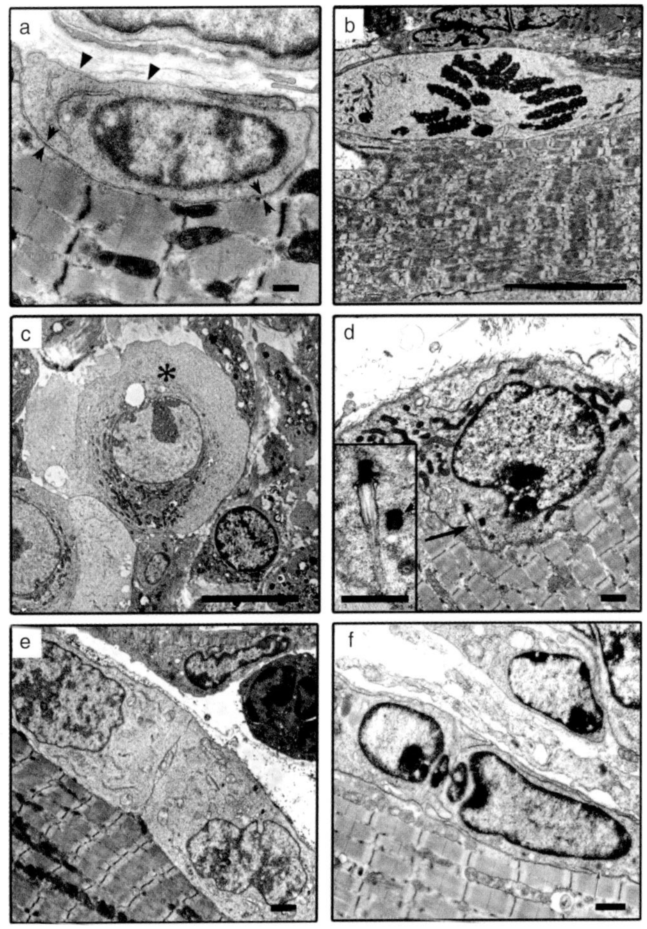

Figure 2.2. Satellite cells identified by electron microscopy. High magnification of satellite cells/myoblasts shown by transmission electron microscopy, in regenerating adult mouse muscle sampled up to 5 days after chemical injury. (a) Classical quiescent satellite cell: note the minimal cytoplasm, the cell membrane surrounding the satellite cell in close proximity to the sarcolemma of the underlying myofiber (short arrows) and the basal lamina of the myofiber enclosing the satellite cell (arrow heads). (b) Activated satellite cell undergoing mitosis; the sarcomere architecture is disturbed in this injured myofiber. Many activated satellite cells remain fusiform often with pseudopodial extensions, but some are spherical with organelles arranged concentrically around the nucleus, similar to (c) spherical myoblasts lying between myofibers: an electron lucent zone can be seen in one of the two cells (asterisk) and phagocytic cells are closely apposed. Cilia are relatively frequent in myoblasts located outside the myofiber although they are rare in satellite cells. (d) An activated satellite cell with cilium (long arrow) with a high power of the cilium and centriole (short arrow) in the insert; the cilia are presumably associated with motility. (e) Two daughter satellite cells following cell division. (f) Two macrophages located between the basal lamina and sarcolemma (distinguished by lysosomes in the cytoplasm), emphasizing the difficulty of precisely identifying satellite cells on the basis of position. Scale bar is 1 μm in (a) and insert in (d); whereas it is 10 μm for all other panels (b, c, d, e, f). All images are from the PhD thesis by Terry Robertson, 1996, the University of Western Australia.

cells cannot be identified until a basal lamina can be detected and this is around 10–15 weeks in utero in humans [8]. Genes and signaling pathways involved in the transition from a population of fetal muscle precursor cells to a self-renewing population of postnatal satellite cells have not yet been characterized.

Source of myoblasts in adult muscle

The source of the myoblasts in adult muscle has been widely debated since the 1800s. The four main possibilities are that myoblasts in adult muscle might originate from: (1) a nucleus within the myofiber, (2) a cell beneath the basal lamina (specialized extracellular matrix) on the surface of the myofiber, (3) local cells in the interstitial connective tissue, possibly perivascular or (4) non-local cells derived from the circulation. In myotubes and myofibers, the nuclei within the sarcoplasm (myonuclei) are generally considered to be postmitotic. In response to injury of adult muscle, the possibility that these postmitotic myonuclei might become sequestered (by new membrane to generate mononucleated cells) to form functional new myoblasts has received little support for mammalian muscle (although this certainly occurs in some other species) but is difficult to completely exclude (reviewed in [9]). Instead, it is now widely accepted that myoblasts are derived mainly from a quiescent myogenic mononucleated precursor cell located on the surface of the myofiber beneath the basal lamina; this was described for frog muscle in 1961 and named the satellite cell purely on the basis of its anatomical position [10] (Figures 2.1 and 2.2). For an excellent description of satellite cells see [11] and for further historical perspectives of satellite cells see [12].

Myogenic cells (myoblasts) extracted from adult skeletal muscle can be grown in tissue culture where they proliferate and form myotubes: it is widely assumed that the myoblasts in such primary muscle cultures originate from satellite cells although it is difficult to exclude the contribution of other cells within the interstitial tissue (e.g., associated with blood vessels or circulating cells). Satellite cells are now widely held to be the main source of myoblasts and may have stem-cell-like properties in postnatal skeletal muscle. Recently, the revived idea that myoblasts can also arise from other sources of cells (points 3 and 4 above) has attracted intense interest as part of the stem cell debate as discussed below (see "Cell therapy: stem cells and other sources of myoblasts").

Postnatal muscle: satellite cells and their control

Genetic hierarchies operating in postnatal satellite cells

Unraveling the complex regulation of muscle formation is a challenging task. Despite recent progress in the field using large-scale genomic approaches, little is known about the genetic regulation that leads to the specificity of distinct myogenic programs, and how these programs are regulated by extracellular signaling pathways. Another issue awaiting elucidation at molecular and cellular levels is the observation that specific defects in genes expressed in all skeletal muscles can lead to phenotypes affecting only some groups of muscles (this has many clinical manifestations). Muscle progenitor cells depend upon Pax3 and Pax7 [7], while myogenesis and the formation of myofibers depend upon expression of the myogenic regulatory factors (MRFs), Myf5, Mrf4 and MyoD. Targeted disruption of *Myf5*, *Mrf4* and *MyoD* genes in the mouse (so that they are no longer expressed) suggests that these three MRFs independently determine muscle identity, since in triple mutant mice (where all three gene products are absent) myoblasts and skeletal muscles are missing at all myogenic sites and the progenitor cells remain undetermined [1, 13, 14]. While Pax3 is a specific marker for early and fetal embryonic muscle precursors [3, 7] nearly all postnatal quiescent satellite cells are identified by the presence of Pax7 protein [15]; *Pax3* expression, unlike that of *Pax7*, is not uniformly maintained in adult satellite cells [2]. Expression of the MRF proteins is not detected in quiescent satellite cells, however a Myf5-driven reporter labels almost all satellite cells, reflecting either the self-renewing mechanism of satellite cells (Figure 2.3) or that Myf5 can be expressed at a low level in quiescent satellite cells. During postnatal muscle growth and after injury, satellite cells are activated and proliferate. Activated satellite cells maintain the expression of the *Pax* genes, and show robust expression of Myf5 and MyoD. Myogenin and MRF4 are only detected in terminally differentiating satellite cells undergoing cell cycle exit. Studies performed ex vivo and in vivo have led to different models where activated satellite cells can undergo asymmetric division, as a means of providing fate diversification allowing self-renewal as well as contributing to muscle repair or growth (Figure 2.3).

As observed during embryonic development, the interplay between the *Pax* and *MRF* genes is important for self-renewal and differentiation of satellite cells: genetic hierarchies at work during embryonic muscle formation are redeployed in adult myogenesis [2], with Pax7 regulating MyoD expression during satellite cell activation [2]. Furthermore, failure of downregulation of Pax7 as activated satellite cells undergo terminal differentiation leads to delayed myogenin expression [3]. While Pax7-deficient mice have a nearly normal content of satellite cells at birth, the population is progressively depleted as a result of increased apoptosis and cell cycle defects [2].

Cell fate decisions in the satellite cells are controlled by Notch signaling [16], as well as asymmetric distribution of Numb, an inhibitor of Notch [17] that segregates with Pax7. The link between Notch signaling and transcriptional regulation has yet to be made.

Markers for satellite cells

Satellite cells were classically identified by their anatomical position using electron microscopy (Figure 2.2). Even this can be difficult since pericytes can resemble satellite cells, and macrophages, neutrophils and other cells can infiltrate and lie beneath the basal lamina of myofibers [11] (Figure 2.2). Now, satellite cells can also be visualized on the surface of myofibers by light microscopy (aided by confocal microscopy) using combinations of specific antibodies to immunostain components of the basal lamina (e.g., laminin or collagen IV) and the sarcolemma (e.g., dystrophin or spectrin). Beyond this approach, quiescent satellite cells are very difficult to observe in tissue sections because they have little cytoplasm and relatively low levels of gene expression (it is difficult to detect small amounts of key proteins in vivo using routine immunohistochemistry, e.g., Myf5). Activated satellite cells can move out of this classical position beneath the basal lamina (into the extracellular matrix space) and, to further complicate the situation, it is now recognized that myoblasts may be derived from cells other than satellite cells, originating outside the myofiber [18]. In adult muscle, all mononucleated myogenic cells are often widely referred to as myoblasts, regardless of their origin.

One of the most reliable markers for quiescent satellite cells in mouse muscle is the cell surface marker M-cadherin that is located at the interface with the underlying myofiber, although mRNA expression appears to be very low. M-cadherin is also present on myoblasts in culture and on isolated myofibers, where most (but probably not all) mouse satellite cells are positive for M-cadherin protein and it appears that M-cadherin protein may be very low (or absent) in some satellite cells. For human muscle, antibodies to M-CAM (CD56), originally called Leu-19, are a useful marker to identify quiescent and activated satellite cells and give similar results to M-cadherin

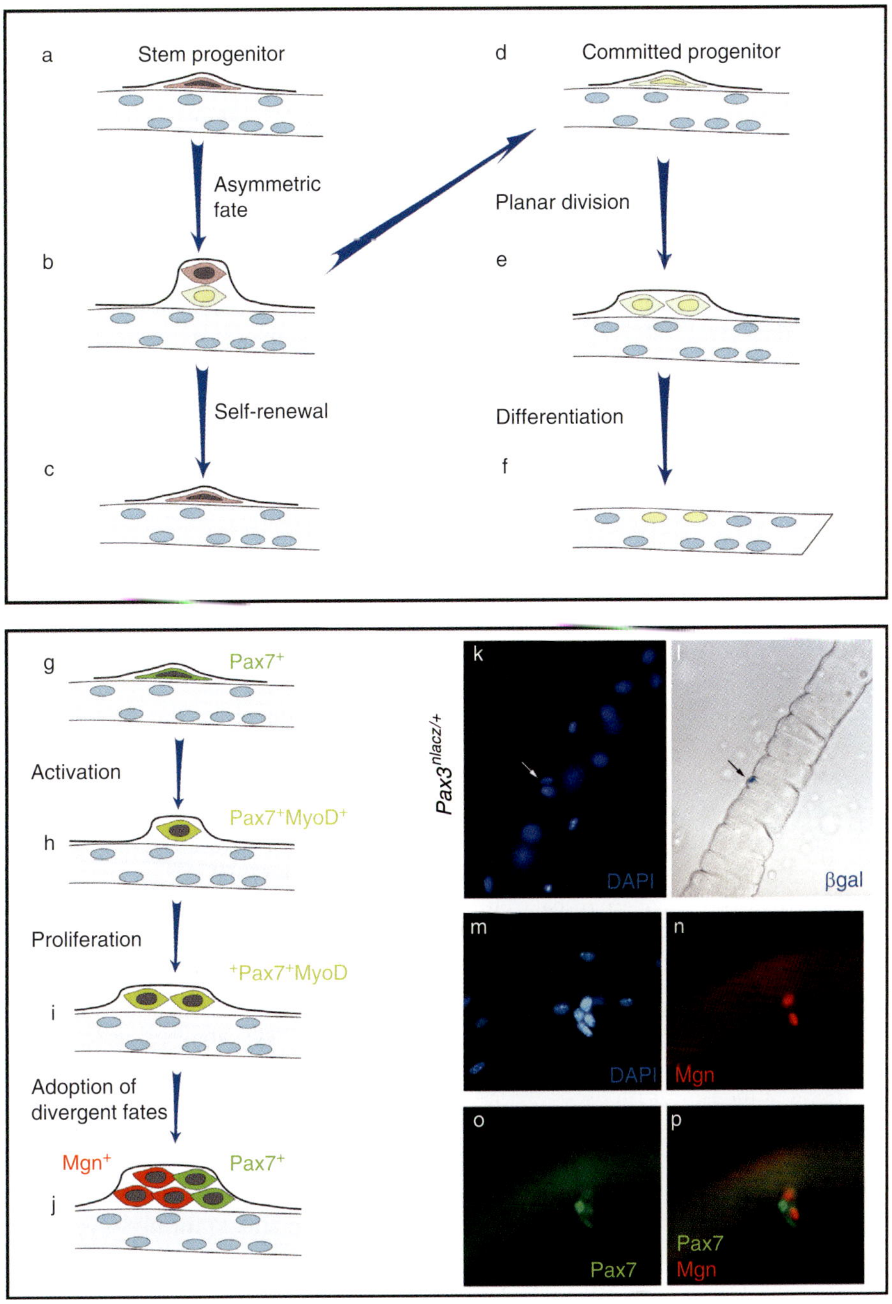

Figure 2.3. Models for satellite cell self-renewal and commitment. (a–f) Satellite cells located under the basal lamina (a) can adopt different fates through asymmetric division (b) by dividing in an apical–basal orientation, which allows self-renewal (c) and specification of committed progenitors (d). Both stem progenitor cells and committed progenitors can also proliferate through planar divisions (e) before differentiation (f) and fusion with the parent myofiber [28]. (g–j) Cultured single mouse myofibers with associated satellite cells allow the visualization of adoption of divergent fates [30]. Quiescent satellite cells are labelled by Pax7 (and Pax3). In floating cultures of intact myofibers, the satellite cells can undergo activation (expressing Pax7 and MyoD; h) before dividing (i). After 3 days of culture, in the clusters formed by the activated satellite cells, divergent fates can be observed: a subset of the cells activates myogenin (Mgn) and undergoes terminal myogenic differentiation while a subset returns to a quiescent-like stage and expresses Pax7. (k, l) Example of cultured single myofibers from *Pax3*$^{nlacZ/+}$ mice. The satellite cells are labeled by gal (l), and represent a subset of the DAPI-positive nuclei (k). (m–p) Example of a cluster of satellite cells on isolated myofibers after 3 days in culture, with asymmetric cell fates. DAPI labeling of the nuclei in shown in (m) (blue), myogenin in (n) (red), Pax7 in (o) (green), and complete absence of co-labeling between Pax7 and myogenin in (p): the images o and p correspond to the diagrams (i) and (j) respectively. (All images provided courtesy of Sonia Alonso-Martin & Relaix.)

antibody [19]. A plethora of molecular markers (cell surface and intracellular) have been described since the early 1990s to help identify satellite cells by light microscopy, using either highly specific antibodies or (in experimental studies) reporter genes such as beta-galactosidase (LacZ) or green fluorescent protein (GFP). Most of these markers are not exclusive to satellite cells (reviewed in [9, 18, 20]). Some that are found only in skeletal muscle cells, e.g., Myf5 and MyoD, are rapidly upregulated in activated satellite cells (Figure 2.3) but are also expressed by differentiated myoblasts and myonuclei (e.g., in denervated muscle). The cytoskeletal protein desmin is a very useful marker for identifying myoblasts [21] but levels are low in quiescent satellite cells and desmin is also expressed by smooth muscle cells of the vasculature and cardiomyocytes. Many other satellite cell markers are less specific since they are also expressed by a variety of other cell types (blood vessels, interstitial or circulating cells) within skeletal muscle tissue, e.g., c-Met (the receptor for hepatocyte growth factor), syndecan-3 and syndecan-4 (proteoglycans that bind many growth factors), and CD34. Other important molecules expressed by satellite cells such as Pax3, Pax7, and nestin are also markers of cells in neural and other tissues. While Pax7 is generally an excellent marker of adult satellite cells (it does not recognize other cell types in skeletal muscle), it is not expressed by many cells lying in the satellite cell position in very old muscle [12, 22]. Combinations of the above markers are often employed. While such molecular markers have been widely used to identify and study isolated cultured muscle precursor cells or satellite cells associated with single myofibers, they do not readily overcome the difficult problem of visualizing all satellite cells in tissue sections, especially of human muscle. Expression of many of these molecular markers has been visualized using reporter genes in experimental animal models. Unfortunately, specific antibodies suitable for immunohistochemistry on sections of human (and mouse) muscle are not readily available for some of these myogenic markers, e.g., Myf5, and thus they cannot be exploited to identify satellite cells in this situation. However, with the development of new antibodies and due care in interpretation, these markers can be useful to identify in tissue sections some (if not all) satellite cells through their expression of Pax7 and nestin [23] and also Myf5. Quiescence is also associated with expression of the truncated form of the cell surface protein CD34 and the β isoform of the forkhead transcription factor MNF (myocyte nuclear factor/FoxK1). When satellite cells are activated (in tissue sections or in culture), Pax7 and nestin expression decreases, whereas levels of Myf5 and/or MyoD increase.

Sca-1 (stem cell antigen-1) is absent from quiescent myoblasts but has been used as a marker of a subpopulation of activated myogenic (putative stem) cells that have a slower rate of proliferation. The expression of Sca-1 demonstrates the heterogeneity of satellite cell/myoblast populations [24] and modulation of Sca-1 by the micro-environment emphasizes the importance of extrinsic factors in the control of myogenesis, a recurring theme throughout this discussion.

Isolated myogenic (or stem) cells extracted from skeletal muscle tissue by enzymatic digestion can be purified by fluorescent activated cell sorting (FACS) using a range of specific antibodies that bind to cell surface markers such as CD34 and CD133 (also known as AC133). It is noted that expression of such cell surface markers may rapidly change once the cells are removed from their normal in vivo environment. Alternatively, side-populations of cells that do not stain with the nuclear dye Hoechst can be isolated and these are widely considered to represent stem cells. None of these markers is exclusive for satellite cells (as indicated above). However, they can be combined for more specific sorting with size and granulosity [25] and are very useful for collecting populations of myogenic (or stem) cells from skeletal muscle for tissue culture studies or for transplantation purposes.

Is there a stem cell subpopulation of satellite cells?

The idea of stem cells was largely motivated by mathematical logic, with little scientific verification for the distinction between stem and precursor cells. The properties of stem cells include longevity, asymmetric cell division, genetic fidelity (immortal DNA strand hypothesis), and plasticity, although many of these also apply to precursor cells.

The first criterion of longevity is clearly met by satellite cells since they are present even in very old muscle, with a capacity to proliferate extensively and to self-renew [22, 26]. The well documented heterogeneity of satellite cells might reflect the presence of a stem cell subpopulation. Asymmetric cell division is a feature of stem cells during embryogenesis, as is preservation of the original strand of DNA (immortal DNA strand hypothesis) throughout many cell divisions, thus providing an unaltered original template for the generation of a replacement stem cell. There is good evidence (using BrdU-labeling of new DNA, as well as lineage studies using genetically controlled reporters) for both the segregation of a template strand of DNA and asymmetric cell division of satellite cells both in tissue culture and in vivo [17, 27, 28, 29] (Figure 2.3). Asymmetric distribution of a range of proteins has been demonstrated in daughter cells after mitosis of satellite cells. One of these is Numb, which is an important marker of asymmetric cell division during development; it also inhibits the transcription factor Notch, which is required for activation of satellite cells in damaged adult muscle (discussed below under *Aging muscle – numbers and function of satellite celles*). Other molecules with demonstrated asymmetric distribution into only one daughter satellite cell are Pax7 and Myf5 (Figure 2.3).

As shown in Figure 2.3, it has been proposed that where a satellite cell divides in a plane where the mitotic spindle is perpendicular to the myofiber (i.e., one daughter cell is in intimate contact with the sarcolemma whereas the other contacts only the basal lamina), this results in asymmetric division to generate one committed ($Pax7^+/Myf5^+$) myoblast (adjacent to the sarcolemma) and one self-renewing ($Pax7^+/Myf5^-$) stem cell (in contact with the basal lamina). In contrast, it is proposed that where the two daughter cells resulting from division of a satellite cell lie parallel to the myofiber (i.e., both have equal exposure to the sarcolemma and the basal lamina) this results in symmetric division with generation of two identical daughter cells (either committed progenitors or stem cells) [28, 29]. Studies performed using floating, isolated, single myofiber cultures have demonstrated that satellite cells can also undergo asymmetric cell fate choice within clusters [30] (Figure 2.3). There are technical issues associated with identification of such asymmetric divisions (that appear to be rare), and the extent to which this might occur in vivo is unclear. That physical contact can determine the lineage fate of cells and generation of stem cells is well established for events during embryogenesis and there is certainly evidence that physical contact is required for non-myogenic cells to convert to a myogenic lineage [18]. One of the key molecules implicated in such myogenic lineage conversion is Notch signaling. Additional studies are required to determine the exact sequence of these events and the molecular pathways involved. Furthermore, the regeneration potential of the different satellite cell populations (i.e., possible stem versus committed progenitors, see Figure 2.3) remains essentially uncharacterized due to the lack of specific markers. In addition, the mechanism determining the consistency of numbers and distribution of satellite cells on different types of myofibers, especially during self-renewal, is not understood and is hardly explained by the current models (Figure 2.3).

With respect to plasticity, there is plenty of evidence that mesenchymal cells such as myoblasts can readily convert into different lineages (adipocytes, fibroblasts, chondrocytes), depending on the precise tissue culture conditions to which they are exposed. Whether this represents a true lineage conversion or a shifting of the molecular and biochemical program within a cell can be debated. Plasticity of satellite cells has clearly been demonstrated experimentally and the impact of a fibrogenic environment that can convert cells from a myogenic to a fibrogenic program in diseased and aged muscle is discussed later.

Overall, the satellite cell population manifests all the properties of stem cells but the question remains as to whether there is a dedicated stem cell subpopulation of satellite cells, or whether the heterogeneous nature of the population means that all satellite cells have the potential to manifest these properties.

Factors controlling satellite cell quiescence, activation, and proliferation in vivo

The factors that maintain the satellite cells in a quiescent state in normal skeletal muscle, as well as the conditions that activate satellite cells from this quiescent state, are not fully understood although there have been intensive studies in tissue culture to try to define the key molecular events involved (reviewed in [18]). With respect to maintenance of quiescence, it seems that the electrical activity (electrical potential) of the sarcolemma may play a role, since silencing neuromuscular transmission (by botulinum toxin or denervation) results in transient activation of satellite cells. However, the precise sequence of membrane-associated signals that results in such activation is not understood. Other situations that alter the status of the sarcolemma are: mechanical tension; growth and hypertrophy that increase myofiber size and stimulate satellite cell proliferation and fusion with the growing myofiber; and physical trauma or muscle diseases that damage the sarcolemma to result in myofiber necrosis that provokes regeneration (with associated inflammation, satellite cell activation, and new muscle formation). All of these situations probably change the response of satellite cells to growth factors (GFs). This involves many different events including modulation of membrane and extracellular matrix components, changes in the availability of GFs stored in the extracellular matrix with conversion from inactive to bioactive forms, possible changes in binding proteins that affect the bioavailability of extracellular GFs, and altered expression of specific GFs and also of receptors for different GFs.

Cell membrane: Sphingolipids are important components of the plasma membrane and sphingolipid signaling may play a central role in maintaining quiescence and in the early events initiating satellite cell activation. Sphingomyelin is located in the inner leaflet of the lipid bilayer of the plasma membrane and, upon activation, is metabolized to form the bioactive sphingolipid, sphingosine-1-phosphate, which binds to a range of cell surface receptors and is mitogenic for many cell types including satellite cells [31]. Differential interactions between the surface of satellite cells and the sarcolemmal or the overlying basement membrane have been proposed as a determinant of asymmetric cell division (in a perpendicular plane compared with symmetric planar division), as a mechanism for possible self-renewal of a stem cell compartment of satellite cells [29].

Extracellular matrix: the cell membrane surface of satellite cells (and myofibers) is in intimate contact with the extracellular matrix (ECM), especially the specialized basement membrane that surrounds the myofiber, and even small changes in this environment will have an impact on the cells. The great complexity of molecular interactions in the ECM that affect satellite and other cells has been recently reviewed with respect to the many events that occur during skeletal muscle regeneration [32]. A brief outline of some of the key molecular interactions involved in normal homeostasis and for activation of satellite cells and all aspects of myogenesis (myoblast proliferation, differentiation, and fusion to form myotubes) follows.

Heparan sulfate (HS) proteoglycans and their modification by sulfation play a crucial role in GF regulation in all tissues. The HS proteoglycans bind to GFs to affect their stability and bioavailability and are also required for the binding of many GFs to their cell surface receptors, e.g., this is especially important for fibroblast growth factors (FGFs) and hepatocyte growth factor (HGF; also known as scatter factor). In skeletal muscle some of the important HS proteoglycans for modulating GF interactions at the satellite cell surface are biglycan, perlecan, syndecans and glycipan-1, with decorin in the interstitial connective tissue playing a role in sequestering GFs such as transforming growth factor beta (TGFβ) and myostatin. The ECM is constantly being modified by myriad enzymes including sulfatases and proteases and their inhibitors, and it is reasonable to conclude that these also play crucial roles in many aspects of myogenesis in muscle tissue. Other ECM molecules such as laminin (in the basement membrane), collagen, fibronectin, and hyaluronan affect different aspects of myogenesis in tissue culture studies, especially myotube formation and maturation, although relatively little is known for many of these regarding their specific importance for satellite cell quiescence, activation, proliferation, and fusion in muscle in vivo. The central importance of the ECM environment in determining the properties and response of satellite cells in vivo is discussed below with respect to the impact of fibrosis in dystrophic, denervated, and aging muscle.

Growth factors and their receptors: growth factors (GFs) are small protein molecules that influence cell behavior, and cytokines are GFs that are produced mainly by inflammatory blood-derived cells (although many are produced by a multitude of other cell types). Many GFs are produced locally to affect the same cell (autocrine action) or an adjacent cell (paracrine effect) but other GFs travel through the bloodstream to affect distant cells (endocrine). Multitudes of GFs play important roles in the complex in vivo milieu to influence many aspects of muscle progenitor behavior including chemotaxis, activation of satellite (and possibly other stem) cells, stimulation of myoblast proliferation and differentiation, and there may be overlapping functions and redundancy. The discussion below focuses on some GFs that are produced by muscle, act locally, and have been extensively studied in cultured muscle cells. The important role of many other GFs (e.g., platelet-derived growth factor, tumor necrosis factor, interleukins, vascular endothelial factor, and hormones) is too broad a subject to be addressed here. Much attention has focused on the role of GFs in all aspects of satellite cell myogenesis, with the vast majority of studies having been carried out using tissue culture and immortalized cell lines, primary cultures of skeletal muscle cells, and isolated myofibers (reviewed in [33]). It can be difficult to translate the results of tissue culture experiments to the in vivo situation due to many factors; for example, the extent to which some of the high doses of GFs used in tissue culture studies reflect normal physiological conditions. Crucial interactions of GFs with many ECM components as occurs in live muscles in vivo [32] also need to be considered, although until recently this was not a feature of most tissue culture studies; however, the importance of heparan sulfate proteoglycans (in the ECM) binding to members of the FGF family and to HGF is now widely recognized (as indicated above). Overall, the availability of the specific heparan sulfate proteoglycans combined with the specific GF receptor and bioavailable GF controls the response of satellite cells. The relative balance between availability and activity of different GFs (and their receptors) determines the final cellular response.

The quiescent state of satellite cells appears to be associated with high levels of the TGFβ superfamily, with decreased activity required for satellite cell activation. In brief, some of the most important GFs involved in the very early events of satellite cell activation and proliferation appear to involve decreased levels of the TGFβ superfamily, combined with increased activity of various FGFs and HGF that are mitogenic for satellite cells (reviewed in [33, 34]).

The TGFβ superfamily has three typical TGFβs that are released as an inactive complex. They are stored in the ECM and have little biological activity until proteinase activity reveals the active domain. It is generally agreed that TGFβ1 suppresses myoblast differentiation and high levels of TGFβ are also strongly associated with fibrosis (the latter is of increasing importance in diseased and aging muscle). There is some dispute over the role of TGFβs in suppressing satellite cell activation and proliferation but this has been overshadowed by the discovery of **myostatin** (GDF8: growth differentiation factor), a member of the TGFβ superfamily that is highly expressed in skeletal muscle. Myostatin attracted huge attention in 1997 when a mouse deficient in myostatin was described with a striking phenotype of massive muscle growth. Such myostatin deficiency associated with "double muscling" has also been identified in cattle, dogs, and humans. It is proposed that myostatin has a negative influence on satellite cell proliferation and that a lack of myostatin leads to increased activation of satellite cells; although evidence is now emerging that postnatal myostatin blockade results in myofiber hypertrophy unaccompanied by any evidence of increased satellite cell activity [35]. The pronounced increase in muscle mass in the absence of myostatin during development is considered to be due to sustained satellite cell proliferation, resulting in additional myofibers (hence the term "double muscling") in addition to myofiber hypertrophy: the relative roles of these two processes during development and in different postnatal muscles lacking myostatin are complex and controversial [36]. Tissue culture studies indicate that the potent effect of myostatin as a suppressor of satellite cell activation and proliferation is mediated by upregulation of p21 (and hence inhibition of cyclin-dependent kinase), which leads to reduced phosphorylation of the retinoblastoma (Rb) protein. Myostatin (like TGFβ1) also prevents myoblast differentiation due to inhibition of MyoD expression and activity: myostatin affects the MyoD promoter via activation of Smad3 signaling. Mighty is a recently characterized gene that appears to play a key role in the signaling cascade between extracellular myostatin and the transcription factors that govern myogenesis [37]. Effects of myostatin on adipocytes and adipogenesis are also of interest [36]. It is important to note that big is not always better: while muscle mass is greatly increased in the absence of myostatin, one group reported no increase in strength [35] and another showed that force production is compromised and muscles are weaker with reduced strength per cross-sectional area of the muscle (specific force) [38]. In addition, dystrophic mdx muscles in which myostatin was inhibited had reduced endurance to treadmill exercise [35]. Furthermore, although overall initial numbers of satellite cells per myofiber are increased in myostatin-null mice, the normal age-related decline in satellite cell numbers appears to occur [33]. There is much interest in the roles that myostatin may play in muscle atrophy and hypertrophy and thus much attention to possible clinical interventions in muscle wasting and disease [36].

The FGF family has over 20 members, which bind to receptors coded for by five different genes (FGFR-1–FGFR-5) with numerous splice forms of these gene products [33]. Of this large GF family, FGF-2 is well recognized as a potent mitogen for satellite cells and myoblasts. Administration of additional FGF-2 to damaged muscles in vivo does not increase myoblast proliferation or improve muscle regeneration, possibly because there is already sufficient FGF-2 available: instead the presence of the FGF-2 receptors and critical

HS proteoglycans may be a limiting factor in vivo. Tissue culture studies show that FGF-1, -2, -4, -6, -9 and HGF all enhance satellite cell proliferation to a similar extent, whereas other FGFs have no effect. High levels of expression of FGF-6 (that correlate with expression of the receptor FGF-4) in developing muscle and also in normal and damaged myofibers suggest that FGF-6 plays a particularly important role in myogenesis of developing and adult muscle. However, studies in FGF-6-null mice are conflicting and it seems likely that there is overlapping function between FGF-2 and FGF-6. Similarly there may be different and overlapping functions between the FGF receptors FGFR1 (present in many cell types) and FGFR4 (high in developing muscle). It is proposed that FGFR1 may maintain myoblast proliferation, whereas FGFR4 may be involved in the transition from proliferation to differentiation [33]. The additive beneficial effects of the FGFs and HGF appear to be critical for satellite cell activation and proliferation but their precise interactions and roles are yet to be fully defined in vivo.

Hepatocyte growth factor (HGF, also called scatter factor, SF) activates quiescent satellite cells and is a potent mitogen for myoblasts but not fibroblasts (in this way it differs from FGF-2), therefore making HGF a very attractive factor for preferentially stimulating myogenesis without fibrosis in vivo. HGF is present in two forms: the inactive monomer (single chain) pro-HGF is secreted and stored in the ECM, where it is cleaved by proteases to form the active heterodimer HGF that has a limited capacity to diffuse in vivo [33]. HGF protein is present in myotubes in vitro and adult myofibers in vivo and the mRNA is produced by myofibers and myoblasts. The receptor for HGF, c-Met, is expressed by quiescent satellite cells and is considered a marker for satellite cells, although c-Met is also expressed on other types of cells present in muscle tissue. Once activated, the satellite cells are kept proliferating and prevented from differentiating by HGF (combined with certain FGFs). The relative importance of HGF compared with FGFs in the early events of satellite cell activation and proliferation is slightly controversial. One very early event that may activate HGF in response to muscle stretch and injury is the release of the enzyme nitric oxide synthase from the basal lamina; this produces nitric oxide that then activates the metalloproteases in the ECM to cleave the pro-HGF to the active form. In addition to their multiple roles in activation, proliferation, and differentiation of muscle cells, both HGF and FGFs are also chemotactic and this may serve to attract satellite (and other) cells to the site of injury to facilitate regeneration. The complexity of in vivo administration of GFs is illustrated by experiments where intramuscular injection of HGF into injured muscles increased myoblast proliferation but did not improve regeneration, whereas sustained administration inhibited myoblast differentiation leading to impaired regeneration. Such studies emphasize the critical importance of the timing of various GF actions that normally occur throughout the process of regeneration, with each GF present in the right amount at the right time.

Insulin-like growth factor-1 (IGF-1) is another important GF that has attracted much attention with respect to skeletal muscle. It is well documented that the IGFs have potent effects on myoblast proliferation and differentiation, and they have recently attracted particular interest due to their anabolic effects which lead to muscle hypertrophy [39]. This has led to suggestions that IGF-I administration might prevent myofiber atrophy and loss of function resulting from aging, disuse, cachexia, and disease as well as reduce the necrosis of dystrophic myofibers (discussed below).

The principles outlined above indicate the complexity of regulating GF activity, with a wealth of different forms of GFs and their receptors, as well as crucial interactions with ECM molecules that determine their bioavailability and bioactivity. Whether administration of exogenous GFs as a therapeutic strategy can significantly enhance clinical muscle function or repair remains to be determined.

Postnatal muscle: response of satellite cells in clinical situations

Satellite cells during muscle regeneration (in response to trauma, disease or transplantation)

Minor trauma or certain stimuli may transiently activate satellite cells; however, if the required conditions are not present, the satellite cells may not proliferate extensively but instead lapse back into a quiescent state. Furthermore, since mature myofibers appear to be refractory to fusion, specific conditions are required to alter the status of the sarcolemma in order for new myoblasts to fuse with the mature parent myofiber: such conditions include significant sarcolemmal/myofiber damage or growth/hypertrophy.

Necrosis and regeneration

Where damage results in myofiber necrosis, the process of regeneration and new muscle formation is initiated. Regeneration involves key early events of inflammation and angiogenesis and then later innervation to restore full function, in addition to actual myogenesis to form the new muscle cells. Muscle damage that leads to necrosis will rapidly alter properties of the sarcolemma. In addition, damage stimulates the rapid accumulation of neutrophils (polymorphonuclear leukocytes) that exit the capillaries at the site of injury within minutes due to the release of cytokines from damaged cells and also from degranulated mast cells. In turn the neutrophils and the damaged myofiber release chemokines that attract macrophages (these predominate by 24 hours) and other cells including myoblasts to the site of injury. The inflammatory cells produce a wealth of proteases (that degrade the ECM) and cytokines, in addition to phagocytosing and removing the necrotic tissue. It is emphasized that the inflammatory cells are of central importance for muscle regeneration yet they are not present throughout myogenesis during development; thus different factors are involved in modulating myogenesis in these two situations, even though the cellular events of muscle formation may be very similar. Autoradiographic studies in vivo show that at least 18–24 hours elapse before satellite cells start to synthesize new DNA in response to muscle injury in mice [40]. Differentiation and fusion of the myoblasts occurs within 3 days, with myotubes first being apparent 2.5–3 days after injury. The wave of myoblast proliferation increases from day 1 to peak by about 3 days and greatly decreases thereafter and is essentially over by 5–6 days in response to cut (minor) or crush (severe) injury in mice [40]. The factors controlling the initiation of activation of satellite cells, and the proliferation, differentiation, and fusion of myoblasts are briefly outlined above although the precise sequence of combined factors controlling these events in vivo remains unclear. Fusion of new myotubes to the ends of the damaged myofibers is delayed until after about a week, further emphasizing the normally refractory nature of the adult myofiber to fusion [41]. It seems likely that similar events occur in human muscle with new muscle formation essentially completed within 1–2 weeks after injury.

While treatments such as low-energy laser irradiation, ultrasound, and hyperbaric (increased) oxygen can activate satellite cells, not all have benefits on skeletal muscle regeneration. Low-energy laser irradiation (LELI) improves muscle regeneration in experimental animal models and these benefits are also demonstrated in tissue culture where LELI increases the survival and also the activation and proliferation of satellite cells via GF-related signaling pathways [42]. In contrast, ultrasound does not seem to improve muscle regeneration as shown by animal experiments: in one study ultrasound produced a marked stimulation of satellite cell proliferation but no overall effect on myotube formation or regeneration [43] and more recent studies confirm no benefit of ultrasound treatment on muscle repair after contusion injury [44]. Hyperbaric oxygen is a therapeutic strategy to improve regeneration of ischemic muscle and it appears to act by increasing expression of FGF and HGF, which activate satellite cells (see above), as well as stimulating the formation of new blood vessels [45].

Fibrosis and impaired regeneration

Repeated cycles of myofiber necrosis occur in Duchenne muscular dystrophy (DMD) and the mdx mouse and dog models of this disease, due to fragility of the sarcolemma resulting from defects in dystrophin. Over time, new muscle formation fails and the muscle is replaced by fibrous fatty connective tissue (this is pronounced in dystrophic humans and dogs). Why does muscle regeneration fail? In part this may be due to different growth parameters and the size of different species [46]. Tissue culture studies of myoblasts from dystrophic mdx muscles report altered kinetics of myoblast proliferation and accelerated differentiation, and that this is influenced by the parent myofiber [47]. Early tissue culture studies which concluded that satellite cell numbers and myogenic capacity are low in dystrophic muscle proposed that this was due to exhaustion of the satellite (stem) cell population by the repeated cycles of damage and regeneration; this is supported by decreased telomere lengths in muscles from DMD boys [48]. However, an alternative explanation that is now gathering favor proposes that an adverse fibrous ECM environment accounts for difficulties in extracting satellite cells for tissue culture studies and adversely affects the myogenic capacity of these cells [49]. Thus an altered ECM environment (that does not favor myogenesis) may be the main problem, rather than the demise or an impaired intrinsic capacity of the satellite (stem) cell population per se.

This explanation also accords with studies of aged (and denervated) muscle where increasing fibrosis in very old muscles (see below) is associated with lineage conversion of myogenic precursors into non-myogenic fibroblasts; both the age-related fibrosis and lineage conversion involve systemic factors and Wnt signaling [50]. With each cycle of myofiber necrosis and regeneration a small amount of fibrous connective tissue (mainly collagens) is deposited around the myofibers and the increasing fibrous connective tissue alters the ECM composition. There is increasing evidence that fibrosis presents unfavorable conditions for myogenesis, with altered gene expression in satellite cells and a lack of myogenic markers on satellite cells from myofibers isolated from old mdx mice, leading to impaired new muscle formation with loss of muscle and replacement by fibrous fatty tissue [49]. It is clearly critical to determine the underlying cellular reasons for the failure of muscle regeneration in DMD (i.e., altered environment versus loss of myogenic capacity), in order to design appropriate therapeutic strategies (e.g., drugs versus stem cells).

Muscle transplantation

Segments or intact whole muscles are transplanted routinely in clinical situations to treat conditions such as incontinence and facial palsy. In muscle that is regenerating after transplantation, a similar sequence of events occurs although here the timing is delayed initially by several days, because the blood vessels are severed during grafting and thus revascularization with formation of new vessels (angiogenesis) is needed (unless vessels are surgically anastomosed). The infiltration of inflammatory cells precedes new vessel formation with macrophages releasing angiogenic factors that stimulate revascularization of the ischemic muscle graft. The importance of angiogenesis for muscle regeneration is emphasized in the situation of ischemic damage of the extremities [51]. Accordingly, administration of the potent angiogenic agent vascular endothelial growth factor (VEGF) accelerated new muscle formation in ischemic muscle grafts in mice [52]: such enhanced angiogenesis might significantly improve new muscle formation and reduce fibrosis in the center of large muscle grafts. Similar viral delivery of VEGF had striking benefits for the pathology of dystrophic muscle in mdx mice, due to effects on angiogenesis and also possible direct effects on satellite cell migration and myogenesis, or recruitment of stem cells into the myogenic lineage [53].

Satellite cell contribution to growing or hypertrophic muscle

In postnatal life, an increase in skeletal muscle mass, due mainly to increased size of the cross-sectional area of individual myofibers, occurs during the growth phase and in response to physical activity (loading). It is widely accepted that the number of myofibers is fixed during development. However, the interpretation of actual myofiber numbers can be complicated by the splitting or branching of (large) myofibers in hypertrophic and aging muscle. Regulation of muscle mass (size) depends on the balance between protein synthesis and degradation, with synthesis exceeding breakdown for mass to increase. Skeletal muscle growth and mass are controlled by nutritional, hormonal, and mechanical factors. While nutrition and hormones are essential during the growth phase, increased mass (hypertrophy) of adult skeletal muscle is primarily driven by mechanical factors (exercise and physical loading). It is important to note that increased muscle size does not always correlate with increased strength (reviewed in [38, 39]). It seems likely that increased net protein synthesis initially drives hypertrophy of (growing and mature) skeletal muscle and this then stimulates activation of the satellite cells that fuse with the growing myofiber: this addition of new myonuclei is required for maintenance of hypertrophy [54]. However, the primary importance of satellite cell proliferation in muscle hypertrophy is still debated [55, 56] and may depend on the growth stimulus (hormonal versus mechanical), age of the muscle (active growth compared with adult), species, and time of sampling [57].

Fate of satellite cells in atrophic myofibers (resulting from disuse, disease, denervation or cachexia)

A wide range of conditions including disuse (e.g., prolonged bed rest or space travel), starvation, disease, and aging lead to a loss of muscle mass (atrophy) and strength [39]. Muscle mass is normally maintained by a balance between protein synthesis and protein degradation and either of these aspects (or both) can be disturbed to result in a net loss of muscle protein. Exercise with muscle activity and loading stimulates the IGF-1 signaling pathway that increases protein synthesis and also inhibits protein degradation, thus leading to hypertrophy. Many factors that cause hypertrophy act through this crucial signaling pathway. Conversely, lack of stimulation, or factors that inhibit the IGF-1 pathway lead to muscle atrophy. For example, inflammatory cytokines such as tumor necrosis factor (TNF) that are elevated in cancer and other disease and also in aging appear to cross-talk and inhibit IGF-1 signaling [58]. Apart from the complexity of molecular mechanisms regulating the size of the myofiber [59], there is considerable interest in the question of what happens to satellite cells when a mature myofiber decreases in size.

This situation has been studied in denervated muscle where experiments in rodents established that denervation initially causes activation and sustained proliferation of satellite cells (for up to one month) followed by a steady decline in the number of satellite cells in long-term-denervated muscle [60]. Autoradiographic studies in mice show progressive loss of labeled nuclei adjacent to muscle fibers (presumed to be replicated satellite cells) in the 1–3 weeks after denervation: it was concluded that these proliferating (labeled) satellite cells migrated out from their original position beneath the basal lamina and did not fuse with the denervated parent myofiber [61]. The nuclear/myofiber ratio remains constant in denervated muscle (at least up to 3 weeks after denervation), indicating that activated satellite cells fail to fuse to the atrophic myofibers (discussed in [62]), supporting the proposal that mature myofibers are generally refractory to fusion. Ultrastructural studies show activated satellite cells and a transient increase in numbers at 2 months but a loss of satellite cells by 18 months after denervation of rat muscles [60, 62].

Elegant ultrastructural examination of short- and long-term-denervated muscles in rodents by the group of Bruce Carlson in the USA [63] and others, as well as in human muscle biopsy samples [64], shows tiny degenerative myotubes/myofibers with minimal cytoplasm and few myofibrils: some of these dwarf myotubes are located beneath the basal lamina whereas others are within the interstitial ECM. Myofiber atrophy is conspicuous by 2 months after denervation and beyond this time there is excessive deposition of fibrous interstitial connective tissue and multiple layers of basal lamina surround the satellite cells [62]. Strong evidence that there is no inherent problem with the myogenic potential of the satellite cells, but that the abortive myogenesis is due to adverse events related to the ECM environment and excessive fibrosis in the denervated muscle is provided by the excellent capacity of the satellite cells to form fully mature myofibers in tissue culture [65]. The tiny thin myotubes in the interstitial connective tissue are presumed to have been formed by satellite cells that have migrated into the interstitial ECM and represent "abortive myogenesis" outside the original myofiber (rather than severely atrophic myofibers) [65], although the contribution of muscle progenitors initially located outside the myofiber is difficult to formally exclude. Interpretation of events in human muscle is complicated in situations of partial denervation where there is a mix of denervated and reinnervated myofibers, especially since nerves can modulate the muscle properties (e.g., satellite cell proliferation, expression of myogenic factors such myogenin and MyoD) by activity-independent mechanisms as well as by nerve activation [66]. The ability of satellite cells to exit the juxtasarcolemmal position beneath the basal lamina means that these cells can no longer be identified using the classic geographic criteria; the extent to which such migration accounts for the decreased number of satellite cells reported in long-term-denervated (and aged) muscle is unknown.

Aging muscle – numbers and function of satellite cells

The progressive loss of muscle mass and function with age is a major problem that has attracted much attention. There are many complex reasons for this including age-related changes in myofiber biochemistry, denervation of myofibers, and an altered ECM environment with increased fibrosis (that also affects blood vessels and innervation) [67, 68], in addition to the issues of possibly decreased satellite (stem) cell numbers, a slightly delayed myogenic response, and possibly impaired new muscle formation (reviewed in [69, 70, 71]. Problems with extracting myogenic cells from aged skeletal muscle for tissue culture studies and a delay in their myogenic response initially led to the conclusion that the number of these cells was reduced in aged muscles and they had impaired replicative capacity and myogenesis [21]. Classical counting of satellite cells in tissue sections using electron microscopy or immunostaining generally concludes that numbers decrease in aged muscles from human and other species [19]; however, Pax7 is downregulated in many apparent satellite cells in aged muscle [22] and this may apply to many other molecular markers with age. Overall there are conflicting data concerning reduced numbers of satellite cells in aged muscles [22]. It has recently been demonstrated that a subpopulation of satellite cells in aged muscles retains excellent myogenic capacity [22] and some decline in satellite cell function may be more important than actual numbers in aging muscles [70]. Proliferation of aged satellite cells is improved by culture under low oxygen conditions and there is increasing evidence that the environment of these cells in vivo plays a major role in influencing their myogenic capacity; this parallels the situation with adverse effects of fibrosis on myogenesis in dystrophic muscle (discussed above). Classical cross-transplantation experiments between old and young rats demonstrated problems with long-term functional restoration of grafted muscles in old hosts (that may mainly reflect issues of reinnervation) and the importance of the systemic host environment in the adverse outcome [72].

Recent experiments using cross-transplantation of whole muscle grafts between young and old (up to 21 months) mice have addressed the effects of aging on the very early events of regeneration (during the first week) and new muscle formation per se [71]. Overall, these studies continue to enforce the idea that excellent new muscle formation can occur in aged muscles. Such studies emphasize that the overall muscle regeneration is influenced by the nature of the injury inflicted (e.g., grafting compared with intramuscular barium chloride injection or cold injury); this may largely reflect problems with the important early events of angiogenesis and inflammation that precede myoblast activation, proliferation, and fusion. Angiogenesis and inflammation are modified by (systemic and local) factors associated with the aged host environment, combined with intrinsic changes within aging muscle cells (e.g., production/availability of angiogenic factors and chemokines) [71]. It is now generally considered that while myogenesis can be slightly delayed in aged muscle, this is not necessarily due to an intrinsic loss of satellite cell numbers or capacity but instead is determined by systemic host factors and can be reversed by exposure to a young environment: again emphasizing the importance of the host environment in the age-related decline in muscle repair (reviewed in [70]). Elegant experiments have started to unravel the molecular events controlling activation of postnatal satellite cells and myogenesis in aged muscle and show that the balance and cross-talk between the signaling pathways for Notch and Wnt orchestrate progression of satellite cells through proliferation and differentiation [50, 70, 73]. In brief, activation of the Notch-1 receptor is necessary during early activation and proliferation of satellite cells and upregulation of Delta-1, the ligand for the Notch receptor, is very low in satellite cells after injury of old (compared with young) muscles. Thus impaired Notch signaling seems to account for the poor myogenic response to some types of injury seen in very old muscles. Notch signaling can also be inhibited by Numb. Members of the Wnt family may antagonize Notch-mediated satellite cell proliferation and inhibition of differentiation, and thus control this process. Notch signaling maintains the activity of GSK3β but this is inhibited by Wnt to result in myoblast differentiation. High levels of Wnt in quiescent or activated satellite cells leads to a loss of myogenic capacity and conversion into a fibrogenic fate in some experimental situations. It is proposed that an unidentified serum factor is associated with the Wnt pathway and is involved in the delayed activation of satellite cells, lineage conversion into non-myogenic cells, and increased fibrosis in aged muscle.

Cell therapy: stem cells and other sources of myoblasts

The transplantation of skeletal muscle progenitor cells is used in a range of clinical situations. Myoblast transfer therapy (MTT) is a strategy for therapeutic gene replacement in human diseases such as DMD, using normal donor nuclei derived from either myoblasts or stem cells. Another use for transplanted myoblasts is to improve the outcome of heart function after ischemic damage [9] and, while the benefits do not seem to depend on fusion of myoblasts with cardiomyocytes, such cardiac therapy shows promise in clinical trials [74]. Myoblasts are also needed for tissue engineering and the construction of muscle tissue ex vivo for potential reconstruction surgery [75]. All of these applications require a good source of autologous donor myoblasts and strategies to enhance their myogenicity and transplantation efficacy. Conventional myoblasts and different non-myogenic (stem) cell sources of myoblasts are discussed below with respect to MTT for dystrophic muscle.

Myoblast transfer therapy relies on the delivery of normal muscle nuclei into the dystrophic muscle fibers by biological fusion, as routinely occurs during muscle repair. Unfortunately, rapid and extensive cell death occurs after

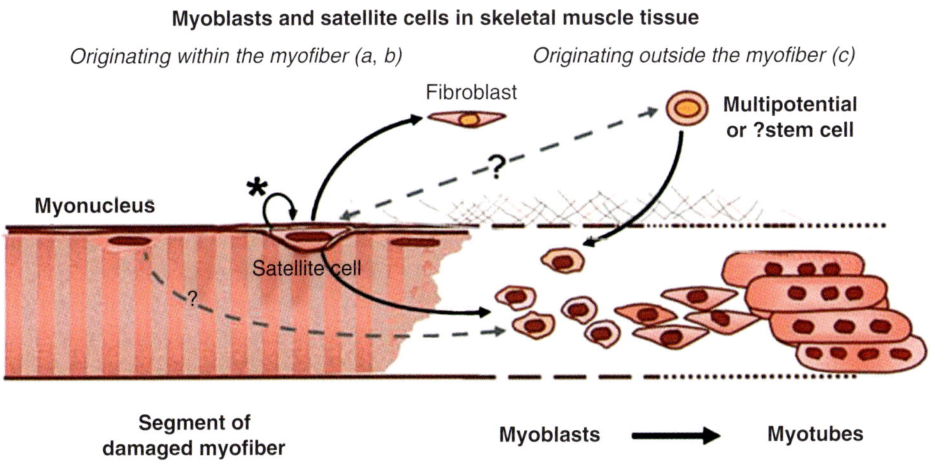

Figure 2.4. Origin and fate of myoblasts and satellite cells in mature muscle in vivo. Diagram of a segment of regenerating adult muscle tissue to indicate that myoblasts are (a) normally derived from satellite cells. The heterogeneity of satellite cells, the possibility of a stem cell subpopulation and replacement of satellite cells after (asymmetric) division (*) are topics of much discussion. The myogenic capacity of satellite cells may also be diverted into a fibroblast-like (or possibly adipogenic) fate in vivo, by alterations to the extracellular matrix (ECM) environment such as fibrosis in diseased and aged muscle. The theoretical possibility that myoblasts might be derived by sequestration of myonuclei after damage (b), is not widely endorsed for mammals but is difficult to test. Much recent attention has focused on myoblasts originating from cells lying beyond the myofiber (c), e.g., from circulating cells, mesenchymal stem cells or blood-vessel-associated cells (such as pericytes, mesangioblasts): the extent to which these may form satellite (stem) cells is unclear. The extent of potential trafficking of myogenic precursor cells between the juxtasarcolemmal satellite cell position and the interstitial connective tissue in damaged or normal tissue is unclear, although emigration of satellite cells is quite widely documented.

intramuscular injection of cultured donor myoblasts (extracted from normal donor muscles) into dystrophic mdx muscles, with about 80% of donor myoblasts dying within days. Trials with transplanted human myoblasts showed a similarly rapid loss of injected myoblasts and were disappointing [76]. Attention then turned to the possibility that there might be a stem cell subpopulation of satellite cells, more suitable for myoblast transplantation. The ideal source of stem cells (often in combination with gene correction) is autologous, i.e., from the patient themselves, to avoid problems of immune rejection. Such autologous myogenic cells would need considerable expansion of numbers in order to effectively repopulate the target muscle [77]. In addition, the ideal delivery system is through the circulation, to reach all muscles. While much research initially focused on bone-marrow-derived stem cells, many different types of stem cells have now been explored for the treatment of muscular dystrophies such as DMD. The great enthusiasm for alternative sources of muscle stem cells was fueled in part by overestimating the promise of tissue culture observations to the in vivo situation, combined with problems and limitations subsequently identified with various markers used to track putative stem cells. However, many valuable ideas have arisen from the stem cell debate, with topics of continuing interest being as follows. Is there a true stem cell subpopulation of satellite cells? Is there a cell population lying outside the myofiber that might be an ongoing source of satellite cells? What is the best source of muscle progenitors for cell therapy? Can the dream of systemic delivery of a myogenic stem cell become a therapeutic clinical reality? Some of these vital issues are discussed with respect to potential applications for cellular therapy (Figure 2.4).

Markers to track donor cells in vivo, conversion of non-myogenic cells into the myogenic lineage, and contribution of bone-marrow derived circulating cells

There was always interest in the idea that, under certain conditions, myoblasts might also be able to arise from other non-myogenic sources of precursor cells, e.g., fibroblasts, macrophages, cells derived from blood vessels such as pericytes, smooth muscle and endothelial cells, myoid cells of the thymus, in addition to circulating cells; in the 2000s there were dozens of reviews on this topic [9, 20, 21, 76, 78, 79].

It is relatively easy to cause cells from different lineages to switch into another cell type (known as plasticity) by manipulating conditions in tissue culture. However, such in vitro observations of plasticity may provide little insight into the capacity of the same cells for self-renewal, a property that is central to the stem cell concept. While such lineage conversion may be readily demonstrated in the artificial conditions of tissue culture (that may bear little resemblance to the in vivo situation), the extent to which this might normally occur in vivo, plus the precise conditions and molecular factors required for recruitment of such cells into the myogenic lineage within skeletal muscle, have barely been investigated. It is a major challenge to clarify these events in living skeletal muscle. One important aspect for conversion of cells into the myogenic lineage in vivo may be physical contact between cells, as illustrated by the need for proximity to a myogenic cell (e.g., myotube) in tissue culture [23]. In order to harness the tantalizing potential of stem cells for clinical myoblast therapy (or other transplantation uses) due consideration should be given to: the complexity of the in vivo environment, the importance of mechanical properties that influence cell behavior in vivo, the interface between the environment and cell behavior (widely referred to as the "stem cell niche") and the ultimate definition of stem cells by the end-point of functionality. The recent recognition that the fibrotic environment in dystrophic muscle can alter the fate of muscle progenitor cells (from myogenic into fibrogenic) emphasizes the importance of an adverse environment and this needs to be considered when contemplating implanting fresh sources of myogenic precursors into dystrophic muscles (see "Fibrosis and impaired regeneration").

It was initially difficult to test the capacity of non-myogenic sources of stem cells to give rise to muscle nuclei in animals due to the lack of good markers to identify donor cells and track their fate in host animals. Some of the best markers available in the 1980s were the different forms (isoenzymes) of enzymes such as glucose-6-phosphate isomerase, a dimer that had different electrophoretic mobility on gels and could be used to distinguish between cells derived from two strains of mice. In 1983, this relatively insensitive cell marker system was used to test the possibility that bone-marrow-derived cells could give rise to myoblasts in vivo and found no evidence to support this notion [80]. Dramatic improvements in cell marker systems to specifically identify transplanted donor cells and especially to visualize them in tissue sections (a very important point) then occurred: there were two major advances. In 1991, highly specific Y-chromosome probes were developed to identify male nuclei transplanted into female hosts (in a range of species). However, the powerful tool that revolutionized the field was the sophisticated genetic engineering of cells and animals (initially mice) with reporter genes that can readily identify (transgenic) donor cells after transplantation. In 1998 a highly significant paper was published (using the transgenic reporter gene technology) that unequivocally demonstrated that bone-marrow-derived cells can indeed give rise to myonuclei in adult skeletal muscle in mice [81]. This heralded in the era of intensive stem cell research at the turn of the century.

To date the huge investment in stem cells as possible therapies for neuromuscular disorders has not converted the much-vaunted promise into reality [78]. Unfortunately, the initial potential contribution of exogenous bone-marrow-derived muscle precursor cells to new myonuclei (and the promise they offered for systemic stem cell therapy) was over-estimated, due in large part to problems with expression of cell markers (used to identify the donor cells), and the phenomenon of fusion of bone marrow cells to myofibers without conversion of donor nuclei into the myogenic lineage (this applied to over 80% of bone-marrow-derived donor nuclei within myofibers) [82]. Thus myogenic conversion of bone-marrow-derived stem cells in vivo is now widely considered to be trivial and of little current interest for cell replacement therapies. Recently, attention has moved to the use of blood-vessel-associated progenitors as an alternative source of myogenic precursors.

Relationship between satellite cells and blood-vessel-associated cells

The intriguing relationship between satellite cells and other cells within skeletal muscle tissue has attracted much attention. This is difficult to investigate because when a satellite cell moves out from the juxtasarcolemmal, classical, position beneath the basal lamina of the myofiber into the interstitial space, it cannot be readily identified. There is certainly evidence that satellite cells can emigrate, but how frequently might this occur? Conversely, how often might the same cells or another incognito myogenic progenitor originating beyond the myofiber migrate into the classical satellite cell position? The dynamics of such potential trafficking in vivo are hard to measure. These issues are central to a putative functional relationship between satellite cells and the blood-vessel-associated cells (mesangioblasts, pericytes, CD133+/AC133+) that have stimulated much recent interest as a promising alternative source of myoblasts for cell therapy.

A significant relationship between myogenic and vascular precursor cells is suggested by the close proximity of satellite cells to endothelial cells of capillaries in postnatal skeletal muscle [11, 83]. In addition, a close proximity of blood vessels and (extrasynaptic) myonuclei (up to 81% in rodent soleus) is emphasized in normal muscle and this is disturbed in denervated muscle [84]. The proximity of these myogenic nuclei to capillaries, combined with the ability of (stem) cell precursors to give rise to both endothelial and myogenic cells under various conditions in tissue culture and in vivo after cell transplantation [79, 85] presents interesting possibilities. Whether these vascular-related myogenic precursors are distinct from (or can give rise to) satellite cells is unclear. Whether the common precursor is a true stem cell is also unclear. Furthermore, the relationship between these vascular precursor (stem) cells, pericytes [86], and mesangioblasts (associated with blood vessels) requires clarification, as does the relationship to DC133+(AC133+) cell populations derived from both skeletal muscle and blood [76, 85]. These vascular-related myogenic cells have attracted much recent interest in cell transplantation experiments to potentially provide healthy donor myonuclei to correct the gene defect in dystrophic mice and dogs. The striking claims of success have attracted controversy [87] but also offer hope for an alternative source of myoblasts that might be delivered through the circulation [88].

Clinical trials using mesangioblasts in boys with DMD have been initiated in Italy, although the scientific basis for this continues to be discussed. Some of the issues that require clarification with respect to blood-vessel-related progenitors as a source of myoblasts to treat DMD are: the best source of the cells (muscle or blood); heterologous cells (with immune issues) or autologous cells (requiring gene correction);

systemic delivery (ideal); amount of muscle formed from donor myonuclei; functional improvement of muscle; longevity of donor nuclei (repeat treatment?); the formation of donor satellite cells (for replenishment of cells in vivo); and the possibility of cancers from bona fide stem cells. If repeated treatments are indeed essential for sustained benefits then blood-derived autologous cells as a source of donor myogenic (stem) cells are preferable, due to issues with repeated biopsies of muscles of DMD boys.

Concluding remarks

The satellite cell has returned to reign as the main source of myogenic precursor cells (myoblasts) in adult muscle and a wealth of new information on myogenic precursors has emerged recently as indicated below.

- Much is now known at the cellular and molecular/gene level about the origins, and factors controlling the development, of myogenic and satellite cells during embryogenesis in various muscles. However, little is known about the clinical consequences of the different sources and patterns of gene expression involved in the formation of the trunk, limb, and head muscles.
- Powerful new molecular and genetics tools have revolutionized the understanding of satellite cells, provided information on the numbers of such cells in diseased and aged muscles, and their capacity to be activated and form new muscle in response to different clinical situations (regeneration, growth and hypertrophy, atrophy, denervation, and aging).
- Factors in adult muscle that control activation of the normally quiescent satellite cells (and subsequent myogenesis) have been elucidated and include molecules associated with the sarcolemma, the crucial importance of the extracellular matrix and interactions with a host of growth factors and their receptors, plus the role of systemic factors.
- The impact of the environment and especially of fibrosis in vivo for altering the fate of myogenic precursor cells has become more widely recognized.
- Whether there is a true stem cell subpopulation of satellite cells to replenish these vital myogenic precursor cells throughout life remains a hot topic.
- Information is emerging on the relationship of satellite cells to other precursors in the interstitial tissue and the possibility of movement of such progenitor cells into and out of the satellite cell compartment.
- The transfer of myogenic (stem) cells for treatment of muscular dystrophy, cardiac damage, and also tissue engineering has continued to attract attention, although the problem of the rapid and massive death of injected myoblasts has not yet been resolved satisfactorily. Intense interest since 1998 has focused on the potential contribution of non-myogenic stem cells to the myogenic lineage with applications to therapeutic cell therapy. Unfortunately disappointing results were obtained with circulating bone-marrow-derived stem cells for systemic delivery of myoblasts. Finally, great progress has been made concerning the possibility that precursor (stem) cells derived from blood vessels might be suitable for clinical applications.

References

1. S. Tajbakhsh, M. Buckingham, The birth of muscle progenitor cells in the mouse: spatiotemporal considerations. *Curr. Top. Dev. Biol.* **48** (2000), 225–268.
2. F. Relaix, D. Montarras, S. Zaffran, *et al.*, Pax3 and Pax7 have distinct and overlapping functions in adult muscle progenitor cells. *J. Cell Biol.* **172**:1 (2006), 91–102.
3. M. Buckingham, F. Relaix, The role of Pax genes in the development of tissues and organs: Pax3 and Pax7 regulate muscle progenitor cell functions. *Annu. Rev. Cell Dev. Biol.* **23** (2007), 645–673.
4. O. Pourquie, The segmentation clock: converting embryonic time into spatial pattern. *Science* **301**:5631 (2003), 328–330.
5. N. Le Douarin, C. Kalcheim, *The Neural Crest.* (Cambridge: Cambridge University Press, 1999.)
6. F. Relaix, Skeletal muscle progenitor cells: from embryo to adult. *Cell. Mol. Life Sci.* **63**:11 (2006), 1221–1225.
7. F. Relaix, D. Rocancourt, A. Mansouri, M. Buckingham, A Pax3/Pax7-dependent population of skeletal muscle progenitor cells. *Nature* **435** (2005), 948–953.
8. M. D. Grounds, Z. Yablonka-Reuveni, Molecular and cell biology of skeletal muscle regeneration. In *Molecular and Cell Biology of Muscular Dystrophy*, ed. T. A. Partridge. (London: Chapman & Hall, 1993), pp. 210–256.
9. M. D. Grounds, J. White, N. Rosenthal, M. A. Bogoyevitch, The role of stem cells in skeletal and cardiac muscle repair. *J. Histochem. Cytochem.* **50**:5 (2002), 589–610.
10. A. Mauro, Satellite cell of skeletal muscle fibers. *J. Biophys. Biochem. Cytol.* **9**:2 (1961), 493–495.
11. R. Mazanet, C. Franzini-Armstrong, The satellite cell. In *Myology*, ed. A. G. Engel, B. Q. Banker. (New York: McGraw-Hill, 1986), pp. 285–307.
12. P. Zammit, The muscle satellite cell: the story of a cell on the edge. In *Skeletal Muscle Repair and Regeneration*, ed. S. Schiaffino, T. Partridge. (New York: Springer, 2008), pp. 45–64.
13. L. Kassar-Duchossoy, B. Gayraud-Morel, D. Gomes, *et al.*, Mrf4 determines skeletal muscle identity in Myf5: Myod double-mutant mice. *Nature* **431**:7007 (2004), 466–471.
14. M. A. Rudnicki, P. N. Schnegelsberg, R. H. Stead, T. Braun, H. H. Arnold, R. Jaenisch, MyoD or Myf-5 is required for the formation of skeletal muscle. *Cell* **75**:7 (1993), 1351–1359.
15. P. Seale, L. A. Sabourin, A. Girgis-Gabardo, A. Mansouri, P. Gruss, M. A. Rudnicki, Pax7 is required for the specification of myogenic satellite cells. *Cell* **102**:6 (2000), 777–786.
16. I. M. Conboy, T. A. Rando, The regulation of Notch signaling controls satellite cell activation and cell fate determination in postnatal myogenesis. *Dev. Cell* **3**:3 (2002), 397–409.

17. V. Shinin, B. Gayraud-Morel, D. Gomes, S. Tajbakhsh, Asymmetric division and cosegregation of template DNA strands in adult muscle satellite cells. *Nat. Cell Biol.* **8**:7 (2006), 677–687.

18. J. Dhawan, T. A. Rando, Stem cells in postnatal myogenesis: molecular mechanisms of satellite cell quiescence, activation and replenishment. *Trends Cell Biol.* **15**:12 (2005), 666–673.

19. V. Renault, L. E. Thornell, P. O. Eriksson, G. Butler-Browne, V. Mouly, Regenerative potential of human skeletal muscle during aging. *Aging Cell* **1**:2 (2002), 132–139.

20. P. S. Zammit, T. A. Partridge, Z. Yablonka-Reuveni, The skeletal muscle satellite cell: the stem cell that came in from the cold. *J. Histochem. Cytochem.* **54**:11 (2006), 1177–1191.

21. V. Mouly, A. Aamiri, A. Bigot, *et al.*, The mitotic clock in skeletal muscle regeneration, disease and cell mediated gene therapy. *Acta Physiol. Scand.* **184**:1 (2005), 3–15.

22. C. A. Collins, P. S. Zammit, A. P. Ruiz, J. E. Morgan, T. A. Partridge, A population of myogenic stem cells that survives skeletal muscle aging. *Stem Cells* **25**:4 (2007), 885–894.

23. Z. Yablonka-Reuveni, K. Day, A. Vine, G. Shefer, Defining the transcriptional signature of skeletal muscle stem cells. *J. Anim. Sci.* **86**:14 Suppl (2008), E207–E216.

24. P. O. Mitchell, T. Mills, R. S. O'Connor, *et al.*, Sca-1 negatively regulates proliferation and differentiation of muscle cells. *Dev. Biol.* **283**:1 (2005), 240–252.

25. D. Montarras, J. Morgan, C. Collins, *et al.*, Direct isolation of satellite cells for skeletal muscle regeneration. *Science* **309** (2005), 2064–2067.

26. C. A. Collins, T. A. Partridge, Self-renewal of the adult skeletal muscle satellite cell. *Cell Cycle* **4**:10 (2005), 1338–1341.

27. M. J. Conboy, A. O. Karasov, T. A. Rando, High incidence of non-random template strand segregation and asymmetric fate determination in dividing stem cells and their progeny. *PLoS Biol.* **5**:5 e102 (2007), 1120–1126.

28. S. Kuang, K. Kuroda, F. Le Grand, M. A. Rudnicki, Asymmetric self-renewal and commitment of satellite stem cells in muscle. *Cell* **129**:5 (2007), 999.

29. G. Cossu, S. Tajbakhsh, Oriented cell divisions and muscle satellite cell heterogeneity. *Cell* **129**:5 (2007), 859–861.

30. P. S. Zammit, J. P. Golding, Y. Nagata, V. Hudon, T. A. Partridge, J. R. Beauchamp, Muscle satellite cells adopt divergent fates: a mechanism for self-renewal? *J. Cell Biol.* **166**:3 (2004), 347–357.

31. Y. Nagata, T. A. Partridge, R. Matsuda, P. S. Zammit, Entry of muscle satellite cells into the cell cycle requires sphingolipid signaling. *J. Cell Biol.* **174**:2 (2006), 245–253.

32. M. D. Grounds, Complexity of extracellular matrix and skeletal muscle regeneration. In *Skeletal Muscle Repair and Regeneration*, ed. S. Schiaffino, T. A. Partridge. (New York: Springer, 2008), pp. 269–302.

33. Z. Yablonka-Reuveni, G. Shefer, Role of growth factors in directing myogenesis of satellite cells. In *Skeletal Muscle Repair and Regeneration*, ed. S. Schiaffino, T. Partridge. (New York: Springer, 2008), pp. 45–54.

34. M. D. Grounds, Muscle regeneration: molecular aspects and therapeutic implications. *Curr. Opin. Neurol.* **12**:5 (1999), 535–543.

35. C. Qiao, J. Li, J. Jiang, *et al.*, Myostatin propeptide gene delivery by adeno-associated virus serotype 8 vectors enhances muscle growth and ameliorates dystrophic phenotypes in mdx Mice. *Hum. Gene Ther.* **19**:3 (2008), 241–254.

36. K. Patel, H. Amthor, The function of myostatin and strategies of myostatin blockade – new hope for therapies aimed at promoting growth of skeletal muscle. *Neuromusc. Disord.* **15** (2005), 117–126.

37. A. Marshall, M. S. Salerno, M. Thomas, *et al.*, Mighty is a novel promyogenic factor in skeletal myogenesis. *Exp. Cell Res.* **314**:5 (2008), 1013–1029.

38. H. Amthor, R. Macharia, R. Navarrete, *et al.*, Lack of myostatin results in excessive muscle growth but impaired force generation. *Proc. Natl. Acad. Sci. U. S. A.* **104**:6 (2007), 1835–1840.

39. T. Shavlakadze, M. D. Grounds, Of bears, frogs, meat, mice and men: insights into the complexity of factors affecting skeletal muscle atrophy/hypertrophy and myogenesis/adipogenesis. *BioEssays* **28**:10 (2006), 994–1009.

40. J. K. McGeachie, M. D. Grounds, Initiation and duration of muscle precursor replication after mild and severe injury to skeletal muscle of mice. *Cell Tissue Res.* **248** (1987), 125–130.

41. T. A. Robertson, J. M. Papadimitriou, M. D. Grounds, Fusion of myogenic cells to the newly sealed region of damaged myofibres in skeletal muscle regeneration. *Neuropathol. Appl. Neurobiol.* **19**:4 (1993), 350–358.

42. G. Shefer, T. A. Partridge, L. Heslop, J. G. Gross, U. Oron, O. Halevy, Low-energy laser irradiation promotes the survival and cell cycle entry of skeletal muscle satellite cells. *J. Cell Sci.* **115**:Pt 7 (2002), 1461–1469.

43. J. Rantanen, O. Thorsson, P. Wollmer, T. Hurme, H. Kalimo, Effects of therapeutic ultrasound on the regeneration of skeletal myofibers after experimental muscle injury. *Am. J. Sports Med.* **27**:1 (1999), 54–59.

44. C. D. Markert, M. A. Merrick, T. E. Kirby, S. T. Devor, Nonthermal ultrasound and exercise in skeletal muscle regeneration. *Arch. Phys. Med. Rehabil.* **86**:7 (2005), 1304–1310.

45. T. Asano, E. Kaneko, S. Shinozaki, *et al.*, Hyperbaric oxygen induces basic fibroblast growth factor and hepatocyte growth factor expression, and enhances blood perfusion and muscle regeneration in mouse ischemic hind limbs. *Circ. J.* **71**:3 (2007), 405–411.

46. M. D. Grounds, Two-tiered hypotheses for Duchenne muscular dystrophy. *Cell Mol. Life Sci.* **65**:11 (2008), 1621–1625.

47. Z. Yablonka-Reuveni, J. E. Anderson, Satellite cells from dystrophic (mdx) mice display accelerated differentiation in primary cultures and in isolated myofibers. *Dev. Dyn.* **235**:1 (2006), 203–312.

48. S. Decary, C. B. Hamida, V. Mouly, J. P. Barbet, F. Hentati, G. S. Butler-Browne, Shorter telomeres in dystrophic muscle consistent with extensive regeneration in young children. *Neuromuscul. Disord.* **10**:2 (2000), 113–120.

49. C. Alexakis, T. Partridge, G. Bou-Gharios, Implication of the satellite cell in dystrophic muscle fibrosis: a self-perpetuating mechanism of collagen overproduction. *Am. J. Physiol. Cell Physiol.* **293**:2 (2007), C661–C669.

50. A. S. Brack, M. J. Conboy, S. Roy, *et al.*, Increased Wnt signaling during aging alters muscle stem cell fate and increases fibrosis. *Science* **317**:5839 (2007), 807–810.

51. P. K. Shireman, The chemokine system in arteriogenesis and hind limb ischemia. *J. Vasc. Surg.* **45** Suppl A (2007), A48–A56.

52. G. M. Smythe, M. C. Lai, M. D. Grounds, P. Rakoczy, Adeno-associated virus-mediated transfer of vascular endothelial growth factor in skeletal muscle prior to transplantation promotes revascularisation of the regenerating skeletal muscle. *Tissue Engineer.* **8**:5 (2002), 871–891.

53. S. Messina, A. Mazzeo, A. Bitto, *et al.*, VEGF overexpression via adeno-associated virus gene transfer promotes skeletal muscle regeneration and enhances muscle function in mdx mice. *FASEB J.* **21**:13 (2007), 3737–3746.

54. G. R. Adams, Satellite cell proliferation and skeletal muscle hypertrophy. *Appl. Physiol. Nutr. Metab.* **31**:6 (2006), 782–790.

55. J. J. McCarthy, K. A. Esser, Counterpoint: Satellite cell addition is not obligatory for skeletal muscle hypertrophy. *J. Appl. Physiol.* **103**:3 (2007), 1100–1102; discussion 2–3.

56. C. Rehfeldt, In response to Point: Counterpoint: "Satellite cell addition is/is not obligatory for skeletal muscle hypertrophy". *J. Appl. Physiol.* **103**:3 (2007), 1104.

57. R. S. O'Connor, G. K. Pavlath, J. J McCarthy, K. A. Esser, Last word on Point: Counterpoint: Satellite cell addition is/is not obligatory for skeletal muscle hypertrophy. *J. Appl. Physiol.* **103**:3 (2007), 1107.

58. M. D. Grounds, H. G. Radley, B. G. Gebski, M. A. Bogoyevitch, T. Shavlakadze, Implications of cross-talk between tumour necrosis factor and insulin-like growth factor-1 signalling in skeletal muscle. *Clin. Exp. Pharmacol. Physiol.* **35**:7 (2008), 846–851.

59. P. G. Arthur, M. D. Grounds, T. Shavlakadze, Oxidative stress as a therapeutic target during muscle wasting: considering the complex interactions. *Curr. Opin. Clin. Nutr. Metab. Care* **11**:4 (2008), 408–416.

60. C. A. Viguie, D. X. Lu, S. K. Huang, H. Rengen, B. M. Carlson, Quantitative study of the effects of long-term denervation on the extensor digitorum longus muscle of the rat. *Anat. Rec.* **248**:3 (1997), 346–354.

61. J. K. McGeachie, M. D. Grounds, Cell proliferation in denervated skeletal muscle: does it provide a pool of potential circulating myoblasts? *Bibl. Anat.* **29** (1986), 173–193.

62. D. X. Lu, S. K. Huang, B. M. Carlson, Electron microscopic study of long-term denervated rat skeletal muscle. *Anat. Rec.* **248**:3 (1997), 355–365.

63. A. B. Borisov, E. I. Dedkov, B. M. Carlson, Abortive myogenesis in denervated skeletal muscle: differentiative properties of satellite cells, their migration, and block of terminal differentiation. *Anat. Embryol. (Berl.)* **209**:4 (2005), 269–279.

64. K. Doppler, M. Mittelbronn, A. Bornemann, Myogenesis in human denervated muscle biopsies. *Muscle Nerve* **37**:1 (2007), 79–83.

65. A. B. Borisov, E. I. Dedkov, B. M. Carlson, Differentiation of activated satellite cells in denervated muscle following single fusions in situ and in cell culture. *Histochem. Cell Biol.* **124**:1 (2005), 13–23.

66. J. P. Hyatt, R. R. Roy, K. M. Baldwin, A. Wernig, V. R. Edgerton, Activity-unrelated neural control of myogenic factors in a slow muscle. *Muscle Nerve* **33**:1 (2006), 49–60.

67. T. Shavlakadze, M. D. Grounds, Therapeutic interventions for age-related muscle wasting: importance of innervation and exercise for preventing sarcopenia. In *Modulating Aging and Longevity*, ed. S. Rattan, (The Netherlands: Kluwer Academic, 2003), pp. 139–166.

68. G. S. Lynch, J. D. Schertzer, J. G. Ryall, Therapeutic approaches for muscle wasting disorders. *Pharmacol. Ther.* **113**:3 (2007), 461–487.

69. M. D. Grounds, Age-associated changes in the response of skeletal muscle cells to exercise and regeneration. *Ann. N. Y. Acad. Sci.* **854** (1998), 78–91.

70. A. Brack, T. A. Rando, Intrinsic changes and extrinsic influences of myogenic stem cell function during aging. *Stem Cell Rev.* **3**:12 (2007), 226–237.

71. G. M. Smythe, T. Shavlakadze, P. Roberts, M. J. Davies, J. K. McGeachie, M. D. Grounds, Age influences the early events of skeletal muscle regeneration: studies of whole muscle grafts transplanted between young (8 weeks) and old (13–21 months) mice. *Exp. Gerontol.* **43**:6 (2008), 550–562.

72. B. M. Carlson, J. A. Faulkner, Muscle transplantation between young and old rats: age of host determines recovery. *Am. J. Physiol.* **256** (1989), 1262–1266.

73. A. Brack, I. M. Conboy, M. J. Conboy, J. Shen, T. A. Rando, A temporal switch from Notch to Wnt signalling in muscle stem cells is necessary for normal adult myogenesis. *Cell Stem Cell* **2** (2008), 50–59.

74. P. Menasche, Skeletal myoblasts and cardiac repair. *J. Mol. Cell Cardiol.* **45**:4 (2008), 545–553.

75. J. Stern-Straeter, F. Riedel, G. Bran, K. Hormann, U. R. Goessler, Advances in skeletal muscle tissue engineering. *In Vivo* **21**:3 (2007), 435–444.

76. L. Boldrin, J. E. Morgan, Activating muscle stem cells: therapeutic potential in muscle diseases. *Curr. Opin. Neurol.* **20**:5 (2007), 577–582.

77. J. P. Tremblay, D. Skuk, Another new "super muscle stem cell" leaves unaddressed the real problems of cell therapy for duchenne muscular dystrophy. *Mol. Ther.* **16**:12 (2008), 1907–1909.

78. T. A. Partridge, Stem cell therapies for neuromuscular diseases. *Acta Neurol. Belg.* **104**:4 (2004), 141–147.

79. B. Peault, M. Rudnicki, Y. Torrente, *et al.*, Stem and progenitor cells in skeletal muscle development, maintenance, and therapy. *Mol. Ther.* **15**:5 (2007), 867–877.

80. M. D. Grounds, Skeletal muscle precursors do not arise from bone marrow cells. *Cell Tissue Res.* **234** (1983), 713–722.

81. G. Ferrari, G. Cusella-De Angelis, M. Coletta, *et al.*, Muscle regeneration by bone marrow-derived myogenic progenitors. *Science* **279** (1998), 1528–1530.

82. G. Wernig, V. Janzen, R. Schafer, *et al.*, The vast majority of bone-marrow-derived cells integrated into mdx muscle fibers are silent despite long-term engraftment. *Proc. Natl. Acad. Sci. U. S. A.* **102**:33 (2005), 11852–11857.

83. C. Christov, F. Chretien, R. Abou-Khalil, *et al.*, Muscle satellite cells and endothelial cells: close neighbors and privileged partners. *Mol. Biol. Cell.* **18**:4 (2007), 1397–1409.

84. E. Ralston, Z. Lu, N. Biscocho, *et al.*, Blood vessels and desmin control the positioning of nuclei in skeletal muscle fibers. *J. Cell. Physiol.* **209**:3 (2006), 874–882.

85. R. Benchaouir, M. Meregalli, A. Farini, *et al.*, Restoration of human dystrophin following transplantation of exon-skipping-engineered DMD patient stem cells into dystrophic mice. *Cell Stem Cell* **1**:6 (2007), 646–657.

86. A. Dellavalle, M. Sampaolesi, R. Tonlorenzi, *et al.*, Pericytes of human skeletal muscle are myogenic precursors distinct from satellite cells. *Nat. Cell. Biol.* **9**:3 (2007), 255–267.

87. K. E. Davies, M. D. Grounds, Treating muscular dystrophy with stem cells? *Cell* **127**:7 (2006), 1304–1306.

88. K. E. Davies, M. D. Grounds, Modified patient stem cells as prelude to autologous treatment of muscular dystrophy. *Cell Stem Cell* **1**:6 (2007), 595–596.

Chapter 3

Biochemical and molecular basis of muscle disease

Susan C. Brown and Cecilia Jimenez-Mallebera

Introduction

The genetic diversity of neuromuscular disorders is far greater than was appreciated at the turn of the century, as exemplified by the number of genes implicated in the muscular dystrophies. These are now known to encode for a broad range of proteins including those associated with the extracellular matrix, sarcolemma, cytoskeleton, contractile apparatus, mitochondria, and nuclear envelope. Whilst identification of the defective gene provides the ultimate diagnosis, the associated protein changes allow insight into the underlying pathogenesis of the disease. The aim of the present chapter is to concentrate on the proteins associated with neuromuscular disease. The main body of this chapter is broadly divided into sections according to the cellular compartment that is predominantly affected. Many of the key proteins that will be discussed are shown schematically in Figure 3.1. It is nonetheless important to recognize that from a functional perspective these are artificial divisions and that muscle is a highly organized structure in which most if not all of the proteins link to one another either through signaling pathways or direct/indirect binding, and it is probably at least partly for this reason that some of the pathologies show a degree of overlap. The best example of this is the dystrophin-associated complex, which encompasses components of the muscle fiber cytoskeleton, sarcolemma, and extracellular matrix, and thus introduces the present chapter.

Dystrophin-associated protein complex

One of the most significant breakthroughs in terms of identifying the genetic basis of neuromuscular disease has been the discovery of dystrophin as the protein missing in Duchenne muscular dystrophy (DMD). This work focused attention on a previously unknown glycoprotein complex now known as the dystrophin-associated glycoprotein complex (DGC), defects in which have subsequently been shown to underlie several other forms of congenital and limb girdle muscular dystrophy. The DGC in skeletal muscle is composed of dystrophin and several subcomplexes, namely: (1) the dystroglycan complex, (2) the sarcoglycan:sarcospan complex, and (3) the cytoplasmic, dystrophin-containing complex [1]. Several other proteins also associate with the DGC at the sarcolemma. These include *dystrobrevin*, neuronal nitric oxide synthase (nNOS), ε-sarcoglycan, and caveolin-3. Some of these associated components are thought to be indicative of a signaling role for the DGC in addition to its well known structural role in linking the extracellular matrix to the actin cytoskeleton of the muscle fiber. A schematic diagram of the DGC is shown in Figure 3.2.

The dystroglycan complex

The dystroglycan complex is thought to play a primary role in the deposition and/or stabilization of basement membranes in addition to being implicated in development, cell adhesion, and signaling in both muscle and nonmuscle tissues. This linkage is disrupted in several forms of muscular dystrophy underscoring its importance in maintaining both structural and functional aspects of striated muscle. A single gene *DAG1* encodes for a polypeptide that is post-translationally modified to yield the two glycoproteins referred to as α- and β-dystroglycan [2] (Figure 3.3).

α-Dystroglycan is a membrane-associated extracellular glycoprotein and binds via glycosylated epitopes to laminin-α2 chain, perlecan, biglycan, neurexin, and agrin within the extracellular matrix whereas β-dystroglycan is transmembrane and links α-dystroglycan to the actin cytoskeleton via either dystrophin or utrophin. α- and β-dystroglycan are tightly associated and form the principal linkage between the fiber cytoskeleton and the surrounding extracellular matrix [3]. The primary sequence of α-dystroglycan predicts a molecular mass of 72 kDa; however, due to extensive glycosylation, the final molecular weight is 156 kDa in skeletal muscle, 140 kDa in cardiac muscle, and 120 kDa in brain and peripheral nerve. These differences in molecular weight are thought to reflect functionally relevant differential glycosylation.

Glycosylation of proteins takes place in the endoplasmic reticulum (ER) and Golgi compartments and involves a complex series of reactions catalyzed by membrane-bound glycosyltransferases and glycosidases. There are two main forms of protein glycosylation, namely N-linked glycosylation in which

Disorders of Voluntary Muscle, 8th edn., eds. George Karpati, David Hilton-Jones, Kate Bushby and Robert C. Griggs. Published by Cambridge University Press.

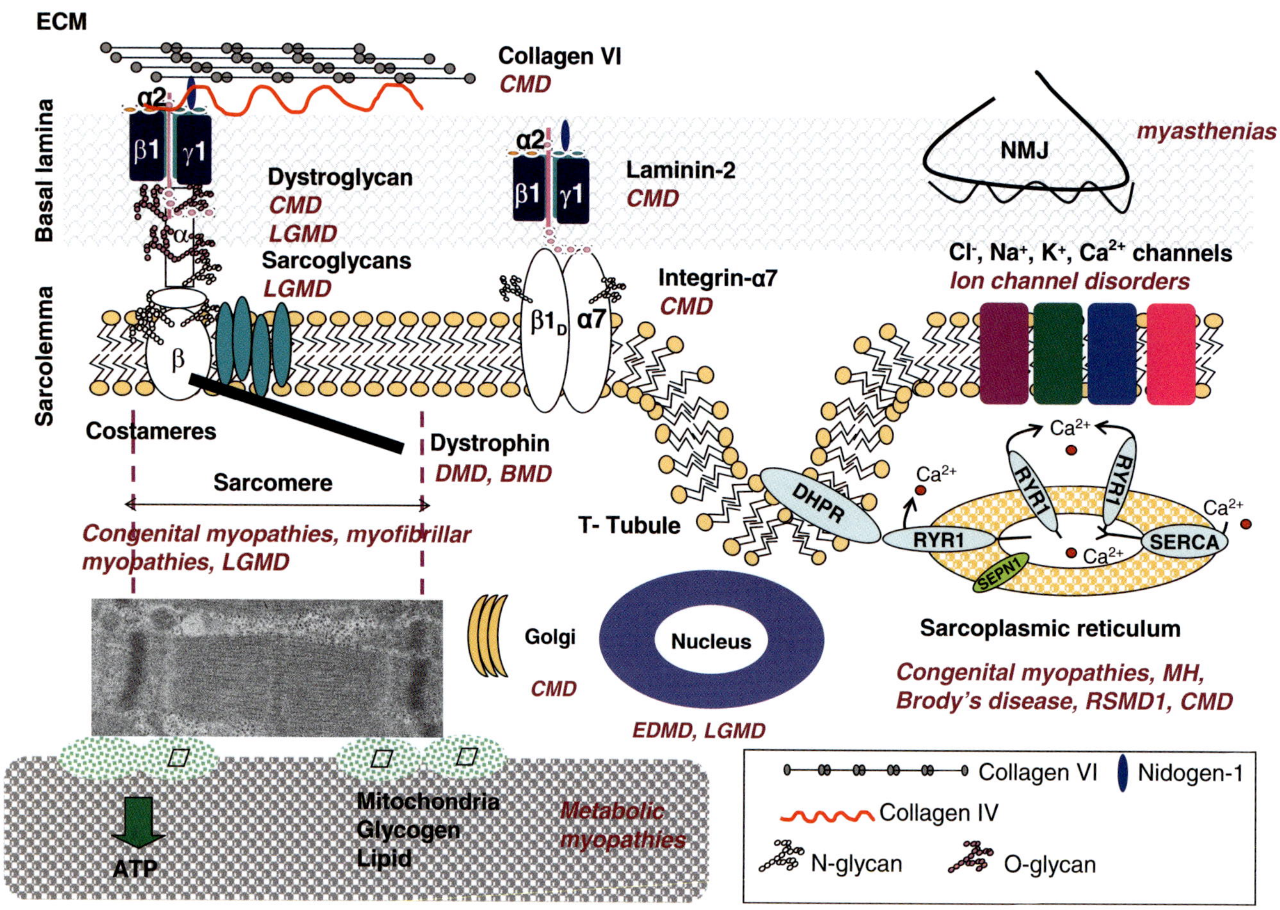

Figure 3.1. Schematic diagram showing the cellular localization and disease association for some of the key proteins associated with neuromuscular disorders. DGC, dystrophin-associated glycoprotein complex; CMD, congenital muscular dystrophy; LGMD, limb-girdle muscular dystrophy; DMD/BMD, Duchenne/Becker muscular dystrophy; MH, malignant hyperthermia; RSMD1, rigid spine syndrome 1; CMD, congenital muscular dystrophy; SEPN1, selenoprotein 1; ECM, extracellular matrix; BM, basement membrane; SERCA, sarcoplasmic reticulum Ca^{2+} ATPases; RYR1, ryanodine receptor type 1; DHP R, dihydropyridine receptor; EDMD, Emery–Dreifuss muscular dystrophy.

the oligosaccharide is added onto an asparagine residue and O-linked glycosylation where the oligosaccharide is attached to a serine or threonine residue. There are more that 200 known glycosyltransferases residing in the Golgi apparatus reflecting the diversity of carbohydrate structures added to proteins and underscoring the biological significance of this form of modification. Electrophoretically α-dystroglycan runs as a broad smear which is not diminished after PNGaseF (N-glycosidase F) treatment suggesting that this band pattern is due to O- rather than N-linked carbohydrate addition. Recent work shows that O-mannosylation within the mucin domain of human dystroglycan occurs preferentially at Thr/Ser residues that are flanked by basic amino acids [4]. O-Mannosyl glycosylation is a rare type of protein modification that is observed only in α-dystroglycan and a limited number of other glycoproteins.

A number of forms of congenital muscular dystrophy and mild limb-girdle muscular dystrophies are now known to be associated with defects in the glycosylation of α-dystroglycan, and are collectively known as the dystroglycanopathies. The dystroglycanopathies are amongst the most common forms of autosomal recessive muscular dystrophies. To date mutations in six genes have been implicated in this group of disorders, namely *Protein O-mannosyl transferase 1* (*POMT1;* OMIM 607423), *Protein O-mannosyl transferase 2* (*POMT2;* OMIM 607439), *Protein O-mannose beta-1, 2-*N*-acetylglucosaminyl-transferase* (*POMGnT1;* OMIM 606822), *Fukutin* (OMIM 607440), *Fukutin-related protein* (*FKRP;* OMIM 606596), and *LARGE* (OMIM 603590). These six genes encode for proteins that are either putative (FUKUTIN and FKRP) or determined glycosyltransferases (POMT1, POMT2, POMGnT1, and LARGE) lending support to the idea that the aberrant post-translational modification of proteins represents a new mechanism of pathogenesis in the muscular dystrophies [5]. A profound reduction in the ligand-binding capacity of α-dystroglycan within the basement membrane is thought to underlie not only the muscular dystrophy of patients with dystroglycanopathy but also the structural brain defects, including cobblestone lissencephaly and hydrocephalus, that are observed at the more severe end of the clinical spectrum.

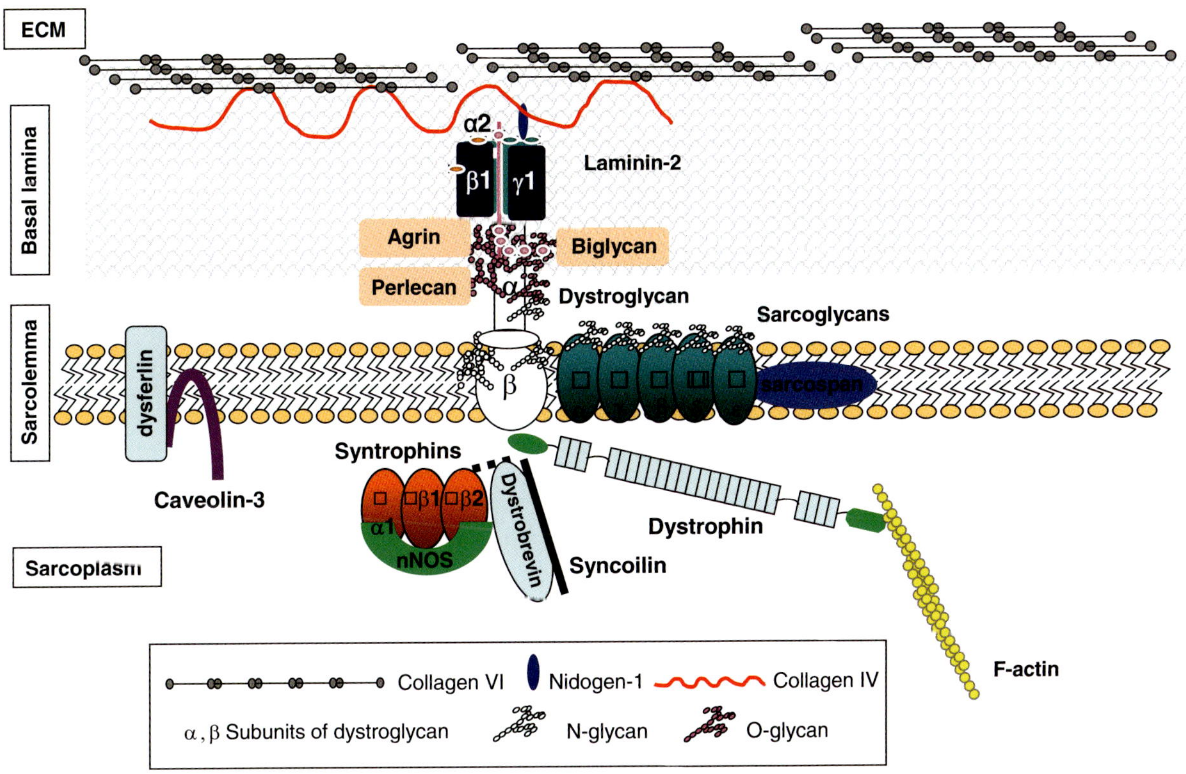

Figure 3.2. Schematic diagram of the dystrophin-associated glycoprotein complex (DGC) and dysferlin. The DGC complex effectively links the extracellular matrix with the actin cytoskeleton of the muscle fiber and consists of several subcomplexes: (1) the dystroglycan complex, which is composed of α-dystroglycan, and which binds to laminin-α2, agrin, and perlecan in the extracellular matrix, and β-dystroglycan, which interacts with the cysteine-rich domain of dystrophin and with the subsarcolemmal actin cytoskeleton; (2) the transmembrane sarcoglycan. sarcospan complex; and (3) the cytoplasmic, dystrophin-containing complex, which consists of the syntrophins, neuronal nitric oxide synthase (nNOS), and dystrobrevin. Additional proteins that associate with the DGC include syncoilin, which via its ability to interact with desmin is thought to link the DGC to the intermediate filament associated cytoskeleton. Dysferlin is not part of the DGC complex but has been shown to interact with caveolin.

POMT1 and POMT2 form a functional complex and are known to be responsible for the first step in *O*-mannosyl glycan synthesis (Figure 3.4). POMGnT1 is responsible for the formation of the GlcNAc-β-1–2Man linkage of *O*-mannosyl glycan, and most mutations have been shown to result in a loss of enzyme activity [6, 7]. A loss in enzymatic activity of POMGnT1 (glycosyltransferase O-linked mannose beta-1,2-*N*-acetylglucosaminyltransferase) is associated with Muscle Eye Brain Disease, strongly suggesting that interference in *O*-mannosyl glycosylation is a pathomechanism for muscular dystrophy, eye defects, and neuronal migration disorders. Regarding fukutin and fukutin-related protein (FKRP), sequence analysis suggests that these two proteins may be involved in the modification of cell-surface glycoproteins or glycolipids [8] but their precise mechanisms of action are currently not known.

LARGE physically interacts with α-dystroglycan (Figure 3.4) and facilitates its proper glycosylation although the precise sugar groups which it adds are currently unclear [9]. The LARGE protein is unusual in that it is predicted to contain two putative catalytic domains both of which seem to be required for its biochemical function [10]. LARGE mutations are extremely rare but have been identified in a novel congenital muscular dystrophy (CMD) variant (MDC1D) [11] and, more recently, in patients with WWS-like syndrome (see following paragraph) [12, 13].

Mutations in the *POMT1*, *POMT2*, *fukutin*, *POMGnT1*, and *FKRP* genes have now been identified in a range of patients, from those with severe structural brain involvement resembling Walker–Warburg syndrome (WWS) and Muscle Eye Brain (MEB) disease to adult-onset limb-girdle muscular dystrophy (LGMD2I) [14, 15, 16, 17], the latter of which represents the most common form of LGMD in Scandinavia and is common in most of northern Europe. As a consequence of this broad range of clinical phenotypes, severity of disease in this group of disorders is thought to be more dependent on the effect of individual gene mutations on protein function rather than the gene primarily involved.

A number of approaches have been used to generate dystroglycanopathy animal models and so provide better insight into the disease process. Dystroglycan-null mice are nonviable due to an early defect in Reichert's membrane, the first basement membrane to form in the embryo, although the phenotype of chimeric mice with a selective deficiency in either

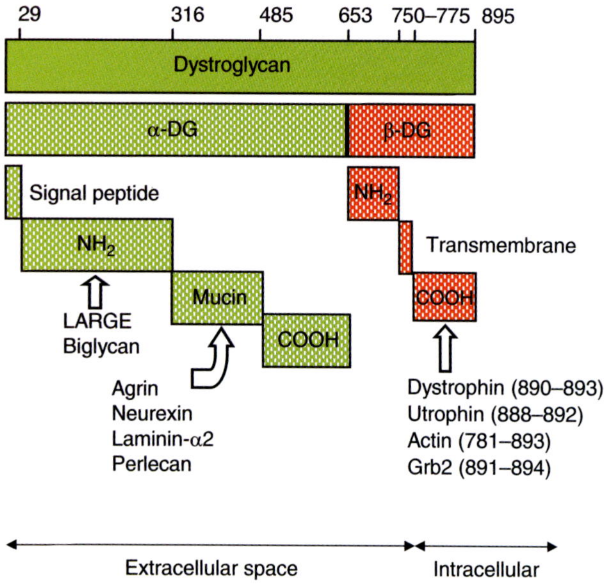

Figure 3.3. Diagram showing the domain organization of the dystroglycan precursor protein, α- and β-dystroglycan (SwissProt Q14118). Numbers refer to the position of the amino acids. The N-terminal region interacts with LARGE and biglycan, whilst the heavily glycosylated mucin-like domain interacts with laminin, agrin, perlecan (in skeletal muscle), and neurexin (in the brain). The C-terminal domain of β-dystroglycan interacts with several proteins including dystrophin, utrophin, Grb2, and actin. The interaction between α- and β-dystroglycan is noncovalent.

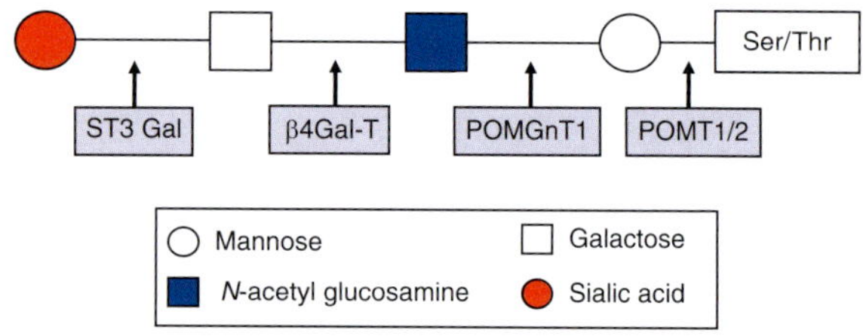

Figure 3.4. Structure of the main *O*-mannosyl glycan modification on α-dystroglycan (Siaα2–3Galβ1–4GlcNac β1–2 mannose). The enzymes involved in the stepwise addition of each of the monosaccharides are protein-mannosyl transferase-1 and -2 (POMT1/2) which function as a heterodimer, protein O-linked mannose beta-1,2-*N*-acetylglucosaminyltransferase (POMGnT1), β1,4-galactosyltransferase II (β4Gal-T), and ST3 beta-galactoside alpha-2,3-sialyltransferase (ST3 Gal). Enzymatic activity has yet to be shown for either fukutin or fukutin-related protein. The sugar groups added by LARGE are also as yet unidentified.

skeletal muscle [18] or neurons [19] demonstrates a crucial role for this complex in both of these cell types. Fukutin and POMT1-null mice also die as embryos due also to defects in the formation of Reichert's membrane [20, 21, 22]. Mice chimeric for fukutin-null and wild-type cells show cortical dysplasia due to a defect in the pial glial limitans [23], and also show defective neuromuscular junction formation and peripheral nerve myelination [24]. The Large^{myd} mouse is a spontaneous mutant with a mutation in the Large gene, and shows a muscle pathology together with defects in neuronal migration and retinal transmission [25, 26]. POMGnT1-null mice are viable and some animals survive into adulthood although they show multiple developmental defects in muscle, eye, and brain [27]. Overall all these animal models demonstrate that basement membrane fragility is a dominant feature of the phenotype although there are important differences between each model which should prove useful in the future to determine if proteins in this group have targets other than α-dystroglycan.

With respect to future therapeutic intervention in the dystroglycanopathies, work in vitro shows that cell lines transduced with LARGE irrespective of whether they are derived from patients with Fukuyama congenital muscular dystrophy (FCMD), MEB disease, WWS or limb-girdle muscular dystrophy 2I (LGMD2I) display a restoration of glycosylation and associated laminin-binding function [9]. This raises the possibility that the upregulation of LARGE or a similar glycosyltransferase may be useful to bypass the defect in glycosylation irrespective of the gene involved.

Sarcoglycan–sarcospan complex

There are six sarcoglycans (namely α, β, γ, δ, ε, and ζ); all are single-pass transmembrane proteins with glycosylation sites and conserved cysteine residues that are required for correct assembly and trafficking through the cell. ε-Sarcoglycan is homologous to α-sarcoglycan, is expressed in other tissues in addition to heart and skeletal muscle [28], and is able to compensate for the absence of α-sarcoglycan in mouse models [29]. ζ-Sarcoglycan is thought to be a functional homologue of γ-sarcoglycan and may play a more important role in the central nervous system [30]. The composition of the sarcoglycan complex varies between tissues but in striated muscle, α-, β-, γ-, and δ-sarcoglycan associate to form a distinct subcomplex of the DGC. The intracellular regions of each of these sarcoglycans have potential tyrosine phosphorylation sites indicating a possible role in signaling. Mutations in α-, β-, γ-, or δ-sarcoglycan genes are responsible for LGMD type 2D, 2E, 2C, and 2F, respectively; thus, the assembly of the entire complex is essential to maintain normal striated muscle physiology [31].

The absence of one sarcoglycan has important consequences for the stability of the remaining sarcoglycan components. This is now thought to be due to the assembly and trafficking to the membrane being initially dependent on β- and δ-sarcoglycan forming a core complex to which α- and γ-sarcoglycan then bind [32]. The presence of a mutant sarcoglycan is thought to prevent the proper insertion of the sarcoglycans into the plasma membrane. Mutations that affect β- or δ-sarcoglycan produce the greatest destabilization of the sarcoglycan complex from the plasma membrane. Whilst exceptions to this do occur [32] this is the case for the majority of patients.

Dystrophin immunolabeling in the muscle of sarcoglycanopathy patients is either normal or only slightly reduced, indicating that the absence of the sarcoglycan complex itself is sufficient to cause a disease phenotype. It is also evident that it stabilizes other components within the DGC such as the interaction between α- and β-dystroglycan, and facilitates the localization of nNOS, which is absent in sarcoglycanopathy patients [33]. The association with the DGC is also thought to be of functional significance by integrating mechanical information between the dystrophin–dystroglycan complex and other transmembrane sensors such as the integrins. Indeed experiments in vitro have suggested that the sarcoglycan complex together with integrin α5 may play a part in bi-directional signaling [34], possibly aided by sarcospan (see below). Interestingly filamin C (FLNC) has been shown to bind γ- and δ-sarcoglycan, which is also suggestive of a mechano-signaling role [35]. In summary therefore one hypothesis is that the deleterious effect of the absence or near-absence of the sarcoglycan complex might be mediated by an uncoupling of the dystrophin–dystroglycan axis from the integrin adhesion system [36].

Sarcospan is a 25-kDa dystrophin-associated protein that is absent from the muscle of DMD patients and sarcoglycanopathy patients [31]. It is structurally related to the tetraspan superfamily of proteins that are attributed with a role in mediating transmembrane protein interactions. In accordance with this, sarcospan forms a tight complex with the sarcoglycans and is an integral component of the DGC. No mutations in this protein have yet been reported in human patients.

The cardiomyopathic hamster (CMH) has a naturally occurring deletion in the δ-sarcoglycan gene and displays both myocardial and skeletal muscle necrosis beginning at 1–2 months of age, resulting in a dystrophic phenotype. The injection of Evans blue dye reveals membrane permeability defects in the CMH that are similar to those seen in the dystrophin-deficient mdx mouse. Stable restoration of the sarcoglycan complex by the injection of a δ-sarcoglycan-containing adenovirus or adeno-associated virus has been reported.

Mice deficient for γ-sarcoglycan show an increase in the rate of myonuclear apoptosis and membrane disruptions, as determined by Evans blue uptake and the levels of serum creatine kinase. The expression of dystrophin, dystroglycan, and laminin appears unaltered by the absence of γ-sarcoglycan [36]. α-Sarcoglycan-deficient mice also show membrane permeability defects that are indicated by an increase in Evans blue uptake, and an elevation of serum pyruvate kinase. However, these mice also show a reduced level of dystrophin and α-dystroglycan, possibly reflecting differences between α- and γ-sarcoglycan with respect to their relationship to dystrophin.

β-Sarcoglycan-null mice also exhibit progressive muscular dystrophy and a loss of other sarcoglycans as well as of sarcospan leading to a destabilization of the dystrophin–dystroglycan complex. Mice with an absence of δ-sarcoglycan develop a muscular dystrophy and cardiomyopathy similar to γ-sarcoglycan nulls. However, unlike the muscle of mice lacking γ-sarcoglycan, δ-sarcoglycan-deficient mice were more sensitive to eccentric contraction-induced damage. The absence of δ-sarcoglycan is also associated with an absence of the other components of the sarcoglycan complex, whereas the absence of γ-sarcoglycan leads to reduced levels of α-, β-, and δ- sarcoglycan at the sarcolemma. These differences are thought to account for the observed differences in resistence to damage by eccentric contraction [37].

In summary all sarcoglycan-null animals display a progressive muscular dystrophy of variable severity, and display a secondary reduction or absence of other members of the sarcoglycan subcomplex. However, recent work has shown that the generation of a knock-in mouse with a missense mutation resulting in an arginine-to-cysteine substitution at position 77 (R77C) in α-sarcoglycan results in a phenotype that does not develop muscular dystrophy, despite the fact that this mutation is a common one in human sarcoglycanopathy patients [38]. Since this mouse expressed the mutant sarcoglycan and other members of the sarcoglycan complex at the sarcolemma, these findings highlight important differences between mice and humans with regard to protein processing and raise a note of caution in assuming that all mouse models accurately represent the human disease.

Sarcospan-deficient mice maintain normal muscle function and do not exhibit any alteration in the DGC [39]. However, the overexpression of sarcospan in mice results in a muscle pathology due to an aggregation of the sarcoglycan complex which leads to destabilization of the dystroglycan complex and an alteration in basement membrane assembly/organization that is similar to that seen in laminin-deficient muscle [40]. These observations implicate sarcospan in the organization of the DGC and components of the basement membrane.

Dystrophin

The gene encoding dystrophin is one of the largest known and extends over 2.5 Mb of DNA and consists of 79 exons [1]. At least seven different dystrophin promoters generate five different protein isoform size classes (Figure 3.5). These promoters are named after their major, though not exclusive, sites of expression. The cortical (C), muscle (M), and Purkinje cell (P) encode full-length forms of dystrophin, consisting of unique first exons spliced to a shared set of 78 exons. Full-length dystrophin is confined to striated muscle (cardiac and skeletal) and the central nervous system. The transcripts from these promoters are approximately 14 kb long and generate a protein of approximately 427 kDa. Several cases of X-linked cardiomyopathy are caused by dystrophin gene mutations. In some of these cases the mutation inactivates the muscle promoter, but a compensatory effect of the C and/or P promoters in skeletal but not cardiac muscle leads to the coexistence of a deleterious heart pathology with relatively mild skeletal muscle pathology [41, 42].

The four internal promoters have unique first exons that splice into exons 30, 45, 56, and 63. These are referred to, respectively, as the retinal (R), brain-3 (B_3), Schwann cell (S), and general (G) promoters and give rise to proteins of

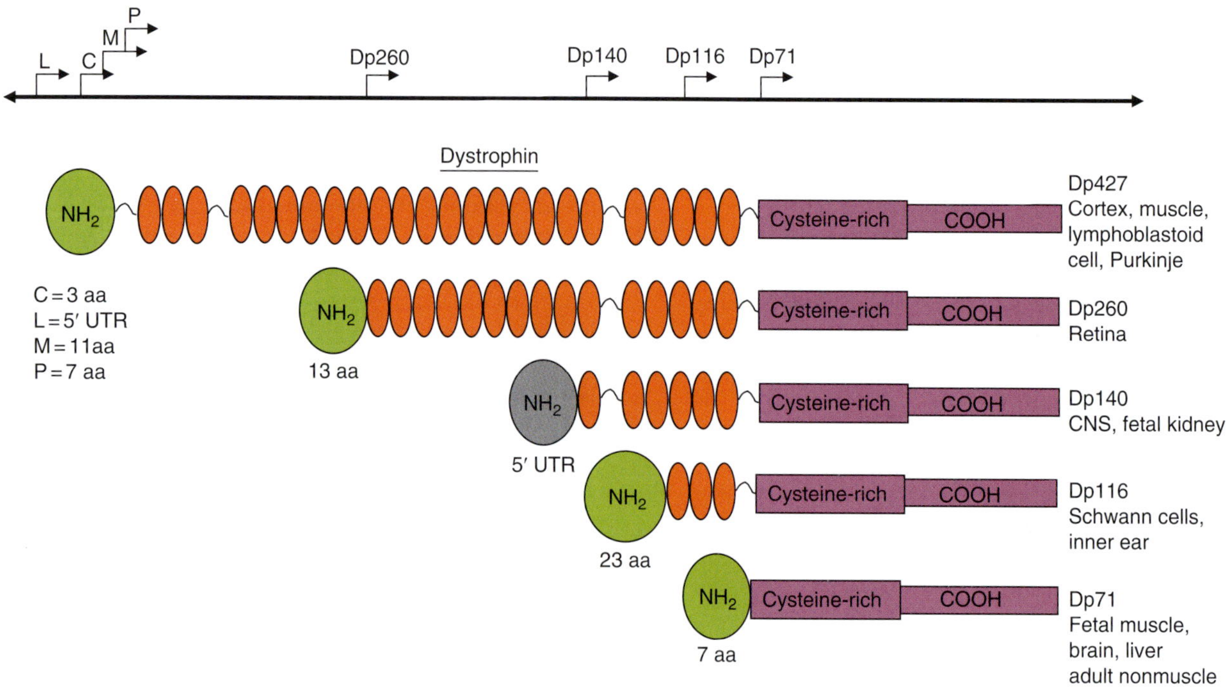

Figure 3.5. Dystrophin isoforms. The line at the top of the figure represents the positions of the transcription start sites of the known dystrophin isoform mRNAs relative to their protein structure shown beneath. The NH_2-terminal domains are colored green to indicate that they contain novel amino acids encoded by the first exon; the remainder are colored gray. The four full-length isoforms are C = cortical; L = lymphoid; M = muscle and P = Purkinje. The L-isoform was identified in lymphoblastoid cells from a DMD patient but no protein has been identified to date for this transcript. The symbol, molecular weight, and major sites of expression of each isoform are indicated. Multiple splice forms have been identified for all the dystrophin transcripts. The most commonly spliced exons are 71 and 78.

260, 140, 116, and 71 kDa (Dp260, Dp140, Dp116, and Dp71). Further diversity is generated by a range of alternative splicing events at the 3′ end of the gene and may reflect the functional adaptation of different isoforms in various locations [1]. Despite the widespread distribution of these isoforms only striated muscle manifests a clear phenotypic consequence of dystrophin gene mutations. However, the degree of mental retardation seen in some DMD patients does appear to be correlated with specific types or locations of dystrophin mutation due to the expression of these smaller isoforms in the brain.

Dystrophin locates to the cytoplasmic face of the normal adult muscle fiber membrane where it associates with the DGC. Sequence analysis indicates that it is composed of four contiguous domains namely (1) an actin-binding N-terminal domain which is similar to the conserved, actin-binding domain of α-actinin, spectrin and *Dictyostelium* actin-binding protein 120, (2) a central rod region composed of 24 spectrin-like repeats interrupted by four proline-rich hinges which fold into a series of triple-helical coils thereby creating a flexible and elastic structure, parts of which also bind actin through a primarily electrostatic interaction, (3) the dystroglycan-binding domain, which is made up of WW, EF hand, and ZZ motifs, and (4) the C-terminal domain, which mediates interactions with dystrobrevin and syntrophin, the latter of which binds to nNOS (Figure 3.2). The assembly and stability of the DGC is dependent on specific domains of the dystrophin protein as discussed above and is severely disrupted in dystrophin-deficient muscle.

Dystrophin is attributed with playing a major role in stabilizing the plasma membrane during contractile activity by providing a structural link between proteins of the extracellular matrix and the actin cytoskeleton of the fiber. There is, in addition, evidence that the DGC mediates signal transduction pathways key to maintaining muscle fiber viability. Indeed a number of signaling pathways have been linked to the dystroglycan axis [43, 44, 45], although their role in the disease process remains to be conclusively shown. Of particular note are the studies showing that the binding of laminin to dystroglycan initiates signaling through dystroglycan-syntrophin-Grb2-SOS1-Rac1-PAK1-JNK [46] and that laminin binding causes recruitment of Src family kinase to the dystrophin glycoprotein complex, activating Rac1 and inducing downstream signaling events [47].

Duchenne (DMD) and Becker muscular dystrophy (BMD) are allelic X-linked muscle wasting disorders caused by mutations in the dystrophin gene. DMD is the most common form with an incidence of 1 in 3500 live male births, whilst BMD has a predicted incidence of 1 in 17 500 live male births [48]. DMD patients are clinically normal at birth, although serum levels of the muscle isoform of creatine kinase are elevated. Muscle degeneration nonetheless ensues and proximal muscle weakness leads to the loss of ambulation around 11 years of age. The regeneration of damaged fibers eventually fails to compensate for the recurrent phases of degeneration, and death due to respiratory or cardiac failure usually occurs by the third decade. By contrast BMD presents a much more varied phenotype with some patients never losing the ability to walk.

In DMD dystrophin is absent, or virtually absent, from the majority of muscle fibers whereas in the milder BMD cases dystrophin is retained to variable degrees. This is mainly due to the effect of the mutation on the reading frame of the dystrophin transcript. In the majority of DMD cases this is disrupted, whereas its maintenance in BMD allows RNA to be transcribed and translated into protein. About 92% of cases conform to this hypothesis but there are some exceptions, which, due to the restoration of the reading frame by splicing, allow some degree of protein expression.

With improvements in molecular techniques the majority of dystrophin mutations can be detected, including point mutations. Mutations may occur in any part of the gene but 2 "hot spots" have been identified. One involves introns 44 and 51; the other, introns 2 and 7. Patients with domain-specific "in frame" deletions show that mutations in the putative actin-binding domain of the N terminus tend to be associated with a severe or intermediate BMD phenotype, whereas the absence of the cysteine-rich and proximal half of the C-terminal domain invariably leads to a severe DMD phenotype [1].

Animal models have made an essential contribution to our understanding of the pathophysiology of DMD and in facilitating the development of novel approaches to treatment; for review see [49]. The *mdx* mouse and Golden Retriever dog (GRMD) are spontaneous dystrophin-deficient mutants. There have also been a number of reports of other breeds of dog and also several cats with dystrophin deficiency. Overall the dogs show a similar phenotype with some suggestion that severity may be increased in the larger breeds. Dystrophin-deficient cats display gross hypertrophy of the tongue and diaphragm and this species has not been widely used.

There are in addition a number of murine models that have been created by exposure to mutagens or genetic manipulation. The spontaneous *mdx* mouse line is deficient in full-length dystrophin due to a premature stop codon in exon 23. This mouse starts to undergo cycles of muscle fiber degeneration and regeneration at around 2–3 weeks of age which then continues up to the age of about 5–6 weeks. The majority of the limb musculature does not show signs of fibrosis although the diaphragm does and so has traditionally been thought of as representative of the human disease. Generally the lifespan and general mobility of the *mdx* mouse is relatively normal, although there can be marked deterioration in older animals. Whilst the relatively mild phenotype in the mouse compared to DMD patients has led to the *mdx* mouse being criticized as a poor model of the disease, it has proved invaluable in evaluations of the structure/function relationships of different elements of dystrophin, as well as in testing the therapeutic potential of recombinant dystrophin, utrophin, and most recently antisense oligonucleotides (AO), which act by directing exon skipping such that the reading frame is restored together with dystrophin expression [49].

A wide variety of other mouse mutants have been generated using ethyl-nitrosourea- (5ENU-) induced mutagenesis; these include the *mdx*2cv, *mdx*3cv, *mdx*4cv, and *mdx*5cv mice, which differ with regard to the expression of the shorter isoforms of dystrophin. The phenotype of the *mdx* is made more severe by crossing with utrophin-null mice and less so by the transgenic overexpression of utrophin, suggesting that utrophin partially compensates for the absence of dystrophin. Crossing the *mdx* with the MyoD knockout leads to impaired muscle regeneration and the development of muscle pathology similar to DMD with premature death at about 1 year. A severe pathology is also obtained following irradiation which impairs regeneration, implying that regeneration is more efficient in the *mdx* than DMD patients.

The closest model to human DMD is the Golden Retriever Muscular Dystrophy (GRMD) dog, which carries a point mutation in the splice acceptor site in intron 6 of the dystrophin gene, leading to the absence of dystrophin in the muscles. The GRMD dog shows clinical signs at 6–9 weeks of age, a marked muscle wasting and skeletal deformity by 6 months of age, and is more vulnerable than normal dogs to muscle damage following eccentric contractions. Some affected pups die shortly after birth with massive necrosis of the respiratory muscles, and there is some considerable variability in severity between dystrophin-negative littermates which could prove to be a disadvantage in terms of therapeutic clinical trials [50].

Dystrobrevin, syntrophin and nitric oxide synthase

A number of proteins associate with the DGC on the cytoplasmic side of the sarcolemma (Figure 3.2). These include the multiple isoforms of α- dystrobrevin and three syntrophin isoforms. To date no human disease has been unequivocally associated with mutations of dystrobrevin genes [51]. Three isoforms of α-dystrobrevin are found at the sarcolemma: α-dystrobrevin-1 and -2, which bind directly to dystrophin and utrophin through the reciprocal coiled-coil regions present in each protein, and α-dystrobrevin-3 which lacks the dystrophin-binding site but is thought to maintain its association with the DGC by binding directly to the sarcoglycan–sarcospan complex [52].

α-Dystrobrevin-null mice exhibit muscle fiber degeneration and abnormalities at the neuromuscular junction although the DGC remains intact leading to the hypothesis that α-dystrobrevin plays a predominant signaling rather than structural role in skeletal muscle [53]. However, more recent work shows that in its absence the biochemical association between dystrophin and β-dystroglycan is compromised [54].

The syntrophins are 59-kDa cytoplasmic proteins thought to serve as adaptor proteins. Each of the five syntrophins (α, β1, β2, γ1, and γ2) consists of two pleckstrin homology

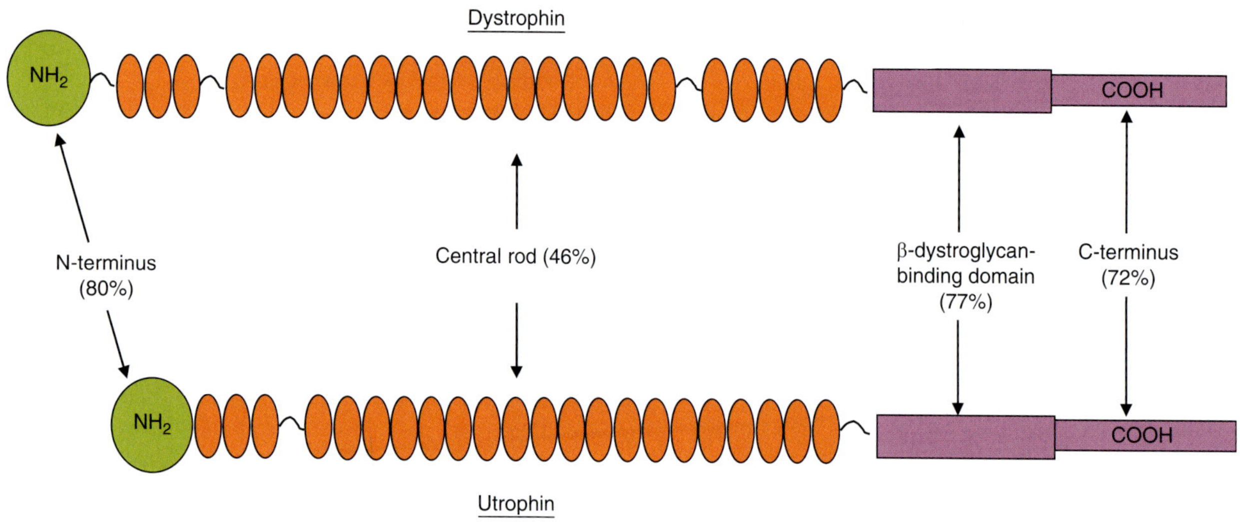

Figure 3.6. A schematic diagram showing the level of amino acid identity (%) between dystrophin and utrophin with respect to the N-terminal, central rod, dystroglycan-binding, and C-terminal domains.

(PH) domains, a postsynaptic density-95/Discs large/zona occludens (PDZ) domain, and a syntrophin unique (SU) region. α-Syntrophin is the major isoform of skeletal and cardiac muscle and binds directly to dystrophin, utrophin, α-dystrobrevin, and nNOS. As a consequence of their domain structure and association with nNOS, aquaporin-4, ion channels, and kinases, the syntrophins are attributed with a role in recruiting signaling proteins to the membrane. In addition recent work suggests that there is an association between TRPC1 channels and α1-syntrophin that may function to anchor store-operated channels to the dystrophin-associated protein complex (DAPC), thus providing a new explanation for the abnormal calcium influx reported by many in dystrophic cells [55].

Recent work reported a missense mutation in α1-syntrophin in a patient with recurrent syncope and markedly prolonged QT interval. However, it remains to be determined if SNTA1 mutations can be considered as a Long QT Syndrome-susceptibility gene [56].

Mice lacking α-syntrophin show no evidence of a muscular dystrophy despite the absence of nNOS and aquaporin-4 in muscle. These mice do, however, have aberrant neuromuscular junctions with reduced levels of acetylcholine receptors (AChRs) and acetylcholinesterase, undetectable postsynaptic utrophin, and altered morphology [57]. Mice null for both α- and β2-syntrophin have a more severe phenotype than mice lacking only one syntrophin, suggesting that each syntrophin may partially compensate for the loss of the other [58].

Neuronal NOS is selectively lost from the plasma membrane of muscle from patients with DMD and from dystrophin-deficient *mdx* mice. Loss of the sarcoglycan–sarcospan complex also causes a dramatic reduction in the levels of nNOS expression at the membrane, even in the presence of normal dystrophin and syntrophin expression [33]. nNOS directly interacts with syntrophin via the PSD-95, Dlg, ZO-1 (PDZ) motif, whilst syntrophin itself interacts with dystrophin. Studies of the muscle from transgenic *mdx* mice and BMD patients indicate that the mid-rod domain of dystrophin also has a profound effect on the localization of nNOS at the sarcolemma. The precise reasons for this are unclear, but may relate to conformational changes induced by mutations in the region of the molecule encompassing exons 45 and 48.

Whilst nNOS-deficient mice display no pathology in their muscle, the absence of nNOS in dystrophin-deficient muscle is thought to contribute to the progression of the dystrophic phenotype [59]. The precise pathways remain to be shown but nNOS is enriched in fast-twitch muscle fibers and nitric oxide (NO) is known to modulate blood flow during exercise by attenuating the sympathetic vasoconstriction that occurs in contracting muscle. Skeletal-muscle-derived NO is also known to modulate several aspects of skeletal muscle physiology, such as exercise-induced glucose uptake and contractile force, and acts upon the calcium-release channel of the sarcoplasmic reticulum.

Dystrophin-related proteins: utrophin

Utrophin is a ubiquitously expressed protein with significant structural and functional similarities to dystrophin. Similarly to dystrophin, utrophin consists of four structurally distinct domains: an actin-binding domain at the N-terminus, a central rod domain of 22 spectrin-like repeats, a cysteine-rich domain and a C-terminal domain. Amino-acid homology with dystrophin is highest in the actin-binding and cysteine-rich domains and lowest in the central rod domain (Figure 3.6). Utrophin also interacts with β-dystroglycan and syntrophin/dystrobrevin via the cysteine-rich and C-terminal domains respectively.

In adult skeletal muscle, full-length utrophin is restricted to the neuromuscular and myotendinous junctions, blood vessels and capillaries, and intramuscular nerves. However, utrophin localizes along the length of the sarcolemma in fetal muscle, regenerating fibers, and sometimes nonregenerating fibers in DMD muscle and other neuromuscular conditions [60]. At the neuromuscular junction utrophin localizes to the peaks of the synaptic folds with acetylcholine receptors, rapsyn, and dystroglycan [61] whereas dystrophia localizes to the troughs where there is a high density of voltage-gated sodium channels. Recently, the utrophin gene (*UTRN*) has been identified as a tumor suppressor gene [62].

The transcriptional regulation of the utrophin gene (6q24) is complex and involves several promoters, two at the 5′ end controlling the transcription of two full-length isoforms (utrophin A and B) and three, possibly four, internal promoters giving rise to short isoforms. B-utrophin is expressed in vascular endothelial cells whilst A-utrophin is expressed at the neuromuscular junction, choroid plexus, pia mater, and renal glomerulus. A- but not B-utrophin is upregulated in dystrophin-deficient muscle but isoform-specific antibodies are required to detect this [63].

The upregulation of utrophin via transgenesis in dystrophin-deficient muscle has been shown to ameliorate the dystrophic pathology in mice, suggesting that the upregulation of endogenous utrophin levels could be a possible form of therapy for DMD [64]. Possible approaches include the systemic delivery of chemical compounds that act upon the utrophin promoter, an approach which, if successful, would be applicable to all DMD patients regardless of their mutation. Indeed the promoter of full-length utrophin A, the isoform normally expressed at the sarcolemma and neuromuscular junction, is well characterized and contains several elements that can be targeted for pharmaceutical intervention. As an example, a small peptide based on the amino acid sequence of the ectodomain of heregulin, a nerve-derived factor which targets the N-box motif in the promoter, has been tested in dystrophin-deficient mice with positive results [65]. Current work includes using high-throughput screening of chemical libraries to identify small molecules that are able to activate the utrophin promoter.

Utrophin-deficient mice display no overt signs of weakness but do have reduced numbers of AChRs and decreased postsynaptic folding. However, this results in only minimal electrophysiological changes. Utrophin is therefore not considered to be essential for AChR clustering at the neuromuscular junction but rather fulfils a function in the development or maintenance of the postsynaptic folds [66].

Sarcolemmal – transmembrane proteins

Integrins constitute a family of transmembrane heterodimers composed of α and β chains which recognize a large number of extracellular ligands through a metal-ion-dependent interaction. Their name reflects their role in integrating cell adhesion and/or migration with the cytoskeleton. Integrins possess no inherent catalytic activity of their own and instead depend upon an extensive array of extracellular and intracellular partners in order to localize to membrane microdomains, recruit signaling molecules, and trigger intracellular signaling cascades.

Integrin α7

α7β1D integrin is the major integrin receptor found in adult skeletal muscle and locates along the entire length of the sarcolemma, but is enriched at the myotendinous and neuromuscular junctions. Integrin α7β1D and α-dystroglycan are the main receptors for laminin-α2 in muscle. Immunolabeling for either α7 or β1D may be secondarily reduced in primary laminin-α2 deficiency as well as in other forms of congenital muscular dystrophy with a secondary reduction of laminin-α2 [67]. Mutations in the gene encoding for integrin α7 (*ITGA7*) underlie a very rare form of congenital myopathy which is associated with a relatively mild muscle pathology without the degeneration and regeneration that is characteristic of most dystrophies [68]. In mice deficient for the α7 chain the structure of the myotendinous junction is severely disrupted with loss of the characteristic digit-like extensions and retraction of the sarcomere from the muscle membrane, suggesting that impairment of force transmission across the myotendinous junction is the basis of muscle weakness in patients [69].

Both the DGC and α7β1D integrin are known to be essential for maintaining myotendinous junction stability and the lateral integrity of the muscle fiber, suggesting that they are independently controlled receptor systems. This is further emphasized by the finding that double-mutant mice lacking both dystrophin and α7 develop a severe dystrophy and die within 4 weeks of birth [70]. However, overexpression of the α7 subunit in these mice results in a threefold increase in life span indicating that increased amounts of integrin $\alpha 7\beta 1_D$ could prove to be beneficial in the muscle of DMD patients [71].

Sarcolemmal – neuromuscular junction

Formation of the neuromuscular junction (NMJ)

Formation of the NMJ depends on agrin, the muscle-specific receptor tyrosine kinase MuSK (which is activated by agrin), the low-density lipoprotein receptor-related protein 4, and two intracellular adaptors, Dok7 and rapsyn, which bind to activated MuSK and the acetylcholine receptor (AChR), respectively. Early events during NMJ formation are a reflection of a complex interaction between the innervating nerve and its target muscle fiber. The "neurocentric model" proposes that agrin released from motor neurons initiates the formation of synaptic AChR clusters; however, AChR clusters are known to form in the absence of the nerve (and agrin) and so the myocentric model proposes that muscle-derived cues spatially restrict the nerve to form synapses by a patterned expression of MuSK (muscle-specific kinase). Recent work now seems to suggest that in those areas of the muscle fiber where MuSK is low, agrin derived from the innervating nerves is required for

MuSK activation, resulting in synapse formation which is consistent with the so-called neurocentric model. However, in areas where there are high levels of MuSK (and also of cofactors such as Dok7 and LRP4), MuSK is autoactivated which results in the formation of aneural AChR clusters. Overall this system means that there is a high probability of motor neurons making contact with a preformed AChR cluster, thus favoring innervation of preformed aneural AChR clusters according to the myocentric model [72].

Neuromuscular transmission

The adult NMJ is a specialized region designed to allow for the rapid transmission of the depolarizing impulse. Neuromuscular transmission depends on both the size and molecular organization of the NMJ. In normal muscle, the postsynaptic membrane is characteristically thrown into numerous folds, the crests of which are adjacent to the nerve terminal and contain the AChRs, at a concentration 1000-fold higher than in the extra-junctional regions of the muscle fiber (Figure 3.7a, b). Five AChR subunits are expressed in skeletal muscle (α1, β1, γ, δ, and ε), two of which (γ and ε) are developmentally regulated (the γ subunit being expressed in embryonic muscle, the ε subunit in adult muscle). Voltage-gated sodium channels (VGSCs) are concentrated at the base of the postsynaptic folds [73, 74]. The role of this arrangement is thought to be to focus endplate current flow on the VGSCs, thereby amplifying the effect of transmitter release and ensuring effective neuromuscular transmission [75].

The complexity of the postsynaptic folds differs with fiber type and in fast-twitch fibers they are usually deeper and more branched. Under the electron microscope regions within the postsynaptic membrane of the nerve terminal may appear darker than others due to the aggregation of the AChRs (Figure 3.7a). A basal lamina, albeit specialized, extends into the folds and anchors NMJ-specific proteins such as acetylcholinesterase, agrin, and neuregulins. The myonuclei around NMJs are also specialized with respect to their transcriptional activity. Defects in the presynaptic nerve terminal, the synaptic cleft or the postsynaptic apparatus underlie congenital myasthenic syndromes (CMS), which define a group of inherited disorders characterized by impaired neuromuscular transmission [76]. Mutations in at least ten genes have now been shown to underlie this group of disorders (Figure 3.8).

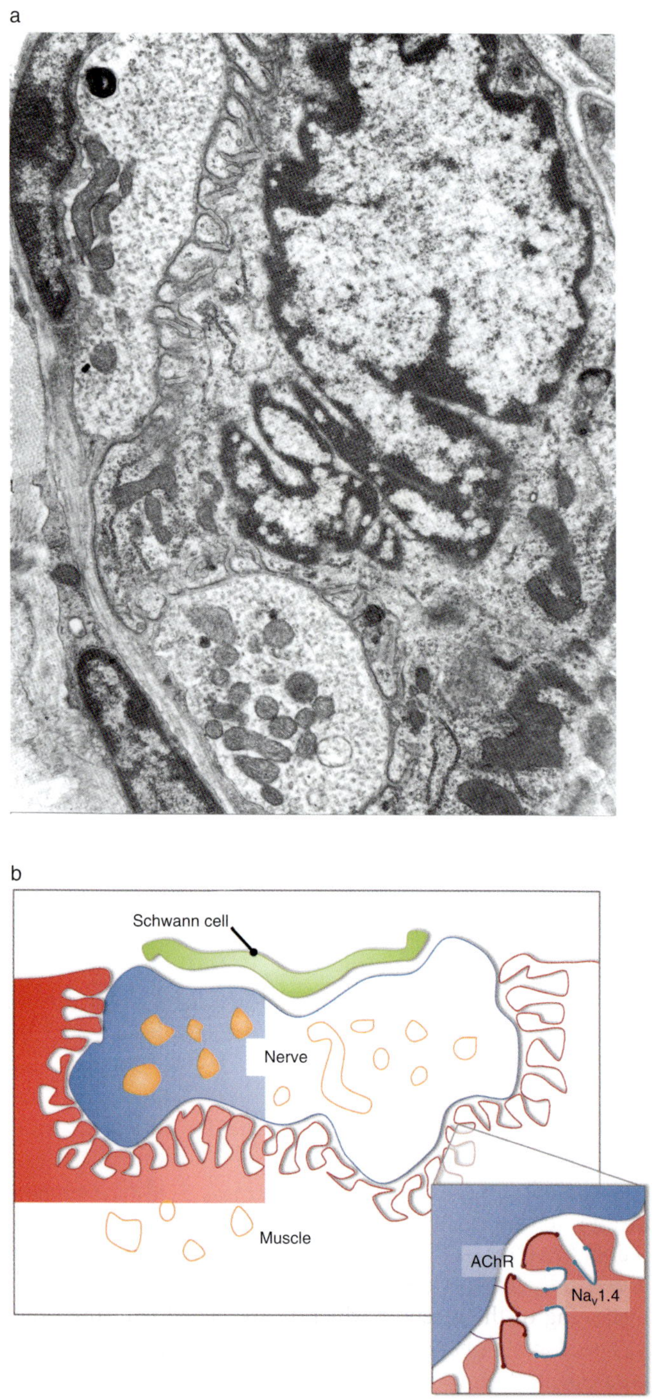

Figure 3.7. (a) Electron micrograph of a mouse neuromuscular junction showing the nerve terminals and characteristic folding of the sarcolemma. Note the high density at the crests of the folds which reflects the localization of the acetylcholine receptors. (b) Schematic showing the localization of the acetylcholine receptors at the crests of the folds and the voltage-gated sodium channels at the base. Figure 3.7b kindly drawn by Mehmet Fidanboylu.

Presynaptic and synaptic defects

To date the only CMS form associated with a presynaptic protein is the one due to mutations in the gene encoding for choline acetyltransferase (ChAT). Mutations in the gene encoding for acetylcholinesterase collagen-like tail subunit (COLQ) represent the only examples of the protein defect localizing to the synapse. A deficiency of this enzyme leads to reduced acetylcholine breakdown and thus an increase in the duration of the endplate current. The associated muscle weakness is thought to arise from a combination of depolarization blockade and desensitization of the AChRs which over an extended time period leads to an endplate myopathy [76].

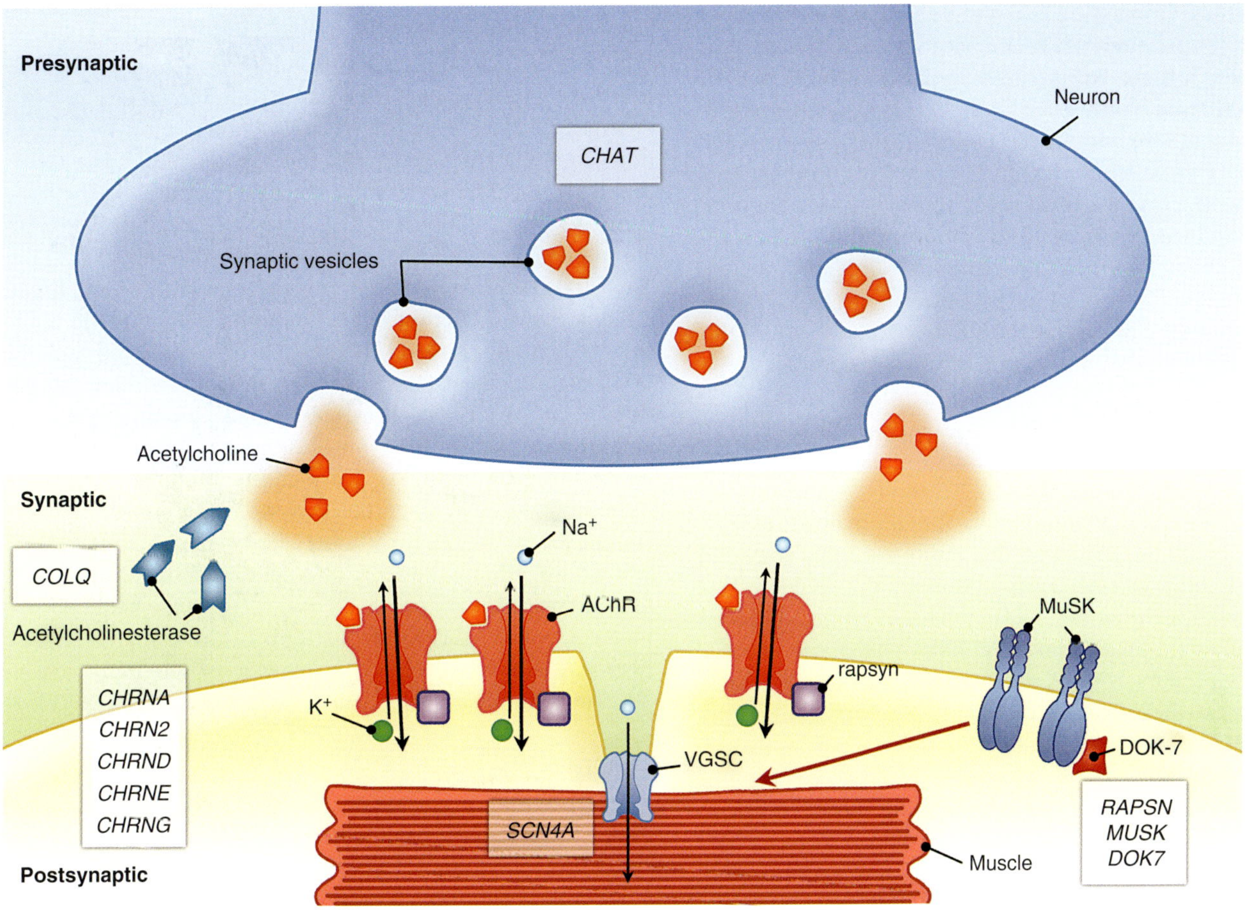

Figure 3.8. A schematic diagram of the neuromuscular junction showing components of the presynaptic, synaptic and postsynaptic compartments that have been associated with congenital myasthenic syndromes. ACh, acetylcholine; CHAT, choline acetyltransferase; AChE, acetylcholinesterase; COLQ, collagen tail attached to acetylcholinesterase; CHRNA-E, subunits of the acetycholine receptor (AChR); MUSK, muscle-specific kinase; DOK7, downstream of tyrosine kinase 7; VGSC, voltage-gated sodium channel; SCN4A, sodium channel α-subunit. Figure kindly drawn by Mehmet Fidanboylu.

Postsynaptic defects

Defects in postsynaptic proteins account for most cases of CMS identified so far. AChR deficiency can arise from mutations in the genes encoding for either an AChR subunit (mainly *CHRNE*) or *RAPSN*. Mutations in the genes encoding for the individual AChR subunits can also lead to abnormal functioning of the receptor which is associated with the slow and fast channel phenotypes. Mutations in the gene encoding for the γ AChR subunit (present during fetal life) underlie fetal akinesia and have most recently been shown to be causative in cases of severe arthrogryposis and multiple pterygium associated with Escobar syndrome in neonates. However, weakness during postnatal life is not a feature due to replacement of the γ with the adult (ε) subunit in utero.

Mutations of the AChR subunits (predominantly ε) cause a recessively inherited receptor deficiency syndrome with onset at birth or infancy. Rapsyn mutations are associated with defective AChR clustering and thus an endplate AChR deficiency. More than 90% of rapsyn CMS patients have at least one copy of the common N88K mutation, which is thought to have derived from a founder in the ancient Indo-European population. Slow channel syndrome is the only CMS that is dominantly inherited. It is associated with mutations in any of the adult AChR subunits (α, β, δ, ε). Fast channel syndrome is, by contrast, recessively inherited and mutations in the AChR α, δ, and ε subunits have been identified. Single case reports of heteroallelic mutations in the postsynaptic sodium channel and in MuSK [77] have also been published [76].

MuSK together with its cytoplasmic activator Dok7 is essential for neuromuscular synaptogenesis. Recessive mutations in DOK7 have been shown to underlie a form of CMS with a highly variable clinical phenotype [78]. However, most of the patients display a characteristic "limb-girdle" pattern of weakness with a waddling gait and ptosis. Patient muscle biopsy samples show small and simplified neuromuscular synapses but normal AChR and acetylcholinesterase function despite defects in neuromuscular transmission [79]. The reason for the smaller endplates and reduced folding is currently unclear although recent electron microscopic studies show evidence of endplate damage and formation of new endplates. Moreover, some patients show normal synaptic folding strongly suggesting that the reduction seen at some NMJs may be a reflection of immaturity of newly formed postsynaptic regions rather than a constitutive reduction [80]. Overall these observations indicate that Dok7 is essential for maintaining size and the structural integrity of the NMJ. The majority of patients with DOK7 mutations have at least one allele with a frameshift mutation resulting in a truncation in the C-terminal region of Dok7, which affects MuSK activation. This is significant in the light of work identifying the N- and C-terminal motifs as key players in Dok7/MuSK signaling during NMJ formation [81]. CMS due to DOK7 mutations are thought to be at present underdiagnosed.

Autoimmune diseases of the neuromuscular junction

Myasthenia gravis (MG) is caused by the failure of neuromuscular transmission mediated by autoantibodies directed against endplate proteins, most commonly the AChRs. This results in weakening of the ocular, bulbar, and limb muscles and produces the characteristic clinical phenotype of MG. Approximately 80%–85% of patients with MG have autoantibodies against the AChR. It is believed that these antibodies reduce the number of AChRs at the endplate by a combination of complement-mediated membrane lysis and acceleration of AChR catabolism by receptor cross-linking. Recent work in rats shows that impaired neuromuscular transmission in MG reflects impaired function of both AChRs and endplate Na^+ channels, although loss of the latter in MG relates to the complement-mediated loss of endplate membrane rather than a direct effect of the acetylcholine antibodies on endplate Na^+ channels [82].

Antibodies against muscle-specific kinase (MuSK) have been found in 30% of MG patients without AChR antibodies. As discussed above MuSK is a tyrosine kinase receptor that plays a fundamental role in NMJ formation during embryonic life. However, more recent studies suggest that MuSK is also important for the maturation and/or maintenance of the adult NMJ. The active immunization of mice with MuSK protein has been shown to lead to MG-like weakness and associated changes in the NMJ suggesting that MuSK is important for maintenance of the adult NMJ.

Whilst previous data questioned the role of MuSK antibodies in the pathogenesis of MuSK-positive MG patients, recent work has shown that the passive transfer of IgG from anti-MuSK-positive MG patients into adult mice reduced the level of AChRs in the postsynaptic membrane and caused changes in the presynaptic and postsynaptic elements of the synapse [83].

There are several other antibody-mediated neuromuscular disorders including Lambert–Eaton syndrome, which is caused by antibodies against voltage-gated calcium channels and often occurs in patients with small cell lung cancer. In addition acquired neuromyotonia is associated with voltage-gated potassium channel antibodies.

Muscle fiber basement membrane

Individual muscle fibers are surrounded by a layer of extracellular matrix called the basement membrane, which is composed of two layers: an internal basal lamina (also referred to as the lamina densa) which directly opposes the plasma membrane, and an external, fibrillar reticular lamina [84]. The basal lamina is secreted by the muscle fiber itself and appears as an amorphous or finely granular layer. It is usually 20–30 nm thick and contains nonfibrillar collagen, in particular collagen IV, a number of glycoproteins (laminins, perlecan, and nidogen), and proteoglycans. The fibrillar reticular layer contains collagen, including type III, and fibronectin, which are embedded in an amorphous proteoglycan-rich ground substance. Collagen IV and laminin form two distinct self assembling networks which are linked via nidogen. Both these networks have multiple binding partners in the basal lamina, reticular lamina, and at the cell membrane thereby effectively forming a link which extends between the cytoskeleton of the muscle fiber to the reticular lamina. Overall this arrangement contributes not only to the tensile strength of the complete muscle fiber but is now recognized as playing an important role in development, regeneration, and synaptogenesis [85].

Collagen VI

Collagen VI consists of three α chains, α1(VI), α2(VI), and α3(VI), encoded by the *COL6A1* and *COL6A2* genes on chromosome 21q22.3 and *COL6A3* gene on chromosome 2q37, respectively (Figure 3.9). Mutations in any of the three collagen VI genes underlie Ullrich congenital muscular dystrophy (UCMD) and Bethlem myopathy (BM) although the degree of genetic heterogeneity in UCMD suggests additional genes may be involved [86].

UCMD is a form of congenital muscular dystrophy which presents during the neonatal period and is characterized by muscle weakness, kyphosis of the spine, joint contractures, torticollis, hip dislocation, and hyperextensibility of the distal joints. Some patients may never achieve ambulation while others will be able to walk independently. Serum creatine kinase levels are usually normal or mildly elevated. Rough skin (follicular hyperkeratosis) is a frequent feature, and impaired wound healing resulting in the formation of keloids is common. Respiratory insufficiency invariably appears in the first or second decade of life and patients may require ventilation. UCMD appears to be the second most common form of CMD after MDC1A in the West and after FCMD in Japan [87].

Bethlem myopathy is characterized by prominent contractures and, compared to UCMD, is associated with a comparatively mild proximal muscle weakness with slower progression. Presentation is sometimes at birth with talipes and torticollis (hip dysplasia is rarely seen), or during childhood, adolescence or adult life. In the early years generalized joint laxity prevails, but contractures of most proximal and also distal joints characterize the later phases of the disorder. The progressive contracture of the long finger flexors, which results in the inability

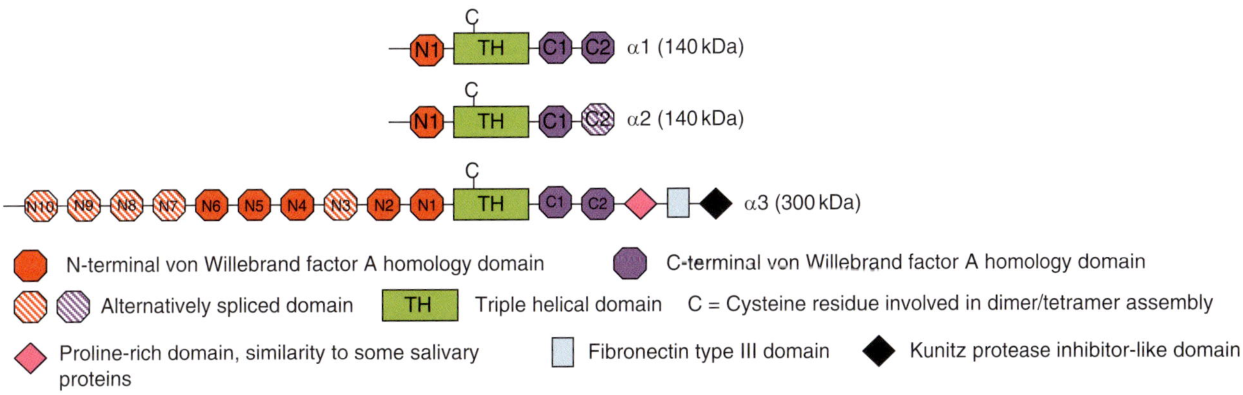

Figure 3.9. Diagram showing the domain structure of the α1, α2, and α3 chains of collagen VI. Each chain consists of a variable number of N-terminal and C-terminal globular domains with homology to von Willebrand factor A. The triple helical (TH) domain contains the Gly-Xaa-Yaa repeats. In addition the α3 chain contains a fibronectin type III domain, a lysine/proline-rich domain found in salivary proteins, and a Kunitz protease inhibitor motif. The hatched domains denote alternative splicing in the α2 and α3 chain. The cysteine residue within the TH domain plays an important role in the dimer and tetramer assembly.

to bring the fingers together in the "prayer sign," is a characteristic feature of this disorder. In addition to the finger contractures, elbow, knee, hip, and ankle contractures also occur in most patients, in association with rigidity of the spine. The muscle weakness affects proximal more than distal muscles, and lower more than upper limbs, and a proportion of patients (~20%) become wheelchair bound in adult life, or very rarely in adolescence.

UCMD can be inherited in a recessive or dominant fashion and de novo mutations are common, which has important implications for prenatal diagnosis and genetic counseling. It has also been recently reported that some null mutations can show variable penetrance [88]. Due to the complexities associated with the genetic analysis of collagen VI genes, in terms of both the size and number of polymorphisms, analysis of collagen VI protein levels in muscle and/or skin fibroblasts can prove to be particularly useful prior to undertaking direct genetic analysis [84, 89]. Collagen VI gene mutations associated with UCMD often result in a partial reduction in the levels of collagen VI in the basal lamina but not endomysial connective tissue as determined with immunohistochemistry. Possible cell surface receptors for collagen VI such as NG2 proteoglycan may also be reduced [90]. In contrast patients with BM, with dominant mutations in collagen VI, display immunolabeling of muscle that is almost always reported as normal although there have been exceptions [91]. Nonetheless a reduction in the immunofluorescent labeling of collagen VI in fibroblast cultures derived from UCMD patients has been shown to be diagnostically useful [92], and more recently this technique has been extended to cases of BM [89].

Most missense mutations in COL6A genes alter amino acids in the triple helical (TH) collagenous domain and the most common amino acid substitution is a glycine to arginine change [93]. It appears that depending on whether the affected glycine is located at the N- or C-terminal ends of the TH domain, the assembly of the tetramer into microfibrils in the extracellular matrix or the binding of the three α chains into the monomer will be affected. The former are the most common type of mutations in BM and are known to result in the introduction of "kinks" in the collagen tetramer impairing the formation of normal microfibrils, exerting a dominant negative effect on the normal collagen [94]. The second most commonly reported mutation in BM patients results in the in-frame deletion of exon 14 of the COL6A1 gene removing a cysteine residue crucial to dimer formation [95, 96] (Figure 3.10).

Missense mutations in the C-terminal end of the triple helical domain of the collagen VI chains are rare compared to mutations in the N-terminus and indeed there is only one reported UCMD patient with a homozygous glycine substitution at the C-terminus of the triple helical (TH) domain. An engineered missense mutation in the C-terminal end of the α3 (VI) chain TH [17] was shown to partially prevent the association of the mutated chain with α1 and α2 chains and the formation of the disulfide bonds that normally stabilize the collagen VI tetramer. Several homozygous in-frame deletions in UCMD patients in the C-terminal end of the TH have been identified which are also predicted to interfere with the assembly of the monomer [93].

Figure 3.10, which is modified from [96], illustrates the mechanism through which two in-frame deletions in the *COL6A1* gene can result in either a severe UCMD phenotype (exerting a dominant negative effect on microfibril formation) or a milder Bethlem phentoype and an overall reduction of collagen VI secretion. Whilst the majority of mutations result in the secretion and deposition of structurally abnormal collagen VI, mutations have been described that do not affect the levels of protein synthesis but rather the interaction of collagen VI with other proteins [97].

Alterations in collagen VI deposition have been reported to alter the organization of fibronectin in fibroblasts derived from UCMD skin [98]. The presence of hypertrophic scars and keloids in both UCMD and Bethlem myopathy has long suggested a defect in the process of wound healing, which is

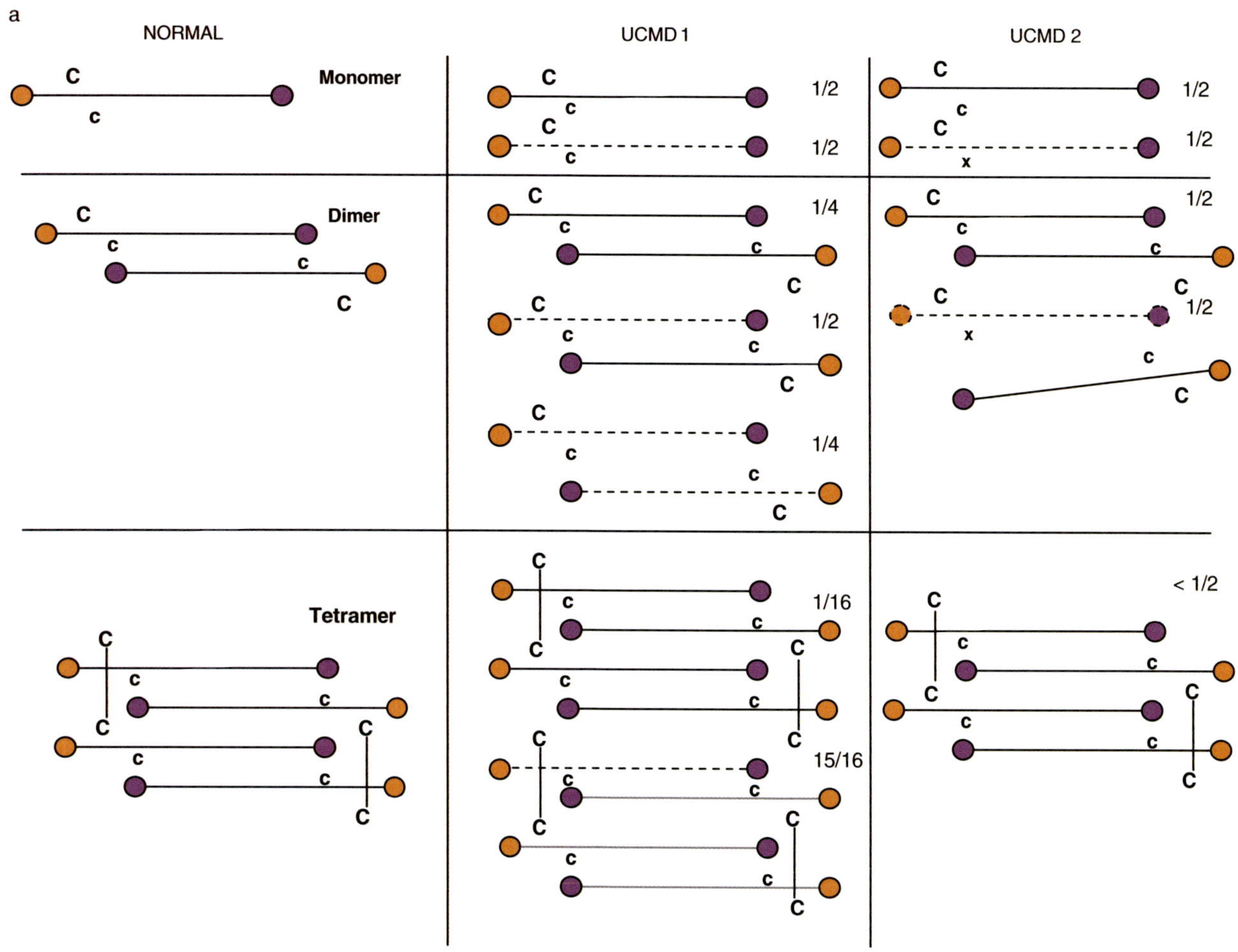

Figure 3.10. (a) Schematic illustrating the mechanism through which two in-frame deletions in the *COL6A1* gene can result in either a severe UCMD phenotype (by exerting a dominant negative effect on microfibril formation) or a milder Bethlem phenotype and an overall reduction of collagen VI secretion. In UCMD 1 a deletion in the N-terminus of the triple helix does not affect the two key cysteine residues involved in either dimer or tetramer assembly, which allows the formation and secretion of tetramers the majority of which are composed of a combination of normal and abnormal chains. These tetramers however cannot associate properly into long microfibrils because they lack the necessary regions within the N-terminus of the triple helix. In contrast, in UCMD 2 the cysteine residue necessary for dimer formation is deleted in half of the α chains. Abnormal monomers are unable to assemble into tetramers and only half of the amount of normal collagen tetramers is secreted into the extracellular matrix. It is possible that a proportion of mutant monomers assemble into dimers which exert a dominant negative effect on the normal dimers resulting in even less than half the amount of normal collagen tetramers being secreted (modified from [96]).

dependent upon the highly coordinated interaction between fibroblasts and components of the matrix which includes collagen VI. The interstitial fibroblasts in muscle are the primary source of collagen VI [99] and this, combined with electron microscopic observations of an absence of collagen VI microfibrils from the area immediately adjacent to the basal lamina in muscle biopsy samples from UCMD patients [84], supports the hypothesis that the underlying pathology of these disorders is related to a defect in adhesion between the muscle fiber and its surrounding matrix.

The consequences of this on the muscle are likely to be severalfold and muscle fibers from the Col6a1 knockout mouse show mitochondrial and sarcoplasmic reticulum ultrastructural abnormalities and increased opening of the permeability transition pore in the mitochondrial membrane [100]. These defects, including the increased incidence of apoptosis, were rescued in vitro by growing the cells on collagen VI and in vivo by ciclosporin treatment, which was accompanied by an amelioration of the contractile strength of the mice, suggesting that pharmacological intervention in UCMD may be possible. Mitochondrial dysfunction has been confirmed in UCMD myoblasts as has an increase in the incidence of apoptosis; ciclosporin has been shown to reverse both these processes [101].

Laminin-α2

Approximately one-third of all CMD cases are due to mutations in the *LAMA2* gene in 6q22, which encodes for the laminin-α2 chain (MDC1A [MIM156225]). Most mutations in the LAMA2 gene result in the complete absence of laminin-α2 protein, which is always associated with a severe phenotype; however, rare allelic mutations can result in partial protein reduction which can give rise to a mild or a severe phenotype depending on the effect of the specific mutation on laminin-α2 function.

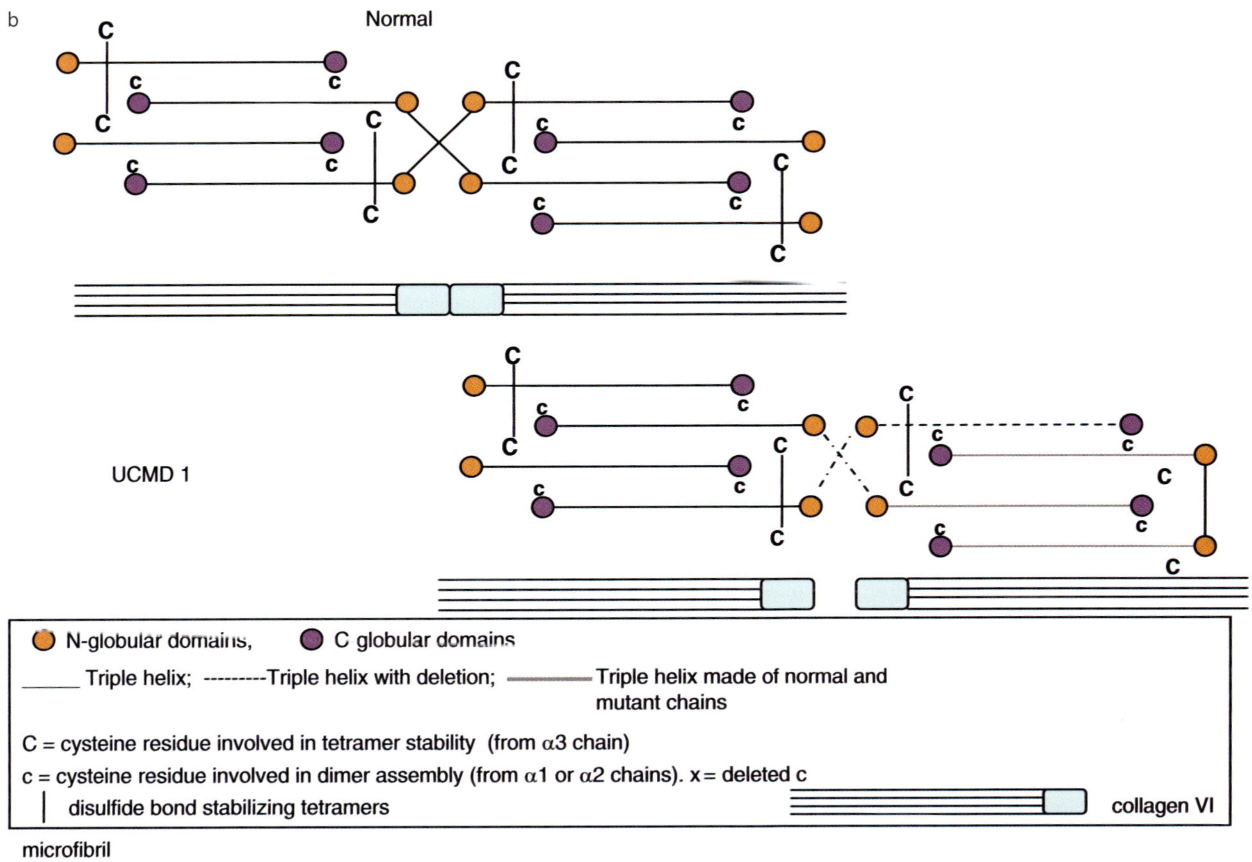

Figure 3.10. *(cont.)*

Presentation is at birth or in the first few weeks of life where hypotonia and muscle weakness may be associated with failure to thrive and respiratory and feeding problems. However, severe respiratory failure at birth is not a feature. Contractures may be present but severe arthrogryposis is rare. Serum CK levels are always elevated consistent with a problem at the interface between the muscle fiber sarolemma and the basement membrane. While cognitive function is usually normal, all patients affected by MDC1A have increased signal intensity in the white matter with T_2-weighted brain magnetic resonance imaging (MRI). Some cases (~5%) also show structural brain changes, such as occipital agyria, which can be accompanied by mental retardation and epilepsy.

The laminins are essential components of basement membranes that provide tissue compartmentalization by acting as barriers to cell penetration and filtration. There are at least 15 different heterotrimers formed from 5α, 3β, and 3γ chains encoded by different genes [102]. The three chains bind together via their central coiled-coiled domains (Figure 3.11). Laminins are able to self-assemble via their short arms and, through multiple interactions with other proteins, play a crucial role in basement membrane integrity both during development and in adult life. Most basement membranes contain more than a single laminin heterotrimer along with type IV collagens, nidogens, perlecan, and agrin. Laminin-211 (α2, β1, and γ1) is the predominant laminin trimer in the skeletal muscle basal lamina although laminin-221 (α2, β2, and γ1) is also present. Laminin-α2 is also expressed in several other tissues including the peripheral nerves and the brain.

Laminins are known to preferentially polymerize when bound to receptors such as dystroglycan and α7β1 integrin in muscle cell cultures. It is this receptor-mediated self-assembly that drives rearrangement of laminin into a cell-associated polygonal network, a process that also involves actin reorganization and tyrosine phosphorylation. This sequence of events causes dystroglycan and integrin to redistribute into a reciprocal network, as do components of the cortical cytoskeleton vinculin and dystrophin [103]. Labeling of teased mouse muscle fibers indicates that the distribution of laminin along the length of the fiber resembles the costameric distribution of α-dystroglycan, an organization that is disrupted in fibers isolated from laminin-α2-deficient dy^{2J} mice. The costameric distribution of dystrophin and vinculin was similarly affected in these mice suggesting that lateral force transmission may be disrupted in the absence of laminin-α2 [104].

There are several mouse models of this disease, namely the *dy/dy* [105], dy^{2J}/dy^{2J} [106], dy^{3K}/dy^{3K} [107], dy^{W}/dy^{W} [108], and dy^{Pas}/dy^{Pas} [109]. The naturally occuring *dy* and dy^{2J} mice both display a reduction in the expression of laminin-α2. The mutation in the *dy/dy* mice has not yet been identified but the

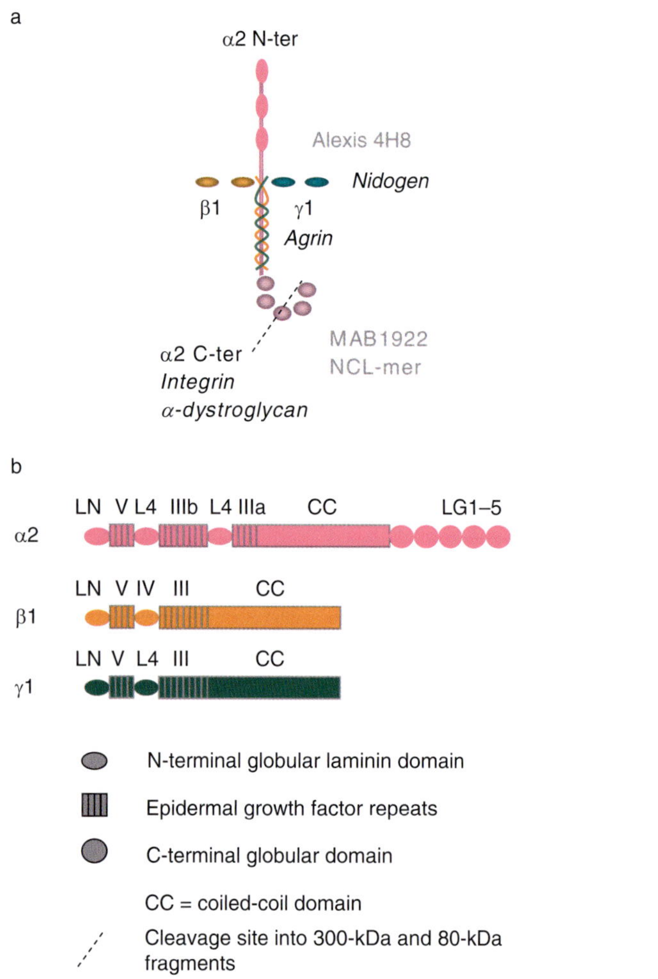

Figure 3.11. (a) Diagram of the laminin-2 heterotrimer composed of laminin-α2, laminin-β1, and laminin-γ1 chains, showing the areas of ligand binding (italics), the epitopes recognized by the three most commonly employed monoclonal antibodies to laminin-α2 (gray text), and the site of autolytic cleavage that gives rise to the 300-kDa and 80-kDa fragments (discontinuous line) (modified from [178]). (b) Domain structure of laminin-α2, -β1 and -γ1. Each chain is composed of a N-terminal short arm of globular domains involved in the formation of laminin polymers, a rod-like domain made of epidermal-growth-factor-like repeats and a coil-coiled domain where the three chains associate. The C-terminal globular domains are only present in the laminin-α2 chain, which is longer than the β1 and γ1 chains (modified from [248]).

dy^{2J}/dy^{2J} mice have a mutation in the *Lama*2 gene that results in abnormal splicing and the production of a laminin-α2 polypeptide that lacks the N-terminal domain VI. This truncated form is expressed in the skeletal muscle of the dy^{2J}/dy^{2J} mice, and the muscular dystrophy is less severe than that of *dy*/*dy* mice. The dy^{Pas}/dy^{Pas} mice are spontaneous mutants that completely lack laminin-α2 due to the insertion of a retrotransposon. dy^{3K}/dy^{3K} and the dy^{W}/dy^{W} are two lines that have been generated by homologous recombination in embryonic stem cells. The dy^{3K}/dy^{3K} mouse is a null mutant, but the dy^{W}/dy^{W} produces low amounts of truncated laminin-α2 in muscle.

Evans blue dye (which accumulates in fibers with membrane damage) does not accumulate inside the muscle fibers of the *dy* and dy^{2J} mice as it does inside *mdx* muscle, suggesting that muscle membrane leakage is not central to the pathogenesis of MDC1A [110]. More recent work using some of the mouse models for laminin-α2 deficiency has shown that muscle-specific overexpression of a miniaturized form of agrin (mini-agrin), which is able to bind to dystroglycan but not α7β1 integrin, substantially ameliorates the dystrophy associated with the absence of laminin-α2 [111, 112]. A chimeric protein containing the dystroglycan-binding domain of perlecan has a similar effect in ameliorating the disease. These experiments suggest that restoring the linkage between the basement membrane and cell membrane could open up new and exciting possibilities for the development of treatment options for this muscular dystrophy.

Perlecan

The role of basement membrane proteoglycans, of which perlecan is one, includes that of being both a structural component and a functional regulator of several growth-factor signaling pathways. Human perlecan is a modular proteoglycan whose protein core is ~470 kDa; however, with the addition of numerous *O*-linked oligosaccharides and as many as four heparan sulfate chains, it has a molecular weight of over 800 kDa.

Missense and splicing mutations in the perlecan gene underlie Schwartz–Jampel syndrome (SJS), a disorder characterized by the association of myotonia with chondrodysplasia. In these patients, only a partially functional form of perlecan is secreted and the neuromyotonia is thought to arise as a consequence of the abnormal anchoring of acetylcholinesterase (AChE; the enzyme that cleaves the main neurotransmitter acetylcholine) at the neuromuscular junction.

However, more recent data obtained from a mouse model carrying hypomorphic mutations of the perlecan gene show that whilst partial endplate AChE deficiency might contribute to SJS muscle stiffness by potentiating muscle force, physiological endplate AChE deficiency is not associated with spontaneous activity at rest on electromyography of the diaphragm, suggesting that additional changes are required to generate the activity characteristic of SJS. Indeed the authors suggest that axonal changes may be a contributory factor since perlecan is present in the axonal basement membrane [113].

Agrin

Agrin is a basal lamina heparan sulfate proteoglycan initially characterized by its ability to induce clustering of AChRs on cultured myotubes. The polypeptide core consists of distinct domains that mediate binding to laminin and α-dystroglycan. A third domain at the C-terminal end of the molecule has been shown to promote agrin-induced activation of the muscle-specific receptor tyrosine kinase (MuSK), which leads to AChR clustering. However, alternative splicing gives rise to a number of functionally diverse isoforms.

The so-called neural isoforms of agrin are unique to neurons and contain inserts of four and eight (and/or 11) amino acids at two sites in the C-terminal fifth of the molecule. Those with inserts of 4 and 8 (and/or 11) amino acids at the C-terminal end are unique to neurons and are referred to as "neural" agrin, whereas those forms lacking the 8/11 inserts are referred to as "muscular" agrin and are expressed in several tissues including muscle and brain [114]. Whilst picomolar concentrations of neural agrin can induce MuSK phosphorylation and AChR clustering on cultured myotubes, muscle agrin is inactive even at 1000-fold higher levels. However, externally applied muscle agrin acts in an activity-dependent and autocrine way to organize the sub-cortical cytoskeleton of skeletal muscle fibers [115] such that the application of muscle agrin at nanomolar concentrations to denervated muscle preserves the normal (transverse) costamere orientation which, in its absence, became disorganized.

One particularly exciting aspect of agrin is the finding that the muscle-specific overexpression of a miniaturized form known as "mini-agrin," which retains the capacity to bind to dystroglycan but not to $\alpha7\beta1$ integrin, is able to substantially ameliorate the disease in mouse models of laminin-$\alpha2$ deficiency [111]. Moreover, the late-onset expression of mini-agrin in these mice is still able to prolong the life span albeit not to the same extent as early expression. Interestingly a chimeric protein containing the dystroglycan-binding domain of perlecan has the same activities as mini-agrin in ameliorating the disease phenotype in this mouse model. This work opens up the possibility for the development of new therapeutic strategies using specifically designed molecules or endogenous ligands that link the basement membrane to dystroglycan [116].

Sarcolemma – proteins involved in trafficking and repair

The movement of proteins and lipids through the cell is important for all cell types but in muscle fibers it is also crucial for the establishment of the neuromuscular junction and the T-tubules and for sarcolemmal repair. This is highlighted by the fact that defects in proteins involved in membrane trafficking underlie several muscle disorders [117].

Dysferlin and other proteins associated with membrane trafficking

Mutations in the dysferlin gene (*DYSF*) result in three clinically distinct phenotypes: LGMD2B, which is characterized by proximal muscle weakness and atrophy; Miyoshi myopathy (MM), which in contrast affects predominantly the distal muscles, in particular the posterior compartment (calf muscle being the most severely affected); and a distal anterior compartment myopathy that progresses rapidly through the anterior tibial muscles. The onset in both LGMD2B and MM is usually in late childhood or adulthood and both are characterized by markedly elevated levels of CK and a slowly progressive course [118].

Dysferlin is a 230-kDa protein member of the ferlin family, which are characterized by the presence of calcium-binding C2 domains. Dysferlin contains seven C2 domains, and missense mutations in any of five of these have been shown to cause muscular dystrophy suggesting that each may fulfil different functions. However, this may also reflect the possibility that alterations in any of these domains leads to protein misfolding and therefore degradation. The dysferlin C2A domain binds phospholipids in a Ca^{2+}-dependent manner. Myoferlin, which is also a member of this family of proteins, is important for myoblast fusion during muscle development. However, to date no mutations have been associated with human disease although mutations or a genetic disruption of myoferlin or dysferlin in mice led to impaired integrity of the sarcolemma.

The sarcolemma undergoes frequent physiological membrane disruptions that in normal circumstances are repaired by a Ca^{2+}-dependent mechanism. Experiments with membrane-impermeable dyes and laser wounding show this repair mechanism is defective in the absence of dysferlin [119]. Consistent with this proposed role dysferlin-deficient human muscle shows sarcolemmal gaps, subsarcolemmal aggregates of small vesicles, and other structural abnormalities of the sarcolemma and basal lamina [120, 121].

Two hypotheses have been proposed to explain membrane repair. The lipid flow promotion hypothesis proposes that lipids at the edge of a membrane lesion flow over to seal the disruption due to their energetically unfavorable status in the aqueous environment. This mechanism may only be applicable to small disruptions. The patch hypothesis suggests that Ca^{2+} enters through the membrane disruption and stimulates fusion between vesicles and the sarcolemma. The model of dysferlin-mediated membrane repair envisages that membrane disruption causes Ca^{2+} to enter the muscle fiber resulting in the activation of proteases such as calpains which cleave cytoskeletal proteins and thus reduce membrane tension. The local elevation in calcium also triggers the aggregation of intracellular vesicles containing dysferlin and promotes their migration to the site of damage, where they fuse with one another and also the plasma membrane creating a "patch" across the damaged area. This process most likely involves other proteins namely soluble NSF attachment protein receptors (SNARE), synaptotagmins, annexins A1 and A2, and affixin [119].

Both caveolin-3 and calpain-3 interact with dysferlin and are probably part of the same pathogenic process. In fact, patients with dysferlin deficiency show reduced calpain-3 expression, and patients with caveolin-3 deficiency show reduced and mislocalized dysferlin.

The SJL mouse line, which was traditionally used as a spontaneous model for autoimmune diseases and muscle regeneration, has an in-frame deletion in the dysferlin gene which leads to the removal of most of the fourth C2 domain and a reduction in dysferlin levels of 15% relative to control mice [122]. The muscle pathology in these mice is compatible with a muscular dystrophy with signs of degeneration and regeneration and fibrosis. Dysferlin-null mice have also been generated by gene targeting [123, 124]. These mice show a progessive muscular dystrophy with loss of sarcolemmal integrity and a preserved dystrophin-associated protein complex. These models have been instrumental in elucidating the role of dysferlin in membrane repair [123]. Dysferlin and dystrophin double-deficient mice develop an early-onset cardiomyopathy suggesting that dysferlin is also important for maintenance of cardiomyocyte integrity [125].

Caveolin-3

One noticeable feature of the sarcolemma under the electron microscope is the number of flask-shaped invaginations 55–65 nm in diameter, known as caveolae. Caveolae are implicated in a variety of processes including sequestration of receptors and their cargo, lipid homeostasis, and cell adhesion. In developing skeletal muscle, they are involved in the formation of the T-tubule system. Caveolins, which are the major protein component of these caveolae, are 21- to 24-kDa integral membrane proteins. The main isoform in skeletal muscle is caveolin-3.

Mutations in the caveolin-3 gene (*CAV3*) can lead to a broad spectrum of clinical phenotypes which include limb-girdle muscular dystrophy, rippling muscle disease, distal myopathy, and a persistently high CK (hyperCKemia). Thus there is a range of skeletal muscle involvement, ranging from LGMD1C to cases with little muscle weakness but persistent hyperCKemia. The main clinical features of LGMD1C are onset in the first decade of life with mild to moderate proximal muscle weakness and calf hypertrophy. Progression is very slow. Cramps following exercise are common and serum CK is moderately to markedly elevated. A significant distal component with intrinsic hand wasting and pes cavus can be present in rare cases. Cardiac involvement is usually absent. The muscle pathology in cases of LGMD1C is consistent with a muscular dystrophy.

In normal muscle caveolin-3 is localized to the caveolae of the sarcolemma, and immunolabeling clearly identifies the sarcolemma. In all other forms of muscular dystrophy immunolabeling is also normal [126], although a secondary reduction may occur in dysferlin deficiency, as caveolin-3 and dysferlin interact [127, 128, 129]. In contrast to most other dominant conditions, patients with a mutation in the caveolin-3 gene may show a reduction in the protein with immunohistochemistry and immunoblotting [129], and this is particularly pronounced in cases of LGMD1C [130, 131, 132, 133]. The mechanism responsible for the reduced or absent protein expression is a dominant negative effect of mutant caveolin, and aggregates of caveolin-3 that are not targeted to the plasma membrane but retained within the Golgi [134]. Internal localization of antibodies to caveolin-3 may be seen in several disorders, particularly in regenerating fibers.

Caveolae appear as small subsarcolemmal vesicles but when caveolin-3 is mutated there is impairment of caveolae formation, discontinuity of the plasma membrane, subsarcolemmal vacuoles, papillary projections, and disorganization of the T-system openings on the plasma membrane [132, 133].

Duchenne muscular dystrophy (DMD) patients and dystrophin-deficient *mdx* mice have increased levels of caveolin-3 expression in their skeletal muscle and the overexpression of caveolin-3 leads to an increase in the number of sarcolemmal muscle cell caveolae, hypertrophic, necrotic, and immature/regenerating fibers, and a downregulation of dystrophin and β-dystroglycan protein expression. These mice also show elevated levels of serum CK.

Myotubularin

The primary function of myotubularin is to dephosphorylate phosphoinositide (PI) residues in various membranous organelles. PI are key regulators of membrane trafficking and therefore myotubularin is thought to be also involved in this process in particular in the movement of vesicles from the endosome to the lysosome. The precise mechanism by which myotubularin deficiency leads to the internalization of nuclei and the other pathological changes is still not fully understood.

Myotubular myopathy is a severe form of congenital myopathy which normally leads to death within the first months of life due to respiratory insufficiency (for a recent review of congenital myopathies see [134, 135]). It is X-linked and although female carriers are often asymptomatic, they can occasionally present in childhood or more commonly in adulthood with mild weakness and progressive ptosis. Myotubular myopathy is caused by mutations in the *MTM1* gene, encoding myotubularin, and at the pathological level it is characterized by the presence of central nuclei in numerous fibers which are surrounded by a pale cytoplasmic halo without myofibrils where various organelles including mitochondria tend to accumulate. These are also features of congenital myotonic dystrophy and other forms of congenital myopathy (see below).

The term myotubular myopathy was assigned because the muscle fibers with central nuclei resemble developing myotubes. However, it is now accepted that these fibers with centrally placed nuclei are not all immature and that nuclei move to their central position after myogenesis has been completed. Analysis of biopsy samples from children with mutations in the *MTM1* gene suggested a role for myotubularin in the maintenance of myofiber diameter and a possible correlation between myofiber size and survival, but the specificity of this finding is not clear [136].

Animal models

Myotubularin-deficient mice develop a progressive myopathy accompanied by the presence of abundant central nuclei in mature fibers as well as atrophy of type 1 fibers similar to patients with myotubular myopathy [137]. Studies of this mouse model support the concept that myotubular myopathy results from a defect in the maintenance of the normal muscle structure rather than a defect of myogenesis, which was normal in these mice. The appearance of centrally located nuclei was progressive and varied between different muscles. By 15 days most nuclei were peripheral but they increased at later stages of the diseases and by 2 months up to 45% of fibers contained central nuclei in the most affected muscles.

The authors showed that some degree of degeneration and regeneration occurred during the course of the disease, which probably accounted for a proportion of the fibers with central nuclei and the expression of histochemical markers of immaturity and regeneration such as embryonic myosin.

Muscle hypotrophy was the earliest and most consistent feature of all muscles studied, in line with results from myotubular myopathy patient muscle, which suggests that a decrease in muscle fiber size is at the center of the pathogenesis and is an indicator of severity and prognosis.

Dynamin-2

Less common than X-linked myotubular myopathy, dominant centronuclear myopathy is caused by mutations in the gene for dynamin 2 (*DNM2*) on 19p13.2 [138]. The disorder involves mainly limb-girdle, trunk, and neck muscles but may also affect distal muscles. Ptosis and limitation of eye movements are common features. In general, patients with dynamin-2 mutations present in adolescence or adulthood with a relatively mild myopathy but more recently mutations have also been described in neonates with generalized muscle weakness including ptosis, and ophthalmoparesis but a tendency to improve [139]. The most prominent histopathological feature is the presence of centrally located nuclei in a large number of fibers but in general these nuclei tend to be small compared to those seen in typical myotubular myopathy. An additional diagnostic feature is the radial arrangement of sarcoplasmic strands around the central nuclei which can be seen with nicotinamide adenine dinucleotide (NADH) and periodic acid Schiff (PAS) stainings.

Dynamins are GTPases involved in membrane fission. Dynamin-2, as opposed to other dynamins, is ubiquitously expressed. It plays a key role in clathrin-mediated endocytosis by triggering coated vesicle scission from the parent membrane. The suggested mechanism of action is that dynamin-2 forms a helical collar around the neck of an invaginating clathrin-coated vesicle which extends and "pinches" the vesicle from the parent membrane. Dynamin-2 is also involved in actin filament reorganization in various processes requiring membrane remodeling including phagocytosis and lamellipodial extension [117].

The mutations described so far in the *DNM2* gene localize to the middle and to the pleckstrin homology (PH) domains and are thought to exert a dominant negative effect impairing normal endocytosis, since no decrease in protein levels has been detected in patients' fibroblasts [138]. Mutations in the PH domain of dynamin-2 are also associated with Charcot–Marie–Tooth disease.

Amphiphysin-2

Mutations in the *BIN1* gene (2q14) have been identified in three consanguineous families with the recessive form of centronuclear myopathy [140]. The age of onset ranged from birth to childhood, the distribution of weakness was proximal, and contractures at birth were noted in one family. Ptosis and ophthalmoplegia, facial weakness, and feeding difficulties were present in some of the cases.

BIN1 encodes amphiphysin-2, a protein with tumor suppressor features which is downregulated in various malignant cell lines and primary breast tumors. Amphiphysins contain a BAR domain which is involved in the regulation of membrane curvature during membrane remodeling, and an SH3 domain which regulates the interaction with other proteins including dynamin-2. The expression of the muscle-specific isoform M-amphiphysin-2 increases during muscle differentiation and is believed to play a key role in the biogenesis of the T-tubules, where it locates via its association with membrane phosphoinositol residues [141].

The mutations identified in the centronuclear myopathy families localize to the N-terminus, the BAR, or to the SH3 domain. Analysis of protein levels in fibroblasts from patients with mutations in the BAR or SH3 domains did not show any alteration in the amount of detectable protein suggesting that the pathogenesis is not related to a reduction in protein levels. Instead missense mutations in the BAR domain abolished the ability of wild-type amphiphysin to promote tubulation in COS cells. The nonsense mutation in the SH3 domain removed part of this domain and abolished its interaction with dynamin-2 and the incorporation of the latter into the tubular system. Therefore, mutations in amphiphysin are likely to disrupt T-tubule biogenesis and endocytosis directly or indirectly by disrupting its interaction with dynamin-2. Although these studies have identified a common pathological mechanism for centronuclear myopathy, the reason why nuclei are displaced to the center of the fiber is still unclear.

Targeted disruption of the amphiphysin gene in drosophila [142] results in flies that are unable to fly. Amphiphysin in drosophila normally localizes to the junctions between the T-tubules and the junctional sarcoplasmic reticulum. In mutant flies, the overall structure of the myofiber was shown to be preserved but there was a reduction in the number of visible T-tubules and SR junctions, and an increase in the diameter of some of the T-tubules and elongation of the junctional SR. Therefore, defects in amphiphysin are associated with structural defects of the T-tubule and SR systems which most likely disturb excitation–contraction coupling.

Bin1 knockout mice develop congenital cardiomyopathy and show abnormal myofibril structure [143]. This differs from patients with centronuclear myopathy in which cardiomyopathy is not a feature. However, it should be noted that mutations in patients do not result in a loss of protein but rather an alteration in its function.

Proteins associated with lysosomes and autophagic vacuoles

The digestion of cellular organelles and large proteins within lysosomes fulfils an important metabolic function and serves several purposes including the recycling of cell components and the cellular response to environmental changes such as nutrient deprivation. Inside the cytoplasm, lysosomes fuse with vesicles carrying either endocytosed or autophagocytosed cargo. There are several human diseases associated with abnormal accumulation of autophagocytic vacuoles but nonproliferative tissues such as muscle and neuronal cells seem particularly sensitive to the accumulation of unwanted material [144].

To date, two neuromuscular disorders are known to be caused by primary defects in lysosomal proteins. One of them is Pompe disease, which is caused by a deficiency of α-glucosidase and is discussed in the context of glycogen metabolism in the section "Sarcoplasm." Danon disease is an X-linked dominant condition caused by mutations in the *LAMP-2* gene (Xq24) encoding a lysosomal membrane protein.

A third disorder, namely X-linked vacuolar myopathy with excessive autophagy (XMEA), overlaps pathologically with Danon disease and although its genetic cause remains to be identified it is likely to be a protein/enzyme related to lysosomes or autophagic vacuoles. The significance of excessive autophagy in the pathogenesis of Pompe and Danon disease and XMEA has recently been reviewed [145].

Accumulation of autophagic vacuoles is also a feature of other myopathies such as distal myopathy with rimmed vacuoles and inclusion body myopathies, which are allelic disorders, and chloroquine-induced myopathy [146]. Mutations in the gene encoding for a chaperone (HspB8) involved in chaperone-mediated macroautophagy of misfolded proteins have been identified in a form of distal hereditary motor neuropathy [147].

LAMP-2

Danon disease is characterized by a combination of cardiomyopathy, myopathy, and mental retardation. However, patients without apparent muscle weakness and/or mental retardation have been reported. When present, muscle weakness affects the neck and shoulder-girdle muscles but distal involvement may also be present. Presentation is usually in childhood/adolescence but female carriers usually present later than male patients and the majority of them do not have mental retardation. Serum CK is always high in males and in the majority of female carriers but not in all. Involvement of liver and retina can also occur.

Accumulation of glycogen is seen in some cases of Danon disease but it is not a constant finding. Lysosomal activity as seen with the acid phosphatase reaction is less pronounced than in Pompe disease or even absent. The most striking pathological feature of Danon disease is the presence of vacuoles that label positively with antibodies for sarcolemmal and basal lamina proteins, giving rise to the term "autophagic vacuoles with sarcolemmal features" (AVSFs) to describe a subgroup of vacuolar myopathies. Those sarcolemmal proteins include acetylcholinesterase, dystrophin, sarcoglycans, and laminin-α2. Double immunofluoresence studies and electron microscopy have shown that some of the smaller autophagic vacuoles and lysosomal granules (identified with markers such as LAMP-1 or microtubule-associated protein light chain 3, LC3-II) are surrounded by the larger vacuoles with sarcolemmal features. The autophagic vacuoles contained myelin figures, cell debris, and electron-dense bodies. A basal lamina is sometimes seen in the inner surface of the larger membrane-bound vacuole.

LAMP-2 is a heavily glycosylated membrane-spanning protein that localizes to lysosomes, endosomes, and late autophagic vacuoles. Studies of *Lamp2* knockout mice showed extensive accumulation of early autophagic vacuoles in many tissues including heart and skeletal muscles [148]. This was linked to a reduction in the degradation rate of proteins and in catabolism in the liver. For these reasons, it was suggested that LAMP-2 is necessary for the maturation of early autophagic vacuoles into late autophagic vacuoles.

Currently available pathological and physiological data suggest that the extensive accumulation of autophagic vacuoles disrupts the normal structure and function of the myocyte and cardiomyocyte leading to impaired contraction and overall function.

In contrast to Danon disease, patients with X-linked vacuolar myopathy with excessive autophagy (XMEA) (Xq28) do not suffer from cardiomyopathy or mental retardation, helping to distinguish both disorders which otherwise have a significant pathological overlap. Although the causative gene in XMEA has not been identified, the pathological similarities of both disorders suggest that it may also be a protein involved in lysosomal degradation or autophagy. The deposition of components of membrane attack complex and calcium and the presence of duplicated basal lamina on and around the vacuoles are thought to be a distinguishing feature of XMEA.

Other vacuolar myopathies with AVSFs include infantile autophagic vacuolar myopathy, adult-onset autophagic vacuolar myopathy with multiorgan involvement, and X-linked congenital autophagic vacuolar myopathy [149]. These forms are still not characterized genetically.

Sarcolemma – ion channels

The sarcolemma consists of several domains, namely the peripheral fiber surface, the transverse (T) tubule network, and the neuromuscular and myotendinous junctions. Despite their continuity the plasma membrane and the T-tubule system maintain distinct protein and lipid compositions. Efficient excitation–contraction coupling is achieved via specific, functional associations that the T-tubule system maintains with regions of the sarcoplasmic reticulum. In human muscle each sarcomere has two tubular networks at the A/I-band junction. The sarcoplasmic reticulum, which is a fenestrated sheath of membranes folded around each myofibril, is responsible for the release and uptake of calcium ions during contraction and relaxation. At the level of the A/I-band interface the sarcoplasmic reticulum forms continuous lateral sacs or terminal cisternae. Two terminal cisternae are in close

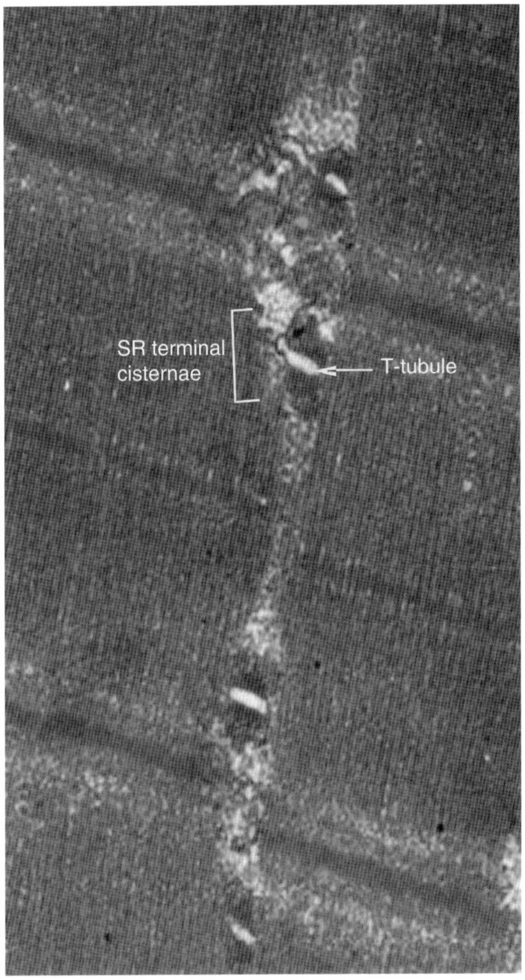

Figure 3.12. Electron micrograph of human skeletal muscle showing several triads each of which consists of a T-tubule flanked by two terminal cisternae of the sarcoplasmic reticulum. Micrograph kindly taken by Dr. Rosalind King.

contact with but separate from a T-system tubule and collectively these form a triad (Figure 3.12). The repetitive arrangement of triads gives a regular pattern at the A/I-band junction along and across the length of the fiber. The T-tubule of the triad is the site of the voltage-gated calcium channel, the dihydropyridine receptor, which is activated by the action potential and induces the ryanodine receptor of the lateral sacs to release calcium (Figure 3.13). At high magnification under the electron microscope the ryanodine receptors can be seen as dense "feet" bridging the junction of the lateral sacs and T-tubules.

Return to the resting potential following activation requires the action of voltage-gated K^+ and Cl^- channels. Mutations in the genes encoding these ion channels result in disturbed excitability, in the form of either hyperexcitability (myotonia) or inexcitability (periodic paralysis). These conditions are collectively referred to as ion channelopathies. There is significant clinical overlap between the different ion channel disorders; in addition, defects in the same gene can give rise to varying phenotypes.

Ion channels are complex multidomain transmembrane proteins and numerous mutations in the corresponding genes have now been identified. The resulting phenotype depends on the type of mutation, the region of the channel affected, and the overall effect on the transport of ions.

Chloride channel

Myotonia congenita is a hereditary muscle disorder characterized by impaired relaxation of skeletal muscle following voluntary contraction (myotonia). The skeletal muscle chloride channel gene *CLCN1* is located on chromosome 7 and encodes a subunit of the skeletal muscle chloride channel, which is almost exclusively expressed in skeletal muscle. CLC-1 channels form dimers with two independent pores. Mutations result in Becker (autosomal recessive) or in Thomsen myotonia (autosomal dominant) [150]. More than 80 different mutations have now been identified. The division into dominant mutations in Thomsen disease and recessive mutations in Becker is now less clear and a particular mutation can be inherited in either a dominant or recessive pattern [151]. This is complicated by the observation of variation of phenotypes/severities between patients with identical mutations and may be explained partly by differences in gender (myotonia manifests more frequently in males but this seems to apply only to recessive cases) and in differential allelic expression (deviation from the expected 1:1 ratio of expression of two alleles).

Chloride conductance ensures the electrical stability of the sarcolemma and remains relatively constant during the action potential, in contrast to the Na^+ and K^+ permeabilities. Indeed the chloride conductance is strictly required to counter the depolarizing effect of K^+ accumulation in the T-tubules during muscle activity. In the muscle fibers of myotonic patients K^+ accumulates in the T-tubular lumen thereby leading to a depolarization of the surface membrane which then initiates a self-sustaining action potential and prolonged (myotonic) contraction. Furthermore, large depolarizations (of 10–20 mV) may cause a number of sodium channels to go into the inactivated state and render the membrane temporarily inexcitable, thus explaining the transient weakness that is sometimes observed in patients with recessive myotonia congenita.

Many of the recessive mutations result in the early truncation of the protein, which results in a nonfunctional subunit. However, the normal wild-type pore in a mutant/wild-type heterodimer is minimally affected. For this reason, two mutant alleles are required to reduce the Cl^- conductance enough to produce myotonia (at least to 30% of the normal conductance). Most of the dominant mutations are missense and exert a dominant negative effect in such a way that the resulting dimers (mutant/mutant or mutant/wild-type) cannot function normally. Many of these missense mutations affect residues close to the channel common gate. The pathomechanism in both recessive and dominant myotonia is a reduced chloride channel conductance of the CLC-1 channel which lowers the threshold for depolarization leading to more action potentials.

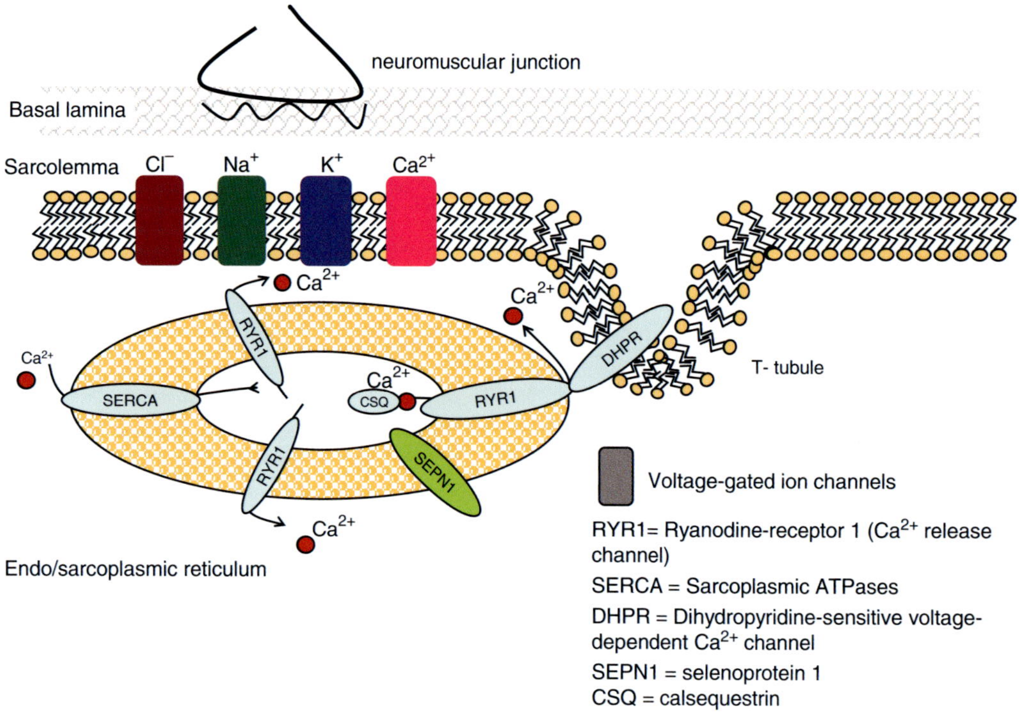

Figure 3.13. Schematic diagram showing the localization of proteins associated with ion channel homeostasis. Those ion channels associated with myotonia (chloride and sodium) and periodic paralysis (sodium and potassium) are shown at the sarcolemma and calcium-regulating proteins in the sarcoplasmic reticulum and T-tubule are shown with arrows depicting the direction of flow of calcium. Selenoprotein 1 is an integral membrane protein of the endoplasmic/sarcoplasmic reticulum.

Chloride and sodium channel myotonia can be treated with drugs that reduce the hyperexcitability of the muscle membrane by interfering with the Na^+ channels.

Sodium channel

Mutations in the *SCN4A* gene (sodium channel) result in potassium-aggravated myotonia and paramyotonia congenita both of which are dominantly inherited. The mutations in the *SCNA4* gene are distributed throughout the various domains of the channel but there appear to be two hot spots for paramyotonia congenita: one in the voltage-sensing transmembrane region (S4) of domain IV and another one in an intracellular loop important for inactivation. The mutations associated with K^+-aggravated myotonia are normally found in intracellular regions. The underlying cause of the myotonia in both paramyotonia and K^+-aggravated myotonia is incomplete or slow inactivation of the sodium channel and therefore increased depolarization. Mutations in this gene also cause hyper- and hypokalemic periodic paralysis syndromes.

Calcium channel

There are two main types of episodic weakness due to inexcitability of ion channels: hyper- and hypokalemic periodic paralysis. They differ in the levels of serum K^+ during the attacks, and in the length and severity of the attacks. The *CACNA1S* gene on chromosome 7 encodes the α1 subunit of the slowly inactivating L-type voltage-sensitive Ca^{2+} channel. This subunit confers the structural features needed for Ca^{2+} channel function and also contains the binding sites for the Ca^{2+} channel blockers such as 1,4-dihydropyridine (DHP). Mutations in this gene cause a proportion of cases of hypokalemic periodic paralysis as well as malignant hyperthermia (MH), which are both dominant traits. The mutations reported for each of these two conditions localize to different parts of the α1 subunit of the channel. MH is characterized by a rapid and sustained rise in temperature during general anesthesia (often as rapid as 1°C every 5 min and going up to 43°C or higher), accompanied by generalized muscle rigidity, tachycardia, tachypnea, and cyanosis. There is also a severe respiratory and metabolic acidosis. Extensive muscle necrosis follows, with subsequent myoglobinuria and renal shutdown. The serum CK is grossly elevated (up to 50 000 iu/liter or more), as is the serum potassium. Anesthetic agents containing halogenated hydrocarbons, such as halothane, and succinylcholine are the ones most frequently involved.

Susceptibility to MH is also a feature of King–Denborough syndrome, which is characterized by the association of a slowly progressive myopathy in young boys with short stature, pectus carinatum, cryptorchidism, kyphoscoliosis, distinctive facial features, and elevated CK in most cases. The syndrome appears to be sporadic rather than familial. All patients with known King–Denborough syndrome should be treated as MH-susceptible, and evaluation of other family members is recommended.

There are five other loci for MH including the locus for the ryanodine receptor type 1 (RYR1), a calcium-release channel that is discussed in the "Sarcoplasmic reticulum" section.

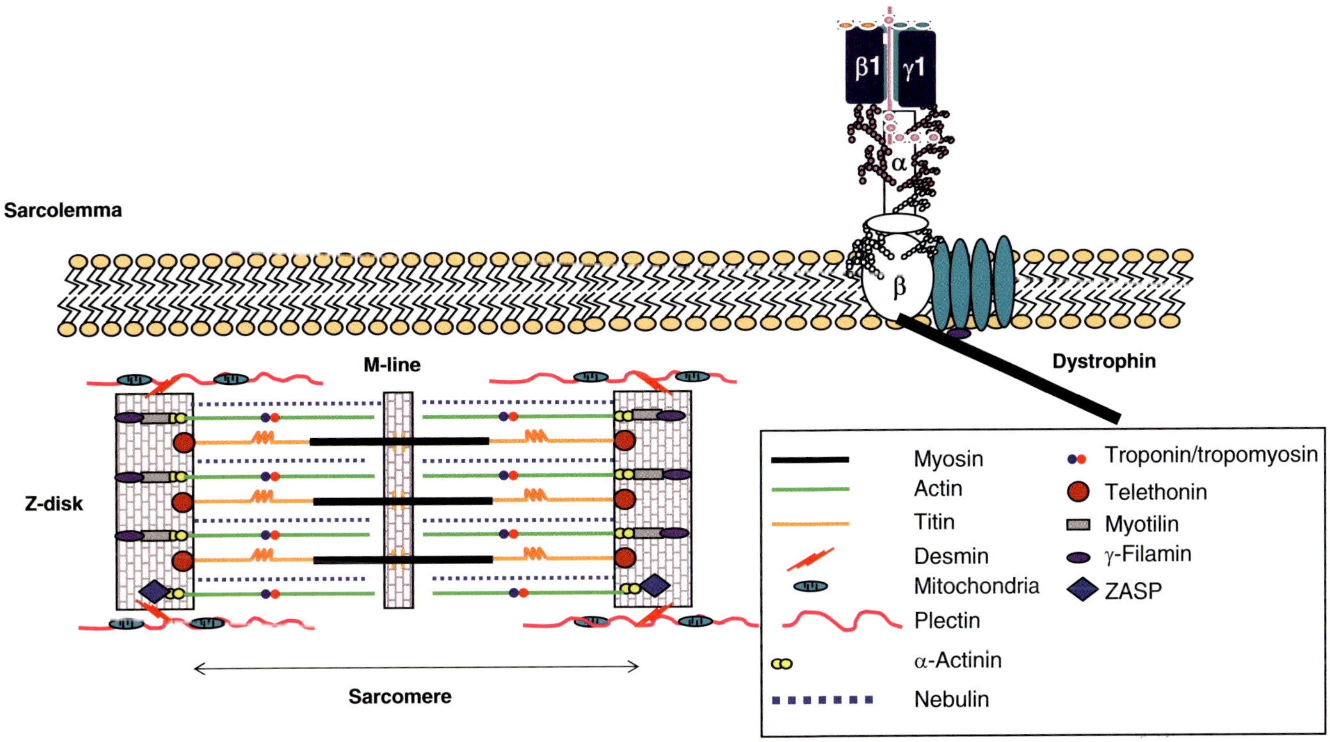

Figure 3.14. Schematic diagram showing the major protein components of the sarcomere. The thin filaments consist of actin, tropomyosin, troponins, and nebulin, and the thick filaments are composed of myosin. Tropomyosin (Tm) locates to the groove formed between actin strands and spans seven actin monomers. Troponin associates with each molecule of tropomyosin. Actin and myosin are crosslinked at the Z-disk and M-band. Myosin filaments in the M-band are crosslinked by a protein network composed of titin and myomesin. Titin and nebulin are two giant proteins attributed with a role in myofibril alignment and elasticity. The N-terminus of titin is embedded in the Z-disk and extends to the M-line. Nebulin has its C-terminus anchored in the Z-line and extends into the I-band. The Z-disk forms a tetragonal network over the actin filament ends from two adjacent sarcomeres. Defects in proteins of the Z-disk give rise to a broad spectrum of clinical phenotypes encompassing congenital myopathies, myofibrillar myopathies, and limb-girdle muscular dystrophies.

Potassium channels

The potassium channel encoded by the *KCNJ2* gene is involved in Andersen syndrome [152] which is characterized by potassium-sensitive periodic paralysis without myotonia indistinguishable from other forms of hyperkalemic periodic paralysis. A proportion of cases with hypokalemic periodic paralysis are caused by mutations in a gene coding for a K^+ channel (*KCNE3 gene*) [153].

Proteins of the sarcomere

The contractile and metabolic components of the fiber occupy approximately 75% of the total volume. Each individual muscle fiber contains many bundles of myofibrils each of which consists of a series of sarcomeres. Sarcomeres are the basic unit of contraction and consist of the thin filaments (actin, tropomyosin, troponins, and nebulin) and the thick filaments (myosin). The *A-band* consists of a hexagonal lattice of thick myosin filaments whilst the *I-band* filaments are chiefly composed of thin, double helical strands of filamentous (F) actin. Tropomyosin (Tm) locates to the groove formed between actin strands and spans seven actin monomers. Troponin associates with each molecule of tropomyosin and comprises a globular complex of three proteins, namely troponin C (TnC, the Ca^{2+}-binding protein), troponin I (TnI, the inhibitory protein), and troponin T (TnT, which binds to Tm). Tm and the troponins (TnI, TnT, and TnC) work cooperatively to regulate muscle contraction by making actin–myosin interactions sensitive to cytosolic calcium levels. Contraction of the muscle fiber is accomplished by the I filaments sliding towards the center of the A-band such that the I-band shortens but the A-band remains at a constant length.

Actin and myosin are crosslinked at the Z-disk and M-band, both of which fulfil a dual structural and signaling role by integrating information relating to mechanical strain, with signaling pathways controlling muscle growth and protein turnover. Myosin filaments in the M-band are crosslinked by a protein network composed of titin and myomesin. The Z-disk forms a tetragonal network over the actin filament ends from two adjacent sarcomeres, an arrangement which not only delineates the sarcomeres but also ensures that tension is transmitted through the Z-disks along the length of the muscle. The width of the Z-disk reflects the mechanical properties of the muscle such that it is narrower in fast compared to slow muscles. Defects in proteins of the Z-disk give rise to a broad spectrum of clinical phenotypes encompassing congenital myopathies, myofibrillar myopathies, and limb-girdle muscular dystrophies. A diagramatic representation of the structure of a sarcomere showing the organization of these proteins is shown in Figure 3.14.

Actin

Mutations in skeletal muscle actin (ACTA-1) are dominantly inherited (and many are de novo). The mutant protein exerts a dominant effect on contractile function although in some cases haploinsufficiency has been demonstrated. Homozygous null mutations have been reported; in these cases there is a complete absence of skeletal muscle α-actin although cardiac actin persists for much longer after birth than in age-matched controls suggesting that an upregulation of cardiac actin may be therapeutic [154]. Mutations in the gene encoding for skeletal α-actin ACTA-1 underlie forms of nemaline myopathy. Nemaline myopathy is a rare, clinically heterogeneous congenital skeletal muscle disease with associated muscle weakness, generally characterized by the presence of nemaline rods (although in actin myopathy the characeristic pathological feature is accumulation of actin filaments without rod formation). Rods are electron-dense structures composed of proteins such as α-actinin which are believed to derive from the Z-disk. In general they are found either within the I-band or between the myofibrils and their size varies and may sometimes extend along the length of several sarcomeres. Interestingly they are sometimes only apparent on the second biopsy after the onset of weakness, suggesting that they are a secondary phenomenon. In some cases with ACTA-1 mutations, rods have been observed inside the nucleus although this is not a common finding. Nuclear rods appear to form from within the nucleus as opposed to forming in the cytoplasm and entering the nucleus afterwards [155].

Actin mutations also underlie a proportion of congenital fiber type disproportion (CFTD) cases where the mutation disrupts the interaction between actin and tropomyosin. CFTD is a heterogeneous congenital myopathy (also caused by mutations in α-tropomyosin and SEPN1).

Myosin

Mutations in the MHY7 gene encoding slow myosin heavy chain cause hyaline body myopathy, Laing myopathy, and myosin storage myopathy (characterized by accumulation of myosin in type 1 fibers). Mutations in the MYHC2A (encoding for fast myosin type IIa) are associated with hereditary inclusion body myopathy. For a recent review of myosin-related myopathies refer to [156].

Thin-filament-associated proteins

An increasing number of proteins that associate with the thin filaments of the sarcomere have now been shown to harbor mutations that result in various forms of neuromuscular disease. These include skeletal muscle α-actin (see above), β-tropomyosin, γ-tropomyosin, fast skeletal muscle troponin I, slow skeletal muscle troponin T, fast skeletal muscle troponin T, and nebulin. The range of diseases with which they are associated includes nemaline myopathy, distal arthrogryposis, cap disease, actin myopathy, congenital fiber-type disproportion, rod-core myopathy, intranuclear rod myopathy, and distal myopathy; with nemaline myopathy the most common [157]. Cofilin-2 is involved in the polymerization of actin, and is the latest protein to be associated with nemaline myopathy [158].

Alternative splicing of four tropomyosin (Tm) genes creates three skeletal muscle isoforms in humans; namely, α-tropomyosin$_{slow}$ (αTm$_{slow}$) encoded by *TPM3*, α-tropomyosin-$_{fast}$ (αTm$_{fast}$) encoded by *TPM1*, and β-tropomyosin (βTm) from *TPM2*. Mutations in three Tm genes have been associated with four different disorders of striated muscle: nemaline myopathy (NM; *TPM2* and *TPM3*), distal arthrogryposis *(TPM2)*, cap disease (*TPM2*), and cardiomyopathy (*TPM1*). Mutations in *TPM3* have been associated with autosomal dominant NM, recessive NM and more recently have been shown to be a relatively common cause of congenital fiber type disproportion (CFTD) [159]. The underlying mechanism of disease is thought to be disruption of α/β-tropomyosin heterodimers which alters sarcomeric thin filament dynamics and thus contributes to muscle weakness [160].

Nebulin has its C-terminus anchored in the Z-line and extends into the I-band. It makes side-to-side contact with titin and is thought to have a role in regulating the length of the actin filaments. Nebulin mutations (nonsense, frameshift or splice site mutations) underlie recessive NM. However, recent work shows that homozygosity for some missense mutations may cause an early-onset mild distal myopathy [161].

Titin and associated proteins

Titin is a giant sarcomeric protein (4 MDa) that extends across the entire half sarcomere from the Z-disk to the M-line, with its N-terminus embedded in the Z-disk. Titin molecules of adjacent sarcomeres overlap in the Z- and M-line. Titin is thought to play a role in the assembly of muscle thick filaments and the maintenance of passive tension [162], the latter being attributed to the highly folded I-band segments which sequentially extend as the muscle sarcomere is stretched thus generating a passive force that helps restore sarcomere length upon relaxation. These properties are conferred on titin's I-band region by multiple segments with tandemly arranged Ig segments and the PEVK segment. Additional spring elements are provided by the N2A segments. By contrast the A-band region and near Z-disk I-band region are inextensible. This system heavily relies on the efficient tethering of titin to the Z-disk.

At least part of this anchoring to the Z-disk is mediated by telethonin, the protein defective in LGMD2H, which binds to two N-terminal titin immunoglobulin-like domains named Z1 and Z2. Crystallographic analysis of this complex shows a novel, palindromic, antiparallel assembly of two titin molecules with telethonin wedged in between [163]. Indeed telethonin appears to distribute the forces between its two joined titin Z2 domains in order to protect the more proximal Z1 domain from bearing excess stress. However, in addition to mediating this very important mechanical linkage this arrangement of proteins is also well placed to act as "stretch sensor" since it is inherently sensitive to variable levels of stretch. Indeed there is now functional evidence that titin and telethonin form a complex with muscle LIM protein, which triggers downstream signaling pathways linked to muscle growth and survival.

Muscle LIM proteins (MLP) contain a cysteine-rich domain and are important for striated muscle differentiation. Cardiac MLP or cysteine-rich protein 3 is encoded by the CSRP3 gene on chromosome 11p15.1 which is mutated in dilated and hypertrophic cardiomyopathy. Some of these patients have been reported to have a mild skeletal muscle myopathy that is similar to what has been seen in MLP-null mice [164]. This may be explained by the expression of this protein in slow muscle fibers. MLP has been proposed to have a role as a mechanosensor in cardiomyocytes, firstly via its interaction with several other proteins and signaling pathways and secondly via its ability to translocate to the nucleus and modify gene expression. MLP protein moves from the nucleus to the cytoplasm where it concentrates in areas of force transmission, i.e., at the costamere, and the Z-disk where it interacts with telethonin and α-actinin.

Titin may also modulate signaling by providing a scaffold for other proteins including muscle ankyrin repeat proteins (MARPs), muscle RING finger proteins (MURFs), sarcomeric-alpha-actinin, obscurin (and obsurin-like protein), and p94/calpain 3. The binding sites for these proteins are centered in the Z-, N2-, and/or M-line regions, leading to the hypothesis that different regions of titin may modulate distinct signaling pathways via the proteins with which they associate [165]. It follows therefore that loss of specific binding sites may underlie certain disease phentypes. Indeed mutations in the last Ig domain of titin have recently been shown to interrupt the interaction between titin and obscurin and obscurin-like protein [166]. Furthermore mutations in the extreme C-terminus of titin, which lies in the M-band, is a hot spot for autosomal dominant and recessive mutations, causing at least three distinct human myopathies, namely tibial muscular dystrophy, childhood-onset limb-girdle muscular dystrophy 2J, and an autosomal recessive cardiac and skeletal titin myopathy.

Additional evidence of the role of the importance of these interactions comes from the finding that mutations in the gene encoding for p94/calpain3, which is a skeletal-muscle-specific calpain, is the primary defect in limb-girdle muscular dystrophy type 2A (LGMD2A, also called "calpainopathy"). The dystrophic phenotype of calpainopathy is caused by the loss of p94 protease activity from skeletal muscle. The phenotypes of transgenic mice in which the p94 protease activity has been manipulated in various ways show that the proteolytic action of p94 is critical for the maintenance of skeletal muscle.

There is a mouse model of muscular dystrophy with myositis (mdm) resulting from an 83-amino-acid deletion in titin that spares the cardiac muscle but affects the skeletal muscle [167]. These observations may in part be related to differences in the binding partners of titin in different muscles [168] or the differential expression of titin isoforms and titin-binding proteins which could confer different functions on titin [169]. Homozygous mdm/mdm mice develop a progressive muscular dystrophy and die at around 2 months of age. The mdm mutation excises the C-terminal portion of titin's N2A region, abolishing its interaction with p94/calpain-3 protease, suggesting that an alteration in the composition of the titin N2A complex is the underlying mechanism of disease in these mice [170].

FHL1 (SLIM1) is an X-chromosome encoded protein of the four-and-a-half LIM domain protein family which has been very recently identified as the major component of reducing bodies, a morphological description of an intracellular inclusion that defines reducing body myopathy (RBM). Mutations in the *FHL1* gene have been identified in several RBM patients as well as in patients with X-linked postural myopathy and with a form of scapuloperoneal myopathy. This protein localizes to the sarcomere, where it interacts with myosin-binding protein C [134, 161]. By immunohistochemistry of isolated fibers it co-localizes with α-actinin in the Z-disk. FHL1 is believed to be important for the assembly of the sarcomere and skeletal muscle growth and differentiation.

There are some general themes that can be drawn for this group of proteins/disorders which are discussed in two reviews [171, 172]. Firstly proteins that are present in both skeletal and cardiac muscle can give rise to both myopathy and cardiac myopathy in the same patient when affected (e.g., desmin). Secondly, myopathies presenting at birth (congenital) will be associated with defects in proteins fundamental to muscle contraction (thin filaments and myosin) whereas defects in the other sarcomeric proteins usually give rise to childhood, juvenile or even adult presentations. Finally, myopathies of the sarcomere are often associated with accumulation of sarcomeric proteins (actin and myosin, desmin, etc.) and can be considered as "protein aggregation myopathies." In fact, the myofibrillar degradation and the pathological protein aggregation and subsequent non-lysosomal protein degradation pathway are believed to be at the center of the pathophysiology of myofibrillar myopathies [174, 176] although some studies indicate that mitochondrial dysfunction may also contribute [173, 174].

Muscle fiber cytoskeleton

The structure of striated muscle is highly dependent on the integrity of a complex cytoskeletal network comprising microtubules, intermediate filaments, and actin filaments. Microtubules are involved in many cell processes; however, perhaps the most relevant with respect to muscle are those relating to intracellular transport and organelle positioning. Microtubules are found between myofibrils at the level of the A–I junction, associated with the sarcolemma, the Golgi complex, and nuclei implying that they participate in the mechanical integration of various organelles. Their orientation may differ between different fiber types, which may be of

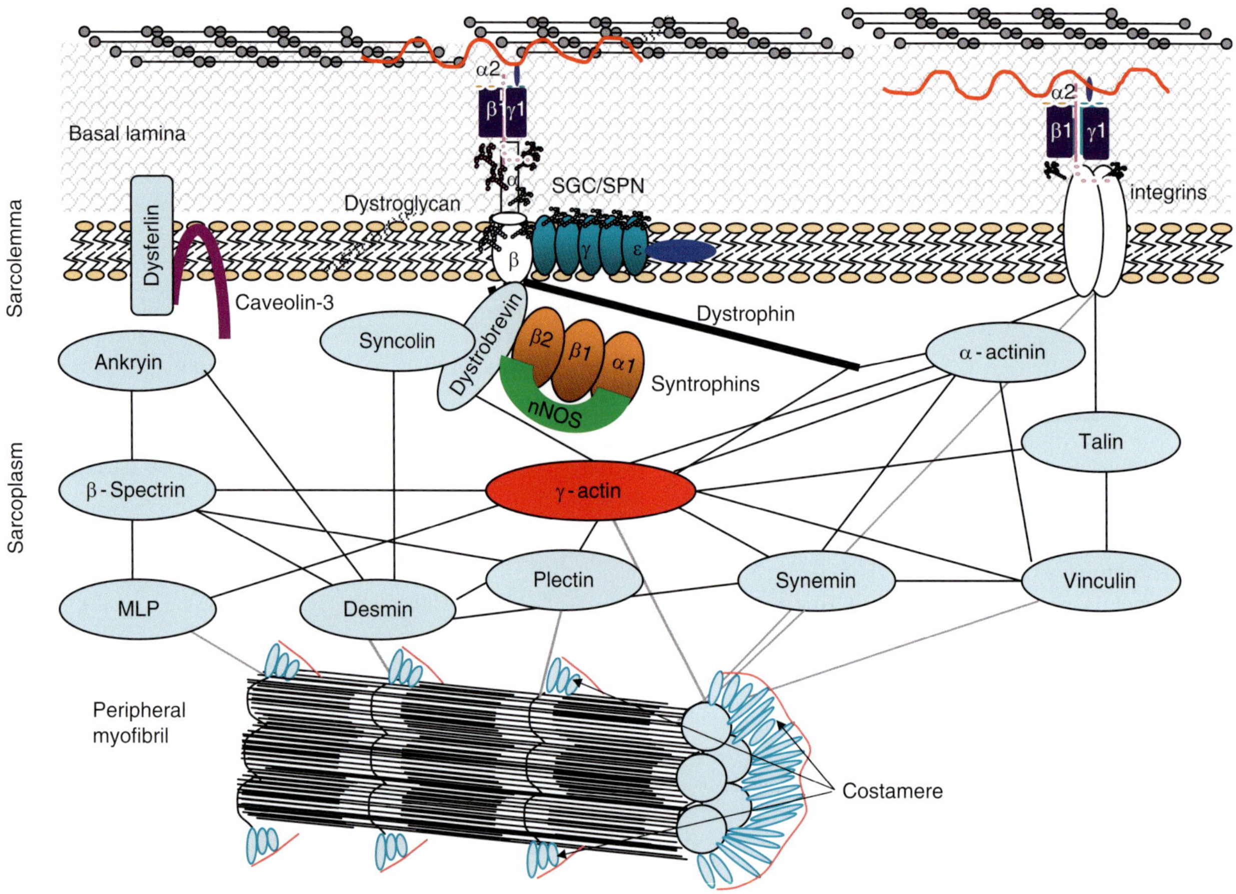

Figure 3.15. Diagram modified from [178] showing some of the costameric proteins and their linkages, either direct or indirect, to a network of cytoskeletal, sarcolemmal, and basement membrane proteins (shown with black lines). Proposed links between these proteins and the myofibrils at the level of the Z-disk are shown as gray lines. Some of the costameric proteins shown also localize to the Z-disk (e.g., MLP and desmin). Dystrophin, ankyrin, MLP, desmin, plectin, and vinculin are primarily affected in various forms of muscular dystrophy and/or cardiomyopathy in humans underscoring the importance of this arrangement.

functional significance (see [175] for review). Roles for the intermediate filament network in myoblast fusion and myofibrillogenesis have been demonstrated; however, this arrangement also plays a crucial role in maintaining muscle fiber integrity by ensuring that adjacent myofibrillar bundles are kept in register and maintain a strong linkage with the sarcolemma/basement membrane at the level of the Z-disk. Whilst cytoplasmic γ-actin is normally expressed at very low levels in skeletal muscle it does localize to costameres, and a muscle-specific knockout in mice is associated with a progressive pattern of muscle fiber necrosis/regeneration and functional deficits [175].

The Z-disk forms a tetragonal network over the actin filament ends from two adjacent sarcomeres, and is at least partly responsible for ensuring that tension is transmitted along the length of the muscle. Indeed the width of the Z-disk reflects the mechanical properties of the muscle and is narrower in fast compared to slow muscles. Defects in proteins of the Z-disk give rise to a broad spectrum of clinical phenotypes encompassing congenital myopathies, myofibrillar myopathies, and limb-girdle muscular dystrophies. The protein assemblies that link the Z-disk and also the M-line to the sarcolemma are referred to as costameres due to their appearance as "rib-like" structures along the length of the muscle fiber upon immunolabeling for key components such as dystrophin, vinculin, talin, α-actinin, and β1 integrins [178] (Figure 3.15). As a consequence of their composition costameres are often thought of as a muscle-specific version of the focal adhesions seen in other cell types.

As might be expected given their role in mediating the transmission of lateral force across the fiber, the composition and organization of the costamere is sensitive to physiological stimuli. For example, talin, vinculin, and filamin C have each been shown to vary as a response to physiological stimuli or disease state. The transverse orientation of the costameric lattice has also been shown to be sensitive to innervation by adopting a more longitudinal rather than transverse array in denervated muscle, an effect that is reversed by electrical stimulation.

Myofibrillar myopathy (MFM) is characterized by focal myofibrillar destruction and cytoplasmic protein aggregations. The underlying causes include mutations in desmin, αB-crystallin, myotilin, Z-band alternatively spliced PDZ motif-containing protein (ZASP) or filamin C.

Desmin and αB-crystallin

The gene encoding for desmin is assigned to human chromosome 2q35. Desmin is the most prominant intermediate filament protein in adult skeletal and heart muscle and forms a three-dimensional scaffold at the level of the Z-disk effectively interconnecting the contractile apparatus with the subsarcolemmal cytoskeleton, myonuclei, and other organelles. Desmin is concentrated at the Z-disk, costameres, and myo tendinous junction [177]. αβ-crystallin is a protein chaperone involved in desmin filament assembly and a member of the small heat shock protein (sHSP) family. It is widely expressed but is present most notably in astrocytes and muscle. Missense mutations in the αB-crystallin gene (*CRYAB*, chromosome 11q22.3–q23.1) are the underlying cause of one form of desmin-related myopathy, now referred to as crystallinopathy.

The ultrastructural findings in both the desminopathies and αB-crystallinopathies are similar and consist of electron-dense granulofilamentous accumulations [178], reflecting the important functional interaction between intermediate filaments and αB-crystallin. Affected individuals all display symmetrical proximal and distal weakness with velopharyngeal involvement, clinical and electrical signs of hypertrophic cardiomyopathy, and opaque lenses.

Desmin knockout mice (Des –/–) develop normally but defects in skeletal, smooth, and cardiac muscles occur postnatally. Weight-bearing muscles such as the soleus and heavily used muscles such as the diaphragm and the heart show the most profound changes and there is evidence that a lack of desmin renders these fibers more susceptible to damage during contraction. Myofibrillogenesis in regenerating fibers appears abnormal, implicating desmin in muscle repair.

Plectin

Plectin is a crosslinker protein that binds to the spectrin–actin cytoskeleton and to various intermediate filaments including desmin, thereby providing mechanical strength. Homozygous mutations in the *PLEC1* gene have been identified in patients with epidermolysis bullosa simplex (EBS) and muscular dystrophy [179]. EBS is a very severe skin blistering condition that results from the disruption of the link between the keratin filament network and the epidermal cells at the level of the hemidesmosomes. EBS can also be found in association with pyloric atresia as opposed to muscular dystrophy.

The age of onset of the muscle weakness ranges from infancy to adulthood and it follows a slowly progressive course [179]. The pathology may vary from mild myopathic changes in the youngest cases to dystrophic changes with necrosis and regeneration in the older cases, in line with the slowly progressive course of the muscle weakness. In normal muscle, by immunohistochemistry, plectin antibodies label the muscle fiber sarcolemma and the cytoplasm with a fiber-type-specific pattern depending on the antibody used. Immunogold labeling of ultrathin sections confirms that desmin and plectin localize between adjacent Z-disks, between peripheral Z-disks and the plasma membrane, and directly beneath the plasma membrane. In EBS-MD patients plectin was reported to be absent at the periphery of all muscle fibers but labeling was retained in the cytoplasm of type II fibers [179]. The pattern of staining of desmin and α-actinin was also disrupted in EBD-MD muscle fibers, consistent with plectin interacting with both of these proteins. Thus the muscle phenotype may be due to the role of plectin in localizing desmin and α-actinin to the periphery of the Z-disk and/or to a wider role in linking intermediate filaments, the spectrin–actin cytoskeleton, and the plasma membrane.

Myotilin

Myotilin is a 57-kDa component of the Z-disk and binds to other proteins including α-actinin, filamin C, F-actin, and FATZ (i.e., filamin actinin and telethonin binding protein of the Z-disk). Mutations in myotilin are associated with limb-girdle muscular dystrophy 1A (LGMD1A) and a subset of myofibrillar myopathies and spheroid body myopathy [180], underscoring its importance in Z-disk maintenance. Myotilin can be detected in nemaline rods and cores with disrupted Z-line material [181].

LGMD1A is characterized by adult onset of proximal weakness, beginning in the hip girdle and progressing later to distal muscles [182]. CK is usually mildly elevated. Several individuals exhibit a distinctive nasal, dysarthric speech. In addition to typical degenerative features of dystrophic muscle, rimmed vacuoles and striking patches of Z-line material occur. There is clinical and pathological overlap between LGMD1A and some cases of myofibrillar myopathy caused by mutations in the same gene [183, 184, 185].

Filamin C

Filamin C (also referred to as γ-filamin) is a myotilin interacting protein that is found both at the periphery of the Z-disk and the sarcolemma where it associates with γ- and δ-sarcoglycans. The interaction of filamin C with both sarcolemmal and myofibrillar proteins associated with limb-girdle muscular dystrophies (LGMD) may indicate that it plays a role in the signaling from sarcolemma to the myofibril. Defects in this protein are responsible for a proportion of cases of myofibrillar myopathy.

The filamin C gene (FLNC) is located on chromosome 7q32.1. A recent study of a group of patients with the same p.W2710X mutation in FLNC showed that the mean age at onset of clinical symptoms ranged between 24 and 57 years [186]. These symptoms included a slowly progressive muscle weakness with a distribution of weakness observed in LGMD. Serum CK levels varied from normal up to 10-fold of the upper limit. The pathological features of this group included an alteration in myofibrillar alignment, accumulation of granulofilamentous material, and intracellular protein deposits which were composed of a variety of proteins, namely desmin, myotilin, Xin, dystrophin, and sarcoglycans.

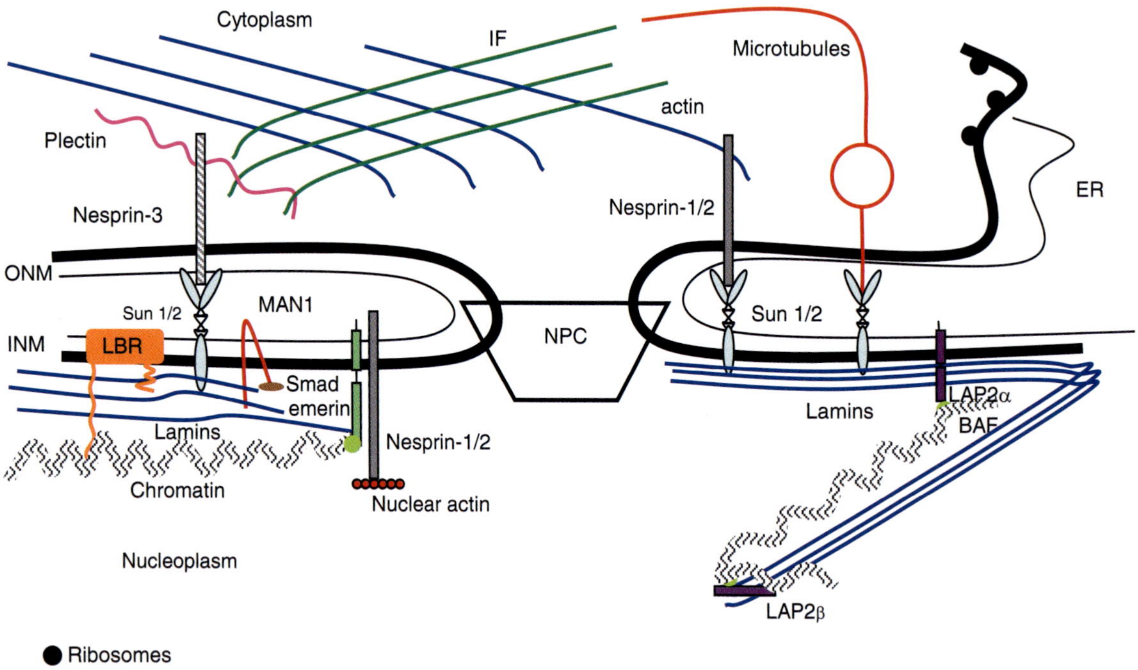

Figure 3.16. Schematic of the protein organization at the nuclear envelope; the inner (INM) and outer (ONM) nuclear membranes are separated by the perinuclear space (PNS) and connected at the sites of the nuclear pore complex (NPC). The ONM is continuous with the membrane of the endoplasmic reticulum (ER); the PNS is an extension of the ER lumen and contains ER-resident proteins. The nuclear lamina is a protein meshwork that associates with both the INM and the chromatin. Main components of the nuclear lamina are lamin-A and lamin-B. SUN proteins and the nesprins are central components of the "linker of nucleoskeleton and cytoskeleton complex" (LINC), which serves to transmit force from the cytoskeleton to nuclear components. Nesprin-1 and -2 bind to actin filaments whereas nesprin-3 binds to intermediate filaments via plectin. Within the nucleoplasm, Sun proteins bind to type A lamins and components of the chromatin. Interactions with the chromatin are mediated by the DNA-binding protein BAF, the LBR, lamins, and emerin. ONM, outer nuclear membrane; INM, inner nuclear membrane; NPC, nuclear pore complex; IF, intermediate filaments; ER, endoplasmic reticulum; MAN1, LEM domain containing protein; LBR, lamin B receptor, which is a transmembrane component of the inner nuclear membrane and which mediates the interaction between the lamin meshwork and the chromatin.

Z-band alternatively spliced PDZ motif-containing protein (ZASP)

Z-band alternatively spliced PDZ motif-containing protein (ZASP) is expressed in the Z-disk of human cardiac and skeletal muscle. Its interaction with α-actinin-2 via its N-terminal PDZ domain suggests that it may aid in anchoring titin at the Z-disk, and a ternary complex between the three proteins has been suggested. The ZASP gene consists of 18 exons, which are differentially spliced to form several isoforms: exon 6 is expressed without exon 4 in skeletal muscle isoforms. Mutations in exon 6 cause a myopathy [187]. The knockout mouse (ZASP orthologue cypher) shows severe congenital myopathy and cardiomyopathy [188].

Nuclear envelope

The nuclear envelope comprises two membranes, which are connected at the sites of the nuclear pores (Figure 3.16). The outermost membrane (ONM) is continuous with the rough endoplasmic reticulum (ER), as is the perinuclear space between the outer and inner membranes. A number of integral membrane proteins locate to the inner nuclear membrane (INM), including members of the LEM domain family named after the founding members, LAP2, emerin, and MAN1. The LEM domain mediates binding to the chromatin-associated protein barrier-to-autointegration factor (BAF) thus recruiting chromatin to the nuclear envelope [189].

A major component of the nuclear lamina which lines the INM is an intermediate filament network composed of lamins A, B, and C. This arrangement is thought to both provide a structural support to the nuclear envelope and maintain the stable localization and retention of inner nuclear membrane proteins. B-type lamins are essential proteins that are expressed in all cells throughout development, whereas lamins A and C tend to be expressed in differentiated cells [190].

Nesprins (nuclear envelope spectrin repeat proteins) are high-molecular-weight cytoskeletal proteins which localize to the ONM and are tethered via transluminal interactions by SUN proteins (which interact with lamin A). Nesprin-1 and -2 bind to actin filaments whereas nesprin-3 binds to intermediate filaments via plectin. This arrangement therefore integrates nuclear and cytoplasmic architecture by connecting the actin cytoskeleton with nuclear components and is referred to as the "linker of nucleoskeleton and cytoskeleton complex" or LINC (Figure 3.16).

Lamins

Lamin A (mol. wt. 72 kDa) and C (mol. wt. 67 kDa) are derived from the alternative splicing of the *LMNA* gene and share a common N-terminal domain, but have unique C-termini. Experimental evidence suggests that the incorporation of lamin A is dependent upon lamin B [191]; however, the presence of lamin A is not essential for the deposition of C since mice expressing only lamin C and not A are essentially normal [192]. The lamins characteristically possess a central α-helical coiled-coil rod domain, flanked by non-helical N-terminal "head" and C-terminal "tail" domains [193, 194]. Lamins form homo- and heteropolymers and associate with a number of other nuclear membrane proteins, properties that enable them to form a network [195] and thus make the nuclear envelope more resilient to mechanical stress relative to the plasma membrane [196]. The lamins have also been attributed with a role in a wide range of functions including nuclear growth and shape, DNA replication, chromatin organization, RNA splicing, cell differentiation, apoptosis, and cell-cycle-dependent control of nuclear architecture. It is now recognized that an increasing number of these functions probably depend on the formation of complexes with other proteins such as LEM-domain proteins, nesprins, and the SUN-domain proteins. Indeed a number of these proteins are dependent on lamin A for their correct organization [197].

Dominant mutations in the *LMNA* gene on chromosome 1q11–23 underlie the autosomal dominant form of Emery–Dreifuss muscular dystrophy (AD EDMD). Mutations in the *LMNA* gene also underlie several allelic conditions, including limb-girdle muscular dystrophy 1B, dilated cardiomyopathy with conduction system disease, familial partial lipodystrophy, Charcot–Marie–Tooth type 2B1, mandibuloacral dysostosis, premature aging disorders, and restrictive dermopathy [198]. These are now often collectively referred to as the "laminopathies," and skeletal muscle is only affected in some (AD EDMD and LGMD1B). Mutations occur throughout the gene although many are found in the common α-helical rod domain of exons 1–10. These mutations result in no detectable alteration in lamin A/C immunolocalization [199]. The reason for the diversity in disease phenotype is not understood. However, recent work suggests that lamin-associated protein complexes may exist at the nuclear envelope and it is possible that tissue-specific differences in these associations underlie some of the tissue specificity of these disorders. Indeed there is considerable interest in other nuclear envelope proteins as candidates for disorders with clinical similarity to the EDMDs and the recent identification of a mutation in LAP2α (lamin-A-associated protein) in a family affected by a form of dilated cardiomyopathy supports this approach [200].

Emerin

The X-linked form of EDMD is caused by mutations in the *STA* gene on chromosome Xq28, which encodes for emerin [201]. Emerin is a 34-kDa nuclear protein which has a hydrophobic C-terminus anchored in the nuclear membrane and a N-terminal tail projecting into the nucleoplasm [201]. The *STA* gene has six exons and mutations have been found throughout the gene with no "hot spots." Most are nonsense or frameshift mutations or occur at splice sites. The majority of mutations result in the absence of localized protein, which can be demonstrated with antibodies [202, 203]. Rare cases have been reported in which emerin expression is reduced rather than absent [204]. Female carriers rarely manifest with muscle weakness but are at risk of cardiac involvement. The absence of emerin in a proportion of nuclei can be detected in carriers in skin and buccal cells [205].

Emerin has been shown to bind to lamin A; it may fulfil several roles and interacts with barrier-to-autointegration factor (BAF), in addition to transcription repressors, an mRNA splicing regulator, nesprin, nuclear myosin I and F-actin [206]. Recent work shows that lamin-A-deficient cells are more fragile than controls and that their signaling responses to mechanical strain are impaired [207]. However, emerin-deficient fibroblasts have less profound deficiencies in strain-induced gene regulation, which suggests that emerin-associated disease is predominantly caused by an impaired signaling response rather than a direct strain-induced injury to the nuclear membrane. Thus whilst the similarity of heart involvement in both autosomal and X-linked forms of EDMD suggests at least one functionally important pathway in common, experimental evidence indicates that this is not directly related to the structural integrity of the nuclear envelope. Nonetheless, both factors act synergistically as the severe clinical phenotype of a patient with a mutation in both emerin and lamin A/C indicates [208].

Lamin, emerin, and muscular dystrophy

The clinical features of the X-linked and autosomal forms of Emery–Dreifuss muscular dystrophy (XL EDMD and AD EDMD, respectively) are similar but often more severe in the latter. EDMD is invariably associated with both cardiac and skeletal muscle involvement. Both disorders present with muscle weakness and early contractures of the elbow, the Achilles tendons, and the spinal extensor muscles. The contractures are progressive and rigidity of the spine often becomes marked. Skeletal muscle involvement typically precedes the cardiac abnormalities, which are evident before the third decade of life and are the most deleterious aspect of both disorders, being characterized by atrioventricular conduction disturbances and heart block. Dilated cardiomyopathy can also be found in AD EDMD.

The skeletal muscle involvement is typically humero-peroneal, also with scapular involvement. Striking wasting of the upper arms and lower legs is often apparent in both, and the two conditions are almost indistinguishable, although subtle differences in the pattern of muscle involvement can be demonstrated using muscle MRI [209]. AD EDMD is more common than the X-linked form and generally more severe, with earlier onset, even congenital in a few instances [210]. With the exception of cases with onset in infancy, ambulation is usually retained for life. Serum CK levels are usually normal, mildly or even moderately elevated, but never in the high range found in Duchenne or Becker muscular dystrophy.

Immunolabeling of emerin and lamin A/C in AD EDMD appears normal but electron microscopy sometimes demonstrates an abnormal aggregation of chromatin and lack of attachment of chromatin to the nuclear membrane [211]. Abnormalities of the nuclear envelope have also been reported in skeletal muscle nuclei and cultured skin fibroblasts [190, 212, 213]. However, the specificity of these findings to EDMD remains to be shown. In the X-linked form emerin is absent from the nuclear membrane or mislocalized to the endoplasmic reticulum.

There are a number of genetically engineered mouse strains with a modified *Lmna* gene, although only two have been shown to be good models for Emery–Dreifuss. The first to be generated was a null phenotype and affected mice displayed a muscular dystrophy, dilated cardiomyopathy (DCM), and death by 8 weeks of age [190]. This model does not generally reflect the situation in patients as to date only one patient has been described with a nonsense mutation (Y259X) that proved to be lethal in the homozygous state and gave rise to a classic LGMD1B phenotype in the heterozygous state [214]. The second mouse model displayed a phenotype similar to that of humans with Hutchinson–Gilford progeria syndrome (HGPS), the reason being that the targeting procedure inadvertently resulted in decreased stability of *lmna* mRNA transcripts and activated a cryptic splice site, causing a possible anomaly in the processing of prelamin A [215]. The third and most accurate model to date carries a missense mutation *Lmna* H222P, originally identified in a family with a typical AD EDMD [216]. These homozygous mice displayed reduced locomotor activity with abnormal stiff walking posture. Their life span did not go beyond 9 months of age and they developed chamber dilation and hypokinesia with conduction defects together with skeletal muscle degeneration and fibrosis. The fourth mouse carries a *Lmna-N195K* mutation which resulted in early death due to arrhythmia, attributed by the authors to a disruption of cardiomyocyte internal organization and/or the expression of transcription factors essential to normal cardiac development, aging or function [217].

Somewhat surprisingly *Emd*-null mice are normal at birth as are their subsequent postnatal growth and locomotion [218]. However, in another line of mice subtle motor coordination abnormalities together with the presence of small vacuoles in the cardiomyocytes and a slight prolongation of atrioventricular conduction time in mice older than 40 weeks of age has been noted [219].

Nucleus

Triple repeat expansion disorders

Myotonic dystrophy is a dominantly inherited multisystemic disorder and is the most common cause of adult-onset muscular dystrophy. Skeletal muscle wasting and cardiac conduction defects are characteristic of this disorder. There are two forms of myotonic dystrophy (DM), both of which are caused by the expansion of repeated DNA sequences. DM1 is the most common and is associated with a CTG repeat located in the 3′ untranslated region of the myotonic dystrophy protein kinase (DMPK) gene. DM2 is associated with a tetranucleotide repeat expansion, CCTG, located in the first intron of zinc finger protein 9 (ZNF9) gene.

The mechanism of disease is thought to be due to the expanded allele being transcribed into RNA, which, due to the unusually long tracts of CUG or CCUG repeats, folds into an unusual hairpin structure. These mutant RNAs then exert a toxic effect, sequestering specific RNA-binding proteins such as Muscleblind and leading to splicing defects in key muscle proteins. Two proteins identified as interacting with CUG RNA repeats, Muscleblind-like 1 (MBNL1) and CUG-binding protein 1 (CUGBP1), play important roles in DM1 pathogenesis.

Disrupted messenger RNA (mRNA) alternative splicing has so far been reported to occur in the genes encoding for cardiac troponin T (*cTnT*), insulin receptor (*IR*), muscle-specific chloride channel (*ClC-1*), *ZASP*, ryanodine receptor 1 (*RYR1*), and sarcoplasmic/endoplasmic reticulum calcium ATPase (*SERCA*). More recently the alternative splicing of α-dystrobrevin has been shown to be dysregulated in muscle, resulting in changes in α-syntrophin binding. These data raise the possibility that splicing may alter protein interactions within the dystrophin-associated glycoprotein complex (DGC) [220].

A recently generated DM1 mouse model with inducible skeletal-muscle-specific expression of large tracts of CTG repeats in the context of *DMPK* exon 15 displays many features associated with DM1 human skeletal muscle, including muscle wasting, CUG RNA foci with Muscleblind-like 1 (MBNL1) protein co-localization, misregulation of developmentally regulated alternative splicing events, myotonia, and increased CUGBP1 levels [221].

Sarcoplasm

The sarcoplasm is filled by the extensive membrane systems of the T-tubule and sarcoplasmic reticulum, but it also contains the mitochondria, Golgi apparatus, glycogen, free ribosomes, lipid droplets, and lipofuscin, an end product of lysosomal activity. Mitochondria are concerned with the energy supply of the fiber and the regulation of intracellular calcium levels. They are found in intermyofibrillar regions adjacent to the I-bands and beneath the sarcolemma and are often more numerous in type 1 fibers. However, in human muscle differences in mitochondrial volume are not a consistent feature distinguishing fiber types. Golgi elements are observed throughout the fiber and are best observed either at the ultrastructural level (Figure 3.17) or following immunolabeling of Golgi proteins in isolated fibers [222]. They undergo dramatic reorganization during muscle development. Glycogen granules, which are visible under the electron microscope, are more

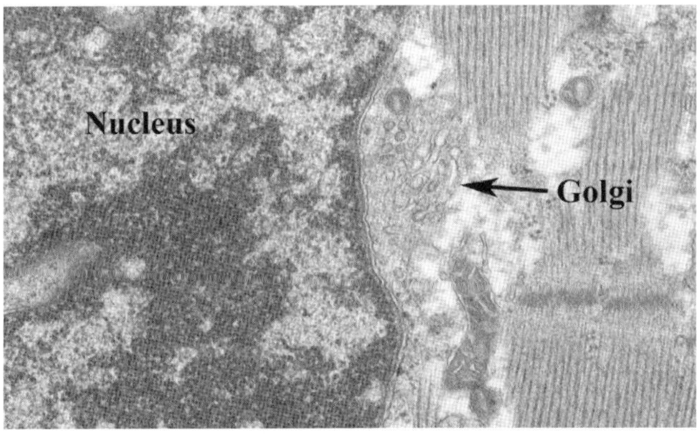

Figure 3.17. Transmission electron micrograph showing the position of Golgi cisternae adjacent to the nuclear envelope.

numerous at the level of the I-band than the A-band. These granules also contain the protein glycogenin and the enzymes responsible for the synthesis, degradation, and control of glycogen metabolism. Free ribosomes are seen in the subsarcolemmal regions and increased numbers are often found in the perinuclear zones, along with Golgi membranes, intermediate filaments, and microtubules.

Type I fibers preferentially express enzymes that oxidize fatty acids, contain slow isoforms of contractile proteins, and are more resistant to fatigue than are glycolytic fibers, whereas type II fibers preferentially metabolize glucose and express the fast isoforms of contractile proteins. Glucose or intramuscular glycogen and fat (through the β-oxidation of fatty acids) provide the substrates for adenosine 5′-triphosphate (ATP) production. An additional source of ATP is creatine phosphate (CrP) and the adenylate kinase reaction, which generates ATP and adenosine monophosphate (AMP) from adenosine diphosphate (ADP). The majority of glucose uptake is thought to be facilitated by the glucose transporter (GLUT4) T-tubule system. Within the muscle glucose is either utilized to yield ATP or stored as glycogen. Glycogen within cells is synthesized as a branching structure composed of long chains of glucose molecules (amylose chains) primarily joined by α-[1–4] linkages interspersed with branching α-[1–6] linkages. Two enzymes play a key process in maintaining appropriate glucose levels in muscle, namely glycogen synthase and glycogen phosphorylase [223]. Both are controlled by hormones in a coordinated manner such that glycogen synthesis and breakdown adapt to the functional requirements of the muscle.

The preferred source of energy that muscle utilizes depends on the type and duration of the exercise. During high-intensity exercise, close to the maximal oxygen uptake or VO_{2max}, or during isometric exercise energy derives from the degradation of glycogen coupled to anaerobic glycolysis. At lower VO_{2max} (70%–80%) the ATP source is also glycogen but this time the glucose produced is metabolized via aerobic glycolysis. During submaximal exercise (<50% VO_{2max}) muscle utilizes the available blood glucose but if the exercise continues it switches to the utilization of fatty acids (via the β-oxidation route).

Disorders that limit the availability of energy to muscle can be broadly divided into those that are characterized by exercise intolerance, cramps, rhabdomyolysis, and myoglobinuria and those that result in fixed weakness as suggested by DiMauro [224].

Glycogen and glucose metabolism

Defects in the enzymes involved in the synthesis and degradation of glycogen and in the metabolism of glucose in the muscle are referred as glycogenoses, each of them associated with a specific enzyme deficiency (at present 15 different subtypes have been described from type 0 to type XIV) (Figure 3.18) and muscle symptoms are apparent in several of these [224]. Inheritance of glycogenoses is usually autosomal recessive. Types I (Gierke disease) and VI (Hers disease) are disorders affecting primarily liver enzymes, glucose 6-phosphatase, and hepatic glycogen phosphorylase and are not included in the diagram.

The synthesis of glycogen is primed by glycogenin, which puts together the first few glucosyl units. This is followed by the action of glycogen synthase (GSD 0), which attaches glucosyl units in an α-[1–4] bond from UDP glucose. The branching enzyme (GSD IV) transfers some of these glucose molecules to nascent lateral chains in an α-[1–6] glucosidic bond.

The process of glycogen degradation to produce glucose is initiated by the release of calcium from the sarcoplasmic reticulum after depolarization of the muscle cell membrane. Calcium binds to the calmodulin subunit of phosphorylase kinase (GSD VIII) and leads to the phosphorylation of the inactive "b" form of phosphorylase to form the active "a" form. Glycogen phosphorylase (GSD V) breaks off the ends of the glycogen chains at the α-[1–4] glucosidic linkages leaving four terminal glucosyl molecules (known as limit dextrin). The debranching enzyme (GSD III) then performs two functions: the first is to transfer three of the remaining glucose molecules to the end of the long amylose chain and the second is to break the α-[1–6] linkage and release the single glucosyl residue left in the branch (Figure 3.19). The glucose-1-phosphate molecules that are released as a result of the combined action of phosphorylase and debranching enzyme enter the glycolytic pathway (glycolysis).

Glycolysis can also take place under anaerobic conditions to generate ATP and bypassing respiratory oxidation, although it is by far a less efficient process than aerobic glycolysis. Anaerobic glycolysis is an important source of energy when oxygen supply to the muscle is reduced such as during extreme and intense exercise. During this process glucose-6-phosphate is transformed to pyruvate. If the oxidative capacity of the cell is impaired, pyruvate may be used as the electron acceptor instead of oxygen giving rise to the lactic acidosis associated with mitochondrial myopathies.

Lipid metabolism

At rest, the major source of fuel is fatty acids, which are taken up by muscle cells into the mitochondria, where they undergo

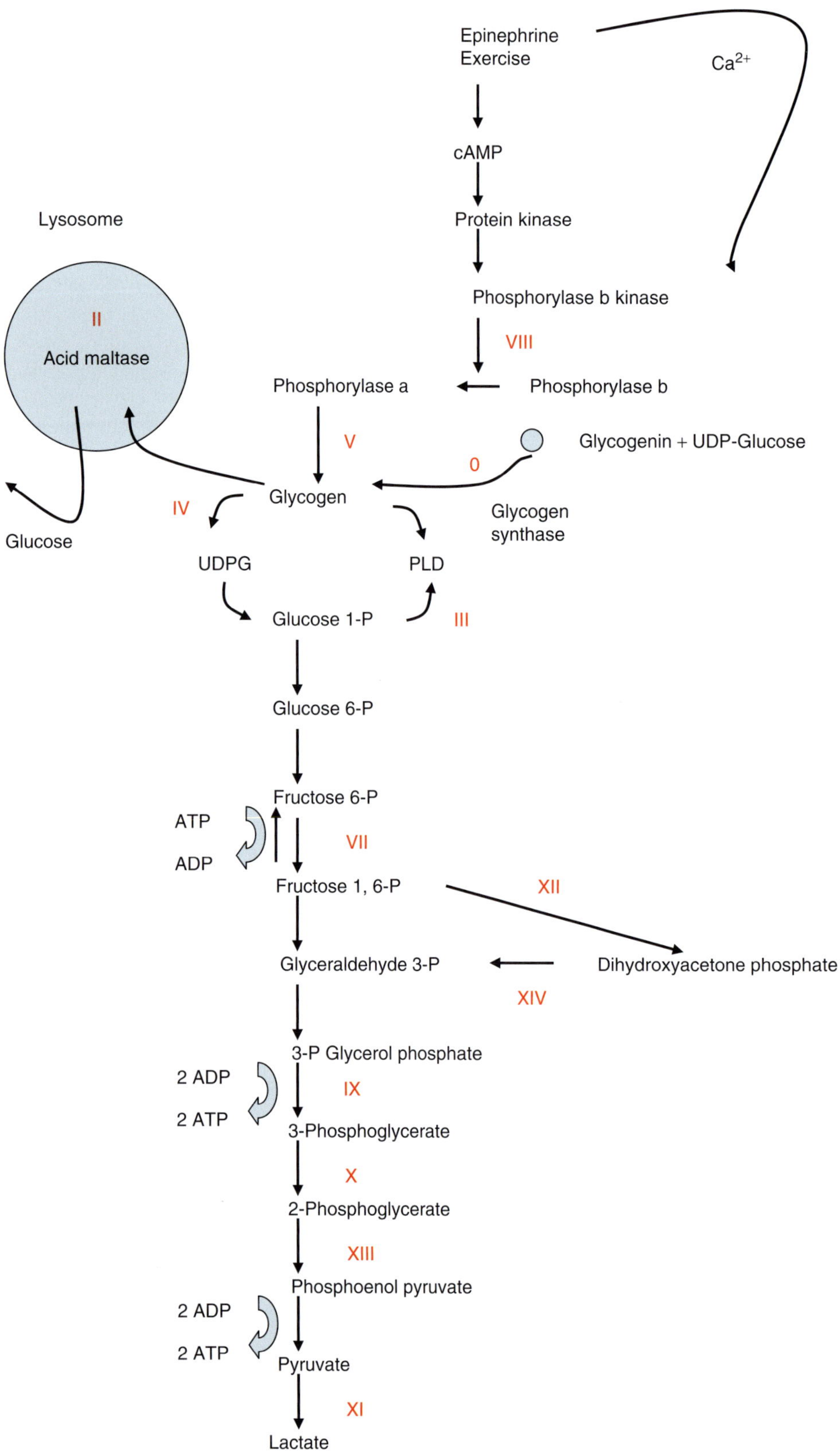

Figure 3.18. Schematic representation of glycogen metabolism and glycolysis indicating, by Roman numerals, the steps implicated in the glycogen storage disorders that affect muscle. The enzymes implicated in each of those are II: acid maltase; III: debrancher enzyme; IV: branching enzyme; V: phosphorylase; VII: phosphofructokinase; VIII: phosphorylase b kinase; X: phosphoglycerate mutase; XI: lactate dehydrogenase; XII: aldolase A; XIII: β-enolase; XIV: triose phosphate isomerase (TPI). PLD, phosphorylase-limit dextrin; UDPG, uridine diphosphate glucose. Modified from [225].

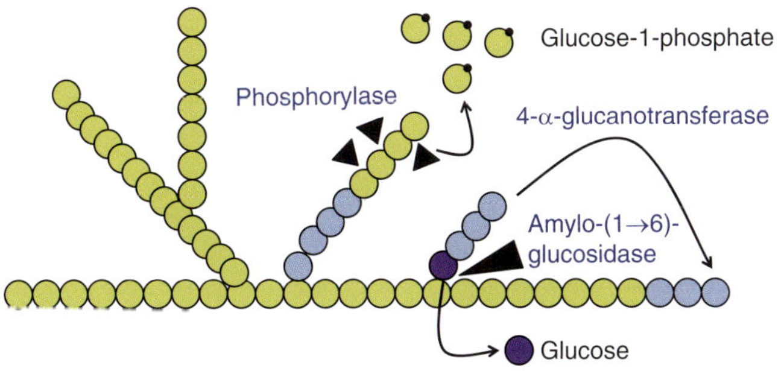

Figure 3.19. Glycogen is progressively degraded by the combined action of *phosphorylase* and the *debranching enzyme*. Phosphorylase removes glucose units from the outer branches, releasing glucose-1-phosphate molecules, but stops four units before a branch point ("limit dextrin"). The glucosyltransferase activity of the debranching enzyme catalyzes the transfer of three glucose units from the end of the branch to form a α [1–4] linkage with another branch. The remaining glucose molecule is hydrolyzed and released in the form of glucose by the glucosidase activity of the debranching enzyme. Phosphorylase and debranching enzyme act simultaneously so that in normal circumstances "limit dextrin" is not produced.

β-oxidation to acetyl-CoA and enter the citric acid cycle. The major steps in fatty acid metabolism, relevant to lipid storage myopathies, are that short- and medium-chain fatty acids enter mitochondria directly and are converted to acyl-CoA esters by acyl-CoA synthetases in the matrix of the mitochondria. In contrast, long-chain fatty acids, such as palmitic acid, are converted to acyl-CoA ester by enzymes in the outer membrane of the mitochondrion and are transported into the matrix in a carnitine-dependent manner, which involves carnitine palmitoyl-transferase (CPT-I and -II) and carnitine–acylcarnitine translocase (CACT). Within the matrix of the mitochondrion, acyl-CoA is converted by β-oxidation to acetyl-CoA, which then enters the citric acid cycle. The first step of the β-oxidation cycle is the dehydrogenation of the acyl-CoA to 2-enoyl-CoA. This reaction is catalyzed by the acyl-CoA dehydrogenases, which differ in their fatty acid chain length specificity and are known as very long, long, medium, and short chain acyl-CoA dehydrogenases (VLCAD, LCAD, MCAD, and SCAD) respectively.

Defects in these pathways lead to a heterogeneous group of disorders. Some of these conditions affect the muscle only whereas others affect other systems/tissues as well, especially the liver and heart. In some cases, muscle is not or only very little affected. The genes affected are encoded by the nuclear genome and these conditions are autosomal recessive.

Those disorders affecting muscle include carnitine, CPT-I and -II and CACT deficiencies. Defects in any of the four acyl-CoA dehydrogenases mentioned above are the commonly diagnosed abnormalities of fatty acid oxidation.

In addition, defects in the mitochondrial trifunctional protein (TFP) (an enzyme with 2-enoyl-CoA hydratase, 3-hydroxyacyl-CoA dehydrogenase, and 3-ketoacyl-CoA thiolase activities) are also associated with weakness and myoglobinuria.

The acyl-CoA dehydrogenases utilize electron transferring flavoprotein (ETF) as the electron acceptor. Abnormalities of ETF or ETF:ubiquinone oxidoreductase (ETF dehydrogenase) lead to a form of lipid myopathy referred to as multiple acyl-CoA dehydrogenation disorder (MADD) since all the dehydrogenases which utilize ETF as an electron acceptor are affected. Because of the presence of glutaric acid in the urine of some patients, this disorder is frequently referred to as glutaric aciduria type II (GA II) to distinguish it from a primary deficiency due to glutaryl-CoA dehydrogenase (GA I).

Excessive lipid accumulation in the muscle biopsy sample is not always a feature in this group of conditions and the overall pathology may be unremarkable or minimally myopathic. In addition, accumulation of lipid may be secondary to a defect in one of the respiratory chain complexes. Biochemical analysis of blood and urine is necessary and measurements of enzymatic activity in fibroblasts or lymphocytes are required to ascertain the specific biochemical defect.

Respiratory chain defects

Mitochondria have a single outer membrane and an inner membrane with deep folds known as cristae. The mitochondrial respiratory chain consists of a group of five enzyme complexes located on the inner mitochondrial membrane. Reduced cofactors [reduced nicotinamide adenine dinucleotide (NADH) and reduced flavin adenine dinucleotide (FADH2)] generated from the intermediary metabolism of carbohydrates, proteins, and fats donate electrons to complex I and complex II. Electrons then flow between the complexes down an electrochemical gradient, shuttled by complexes III and IV and by ubiquinone (ubiquinol-coenzyme Q10), and cytochrome c. The energy is used by complexes I, III, and IV to pump protons out of the mitochondrial matrix into the intermembrane space. This proton gradient is responsible for the bulk of the mitochondrial membrane potential and is harnessed by complex V to synthesize ATP from ADP and inorganic phosphate.

The mitochondrial myopathies are a complex and heterogeneous group of neuromuscular disorders. Many organs may be affected but the major clinical and pathological emphasis is upon skeletal muscle, with or without involvement of the central nervous system [225]. Mitochondrial myopathies can be caused by defects in components of the respiratory chain, mitochondrial tRNA or mitochondrial DNA synthesis. Respiratory chain proteins are synthesized from two distinct genomes, namely mitochondrial DNA (mtDNA) and nuclear DNA (nDNA), making the genetic basis of this group of myopathies complex. mtDNA encodes for 13 respiratory chain polypeptides and nucleic acids (rRNAs and tRNAs) required for intra-mitochondrial protein synthesis. nDNAs encode for the majority of mitochondrial respiratory chain polypeptides.

The overall pathology may be unremarkable or minimally myopathic. Pathological features include subsarcolemmal accumulations of abnormal mitochondria commonly reported as ragged-red fibers (so-called because of their red color with Gomori trichrome stain). Deficiencies in respiratory chain enzymes can be detected using specific histochemical reactions such as the reaction for cytochrome c oxidase (COX, complex IV) and succinate dehydrogenase (SDH), which is part of complex II of the respiratory chain. COX contains subunits encoded by both mtDNA and nDNA, whereas SDH contains subunits encoded only by nDNA. As a result of disrupted mitochondrial function, fatty acids accumulate and in some cases an increase in intracellular lipid and glycogen may be seen.

The biochemical and cellular consequences of specific mtDNA mutations have been studied using transmitochondrial cytoplasmic cybrid cells in which immortalized human cell lines depleted of their endogenous mtDNA are repopulated with exogenous, patient mitochondria. As these cells have no functional respiratory chain and so are dependent on pyruvate and uridine for growth, the loss of either of these two metabolic requirements can be used to select for transformants that harbor complementing (exogenous) mtDNA.

Regarding amino acid metabolism both leucine and isoleucine can be metabolized by muscle to provide energy. Glutamate is used to generate intermediaries of the tricarboxylic acid (TCA) cycle. Other amino acids that can be metabolized by muscle are valine, asparagine, and aspartate. All play a very important role in energy metabolism.

Sarcoplasmic reticulum

Skeletal muscles contract and relax by the fine regulation of calcium release and uptake in specific muscle compartments. Two key players are the skeletal muscle ryanodine receptor (*RYR1*), which comprises four subunits that assemble to form a Ca^{2+} release channel in the junctional cisternae of the sarcoplasmic reticulum, and the dihydropyridine receptor (*DHPR*) which localizes to the T-tubule system. The rapid removal of Ca^{2+} ions from the cytosol following muscle contraction is achieved by the combined work of the sarco/endoplasmic reticulum Ca^{2+}-ATPases (SERCAs), the plasma membrane calcium pumps (PMCA), and mitochondria (Figure 3.13).

Ryanodine receptor

Core myopathies including central core disease (CCD) and multi-minicore disease (MmD) are the most common forms of congenital myopathy. They are typically characterized by areas within the fiber devoid of mitochondria and showing varying degrees of myofibrillar disruption. An absence of oxidative activity as determined by cytochrome oxidase, succinic dehydrogenase or nicotinamide adenine dinucleotide dehydrogenase-tetrazolium reductase gives the appearance of "cores" within the fibers, the number, size, and position of which are variable. A predominance of type 1 fibers is often a feature [226]. The mechanism leading to core formation remains unclear.

RYR1 mutations cause muscle weakness and carry the risk of developing a life-threatening reaction to general anesthesia (malignant hyperthermia susceptibility). Mutations in the *RYR1* gene account for most (~90%) cases of CCD and ~40% of MmD cases, while mutations in the gene encoding for selenoprotein 1 (*SEPN1*) account for ~50% of other MmD. However, screening of these genes in some cases has not identified any mutations, suggesting further genetic heterogeneity. Genotype–phenotype correlations associated with RYR1 mutations are complicated by the involvement of dominant and recessive mutations. Functional studies have shown some physiological differences between dominant and recessive RYR1 mutations [227, 228, 229], and a full understanding of the consequences of the mutant protein could provide a basis for targeted therapeutic intervention.

The spectrum of *RYR1* mutations, the clinical phenotypes, and the associated pathological changes is now much wider than originally thought and recessive *RYR1* mutations have been identified in patients with a core-like myopathy and weakness of the eye muscles, and in individuals with features of centronuclear myopathy.

The inheritance of most *RYR1* mutations is autosomal dominant and several sporadic de novo dominant cases have also been reported. In addition some recessive cases [230] epigenetic silencing of *RYR1* has been shown, where it appears that the mutated but not the normal allele is expressed in muscle. The human *RYR1* gene is large with 106 exons, two of which are alternatively spliced to produce two isoforms of proteins. Although mutations in the *RYR1* gene are known to occur across the gene, mutations associated with central core disease are often, but not exclusively, in the C-terminal exons, whilst those associated with MH are often in the cytoplasmic domain [231, 232, 233] which interacts with the cytosolic region of the α1-subunit of the DHPR.

The identification of a wide range of mutations across the *RYR1* gene and the appreciation of the wider spectrum of associated clinical phenotypes has led to a better understanding of the pathogenesis of core myopathies due to defects in RYR1 and has made possible phenotype–genotype correlations [234, 235, 236].

The main mechanisms thought to be involved are:

1. Leaky channel resulting in a depletion of Ca^{2+} sarcoplasmic reticulum stores.
2. Impaired transmission of the depolarization signal from the sarcolemma to the ryanodine receptor, i.e., "excitation-contraction (EC) uncoupling."

Both these mechanisms would be expected to result in reduced Ca^{2+} release upon excitation and are the most likely mechanisms of disease in patients with dominant mutations mostly located in the C-terminal, pore-forming part of the molecule, a typical central core disease phenotype and normal ryanodine receptor protein levels.

The functional consequences of recessive mutations are less well understood but the following mechanisms have been proposed:

1. A reduction in RYR1 protein levels. This has been shown by Western blotting analysis of muscle from patients with multi-minicores and a more severe phenotype with generalized weakness and ophthalmoplegia [237].

This group included patients who were heterozygous at the genomic level but in whom the normal allele was silenced in skeletal muscle [230] resulting in the exclusive expression of the mutant allele (acting as a homozygous mutation).

2. A reduced ability of the RYR1 channel to transport Ca^{2+} upon activation [227, 230].
3. Reduced Ca^{2+} release due to instability of the RYR1 macromolecular complex [235].
4. An increase in the sensitivity to depolarization-induced Ca^{2+} release. This was shown by a missense mutation in the *RYR1* gene responsible for the centronuclear myopathy phenotype [238].

Slow fiber predominance is one of the most common pathological findings in core myopathies associated with defects in RYR1 and may precede the appearance of cores. The reason for this switch in fiber type profile is not entirely understood but studies in isolated chicken myoblasts suggest that RYR1 activity regulates Ca^{2+} transients in a fiber-type-specific manner and that this in turn controls the expression of slow myosin and other fiber-type-specific genes. Those pathways involve the phosphatase calcineurin, the transcription factors nuclear factor activated T cell (NFAT) and myocyte enhancing factor 2 (MEF2) and protein kinase C. Inhibition of RYR activity using ryanodine induced the expression of slow myosin (MyHC2) in myoblasts from pectoralis major muscles, which normally do not express slow myosin as determined by immunohistochemistry.

Regarding the mechanism of disease in these disorders recent work using mice carrying a malignant hyperthermia mutation (Y522S) in RyR1 shows that this mutation causes a Ca^{2+} leak, which results in an increase in the generation of reactive nitrogen species. The ensuing S-nitrosylation of the mutant RyR1 further enhances Ca^{2+} leak and increases susceptibility to heat-induced sudden death in these mice [239]. A Zebrafish spontaneous mutant has also recently been characterized which provides a good model to study the effect of recessive mutations in the *RYR1* gene. The "relatively relaxed" phenotype was found to have a homozygous insertion in the ryr1b gene, encoding for the ryr1b isoform which is expressed in zebrafish fast muscles. This resulted in slow swimming due to EC uncoupling. The insertion was shown to result in reduced levels of normal mRNA and a significant reduction of RYR1 (and DHPR) labeling in fast fibers. The phenotype could be rescued transiently using antisense oligonucleotides which restored normal splicing [240].

SERCA1

SERCA1 is encoded by the *ATP2A1* gene on chromosome 16p12 and is expressed almost exclusively in type 2 fibers (fast twitch) whereas a second isoform SERCA2 (encoded by the *ATP2A2* gene on chromosome 12q23) is expressed in cardiac and type 1 (slow) muscle fibers. Mutations in the *ATP2A1* gene are responsible for Brody disease [241], a recessive disorder characterized by painless cramps and impairment of muscle relaxation. Three nonsense and one missense mutation have been identified to date. Muscle contraction is normal but the relaxation phase becomes increasingly slow during exercise. Administration of dantrolene and verapamil can ameliorate the symptoms of Brody disease [242].

An absence of SERCA1 protein from fast fibers has been noted in some, but not all, patients with an *ATP2A1* mutation. Whilst this was associated with a total loss of enzymatic activity other studies have shown reduced ATPase activity (up to 50% reduction) and expression of a nonfunctional protein [243]. Therefore, the presence of SERCA1-positive fibers does not exclude Brody disease.

Patients with some features in common with Brody disease but with no mutations in the *ATP2A1* gene are described as having Brody syndrome. Various candidate genes have been excluded, including the *ATP2A2* gene encoding SERCA2 in slow fibers.

Selenoprotein

Selenoproteins are a family of enzymes that contain a selenium atom in the form of a seleno-cysteine in the catalytic site and they are involved in oxidation-reduction reactions. Selenoprotein-1 (SEPN1) is a 70-kDa glycoprotein localizing to the rough endoplasmic reticulum in several tissues including skeletal muscle, heart, brain, lung, and placenta [244]. Levels of SEPN1 are higher in fetal tissues relative to adult tissues suggesting a role for SEPN1 in early development and in cell proliferation or regeneration.

Mutations in the gene encoding for selenoprotein-1 (*SEPN1*) are associated with rigid spine muscular dystrophy 1 (RSMD1), multi-minicore myopathy (both of which are part of the same phenotypic spectrum), congenital fiber type disproportion (CFTD), and Mallory body myopathy. Clinically, these phenotypes are rather homogeneous and are characterized by severe axial weakness, scoliosis, respiratory insufficiency requiring ventilation, rigidity of the spine, and mild proximal weakness. The severity is variable but most patients achieve and maintain ambulation. The protein is found at high levels in the diaphragm, which could explain the respiratory impairment in patients. Levels of serum CK are normal or mildly elevated. RSMD1 patients have a characteristic nasal speech due to palatal weakness. The pathology is, in contrast, variable, ranging from mild myopathic changes with and without minicores, to dystrophic features including connective and adipose tissue proliferation, to the presence of Mallory body-like inclusions and fiber type disproportion, although the latter is not a specific feature [245].

Although the role of *SEPN1* in the pathogenesis of muscle disease in humans is still largely still unknown, studies in zebrafish have produced important clues. Firstly, a knockdown zebrafish model [246] showed significant disorganization of the muscle architecture and ultrastructure and reduced mobility suggesting a role for SEPN1 in early myogenesis, which is in line with the higher expression of SEPN1 in fetal human muscle and other tissues. More recent work has now shown that zebrafish completely depleted of all SepN transcripts display significant myofibril disorganization, Z-disk defects, and hypotrophy of slow fibers [247]. Defects in SEPN and RYR1 in humans can result in the same clinicopathological phenotype (multi-minicore disease). The SepN-depleted zebrafish model now provides evidence that the two proteins may act in the same biochemical pathway by showing that SepN is a modulator of RyR activity, and affects the ability of the ryanodine receptor to function as a redox sensor, the latter property being important in maintaining the correct function of the channel and the control of Ca^{2+} flow.

In summary it appears that SEPN and RYR are physically and functionally linked (Figure 3.13) and that SEPN may have a role in the early development of muscle and in the modulation of ryanodine receptor function.

References

1. D. J. Blake, A. Weir, S. E. Newey, K. E. Davies, Function and genetics of dystrophin and dystrophin-related proteins in muscle. *Physiol. Rev.* **82**:2 (2002), 291–329.
2. O. Ibraghimov-Beskrovnaya, A. Milatovich, T. Ozcelik, *et al.*, Human dystroglycan: skeletal muscle cDNA, genomic structure, origin of tissue specific isoforms and chromosomal localization. *Hum. Mol. Genet.* **2**:10 (1993), 1651–1657.
3. R. D. Cohn, K. P. Campbell, Molecular basis of muscular dystrophies. *Muscle Nerve* **23**:10 (2000), 1456–1471.
4. I. Breloy, T. Schwientek, B. Gries, H. Razawi, M. Macht, C. Albers, *et al.*, Initiation of mammalian O-mannosylation in vivo is independent of a consensus sequence and controlled by peptide regions within and upstream of the alpha-dystroglycan mucin domain. *J. Biol. Chem.* **283**:27 (2008), 18832–18840.
5. F. Muntoni, M. Brockington, S. Torelli, S. C. Brown, Defective glycosylation in congenital muscular dystrophies. *Curr. Opin. Neurol.* **17**:2 (2004), 205–209.
6. H. Manya, K. Sakai, K. Kobayashi, K. Taniguchi, M. Kawakita, T. Toda, *et al.*, Loss-of-function of an *N*-acetylglucosaminyltransferase, POMGnT1, in muscle-eye-brain disease. *Biochem. Biophys. Res. Commun.* **306**:1 (2003), 93–97.
7. A. Yoshida, K. Kobayashi, H. Manya, K. Taniguchi, H. Kano, M. Mizuno, *et al.*, Muscular dystrophy and neuronal migration disorder caused by mutations in a glycosyltransferase, POMGnT1. *Dev. Cell.* **1**:5 (2001), 717–724.
8. L. Aravind, E. V. Koonin, The fukutin protein family – predicted enzymes modifying cell-surface molecules. *Curr. Biol.* **9**:22 (1999), R836–R837.
9. R. Barresi, D. E. Michele, M. Kanagawa, H. A. Harper, S. A. Dovico, J. S. Satz, *et al.*, LARGE can functionally bypass alpha-dystroglycan glycosylation defects in distinct congenital muscular dystrophies. *Nat. Med.* **10**:7 (2004), 696–703.
10. M. Brockington, S. Torelli, P. Prandini, C. Boito, N. F. Dolatshad, C. Longman, *et al.*, Localization and functional analysis of the LARGE family of glycosyltransferases: significance for muscular dystrophy. *Hum. Mol. Genet.* **14**:5 (2005), 657–665.
11. C. Longman, M. Brockington, S. Torelli, C. Jimenez-Mallebrera, C. Kennedy, N. Khalil, *et al.*, Mutations in the human LARGE gene cause MDC1D, a novel form of congenital muscular dystrophy with severe mental retardation and abnormal glycosylation of alpha-dystroglycan. *Hum. Mol. Genet.* **12**:21 (2003), 2853–2861.
12. C. Godfrey, E. Clement, R. Mein, M. Brockington, J. Smith, B. Talim, *et al.*, Refining genotype phenotype correlations in muscular dystrophies with defective glycosylation of dystroglycan. *Brain* **130** (2007), 2725–2735.
13. J. van Reeuwijk, P. K. Grewal, M. A. Salih, D. Beltran-Valero de Bernabe, J. M. McLaughlan, C. B. Michielse, *et al.*, Intragenic deletion in the LARGE gene causes Walker-Warburg syndrome. *Hum. Genet.* **121**:6 (2007), 685–690.
14. D. B. Beltran-Valero, T. Voit, C. Longman, A. Steinbrecher, V. Straub, Y. Yuva, *et al.*, Mutations in the FKRP gene can cause muscle-eye-brain disease and Walker-Warburg syndrome. *J. Med. Genet.* **41**:5 (2004), e61.
15. N. Louhichi, C. Triki, S. Quijano-Roy, P. Richard, S. Makri, M. Meziou, *et al.*, New FKRP mutations causing congenital muscular dystrophy associated with mental retardation and central nervous system abnormalities. Identification of a founder mutation in Tunisian families. *Neurogenetics* **5**:1 (2004), 27–34.
16. E. Mercuri, H. Topaloglu, M. Brockington, A. Berardinelli, A. Pichiecchio, F. Santorelli, *et al.*, Spectrum of brain changes in patients with congenital muscular dystrophy and FKRP gene mutations. *Arch Neurol.* **63**:2 (2006), 251–257.
17. H. Topaloglu, M. Brockington, Y. Yuva, B. Talim, G. Haliloglu, D. Blake, *et al.*, FKRP gene mutations cause congenital muscular dystrophy, mental retardation, and cerebellar cysts. *Neurology* **60**:6 (2003), 988–992.
18. P. D. Cote, H. Moukhles, M. Lindenbaum, S. Carbonetto, Chimaeric mice deficient in dystroglycans develop muscular dystrophy and have disrupted myoneural synapses. *Nat. Genet.* **23**:3 (1999), 338–342.
19. S. A. Moore, F. Saito, J. Chen, D. E. Michele, M. D. Henry, A. Messing, *et al.*, Deletion of brain dystroglycan recapitulates aspects of congenital muscular dystrophy. *Nature* **418**:6896 (2002), 422–425.
20. S. Takeda, M. Kondo, J. Sasaki, H. Kurahashi, H. Kano, K. Arai, *et al.*, Fukutin is required for maintenance of muscle integrity, cortical histiogenesis and normal eye development. *Hum. Mol. Genet.* **12**:12 (2003), 1449–1459.
21. T. Willer, B. Prados, J. M. Falcon-Perez, I. Renner-Muller, G. K. Przemeck, M. Lommel, *et al.*, Targeted disruption of the Walker-Warburg syndrome gene Pomt1 in mouse results in embryonic lethality. *Proc. Natl. Acad. Sci. U. S. A.* **101**:39 (2004), 14126–14131.
22. R. A. Williamson, M. D. Henry, K. J. Daniels, R. F. Hrstka, J. C. Lee, Y. Sunada, *et al.*, Dystroglycan is essential for early embryonic development: disruption of Reichert's membrane in Dag1-null mice. *Hum. Mol. Genet.* **6**:6 (1997), 831–841.
23. T. Chiyonobu, J. Sasaki, Y. Nagai, S. Takeda, H. Funakoshi, T. Nakamura, *et al.*, Effects of fukutin deficiency in the developing mouse brain. *Neuromuscul. Disord.* **15**:6 (2005), 416–426.

24. F. Saito, T. Masaki, Y. Saito, A. Nakamura, S. Takeda, T. Shimizu, *et al.*, Defective peripheral nerve myelination and neuromuscular junction formation in fukutin-deficient chimeric mice. *J. Neurochem.* **101**:6 (2007), 1712–1722.

25. P. J. Holzfeind, P. K. Grewal, H. A. Reitsamer, J. Kechvar, H. Lassmann, H. Hoeger, *et al.*, Skeletal, cardiac and tongue muscle pathology, defective retinal transmission, and neuronal migration defects in the Large(myd) mouse defines a natural model for glycosylation-deficient muscle–eye–brain disorders. *Hum. Mol. Genet.* **11**:21 (2002), 2673–2687.

26. P. K. Grewal, P. J. Holzfeind, R. E. Bittner, J. E. Hewitt, Mutant glycosyltransferase and altered glycosylation of alpha-dystroglycan in the myodystrophy mouse. *Nat. Genet.* **28**:2 (2001), 151–154.

27. J. Liu, S. L. Ball, Y. Yang, P. Mei, L. Zhang, H. Shi, *et al.*, A genetic model for muscle-eye-brain disease in mice lacking protein O-mannose 1,2-N-acetylglucosaminyltransferase (POMGnT1). *Mech. Dev.* **123**:3 (2006), 228–240.

28. E. M. McNally, C. T. Ly, L. M. Kunkel, Human epsilon-sarcoglycan is highly related to alpha-sarcoglycan (adhalin), the limb girdle muscular dystrophy 2D gene. *FEBS Lett.* **422**:1 (1998), 27–32.

29. M. Imamura, Y. Mochizuki, E. Engvall, S. Takeda, Epsilon-sarcoglycan compensates for lack of alpha-sarcoglycan in a mouse model of limb-girdle muscular dystrophy. *Hum. Mol. Genet.* **14**:6 (2005), 775–783.

30. K. Shiga, H. Yoshioka, T. Matsumiya, I. Kimura, S. Takeda, M. Imamura, zeta-sarcoglycan is a functional homologue of gamma-sarcoglycan in the formation of the sarcoglycan complex. *Exp. Cell Res.* **312**:11 (2006), 2083–2092.

31. G. E. Crawford, J. A. Faulkner, R. H. Crosbie, K. P. Campbell, S. C. Froehner, J. S. Chamberlain, Assembly of the dystrophin-associated protein complex does not require the dystrophin COOH-terminal domain. *J. Cell. Biol.* **150**:6 (2000), 1399–1410.

32. R. H. Crosbie, L. E. Lim, S. A. Moore, M. Hirano, A. P. Hays, S. W. Maybaum, *et al.*, Molecular and genetic characterization of sarcospan: insights into sarcoglycan-sarcospan interactions. *Hum. Mol. Genet.* **9**:13 (2000), 2019–2027.

33. R. H. Crosbie, R. Barresi, K. P. Campbell, Loss of sarcolemma nNOS in sarcoglycan-deficient muscle. *FASEB J.* **16**:13 (2002), 1786–1791.

34. T. Yoshida, Y. Pan, H. Hanada, Y. Iwata, M. Shigekawa, Bidirectional signaling between sarcoglycans and the integrin adhesion system in cultured L6 myocytes. *J. Biol. Chem.* **273**:3 (1998), 1583–1590.

35. T. G. Thompson, Y. M. Chan, A. A. Hack, M. Brosius, M. Rajala, H. G. Lidov, *et al.*, Filamin 2 (FLN2): a muscle-specific sarcoglycan interacting protein. *J. Cell. Biol.* **148**:1 (2000), 115–126.

36. A. A. Hack, M. E. Groh, E. M. McNally, Sarcoglycans in muscular dystrophy. *Microsc. Res. Tech.* **48**:3–4 (2000), 167–180.

37. A. A. Hack, M. Y. Lam, L. Cordier, D. I. Shoturma, C. T. Ly, M. A. Hadhazy, *et al.*, Differential requirement for individual sarcoglycans and dystrophin in the assembly and function of the dystrophin-glycoprotein complex. *J. Cell Sci.* **113**:Pt 14 (2000), 2535–2544.

38. K. Kobuke, F. Piccolo, K. W. Garringer, S. A. Moore, E. Sweezer, B. Yang, *et al.*, A common disease-associated missense mutation in alpha-sarcoglycan fails to cause muscular dystrophy in mice. *Hum. Mol. Genet.* **17**:9 (2008), 1201–1213.

39. C. S. Lebakken, D. P. Venzke, R. F. Hrstka, C. M. Consolino, J. A. Faulkner, R. A. Williamson, *et al.*, Sarcospan-deficient mice maintain normal muscle function. *Mol. Cell. Biol.* **20**:5 (2000), 1669–1677.

40. A. K. Peter, G. Miller, R. H. Crosbie, Disrupted mechanical stability of the dystrophin-glycoprotein complex causes severe muscular dystrophy in sarcospan transgenic mice. *J. Cell Sci.* **120**: Pt 6 (2007), 996–1008.

41. M. Neri, S. Torelli, S. Brown, I. Ugo, P. Sabatelli, L. Merlini, *et al.*, Dystrophin levels as low as 30% are sufficient to avoid muscular dystrophy in the human. *Neuromuscul. Disord.* **17**:11–12 (2007), 913–918.

42. F. Muntoni, M. A. Melis, A. Ganau, V. Dubowitz, Transcription of the dystrophin gene in normal tissues and in skeletal muscle of a family with X-linked dilated cardiomyopathy. *Am. J. Hum. Genet.* **56**:1 (1995), 151–157.

43. S. A. Oak, Y. W. Zhou, H. W. Jarrett, Skeletal muscle signaling pathway through the dystrophin glycoprotein complex and Rac1. *J. Biol. Chem.* **278**:41 (2003), 39287–39295.

44. S. A. Oak, K. Russo, T. C. Petrucci, H. W. Jarrett, Mouse alpha1-syntrophin binding to Grb2: further evidence of a role for syntrophin in cell signalling. *Biochemistry* **40**:37 (2001), 11270–11278.

45. H. J. Spence, A. S. Dhillon, M. James, S. J. Winder, Dystroglycan, a scaffold for the ERK-MAP kinase cascade. *EMBO Rep.* **5**:5 (2004), 484–489.

46. Y. W. Zhou, D. B. Thomason, D. Gullberg, H. W. Jarrett, Binding of laminin alpha1-chain LG4–5 domain to alpha-dystroglycan causes tyrosine phosphorylation of syntrophin to initiate Rac1 signaling. *Biochemistry* **45**:7 (2006), 2042–2052.

47. Y. Zhou, D. Jiang, D. B. Thomason, H. W. Jarrett, Laminin-induced activation of Rac1 and JNKp46 is initiated by Src family kinases and mimics the effects of skeletal muscle contraction. *Biochemistry* **46**:51 (2007), 14907–14916.

48. A. E. Emery, Population frequencies of inherited neuromuscular diseases – a world survey. *Neuromuscul. Disord.* **1**:1 (1991), 19–29.

49. D. J. Wells, K. E. Wells, What do animal models have to tell us regarding Duchenne muscular dystrophy? *Acta Myol.* **24**:3 (2005), 172–180.

50. C. E. Ambrosio, M. C. Valadares, E. Zucconi, R. Cabral, P. L. Pearson, T. P. Gaiad, *et al.*, Ringo, a Golden Retriever Muscular Dystrophy (GRMD) dog with absent dystrophin but normal strength. *Neuromuscul. Disord.* **18**:11 (2008), 892–893.

51. M. L. Rees, C. F. Lien, D. C. Gorecki, Dystrobrevins in muscle and non-muscle tissues. *Neuromuscul. Disord.* **17**:2 (2007), 123–134.

52. D. J. Blake, Dystrobrevin dynamics in muscle-cell signalling: a possible target for therapeutic intervention in Duchenne muscular dystrophy? *Neuromuscul. Disord.* **12** Suppl 1(2002), S110–S117.

53. R. M. Grady, R. W. Grange, K. S. Lau, M. M. Maimone, M. C. Nichol, J. T. Stull, *et al.*, Role for alpha-dystrobrevin in the pathogenesis of dystrophin-dependent muscular dystrophies. *Nat. Cell Biol.* **1**:4 (1999), 215–220.

54. T. M. Bunnell, M. A. Jaeger, D. P. Fitzsimons, K. W. Prins, J. M. Ervasti, Destabilization of the dystrophin-glycoprotein complex without functional deficits in alpha-dystrobrevin null muscle. *PLoS ONE* **3**:7 (2008), e2604.

55. A. Vandebrouck, J. Sabourin, J. Rivet, H. Balghi, S. Sebille, A. Kitzis, *et al.*, Regulation of capacitative calcium entries by alpha1-syntrophin: association of TRPC1 with dystrophin complex and the PDZ domain of alpha1-syntrophin. *FASEB J.* **21**:2 (2007), 608–617.

56. K. Ueda, C. Valdivia, A. Medeiros-Domingo, D. J. Tester, M. Vatta, G. Farrugia, *et al.*, Syntrophin mutation associated with long QT syndrome through activation of the nNOS-SCN5A macromolecular complex. *Proc. Natl. Acad. Sci. U. S. A.* **105**:27 (2008), 9355–9360.

57. M. E. Adams, N. Kramarcy, S. P. Krall, S. G. Rossi, R. L. Rotundo, R. Sealock, *et al.*, Absence of alpha-syntrophin leads to structurally aberrant neuromuscular synapses deficient in utrophin. *J. Cell. Biol.* **150**:6 (2000), 1385–1398.

58. M. E. Adams, N. Kramarcy, T. Fukuda, A. G. Engel, R. Sealock, S. C. Froehner, Structural abnormalities at neuromuscular synapses lacking multiple syntrophin isoforms. *J. Neurosci.* **24**:46 (2004), 10302–10309.

59. D. S. Bredt, Knocking signalling out of the dystrophin complex. *Nat. Cell Biol.* **1**:4 (1999), E89–E91.

60. A. Clerk, G. E. Morris, V. Dubowitz, K. E. Davies, C. A. Sewry, Dystrophin-related protein, utrophin, in normal and dystrophic human fetal skeletal muscle. *Histochem. J.* **25**:8 (1993), 554–561.

61. R. M. Grady, H. Zhou, J. M. Cunningham, M. D. Henry, K. P. Campbell, J. R. Sanes, Maturation and maintenance of the neuromuscular synapse: genetic evidence for roles of the dystrophin–glycoprotein complex. *Neuron* **25**:2 (2000), 279–293.

62. Y. Li, J. Huang, Y. L. Zhao, J. He, W. Wang, K. E. Davies, *et al.*, UTRN on chromosome 6q24 is mutated in multiple tumors. *Oncogene* **26**:42 (2007), 6220–6228.

63. A. P. Weir, E. A. Burton, G. Harrod, K. E. Davies, A- and B-utrophin have different expression patterns and are differentially up-regulated in mdx muscle. *J. Biol. Chem.* **277**:47 (2002), 45285–45290.

64. P. Miura, B. J. Jasmin, Utrophin upregulation for treating Duchenne or Becker muscular dystrophy: how close are we? *Trends Mol. Med.* **12**:3 (2006), 122–129.

65. T. O. Krag, S. Bogdanovich, C. J. Jensen, M. D. Fischer, J. Hansen-Schwartz, E. H. Javazon, *et al.*, Heregulin ameliorates the dystrophic phenotype in mdx mice. *Proc. Natl. Acad. Sci. U. S. A.* **101**:38 (2004), 13856–13860.

66. A. E. Deconinck, A. C. Potter, J. M. Tinsley, S. J. Wood, R. Vater, C. Young, *et al.*, Postsynaptic abnormalities at the neuromuscular junctions of utrophin-deficient mice. *J. Cell. Biol.* **136**:4 (1997), 883–894.

67. E. Pegoraro, F. Cepollaro, P. Prandini, A. Marin, M. Fanin, C. P. Trevisan, *et al.*, Integrin alpha 7 beta 1 in muscular dystrophy/myopathy of unknown etiology. *Am. J. Pathol.* **160**:6 (2002), 2135–2143.

68. Y. K. Hayashi, F. L. Chou, E. Engvall, M. Ogawa, C. Matsuda, S. Hirabayashi, *et al.*, Mutations in the integrin alpha7 gene cause congenital myopathy. *Nat. Genet.* **19**:1 (1998), 94–97.

69. U. Mayer, G. Saher, R. Fassler, A. Bornemann, F. Echtermeyer, K. von der Mark, *et al.*, Absence of integrin alpha 7 causes a novel form of muscular dystrophy. *Nat. Genet.* **17**:3 (1997), 318–323.

70. U. Mayer, Integrins: redundant or important players in skeletal muscle? *J. Biol. Chem.* **278**:17 (2003), 14587–14590.

71. D. J. Burkin, G. Q. Wallace, K. J. Nicol, D. J. Kaufman, S. J. Kaufman, Enhanced expression of the alpha 7 beta 1 integrin reduces muscular dystrophy and restores viability in dystrophic mice. *J. Cell. Biol.* **152**:6 (2001), 1207–1218.

72. S. Lin, L. Landmann, M. A. Ruegg, H. R. Brenner, The role of nerve- versus muscle-derived factors in mammalian neuromuscular junction formation. *J. Neurosci.* **28**:13 (2008), 3333–3340.

73. G. S. Bewick, L. V. Nicholson, C. Young, E. O'Donnell, C. R. Slater, Different distributions of dystrophin and related proteins at nerve-muscle junctions. *Neuroreport* **3**:10 (1992), 857–860.

74. R. Sealock, M. H. Butler, N. R. Kramarcy, K. X. Gao, A. A. Murnane, K. Douville, *et al.*, Localization of dystrophin relative to acetylcholine receptor domains in electric tissue and adult and cultured skeletal muscle. *J. Cell. Biol.* **113**:5 (1991), 1133–1144.

75. S. J. Wood, C. R. Slater, Safety factor at the neuromuscular junction. *Prog. Neurobiol.* **64**:4 (2001), 393–429.

76. D. Beeson, R. Webster, J. Cossins, D. Lashley, H. Spearman, S. Maxwell, *et al.*, Congenital myasthenic syndromes and the formation of the neuromuscular junction. *Ann. N. Y. Acad. Sci.* **1132** (2008), 99–103.

77. F. Chevessier, B. Faraut, A. Ravel-Chapuis, P. Richard, K. Gaudon, S. Bauche, *et al.*, MUSK, a new target for mutations causing congenital myasthenic syndrome. *Hum. Mol. Genet.* **13**:24 (2004), 3229–3240.

78. J. Palace, D. Lashley, J. Newsom-Davis, J. Cossins, S. Maxwell, R. Kennett, *et al.*, Clinical features of the DOK7 neuromuscular junction synaptopathy. *Brain* **130**:Pt 6 (2007), 1507–1515.

79. C. R. Slater, P. R. Fawcett, T. J. Walls, P. R. Lyons, S. J. Bailey, D. Beeson, *et al.*, Pre- and post-synaptic abnormalities associated with impaired neuromuscular transmission in a group of patients with 'limb-girdle myasthenia'. *Brain* **129**:Pt 8 (2006), 2061–2076.

80. D. Selcen, M. Milone, X. M. Shen, C. M. Harper, A. A. Stans, E. D. Wieben, *et al.*, Dok-7 myasthenia: phenotypic and molecular genetic studies in 16 patients. *Ann. Neurol.* **64**:1 (2008), 71–87.

81. J. Hamuro, O. Higuchi, K. Okada, M. Ueno, S. Iemura, T. Natsume, *et al.*, Mutations causing DOK7 congenital myasthenia ablate functional motifs in Dok-7. *J. Biol. Chem.* **283**:9 (2008), 5518–5524.

82. R. L. Ruff, V. A. Lennon, How myasthenia gravis alters the safety factor for neuromuscular transmission. *J. Neuroimmunol.* **201–202** (2008), 13–20.

83. R. N. Cole, S. W. Reddel, O. L. Gervasio, W. D. Phillips, Anti-MuSK patient antibodies disrupt the mouse neuromuscular junction. *Ann. Neurol.* **63**:6 (2008), 782–789.

84. C. Jimenez-Mallebrera, S. C. Brown, C. A. Sewry, F. Muntoni, Congenital muscular dystrophy: molecular and cellular aspects. *Cell. Mol. Life Sci.* **62**:7–8 (2005), 809–823.

85. J. R. Sanes, The basement membrane/basal lamina of skeletal muscle. *J. Biol. Chem.* **278**:15 (2003), 12601–12604.

86. S. Petrini, A. D'Amico, P. Sale, L. Lucarini, P. Sabatelli, A. Tessa, *et al.*, Ullrich myopathy phenotype with secondary ColVI defect identified by confocal imaging and electron microscopy analysis. *Neuromuscul. Disord.* **17**:8 (2007), 587–596.

87. R. A. Peat, J. M. Smith, A. G. Compton, N. L. Baker, R. A. Pace, D. J. Burkin, *et al.*, Diagnosis and etiology of congenital muscular dystrophy. *Neurology* **71**:5 (2008), 312–321.

88. R. A. Peat, N. L. Baker, K. J. Jones, K. N. North, S. R. Lamande, Variable penetrance of COL6A1 null mutations: implications for prenatal diagnosis and genetic counselling in Ullrich congenital muscular dystrophy families. *Neuromuscul. Disord.* **17**:7 (2007), 547–557.

89. D. Hicks, A. K. Lampe, R. Barresi, R. Charlton, C. Fiorillo, C. G. Bonnemann, *et al.*, A refined diagnostic algorithm for Bethlem myopathy. *Neurology* **70**:14 (2008), 1192–1199.

90. S. Petrini, A. Tessa, W. B. Stallcup, P. Sabatelli, M. Pescatori, B. Giusti, *et al.*, Altered expression of the MCSP/NG2 chondroitin sulfate proteoglycan in collagen VI deficiency. *Mol. Cell. Neurosci.* **30**:3 (2005), 408–417.

91. E. Mercuri, Y. Yuva, S. C. Brown, M. Brockington, M. Kinali, H. Jungbluth, *et al.*, Collagen VI involvement in Ullrich syndrome: a clinical, genetic, and immunohistochemical study. *Neurology* **58**:9 (2002), 1354–1359.

92. C. Jimenez-Mallebrera, M. A. Maioli, J. Kim, S. C. Brown, L. Feng, A. K. Lampe, *et al.*, A comparative analysis of collagen VI production in muscle, skin and fibroblasts from 14 Ullrich congenital muscular dystrophy patients with dominant and recessive COL6A mutations. *Neuromuscul. Disord.* **16**:9–10 (2006), 571–582.

93. A. K. Lampe, K. M. Bushby, Collagen VI related muscle disorders. *J. Med. Genet.* **42**:9 (2005), 673–685.

94. S. R. Lamande, M. Morgelin, C. Selan, G. J. Jobsis, F. Baas, J. F. Bateman, Kinked collagen VI tetramers and reduced microfibril formation as a result of Bethlem myopathy and introduced triple helical glycine mutations. *J. Biol. Chem.* **277**:3 (2002), 1949–1956.

95. G. Pepe, B. Giusti, E. Bertini, T. Brunelli, B. Saitta, P. Comeglio, *et al.*, A heterozygous splice site mutation in COL6A1 leading to an in-frame deletion of the alpha1(VI) collagen chain in an Italian family affected by Bethlem myopathy. *Biochem. Biophys. Res. Commun.* **258**:3 (1999), 802–807.

96. T. C. Pan, R. Z. Zhang, D. G. Sudano, S. K. Marie, C. G. Bonnemann, M. L. Chu, New molecular mechanism for Ullrich congenital muscular dystrophy: a heterozygous in-frame deletion in the COL6A1 gene causes a severe phenotype. *Am. J. Hum. Genet.* **73**:2 (2003), 355–369.

97. N. L. Baker, M. Morgelin, R. A. Pace, R. A. Peat, N. E. Adams, R. J. Gardner, *et al.*, Molecular consequences of dominant Bethlem myopathy collagen VI mutations. *Ann. Neurol.* **62**:4 (2007), 390–405.

98. P. Sabatelli, P. Bonaldo, G. Lattanzi, P. Braghetta, N. Bergamin, C. Capanni, *et al.*, Collagen VI deficiency affects the organization of fibronectin in the extracellular matrix of cultured fibroblasts. *Matrix Biol.* **20**:7 (2001), 475–486.

99. Y. Zou, R. Z. Zhang, P. Sabatelli, M. L. Chu, C. G. Bonnemann, Muscle interstitial fibroblasts are the main source of collagen VI synthesis in skeletal muscle: implications for congenital muscular dystrophy types Ullrich and Bethlem. *J. Neuropathol. Exp. Neurol.* **67**:2 (2008), 144–154.

100. W. A. Irwin, N. Bergamin, P. Sabatelli, C. Reggiani, A. Megighian, L. Merlini, *et al.*, Mitochondrial dysfunction and apoptosis in myopathic mice with collagen VI deficiency. *Nat. Genet.* **35**:4 (2003), 367–371.

101. L. Merlini, A. Angelin, T. Tiepolo, P. Braghetta, P. Sabatelli, A. Zamparelli, *et al.*, Cyclosporin A corrects mitochondrial dysfunction and muscle apoptosis in patients with collagen VI myopathies. *Proc. Natl. Acad. Sci. U. S. A.* **105**:13 (2008), 5225–5229.

102. M. Aumailley, L. Bruckner-Tuderman, W. G. Carter, R. Deutzmann, D. Edgar, P. Ekblom, *et al.*, A simplified laminin nomenclature. *Matrix Biol.* **24**:5 (2005), 326–332.

103. H. Colognato, D. A. Winkelmann, P. D. Yurchenco, Laminin polymerization induces a receptor-cytoskeleton network. *J. Cell. Biol.* **145**:3 (1999), 619–631.

104. P. D. Yurchenco, Y. S. Cheng, K. Campbell, S. Li, Loss of basement membrane, receptor and cytoskeletal lattices in a laminin-deficient muscular dystrophy. *J. Cell Sci.* **11**:Pt 5 (2004), 735–742.

105. A. M. Michelson, E. S. Russell, P. J. Harman, Dystrophia muscularis: a hereditary primary myopathy in the house mouse. *Proc. Natl. Acad. Sci. U. S. A.* **41**:12 (1955), 1079–1084.

106. H. Meier, J. L. Southard, Muscular dystrophy in the mouse caused by an allele at the dy-locus. *Life Sci.* **9**:3 (1970), 137–144.

107. Y. Miyagoe, K. Hanaoka, I. Nonaka, M. Hayasaka, Y. Nabeshima, K. Arahata, *et al.*, Laminin alpha2 chain-null mutant mice by targeted disruption of the Lama2 gene: a new model of merosin (laminin 2)-deficient congenital muscular dystrophy. *FEBS Lett.* **415**:1 (1997), 33–39.

108. W. Kuang, H. Xu, P. H. Vachon, L. Liu, F. Loechel, U. M. Wewer, *et al.*, Merosin-deficient congenital muscular dystrophy. Partial genetic correction in two mouse models. *J. Clin. Invest.* **102**:4 (1998), 844–852.

109. S. Besse, V. Allamand, J. T. Vilquin, Z. Li, C. Poirier, N. Vignier, *et al.*, Spontaneous muscular dystrophy caused by a retrotransposal insertion in the mouse laminin alpha2 chain gene. *Neuromuscul. Disord.* **13**:3 (2003), 216–222.

110. V. Straub, J. A. Rafael, J. S. Chamberlain, K. P. Campbell, Animal models for muscular dystrophy show different patterns of sarcolemmal disruption. *J. Cell. Biol.* **139**:2 (1997), 375–385.

111. J. Moll, P. Barzaghi, S. Lin, G. Bezakova, H. Lochmuller, E. Engvall, *et al.*, An agrin minigene rescues dystrophic symptoms in a mouse model for congenital muscular dystrophy. *Nature* **413**:6853 (2001), 302–307.

112. C. F. Bentzinger, P. Barzaghi, S. Lin, M. A. Ruegg, Overexpression of mini-agrin in skeletal muscle increases muscle integrity and regenerative capacity in laminin-alpha2-deficient mice. *FASEB J.* **19**:8 (2005), 934–942.

113. M. Stum, E. Girard, M. Bangratz, V. Bernard, M. Herbin, A. Vignaud, *et al.*, Evidence of a dosage effect and a physiological endplate acetylcholinesterase deficiency in the first mouse models mimicking Schwartz-Jampel syndrome neuromyotonia. *Hum. Mol. Genet.* **17**:20 (2008), 165–181.

114. G. Bezakova, M. A. Ruegg, New insights into the roles of agrin. *Nat. Rev. Mol. Cell. Biol.* **4**:4 (2003), 295–308.

115. G. Bezakova, T. Lomo, Muscle activity and muscle agrin regulate the organization of cytoskeletal proteins and attached acetylcholine receptor (AchR) aggregates in skeletal muscle fibers. *J. Cell. Biol.* **153**:7 (2001), 1453–1463.

116. S. Meinen, P. Barzaghi, S. Lin, H. Lochmuller, M. A. Ruegg, Linker molecules between laminins and dystroglycan ameliorate laminin-alpha2-deficient muscular dystrophy at all disease stages. *J. Cell. Biol.* **176**:7 (2007), 979–993.

117. J. J. Dowling, E. M. Gibbs, E. L. Feldman, Membrane traffic and muscle: lessons from human disease. *Traffic* **9**:7 (2008), 1035–1043.

118. K. M. Bushby, Dysferlin and muscular dystrophy. *Acta Neurol. Belg.* **100**:3 (2000), 142–145.

119. R. Han, K. P. Campbell, Dysferlin and muscle membrane repair. *Curr. Opin. Cell. Biol.* **19**:4 (2007), 409–416.

120. D. Selcen, G. Stilling, A. G. Engel, The earliest pathologic alterations in dysferlinopathy. *Neurology* **56**:11 (2001), 1472–1481.

121. G. Cenacchi, M. Fanin, L. B. Giorgi, C. De Angelini, Ultrastructural changes in dysferlinopathy support defective membrane repair mechanism. *J. Clin. Pathol.* **58**:2 (2005), 190–195.

122. R. E. Bittner, L. V. Anderson, E. Burkhardt, R. Bashir, E. Vafiadaki, S. Ivanova, *et al.*, Dysferlin deletion in SJL mice (SJL-Dysf) defines a natural model for limb girdle muscular dystrophy 2B. *Nat. Genet.* **23**:2 (1999), 141–142.

123. D. Bansal, K. Miyake, S. S. Vogel, S. Groh, C. C. Chen, R. Williamson, *et al.*, Defective membrane repair in dysferlin-deficient muscular dystrophy. *Nature* **423**:6936 (2003), 168–172.

124. M. Ho, C. M. Post, L. R. Donahue, H. G. Lidov, R. T. Bronson, H. Goolsby, *et al.*, Disruption of muscle membrane and phenotype divergence in two novel mouse models of dysferlin deficiency. *Hum. Mol. Genet.* **13**:18 (2004), 1999–2010.

125. R. Han, D. Bansal, K. Miyake, V. P. Muniz, R. M. Weiss, P. L. McNeil, *et al.*, Dysferlin-mediated membrane repair protects the heart from stress-induced left ventricular injury. *J. Clin. Invest.* **117**:7 (2007), 1805–1813.

126. R. H. Crosbie, H. Yamada, D. P. Venzke, M. P. Lisanti, K. P. Campbell, Caveolin-3 is not an integral component of the dystrophin glycoprotein complex. *FEBS Lett.* **427**:2 (1998), 279–282.

127. C. Matsuda, Y. K. Hayashi, M. Ogawa, M. Aoki, K. Murayama, I. Nishino, *et al.*, The sarcolemmal proteins dysferlin and caveolin-3 interact in skeletal muscle. *Hum. Mol. Genet.* **10**:17 (2001), 1761–1766.

128. M. C. Walter, C. Braun, M. Vorgerd, M. Poppe, C. Thirion, C. Schmidt, *et al.*, Variable reduction of caveolin-3 in patients with LGMD2B/MM. *J. Neurol.* **250**:12 (2003), 1431–1438.

129. C. Minetti, F. Sotgia, C. Bruno, P. Scartezzini, P. Broda, M. Bado, *et al.*, Mutations in the caveolin-3 gene cause autosomal dominant limb-girdle muscular dystrophy. *Nat. Genet.* **18**:4 (1998), 365–368.

130. R. Herrmann, V. Straub, M. Blank, C. Kutzick, N. Franke, E. N. Jacob, *et al.*, Dissociation of the dystroglycan complex in caveolin-3-deficient limb girdle muscular dystrophy. *Hum. Mol. Genet.* **9**:15 (2000), 2335–2340.

131. F. Galbiati, D. Volonte, C. Minetti, J. B. Chu, M. P. Lisanti, Phenotypic behavior of caveolin-3 mutations that cause autosomal dominant limb girdle muscular dystrophy (LGMD-1C). Retention of LGMD-1C caveolin-3 mutants within the Golgi complex. *J. Biol. Chem.* **274**:36 (1999), 25632–25641.

132. C. Minetti, M. Bado, P. Broda, F. Sotgia, C. Bruno, F. Galbiati, *et al.*, Impairment of caveolae formation and T-system disorganization in human muscular dystrophy with caveolin-3 deficiency. *Am. J. Pathol.* **160**:1 (2002), 265–270.

133. C. Kubisch, B. G. Schoser, M. von During, R. C. Betz, H. H. Goebel, S. Zahn, *et al.*, Homozygous mutations in caveolin-3 cause a severe form of rippling muscle disease. *Ann. Neurol.* **53**:4 (2003), 512–520.

134. N. G. Laing, Congenital myopathies. *Curr. Opin. Neurol.* **20**:5 (2007), 583–589.

135. C. A. Sewry, C. Jimenez-Mallebrera, F. Muntoni, Congenital myopathies. *Curr. Opin. Neurol.* **21**:5 (2008), 569–575.

136. C. R. Pierson, P. B. Agrawal, J. Blasko, A. H. Beggs, Myofiber size correlates with MTM1 mutation type and outcome in X-linked myotubular myopathy. *Neuromuscul. Disord.* **17**:7 (2007), 562–568.

137. A. Buj-Bello, V. Laugel, N. Messaddeq, H. Zahreddine, J. Laporte, J. F. Pellissier, *et al.*, The lipid phosphatase myotubularin is essential for skeletal muscle maintenance but not for myogenesis in mice. *Proc. Natl. Acad. Sci. U. S. A.* **99**:23 (2002), 15060–15065.

138. M. Bitoun, S. Maugenre, P. Y. Jeannet, E. Lacene, X. Ferrer, P. Laforet, *et al.*, Mutations in dynamin 2 cause dominant centronuclear myopathy. *Nat. Genet.* **37**:11 (2005), 1207–1209.

139. M. Bitoun, J. A. Bevilacqua, B. Prudhon, S. Maugenre, A. L. Taratuto, S. Monges, *et al.*, Dynamin 2 mutations cause sporadic centronuclear myopathy with neonatal onset. *Ann. Neurol.* **62**:6 (2007), 666–670.

140. A. S. Nicot, A. Toussaint, V. Tosch, C. Kretz, C. Wallgren-Pettersson, E. Iwarsson, *et al.*, Mutations in amphiphysin 2 (BIN1) disrupt interaction with dynamin 2 and cause autosomal recessive centronuclear myopathy. *Nat. Genet.* **39**:9 (2007), 1134–1139.

141. E. Lee, M. Marcucci, L. Daniell, M. Pypaert, O. A. Weisz, G. C. Ochoa, *et al.*, Amphiphysin 2 (Bin1) and T-tubule biogenesis in muscle. *Science* **297**:5584 (2002), 1193–1196.

142. A. Razzaq, I. M. Robinson, H. T. McMahon, J. N. Skepper, Y. Su, A. C. Zelhof, *et al.*, Amphiphysin is necessary for organization of the excitation-contraction coupling machinery of muscles, but not for synaptic vesicle endocytosis in Drosophila. *Genes Dev.* **15**:22 (2001), 2967–2979.

143. A. J. Muller, J. F. Baker, J. B. DuHadaway, K. Ge, G. Farmer, P. S. Donover, *et al.*, Targeted disruption of the murine Bin1/Amphiphysin II gene does not disable endocytosis but results in embryonic cardiomyopathy with aberrant myofibril formation. *Mol. Cell. Biol.* **23**:12 (2003), 4295–4306.

144. T. Shintani, D. J. Klionsky, Autophagy in health and disease: a double-edged sword. *Science* **306**:5698 (2004), 990–995.

145. M. C. Malicdan, S. Noguchi, I. Nonaka, P. Saftig, I. Nishino, Lysosomal myopathies: an excessive build-up in autophagosomes is too much to handle. *Neuromuscul. Disord.* **18**:7 (2008), 521–529.

146. N. Kimura, T. Kumamoto, Y. Kawamura, T. Himeno, K. I. Nakamura, H. Ueyama, *et al.*, Expression of autophagy-associated genes in skeletal muscle: an experimental model of chloroquine-induced myopathy. *Pathobiology* **74**:3 (2007), 169–176.

147. R. Benndorf, M. J. Welsh, Shocking degeneration. *Nat. Genet.* **36**:6 (2004), 547–548.

148. Y. Tanaka, G. Guhde, A. Suter, E. L. Eskelinen, D. Hartmann, R. Lullmann-Rauch, *et al.*, Accumulation of autophagic vacuoles and cardiomyopathy in LAMP-2-deficient mice. *Nature* **406**:6798 (2000), 902–906.

149. D. Kaneda, K. Sugie, A. Yamamoto, H. Matsumoto, T. Kato, I. Nonaka, *et al.*, A novel form of autophagic vacuolar myopathy with late-onset and multiorgan involvement. *Neurology* **61**:1 (2003), 128–131.

150. E. Colding-Jorgensen, Phenotypic variability in myotonia congenita. *Muscle Nerve* **32**:1 (2005), 19–34.

151. N. P. Davies, M. G. Hanna, The skeletal muscle channelopathies: basic science, clinical genetics and treatment. *Curr. Opin. Neurol.* **14**:5 (2001), 539–551.

152. G. Andelfinger, A. R. Tapper, R. C. Welch, C. G. Vanoye, A. L. George, Jr., D. W. Benson, KCNJ2 mutation results in Andersen syndrome with sex-specific cardiac and skeletal muscle phenotypes. *Am. J. Hum. Genet.* **71**:3 (2002), 663–668.

153. G. W. Abbott, M. H. Butler, S. Bendahhou, M. C. Dalakas, L. J. Ptacek, S. A. Goldstein, MiRP2 forms potassium channels in skeletal muscle with Kv3.4 and is associated with periodic paralysis. *Cell* **104**:2 (2001), 217–231.

154. K. J. Nowak, C. A. Sewry, C. Navarro, W. Squier, C. Reina, J. R. Ricoy, *et al.*, Nemaline myopathy caused by absence of alpha-skeletal muscle actin. *Ann. Neurol.* **61**:2 (2007), 175–184.

155. A. Domazetovska, B. Ilkovski, S. T. Cooper, M. Ghoddusi, E. C. Hardeman, L. S. Minamide, *et al.*, Mechanisms underlying intranuclear rod formation. *Brain* **130**:Pt 12 (2007), 3275–3284.

156. A. Oldfors, Hereditary myosin myopathies. *Neuromuscul. Disord.* **17**:5 (2007), 355–367.

157. J. Ochala, Thin filament proteins mutations associated with skeletal myopathies: defective regulation of muscle contraction. *J. Mol. Med.* **17**:5 (2008), 355–367.

158. P. B. Agrawal, R. S. Greenleaf, K. K. Tomczak, V. L. Lehtokari, C. Wallgren-Pettersson, W. Wallefeld, *et al.*, Nemaline myopathy with minicores caused by mutation of the CFL2 gene encoding the skeletal muscle actin-binding protein, cofilin-2. *Am. J. Hum. Genet.* **80**:1 (2007), 162–167.

159. N. F. Clarke, H. Kolski, D. E. Dye, E. Lim, R. L. Smith, R. Patel, *et al.*, Mutations in TPM3 are a common cause of congenital fiber type disproportion. *Ann. Neurol.* **63**:3 (2008), 329–337.

160. M. A. Corbett, P. A. Akkari, A. Domazetovska, S. T. Cooper, K. N. North, N. G. Laing, *et al.*, An alpha-tropomyosin mutation alters dimer preference in nemaline myopathy. *Ann. Neurol.* **57**:1 (2005), 42–49.

161. N. G. Laing, More surprises in sarcomeric protein diseases. *Brain* **130**:Pt 6 (2007), 1453–1455.

162. L. Tskhovrebova, J. Trinick, Titin: properties and family relationships. *Nat. Rev. Mol. Cell. Biol.* **4**:9 (2003), 679–689.

163. P. Zou, N. Pinotsis, S. Lange, Y. H. Song, A. Popov, I. Mavridis, *et al.*, Palindromic assembly of the giant muscle protein titin in the sarcomeric Z-disk. *Nature* **439**:7073 (2006), 229–233.

164. C. Geier, K. Gehmlich, E. Ehler, S. Hassfeld, A. Perrot, K. Hayess, *et al.*, Beyond the sarcomere: CSRP3 mutations cause hypertrophic cardiomyopathy. *Hum. Mol. Genet.* **17**:18 (2008), 2753–2765.

165. K. Ojima, Y. Ono, S. Hata, S. Koyama, N. Doi, H. Sorimachi, Possible functions of p94 in connectin-mediated signaling pathways in skeletal muscle cells. *J. Muscle Res. Cell Motil.* **26**:6–8 (2005), 409–417.

166. A. Fukuzawa, S. Lange, M. Holt, A. Vihola, V. Carmignac, A. Ferreiro, *et al.*, Interactions with titin and myomesin target obscurin and obscurin-like 1 to the M-band – implications for hereditary myopathies. *J. Cell Sci.* **121**:Pt 11 (2008), 1841–1851.

167. S. M. Garvey, C. Rajan, A. P. Lerner, W. N. Frankel, G. A. Cox, The muscular dystrophy with myositis (mdm) mouse mutation disrupts a skeletal muscle-specific domain of titin. *Genomics* **79**:2 (2002), 146–149.

168. S. Lange, F. Xiang, A. Yakovenko, A. Vihola, P. Hackman, E. Rostkova, *et al.*, The kinase domain of titin controls muscle gene expression and protein turnover. *Science* **308**:5728 (2005), 1599–1603.

169. S. Weinert, N. Bergmann, X. Luo, B. Erdmann, M. Gotthardt, M line-deficient titin causes cardiac lethality through impaired maturation of the sarcomere. *J. Cell. Biol.* **173**:4 (2006), 559–570.

170. C. C. Witt, Y. Ono, E. Puschmann, M. McNabb, Y. Wu, M. Gotthardt, *et al.*, Induction and myofibrillar targeting of CARP, and suppression of the Nkx2.5 pathway in the MDM mouse with impaired titin-based signalling. *J. Mol. Biol.* **336**:1 (2004), 145–154.

171. N. G. Laing, K. J. Nowak, When contractile proteins go bad: the sarcomele and skeletal muscle disease. *Bioessays.* **27**:8 (2005), 809–822.

172. K. A. Clark, A. S. McElhinny, M. C. Beckerle, C. C. Gregorio, Striated muscle cytoarchitecture: an intricate web of form and function. *Annu. Rev. Cell. Dev. Biol.* **18** (2002), 637–706.

173. J. Reimann, W. S. Kunz, S. Vielhaber, K. Kappes-Horn, R. Schroder, Mitochondrial dysfunction in myofibrillar myopathy. *Neuropathol. Appl. Neurobiol.* **29**:1 (2003), 45–51.

174. M. Olivé, F. W. van Leeuwen, A. Janué, D. Moreno, B. Torrejon-Escribano, I. Ferrer, Expression of mutant ubiquitin (UBB+1) and p62 in myotilinopathies and desminopathies. *Neuropathol. Appl. Neurobiol.* **34**:1 (2008), 76–87.

175. K. J. Sonnemann, D. P. Fitzsimons, J. R. Patel, Y. Liu, M. F. Schneider, R. L. Moss, *et al.*, Cytoplasmic gamma-actin is not required for skeletal muscle development but its absence leads to a progressive myopathy. *Dev. Cell.* **11**:3 (2006), 387–397.

176. J. M. Ervasti, Costameres: the Achilles' heel of Herculean muscle. *J. Biol. Chem.* **278**:16 (2003), 13591–13594.

177. D. Paulin, Z. Li, Desmin: a major intermediate filament protein essential for the structural integrity and function of muscle. *Exp. Cell Res.* **301**:1 (2004), 1–7.

178. K. G. Claeys, M. Fardeau, R. Schroder, T. Suominen, K. Tolksdorf, A. Behin, *et al.*, Electron microscopy in myofibrillar myopathies reveals clues to the mutated gene. *Neuromuscul. Disord.* **18**:8 (2008), 656–666.

179. J. R. McMillan, M. Akiyama, F. Rouan, J. E. Mellerio, E. B. Lane, I. M. Leigh, *et al.*, Plectin defects in epidermolysis bullosa simplex with muscular dystrophy. *Muscle Nerve* **35**:1 (2007), 24–35.

180. T. Foroud, N. Pankratz, A. P. Batchman, M. W. Pauciulo, R. Vidal, L. Miravalle, *et al.*, A mutation in myotilin causes spheroid body myopathy. *Neurology* **65**:12 (2005), 1936–1940.

181. R. Schroder, J. Reimann, P. Salmikangas, C. S. Clemen, Y. K. Hayashi, I. Nonaka, *et al.*, Beyond LGMD1A: myotilin is a component of central core lesions and nemaline rods. *Neuromuscul. Disord.* **13**:6 (2003), 451–455.

182. M. A. Hauser, C. B. Conde, V. Kowaljow, G. Zeppa, A. L. Taratuto, U. M. Torian, *et al.*, Myotilin mutation found in second pedigree with LGMD1A. *Am. J. Hum. Genet.* **71**:6 (2002), 1428–1432.

183. D. Selcen, K. Ohno, A. G. Engel, Myofibrillar myopathy: clinical, morphological and genetic studies in 63 patients. *Brain* **127**:Pt 2 (2004), 439–451.

184. M. A. Hauser, S. K. Horrigan, P. Salmikangas, U. M. Torian, K. D. Viles, R. Dancel, *et al.*, Myotilin is mutated in limb girdle muscular dystrophy 1A. *Hum. Mol. Genet.* **9**:14 (2000), 2141–2147.

185. M. Olive, L. G. Goldfarb, A. Shatunov, D. Fischer, I. Ferrer, Myotilinopathy: refining the clinical and myopathological phenotype. *Brain* **128**:Pt 10 (2005), 2315–2326.

186. R. A. Kley, Y. Hellenbroich, P. F. van der Ven, D. O. Fürst, A. Huebner, V. Bruchertseifer, *et al.*, Clinical and morphological phenotype of the filamin myopathy: a study of 31 German patients. *Brain* **130**:Pt 12 (2007), 3250–3264.

187. D. Selcen, A. G. Engel, Mutations in ZASP define a novel form of muscular dystrophy in humans. *Ann. Neurol.* **57**:2 (2005), 269–276.

188. Q. Zhou, P. H. Chu, C. Huang, C. F. Cheng, M. E. Martone, G. Knoll, *et al.*, Ablation of Cypher, a PDZ-LIM domain Z-line protein, causes a severe form of congenital myopathy. *J. Cell. Biol.* **155**:4 (2001), 605–612.

189. B. Burke, C. L. Stewart, Life at the edge: the nuclear envelope and human disease. *Nat. Rev. Mol. Cell. Biol.* **3**:8 (2002), 575–585.

190. T. Sullivan, D. Escalante-Alcalde, H. Bhatt, M. Anver, N. Bhat, K. Nagashima, *et al.*, Loss of A-type lamin expression compromises nuclear envelope integrity leading to muscular dystrophy. *J. Cell. Biol.* **147**:5 (1999), 913–920.

191. J. A. Dyer, B. E. Lane, C. J. Hutchison, Investigations of the pathway of incorporation and function of lamin A in the nuclear lamina. *Microsc. Res. Tech.* **45**:1 (1999), 1–12.

192. L. G. Fong, J. K. Ng, J. Lammerding, T. A. Vickers, M. Meta, N. Cote, *et al.*, Prelamin A and lamin A appear to be dispensable in the nuclear lamina. *J. Clin. Invest.* **116**:3 (2006), 743–752.

193. F. D. McKeon, M. W. Kirschner, D. Caput, Homologies in both primary and secondary structure between nuclear envelope and intermediate filament proteins. *Nature* **319**:6053 (1986), 463–468.

194. J. Lammerding, P. C. Schulze, T. Takahashi, S. Kozlov, T. Sullivan, R. D. Kamm, *et al.*, Lamin A/C deficiency causes defective nuclear mechanics and mechanotransduction. *J. Clin. Invest.* **113**:3 (2004), 370–378.

195. J. L. Broers, F. C. Ramaekers, G. Bonne, R. B. Yaou, C. J. Hutchison, Nuclear lamins: laminopathies and their role in premature ageing. *Physiol. Rev.* **86**:3 (2006), 967–1008.

196. K. N. Dahl, S. M. Kahn, K. L. Wilson, D. E. Discher, The nuclear envelope lamina network has elasticity and a compressibility limit suggestive of a molecular shock absorber. *J. Cell Sci.* **117**: Pt 20 (2004), 4779–4786.

197. Y. Gruenbaum, A. Margalit, R. D. Goldman, D. K. Shumaker, K. L. Wilson, The nuclear lamina comes of age. *Nat. Rev. Mol. Cell. Biol.* **6**:1 (2005), 21–31.

198. R. Somech, S. Shaklai, N. Amariglio, G. Rechavi, A. J. Simon, Nuclear envelopathies – raising the nuclear veil. *Pediatr. Res.* **57**:5 Pt 2 (2005), 8R–15R.

199. C. A. Sewry, S. C. Brown, E. Mercuri, G. Bonne, L. Feng, G. Camici, *et al.*, Skeletal muscle pathology in autosomal dominant Emery-Dreifuss muscular dystrophy with lamin A/C mutations. *Neuropathol. Appl. Neurobiol.* **27**:4 (2001), 281–290.

200. M. R. Taylor, D. Slavov, A. Gajewski, S. Vlcek, L. Ku, P. R. Fain, *et al.*, Thymopoietin (lamina-associated polypeptide 2) gene mutation associated with dilated cardiomyopathy. *Hum. Mutat.* **26**:6 (2005), 566–574.

201. A. Nagano, K. Arahata, Nuclear envelope proteins and associated diseases. *Curr. Opin. Neurol.* **13**:5 (2000), 533–539.

202. S. Manilal, T. M. Nguyen, C. A. Sewry, G. E. Morris, The Emery-Dreifuss muscular dystrophy protein, emerin, is a nuclear membrane protein. *Hum. Mol. Genet.* **5**:6 (1996), 801–808.

203. C. Di Blasi, L. Morandi, M. Raffaele di Barletti, S. Bione, P. Bernasconi, M. Cerletti, *et al.*, Unusual expression of emerin in a patient with X-linked Emery-Dreifuss muscular dystrophy. *Neuromuscul. Disord.* **10**:8 (2000), 567–571.

204. L. Cartegni, M. R. di Barletta, R. Barresi, S. Squarzoni, P. Sabatelli, N. Maraldi, *et al.*, Heart-specific localization of emerin: new insights into Emery-Dreifuss muscular dystrophy. *Hum. Mol. Genet.* **6**:13 (1997), 2257–2264.

205. P. Sabatelli, S. Squarzoni, S. Petrini, C. Capanni, A. Ognibene, L. Cartegni, *et al.*, Oral exfoliative cytology for the non-invasive diagnosis in X-linked Emery-Dreifuss muscular dystrophy patients and carriers. *Neuromuscul. Disord.* **8**:2 (1998), 67–71.

206. L. Bengtsson, K. L. Wilson, Multiple and surprising new functions for emerin, a nuclear membrane protein. *Curr. Opin. Cell. Biol.* **16**:1 (2004), 73–79.

207. J. Lammerding, P. C. Schulze, T. Takahashi, S. Kozlov, T. Sullivan, R. D. Kamm, *et al.*, Lamin A/C deficiency causes defective nuclear mechanics and mechanotransduction. *J. Clin. Invest.* **113**:3 (2004), 370–378.

208. F. Muntoni, G. Bonne, L. G. Goldfarb, E. Mercuri, R. J. Piercy, M. Burke, *et al.*, Disease severity in dominant Emery Dreifuss is increased by mutations in both emerin and desmin proteins. *Brain* **129**:5 (2006), 1260–1268.

209. E. Mercuri, S. Counsell, J. Allsop, H. Jungbluth, M. Kinali, G. Bonne, *et al.*, Selective muscle involvement on magnetic resonance imaging in autosomal dominant Emery-Dreifuss muscular dystrophy. *Neuropediatrics* **33**:1 (2002), 10–14.

210. E. Mercuri, S. C. Brown, P. Nihoyannopoulos, J. Poulton, M. Kinali, P. Richard, *et al.*, Extreme variability of skeletal and cardiac muscle involvement in patients with mutations in exon 11 of the lamin A/C gene. *Muscle Nerve* **31**:5 (2005), 602–609.

211. S. C. Brown, F. Muntoni, C. A. Sewry, Non-sarcolemmal muscular dystrophies. *Brain Pathol.* **11**:2 (2001), 193–205.

212. A. Fidzianska, D. Toniolo, I. Hausmanowa-Petrusewicz, Ultrastructural abnormality of sarcolemmal nuclei in Emery-Dreifuss muscular dystrophy (EDMD). *J. Neurol. Sci.* **159**:1 (1998), 88–93.

213. A. Ognibene, P. Sabatelli, S. Petrini, S. Squarzoni, M. Riccio, S. Santi, *et al.*, Nuclear changes in a case of X-linked Emery-Dreifuss muscular dystrophy. *Muscle Nerve* **22**:7 (1999), 864–869.

214. B. G. van Engelen, A. Muchir, C. J. Hutchison, A. J. van der Kooi, G. Bonne, M. Lammens, The lethal phenotype of a homozygous nonsense mutation in the lamin A/C gene. *Neurology* **64**:2 (2005), 374–376.

215. L. C. Mounkes, S. Kozlov, L. Hernandez, T. Sullivan, C. L. Stewart, A progeroid syndrome in mice is caused by defects in A-type lamins. *Nature* **423**:6937 (2003), 298–301.

216. T. Arimura, A. Helbling-Leclerc, C. Massart, S. Varnous, F. Niel, E. Lacene, *et al.*, Mouse model carrying H222P-Lmna mutation develops muscular dystrophy and dilated cardiomyopathy similar to human striated muscle laminopathies. *Hum. Mol. Genet.* **14**:1 (2005), 155–169.

217. L. C. Mounkes, S. V. Kozlov, J. N. Rottman, C. L. Stewart, Expression of an LMNA-N195K variant of A-type lamins results in cardiac conduction defects and death in mice. *Hum. Mol. Genet.* **14**:15 (2005), 2167–2180.

218. G. Melcon, S. Kozlov, D. A. Cutler, T. Sullivan, L. Hernandez, P. Zhao, *et al.*, Loss of emerin at the nuclear envelope disrupts the Rb1/E2F and MyoD pathways during muscle regeneration. *Hum. Mol. Genet.* **15**:4 (2006), 637–651.

219. R. Ozawa, Y. K. Hayashi, M. Ogawa, R. Kurokawa, H. Matsumoto, S. Noguchi, *et al.*, Emerin-lacking mice show minimal motor and cardiac dysfunctions with nuclear-associated vacuoles. *Am. J. Pathol.* **168**:3 (2006), 907–917.

220. M. Nakamori, T. Kimura, T. Kubota, T. Matsumura, H. Sumi, H. Fujimura, *et al.*, Aberrantly spliced alpha-dystrobrevin alters alpha-syntrophin binding in myotonic dystrophy type 1. *Neurology* **70**:9 (2008), 677–685.

221. J. P. Orengo, P. Chambon, D. Metzger, D. R. Mosier, G. J. Snipes, T. A. Cooper, Expanded CTG repeats within the DMPK 3′ UTR causes severe skeletal muscle wasting in an inducible mouse model for myotonic dystrophy. *Proc. Natl. Acad. Sci. U. S. A.* **105**:7 (2008), 2646–2651.

222. Z. Lu, D. Joseph, E. Bugnard, K. J. Zaal, E. Ralston, Golgi complex reorganization during muscle differentiation: visualization in living cells and mechanism. *Mol. Biol. Cell.* **12**:4 (2001), 795–808.

223. T. N. Devlin, *Textbook of Biochemistry with Clinical Correlations*, 2nd edn. (New York: John Wiley, 1982).

224. S. DiMauro, Muscle glycogenoses: an overview. *Acta Myol.* **26**:1 (2007), 35–41.

225. S. DiMauro, Mitochrondrial myopathies. *Curr. Opin. Rheumatol* **18**:6 (2006), 636–641.

226. C. A. Sewry, C. Muller, M. Davis, J. S. Dwyer, J. Dove, G. Evans, *et al.*, The spectrum of pathology in central core disease. *Neuromuscul. Disord.* **12**:10 (2002), 930–938.

227. H. Zhou, N. Yamaguchi, L. Xu, Y. Wang, C. Sewry, H. Jungbluth, *et al.*, Characterization of recessive RYR1 mutations in core myopathies. *Hum. Mol. Genet.* **15**:18 (2006), 2791–2803.

228. H. Jungbluth, C. R. Muller, B. Halliger-Keller, M. Brockington, S. C. Brown, L. Feng, *et al.*, Autosomal recessive inheritance of RYR1 mutations in a congenital myopathy with cores. *Neurology* **59**:2 (2002), 284–287.

229. A. Ferreiro, N. Monnier, N. B. Romero, J. P. Leroy, C. Bonnemann, C. A. Haenggeli, *et al.*, A recessive form of central core disease, transiently presenting as multi-minicore disease, is associated with a homozygous mutation in the ryanodine receptor type 1 gene. *Ann. Neurol.* **51**:6 (2002), 750–759.

230. H. Zhou, M. Brockington, H. Jungbluth, D. Monk, P. Stanier, C. A. Sewry, *et al.*, Epigenetic allele silencing unveils recessive RYR1 mutations in core myopathies. *Am. J. Hum. Genet.* **79**:5 (2006), 859–868.

231. M. R. Davis, E. Haan, H. Jungbluth, C. Sewry, K. North, F. Muntoni, *et al.*, Principal mutation hotspot for central core disease and related myopathies in the C-terminal transmembrane region of the RYR1 gene. *Neuromuscul. Disord.* **13**:2 (2003), 151–157.

232. N. Tilgen, F. Zorzato, B. Halliger-Keller, F. Muntoni, C. Sewry, L. M. Palmucci, *et al.*, Identification of four novel mutations in the C-terminal membrane spanning domain of the ryanodine receptor 1: association with central core disease and alteration of calcium homeostasis. *Hum. Mol. Genet.* **10**:25 (2001), 2879–2887.

233. N. Monnier, N. B. Romero, J. Lerale, P. Landrieu, Y. Nivoche, M. Fardeau, *et al.*, Familial and sporadic forms of central core disease are associated with mutations in the C-terminal domain of the skeletal muscle ryanodine receptor. *Hum. Mol. Genet.* **10**:22 (2001), 2581–2592.

234. S. Treves, H. Jungbluth, F. Muntoni, F. Zorzato, Congenital muscle disorders with cores: the ryanodine receptor calcium channel paradigm. *Curr. Opin. Pharmacol.* **8**:3 (2008), 319–326.

235. F. Zorzato, H. Jungbluth, H. Zhou, F. Muntoni, S. Treves, Functional effects of mutations identified in patients with multiminicore disease. *IUBMB Life* **59**:1 (2007), 14–20.

236. H. Zhou, H. Jungbluth, C. A. Sewry, L. Feng, E. Bertini, K. Bushby, *et al.*, Molecular mechanisms and phenotypic variation in RYR1-related congenital myopathies. *Brain* **130**:Pt 8 (2007), 2024–2036.

237. N. Monnier, A. Ferreiro, I. Marty, A. Labarre-Vila, P. Mexin, J. Lunardi, A homozygous splicing mutation causing a depletion of skeletal muscle RYR1 is associated with multi-minicore disease congenital myopathy with ophthalmoplegia. *Hum. Mol. Genet.* **12**:10 (2003), 1171–1178.

238. H. Jungbluth, H. Zhou, C. A. Sewry, S. Robb, S. Treves, M. Bitoun, *et al.*, Centronuclear myopathy due to a de novo dominant mutation in the skeletal muscle ryanodine receptor (RYR1) gene. *Neuromuscul. Disord.* **17**:4 (2007), 338–345.

239. W. J. Durham, P. Racena-Parks, C. Long, A. E. Rossi, S. A. Goonasekera, S. Boncompagni, *et al.*, RyR1 S-nitrosylation underlies environmental heat stroke and sudden death in Y522S RyR1 knockin mice. *Cell.* **133**:1 (2008), 53–65.

240. H. Hirata, T. Watanabe, J. Hatakeyama, *et al.*, Zebrafish relatively relaxed mutants have a ryanodine receptor defect, show slow swimming and provide a model of multi-minicore disease. *Development* **134**:15 (2007), 2771–2781.

241. A. Odermatt, P. E. Taschner, V. K. Khanna, H. F. Busch, G. Karpati, C. K. Jablecki, *et al.*, Mutations in the gene-encoding SERCA1, the fast-twitch skeletal muscle sarcoplasmic reticulum Ca^{2+} ATPase, are associated with Brody disease. *Nat. Genet.* **14**:2 (1996), 191–194.

242. A. A. Benders, J. H. Veerkamp, A. Oosterhof, P. J. Jongen, R. J. Bindels, L. M. Smit, *et al.*, Ca^{2+} homeostasis in Brody's disease. A study in skeletal muscle and cultured muscle cells and the effects of dantrolene an verapamil. *J. Clin. Invest.* **94**:2 (1994), 741–748.

243. A. Odermatt, K. Barton, V. K. Khanna, J. Mathieu, D. Escolar, T. Kuntzer, *et al.*, The mutation of Pro789 to Leu reduces the activity of the fast-twitch skeletal muscle sarco(endo) plasmic reticulum Ca^{2+} ATPase (SERCA1) and is associated with Brody disease. *Hum. Genet.* **106**:5 (2000), 482–491.

244. N. Petit, A. Lescure, M. Rederstorff, A. Krol, B. Moghadaszadeh, U. M. Wewer, *et al.*, Selenoprotein N: an endoplasmic reticulum glycoprotein with an early developmental expression pattern. *Hum. Mol. Genet.* **12**:9 (2003), 1045–1053.

245. U. Schava, W. Kress, C. G. Bönnemann, *et al.*, The phenotype and long-term follow-up in patients with Juvenille selenoprotein n1-related myopathy. *Eur. J. Paediatr Neurol* **12**:3 (2008), 224–230.

246. M. Deniziak, C. Thisse, M. Rederstorff, C. Hindelang, B. Thisse, A. Lescure, Loss of selenoprotein N function causes disruption of muscle architecture in the zebrafish embryo. *Exp. Cell Res.* **313**:1 (2007), 156–167.

247. M. J. Jurynec, R. Xia, J. J. Mackrill, D. Gunther, T. Crawford, K. M. Flanigan, *et al.*, Selenoprotein N is required for ryanodine receptor calcium release channel activity in human and zebrafish muscle. *Proc. Natl. Acad. Sci. U. S. A.* **105**:34 (2008), 12485–12490.

Section 2 Chapter 4

Investigation of muscle disease

Electrophysiological evaluation of suspected myopathy

Eric Logigian and Emma Ciafaloni

Introduction

Patients with suspected muscle disease are often referred for electrodiagnostic evaluation to help localize the lesion to muscle, muscle membrane, or neuromuscular junction; to determine etiology, disease severity, response to treatment; or to select a muscle for biopsy. The electrophysiological study is an extension of the history and neuromuscular examination. This clinical information is required to focus and plan the electrodiagnostic testing in order to best narrow the list of competing neuromuscular diagnoses, and to place the electrophysiological results in clinical context when drawing conclusions.

Typically, nerve conduction studies are carried out first to help exclude peripheral neuropathies or those myopathies with low-amplitude motor responses. Needle electromyography (EMG), by far the most useful electrodiagnostic tool in the evaluation of suspected myopathy, is performed to help confirm the presence, distribution, and activity of an underlying myopathy. In the appropriate clinical setting, repetitive stimulation of nerves innervating symptomatic muscles may also be carried out to confirm the presence of a neuromuscular junction disorder. Occasionally, other techniques are performed such as single-fiber EMG (SFEMG) to demonstrate subtle disorders of neuromuscular transmission, or exercise testing to help corroborate the diagnosis of muscle membrane disorders such as periodic paralysis or to differentiate among various myotonic myopathies. Still other testing including quantitative EMG, macro EMG, or quantitative muscle strength assessment is also sometimes performed particularly in research or clinical trial settings.

At the end of the studies, the consultant synthesizes the clinical and electrophysiological data to reach a tentative neuromuscular diagnosis, syndrome or category of disease that best explains the symptoms, signs, and laboratory abnormalities. This chapter will review the major electrophysiological testing procedures, and the electrodiagnostic "signature" of the various muscle diseases.

Electrophysiological tests

Motor nerve conduction studies

Compound muscle action potentials (CMAPs) recorded with surface electrodes over the target muscle are evoked by supramaximal percutaneous electrical stimulation of the target peripheral nerve at distal and proximal sites. This allows calculation of CMAP amplitude and area evoked from distal and proximal sites, distal motor latency, and motor conduction velocity (Figure 4.1). The CMAP is a population response – an electrical summation of action potentials from all muscle fibers of all motor units innervating the recorded muscle. Disease of the motor neuron, motor axon, neuromuscular junction or the muscle fiber itself may result in a reduction of CMAP amplitude proportional to the number of muscle fiber action potentials that are lost from the disease process. Distal latency and conduction velocity are usually normal, but latency may be slightly prolonged or velocity slowed when CMAP amplitude is moderately to severely reduced.

Thus, low-amplitude motor responses with relative preservation of latency and velocity can be seen in myopathy, and when present should bring to mind Lambert–Eaton myasthenic syndrome (LEMS), botulism, critical illness myopathy, and distal myopathy, among other less common diagnostic possibilities.

By contrast, diseases primarily affecting myelin of motor nerve fibers result in significant prolongation of distal latency and slowing of velocity, as may be seen in a patient with proximal and distal muscle weakness due to chronic inflammatory demyelinating polyneuropathy (CIDP) for example. CMAP amplitude and area may also decline in demyelinative neuropathies in which a demyelinative lesion is interposed between the stimulating and recording electrodes (e.g., conduction block). In patients with suspected myopathy, usual practice is to perform at least two motor conduction studies, one in the arm (e.g., ulnar nerve) and one in the leg (e.g., tibial nerve), along with late responses. If abnormalities are found, further motor studies may be required.

Disorders of Voluntary Muscle, 8th edn., eds. George Karpati, David Hilton-Jones, Kate Bushby and Robert C. Griggs. Published by Cambridge University Press.

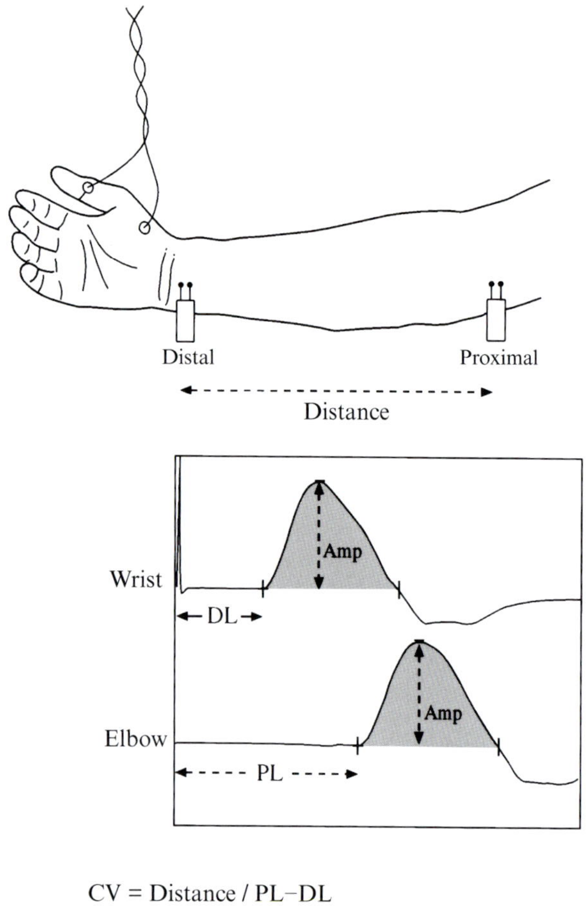

Figure 4.1. Compound muscle action potentials (CMAPs) evoked from the abductor pollicis brevis muscle after percutaneous, supramaximal median nerve stimulation at the wrist (distal site) and elbow (proximal site). The measurements of interest are the distal and proximal amplitude (Amp), distal motor latency (DL), proximal motor latency (PL), distance between the two stimulation sites, and calculated forearm conduction velocity (CV, formula shown). Also shown is the area of the negative phase of the CMAPs (shaded).

Sensory nerve conduction studies

Orthodromic or antidromic compound sensory nerve action potentials (SNAPs) are usually recorded with surface electrodes over the target cutaneous nerve evoked by supramaximal percutaneous electrical stimulation of the target peripheral nerve. There are important differences between sensory and motor conduction studies. Sensory responses are nerve action potentials without a neuromuscular junction interposed between the stimulating and recording electrodes. Therefore, they are approximately 1000 times smaller in amplitude than motor responses and signal averaging is often required to evoke SNAPs with clear onset and amplitude. Another difference is that the physiological drop in amplitude that occurs with increasing distance between stimulation and recording sites is much greater for sensory than for motor nerve conduction studies. As a result, sensory nerve conduction studies are typically performed utilizing one distal stimulation and one recording site. This allows calculation of distal SNAP amplitude, peak and onset latencies, and an approximate sensory conduction velocity. In patients with suspected myopathy, it is wise to perform at least two sensory conduction studies, one in the arm (e.g., ulnar SNAP) and one in the leg (e.g., sural SNAP). If abnormalities are found, further sensory studies may be required.

In most myopathies, sensory nerve conduction studies are normal, but there are some that have an associated polyneuropathy manifested by reduction in sensory response amplitudes evoked from distal nerve segments in the foot or hand. A smaller subgroup of myopathies even has evidence of a coexistent polyneuropathy affecting motor fibers. Therefore, the presence of a polyneuropathy does not necessarily mean that muscle weakness is also on a neuropathic basis. A coexistent sensory or sensorimotor polyneuropathy can in fact be seen in a number of toxic, inflammatory, distal, and metabolic myopathies.

Needle electromyography

Spontaneous muscle activity and voluntary motor unit potentials (MUPs) can be recorded with various intramuscular, extracellular electrodes. For routine EMG, most electrodiagnostic laboratories use disposable concentric needle electrodes consisting of a small platinum wire (recording electrode) surrounded by insulating material and a cannula of variable diameter (reference electrode), each connected to one of the two inputs to the differential amplifier.

For most primary disorders of muscle, needle EMG is the most sensitive electrodiagnostic procedure. Symptomatic muscles should be specifically examined, which in most cases means the proximal girdle muscles of the upper and lower limbs along with the paraspinal muscles. However, distal muscles in the forearm and hand and below the knee should be targeted in patients with suspected distal myopathy. Some proximal limb muscles are more informative than others. For example, in inflammatory myopathy, in the arms, the spinati are more likely to yield abnormalities than are the deltoid or biceps, while in the legs, the iliaci and glutei may be more revealing than the quadriceps [1].

During routine needle EMG the following three components are examined: insertional and spontaneous muscle activity, motor unit morphology during submaximal voluntary muscle contraction, and electromyographic interference pattern during a maximum voluntary muscle contraction.

Insertional and spontaneous activity

In normal subjects, brief insertions of the needle electrode into relaxed muscle typically produce bursts of electrical activity lasting 50–100 ms [2]. In myopathy with muscle fiber irritability, insertional bursts increase in duration. More severe irritability gives rise to runs of positive sharp waves and fibrillation potentials that persist with the needle stationary in the muscle (Figure 4.2b). These potentials must be distinguished from end-plate noise or end-plate spikes, a normal

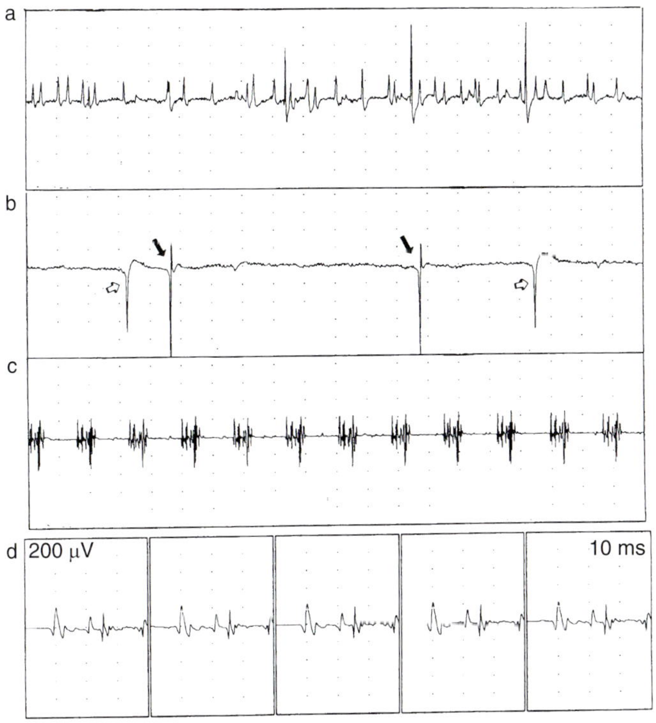

Figure 4.2. Several kinds of spontaneous electromyographic (EMG) activity in a patient with polymyositis. (a) Normal spontaneous activity: end-plate spikes composed of biphasic, negative (up-going), brief duration (1–2 ms) potentials. (b) Abnormal spontaneous activity: brief duration triphasic fibrillation potentials (closed arrows) with an initial positive (down-going) phase, and longer duration, biphasic positive sharp waves (open arrows). (c) and (d) Complex, repetitive discharge (CRD) with regular *inter*-burst and *intra*-burst discharge frequencies. Sweep speed 10 ms/division in (a, b, d); 50 ms/division in (c). Sensitivity 100 μV/division in (a, b); 200 μV/division in (c, d).

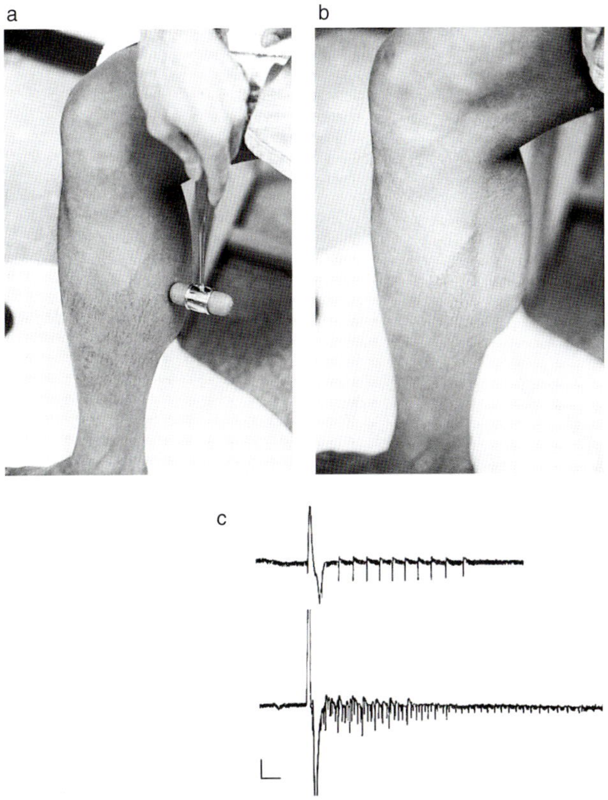

Figure 4.3. Percussion myotonia in a patient with dominantly inherited myotonia congenita. Percussion of the hypertrophied medial gastrocnemius muscle (a) results in a large depression in the muscle (b). (c) Waning myotonic discharges are shown recorded from the muscle in (a) and (b). Light tap produces a repetitive single muscle fiber discharge (top trace); stronger tap results in a longer, repetitive discharge of several muscle fibers (bottom trace).

form of persistent spontaneous activity observed when the needle electrode is inadvertently placed in the region of the muscle end plate (Figure 4.2a). Although fibrillation potentials and sharp waves are most commonly observed in neurogenic disorders, they are also seen in various muscle diseases. In myopathy, the fibrillations result from segmental necrosis of muscle fibers with a portion of the fiber deprived of its end-plate [3]. At the other end of the spectrum, patients with severe, chronic muscle disease and replacement of skeletal muscle with fibrous and adipose tissue will have increased resistance to needle insertion and reduced insertional activity.

Chronic "denervation" of muscle fiber segments may lead to groups of denervated fiber segments in close proximity, each fiber segment being activated ephaptically by its neighbor in a fairly fixed sequence beginning with the fiber segment that serves as a pacemaker. This circular current results in a spontaneous, complex repetitive discharge (CRD) (Figure 4.2c, d), which tends to stop and start abruptly and is so regular that it sounds like a monotonous machine over the audio. Because transmission occurs through ephapses rather than neuromuscular junctions, there is very little jitter (see below) between the various muscle fibers that participate in a CRD [4]. Again, like fibrillations and positive sharp waves in active neuropathy, neuronopathy or myopathy, CRDs can be seen as a manifestation of chronic denervation resulting from motor neuron, nerve, or muscle disease. They are commonly seen in patients with subacute or chronic myopathy, particularly inflammatory myopathy.

Myotonic discharges (Figure 4.3) consist of trains of positive waves or fibrillation potentials that wax and wane in frequency and amplitude, and sound like a decelerating and accelerating motorcycle. They are elicited by needle movement, by voluntary muscle activation or muscle percussion [5], and represent repetitive, spontaneous muscle fiber action potentials. They may be present in the absence of clinical myotonia. Detecting the presence of electrical myotonia is a major diagnostic clue, since it is far more common in muscle than nerve disease, and its presence can narrow the differential diagnosis considerably (see below). Depending on the disease, some muscles are more likely to show electrical myotonia than others. For example, in adults with myotonic dystrophy (DM), myotonic discharges are more likely to be found in distal upper extremity or facial muscles [6] and they are more easily evocable in DM1 than DM2 [7]. In congenital myotonic dystrophy, acid maltase deficiency, and toxic myopathies, myotonic discharges should be sought in proximal and paraspinal muscles.

Motor unit morphology

Just as the CMAP is an electrical summation of motor units, the motor unit potential (MUP) is an electrical summation of its constituent muscle fiber action potentials. Since the MUP is an extracellular recording made in a volume conductor, the shape of the MUP generally has two to three phases, as does that of each muscle fiber. There is often an initial positive phase generated by approaching action potentials, a negative phase whose onset corresponds to action potentials in closest proximity to the recording surface of the electrode, and a terminal positive phase generated by the receding muscle fiber action potentials (Figure 4.4). The primary measurements of interest are: (1) the duration of the MUP, measured from the onset of the initial positive phase to the terminus of the final phase, (2) the amplitude, measured from the lowest positive peak to the highest negative peak, and (3) the total number of phases above and below the baseline (Figure 4.4). The number of turns, or serrations, that do not cross the baseline in the MUP profile is another quantifiable parameter related to and correlated with the number of phases.

Motor unit potential duration is determined by the number and firing synchrony of muscle fibers within about 2.5 mm of the recording surface of the needle electrode [8]. The number of MUP phases and turns is largely dependent on the firing synchrony of its constituent muscle fiber action potentials. Firing synchrony increases with greater homogeneity in terminal axon length and conduction velocity, neuromuscular junction delay, and muscle fiber size and propagation velocity [9]. The greater the synchrony, the shorter the MUP duration and the fewer the phases and turns. The MUP amplitude is dependent on a much smaller subset of muscle fibers than MUP duration, i.e., those in closest proximity (about 0.5 mm) to the tip of the needle electrode [8, 10]. The amplitude and rise time of the negative phase of the MUP are therefore far more sensitive to slight movements of the electrode than is duration. The main difficulty in evaluating MUP morphology in a patient with neuromuscular symptoms is that the range of normal values is wide. For example, in the normal biceps brachii, MUP duration varies from about 3 to 17 ms and amplitude from about 50 to 1000 μV [9]. Moreover, the ranges of these parameters are slightly different for different muscles, and all, i.e., MUP duration, amplitude, and phases, slowly increase with age [11].

In general, patients with acute or subacute myopathy show a reduction in MUP duration (Figure 4.5a), and an increase in MUP phases and turns. Decrease in MUP amplitude is a later finding. MUP duration declines mainly because the disease process reduces the total number of muscle fiber action potentials. In contrast, the number of MUP phases and turns increases, because the remaining muscle fibers fire less synchronously. Muscle fiber conduction velocity, being proportional to fiber size, is more variable in muscle disease with variation in fiber size. Increased variation in muscle fiber conduction velocity decreases firing synchrony and thus increases the number of phases and turns. It also follows that these abnormalities are not specific for diseases that target the muscle fiber or neuromuscular junction, but also occur in those that affect the distal axon terminals [12]. The other condition associated with brief-duration, low-amplitude MUPs is the early recovery stage of a severe axon loss neuropathy, at a time when nerve regeneration and muscle reinnervation have proceeded to a point where motor units consist of only a few muscle fibers [13].

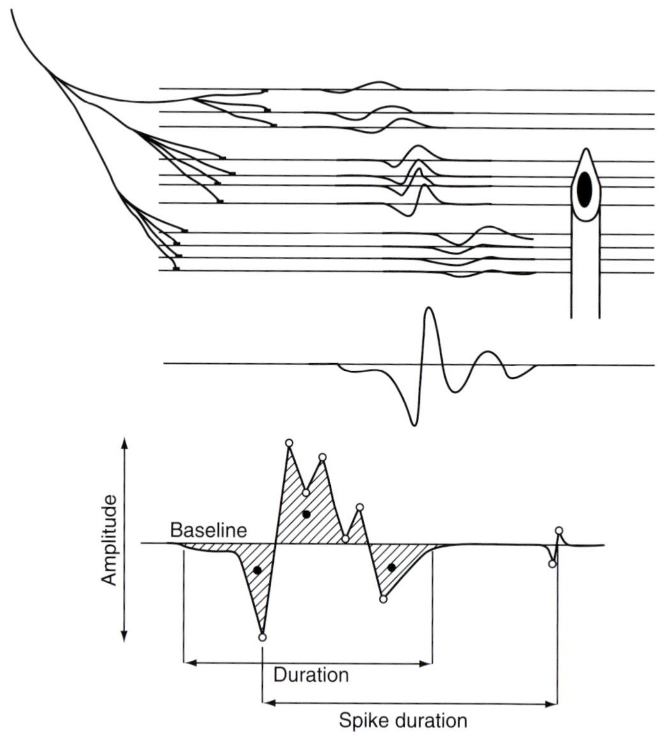

Figure 4.4. Schematic representation of motor unit potential parameters. (Reprinted from Stålberg and Trontelj, in: Vinken, P. *et al.*, (eds.) *Handbook of Clinical Neurology,* copyright (1992), Vol. 62, pp. 49–84, with permission from Elsevier Science. © Elsevier 1992).

In more indolent myopathy, the aforementioned MUP abnormalities may become less clear-cut, with an increasing number of MUPs with prolonged duration and even high amplitude. The explanation for these findings is that muscle disease results in split muscle fibers, or denervated or regenerating fibers that may over time become reinnervated by other motor units. The resultant remodeled MUPs have decreased fiber firing synchrony, perhaps an increased complement of muscle fibers, and are therefore of higher amplitude and longer duration than those of age-matched controls [14]. These morphological changes are also not specific for chronic muscle disease, and are typical of chronic, partial motor axon or neuron loss in which reinnervation of denervated muscle fibers by remaining axons compensates for loss of other axons or neurons (Figure 4.5b). In such patients, needle EMG distinguishes chronic myopathy from neuropathy either by the presence of two populations of MUPs, i.e., those with short

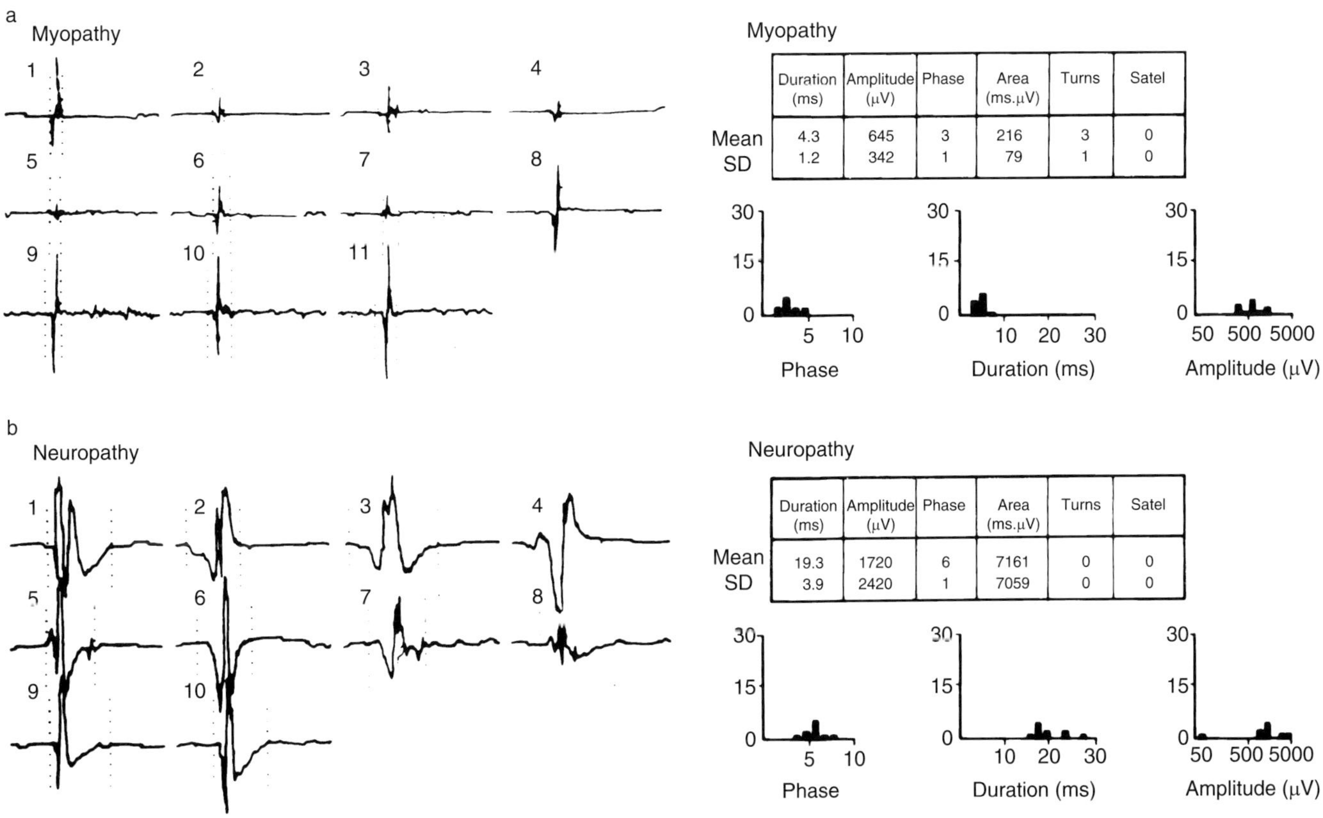

Figure 4.5a, b. Motor unit potentials (MUP) from the vastus medialis in a patient with polymyositis (a), and in a patient with diabetic neuropathy (b). MUP duration is far briefer and on average lower in amplitude in the patient with myopathy than in the patient with neuropathy.

and those with long duration, in the same muscle, or by the presence of some muscles whose MUPs are predominantly brief in duration.

Motor unit recruitment

The first concentric needle electromyographic studies of human skeletal muscle showed that muscle force increases as a result of increasing motor unit firing frequency and through recruitment of new motor units [15]. In a slowly increasing ramp contraction of muscle, motor units are generally recruited according to the size principle [16] with the smaller followed by the larger. When first recruited, motor units fire pseudo-regularly at about 4–6 Hz, but then steadily increase to much higher rates. At maximum voluntary force, firing frequencies vary depending on the muscle, but are in the range of 30 Hz for the biceps brachii and adductor pollicis in the upper extremity, and 11 Hz for the soleus in the lower extremity [17]. The MU spike density and amplitude of the interference pattern increase as force increases so that at maximum force the pattern is fully developed.

In myopathy, a so-called *early recruitment* pattern may be observed, in which the interference pattern is fuller than expected for the level of force generated [18] (Figure 4.6a). The explanation offered for this phenomenon is that in myopathy, the force generated per motor unit is reduced, and therefore a greater number of motor unit discharges is required to maintain a given target force. By contrast, in severe muscle disease, motor unit recruitment may be reduced; that is, the interference pattern shows a reduced number of rapidly firing motor units for the level of force generated. This *reduced recruitment* pattern is typical for patients with motor neuron or axon loss, but it can also be seen with severe muscle disease in which all constituent muscle fibers from a significant proportion of the motor unit population are destroyed, thus effectively reducing the number of motor units. In this situation, the nervous system cannot compensate for muscle weakness by early recruitment of motor units, so it compensates to some degree by an increasing firing frequency of the few remaining units. Inevitably though, throughout the range of force generated by the muscle, the motor unit spike interference pattern is less dense or full than normal.

Repetitive nerve stimulation (RNS)

In this technique, a series of supramaximal CMAPs recorded from a target muscle is evoked by RNS of the target nerve. Decline in CMAP amplitude and area, compared to the initial baseline CMAP, is referred to as a decrement whereas an increase in these measurements is an increment. Decrements are seen more often with low rates of stimulation of 1–3 Hz and, when not present in rested muscle, may be amplified

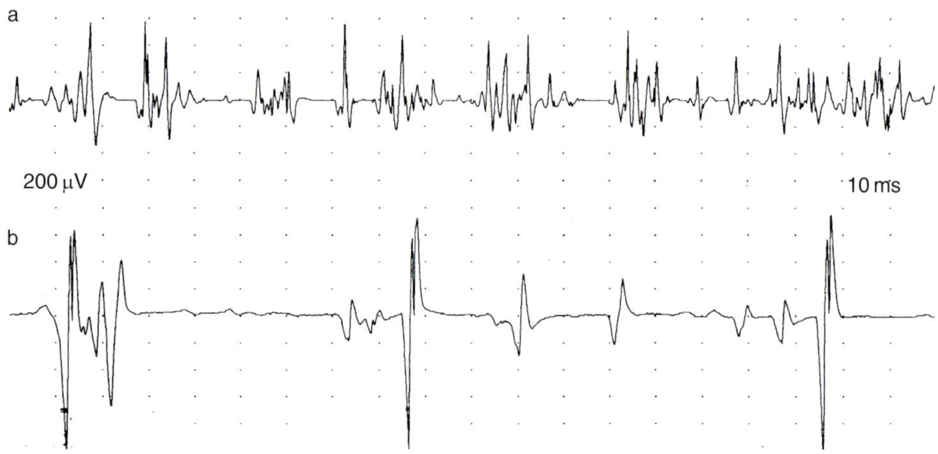

Figure 4.6a, b. Motor unit recruitment pattern in the extensor indicis proprius muscle in a patient with distal myopathy (a), and a normal subject (b). Each elevates the index finger against a 200-g weight. The recruitment is early in the patient with myopathy in whom the interference pattern is nearly filled with brief duration motor units compared to only a few units in the normal subject.

2–4 min after fatiguing exercise of 30–60 s duration (i.e., post-exercise exhaustion [19, 20]). Decrements can be seen in both postsynaptic disorders of the neuromuscular junction (e.g., myasthenia gravis, Figure 4.7) and presynaptic disorders, particularly Lambert–Eaton myasthenic syndrome (LEMS, Figure 4.8) [21, 22, 23]. LEMS is usually easily distinguished from myasthenia gravis by low-amplitude resting motor responses and by a large increment in motor response amplitude of over 100% after exercise or high-frequency RNS [24, 25].

Repetitive nerve stimulation at higher rates of 20–50 Hz is generally required to demonstrate increments. But in cooperative patients, an alternative (and essentially painless) method to demonstrate an increment is to show a post-exercise increase in CMAP amplitude and area in response to a single supramaximal percutaneous stimulus delivered before and just after a brief 10- to 30-s period of exercise. Increments can also be seen in both post- and presynaptic disorders [23], but in myasthenia gravis the increment is only rarely over 100% [23, 26, 27] whereas the increment in LEMS is rarely under 100% (mean increment 890% [25], Figure 4.8). The increment in botulism, another presynaptic disorder of the neuromuscular junction, is, however, less dramatic than that in LEMS being frequently under 100% (Figure 4.9), although more long lasting. Resting motor responses in botulism are also typically of low amplitude, but, in contrast to LEMS, weak muscles demonstrate increased insertional activity.

Obtaining meaningful data from RNS studies requires attention to a number of technical and physiological details: (1) the muscle should be immobilized in order to avoid movement artifact; (2) the temperature of the recorded muscle should be maintained at or above 34°C; (3) in patients with suspected myasthenia gravis, symptomatic proximal or facial muscles should be studied, before and after fatiguing exercise; (4) in patients with suspected LEMS or botulism and low (or borderline) resting CMAP amplitude, an increment should be sought after a 15- to 30-s maximum voluntary contraction (Figure 4.8), or, in uncooperative patients, after high-frequency RNS (Figure 4.9); (5) standard needle EMG examination should be performed to help exclude neuromuscular

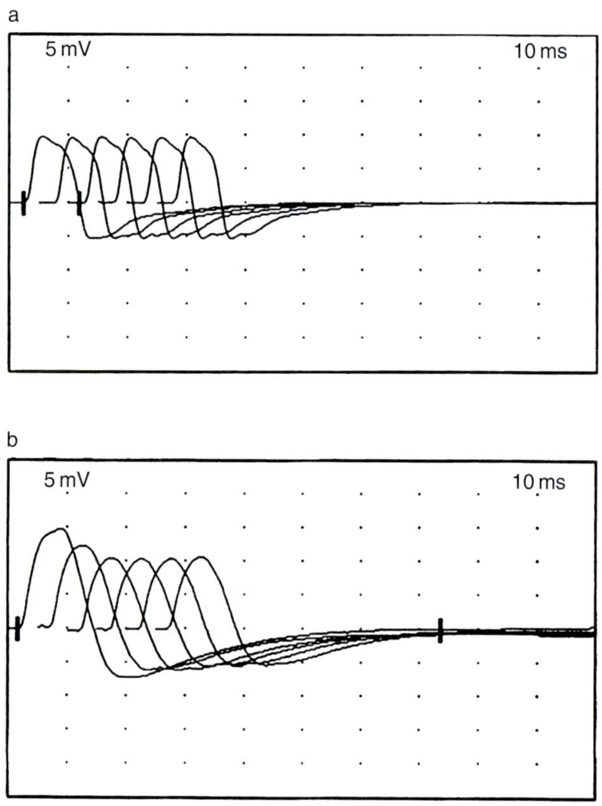

Figure 4.7a, b. (a) Normal response to repetitive stimulation (3 Hz); (b) decremental response to repetitive stimulation (3 Hz) in myasthenia gravis.

diseases such as motor neuron disease or myotonic myopathy that do not primarily affect the neuromuscular junction but may be associated with abnormal decrements on RNS.

In general, the decrement in CMAP amplitude and area seen in primary disorders of neuromuscular transmission is reproducible, is at least 10% in magnitude [20], shows the greatest decline from the first to the second CMAP, and gradually plateaus with each successive stimulus. In myasthenia gravis, the plateau is usually reached by the fourth or fifth potential [28] (Figure 4.7). Thereafter, the CMAP may

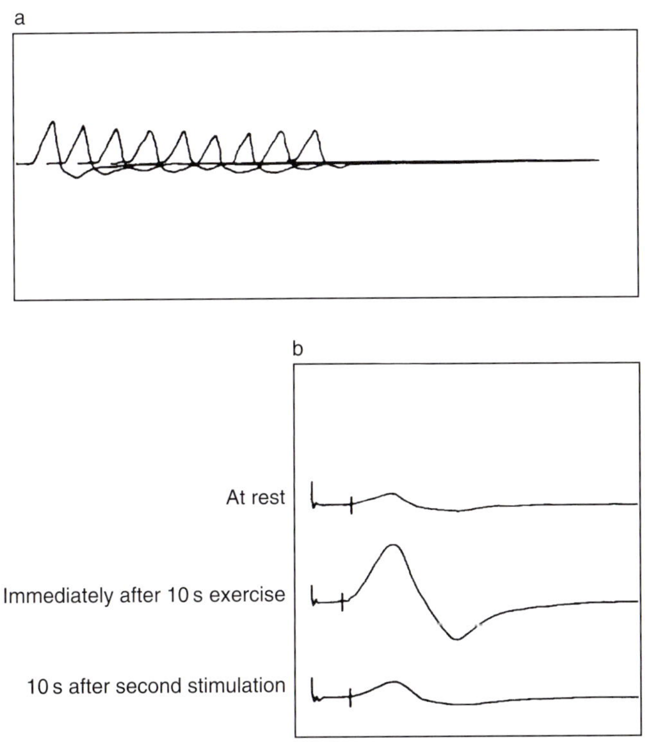

Figure 4.8a, b. Patient with Lambert–Eaton myasthenic syndrome (LEMS). (a) Baseline CMAP is of very low amplitude (1.2 mV). RNS at 2 Hz results in a 27% decrement in CMAP amplitude. (b) Baseline CMAP of very low amplitude (top trace); 790% increment in CMAP amplitude within a few seconds of voluntary activation (middle trace). Ten seconds later, the CMAP has returned to baseline low amplitude level (bottom trace).

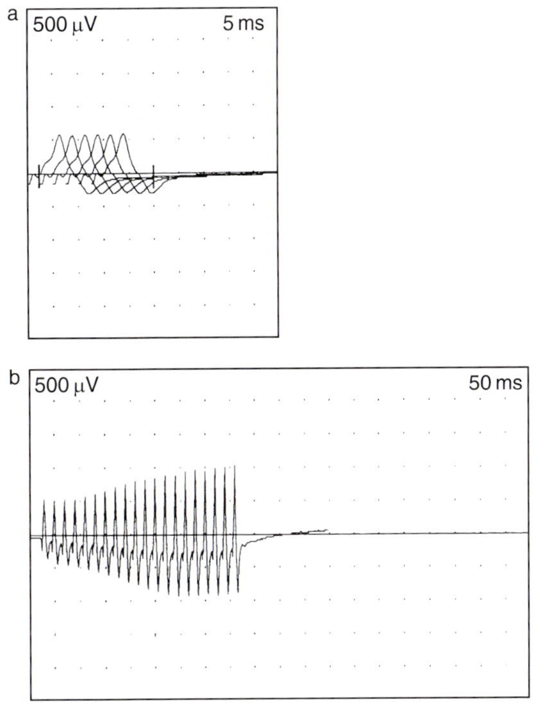

Figure 4.9. Repetitive nerve stimulation (RNS) of the ulnar nerve recording from abductor digiti minimi (ADM) in an infant with culture-proven botulism. (a) Baseline amplitude of the ADM CMAP is low (580 µV), and there is no significant decrement or increment on 2 Hz RNS. (b) Progressive increment of the ADM CMAP after 50 Hz RNS. When the CMAP plateaus, the increment is 94% for amplitude and 61% for area.

occasionally begin to increase. This pattern is nonspecific, however. It may be seen occasionally in patients with severe denervation such as active motor neuron disease [29, 30, 31]. A decrement may also be seen in some myotonic myopathies, but in this group, it is typically progressive or continuous, does not plateau after four to five stimuli, and may not be reproducible [28, 32]. Although such progressive *decrements* are unusual in primary disorders of the neuromuscular junction, patients with presynaptic disorders of neuromuscular transmission may show progressive *increments* with high-frequency RNS. Such patients may have a slow, continuous rise in CMAP amplitude that may not plateau for 10–100 stimuli (Figure 4.9).

Single-fiber electromyography (SFEMG)

Using a needle with a small recording surface and a high-frequency, high-pass filter setting, SFEMG [4, 33, 34] selectively records muscle fiber action potentials from a single motor unit. Only a small portion of the motor unit is observed with this technique, since the SFEMG electrode records electrical activity within about 300 µm of the recording surface. The two parameters of interest are the determination of jitter, a measure of the safety factor of neuromuscular junction transmission, and of fiber density, a measurement of the spatial organization of the muscle fibers within the motor unit.

Jitter can be measured during voluntary activation of a muscle, or during nerve stimulation. In the voluntary condition, the SFEMG needle electrode is positioned such that it optimally records from two or more fibers from the same motor unit. Using one fiber as the stable triggering potential, the variation in the time interval between the triggering potential and the second muscle fiber potential is measured over at least 50 motor unit discharges. The variation in intervals is a measure of jitter and is expressed statistically as the mean consecutive difference (MCD) or mean sorted difference (MSD). This process is then repeated for a total of 20 separate muscle fiber pairs and the mean and range of MCDs or MSDs are calculated. The results are interpreted using age-dependent normal values that are available for a number of limb and cranial muscles [35].

Disease of the neuromuscular junction is associated with increased jitter (Figure 4.10). When severe enough to produce muscle weakness, the neuromuscular junction disorder is associated with both increased jitter and blocking of the second potential. The physiological explanation for increased jitter and blocking is as follows. The more severe the disorder of neuromuscular transmission, the more variable is the end-plate potential (EPP) amplitude from one discharge to the next. Because the rate of rise of the muscle fiber EPP is proportional to its amplitude, the more variable the amplitude, the more variable the rate of rise of the EPP, and thus the more

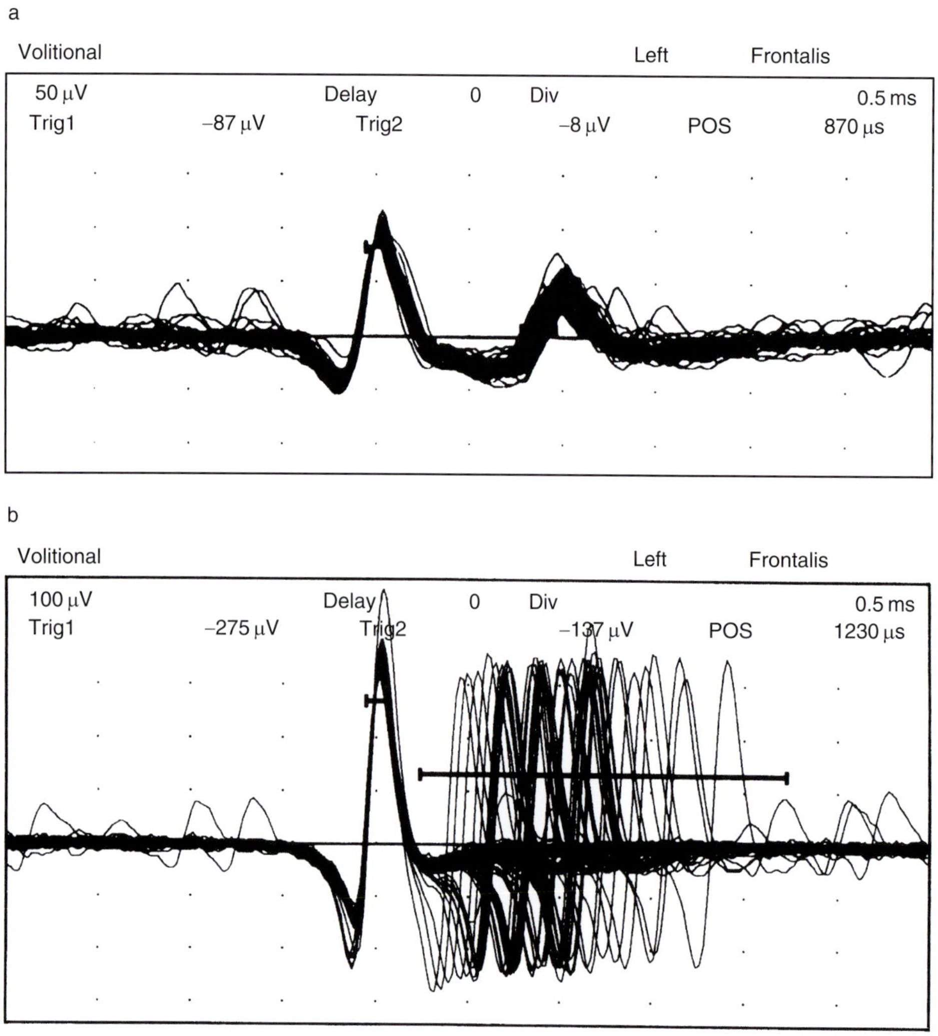

Figure 4.10. Single-fiber EMG study in a normal subject (a) and a patient with myasthenia gravis (b). Each trace represents 100 superimposed recordings from two muscle fibers of a frontalis motor unit, with the first fiber serving as a "trigger." One can see that the variability in inter-spike latency between the first and second muscle fiber potentials (e.g., jitter) is much greater in the patient than in the normal subject.

variable the synaptic delay, and the larger the jitter. In more severe disease, the EPP is not only quite variable, but it is also intermittently subthreshold for generation of a muscle fiber action potential, and "blocking" is seen on SFEMG. Increased jitter and blocking are characteristic of neuromuscular junction disease, but they can also be seen occasionally in patients with neuropathy or motor neuronopathy, particularly during the early stages of reinnervation, and to a lesser extent with primary disorders of muscle. One interesting feature of myopathy is the presence of occasional fiber pairs with very low jitter, due to muscle fiber splitting, both fragments innervated by the same endplate.

Fiber density is the mean number of muscle fiber potentials seen by the SFEMG electrode on 20 separate insertions, each optimally positioned to record the first visible muscle fiber action potential. Fiber density increases with age, and varies among muscles, but is normally between 1.5 and 2.5 [36]. Fiber density is particularly increased in neuropathy as a result of collateral sprouting of nerve fibers and reinnervation of denervated muscle fibers. Fiber density is increased in most myopathies as well, but usually to a lesser extent, and is due to several mechanisms including muscle fiber splitting [33].

Macro EMG

This technique uses a modified SFEMG electrode in which the recording surface is the distal 15 mm of the needle electrode cannula. In contrast to the concentric or monopolar EMG needle electrode, the large recording surface picks up electrical activity from all muscle fibers from a single motor unit that are distributed over a 5- to 15-mm region of muscle. This technique averages successive motor unit discharges using one of its fibers as a trigger, thereby recording the electrical activity of only the one motor unit whose muscle fibers fire in a roughly time-locked fashion to the triggering potential. In general, macro EMG MUP amplitude and area correlate with motor unit muscle fiber number [37], being low in myopathy due to muscle fiber drop out, and high in neuropathy or neuronopathy due to reinnervation. These macro EMG findings suggest that the increased fiber density seen in neuropathy and myopathy have different explanations. In neuropathy, the process of reinnervation increases the total number of muscle fibers in the remaining motor units, whereas in myopathy, the total number of intact fibers per motor unit is the same or less, but in places they are split, or grouped together [38].

Quantitative EMG

Routine EMG includes a qualitative assessment of spontaneous activity, motor unit morphology, and the interference pattern. There are also quantitative methods that may be useful when the qualitative studies are not clearly diagnostic, or when serial studies are contemplated. Motor unit morphology can be quantified by analyzing duration, amplitude, phases, turns, area, or area/amplitude ratio for 20 or more randomly selected simple MU (e.g., fewer than five phases) from a given muscle and comparing the results to age-matched normative data. This kind of analysis can be performed manually [10], using spike-triggered averaging techniques [39], or now using various semi-automated computerized techniques [40, 41]. The most sensitive parameters for myopathy seem to be motor unit duration and the motor unit area/amplitude ratio. Both parameters measure the thinness of the motor unit, which correlates with the loss of muscle fiber action potentials seen in many myopathies.

There are also computerized methods to analyze quantitatively the EMG interference pattern from a given muscle using age- and gender-matched normative data [37, 42]. One parameter of interest is the turns/amplitude ratio, which can be measured at a single, standardized level of muscle force [43], or over the range of forces generated by the muscle [37, 42]. Patients with muscle disease have an elevated turns/amplitude ratio, while those with neuropathy have a reduced ratio [37, 42]. Some studies have shown that quantitative analysis of the interference pattern is more sensitive for muscle disease than is quantitative analysis of motor unit morphology [44].

There are clearly some patients with evidence of myopathy on one or more of the quantitative techniques whose routine qualitative EMG study is normal. On the other hand, the overall sensitivity of the quantitative studies is not always higher than routine EMG [39, 42]. Whether quantitative techniques significantly increase the diagnostic sensitivity or specificity for myopathy is not yet clear. In any case, using histology as a gold standard, the diagnostic sensitivity of careful EMG in muscle disease in general is, according to some experts, in the range of 80%–90% [45, 46].

Exercise testing – short and long exercise tests

The effect of exercise on neuromuscular junction physiology and its importance in the diagnosis of neuromuscular transmission defects is described above. Exercise also produces characteristic changes in CMAP amplitude in patients with myotonias and periodic paralysis [5, 47, 48, 49, 50]. In patients with myotonic dystrophy type 1 (DM1), myotonia congenita (particularly the recessive form), and paramyotonia congenita, brief exercise for 5–10 s will produce an immediate drop in the amplitude of the CMAP followed by prompt recovery within about 2 min. If the test is repeated, a drop in CMAP amplitude is reproducible in paramyotonia congenita, and possibly the recessive form of myotonia congenita, but not in DM1. In one small series [51], drop in postexercise CMAP amplitude and area was seen in DM1, but not in proximal myotonic myopathy (PROMM, or DM2), but whether DM1 can be distinguished from DM2 by exercise testing awaits confirmation.

A long exercise test of 2–5 min, with periodic breaks to prevent muscle ischemia, is useful in the diagnosis of patients with periodic paralysis, in whom the short exercise test is usually negative. After an initial increment in amplitude during the exercise phase of the test, patients with acquired or inherited periodic paralysis show a progressive long-lasting drop in CMAP amplitude (and area) by more than 30%–40% from peak intra-exercise amplitude typically occurring about 20–40 min after exercise [47, 52]. The CMAP slowly recovers thereafter (Figure 4.11). This phenomenon can also be seen in some patients with paramyotonia congenita, but, typically, the postexercise decline in CMAP amplitude in patients with this disorder reaches the nadir more quickly after completion of the exercise test [47, 50].

Electrophysiological signatures of muscle disease

After completion of the motor and sensory nerve conduction studies and needle EMG in patients with suspected myopathy, the results typically fall into one of several electrophysiological categories, each with its own differential diagnosis. It is important to recognize, however, that there is significant overlap in these categories in that mild and severe forms of the same myopathy may be placed in different categories.

1. Low-amplitude distal CMAPs, normal sensory responses (typically); needle EMG findings of normal or increased insertional activity, and brief duration, polyphasic or low amplitude motor units

This electrophysiological scenario is most commonly seen in one of four conditions: LEMS, botulism, critical illness myopathy [53], or one of the distal myopathies. The former two presynaptic neuromuscular junction disorders can usually be distinguished from the others by demonstration of an increment in baseline CMAP amplitude either with 50 Hz RNS or immediately after a 10- to 20-s maximal voluntary muscle contraction.

2. Normal motor responses, normal sensory responses (typically); needle EMG findings of increased insertional activity with persistent fibrillation potentials, positive waves, or CRDs; brief duration, polyphasic or low-amplitude motor units.

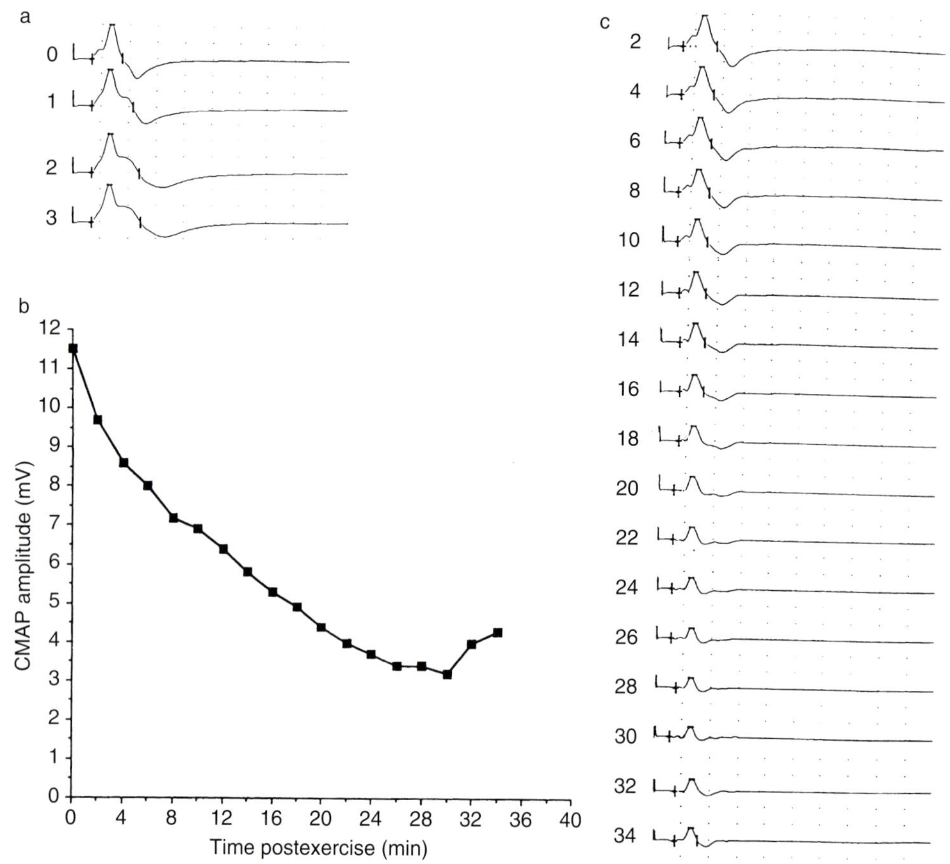

Figure 4.11a–c. Long exercise test in a patient with hypokalemic periodic paralysis. CMAPs evoked from the abductor digiti minimi during brief pauses in 3 min of exercise (a) show a transient increase in amplitude (17%) and area (81%). After exercise, there is gradual 70% decrease in CMAP amplitude with the nadir at 30 min (b, c).

This scenario is typical of any active myopathy with significant ongoing muscle fiber necrosis or degeneration. It is most commonly observed in the inflammatory or toxic myopathies, but can also be seen in some metabolic myopathies (e.g., acid maltase deficiency) or muscular dystrophies (e.g., dystrophinopathy). This pattern is sometimes referred to as myopathy with muscle fiber irritability.

3. Normal motor responses, normal sensory responses (typically); needle EMG findings of normal insertional activity, but brief duration, polyphasic or low-amplitude motor units.

This pattern, sometimes referred to as a "nonirritable" myopathy, is seen in many mild, or more slowly progressive myopathies typically with less vigorous ongoing muscle fiber necrosis or degeneration than in patients who fall in category 2. This pattern is also observed in patients with inflammatory myopathies who have been adequately treated with immunosuppressive agents.

4. Normal motor responses, normal sensory responses (typically); needle EMG findings of increased insertional activity, but normal motor unit morphology.

This nonspecific category includes: (1) a small percentage of normal subjects with isolated increased insertional activity (presumably due to abnormal muscle membrane excitability) but without clinical evidence of neuromuscular disease; (2) patients with active myopathy in whom some muscles have only muscle fiber irritability, while others have irritability accompanied by typical "myopathic" changes of motor unit morphology (e.g., brief duration motor units, etc.); and (3) patients with denervating conditions in whom some muscles have only muscle fiber irritability, while others have irritability accompanied by typical "neuropathic" changes of motor unit morphology (e.g., prolonged duration motor units, etc.).

5. Normal motor responses, normal sensory responses (typically); needle EMG findings of increased insertional activity with prominent myotonic discharges; normal or brief duration, polyphasic or low-amplitude motor units.

This electrophysiological pattern is most commonly observed in patients with myotonic myopathy and clinically demonstrable myotonia such as Type 1 or 2 myotonic dystrophy, recessive or dominant myotonia congenita, paramyotonia congenita, and hyperkalemic periodic paralysis. Electrical myotonia without clinical myotonia can also be observed in some metabolic and toxic myopathies, as well as in hypothyroid, centronuclear (myotubular), and occasionally even inflammatory myopathy.

6. Normal motor responses, normal sensory responses (typically); needle EMG findings of normal or increased

insertional activity, population of polyphasic MUPs with broad duration in some muscles, occasional high-amplitude MUPs.

This constellation of findings can be observed in more indolent, long-standing, moderate to severe myopathy (e.g., inclusion body myositis) in which motor unit "remodeling" occurs [54]. There is the potential to misdiagnose such patients with polyneuropathy, particularly when distal muscles are affected, but when mean motor unit duration is actually carefully quantitated in such patients, it is usually not prolonged [55].

7. Normal motor and sensory nerve conduction studies; needle EMG findings of normal insertional activity and normal motor unit morphology.

This signature is also not uncommon in long-standing congenital, metabolic, mitochondrial or dystrophic myopathies or in mild toxic myopathy. Patients with myasthenia gravis or periodic paralysis may also fall into this category. Therefore, in the appropriate clinical setting, these latter disorders can be further pursued electrophysiologically with RNS, single-fiber EMG, and long exercise testing.

8. Normal motor and sensory nerve conduction studies; needle EMG findings of reduced insertional activity with increased tissue resistance to needle insertion, few or no recruitable motor units evident, motor units if present are usually brief, low amplitude and polyphasic.

This pattern is typical of end-stage muscle disease in which the muscle is largely replaced by fibrous and adipose tissue. It can be observed in any severe myopathy, and in the absence of recruitable motor units may only be distinguishable from severe denervating disease by EMG sampling of other less affected muscles.

References

1. A. Wilbourn, The electrodiagnostic examination with myopathies. *J. Clin. Neurophysiol.* **10** (1993), 132–148.
2. F. Buchthal, P. Rosenfalk, Spontaneous electrical activity of human muscle. *Electroencephalogr. Clin. Neurophysiol.* **20** (1966), 321–326.
3. J. E. Desmedt, S. Borenstein, Relationship of spontaneous fibrillation potentials to muscle fibre segmentation in human muscular dystrophy. *Nature* **258** (1975), 531–534.
4. E. Stålberg, J. V. Trontelj, *Single Fibre Electromyography.* (Old Woking: Mirvalle Press Ltd, 1979.)
5. E. W. Streib, AAEE Minimonograph #27: Differential diagnosis of myotonic syndromes. *Muscle Nerve* **10** (1987), 603–615.
6. E. W. Streib, S. F. Sun, Distribution of electrical myotonia in myotonic muscular dystrophy. *Ann. Neurol.* **14** (1983), 80–82.
7. E. L. Logigian, E. Ciafaloni, C. Quinn, N. Dilek, S. Pandya, R. T. Moxley, C. A. Thornton, Severity, type and distribution of myotonic discharges are different in type 1 versus type 2 myotonic dystrophy. *Muscle Nerve* **35**:4 (2007), 479–485.
8. S. D. Nandedekar, P. E. Barkhaus, D. B. Sanders, E. V. Stålberg, Analysis of amplitude and area of concentric needle EMG motor unit action potentials. *Electroencephalogr. Clin. Neurophysiol.* **69** (1988), 561–567.
9. F. Buchthal, C. Guld, P. Rosenfalck, Action potential parameters in normal human muscle and their dependence on physical variables. *Acta Physiol. Scand.* **32** (1954), 200–218.
10. P. Rosenfalck, A. Rosenfalck, *Electromyography and Sensory/Motor conduction: Findings in Normal Subjects.* (Rigshospitalet, Copenhagen: Laboratory of Clinical Neurophysiology, 1975.)
11. F. Buchthal, P. Pinelli, P. Rosenfalck, Action potential parameters in normal human muscle and their physiological determinants. *Acta Physiol. Scand.* **32** (1954), 219–229.
12. W. K. Engel, "Myopathic EMG" – nonesuch animal. *New Engl. J. Med.* **289** (1973), 485–486.
13. G. Weddell, B. Feinstein, R. E. Pattle, The electrical activity of voluntary muscle in man under normal and pathological conditions. *Brain* **67** (1944), 178–257.
14. A. Uncini, D. J. Lange, R. E. Lovelace, M. Solomon, A. P. Hays, Long-duration polyphasic motor unit potentials in myopathies: a quantitative study with pathological correlation. *Muscle Nerve* **13** (1990), 263–267.
15. E. D. Adrian, D. W. Bronk, The discharge of impulses in motor nerve fibers. Part II. The frequency of discharge in reflex and voluntary contractions. *J. Physiol. (Lond.)* **67** (1929), 119–151.
16. E. Henneman, Relation between size of neurones and their susceptibility to discharge. *Science* **126** (1957), 1345–1347.
17. F. Bellemare, J. J. Woods, R. Johansson, B. Biglan-Ritchie, Motor-unit discharge rates in maximal voluntary contractions of three human muscles. *J. Neurophysiol.* **50**:6 (1983), 1380–1392.
18. J. R. Daube, AAEM Minimonograph #11: Needle examination in clinical electromyography. *Muscle Nerve* **14** (1991), 685–700.
19. J. E. Desmedt, The neuromuscular disorder in myasthenia gravis. I. Electrical and mechanical responses to nerve stimulation in hand muscles. In *New Developments in Electromyography and Clinical Neurophysiology*, Vol 1, ed. J. E. Desmedt. (Basel: S. Karger, 1973), pp. 241–304.
20. J. E. Desmedt, S. Borenstein, Diagnosis of myasthenia gravis by nerve stimulation. *Ann. N. Y. Acad. Sci.* **274** (1976), 174–188.
21. E. H. Lambert, L. M. Eaton, E. D. Rooke, Defect of neuromuscular conduction associated with malignant neoplasms. *Am. J. Physiol.* **187** (1956), 612–613.
22. E. H. Lambert, Defects in neuromuscular transmission in syndromes other than myasthenia gravis. *Ann. N. Y. Acad. Sci.* **135** (1966), 367–384.
23. R. W. Tim, D. B. Sanders, Repetitive nerve stimulation studies in the Lambert-Eaton myasthenic syndrome. *Muscle Nerve* **17** (1994), 995–1001.
24. E. H. Lambert, E. D. Rooke, L. M. Eaton C. H. Hodgson, Myasthenic syndrome occasionally associated with bronchial neoplasm: neurophysiologic studies. In *Myasthenia Gravis*, ed. H. R. Viets. (Springfield, IL: C. C. Thomas, 1961), pp. 362–410.
25. J. H. O'Neill, N. M. F. Murray, J. Newsome-Davis, The Lambert-Eaton myasthenic syndrome, a review of 50 cases. *Brain* **111** (1988), 577–596.

26. R. F. Mayer, I. R. Williams, Incrementing responses in myasthenia gravis. *Arch. Neurol.* **31** (1974), 24–26.
27. W. S. Musser, R. L. Barbano, C. A. Thornton, R. T. Moxley, D. N. Herrmann, E. L. Logigian, Distal myasthenia gravis with a decrement, an increment and denervation. *J. Clin. Neuromusc. Dis.* **3** (2001), 16–19.
28. C. Ozdemir, R. R. Young, The results to be expected from electrical testing in the diagnosis of myasthenia gravis. *Ann. N. Y. Acad. Sci.* **274** (1976), 203–222.
29. L. P. Berstein, J. P. Antel, Motor neuron disease: decremental responses to repetitive nerve stimulation. *Neurology* **31** (1981), 202–204.
30. E. H. Denys, F. H. Norris, Amyotrophic lateral sclerosis: impairment of neuromuscular transmission. *Arch. Neurol.* **36** (1979), 202–205.
31. R. D. Henderson, J. R. Daube, Decrement in surface-recorded motor unit potentials in amyotrophic lateral sclerosis. *Neurology* **63** (2004), 1670–1674.
32. M. J. Aminoff, R. B. Layzer, S. Satya-Murti, A. I. Faden, The declining electrical response of muscle to repetitive nerve stimulation in myotonia. *Neurology* **27** (1977), 812–816.
33. D. B. Sanders, E. V. Stålberg, AAEM Minimonograph #25: Single-fiber electromyography. *Muscle Nerve* **19** (1996), 1069–1083.
34. E. Stålberg, J. V. Trontelj, *Single Fiber Electromyography. Studies in Healthy and Diseased Muscle*, 2nd edn. (New York: Raven Press, 1994.)
35. J. M. Gilchrist, and ad hoc committee, Single fiber EMG reference values: a collaborative effort. *Muscle Nerve* **15** (1992), 151–161.
36. M. B. Bromberg, D. M. Scott, Single fiber EMG reference values: reformatted in tabular form. *Muscle Nerve* **17** (1994), 820–821.
37. E. Stålberg, Macro EMG. *Muscle Nerve* **6** (1983), 619–630.
38. E. Stålberg, Invited Review: Electrodiagnostic assessment and monitoring of motor unit changes in disease. *Muscle Nerve* **14** (1991), 293–303.
39. C. R. Stewart, S. D. Nandedekar, J. M. Massey, J. M. Gilchrist, P. E. Barkhaus, D. B. Sanders, Evaluation of an automatic method of measuring features of motor unit action potentials. *Muscle Nerve* **12** (1989), 141–148.
40. L. Dorfman, J. Howard, K. McGill, Clinical studies using automatic decomposition electromyography (ADEMG) in needle and surface EMG. In *Computer-Aided Electromyography and Expert Systems*, ed. J. Desmedt. (New York: Elsevier, 1989), pp. 189–204.
41. S. D. Nandedkar, P. E. Barkhaus, C. Charles, Multi-motor unit action potential analysis (MMA). *Muscle Nerve* **18** (1995), 1155–1166.
42. J. M. Gilchrist, S. D. Nandedekar, C. R. Stewart, J. M. Massey, D. B. Sanders, P. E. Barkhaus, Automatic analysis of the interference pattern using the turns:amplitude ratio. *Electroencephalogr. Clin. Neurophysiol.* **70** (1988), 534–540.
43. A. Rose, R. Willison, Quantitative electromyography using automatic analysis: studies in healthy subjects and patients with primary muscle disease. *J. Neurol. Neurosurg. Psychiatry* **30** (1967), 403–410.
44. P. E. Barkhaus, S. D. Nandedekar, D. B. Sanders, Quantitative EMG in inflammatory myopathy. *Muscle Nerve* **13** (1990), 247–253.
45. F. Buchthal, Z. Kamieniecka, The diagnostic yield of quantified electromyography and quantified muscle biopsy in neuromuscular disorders. *Muscle Nerve* **5** (1982), 265–280.
46. I. Hausmanowa-Petrucewicz, H. Jedrezejowska, Correlation between electromyographic findings and muscle biopsy in cases of neuromuscular disease. *J. Neurol. Sci.* **13** (1971), 85–106.
47. P. G. McManis, E. H. Lambert, J. R. Daube, The exercise test in periodic paralysis. *Muscle Nerve* **9** (1986), 704–710.
48. E. W. Streib, S. F. Sun, T. Yarkowski, Transient paresis in myotonic syndromes: a simplified electrophysiologic approach. *Muscle Nerve* **5** (1982), 719–723.
49. T. Kuntzer, F. Flocard, C. Vial, *et al.*, Exercise test in muscle channelopathies and other muscle disorders. *Muscle Nerve* **23** (2000), 1089–1094.
50. E. Fournier, M. Arzel, D. Sternberg, S. Vicart, P. Laforet, B. Eymard, J-C. Willer, N. Tabti, B. Fontaine, Electromyography guides toward subgroup of mutations in muscle channelopathies. *Ann. Neurol.* **56** (2004), 650–661.
51. H. W. Sander, G. P. Tavoulareas, C. M. Quinto, D. M. Menkes, S. Chokroverty, The exercise test distinguishes proximal myotonic myopathy from myotonic dystrophy. *Muscle Nerve* **20** (1997), 235–237.
52. C. H. Tengan, A. C. Antunes, A. A. Gabbai, G. M. Manzano, The exercise test as a monitor of disease status in hypokalemic periodic paralysis. *J. Neurol. Neurosurg. Psychiatry* **75** (2004), 497–499.
53. D. Lacomis, M. Giuliani, A. Van Cott, D. Kramer, Acute myopathy of intensive care: clinical, electromyographic, and pathological aspects. *Ann. Neurol.* **40** (1996), 645–654.
54. A. Eisen, K. Berry, G. Gibson, Inclusion body myositis (IBM): myopathy or neuropathy. *Neurology* **33** (1983), 1109–1114.
55. P. E. Barkhaus, M. I. Periquet, S. D. Nandedkar, Quantitative electrophysiologic studies in sporadic inclusion body myositis. *Muscle Nerve* **22** (1999), 480–487.

Chapter 5

Histopathology and immunoanalysis of muscle

Caroline A. Sewry and Maria J. Molnar

Introduction

Muscle pathology has an increasing role in the diagnosis of neuromuscular disorders, and there is now a greater appreciation of the pathological features associated with particular clinical features, and their underlying molecular causes. With the wide genetic diversity of neuromuscular disorders and numerous defective genes responsible, muscle pathology can help to direct molecular analysis. This chapter aims to highlight the most relevant techniques for diagnosis, in particular histological, histochemical, and immunoanalytical methods, and the interpretation of the features. Ultrastructural studies are described in Chapter 6. It is essential, however, to assess all the pathological findings together, and to correlate them with all the clinical features, and the results of any special investigations, such as serum enzymes, serum antibodies, lactate levels, magnetic resonance imaging (MRI) of muscle and brain, muscle ultrasound, and electrophysiology.

In some conditions molecular analysis is now so reliable that muscle pathology often provides little additional diagnostic information, and muscle biopsies are now rarely performed. In particular, molecular analysis is now the test of choice for the diagnosis of spinal muscular atrophy (SMA), myotonic muscular dystrophy (DM1), and facioscapulohumeral muscular dystrophy (FSHD). Similarly, in myasthenic syndromes and ion channel disorders muscle pathology may be minimal or nonspecific and the combination of careful clinical and electrophysiological studies often provides the diagnosis. In most of the remaining conditions, however, muscle pathology has an important role both in directing molecular analysis and in identifying morphological defects associated with certain symptoms.

The identification of defects in a number of interacting proteins and the overlap of clinico-pathological features have challenged the traditional clinical classification. In addition, the same morphological feature can result from defects in more than one gene, and defects in the same gene can result in a variety of morphological defects. The traditional clinical classifications, however, still have merit as it is the clinical symptoms that lead to referral, and to the need for a muscle biopsy. Molecular analysis and identification of the defective gene provide the ultimate diagnosis, but in most disorders this is not usually the starting point.

Selection of muscle

The selection of the site for a muscle biopsy is determined by the distribution of muscle weakness and the degree of involvement. It is important not to select a muscle that is so severely involved that it is replaced by fat or connective tissue and contains few muscle fibers for assessment, or to choose a muscle that is so little affected that it does not show sufficient change. Focal pathology may be missed in a single sample and some centers therefore take samples from more than one site. Differential involvement of muscle occurs in several disorders and ultrasound and MRI of muscle can reveal patterns associated with individual diseases and aid the choice for sampling [1, 2]. In general, the quadriceps, biceps, deltoid, and gastrocnemius are appropriate muscles to sample, and their fiber type composition and range of fiber sizes are well characterized. It is important to avoid sampling at the site of either electromyography (EMG) or any form of injection, as needling of any kind can produce changes in the muscle [3]. Injection of vaccines can result in focal macrophage fasciitis [3]. Sites of myotendinous junctions should also be avoided as these commonly show internal nuclei, fiber branching, and higher levels of several proteins including those of the dystrophin-associated complex, integrins, and cadherins. In addition, sports injuries or other traumas, the use or disuse of the muscle, aging, and any possible effect of contractures also need to be taken into account when drawing conclusions from a biopsy.

Biopsy method and tissue preparation

Muscle biopsies can be obtained by an open or needle technique, provided a suitable instrument is used. The type of technique is a matter of choice of the physician. The author (C. A. S.) has over 30 years' experience of the pathological value of needle biopsies taken with an instrument devised by Bergström [3]. It provides sufficient material for a variety of

Disorders of Voluntary Muscle, 8th edn., eds. George Karpati, David Hilton-Jones, Kate Bushby and Robert C. Griggs. Published by Cambridge University Press.

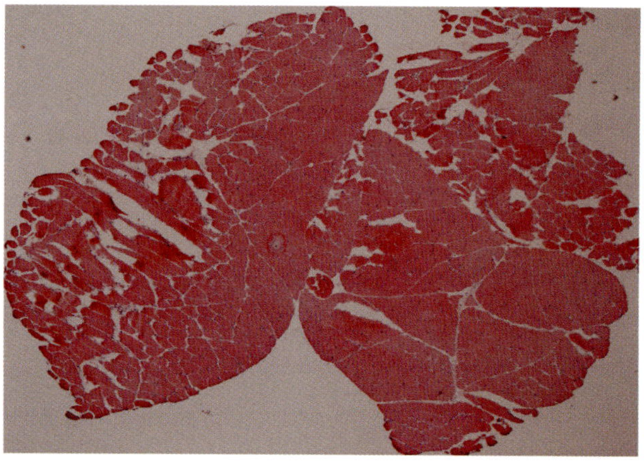

Figure 5.1. Low-power view of a whole needle muscle biopsy taken with a Bergström needle. H&E.

morphological and biochemical techniques, and is a safe, rapid procedure that requires only a small incision and does not involve the use of stitches. It leaves only a small scar that often becomes almost invisible. Samples using a conchotome, alligator-type forceps can also provide adequate samples [4]. It is essential that samples are orientated under a dissection microscope before freezing, to obtain good transverse orientation, as this provides the most information. Figure 5.1 shows the quality of a typical needle biopsy obtained using the Bergström needle. In comparison with needle biopsies, open biopsies provide a larger sample, which may be necessary for some biochemical studies, but in most situations the same diagnostic conclusion can be reached from a needle sample. Developments in the sensitivity of biochemical and immunoblotting techniques have also reduced the need for large samples [5].

All histological, histochemical, and immunohistochemical studies of muscle are performed on frozen material. This avoids the distortion caused by fixatives and wax-embedding, and is essential for preserving enzyme activity. Some immunohistochemistry is possible on wax-embedded material, depending on the antibody, but a full panel of immunohistochemical and enzyme histochemistry studies is not possible. Fixation is used for preparation of samples for electron microscopy.

Fetal muscle biopsy

Although rarely performed, muscle can be obtained from fetuses in utero using a needle under ultrasound guidance [6]. In Duchenne muscular dystrophy (DMD), for example, expression of dystrophin can be assessed when DNA from the proband is not available, or is noninformative. Theoretically, fetal muscle samples can be used in any situation where the expression of the relevant protein is sufficiently abnormal for it to be detected immunohistochemically, or a structural feature is likely to be present. In practice, DNA and/or protein assessment of chorionic villus samples is preferred. There is insufficient information on the presence of structural changes (such as nemaline rods) in utero for fetal sampling to be diagnostically reliable, but they are known to be present early in fetal development.

Immunohistochemistry of samples from aborted fetuses at risk for DMD can be useful for prenatal diagnosis of subsequent pregnancies, as dystrophin expression can be assessed, and the DNA analyzed. Dystrophin can be detected from at least 9 weeks of gestation and a significant reduction, or absence, occurs in affected DMD fetuses [7, 8].

Other tissues for diagnosis

Although muscle is the tissue of choice, useful diagnostic information on the immunolocalization of some proteins can be obtained from other tissues, particularly when muscle wasting is extensive. For example, skin biopsies can be used to assess laminin-α2, emerin collagen VI, and plectin [9, 10, 11, 12]. Emerin, which is expressed in the nuclei of many tissues, can also be assessed in the viable oral foliate cells [13].

Prenatal diagnosis can be aided by studies of the immunolabeling of proteins in chorionic villi, for example in congenital muscular dystrophy (CMD) caused by a primary deficiency of the laminin-α2 chain ("merosin-deficient" CMD) [14], or the Ullrich form of CMD caused by mutations in collagen VI [15, 16].

Cultured fibroblasts from skin biopsies can be useful for mitochondrial and metabolic studies, and studies suggest they are also useful for assessing collagen VI in some patients with Ullrich CMD or Bethlem myopathy [17, 18].

Histological and histochemical abnormalities

A wide variety of histological and histochemical stains have been used to reveal abnormalities in skeletal muscle in neuromuscular disorders. We summarize here the most important stains and information that can be obtained from them [3, 19].

Hematoxylin and eosin (H&E) provides an excellent overview of a sample, revealing the size and shape of fibers, the presence of necrotic and regenerating fibers, excess fibrous and adipose tissue, the position of nuclei, and the presence of inflammatory cells and vacuoles, and identifies the vascular and neural components. Areas with pale staining may reflect accumulation of a protein such as actin, whereas enhanced eosinophilia may be seen in the myofibrillar myopathies caused by mutations in the genes for desmin, myotilin, αB-crystallin, and filamin C (see below).

The modified Gömöri trichrome technique is also useful as, in addition to the general features of the fibers, it can demonstrate the presence of red-stained inclusions such as nemaline rods, abnormal mitochondria, cytoplasmic bodies, tubular aggregates, and membranous myelin-like whorls associated with vacuoles. Abnormal accumulations of myofibrillar material stain more darkly and are a feature of myofibrillar

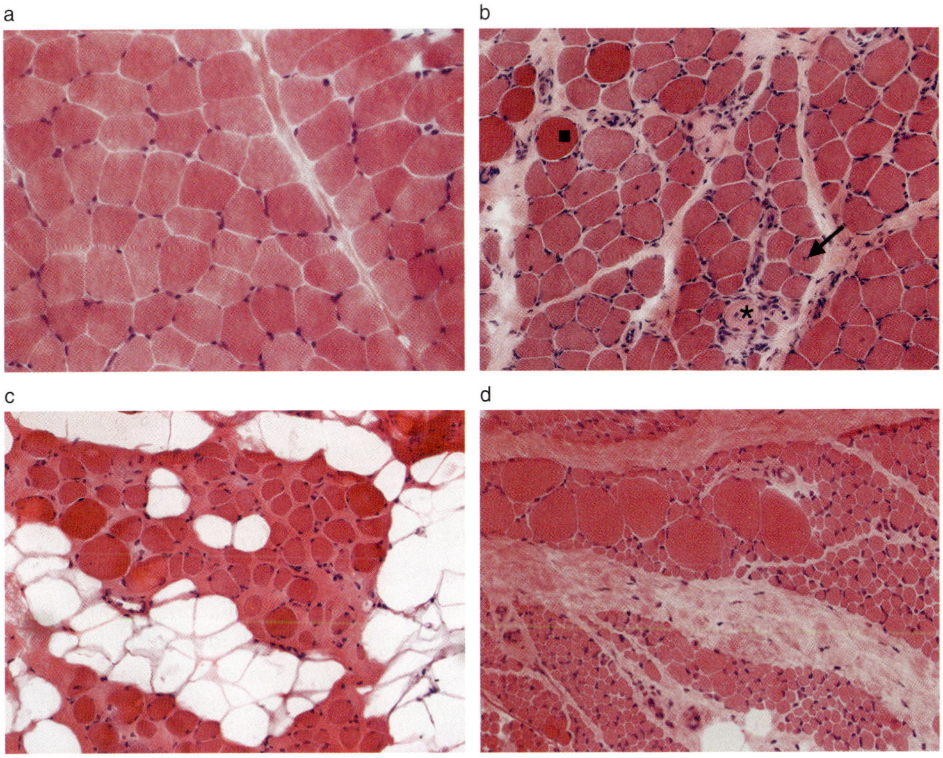

Figure 5.2a–d. (a) Normal muscle showing closely packed polygonal fibers with peripheral nuclei; (b) case of Duchenne muscular dystrophy showing a diffuse wide variation in fiber size, rounded fibers, hypercontracted fibers (black square), necrotic fibers (*), excess connective tissue and fat, and several internal nuclei (arrow); (c) case of congenital muscular dystrophy showing pronounced fibrous and adipose tissue; (d) case of spinal muscular atrophy (SMA 1) with groups of atrophic and hypertrophic fibers.

myopathies (see below). The presence or absence of glycogen is usually shown with the periodic acid Schiff (PAS) technique, and the excess intracellular lipid seen in carnitine deficiency and some mitochondrial disorders, with Oil Red O or Sudan Black.

Normal muscle fibers are polygonal in shape when sectioned transversely (Figure 5.2), and are closely packed together. They show only a little variation in size (approximately 40–80 μm for adult males, and 30–70 μm for adult females), with a statistically normal distribution. The number of fibers is set by birth, or soon after, but their size is age-dependent, and adult size is usually achieved by puberty. In neonatal muscle some larger rounded fibers, resembling Wohlfart B fibers, are often present and may give a false impression of fiber size variability.

In dystrophic or myopathic conditions fibers often appear round in shape (Figure 5.2b, c). Atrophic, denervated fibers, in contrast, may be angular, except in SMA where the grouped atrophic fibers are often round (Figure 5.2d). Assessment of changes in fiber size and the distribution of the changes is fundamental to interpretation. Myopathic conditions are characterized by diffuse changes throughout the sample, whereas in neurogenic disorders there is grouping of affected fibers (see below; Figure 5.2). Fiber size variation is often obvious, but it can be informative to measure the smallest and largest fiber in a sample to establish if the range is appropriate for age. It is common to rely on published morphological data (see [3]) but it must be remembered that samples may not have been from unequivocally normal individuals, and measurements made with modern computer systems may differ slightly from those using an eye-piece micrometer scale.

In addition to innervation, fiber size is also influenced by other factors including growth factors, aging, and work load. Excessive load on a muscle results in an increase in fiber size (hypertrophy), whereas disuse and denervation cause a decrease in size (atrophy). Longitudinal splitting and branching of fibers occurs under certain pathological circumstances and can contribute to the appearance of fiber size variation in cross-section. Occasionally multiple splitting may result in the appearance in transverse section of a small cluster of fibers. This multiple splitting is common near myotendinous junctions but it is not clear if this always accounts for their presence.

Nuclei are usually peripherally situated beneath the sarcolemma in normal fibers, but nuclei internal within a fiber are a common finding, particularly in myopathic disorders (Figure 5.2). They can, however, also occur in chronic neuropathies. It is often stated that the number of internal nuclei is not significant unless more than 3% of fibers in transverse section show one. In pediatric muscle this is probably an overestimate, and in the authors' experience even a few internal nuclei in pediatric muscle are probably significant. In normal adults internal nuclei are more common, particularly in individuals involved in sporting activities. In myotonic dystrophies (DM1 and DM2) and myofibrillar myopathies multiple internal nuclei are often particularly abundant.

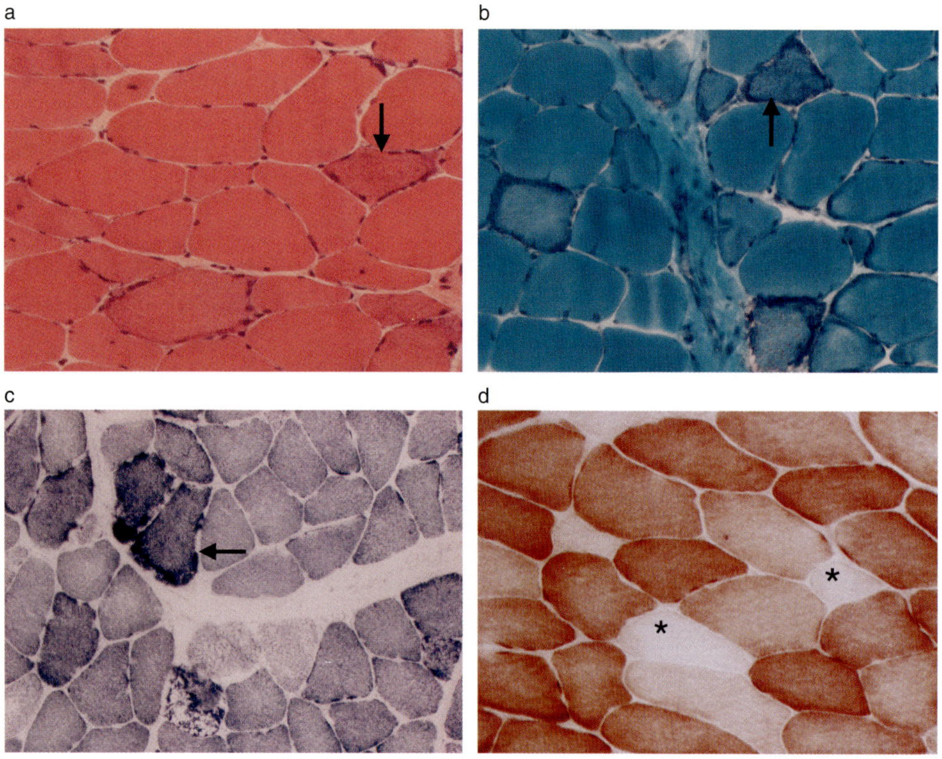

Figure 5.3a–d. Muscle biopsy from a case with a mitochondrial myopathy showing (a) granular basophilic fibers (arrow) stained with H&E, (b) ragged-red fibers with Gömöri trichrome (arrow), (c) enhanced SDH activity in ragged fibers (arrow), and (d) fibers devoid of COX activity (*).

Occasional internal nuclei occur in normal muscle, and they are common near myotendinous junctions, and care in interpretation of such regions is needed. In some conditions the nuclei may be central within the fiber, and in regenerating fibers in longitudinal section they may form a chain down the center of the fiber. In some conditions central nuclei are a characteristic feature, for example myotubular and centronuclear myopathies and CMD, where they are regularly spaced down the fiber. Central nuclei also occur in central core disease associated with defects in ryanodine receptor 1. In other situations, internal nuclei are scattered within the myofibrils. In split fibers they often occur along the internal membrane; some of these relate to nuclei of the capillary endothelial cells.

Necrosis, regeneration, and an increase in connective tissue and adipose tissue are key features of dystrophic muscle (Figure 5.2). Necrosis, however, is segmental and may not always be apparent in the plane of section. The amount of fibrous and adipose tissue is minimal in endomysial areas of normal muscle but the width of perimysial bands varies with age, and is wider in neonates than adults. In dystrophic muscle the amount of connective tissue is variable and it separates the individual fibers (Figure 5.2). A significant amount may also be seen in other conditions; for example, in central core disease, in which differential muscle involvement is a feature. This may cause diagnostic confusion with CMDs, where connective tissue is often particularly excessive (Figure 5.2).

Necrotic fibers can be identified by their pale staining with H&E and Gömöri trichrome, and may be associated with phagocytes, and fibrosis (Figure 5.2). Their fiber type profile, however, with regard to myosin isoforms is often retained. Hypercontracted fibers stain intensely with most stains and represent damaged or necrotic fibers, and are more common in DMD and Becker muscular dystrophy (BMD). Regenerating fibers are distinguished by their basophilia, but this only represents the early stages of regeneration, and antibodies to developmental myosins more accurately identify fibers at varying stages of maturity. Histochemically regenerating fibers have a profile of type 2C fibers (see below), and at early stages of maturity they are not innervated and therefore show extrajunctional neuronal cell adhesion molecule (N-CAM). Basophilic fibers also have a high RNA and acid phosphatase content, and show enhanced sarcolemmal, and sometimes internal, labeling with antibodies to several proteins, including desmin, vimentin, utrophin, caveolin-3, dysferlin, and major histocompatibility complex class I (MHC-1); but they lack neuronal nitric oxide synthase (nNOS) and β-spectrin may be reduced. In addition, they may show enhanced labeling of basal lamina proteins, probably resulting from duplication of the basal lamina (i.e., that of the original fiber together with that of the regenerating fiber).

Basophilia may also be seen in split fibers and non-regenerating fibers. Granular fibers with abnormal mitochondria also appear basophilic, and may appear red with the modified Gömöri trichrome stain (see Figure 5.3). These are often referred to as "ragged-red fibers." They occur in some mitochondrial disorders, and as an incidental feature in several disorders, or as a consequence of aging.

Table 5.1. Main characteristics of the different fiber types in human muscle. NADH-TR, reduced nicotinamide adenine dehydrogenase tetrazolium reductase; PAS, periodic acid Schiff

	Type 1	Type 2A	Type 2B	Type 2C
ATPase pH 9.4	+	+++	+++	+++
ATPase pH 4.6	+++	−	++	+++
ATPase 4.3	+++	−	−	++ or +++
NADH-TR	+++	++	+	++ or +++
Cytochrome oxidase	+++	++	+	+
Succinic dehydrogenase	+++	++	+	++
Phosphorylase	− or +	+++	+++	+++
PAS	+ or ++	+++	++	++
Lipid droplets	+++	++ or +++	+	
Antibodies to fast myosin heavy chain	−	+++	+++	++ or +++
Antibodies to slow myosin heavy chain	+++	-	-	−+ or ++

Keys: −, +, ++, +++ represent increasing intensity of stain.

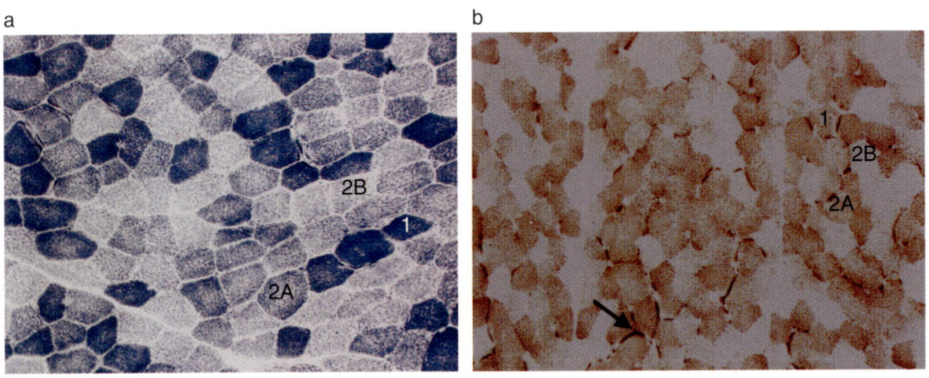

Figure 5.4a, b. Transverse section stained for nicotinamide adenine dinucleotide dehydrogenase tetrazolium reductase (NADH-TR) (a) and cytochrome oxidase (COX) (b) showing highest oxidative activity in type 1 fibers, pale staining of 2B fibers and an intermediate intensity of 2A fibers. Note the normal peripheral clusters of mitochondria (arrow).

Damaged fibers or necrotic fibers may lose glycogen, and appear as white fibers with the PAS stain, in contrast to the variable pink color of the other fibers. This is a nonspecific finding but a variable number is quite common in DMD. When present they suggest fiber damage; loss of glycogen may also occur if there is long delay before freezing, or as a result of denervation.

The PAS stain is also useful for revealing the varying glycogen content in the different fiber types (see below), and excess storage of glycogen in glycogen storage disorders (see "Metabolic myopathies"). It also reveals defects such as ring fibers (with a peripheral band of myofibrils at 90° to the rest of the fiber), and the spoke-like distribution of glycogen in some cases of centronuclear myopathy with dynamin 2 mutations [20].

Enzyme histochemistry has an essential role in identifying the different fiber types in muscle, and can also identify or suggest enzyme deficiencies. The differences in staining of fiber types reflect physiological differences, and differences in metabolism and the number of mitochondria (Table 5.1). Defining fiber types is essential in the analysis of muscle and there is a reciprocal relationship between type 1 and type 2 fibers: in general type 1 fibers have a slow phenotype and a high oxidative enzyme activity with more mitochondria than type 2 fibers (Figure 5.4). This is revealed by staining for nicotinamide adenine dinucleotide dehydrogenase tetrazolium reductase (NADH-TR), cytochrome oxidase (COX), and succinic dehydrogenase (SDH). This is in contrast to type 2 fibers, which have a higher glycolytic metabolism. Type 2 fibers can be subdivided into 2A, 2B and 2C fibers. Type 2A fibers have higher oxidative enzyme content than type 2B, and therefore have a staining intensity intermediate between types 1 and 2B with oxidative enzyme stains. In contrast, type 2B fibers have an intermediate staining intensity with adenosine triphosphatase (ATPase) preincubated a pH 4.6 (Figure 5.5). With preincubation at pH 4.3 the ATPase stain gives a reciprocal pattern to that at the routine pH of 9.4, and type 1 fibers are dark at pH 4.3 but light at pH 9.4 (Table 5.1, Figure 5.5). A third type of type 2 fiber (2C) stains for ATPase at all pH, sometimes with varying intensity. Some of these fibers are

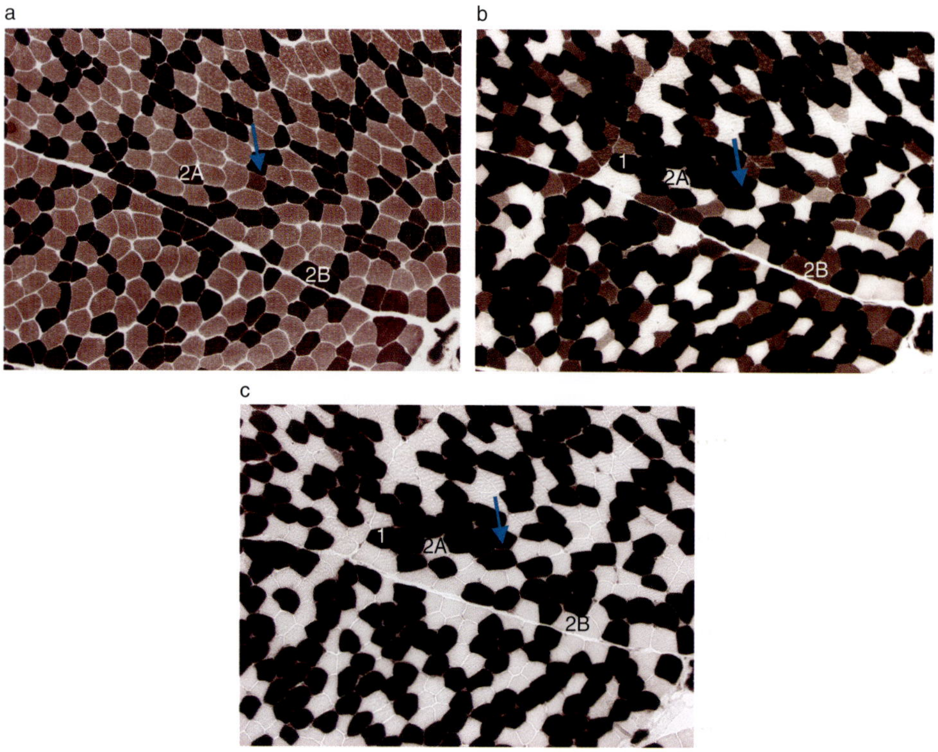

Figure 5.5a–c. Serial sections stained for ATPase at pH 9.4 (a) and following preincubation at pH 4.7 (b) and pH 4.3 (c) showing a normal fiber type pattern and the subdivision of type 2 fibers into 2A and 2B. Note the occasional 2C fiber that stains at all pH (arrow).

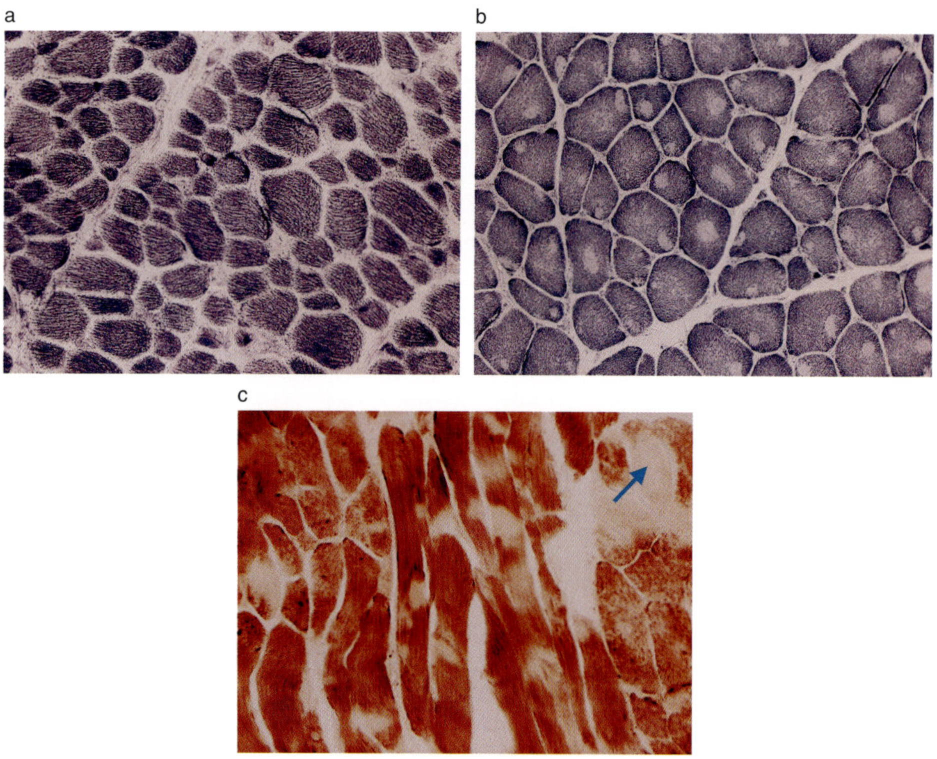

Figure 5.6a–c. Muscle biopsies from three cases with a mutation in the *RYR1* gene stained for NADH-TR (a, b) and COX (c) showing the variability in staining associated with defects in this gene. Note the absence of cores in (a) (2 months old) but classical central cores in the 3-year-old sibling (b). (c) Longitudinal and transversely sectioned fibers show multiple large cores with some fibers with a "wiped out" appearance. Note also the fiber type uniformity in all.

regenerating fibers, but some reflect the coexpression of myosin isoforms and are hybrid fibers (see below; Sewry and Costin-Kelly, unpublished observations).

In addition to fiber typing, oxidative enzyme staining reveals the distribution of mitochondria, and an absence or excess staining in relation to mitochondrial defects. In normal muscle mitochondria are evenly distributed through the fiber, although small clusters are often seen peripherally, particularly near capillaries (Figure 5.4b). In core myopathies areas devoid of mitochondria are seen with oxidative enzyme stains (see Figure 5.6).

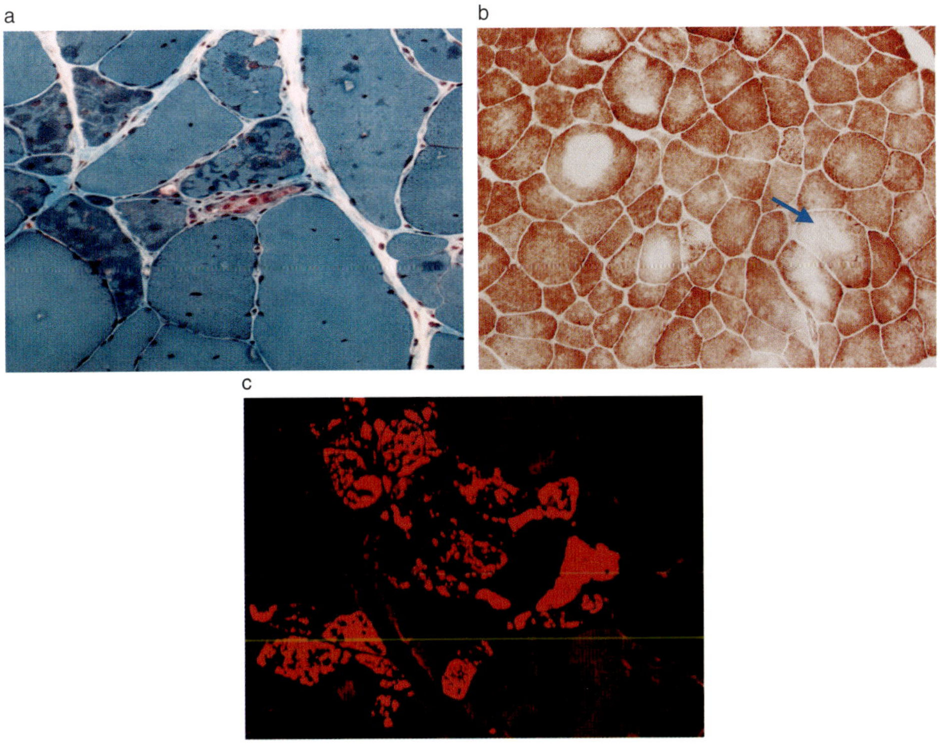

Figure 5.7a–c. Muscle biopsy from a case with a myofibrillar myopathy with a mutation in the gene encoding myotilin stained with Gömöri trichrome (a), for COX activity (b) and immunolabeled for myotilin (c). Note the dark green areas in (a) and multiple internal nuclei, the large "wiped out" areas devoid of COX activity in (b) (arrow), and the pronounced accumulation of myotilin in (c).

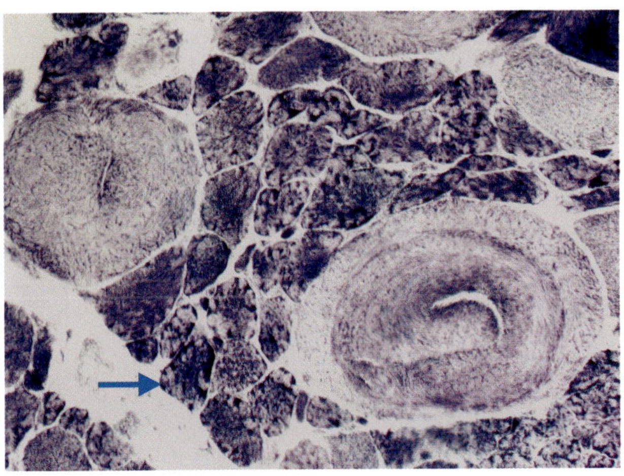

Figure 5.8. Lobulated fibers (arrow) and hypertrophic split and whorled fibers in a biopsy from a case of limb-girdle muscular dystrophy. NADH-TR.

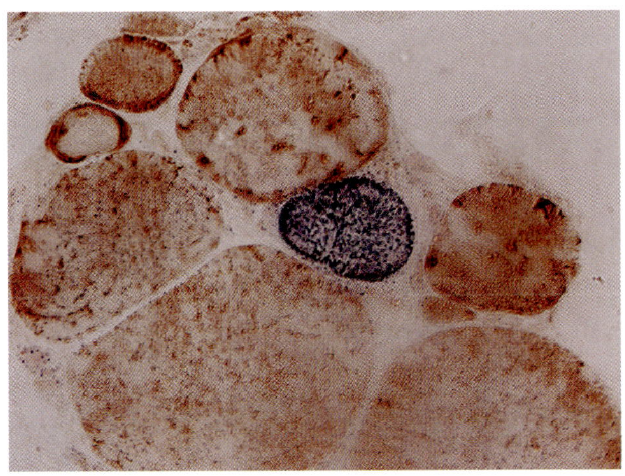

Figure 5.9. A blue-stained fiber devoid of cytochrome oxidase activity. Combined COX-SDH.

These areas may be large and central (central cores) or multiple and focal (minicores), as seen in some congenital myopathies (see below). In myofibrillar myopathies areas of accumulated myofibrillar material are devoid of mitochondria and may be extensive within a fiber ("wiped out" areas; see Figure 5.7b). Target fibers in neurogenic disorders have a central area devoid of oxidative enzyme activity that is surrounded by a dark staining zone. Lobulated fibers (Figure 5.8) have prominent peripheral clusters of small mitochondria. These are often triangular in shape and the fibers are smaller in size. These are a nonspecific feature but are rare in pediatric muscle. They have been noted in cases with a defect in the calpain-3 gene (LGMD2A). In some mitochondrial disorders fibers with enhanced oxidative enzyme activity may be seen, or there may be an absence of COX. The combined method for COX and SDH is particularly useful for revealing fibers without COX that retain SDH activity, as they stain blue (Figure 5.9), and also with modification of the SDH reaction by addition of phenazine methosulfate.

Immunohistochemical detection of different isoforms of myosin is also highly reliable for identifying fiber types and has certain advantages over enzyme histochemistry [3, 21]. In normal muscle most fibers express either fast or slow myosin, and only a few hybrid fibers co-express more than one isoform. In diseased muscle there is an increase in

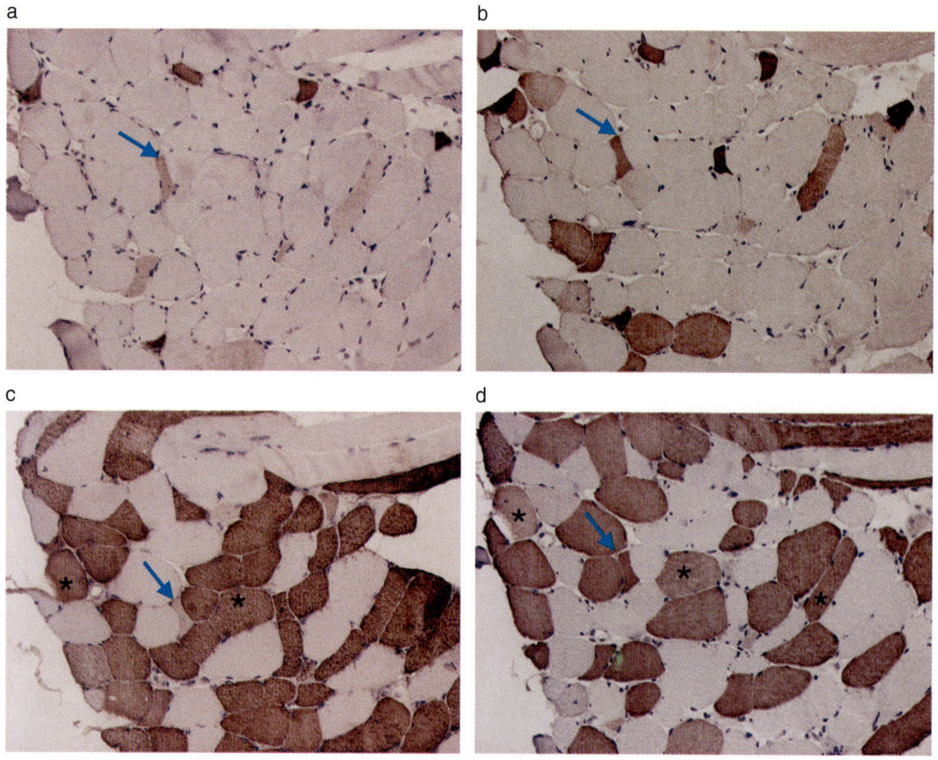

Figure 5.10a–d. Serial sections of a muscle biopsy from a case of myositis immunolabeled with antibodies to developmental (a), neonatal (b), fast (c), and slow (d) myosin. Note the number of hybrid fibers co-expressing more than one isoform (*) and fibers that label with all four antibodies (arrow). Fibers labeled with both developmental myosin and neonatal myosin are probably regenerating.

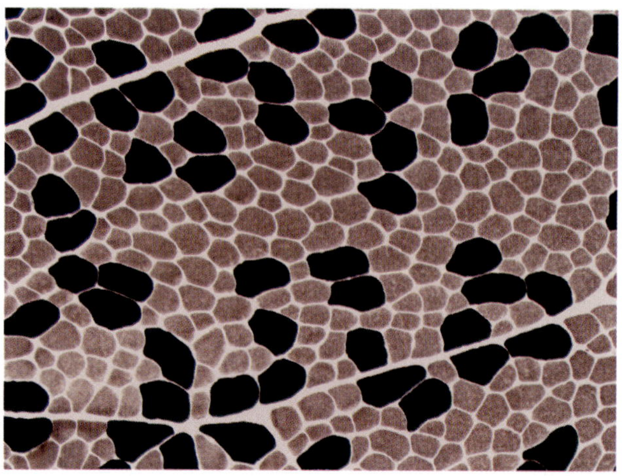

Figure 5.11. Muscle biopsy from a case with a mutation in the *ACTA1* gene stained for ATPase at pH 9.4 showing fiber type disproportion with a predominance of small pale type 1 fibers.

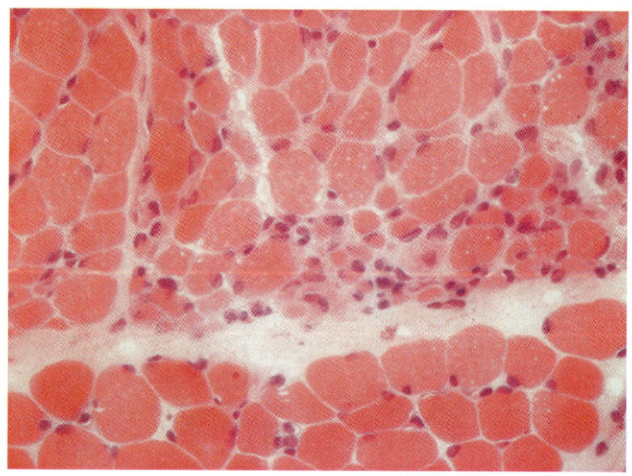

Figure 5.12. Atrophic fibres at the periphery of a fascicle in a biopsy from a case of juvenile dermatomyositis. H&E.

the number of the hybrid fibers, and sometimes an increase in fibers expressing developmental isoforms of myosin (see Figure 5.10). Hybrid fibers are not easily detected with ATPase staining. The co-expression of more than one isoform accounts for the poor distinction of fiber types sometimes seen in diseased muscle with the ATPase method. In addition, several commercial antibodies to myosin isoforms can be applied to wax-embedded material using antigen retrieval techniques, and can be used to reveal fiber types in postmortem material, when enzyme activity may be lost.

Specific involvement of one fiber type can occur in some disorders, for example atrophy of type 2 fibers is a common nonspecific feature. In dystrophic disorders atrophy and hypertrophy of both fiber types occurs. Type 1 atrophy occurs in several congenital myopathies (see Figure 5.11), often with type 2 hypertrophy, and is also a feature of DM1. In denervation the groups of atrophic fibers are of both types, and a perifascicular distribution of atrophic fibers is a characteristic of dermatomyositis (Figure 5.12). In chronic conditions atrophy of a fiber may be so severe that only a clump of nuclei remains (Figure 5.13). These often express fast and/or neonatal myosin. Exercise can induce type 2 hypertrophy, and marked fiber hypertrophy can be seen in some cases of myasthenia caused by mutations in genes associated with proteins at the neuromuscular junction. In the childhood forms of SMA (SMA1 and 2) the hypertrophic fibers are frequently type 1/slow (see Figure 5.14).

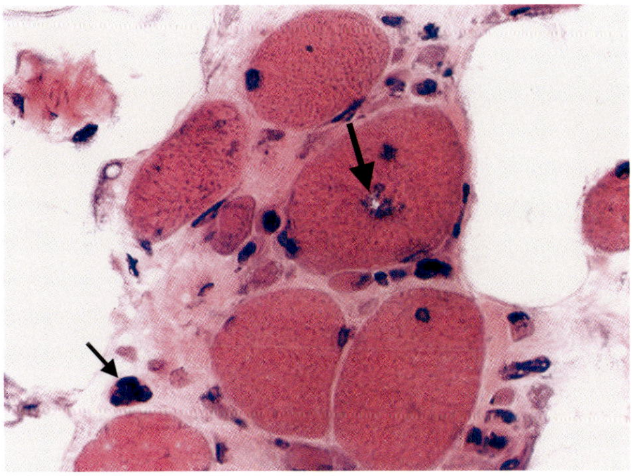

Figure 5.13. Rimmed vacuole (large arrow) and nuclear clumps (small arrow) in a biopsy from a case of inclusion body myositis. H&E.

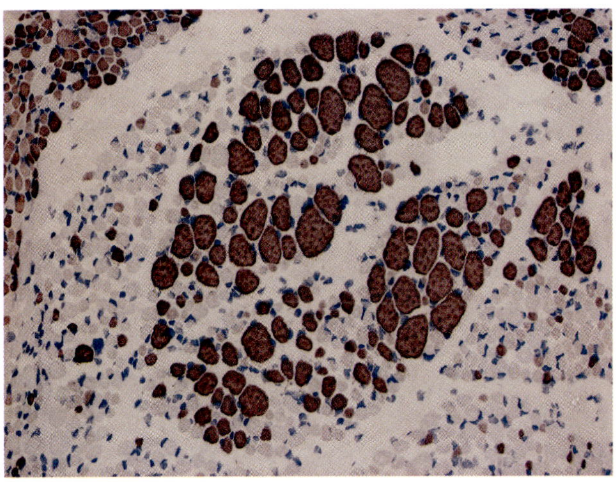

Figure 5.14. Muscle biopsy of a case of SMA1 immunolabeled with an antibody to slow myosin showing fiber type grouping. Note the groups of positive and negative fibers; the atrophic fibers are of both types but often negative (fast), and the hypertrophied fibers have slow myosin.

The proportion of fiber types varies in different muscles, and it is therefore important to know the muscle that has been sampled. Published data are often relied on as a baseline (see [3]). Alterations in fiber type proportions frequently occur in pathological situations, and in myopathic disorders type 1 fiber predominance is common. Following spinal cord injury, type 2 predominance occurs. It is important not to confuse fiber type predominance with fiber type grouping that arises from collateral sprouting of surviving nerves following denervation.

The number of capillaries relates to fiber type and is also age dependent, with a smaller network of capillaries being apparent with most techniques in muscle from neonates.

Other enzyme techniques that may need to be applied include phosphorylase, phosphofructokinase, acid phosphatase, myoadenylate deaminase (MAD), and menadione-linked α-glycerophosphate dehydrogenase. Phosphorylase activity is absent in McArdle disease (see "Metabolic myopathies"). The only other disorder where this is seen is when muscle glycogen synthase is mutated and glycogen is absent from the muscle [22]. The phosphorylase technique requires endogenous glycogen, thus the enzyme is not revealed in the absence of endogenous glycogen. Similarly, the fibers in dystrophic muscle, or areas such as cores, that lack endogenous glycogen do not stain for phosphorylase. Phosphofructokinase deficiency can be detected histochemically but it is more reliably determined biochemically. The lysosomal enzyme acid phosphatase is high in necrotic fibers but its major uses are in revealing the presence of macrophages and high activity in vacuoles, particularly those associated with acid maltase deficiency (see Figure 5.15). It also highlights autofluorescent deposits seen in vitamin E deficiency and Batten disease. Demonstration of MAD is favored by some but interpretation is hampered by the presence of a common mutation in the normal population that obliterates the enzyme. The only diagnostic role of menadione-linked α-glycerophosphate dehydrogenase is in the identification of reducing bodies that characterize the congenital myopathy named after them. Reducing bodies stain intensely with this method but substrate is not required to reveal them, as they reduce the menadione nitroblue tetrazolium (NBT). With the identification of *FHL1* as the gene responsible for reducing body myopathy [23], and

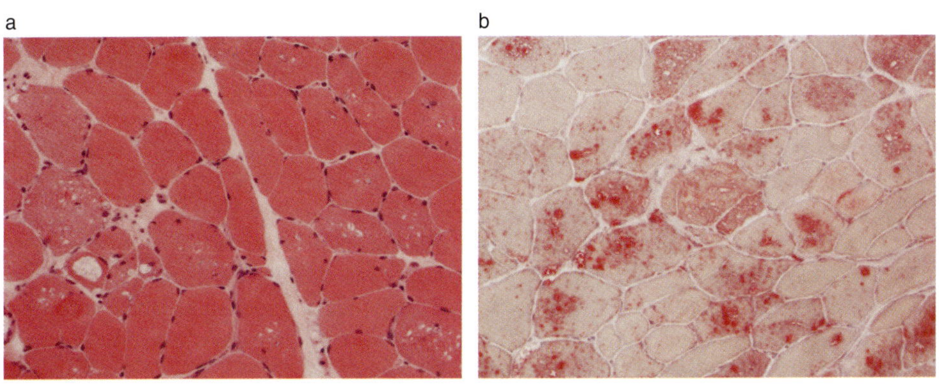

Figure 5.15a, b. Muscle biopsy from a case of acid maltase deficiency stained with H&E (a) and for acid phosphatase (b) activity showing multiple vacuoles containing acid phosphatase.

the wide clinical spectrum associated with mutations [24, 25], the importance of this technique is increasing.

Vacuoles can occur in several conditions and they are of different types. They are a feature of distal myopathies, inclusion body myositis, the myofibrillar myopathies, glycogenoses, and periodic paralyses, although absence of vacuoles in a sample does not exclude these diagnoses. Vacuoles rimmed by basophilia and red-staining material with Gömöri trichrome are typical of distal myopathies, inclusion body myositis, and myofibrillar myopathies (Figure 5.13). Some vacuoles have detectable material within them, others appear as empty spaces. It is important not to interpret the presence of excess lipid droplets as vacuoles, as lipid appears unstained with many techniques. Autophagic vacuoles lined by membrane expressing sarcolemmal proteins are seen in two X-linked conditions, one linked to Xq28 [26] and the other caused by mutations in the LAMP-2 (i.e., lysosomal-associated membrane-2 protein) gene, also on the X chromosome [27]. Indentations of the sarcolemma also show sarcolemmal proteins and when sectioned transversely they may appear as vacuoles. This is common at myotendinous junctions.

A variety of cellular reactions may be present in a biopsy. These can be seen with routine histological stains such as H&E, and defined with specific cellular differentiation markers (Figure 5.16). Macrophages are the most common infiltrating cells seen, which may be present both within necrotic fibers and in the interstitial tissue. Inflammatory cellular reactions can occur to varying degrees in various forms of muscular dystrophy, including DMD, FSHD, and LGMD2B, and they are a feature of the inflammatory myopathies. They are not a universal feature in all cases of inflammatory myopathies, however, and absence of a cellular infiltrate does not exclude the diagnosis. The distribution of inflammatory cells may be predominantly perivascular or endomysial, and the cell type may vary with the acuteness of the condition.

Immunohistochemistry

Immunohistochemical assessment of various proteins is now an essential part of the assessment of a muscle biopsy [3, 28]. Antibodies to most cellular components and organelles are now available but not all are relevant to diagnosis and we will therefore confine details here to those relevant to pathological assessment.

Developmental regulation of proteins

It is not only essential to know the localization of a protein in normal muscle but also how it varies during development, as samples from fetuses and neonates may have to be assessed, as well as samples containing regenerating fibers at varying stages of maturity. Several proteins in skeletal muscle are developmentally regulated and the level of detectable protein may be either higher or lower than in mature muscle, and its localization may alter (Table 5.2). In addition, a different isoform of a protein may be present at different stages of development (Table 5.2). It is also important, as with all immunohistochemical studies, to consider the varying affinity of antibodies, and that the absence of detectable labeling could be due to conformational masking of the epitope of the antibody.

Studies of developmental isoforms of myosin are useful for assessing immaturity and can help to distinguish an atrophic fiber from one that is small because it is regenerating. Neonatal myosin is detectable in muscle fibers of neonates. The number declines with age, with a large number of positive fibers being

Table 5.2. Proteins relevant to pathological assessment whose expression changes during development. MHC, major histocompatibility complex; N-CAM, neuronal cell adhesion molecule; nNOS, neuronal nitric oxide synthase

Change of isoform	
Actin	Cardiac → skeletal
Myosin	Embryonic → neonatal → fast or slow
Low expression on immature and regenerating fibers	
β-spectrin low round small regenerating fibers	
C-terminal dystrophin (sometimes)	
Some dystrophin-associated proteins	
nNOS	
High expression on/in regenerating fibers	
Utrophin	
Laminin-α5	
N-CAM	
Caveolin-3	
Dysferlin	
Vimentin	
Desmin	
MHC class I	

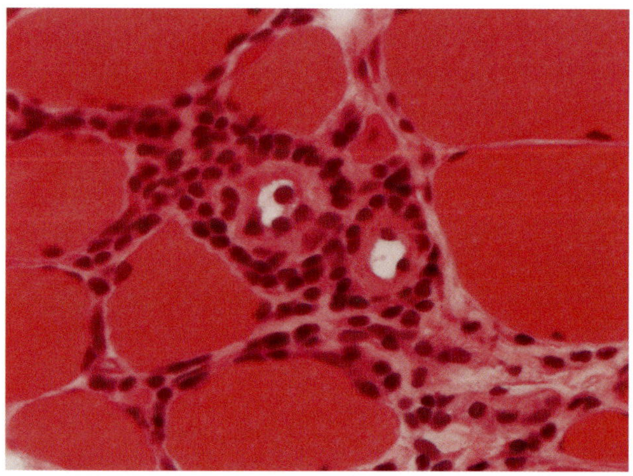

Figure 5.16. Inflammatory cells around blood vessels and fibers in a biopsy from a case of myositis. H&E.

Table 5.3. Primary protein defects in neuromuscular disorders where immunoanalysis can be informative

Sarcolemma	
Dystrophin	Xp21 muscular dystrophies (usually absent in Duchenne, reduced in Becker)
Sarcoglycans	Limb-girdle muscular dystrophies 2C–F
Dysferlin	Limb-girdle muscular dystrophy 2B
Caveolin-3	Limb-girdle muscular dystrophy 1A, rippling muscle disease, hyperCKemia, autoimmune caveolin-3
Laminin-α2	MDC1A ("merosin-deficient" congenital muscular dystrophy)
Collagen VI	Ullrich congenital muscular dystrophy (no detectable change in Bethlem myopathy)
Integrin-α7	Mild congenital dystrophy/myopathy (*no commercial antibody*)
Nuclear membrane	
Emerin	X-linked Emery–Dreifuss muscular dystrophy
Sarcoplasmic reticulum	
SERCA1	Brody disease
Cytoskeleton	
Plectin	Epidermolysis bullosa with muscular dystrophy
Enzymes	
Calpain-3	This has mainly be assessed on immunoblots and may show an absence in LGMD2A
Accumulation of proteins	
Actin	Congenital actinopathy/nemaline myopathy
Myosin	Hyaline body myopathy
Desmin	Desmin-related myopathies
Myotilin	Myofibrillar myopathy

present at birth and relatively few after 6 months of age. Some positive fibers may be seen up to 2 years of age but it is not yet clear if this is within the normal spectrum of expression, or if it is pathological. Although the presence of neonatal myosin can reflect immaturity, its presence in some situations may relate to noninnervation of a fiber, or to a nonspecific pathological response. In disorders such as motor neuron disease and SMA several of the small fibers usually considered to be noninnervated fibers show neonatal myosin, and may also show additional developmentally regulated proteins. It is not known if this could reflect regeneration induced by denervation, and/or arrest in maturation, and/or the re-expression of neonatal myosin induced by the pathological state. Nevertheless, studies of neonatal myosin are important for the assessment of other developmentally regulated proteins and for identifying different patterns of expression that are associated with different disorders (see below).

Actin is also an important myofibrillar muscle protein that changes isoform during development. In fetal skeletal muscle the isoform found in adult cardiac muscle is predominant and this is then replaced by the isoform of skeletal muscle by the late stages of gestation [29]. Thus by birth very few fibers show cardiac actin, but it is present in regenerating fibers.

Primary protein defects in muscle detectable with immunohistochemistry

Detectable abnormalities in protein localization caused by a defect in the corresponding gene are summarized in Table 5.3. The proteins are localized to diverse subcellular components and whether a change is seen depends on the nature of the mutation, its effect on the protein product, and its mode of inheritance. In recessive disorders, if the mutations result in a stop codon, an absence of protein can be seen, but if the mutations are missense, an alteration in protein may not be apparent with immunohistochemistry. In some instances a reduction in the amount or molecular mass of protein may be visible on immunoblots (see below). In dominant disorders, the expression of protein from the normal allele may mask the alteration from the abnormal allele. An exception to this is dominant mutations of the caveolin-3 gene where reduction of protein can be seen (see "Limb-girdle muscular dystrophies" below) [30, 31].

In assessment of some proteins it is important to use more than one antibody, for example dystrophin and laminin-α2 (see "Duchenne and Becker muscular dystrophy" and "Congenital muscular dystrophies"). In some conditions the

Table 5.4. Secondary abnormalities in protein expression useful for assessment of pathological muscle. AD EDMD, autosomal dominant form of Emery–Dreifuss muscular dystrophy; CMDs, congenital muscular dystrophies; LGMDs, limb-girdle muscular dystrophies; MHC, major histocompatibility complex; nNOS, neuronal nitric oxide synthase

Protein	Disorder where useful
Utrophin	Xp21 and LGMDs
Sarcoglycans	LGMDs 2C–F, Xp21
β-dystroglycan	Xp21 (normal in CMDs and LGMDs)
α-dystroglycan hypoglycosylation	CMDs and LGMD2I
nNOS	Xp21 & disorders with denervation
Laminin-α2	CMDs
Laminin-β1	LGMD2I, AD EDMD, Bethlem myopathy
Laminin-α5	CMDs and denervation
MHC class I	All inflammatory myopathies, LGMD2B
Myosin isoforms	Hybrid fibers in most disorders (*good alternative to ATPase)*
Desmin accumulation	Cores, myofibrillar myopathies
Myotilin accumulation	Myofibrillar myopathies
Phosphorylated Tau accumulation	Inclusion body myositis, myofibrillar myopathies

alteration in immunolabeling may be subtle, for example collagen VI in Ullrich CMD (see "Congenital muscular dystrophies"). In these situations labeling of an additional protein to control for good preservation of the basement membrane is important, such as with an antibody to perlecan or collagen V. Good preservation of the sarcolemma is also important when assessing dystrophin and laminin-α2. Antibodies to β-spectrin and laminin-γ1 are used for this.

Secondary defects

Alterations in protein expression and localization that are a secondary consequence of a primary defect in another gene are also useful in pathological studies. Each pathologist often has their own preference for a panel of antibodies, but we summarize in Table 5.4 those that we find helpful in the study of pathological samples and in differential diagnosis. Secondary reductions can occur if proteins interact, and both immunohistochemistry and immunoblots are then useful.

Studies of β-spectrin are useful for assessing the integrity of the plasmalemma, either artifactually or pathologically induced. This is particularly important in studies of many sarcolemmal proteins. As it labels the periphery of the fibers, β-spectrin can sometimes give a clearer indication of fiber size variability than routine histological stains. Beta-spectrin is lost from the sarcolemma of necrotic fibers, and labeling can appear weaker on regenerating fibers. Internal labeling is seen on the membranes of splits, invaginations and branched fibers, and some types of vacuoles. Neuromuscular and myotendinous junctions are more intensely labeled with antibodies to several plasmalemmal and basal lamina proteins because of membrane folding. Invaginations of the sarcolemma – when sectioned transversely, for example at myotendinous junctions – may sometimes be confused with vacuoles. Some vacuoles of lysosomal origin, such as in acid maltase deficiency or those derived from the sarcoplasmic reticulum, may label with β-spectrin but not with antibodies to basal lamina proteins. Autophagic vacuoles in Danon disease (LAMP-2 mutation) and the other X-linked disorder with similar pathology (X-linked myopathy with excessive autophagy), in contrast, show the presence of sarcolemmal proteins on most vacuoles and of basal lamina proteins on some [26, 27].

Dystrophin rarely shows a secondary reduction in well-preserved muscle, except in recessive LGMD2E, caused by a defect in the gene encoding β-sarcoglycan [32]. A reduction in dystrophin may occasionally be seen in other LGMDs and occasionally in some cases of CMD [33], but in most disorders other than Xp21, immunolabeling is indistinguishable from normal. If dystrophin is reduced in a female patient careful distinction from a Duchenne carrier is needed. Weak labeling with antibodies to the C-terminus of dystrophin may be seen in some neonatal samples, possibly because of differential splicing at the C-terminus of the gene.

Dystrophin is associated with a complex of proteins at the sarcolemma, the dystrophin-associated complex (DAPC; see Chapter 3). In Xp21 muscular dystrophies, when dystrophin is absent or reduced, most proteins of the DAPC are also reduced, and assessment can be useful in differential diagnosis (see "Duchenne and Becker muscular dystrophy"). In addition to studies of muscular dystrophies, labeling of nNOS can be useful in the assessment of neurogenic disorders, as denervated fibers lose sarcolemmal nNOS [34].

The sarcoglycans (α, β, γ, δ) act as a complex such that a primary mutation affecting one of the genes results in a

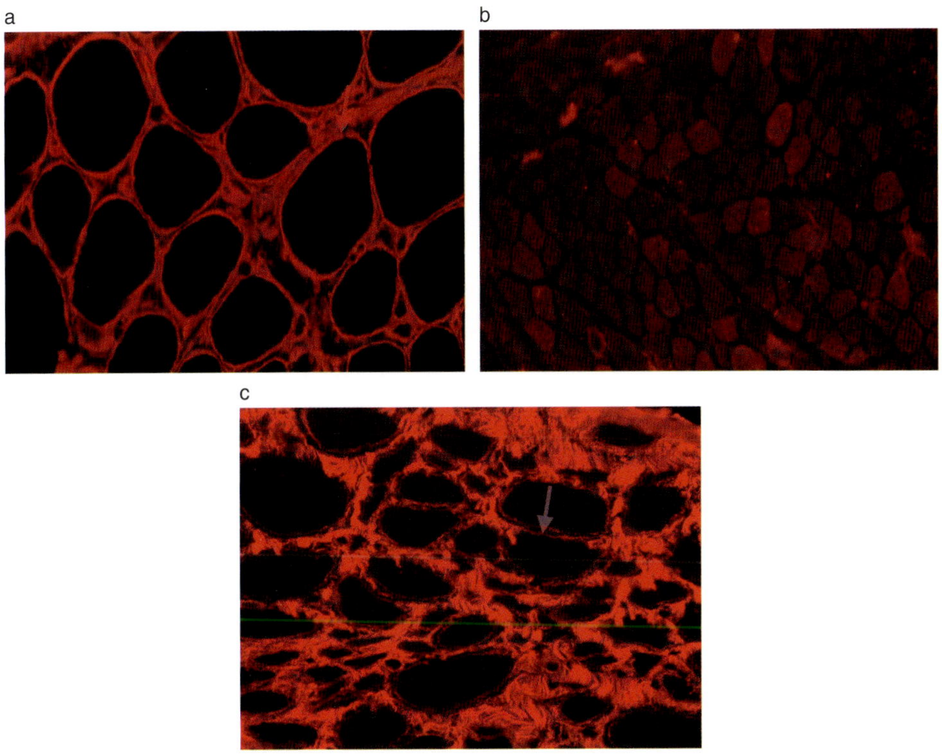

Figure 5.17a–c. Immunolabeling of collagen VI in muscle biopsies from a dystrophic control (a), and two cases of Ullrich congenital muscular dystrophy (b, c). In the control sample labeling of the sarcolemma is enhanced compared with the endomysium (arrow) but there is an absence in case (b) but reduced sarcolemmal labelling in (c) (arrow).

secondary reduction in the others, and cause forms of LGMD. All four are reduced to a variable extent in Xp21 disorders, and in LGMDs it can be difficult to determine where the primary defect lies. Two other sarcoglycans, ε- and ζ-sarcoglycan, have also been identified and are thought to have a greater role in smooth muscle [35, 36, 37]. In smooth muscle ε-sarcoglycan replaces α-sarcoglycan and forms a different complex with β- and δ-sarcoglycan; ζ-sarcoglycan may replace γ-sarcoglycan, but the exact relationships are not clear. Mutations in the gene for ε-sarcoglycan cause myoclonus-dystonia syndrome [38], but no pathogenic mutations have been found in ζ-sarcoglycan or in sarcospan, another component of the DAPC that is thought to be associated with the sarcoglycans.

Utrophin is developmentally regulated in muscle. In addition to regenerating fibers in all disorders, utrophin is prominent on the sarcolemma of mature fibers (without neonatal myosin) in DMD, BMD, and inflammatory myopathies, although in young cases of DMD only a few mature fibers are labeled. Manifesting carriers of DMD also show overexpression, on fibers with and without dystrophin. Overexpression of utrophin is not specific to Xp21 disorders, and low levels can be detected in neonatal muscle, in a variety of disorders, and on muscle fibers adjacent to tumors. The highest levels, however, are seen in Xp21 dystrophies [3, 19].

A secondary modification in the O-glycosylation of α-dystroglycan, a DAPC protein, is now recognized as an important pathogenic mechanism, particularly in various forms of CMD [39, 40]. Mutations in several genes encoding proven or putative glycosyltransferases result in abnormal glycosylation of α-dystroglycan (see "Congenital muscular dystrophies"). Caution and carefully controlled studies are needed for the interpretation of results with current commercial antibodies to α-dystroglycan, as different batches can give variable results. Despite this, different disease-associated patterns of dystroglycan expression are emerging. In Xp21 disorders labeling of both the glycosylated epitope of α-dystroglycan and β-dystroglycan show a reduction, in common with other proteins of the DAPC. In the various forms of CMD β-dystroglycan usually shows normal sarcolemmal localization, when the plasmalemma is well preserved, but variable degrees of reduced α-dystroglycan are seen (see "Congenital muscular dystrophies").

The increased connective tissue in the perimysium and endomysium that occurs in several disorders shows the presence of several extracellular matrix proteins. These include various types of collagen, such as types III, V and VI, and fibronectin. In normal muscle several collagen types are constituents of the basement membrane and appear around each fiber at the sarcolemma. In normal muscle the periphery of each fiber is clearly delineated by antibodies to proteins such as collagen types IV, V, VI, laminins, perlecan, and nidogen. They are also seen in the extracellular matrix around blood vessels. When connective tissue is excessive the sarcolemmal labeling of collagen types V and VI is usually more prominent than that of the adjacent endomysium (see Figure 5.17 and "Congenital muscular dystrophies").

Secondary changes in some laminin chains are seen in various muscular dystrophies. In various forms of CMD and LGMD2I laminin-α2, a receptor for α-dystroglycan, may show a secondary reduction [41]. A reduction of laminin-β1 on the

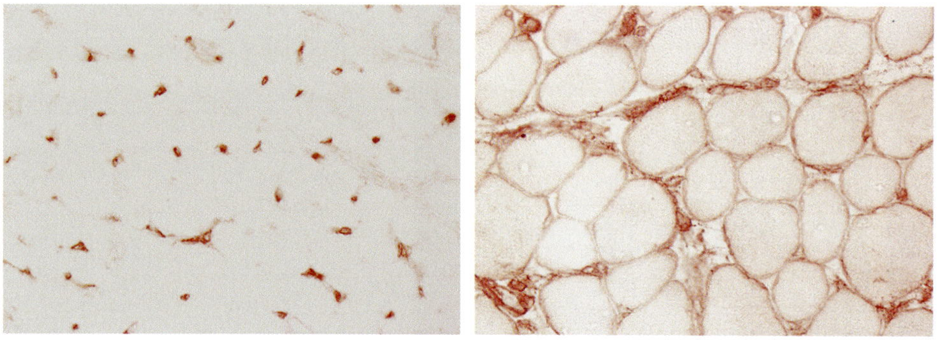

Figure 5.18a, b. MHC class 1 immunolabeling of normal muscle (a) and a biopsy from a case of juvenile dermatomyositis (b). Note the normal labeling of blood vessels in both but the abnormal sarcolemmal labeling and reduced number of capillaries in (b).

sarcolemma, but not the blood vessels, can be seen in some conditions such as Bethlem myopathy and autosomal dominant Emery–Dreifuss muscular dystrophy [42]. This, however, is not specific and has been observed in a variety of myopathies (R. Charlton, personal observation). The reduction in sarcolemmal laminin-β1 appears to be age dependent; it is seen in affected adults and adolescents, but rarely in biopsies from children.

Laminin-α5 on the sarcolemma is higher in cases with a primary defect in laminin-α2 (MDC1A) and is often higher than in normal muscle in Xp21 dystrophies and inflammatory myopathies. As expression of laminin-α5 is developmentally regulated, some of this may relate to regeneration and immaturity, and careful correlation with neonatal myosin is needed.

Assessment of major histocompatibility class I antigens (MHC-1) is essential for the assessment of all inflammatory myopathies. Normal mature muscle fibers express minimal or no detectable MHC-1, but it is seen on endothelial cells of blood vessels, and the capillary network is clearly visible (Figure 5.18). MHC-1 is high on regenerating fibers in all disorders, but not fetal fibers, and comparisons with neonatal myosin are then important for distinguishing the abnormal MHC-1 from that related to regeneration. In inflammatory myopathies overexpression of MHC-1 can be detected on the sarcolemma, and sometimes also internally in the fibers, in all forms of inflammatory myopathy (Figure 5.18), even when there is minimal pathology and no significant inflammatory cellular reaction [43]. As with utrophin, however, overexpression of MHC-1 is not specific to inflammatory myopathies and it may also be seen in Xp21 muscular dystrophies [3], and in LGMD2B with a defect in the gene for dysferlin [44], in which inflammatory cells may be present.

Studies of myosin heavy chain isoforms are informative in the assessment of fiber types in most biopsies. In normal human muscle the majority of fibers express either a slow or fast myosin heavy chain isoform, corresponding to the histochemical fiber types 1 and 2, respectively. The slow isoform is the same as the beta cardiac isoform and in human muscle the fast 2A and 2X heavy chains are expressed. The 2B myosin isoform has not been detected in human muscles. Thus a fiber defined by ATPase staining as 2B does not express 2B myosin, but 2X. In diseased muscle hybrid fibers expressing more than one isoform are common, and an excessive number can be used as a marker of abnormality (Figure 5.10).

As embryonic and neonatal myosin heavy chains are abundant in regenerating fibers their presence is often a reflection of immaturity, as discussed above. In addition to regenerating fibers, however, neonatal myosin is also expressed in nuclear clumps and an appreciable number of nonbasophilic fibers in the muscular dystrophies. It is frequently co-expressed with fast and/or slow isoforms in a variety of disorders. Although some of this may relate to regenerated fibers at different stages of maturity, some is probably a nonspecific pathological response. There is also evidence that denervation can result in the re-expression of neonatal myosin. If a small fiber shows neonatal myosin it may be difficult to determine if it is denervated or regenerating. Nevertheless, the size and number of fibers with neonatal myosin in pathological muscle vary and the different patterns of their distribution in different disorders can be useful to assess. In severe muscular dystrophies, such as DMD, a large diffuse population of fibers of variable size and intensity of labeling is often seen; in BMD clusters of positive fibers may occur in some areas with very small positive fibers diffusely distributed elsewhere; whereas in congenital myopathies relatively few fibers with neonatal myosin are seen, and those present are often only a few microns in diameter and diffusely distributed.

Abnormal accumulation of a protein occurs in some disorders [45]. In both myofibrillar myopathies and inclusion body myositis a variety of the same proteins accumulate, which can cause diagnostic difficulties. These include desmin, myotilin, αB-crystallin, filamin-C, phosphorylated neurofilaments (Tau), ubiquitin, β-amyloid precursor protein, prion protein, and presenilin, as well as accumulation of amyloid-β [46, 47]. Cores with disruption of myofibrils show accumulation of several proteins including heat shock proteins, filamin-C, myotilin, and ubiquitin [48].

Myosin heavy chain accumulation has been localized to the hyaline bodies in cases with a mutation in the *MYH7* gene [49] and actin filaments may accumulate in some severe neonatal cases of nemaline myopathy, caused by a mutation in the *ACTA1* gene. There are no commercial antibodies that specifically recognize skeletal muscle actin but accumulation of actin

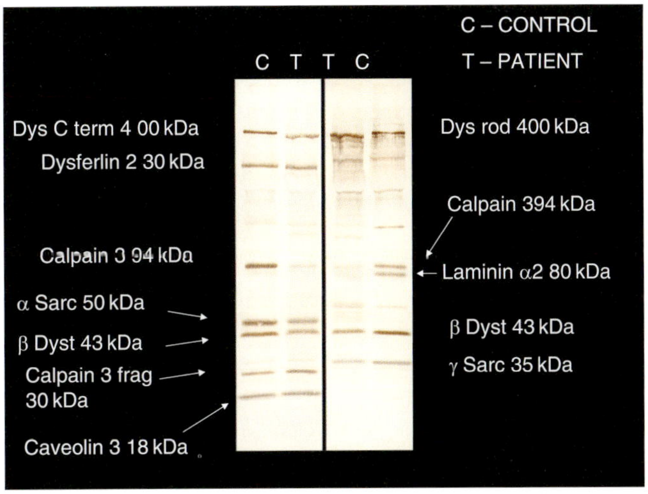

Figure 5.19. A multiplex immunoblot of several proteins in control (C) and a case of LGMD 2I (T). Note the slight reduction of dystrophin in this case which led to the suggestion that this case might have Becker dystrophy but laminin-α2 is reduced; calpain-3 (94 kDa) is also reduced. (Courtesy of the late Dr. Louise V. B. Anderson.)

can be suspected by the presence of weak areas of eosin staining, and labeling with phalloidin.

Immunoblot analysis in the diagnosis of muscle disorders

Immunohistochemical studies are complemented by immunoblot analysis (Western blot). Immunoblotting is a method for detecting specific proteins in a muscle homogenate or extract. It uses polyacrylamide gel electrophoresis (PAGE) to separate denatured proteins according to the length of the polypeptide. The separated proteins are then transferred to a membrane (usually nitrocellulose), where each protein is detected by an antibody specific to the target protein. The advantages of immunoblotting are: (1) quantitative estimation of the amount of a protein present, (2) determination of the molecular mass of the protein, and (3) several proteins can be examined on the same blot to examine secondary changes, particularly in interacting proteins (Figure 5.19). Quantification requires reference to a control/reference sample with equal loading of total protein. Some antibodies that are suitable for use in microscopic immunohistochemistry are not useful for immunoblot, and vice versa.

Immunoblotting is time consuming and more costly than immunohistochemistry, and not necessary for all proteins on a routine basis. All results are related to those from immunohistochemistry and the clinical phenotype, and these often determine the need for immunoblotting. Creatine kinase levels can be a useful guide, as many of the disorders where immunoblotting is helpful are associated with a significantly raised level.

It is not necessary to determine the absence of protein such as dystrophin by immunoblotting in a case of DMD, as this is easily seen on sections; but examining the quantity and the molecular mass of dystrophin in a possible case of BMD can be informative, particularly in cases where a deletion has not been detected by routine analysis. Detection of a lower molecular mass will only be observed if there is a deletion of one or more exons, and not if there is a point mutation. A reduction in quantity, however, may occur if there is point mutation.

In sarcoglycanopathies, where the primary loss or deficiency of one of the four sarcoglycans (α, β, γ, δ) leads to a secondary deficiency of the whole subcomplex, examining all four proteins on a multiplex blot can sometimes help to direct molecular analysis [50].

In assessment of some disorders, immunoblotting is essential as the antibody gives a clearer result on immunoblots, and differences in interacting proteins must be examined. For example, the deficiency of the enzyme calpain-3 in LGMD2A requires immunoblots as it is important to distinguish a pathogenic deficiency from that caused by degradation. The commercial antibodies to calpain-3 deficiency can identify the absence of native protein in a section [51], but a reduction is more difficult to determine and requires immunoblotting, although recent data have shown the value of labeling of sections [52]. Similarly, dysferlin can be detected on sections but a clearer result is obtained on immunoblots. In addition, it is important to compare dysferlin, calpain-3, and caveolin-3 simultaneously on a multiplex blot, as secondary reductions can occur when there is a primary defect in any of these [53, 54]. A secondary reduction in calpain-3 also occurs in tibial muscular dystrophy caused by M-line titin mutations [55]. Detection of a normal quantity of calpain-3 does not exclude a molecular defect [56], because immunoblotting only detects the presence of the protein, not enzyme activity.

Other proteins may also show no detectable abnormality on immunoblots or sections, but molecular analysis reveals a defect. For example, in a family with a late-onset distal myopathy caused by a ZASP gene mutation, the 32-kDa and 78-kDa bands of ZASP on immunoblotting appeared normal, and immunohistochemistry in muscle revealed normal Z-disk localization of ZASP [57]. There were, however, moderate accumulations of myotilin, desmin, αB-crystallin, and α-actinin on sections.

Immunoblotting can complement the detection of reduced glycosylation of α-dystroglycan observed by immunohistochemistry in various forms of CMD. The reduction in glycosylation is seen on blots as a narrowing and lowering of the normal broad band. Correlative studies of the core protein of α-dystroglycan are currently hampered by the lack of suitable antibodies that detect both native protein on sections and denatured protein on blots.

In glycosylation deficiencies a variable secondary reduction of both laminin-α2 and α-dystroglycan is seen [58], and immunohistochemical staining and immunoblot analysis may give rise to conflicting results. For example, LGMD2I immunostaining for laminin-α2 (using an antibody directed against the 80-kDa fragment) may show normal labeling on sections but an absence on immunoblots [59] (Figure 5.19).

Histochemical and immunochemical changes in specific disorders

The details relating to specific disorders should be read in conjunction with the sections above and other relevant chapters.

Neurogenic disorders

Neurogenic disorders are caused by defective function or damage of lower motor neurons or peripheral nerves. Characteristic changes are seen in muscle biopsies but it is not usually possible to determine the site of the lesion, or whether the denervation is active or progressive, or how recently it occurred. The lower motor neuron is damaged in amyotrophic lateral sclerosis (ALS) and various forms of inherited SMA. These include the common 5q-linked form, the late-onset X-linked bulbospinal form (Kennedy disease), and a form with severe respiratory distress (SMARD) on chromosome 11. Disorders of the peripheral nerves may be divided into genetic and nongenetic, acquired forms.

Denervation means anatomical uncoupling of muscle fibers from their motor nerves. The most striking morphological change is shrinkage of fiber cross-sectional area. These are often in groups but may also be isolated. In adults the atrophic fibers are often angulated but in childhood disorders such as SMA they are round in shape (see Figure 5.2). The degree of atrophy appears to be determined by at least two factors: the duration of the denervated state and the histochemical fiber type. The longer denervation lasts, the more atrophic a fiber becomes. The type 2 fibers appear to shrink at a faster rate than type 1. Most muscle biopsies show a state of partial denervation with only a proportion of denervated, atrophic fibers. The groups of atrophic, denervated fibers are of both histochemical types but they often show as type 2 more than type 1. In some denervating situations most muscle fibers may be type 2 and in such cases it is difficult to distinguish it from type 2 fiber atrophy. The atrophic fibers tend to show higher than normal levels of oxidative enzymes and nonspecific esterase activity, and denervated fibers may also lose their glycogen content, and show extrajunctional N-CAM immunolabeling.

Neuronal NOS is lost from denervated fibers but it reappears when a fiber is reinnervated. Angulated fibers are particularly darkly stained with NADH-TR, but ATPase and myosin immunostaining show that these are of both types. Atrophic, denervated muscle fibers retain their internal architecture until late in the atrophic process, when all that may remain is a clump of nuclei, which may be pyknotic (see Figure 5.13). The groups of atrophic fibers are often accompanied by groups of hypertrophied fibers, or fibers of normal size. Fibers supplied by an intact motor nerve retain their normal size, or undergo compensatory hypertrophy, or surviving nerves (terminal nerves or collaterals) sprout and reinnervate clusters of denervated fibers, causing them to enlarge again. This collateral sprouting results in groups of fibers of the same type, creating type grouping (Figure 5.14). In severe childhood cases of SMA the groups of hypertrophic fibers are usually type1/slow. It is important to distinguish fiber type predominance from fiber type grouping, especially in a small sample, and groups of both types should be present to make the diagnosis of denervation. Co-expression of myosin isoforms may make fiber types and grouping difficult to define in sections stained for ATPase, and some angulated fibers show neonatal myosin and may co-express fast myosin.

Another characteristic of denervated muscle is the presence of target fibers, particularly in chronic disorders. They are rarely seen in the severe childhood forms of SMA. In some biopsies the dark rim of the target surrounding the pale zone devoid of oxidative enzyme activity may not be prominent and the fibers then have an appearance similar to that of a fiber with a central core. Core-like areas can occur in fibers of varying size and, like targets, are usually focal lesions, rarely extending down the whole length of a fiber. Other architectural changes such as moth-eaten fibers and whorled fibers may occasionally be seen with oxidative enzyme stains. Internal nuclei may be seen in some hypertrophic fibers, and these features, in the absence of fiber type grouping, may make it difficult to distinguish from a "myopathic" appearance. This is also enhanced by the occasional necrosis that develops in hypertrophied fibers. The appearance of intramuscular nerves may also reflect axonal loss but Wallerian degeneration is rare in intramuscular nerves. The density of endomysial capillaries tends to become reduced in chronic denervation. In denervation caused by diabetic neuropathy the endomysial capillaries show thickening of their basal lamina.

The muscular dystrophies and allied disorders

The muscular dystrophies have traditionally been defined as inherited disorders with progressive weakness and wasting of skeletal muscle. Dramatic advances have been made in our understanding of the pathological changes in the muscular dystrophies with identification of causative gene defects, and their associated alterations in protein expression. This has led to a trend in classifying patients according to their protein defect, for example dystrophinopathies and sarcoglycanopathies [60]. Most histological or histochemical features are nonspecific and can occur in more than one clinical condition. Patterns, however, have long been known. A deficiency of the affected protein can often be identified in recessive muscular dystrophies, in association with a variety of secondary changes which can both aid and confuse interpretation.

Duchenne and Becker muscular dystrophy (DMD, BMD)

The pathology in DMD and BMD shows a diffuse pattern with increased variability in fiber size, degeneration, and

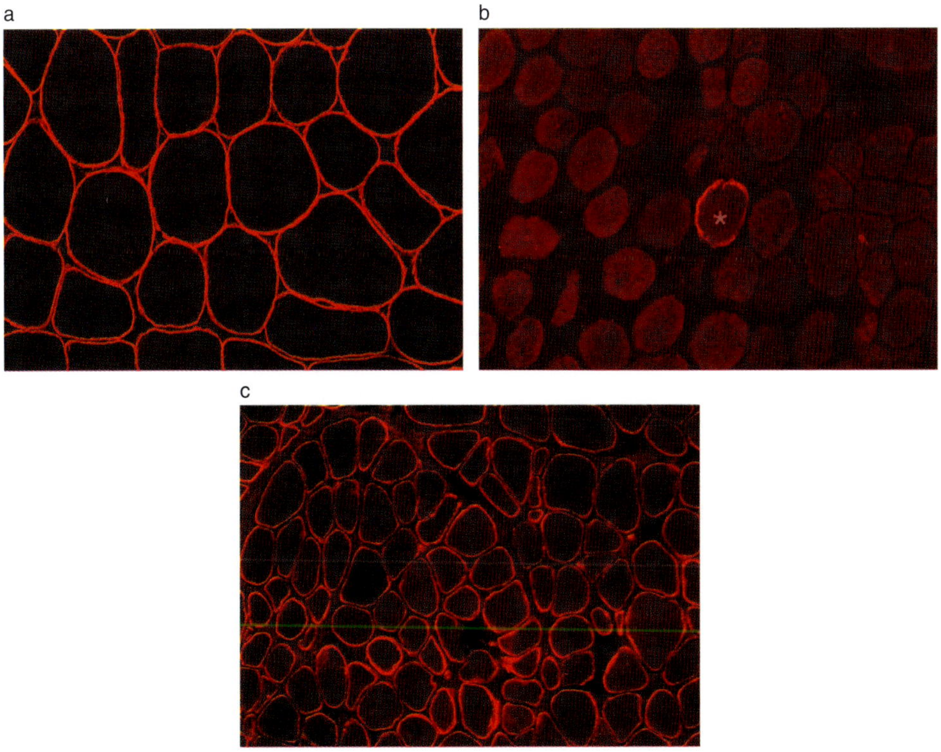

Figure 5.20a–c. Immunolabeling of dystrophin in muscle biopsies from a control (a), a case of Duchenne muscular dystrophy (b), and a case of Becker muscular dystrophy (c). Note the normal sarcolemmal labeling in the control, the absence of dystrophin from most fibers except one revertant fiber (*) in the Duchenne case, and the reduced labeling of several fibers in the Becker case.

regeneration of muscle fibers, and an increase in endomysial and perimysial fibrous tissue and of adipose tissue (see Figure 5.2). The variation in fiber size may be very wide, and some results from fiber splitting or branching. The degree of pathology is variable, particularly in BMD, and there is often no correlation with clinical severity. There is sometimes an increase in cellularity, often near the regions of necrosis. Other features include an increase in internal nuclei, internal splits, and varying degrees of myofibrillar disruption, such as that seen in whorled fibers. Unevenness of oxidative enzyme staining and moth-eaten fibers occur but are less common in DMD than in some other dystrophies. Hypercontracted fibers, necrotic fibers, and phagocytosis are common features, and fibers that are unstained with PAS may be frequent.

Both major fiber types show a wide variation in fiber size, although fiber typing may be indistinct in DMD, and predominance of type 1/slow fibers is common. The differentiation into type 1 and type 2 fibers with the ATPase technique at pH 9.4 is probably indistinct because of co-expression of myosin isoforms. Thus defining the fiber type may be difficult. Developmental isoforms of myosin are expressed not only in the basophilic regenerating fibers, but also in nonbasophilic fibers of varying size and number (see Figure 5.10); in DMD they are numerous. Regenerating fibers (see above) may be isolated, but often occur in clusters.

Dystrophin expression in Duchenne and Becker muscular dystrophy

Localization of dystrophin to the sarcolemma and its identification as the defective gene product in DMD/BMD led the way to the revolution in muscle pathology. In most cases of DMD dystrophin is not detected on the majority of fibers. In contrast, cases of BMD show reduced and/or uneven labeling of muscle fibers (Figure 5.20). This difference is explained by deletions that disrupt the reading frame, resulting in no protein and a severe Duchenne phenotype; whereas those that maintain the reading frame lead to some expression of the protein and give rise to the milder Becker dystrophy [61]. Although about 95% of cases conform to this dogma, there are exceptions. Notable exceptions are cases with a deletion of exons 3–7, which is a frame-shift deletion and should result in no expression of dystrophin and a severe phenotype. These cases, however, show some expression of protein because of a splicing event around the deletion; they often have a phenotype intermediate between DMD and BMD. Other exceptions also involve mutations around exon 3, and cases with very large deletions [62]. In general, most cases of DMD show an absence of C-terminal dystrophin, while in most cases of BMD it is preserved [28, 41]. Exceptions, however, have been reported [63]. The degree of immunolabeling of dystrophin in cases of BMD is variable, and can range from a pronounced to mild reduction, or labeling that is indistinguishable from normal. Immunoblot analysis can be informative in these cases. It is important to distinguish cases of BMD with near-normal expression of dystrophin from cases of LGMD2I, as these can often clinically resemble BMD. Studies of secondary abnormalities are then useful (see below).

Low levels of dystrophin expression can be detected in some cases of DMD, and dystrophin is particularly prominent on fibers known as "revertant" fibers (Figure 5.20). The expression on these fibers is of normal intensity and arises

a b

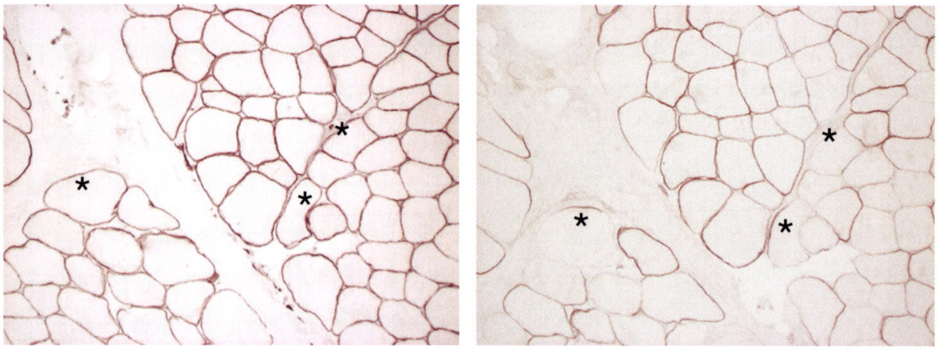

Figure 5.21a, b. Serial sections of a muscle biopsy from a manifesting carrier of Duchenne muscular dystrophy immunolabeled with antibodies to β-spectrin (a) and dystrophin (b) showing several fibers that are not labeled, or weakly labeled, with dystrophin but with normal labeling of β-spectrin (*).

from restoration of the reading frame. The truncated dystrophin of revertant fibers may be of variable size, depending on the exons used in restoration of the reading frame. The number of revertant fibers in a biopsy is variable: some have none, others a few isolated ones, and others have several in clusters. The number shows no correlation with severity, but sampling is a problem that makes this difficult to address.

As the position and size of the mutations in the dystrophin gene vary it is essential to use antibodies that correspond to more than one domain. In practice, antibodies to an N-terminal, rod, and C-terminal domain are used. The importance of this is illustrated in cases with large deletions, as one antibody (to an epitope in the deleted region) may show an absence whereas another reveals its presence. An important role of immunohistochemistry is shown in DMD cases with a point mutation where the deletion cannot easily be detected by routine molecular techniques, but is easily detected with immunohistochemistry.

Secondary abnormalities in protein expression in Duchenne and Becker dystrophy

Abnormal expression of dystrophin in Xp21 dystrophies is associated with secondary abnormalities in the expression of several other proteins. The proteins associated with dystrophin in the sarcolemmal DAPC show reduced sarcolemmal expression [19, 28]. This includes all the sarcoglycans, dystroglycans, syntrophins, dystrobrevin, and nNOS, which is usually absent from the majority of fibers in DMD. In BMD with a mutation in the common rod domain "hotspot" nNOS is also absent and is a useful marker for such cases [41]. Utrophin, in contrast, is overexpressed in both DMD and BMD and is a useful diagnostic aid in cases of Becker dystrophy where dystrophin may show minimal reduction.

Abnormal sarcolemmal utrophin expression is related to age, and cases of Xp21 dystrophies less than about 2 years of age show very little sarcolemmal expression on mature fibers, in contrast to older cases where it is usually abundant. As utrophin is also expressed on regenerating fibers careful correlation with the expression of developmental myosins is often needed. Similarly, immaturity has to be taken into account in the assessment of MHC-1 overexpression in cases of Xp21 dystrophy.

In common with other proteins of the DAPC both β- and α-dystroglycan are reduced in DMD and BMD. This can be useful in the differential diagnosis of BMD from cases of LGMD2I, as β-dystroglycan is usually normal in LGMD2I, but the gene defect causes hypoglycosylation of α-dystroglycan, which can be detected with immunohistochemistry [64].

Carriers of Duchenne and Becker muscular dystrophy

Muscle biopsies from some carriers show morphological abnormalities, particularly manifesting carriers of DMD and BMD. Changes include variation in fiber size, increase in internal nuclei, and patchiness or moth-eaten fibers as revealed with oxidative enzyme techniques. Immunohistochemical studies of carriers of DMD and BMD have mainly been confined to studies of the expression of myosin isoforms, dystrophin, and utrophin. As in many myopathic conditions fibers expressing slow myosin are often predominant, and cases with marked pathological changes have fibers that co-express the fast and slow, and/or fetal isoforms.

Dystrophin analysis has an essential role in differentiating between a manifesting carrier and autosomal forms of muscular dystrophy in which dystrophin expression is often normal. Many manifesting carriers show a "mosaic" pattern of dystrophin-positive and dystrophin-negative or deficient fibers, although the pattern of dystrophin expression may vary along the length of the fiber. This is in contrast to normal labeling of β-spectrin (Figure 5.21). The mosaic pattern results from skewing of the active X-chromosomes and the proportion of nuclei with a normal active X-chromosome compared to those carrying a mutation in the DMD gene. If a biopsy from a young female is unequivocally dystrophic and dystrophin expression appears normal, it is unlikely that she is a manifesting carrier. This may not be the case in older females as the number of dystrophin-negative fibers may change. The number of dystrophin-negative fibers may also vary between muscles. Asymptomatic carriers usually show only subtle changes in dystrophin immunolabeling and only occasional dystrophin-negative fibers, and/or reduced abundance of dystrophin on immunoblots. Utrophin can be expressed on both dystrophin-positive and -negative fibers in carriers, and in asymptomatic carriers with minimal alterations in dystrophin utrophin can be a useful additional marker of abnormality.

Females with an Xp21 translocation

Females with a chromosomal translocation affecting the dystrophin gene manifest the disease and can be as severe as affected boys. The morphological features in these females are similar to those of affected boys, and dystrophin is usually absent from the sarcolemma, as the X-chromosome carrying the translocation is usually predominantly the active chromosome.

X-linked cardiomyopathy

Cases of cardiomyopathy with minimal skeletal muscle weakness caused by mutations in the dystrophin gene have been identified. Skeletal muscle biopsies from these cases show near-normal immunolabeling of dystrophin but it is abnormal in cardiac muscle. The difference in dystrophin expression in these cases has been explained by differential splicing in skeletal and cardiac tissue [65].These cases of X-linked cardiomyopathy are rare, and the mutations seem to be of Italian origin.

Limb-girdle muscular dystrophies

The limb-girdle muscular dystrophies (LGMDs) are clinically and molecularly heterogeneous, and are dominantly (LGMD1) or recessively (LGMD2) inherited [66]. The defective proteins localize to various compartments of the muscle fiber, including the sarcolemma, nuclear envelope, sarcoplasm, membrane systems of the fibers, and components of the sarcomere, and are associated with a wide clinical spectrum ranging from a LGMD phenotype to a severe phenotype of a CMD, or a disorder classified as a myofibrillar myopathy. Some of these conditions are considered allelic.

The histological and histochemical features of the LGMDs are those associated with all muscular dystrophies with necrosis and fibrosis (see above). The degree of abnormality is variable and does not reflect clinical severity; fiber size variation may be extreme. In contrast to DMD fiber typing with the ATPase pH 9.4 techniques is often more distinct, and hypercontracted fibers are less common. Internal nuclei are often abundant, and multiple within one fiber. Nuclear clumps are common in chronic conditions. In addition to the presence of moth-eaten or whorled fibers oxidative enzyme stains may show the presence of lobulated fibers (see Figure 5.8). These can be a feature of LGMD2A (calpain-3 deficiency), particularly in adults, but are not specific and occur in a number of other myopathies and dystrophies. Inflammatory cells may be present, and in cases of LGMD2B (dysferlin deficiency) this has sometimes resulted in misdiagnosis. Eosinophils can be a feature of LGMD2A but are rare in other forms. Occasional rimmed vacuoles occur in a variety of LGMDs.

It is rarely possible to identify the defective gene from histological and histochemical studies. Immunohistochemistry and immunoblotting (summarized below) have an important role in directing molecular analysis, particularly in the recessive forms of LGMD.

Dominant limb-girdle muscular dystrophies

LGMD1A. Mutations in the gene for myotilin are responsible for this disorder and there is clinical and pathological overlap with the myofibrillar myopathy associated with the same gene (see below); they are probably allelic. Myotilin accumulation occurs in both [67].

LGMD1B. Although histopathology can help to exclude other conditions, there are no specific markers to identify the defect in the nuclear membrane lamin A/C protein. The clinical phenotype associated with lamin A/C mutations is wide and diagnosis relies on molecular analysis and careful clinical observations. Immunolabeling of the nuclear membrane proteins emerin and lamins is indistinguishable from normal (see "Emery–Dreifuss muscular dystrophies").

LGMD1C. In addition to LGMD1C, mutations in the gene encoding caveolin-3 are also responsible for rippling muscle disease and cases with little muscle weakness but persistently high creatine kinase (CK) (hyperCKaemia). In normal muscle caveolin-3 is localized to the sarcolemma, but patients with a mutation in the caveolin-3 gene show a reduction in the protein with immunohistochemistry and immunoblotting [31]. Detectable abnormalities in the primary defective protein are rare in dominantly inherited defects but caveolin-3 is an exception. The reduced or absent protein expression is due to a dominant negative effect of mutant caveolin, and aggregates of caveolin-3 that are not targeted to the plasma membrane but retained within the Golgi. Internal localization of antibodies to caveolin-3 may be seen in several disorders, particularly in regenerating fibers. In addition, a mosaic pattern of caveolin-3 labeling, with positive and negative fibers, can be seen in cases without mutations in the gene, which are thought to be of autoimmune origin [68].

LGMD1D–1G. The proteins responsible for these forms have not yet been identified and histopathology does not contribute to the diagnosis of these forms.

Recessive limb-girdle muscular dystrophies

The recessive forms of LGMD are more frequent than the dominant forms, in particular LGMD2A and LGMD2I in the Caucasian population, although there are geographic differences. LGMD2G, 2H and 2J are rare and have only been described in a few families. The general histopathological features are similar to those seen in other muscular dystrophies, but the gene mutations result in detectable alterations in the expression of the primary protein, as well as secondary alterations in protein expression, which aid diagnosis.

LGMD2A. Studies of the defective enzyme, calpain-3, are possible on sections [52] but most studies have been performed on immunoblots, where the secondary changes that can occur when the primary defect is in dysferlin or another protein, and those resulting from autolysis, can be assessed [51, 53, 56]. A normal quantity of calpain-3 on an immunoblot, which cannot assess enzyme activity, does not exclude a defect in the gene.

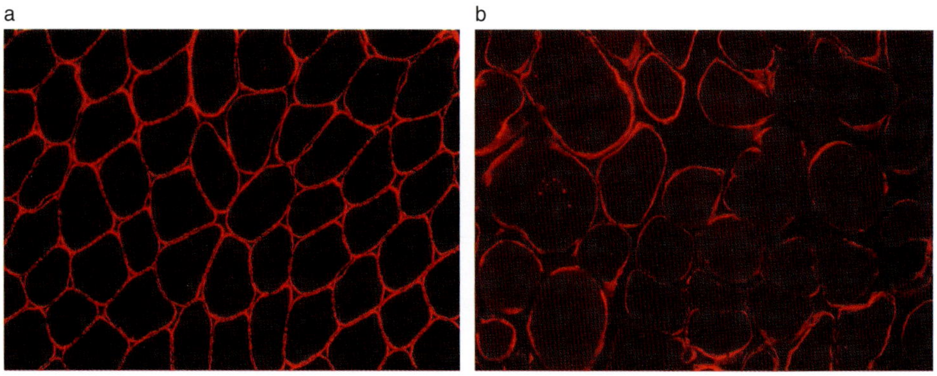

Figure 5.22a, b. Muscle biopsies from a control (a), and a case of LGMD 2I (b) immunolabeled with antibodies to α-dystroglycan. Note the uneven and reduced labeling in the case of LGMD2I compared with the control.

LGMD2B and Myoshi myopathy. These are clinically distinct disorders but defects in the gene for dysferlin are responsible for both. In addition to degenerative dystrophic changes, inflammatory infiltrates are common, as well as overexpression of sarcolemmal MHC-class I antigens on mature fibers. In normal muscle dysferlin is localized to the sarcolemma and an absence or reduction in intensity of labeling can be seen with immunohistochemistry in both LGMD2B and Miyoshi myopathy [69]. Internal labeling of a population of fibers, and regenerating fibers may also occur. The use of two commercial antibodies on immunoblots that recognize different epitopes at different ends of the protein, however, gives a clearer indication of quantity. Immunoblots are also important for distinguishing the secondary reduction in dysferlin that can occur when the gene for either calpain-3 or caveolin-3 is defective [53, 54], and occasionally in other muscular dystrophies including sarcoglycanopathies and dystrophinopathies [70, 71].

LGMD2C–2F. These forms are often collectively referred to as the "sarcoglycanopathies," as each one is caused by a defect in a member of the sarcoglycan complex (α, β, γ, δ), associated with the dystrophin [66]. The expression of each sarcoglycan in affected patients can vary from absence, to traces, to a mild reduction; an abnormality in one results in a secondary reduction of the other members of the complex. An absence of one in association with a reduction of the others is highly suggestive of the primary defect in the corresponding gene. Absence of all sarcoglycans can occur, and is often caused by mutations in the gene encoding β-sarcoglycan. Dystrophin expression is often normal but a secondary reduction can occur in some sarcoglycanopathies (LGMD2C–2F), in particular LGMD2E (β-sarcoglycan) [32]. A secondary reduction of sarcoglycans occurs in DMD and BMD, and in male patients studies of utrophin can be helpful in distinguishing between LGMD and BMD. Patients with the former usually have normal or only low expression of utrophin, in contrast to the marked overexpression in BMD.

LGMD2G is very rare and so far has only been identified in a few families. It is caused by a defect in the gene encoding telethonin. Rimmed vacuoles were reported in some of the cases studied [72] and telethonin immunolabeling was absent in the patients studied. No secondary defects have been reported.

LGMD2H is also very rare and so far has only been described in the Hutterite Canadian population [73]. There are no reported studies of the expression of the defective protein TRIM 32, a putative E3 ubiquitin ligase that is possibly involved in tagging of target proteins with ubiquitin, ready for degradation. The same gene is also responsible for cases of sarcotubular myopathy [74], who had ancestral links to the Hutterites.

LGMD2I is a common LGMD variant in some Caucasian populations, caused by defects in the gene encoding the fukutin-related protein (FKRP) [40]. Allelic mutations are also responsible for a severe form of CMD (MDC1C; see "Congenital muscular dystrophies") [40, 64]. FKRP is named after its sequence homology to fukutin, the defective protein in Fukuyama CMD [75]. The sequence homology suggests it is a member of the glycosyltransferase family, and that it has a role in glycosylation, in particular of α-dystroglycan.

The histological and histochemical changes in muscle in LGMD2I are variable in severity, but are similar to those of other muscular dystrophies. There are no commercial antibodies to FKRP but studies of secondary changes can be helpful in differential diagnosis. The distinction between BMD and LGMD2I is sometimes difficult, especially in cases with no detectable change in dystrophin. Immunolabeling on nNOS, however, can be useful, as many cases of BMD have a mutation in the rod domain hot spot and lack sarcolemmal nNOS, in contrast to LGMD2I in which nNOS is present. Another important secondary change in LGMD2I is the reduction in labeling of the glycosylated epitope of α-dystroglycan [64]. This is a common finding but the degree of reduction is variable; in some cases it is unequivocal but in others, especially patients at the mild end of the clinical spectrum, it may be subtle (Figure 5.22). There are currently no commercial antibodies to the core protein of α-dystroglycan but research studies have shown that it is retained in LGMD2I.

Another common secondary protein deficiency associated with mutations in the FKRP gene is a reduction of laminin-α2, but this may only be apparent on immunoblots [59, 64]. Sarcolemmal labeling of laminin-β1 may also be reduced, especially in adults, in contrast to that on blood vessels, but this is nonspecific and has been observed in other conditions. Upregulation of utrophin can also occur on mature fibers in

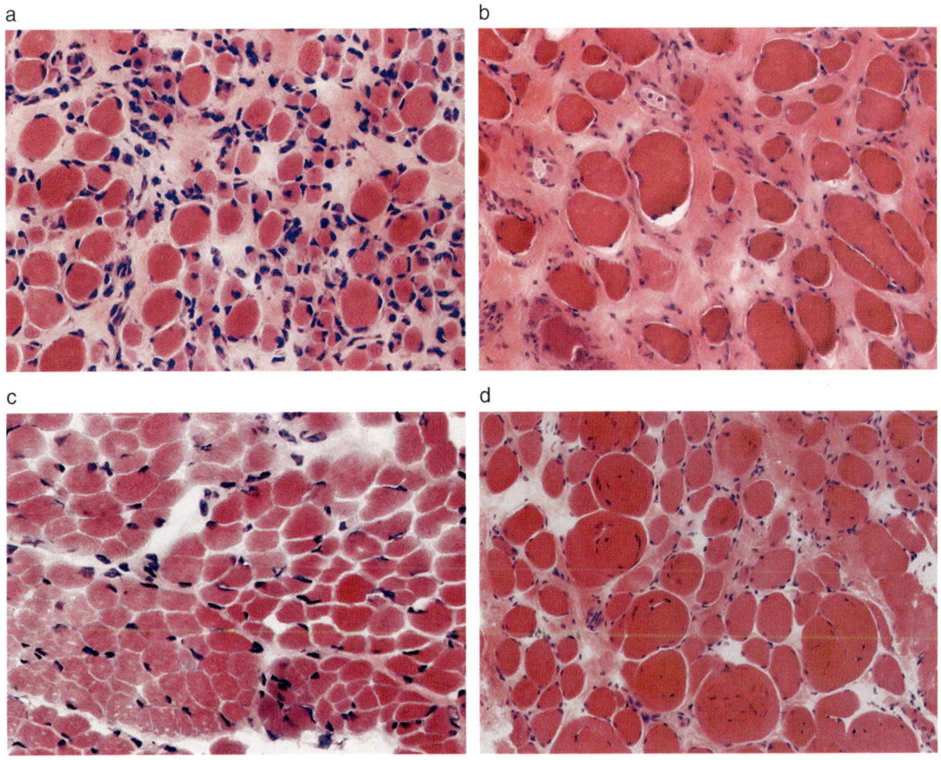

Figure 5.23a–d. Muscle biopsies of four cases (a–d) of congenital muscular dystrophy with molecular defects in the genes that affect glycosylation of α-dystroglycan showing variable degrees of pathology. H&E.

LGMD2I, although it is usually less pronounced than in DMD and BMD [76].

LGMD2J is a rare form of LGMD described in the Finnish population with distal muscle involvement, limited to the anterior compartment of the leg. It is caused by recessive mutations in the gene for titin [77]. Dominant mutations in titin result in isolated cardiomyopathy. They can also give rise to a later onset tibial muscular dystrophy that is often grouped with other distal myopathies, including Welander myopathy and the Nonaka type, allelic to hereditary inclusion body myositis [78, 79, 80]. Rimmed vacuoles may be present in titin-related disorders but not universally, and accumulation of tau or amyloid-β, often associated with such vacuoles in other conditions, is not a feature. Rimmed vacuoles are not a feature of the recessive cases. Titin is still detectable with commercial antibodies but an antibody raised specifically against the mutated last exon of this giant gene shows an absence [55]. Titin has binding sites for calpain-3 and telethonin and a secondary reduction in calpain-3 is associated with titin mutations [81].

LGMD2K, 2L, 2M, 2N, 2O. These are rare variants caused by mutations in different genes (e.g., *POMT1*, *Fukutin*, *POMT2*, and *POMGnT1*) which are also responsible for severe forms of CMD (see below) [40]. The muscle pathology is variable and shows the typical features of a muscular dystrophy. As in LGMD2I immunolabeling of α-dystroglycan can be helpful, but the degree of reduced labeling is variable and may be subtle or absent [58].

Congenital muscular dystrophies

Major advances in the understanding of CMD have been made in recent years, and the genetic defects of 10 variants have been identified [40, 82]. The clinical spectrum associated with the defective genes is wide, ranging from severe, early-onset forms of CMD to milder variants with a limb-girdle phenotype (see above). A variable degree of brain and central nervous system involvement is common, and correct post-translational glycosylation of α-dystroglycan underlies the pathogenesis of several forms [39, 40].

The classification of the CMDs was initially based on clinical features [83, 84, 85, 86, 87] but with increasing knowledge of their underlying molecular cause and abnormalities in protein expression, a classification that also takes into account the primary biochemical defect has been proposed [88].

All variants of CMD share common pathological features, although the degree of abnormality is variable. The general features are similar to those seen in other muscular dystrophies, and may appear considerably worse than the clinical picture. The degree of pathology cannot be used as an indication of severity or prognosis, and the amount of fibrosis and adipose tissue may be marked (Figure 5.23). An inflammatory infiltrate may sometimes be present. Areas of mitochondrial depletion (cores), aggregation, and myofibrillar disruption may be seen with oxidative enzyme stains, and some fibers resemble lobulated fibers but are usually not as distinctive as in adults. As some of these features also occur in some congenital myopathies (see below), and there can be clinical similarities, congenital

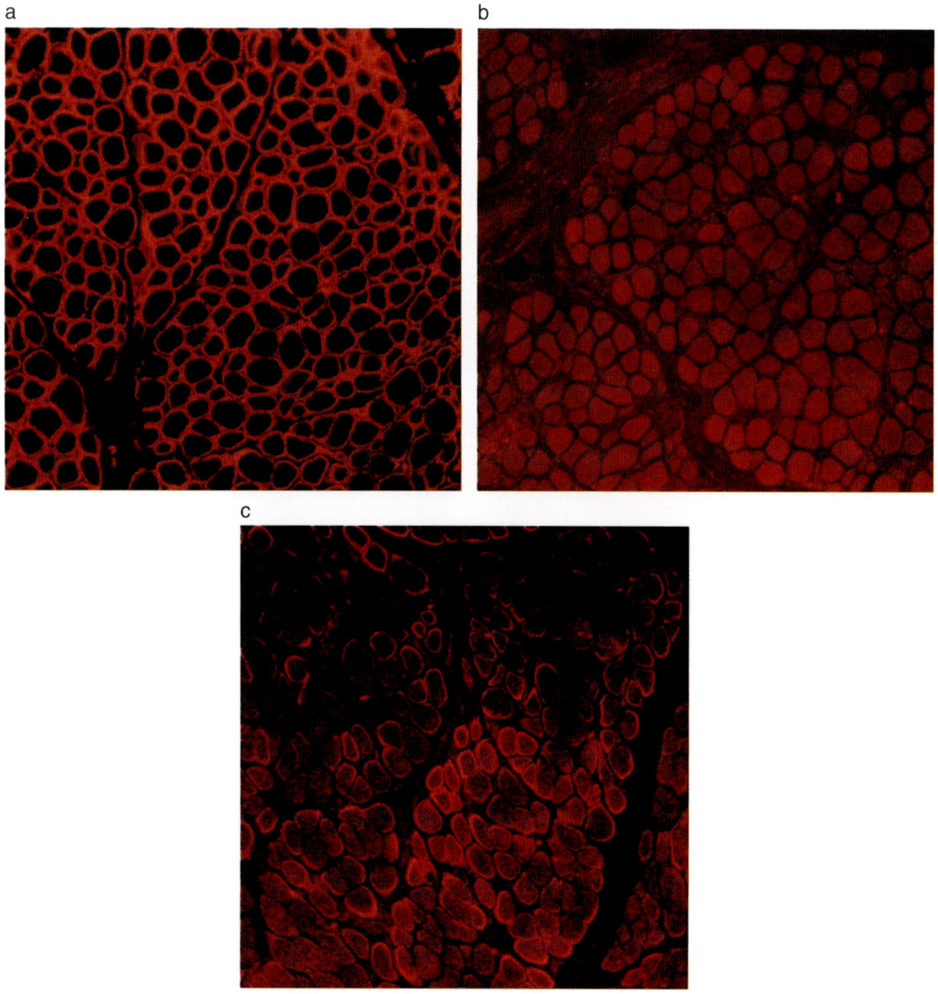

Figure 5.24a–c. Immunolabeling of laminin-α2 in muscle biopsies from a control (a), and two severely affected cases of MDC1A with molecular defects in the *LAMA2* gene (b, c). Note the absence of laminin-α2 in (b) but traces on several fibers in (c).

myopathies may have to be considered in the differential diagnosis. Muscle fiber necrosis and regeneration are not striking features in all variants, and in some the overall pathology may resemble a myopathy rather than a dystrophic process with necrosis. It is not possible to identify a particular form of CMD from the histological and histochemical features alone, but immunohistochemistry can be useful for directing molecular analysis.

Congenital muscular dystrophies due to defects in extracellular matrix proteins

Laminin-α2 deficient CMD (merosin-deficient CMD, MDC1A). This form of CMD (MDC1A) is caused by mutations in the *LAMA 2* gene on chromosome 6q22. Affected cases present at birth, or in the first few weeks of life, with hypotonia and muscle weakness [82]. Serum CK levels are always elevated and increased signal intensity in the white matter with T_2-weighted brain MRI is a common feature that is clearly visible by the age of 6 months. Most mutations result in complete absence of laminin-α2 protein, or only traces of detectable protein, and these are always associated with a severe phenotype, with patients rarely achieving the ability to stand independently (Figure 5.24). Some *LAMA 2* mutations result in partial protein reduction, and are usually associated with a milder phenotype, which can resemble a LGMD. This partial reduction of laminin-α2 is more easily seen on sections with antibodies to the 300-kDa fragment than to the 80-kDa fragment [89]. Western blotting can also be used to detect laminin-α2 defects but not all commercial antibodies are suitable. The one commonly used from Chemicon recognizes the 80-kDa fragment, which in normal muscle appears as a single or double band, but those to the 300-kDa fragment (from Alexis) are not suitable for immunoblotting. The fragment recognized by the antibody from Novocastra is not known but it reveals a partial reduction on sections better than the one from Chemicon.

Laminin-α2 labeling of intramuscular nerves is also absent in cases of MDC1A. In skin, which can be used as an alternative to muscle in cases where no muscle is available or is difficult to obtain, laminin-α2 is absent at the epidermal–dermal junction, on the sensory nerves and glands in MDC1A patients. Laminin-α2 is absent from all blood vessels of skin and muscle, but is present on blood vessels in the brain.

Several proteins are secondarily affected in MDC1A. Laminin-β2 and α7-integrin are reduced on the sarcolemma but laminin-α5 and -α4 chains are overexpressed. Age and developmental regulation of these proteins must be taken into account when assessing all these proteins. α-Dystroglycan may also be reduced in MDC1A, and in cases with a partial reduction of laminin-α2 it may be difficult to distinguish between a primary and secondary deficiency CMD (see below).

As laminins are expressed in chorionic villi (CV) on the basal lamina beneath the trophoblast, immunohistochemical studies of CV samples can be useful for prenatal diagnosis. Absence of laminin-α2 from trophoblast is highly suggestive of a fetus affected by MDC1A and is accompanied by a reduction in laminin-β2, but a combined molecular genetic approach is recommended [90]. The reliability of immunohistochemical studies of CV in cases with a primary partial deficiency, or in cases with secondary deficiency, is unknown. It is therefore important to establish the laminin-α2 status in the proband before assessing the immunohistochemistry of CV samples.

Integrin-α7-deficient CMD. This is a very rare form of CMD [91]. Immunohistochemical studies identified an absence of integrin-α7 from the sarcolemma, and mutations in the corresponding gene (*ITGA7*) were found. The morphological changes in the muscle were mild and necrosis was not a feature, although regenerating fibers were seen in one patient. Integrin-β1D was also slightly reduced; laminin-α2 was normal. Analysis of integrin-α7 localization in CMD muscle is limited by the availability of antibodies.

Ullrich congenital muscular dystrophy (UCMD). UCMD is one of the most common forms of CMD and mutations in one of the three collagen 6A genes that encode α1(VI), α2(VI), and α3(VI) chains have been identified [92]. The involvement of three other recently identified collagen VI chains encoded by genes at a locus on chromosome 3q.22.1, α4 (VI), α5 (VI), and α6 (VI), is not yet known. Collagen VI is a major extracellular matrix protein which is localized to the perimysium and endomysium, with enhanced labeling at the sarcolemmal basement membrane (Figure 5.17). A reduction in immunohistochemical labeling can be seen in UCMD but normal labeling does not exclude a defect. Some cases show a complete absence or an unequivocal reduction; whilst in others the reduction is subtle and may only be apparent at the sarcolemma, with normal labeling of the endomysium (Figure 5.17). The absence or reduction of collagen VI around axons and blood vessels may also be apparent but this is not a universal feature. Comparison with double labeling of another protein, such as perlecan, collagen IV or V, to assess the integrity of the basal lamina may be necessary to identify a subtle reduction.

Skin may also be used to identify an absence of collagen VI, but the majority of patients have residual expression of collagen VI and any abnormality is more difficult to assess than in muscle [11]. Studies of collagen VI expression in cultures of UCMD skin fibroblasts suggest subtle alterations in collagen VI production, as has been shown for patients with Bethlem myopathy [17, 18].

An absence of immunolabeling of collagen VI in CV samples can also be useful for prenatal diagnosis of UCMD [15], but experience so far is limited to patients in whom muscle of the proband showed absent immunolabeling of collagen VI.

Congenital muscular dystrophies associated with abnormal glycosylation of α-dystroglycan

Hypoglycosylation of α-dystroglycan is a secondary abnormality responsible for several variants of CMD, often collectively referred to as the "dystroglycanopathies" [40]. The clinical spectrum is broad, and varying degrees of brain and eye involvement are common. Mutations in six genes have been identified in a proportion of patients, but undoubtedly further genes will be identified in phenotypically similar cases not linked to the known loci.

Immunohistochemistry and immunoblotting of muscle biopsy reveal a reduction in labeling of glycosylated epitopes of α-dystroglycan but β-dystroglycan is often normal (in contrast to DMD/BMD in which both α- and β-dystroglycan are reduced). The two commercially available monoclonal antibodies to the glycosylated epitopes of α-dystroglycan (clones IIH6 and VIA4–1, Upstate Biotechnologies) show significant variability between batches and carefully controlled studies are required to assess α-dystroglycan immunolabeling. Research studies using antibodies to the primary core amino acid sequence of α-dystroglycan have also revealed changes in the amount of core α-dystroglycan protein [58].

The extent of the reduction of α-dystroglycan immunolabeling is variable both within and between cases. It ranges from absent, or traces, to a mild or minimal reduction (Figure 5.25). It is not yet clear if epitope masking may account for some of this variability. There is some correlation between reduced α-dystroglycan and clinical severity in patients with mutations in *POMT1*, *POMT2*, and *POMGnT1*, but this is not always the case in patients with defects in the *fukutin* and *FKRP* genes [58]. It is not possible to identify the defective gene from immunohistochemistry.

Laminin-α2 is a ligand for α-dystroglycan, and a reduction of laminin-α2 can be detected in both muscle and skin biopsies when α-dystroglycan is hypoglycosylated. The extent of the immunohistochemical reduction of laminin-α2 is variable but complete absence is never observed, in contrast to cases with a primary laminin-α2 defect. Other proteins show a secondary reduction in some of these forms of CMD, including laminin-β2, perlecan, P180, integrin-α7 and -β1D chains, but the expression related to maturation of some of these proteins has not always been taken into account.

Enzyme activity of POMGnT1 can be assessed and is reduced in muscle and cultured fibroblasts from patients with a mutation in the corresponding gene, and suggests this may be of diagnostic value [93].

Proteins of the sarcoplasmic reticulum

Rigid spine muscular dystrophy (RSMD1). Rigidity of the spine is an associated feature of several neuromuscular disorders, but

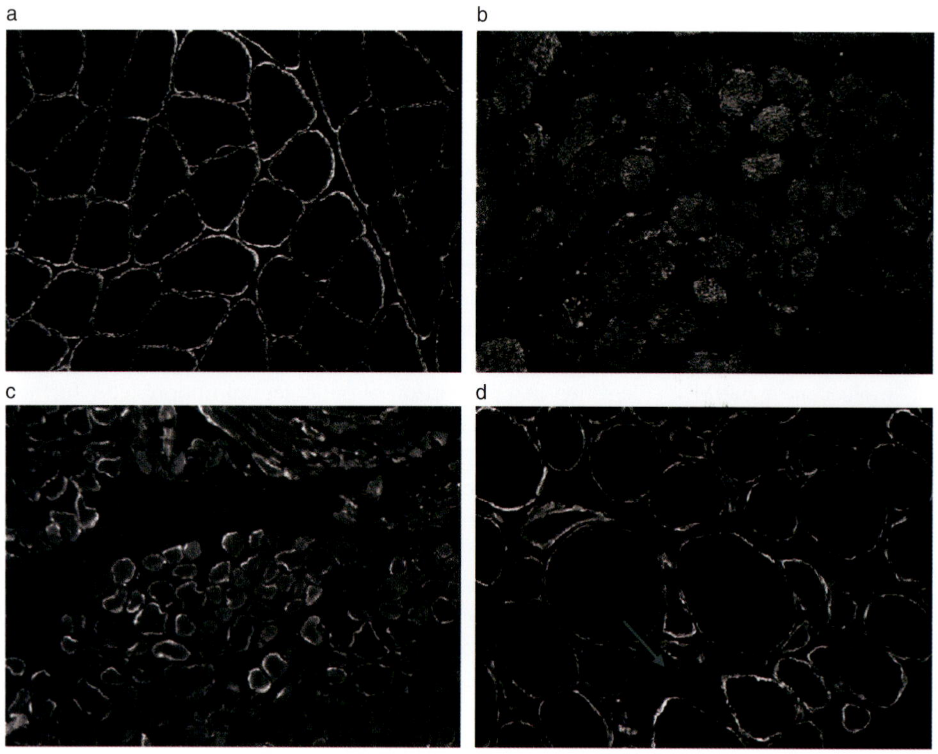

Figure 5.25a–d. Immunolabeling of α-dystroglycan in muscle biopsies from a control (a) and three molecularly proven cases of congenital muscular dystrophy (b–d) related to glycosylation defects showing the variability that can range from absent (b), to traces (c), to mild reduction on some fibers only (d, arrow).

it is an invariable complication in one form of CMD, RSMD1, caused by recessive mutations in the gene encoding selenoprotein N (*SEPN1*) on chromosome 1p35–36. Mutations in the *SEPN1* gene are also responsible for forms of congenital myopathies, in particular multi-minicore disease. There is considerable clinical and pathological overlap between these disorders and many consider that they represent a clinicopathological spectrum instead of distinct entities. In addition to variation in fiber size, the muscle pathology may show a mild increase in endomysial connective tissue and an increase in internal nuclei, although these are not usually abundant. Unevenness of oxidative enzyme stain, in the form of multiple core-like lesions in both fiber types, is often a feature associated with mutations in the *SEPN1* gene. Multiple cores, however, may also be seen in cases with a mutation in the *RYR1* gene, which may cause diagnostic confusion (see below). Antibodies to SEPN1 used in research studies have shown absence of the 70-kDa SEPN1 band on immunoblots of fibroblasts cultured from a RSMD1 patient [94]. At present, changes in SEPN1 levels cannot be ascertained on sections by immunohistochemistry, and there are no reported secondary protein abnormalities.

Emery–Dreifuss muscular dystrophy

The X-linked and autosomal forms of Emery–Dreifuss muscular dystrophy (XL EDMD and AD EDMD respectively) share some similar clinical and pathological features [42]. The clinical spectrum, particularly of forms caused by mutations in the lamin A/C gene, is wide, and cases resembling CMD have been identified. In quadriceps biopsies the abnormal variation in fiber size is not usually marked. Occasional atrophic fibers are common and some fibers may be hypertrophic. Internal nuclei may be occasional or numerous, with more than one per fiber. Necrosis is rare and there is usually only a mild, or little, increase in adipose or connective tissue. Similarly, there is little ongoing muscle fiber regeneration and only a few fibers express neonatal myosin. A few small basophilic fibers, however, with a slightly granular appearance and aggregation of NADH-TR stain may be present, and may be regenerating fibers as they show neonatal myosin and increased desmin. A two-fiber-type pattern is usually maintained, with a tendency for the type 1 fibers to be smaller. A predominance of type 1 fibers may also occur. Nonspecific structural changes such as cores can also occur.

In the X-linked form caused by mutations in the gene encoding the nuclear membrane protein emerin, the majority of mutations result in absence of protein; this is easily demonstrated with antibodies. Rare cases have been reported in which emerin expression is reduced rather than absent. Female carriers rarely manifest with muscle weakness but are at risk of cardiac involvement. The absence of emerin in a proportion of nuclei can be detected in carriers in skin and viable buccal cells. Immunolabeling of lamins in XL EDMD appears normal in sections.

In AD EDMD, caused by dominant mutations in the *LMNA* gene on chromosome 1q11–23, immunolabeling of emerin and lamin A/C appears normal. Some antibodies that specifically detect lamin A, but not the spliced C lamin isoform, show labeling of very few nuclei in mature human muscle; this is thought to be due to epitope masking as it is not seen with all the antibodies. Similarly, differences in the immunolabeling of lamin B1 with different antibodies are thought to be due to epitope masking [3].

There is considerable interest in other nuclear envelope proteins as candidates for disorders with clinical similarly to the EDMD, such as LAP2, SUN1, and nesprins. A mutation in LAP2α (lamin-A-associated protein) has been identified in a family affected by a form of dilated cardiomyopathy and a reduction in protein in cardiac tissue was reported [95].

Immunolabeling of all proteins associated with the sarcolemma is normal in both forms of EDMD, with the exception of laminin-β1. Reduced laminin-β1 labeling on the sarcolemma may be apparent in some cases but all blood vessels, including the capillary network, show a normal intensity. This reduced sarcolemmal laminin-β1 labeling is not specific for the Emery–Dreifuss muscular dystrophies and may also be seen in cases of Bethlem myopathy and a variety of other myopathies, including LGMD2I. It is an age-related phenomenon, observed in adult and adolescent cases, but rarely in young children [42].

Bethlem myopathy

Bethlem myopathy results from dominant mutations in the genes encoding collagen VI, as in UCMD (in which mutations are, however, more commonly recessive). It is increasingly apparent that severe dominant mutations can result in UCMD, suggesting that the distinction between these conditions is clinical, and dependent on the effect of the mutation(s) on collagen assembly, secretion, and function [92]. Abnormalities in muscle biopsies are usually mild and nonspecific, with mild to moderate variation in fiber size, sometimes with fiber hypertrophy. There is usually little, or no, increase in connective and adipose tissues and internal nuclei are not usually abundant. Enzyme histochemistry shows retention of a two-fiber-type pattern, although some cases may show type 1 fiber predominance. Structural changes such as core-like lesions or whorled fibers are not usually present but some unevenness of oxidative enzyme stain may be apparent. In contrast to UCMD, immunolabeling of collagen VI in muscle sections from most cases is usually indistinguishable from normal. Studies of collagen VI in cultured skin fibroblasts, however, are proving to be useful [18]. Labeling of sarcolemmal proteins is normal except for a nonspecific reduction in sarcolemmal laminin-β1 in some adult and adolescent cases.

Disorders associated with deletions or expansion of repeated sequences

These conditions include facioscapulohumeral muscular dystrophy (FSHD), myotonic muscular dystrophies, and oculopharyngeal muscular dystrophy. With the advent of reliable molecular testing for FSHD and myotonic dystrophies, muscle biopsies are less often performed and the role of muscle pathology has diminished. We summarize here, however, the features associated with these disorders that may alert the pathologist.

Facioscapulohumeral muscular dystrophy (FSHD)

The abnormalities in FSHD are nonspecific, and the degree of change is variable. They may be influenced by the clinical involvement of the muscle that is sampled. Variation in the size of both fiber types is common but some biopsies from minimally involved muscles may only show scattered, very small fibers. These fibers have been described as atrophic but the expression of developmentally regulated proteins in them raises the possibility that they may represent attempts at regeneration [3]. Fiber type grouping is not a feature but clusters of small fibers, as in BMD, have been put forward as evidence of denervation. These fibers, however, also show proteins associated with immaturity and there are no electrophysiological data to support the proposal of denervation. An increase in fibrous and adipose tissue may be seen and necrosis is not usually a marked feature, but can occur. Internal nuclei may be numerous but they are often not increased. A frequent finding, however, is an inflammatory response which may vary from mild to profuse. In contrast to inflammatory myopathies (see below) and LGMD2B, overexpression of sarcolemmal MHC-1 is rarely observed in cases of FSHD. There are no specific, consistent immunohistochemical abnormalities.

Myotonic dystrophies (DM1 and DM2)

DM1 is a common disorder, while DM2 is rarer. There are no reported congenital cases of DM2 but congenital presentation of DM1 is well recognized. One of the earliest changes in DM1 is atrophy of type 1 fibers and hypertrophy of the type 2 fibers. In DM2 the atrophy affects type 2 more than type 1 fibers in some cases, and the prominent nuclear clumps label with antibodies to fast and immature myosin isoforms [96]. Type 1 fiber predominance may occur but it is not usually pronounced. Numerous internal nuclei, often in long chains, are a particular feature in DM1. There is a higher incidence of ring fibers in DM1 than in other chronic dystrophies, and dark-staining sarcoplasmic masses with disorganized myofibrillar material and dilated SR are a typical feature. Congenital forms of DM1 may show many central nuclei, and the pathology is difficult to distinguish from myotubular myopathy (see below), although differences in contractile protein profiles have been reported. Molecular analysis of the DM1 locus is therefore essential in all neonates with abundant central nuclei. The sequestration of muscleblind1 protein to nuclear foci in DM1 and DM2 has also been reported and may be of diagnostic value [97].

Oculopharyngeal muscular dystrophy (OPMD)

The pathological feature of note in OPMD is the presence of rimmed vacuoles that are often more common in type 1 than type 2 fibers. The vacuoles often contain acid phosphatase and electron microscopy shows that they are autophagic and contain osmiophilic, membranous myelin-like whorls and cytoplasmic debris. Electron microscopy reveals characteristic intranuclear tubular filaments, about 2.5 µm in length, with an outer diameter of 8.5 nm and an inner diameter of 3 nm. They are only seen in muscle nuclei and never in the cytoplasm or nuclei of other cell types, such as satellite cells, endothelial or interstitial cells. Thus the nuclear inclusions of OPMD are distinct from the 15- to 18-nm-long filaments seen in inclusion body myositis and distal myopathies with rimmed vacuoles, which can occur in both nuclei and the cytoplasm. Antibodies to PABPN1 localize to the nuclear inclusions, and poly (A) RNA can be detected in them with *in situ* hybridization [98]. They are also recognized by antibodies to ubiquitin and proteasomal subunits [99].

Congenital myopathies

Muscle pathology has a major role in these early-onset disorders, and many are named after a characteristic morphological feature. They show a wide spectrum of clinicopathological features and the boundaries between congenital myopathies and the dominantly inherited distal arthrogrypotic syndromes are not clear. There is significant overlap between the disorders, with defects in the same gene giving rise to a congenital, or a late-onset myopathy. Similarly, defects in the same gene can give rise to different pathologies, and the same pathological defect can arise from defects in more than one gene [100].

Variation in fiber size may be pronounced, especially in severe neonatal cases, or minimal, but necrosis and regeneration are rare. Scattered, very small fibers containing neonatal myosin, however, are often seen, but it is not clear if these represent attempts at regeneration. Fibrosis is not usually a feature but can be marked, especially in disorders with pronounced differential involvement of muscles, such as central core disease. Hypotrophy of type 1 fibers is common, and there is often a pronounced predominance or uniformity of type 1 fibers. In neonatal cases the muscle is often immature and fibers with developmental myosins persist. Centrally placed nuclei are a particular feature of myotubular and centronuclear myopathies but can also be common in association with mutations in the *RYR1* gene.

Nemaline myopathies

These are identified by the red-staining, rod-shaped structures seen with the Gömöri trichrome technique (Figure 5.26). Rods have a similar lattice structure to the Z-line and contain similar proteins. The spectrum of clinical severity is broad, and six causative genes encoding thin filament proteins have been identified, with defects in *ACTA1* (skeletal actin) and *NEB* (nebulin) being the most common. The number of rods does not correlate with clinical severity, and varies between fibers and muscles, but they are usually abundant. They may be present in prominent peripheral clusters, in lines, or diffusely distributed through the fiber. In rare cases rods occur in, or are restricted to, nuclei, but in most cases they are only seen in the sarcoplasm. In some cases they are restricted to type 1 fibers; they are not a feature of the intrafusal fibers of spindles. Additional structural features such as cores or concentric laminated whorls can also occur in association with rods in various nemaline myopathies. Other myopathies may show occasional or abundant rods but with a phenotype that is not typical of childhood nemaline myopathy; these are better considered as "myopathies with rods" rather than nemaline myopathy. These include cases with dual pathology and cases where mutations in the same gene result in two pathologies in different members of the same family [100].

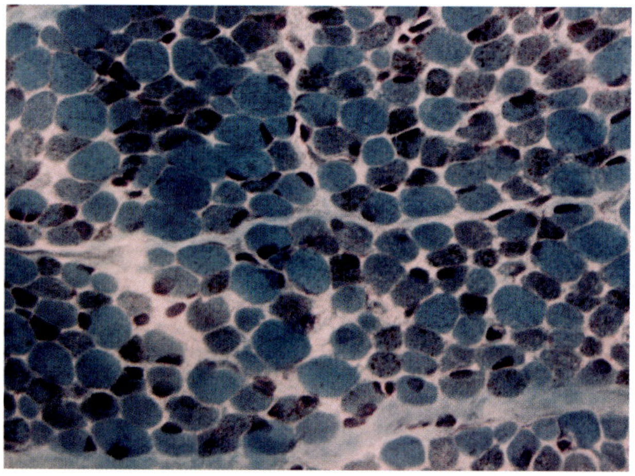

Figure 5.26. Muscle biopsy from a case of nemaline myopathy with a mutation in the *ATCA1* gene stained with the Gömöri trichrome method and abundant red-stained rods in many fibers.

Accumulation of actin thin filaments is seen in some cases as pale staining areas with H&E and the Gömöri trichrome stain. This, and the presence of nuclear rods, is associated with defects in *ACTA1*, but it is rarely possible to identify the defective gene from the pathology. Rods and Z-line abnormalities are also seen in these cases with actin accumulation, and they should therefore be considered to be at the severe end of the "ACTA1" spectrum, rather than as a separate disease entity. Mutations in *ACTA1* have not been identified in all cases with accumulation of skeletal actin, suggesting further genetic heterogeneity. There are no commercial antibodies available that specifically label the skeletal muscle isoform of actin, but fluorescently labeled phalloidin that binds to filamentous actin can be useful. Rare cases with null mutations in *ACTA1* have no skeletal actin, but all fibers express the cardiac actin isoform. The cardiac isoform is present in all fetal muscles and is replaced in most fibers by the skeletal isoform before birth. In most forms of nemaline myopathy fibers with the cardiac actin are rare but a population may be seen in some neonatal cases; the relationship to immaturity in these is not yet clear.

Core myopathies

Cores are areas devoid of mitochondria and thus oxidative enzyme stain; ultrastructurally they show varying degrees of myofibrillar disruption. The size and distribution of cores are variable; they may be extensive and extend down a long length of a fiber, or be focal and multiple affecting only a few sarcomeres. Large cores, that may be central or peripheral, define central core disease caused by mutations in the *RYR1* gene (Figure 5.6). Not all cases with *RYR1* mutations, however, show these large cores and they may be absent (possibly an age-related feature), or focal and multiple (Figure 5.6). Multiple cores can be associated with defects in the *RYR1*, *SEPN1*, *TTN* (titin) genes, and sometimes *COL6* in cases of UCMD. Core formation can also occur in association with other defective genes including *CFL2* (cofilin), *MYH7* (myosin heavy chain 7), *ACTA1*, as well as in a variety of myopathic and neurogenic conditions. In addition, a molecular defect has not been identified in some cases with cores. As there can be considerable clinical and pathological overlap associated with *RYR1* and *SEPN1* mutations, and the cores can evolve with time, it is useful to collectively refer to this group of conditions with a clinical phenotype of a congenital myopathy as "core myopathies," rather than the original distinction of central core disease and multi-minicore disease.

In cases with *RYR1* mutations fiber size variation is often mild, but fiber hypertrophy is common, particularly in adults. If fiber typing is retained the cores have a predilection for type 1 fibers, but fiber type uniformity is common, with most staining as type 1 with the associated phenotype of slow fibers (Figure 5.6). A few fibers may co-express fast myosin and there may be a few very small fibers with neonatal myosin scattered through the biopsy. Some biopsies may show rods and cores in a few fibers, and occasionally the rods are a particular feature. The co-existence of rods and cores is likely to be genetically heterogeneous as there are examples of cases where linkage to *RYR1* and the loci of nemaline myopathy have been excluded.

Internal nuclei may be numerous in *RYR1* cases, and several may be in a central position, and even resemble centronuclear myopathy. In some samples adipose tissue and fibrous tissue are extensive and cause diagnostic confusion with a muscular dystrophy. Some of these samples may show only subtle unevenness of oxidative enzyme stains. Cores lack glycogen but some may be delineated by glycogen and by various proteins, such as desmin and calsequestrin. Accumulations of proteins are also seen within some cores; these include desmin, myotilin, ryanodine receptor 1, calsequestrin, filamin C, small heat shock proteins, and αB-crystallin. Accumulation of proteins is not usually a feature of minicores. Phosphorylase is not demonstrated within large cores associated with *RYR1* mutations, probably because of the absence of glycogen.

The inheritance of *RYR1*-related myopathies is usually autosomal dominant but a significant number of recessively inherited cases have been identified, including severely affected neonates with the fetal akinesia sequence. Recessive cases show considerable clinical and pathological overlap with cases with *SEPN1* mutations and, like them, tend to have more axial involvement; muscle biopsies usually show multiple minicores rather than extensive central cores. Many *RYR1* mutations are de novo and quite common; the possibility of these in association with a mutation in a second gene ("double trouble") can occur and should be considered, especially in clinically atypical cases.

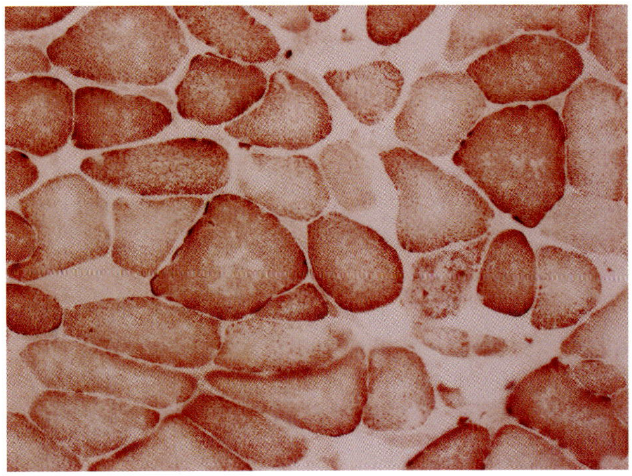

Figure 5.27. Muscle biopsy from a case with a mutation in the *SEPN1* gene stained for COX showing multiple cores devoid of activity in both fiber types and retention of a two-fiber pattern.

Useful histopathological aids for the differential diagnosis of *RYR1* and *SEPN1* cases are the preservation of fiber typing in *SEPN1* cases, in contrast to uniformity or marked type 1 predominance in *RYR1* cases, and the presence of central nuclei in *RYR1* cases (Figures 5.6 and 5.27). These features, however, are not specific for *RYR1* cases and can also occur in neonatal cases with mutations in the titin gene. Very small fibers expressing neonatal myosin may be a feature of *RYR1* cases, but little neonatal myosin is usually present in *SEPN1* cases. Mallory bodies and desmin accumulation have also been observed in some cases with *SEPN1* mutations, but not in any cases with *RYR1* mutations, except desmin in the cores.

Myotubular and centronuclear myopathies

Early descriptions of muscle biopsies with abundant central nuclei led to the introduction of the terms "myotubular myopathy," (because central nuclei are a feature of fetal myotubes) and "centronuclear myopathy." The term myotubular myopathy is now often reserved for the X-linked disorder caused by mutations in the myotubularin gene (*MTM1*), and the term centronuclear myopathy for the molecularly heterogeneous group of autosomal disorders characterized by central nuclei.

The characteristic pathological feature is centrally placed nuclei that occupy a large volume of the fiber (Figure 5.28) and are regularly spaced down the fiber, not in chains as in regenerating fibers; thus the plane of section influences the number of central nuclei observed in transverse section. The central nuclei may be surrounded by an area devoid of myofibrils and organelles that appears as a space when sectioned (Figure 5.28). The number of central nuclei is variable between muscles and they may not be numerous at birth. Central nuclei

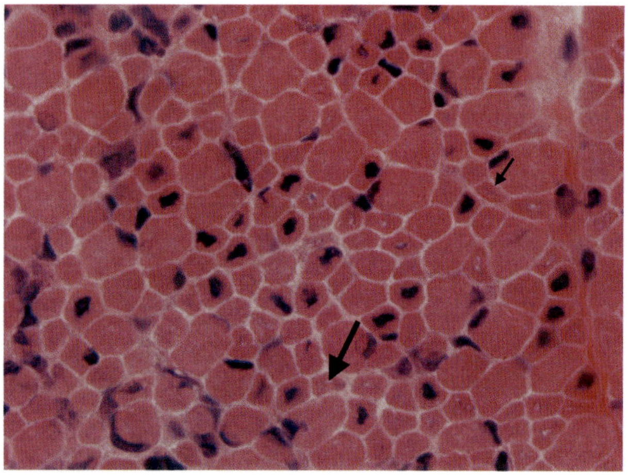

Figure 5.28. Muscle biopsy from a case of severe X-linked myotubular myopathy showing several prominent central nuclei, central areas devoid of stain (large arrow) or with granular basophilia (small arrow). H&E.

are present in both fiber types, and in fibers with and without neonatal myosin. As in other congenital myopathies type 1 fibers may be predominant and/or hypotrophic. The centers of the fiber are often granular and basophilic, and contain an accumulation of mitochondria and glycogen, whilst the peripheries of the fibers may appear as a pale halo. Some fibers may show high desmin and vimentin levels. Female carriers can occasionally present in childhood if X-inactivation is skewed, or more commonly in adulthood with mild weakness and progressive ptosis, but most often they are asymptomatic.

In addition to the similar histological and histochemical pattern in congenital myotonic dystrophy, some cases with *RYR1* mutations can pathologically resemble a myotubular/centronuclear myopathy, and cores may not always be apparent, particularly in very young cases.

Autosomal cases of centronuclear myopathy are more rare than X-linked *MTM1* cases, and molecularly heterogeneous; mutations identified so far are in the genes for dynamin 2 (*DNM2*) or amphiphysin 1/BIN1, which interacts with dynamin 2. In addition to the features described above, cases with *DMN2* mutations show a spoke-like pattern radiating from the center with oxidative enzyme stains and PAS. It is not yet clear if this is a specific feature associated with *DNM2* mutations. These cases have not been reported to show pale peripheral halos with oxidative enzyme stains, and it has not been established if this appearance is related to age, as some molecularly unresolved autosomal infants with centronuclear myopathy do show halos.

Congenital fiber type disproportion (CFTD)

This is a pathological description rather than a disease, in which type 1 fibers are at least 12% smaller than type 2 fibers (later revised to 25%), and show no other pathological features (Figure 5.11). Mutations in *ACTA1*, *SEPN1*, and *TPM3* have been identified, all of which can also be associated with other features such as rods and cores.

Hereditary myosin myopathies

Disorders resulting from mutations in various myosin genes, including *MYH2*, *MYH3*, *MYH7*, and *MHY8*, are an emerging group of disorders that can present during fetal development, childhood or adulthood [49]. Mutations in the same genes can result in a very variable phenotype, including cardiomyopathies. Muscle pathology can show some overlap with congenital myopathies, and in hyaline myopathy (*MYH7* mutations) myosin storage in type 1 fibers is the characteristic feature.

Congenital myopathies characterized by other structural defects

Several myopathies have been defined by the abundance of an unusual structure. It is not clear if all these are genetic entities but gene mutations have now been associated with several of them. Many of these structures are highlighted by the Gömöri trichrome stain, or stains that use tetrazolium salts, and their detail visualized with electron microscopy.

Reducing bodies that characterize the severe X-linked dominant disorder named after them result from mutations in the gene encoding the four and half lim domain 1 protein (*FHL1*) [23], but they are not seen in all cases, and there is a wide clinical spectrum associated with *FHL1*, including adult variants with a limb-girdle phenotype [24, 25]. They can be seen with H&E and trichrome staining and specifically with menadione NBT. In addition, structures resembling reducing bodies can occur in association with acid maltase deficiency.

The structural feature that characterizes *cap disease* is focal, peripheral hyaline areas composed of disrupted myofibrillar material with thickened Z-lines. Mutations in the β-tropomyosin *TPM2* gene are responsible, which is also responsible for a form of nemaline myopathy, and both pathologies have been identified in different members of the same family [100].

Any possible genetic basis for the presence of other structures such as fingerprint bodies, zebra bodies, cylindrical spirals, concentric laminate whorls, and tubular aggregates has not been determined.

Metabolic myopathies

This description includes only hereditary metabolic myopathies caused by enzymatic defects, where pathology has a role. Most recognized metabolic myopathies are considered primary inborn errors of metabolism and many forms are associated with known or postulated enzymatic defects that affect the ability of muscle fibers to maintain adequate ATP concentrations. Traditionally, these diseases are grouped into abnormalities of glycogen, lipid, purine metabolism, or mitochondrial biochemistry. While the use of histochemistry can be helpful for initial guidance, the definitive diagnosis of these conditions relies on specialized biochemical techniques and confirmatory genetic testing. For a detailed description of metabolic diseases affecting muscle and their biochemical diagnosis, the reader is referred to various reviews [101, 102].

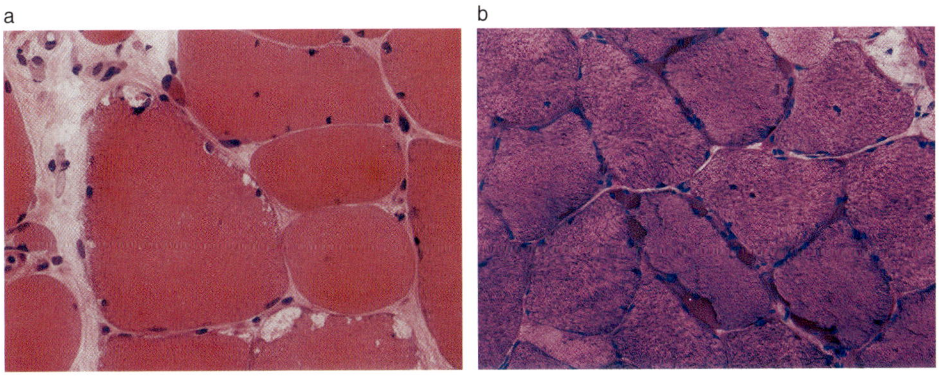

Figure 5.29a, b. Muscle biopsy from a case of McArdle disease stained with H&E (a) and PAS (b) showing peripheral vacuolar areas containing excess glycogen.

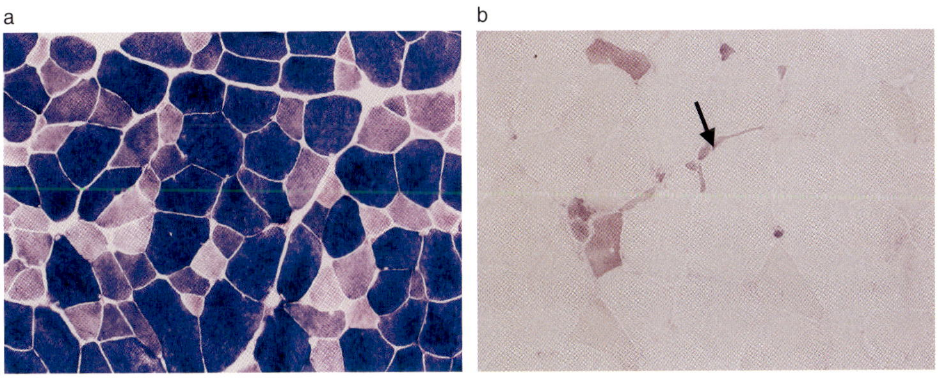

Figure 5.30a, b. Staining for phosphorylase activity in a control muscle sample with a normal checkerboard pattern (a) and the same case of McArdle disease as Figure 5.29 showing an absence of activity in the majority of fibers except some regenerating fibers containing a different isoform (b, arrow).

Disorders of glycogen metabolism and glycolysis

There are two major groups of diseases in this category. First, disorders of anaerobic glycolysis (McArdle and Tauri are the most important prototypes); these disorders cause exercise intolerance and cytosolic storage of glycogen. Second, lysosomal disorders of glycogen catabolism that result in massive accumulation of lysosomal glycogen, such as Pompe disease (infantile and adult, acid maltase deficiency) and Danon disease, in which excess glycogen is related to the deficiency of a lysosomal membrane protein (LAMP-2). In these diseases there is no exercise intolerance.

Disorders of anaerobic glycolysis

Type V glycogenosis (McArdle disease). The muscle isoform of phosphorylase (myophosphorylase) is defective in this recessive disease. Muscle biopsies may show relatively little change on light microscopy. There may be a few degenerating or necrotic fibers, accompanied by regeneration, but the most consistent finding is the presence of subsarcolemmal vacuole-like areas or blebs (which are not membrane bound) containing PAS-positive glycogen, provided it is retained (Figure 5.29). The excess glycogen may only be apparent in these peripheral areas but may be more apparent at the ultrastructural level. The absence of phosphorylase can be demonstrated readily with the histochemical reaction but must always be performed with a positive control to avoid false-negative results. The result is unequivocal and McArdle disease is the only disorder to show this absence of enzyme activity, with the exception of the disorder caused by a mutation in muscle glycogen synthase when glycogen is absent from the muscle (see above). Phosphorylase activity, however, is demonstrated in McArdle disease in intrafusal fibers of spindles, smooth muscle cells of arteries, and regenerating fibers, if present, because of the presence of two other isoforms of phosphorylase (brain or liver isoforms) encoded by different genes (Figure 5.30).

Type VII glycogenosis (Tarui disease). Phosphofructokinase (PFK) catalyzes the conversion of fructose-6-phosphate to fructose-1,6-diphosphate and its absence inhibits the utilization of glucose from either glycogen or glucose metabolism. Muscle biopsies show nonspecific changes on light microscopy and excessive glycogen at the electron microscopic level, although this may not be pronounced. PAS-positive diastase-resistant polyglucosan deposits may also be present, which accumulate with age. Absence of PFK activity can be detected histochemically but the reduction is more reliably determined biochemically. Both adult and severe infantile forms occur, and the absence of the enzyme in erythrocytes probably accounts for the associated hemolytic anemia.

Lysosomal disorders of glycogen catabolism

Type II glycogenosis (Pompe disease). Acid maltase (acid α-glucosidase) is a lysosomal enzyme that degrades glycogen by hydrolyzing the 1,4-links. Absence of this enzyme results in glycogen accumulation in membrane-bound areas of lysosomal origin in several tissues, but predominantly in muscle. Severe infantile (Pompe disease), juvenile, and adult-onset forms can be distinguished. Muscle biopsies from severe cases of Pompe disease show a pronounced vacuolar appearance with large PAS-positive deposits of glycogen in most fibers. The glycogen is digested by diastase but some resistant material may remain. Ultrastructurally, the glycogen is characteristically in membrane-bound areas as well as in large lakes of freely dispersed granules. Glycogen is easily lost during processing and the excess may not always be apparent. In some cases so few myofibrils or glycogen may remain that only the subsarcolemmal regions are spared. As the enzyme is lysosomal, there is also abundant acid phosphatase activity in the vacuoles. The muscle pathology in milder cases is variable, and increased glycogen is usually apparent. The vacuolation may be extensive, or minimal, or may be mainly confined to type 1 fibers, and they contain acid phosphatase (Figure 5.15). The vacuoles may be lined by dystrophin or spectrin but not laminins. MHC-1 may also be associated with the vacuoles, and be overexpressed on the sarcolemma and internally in the fiber.

Lysosomal glycogen storage with normal acid maltase (Danon disease). Danon disease is an X-linked vacuolar myopathy with normal acid maltase levels caused by mutations in the gene encoding the lysosomal-associated membrane-2 protein (LAMP-2) [27]. Not all cases show glycogen storage and the disorder is frequently now referred to as "X-linked vacuolar myopathy." In addition to abnormal variation in the size of both fiber types, the striking feature is the presence of numerous vacuoles containing granular osmiophilic material. In contrast to the vacuoles in acid maltase deficiency, acid phosphatase in the vacuoles is reported to be minimal or absent. The vacuoles are lined by a membrane that shows dystrophin, β-spectrin, laminin chains, and other sarcolemmal proteins. Acetylcholinesterase activity and nonspecific esterases have also been demonstrated on the vacuoles. The membrane and content of the vacuoles are labeled with some lectins; this can help distinguish the vacuoles from those seen in acid maltase deficiency, which show little or no labeling with lectins. Immunohistochemistry and immunoblots show a virtual absence of LAMP-2 protein. The pathology in Danon disease is remarkably similar to that in the X-linked myopathy with excessive autophagy (XMEA, gene locus Xq28) [26], in which sarcolemmal proteins are also found on vacuoles. Calcium deposits can be detected in subsarcolemmal areas, and complement C5b-9 (membrane attack complex, MAC) can be demonstrated on the sarcolemma of XMEA [3, 19]. An additional difference between these two conditions is the abundant duplication of the basal lamina and debris that occurs between the plasma membrane and basal lamina in XMEA.

Disorders of fatty acid metabolism

The oxidation of fatty acids is a major source of energy and a heterogeneous group of disorders are caused by defects in the β-oxidation metabolic pathway. The most common forms of β-oxidation deficiency are carnitine deficiency and deficiencies of carnitine palmitoyltransferases (CPT) I and II. Carnitine deficiency falls into two broad groups: those in which muscle symptoms are the predominant complaint, and those in which muscle involvement is part of a systemic condition. Both myopathic and systemic carnitine deficiencies cause marked excess of lipid globules in muscle which can be demonstrated with the Oil Red O or Sudan Black stains. In some biopsies an excess of enlarged mitochondria with abnormal shape can be seen. The contribution of muscle pathology has diminished in these disorders with advances in molecular analysis and biochemical assays. In patients with CPT deficiencies, however, the amount of lipid may not be increased, and the overall pathology is minimal or absent. If a muscle biopsy is taken soon after an episode of myoglobinuria in CPT deficiency, necrotic and/or regenerating fibers may be present.

Disorders of purine nucleotide metabolism

Adenylate deaminase is an enzyme that catalyzes transformation of adenosine monophosphate to inosine monophosphate and ammonia. This reaction mainly occurs during anaerobic exercise to replenish ATP, which is an essential source of energy for the muscles. Myoadenylate deaminase (MAD) deficiency is the result of a relatively common mutant allele with a heterogeneous clinical presentation. The significance of absent enzyme activity has therefore been questioned. The histochemical reaction for MAD is negative in affected individuals, but symptoms are mild and nonspecific.

Mitochondrial myopathies

The mitochondrial myopathies are a heterogeneous group of multisystem disorders which often affect skeletal muscle and the nervous system. They are mostly due to dysfunction of the mitochondrial respiratory chain. A variety of organs may be affected by mitochondrial dysfunction. The disorders are caused either by mutations of the maternally inherited mitochondrial genome or by nuclear DNA (nDNA) mutations. Today approximately 200 different disease-causing mutations of mitochondrial DNA (mtDNA), and several mutations of nDNA are known. The pathological changes in muscle biopsies are variable and range from striking abnormalities, highly evocative of a mitochondrial disease, to those that are nonspecific or minimal. The absence of pathological changes does not exclude a mitochondrial problem. The most valuable pathological tools are the oxidative enzyme stains (NADH-TR, SDH, COX), the Gömöri trichrome, and Oil Red O or Sudan Black. The Gömöri trichrome stain identifies well-developed ragged red fibers with structurally abnormal mitochondria, but these are not a feature of all mitochondrial myopathies (Figure 5.3). With H&E granular fibers with basophilia react intensely for SDH and NADH-TR (Figure 5.3). Modification of the SDH reaction by addition of phenazine methosulfate is useful because it suppresses the reactivity of normal mitochondria. It shows both ragged red fibers and ragged red equivalents. Fibers devoid of COX activity are easily seen as blue fibers when the techniques for COX and SDH are combined (Figures 5.3 and 5.9). Lipid is often increased in fibers with abnormal mitochondria but in some cases the changes are subtle and are only reflected in varying size of the lipid droplets. Other pathological features include variation in fiber size, with atrophy but little or no hypertrophy, an increase in internal nuclei, and necrosis and regeneration in cases with myoglobinuria. In conditions in which there is associated peripheral nerve involvement there may be associated fiber type grouping. Electron microscopy reveals the structural alterations to the mitochondria, myofibrillar loss and disruption, and an increase in intracellular lipid. Ultrastructural changes are rarely seen if there are no abnormalities seen at the light level. Ragged red and COX-negative fibers are not specific for mitochondrial myopathies and may be a secondary feature in some muscular dystrophies and inflammatory myopathies, in particular inclusion body myositis (see below). As the number of COX-negative fibers increases with age the presence of two to three in a sample from an elderly patient has to be interpreted with caution.

Myofibrillar myopathies

Histopathology has an important role in the diagnosis of myofibrillar myopathies. These are an expanding group of disorders associated with disintegration of the Z-line, and are often of late onset. Defects in the genes for desmin, αB-crystallin, myotilin, filamin C, Bag3 (bcl-2-associated athanogene gene 3) and ZASP (Z-line alternatively spliced PDZ protein) have been identified, and other candidates are under investigation [46, 57]. In addition to nonspecific pathological features, such as fiber atrophy and hypertrophy, fiber splitting, excess internal nuclei (often multiple), and proliferation of endomysial connective tissue and adipose tissue, a characteristic feature is rimmed vacuoles and eosinophilic areas on H&E, but these may not be present in all cases. These eosinophilic hyaline areas are darkly stained with the Gömöri trichrome stain and they lack mitochondria and appear "wiped out" with oxidative enzyme stains (Figure 5.7). A predominance of type 1 fibers may occur, and fiber type grouping and groups of atrophic fibers of both types may be present, consistent with the peripheral neuropathy in some cases. Red-stained cytoplasmic bodies and spheroid bodies are also common, and congophilia, indicating the presence of amyloid-β. Immunohistochemistry shows the accumulation of several proteins, including desmin, αB-crystallin, syncoilin, ubiquitin, myotilin, dystrophin, β-amyloid precursor protein, filamentous actin, neural cell adhesion molecule (NCAM), phosphorylated tau, and prion protein, several of which are also seen in inclusion body myositis (IBM), causing diagnostic difficulties (Figure 5.7). Inflammation is usually minimal or only focal, in contrast to IBM. The sarcolemma of some mature fibers may express MHC-1 but not on all fibers, as occurs in IBM. Cardiomyopathy is present in some cases, particularly those with mutations in the gene for desmin. Desmin accumulation is often seen but the degree variable and sometimes minimal. Characteristic granulofilamentous material is seen ultrastructurally, and, although more often associated with mutations in the genes for desmin and αB-crystallin, it can also occur in other myofibrillar myopathies. It is rarely possible to predict the gene defect from the pathology.

In addition to IBM similar pathological features are also seen in the hereditary forms of inclusion body myopathy, including the "quadriceps sparing" myopathy caused by mutations in the gene encoding UDP-*N*-acetylglucosamine-2 epimerase/*N*-acetylmannosamine kinase (*GNE*). This is allelic to the "distal myopathy with rimmed vacuoles" described by Nonaka. Other distal myopathies also show rimmed vacuoles [79, 80].

A dominantly inherited form of inclusion body myopathy that presents with Paget disease and fronto-temporal dementia is caused by missense mutations encoding p97/VCP (vasolin-containing protein) [103]. Immunohistochemistry of the VCP protein shows cytoplasmic and nuclear accumulation of this chaperone protein, and can be informative in these cases.

Inflammatory myopathies

The inflammatory disorders that affect muscle are polymyositis (PM), adult and juvenile dermatomyositis, IBM, and those induced by viruses, and more rarely by bacteria and fungi [104]. Defining the type of inflammatory disorder is important for management as not all are responsive to drug therapy, such as IBM. There is a well-established association between malignancy and dermatomyositis in adults, and the myopathy can precede the diagnosis of the tumor, although they usually present within a short time of each other. Although the underlying pathogenesis of PM is different to that of dermatomyositis, which influences some of the pathological features, muscle fiber necrosis and the presence of inflammatory cells are common to all the inflammatory myopathies. The degree of these, however, is variable, and the absence of inflammation does not exclude the diagnosis. Some biopsies may show very little change, and immunohistochemistry is then particularly useful, in particular the presence of sarcolemmal MHC-1 on mature fibers. As inflammation can occur in other disorders (see above), clinical presentation is important for diagnosis.

Abnormal variation in fiber size is often present but hypertrophy is usually less pronounced, or absent, compared with muscular dystrophies. Other variable features include an increase in internal nuclei, basophilic fibers, moth-eaten fibers or fibers with core-like areas, and fiber splitting. The amount of connective tissue is also variable, but often less compared to muscular dystrophy. There may also be a loose edematous separation of the muscle fibers with interspersed fibrous tissue. Perifascicular atrophy is a particular feature of dermatomyositis that is not seen in PM (see Figure 5.12). Histochemically these perifascicular fibers are of both types and NADH-TR activity often aggregated. Co-expression of more than one isoform of myosin occurs and they express proteins associated with immaturity, such as neonatal myosin, desmin, and N-CAM. Differentiating them from regenerating fibers is then difficult.

Necrosis and regeneration and a characteristic vacuolar degeneration may be extensive. Necrotic fibers may show a peripheral basophilic regenerative cuff, a feature rarely seen in the muscular dystrophies. The necrosis may be segmental and involve clusters or single muscle fibers. In dermatomyositis areas of infarction with groups of pale-staining fibers may be seen. There is frequently a granular basophilia with H&E stain that is red with trichrome staining. Acid phosphatase activity is associated with the infiltrating cells, and is also increased in the muscle fibers.

The principal cell types in the infiltrating cells, identified with specific antibodies to cluster of differentiation markers (CD markers), are T-lymphocytes, B-cells, dendritic cells, and macrophages. They occur in the perimysium and endomysium, and are often perivascular (see Figure 5.16), and may invade the blood vessel walls. Eosinophils are not usually seen. The proportion and distribution of the various inflammatory cell types differ in PM and dermatomyositis. In PM the infiltrate is predominately endomysial with a high number of $CD8^+$ T-lymphocytes. These are seen surrounding and invading non-necrotic muscle fibers, but this is not a feature of dermatomyositis. B-cells, in contrast, are predominantly perivascular and rare in the endomysium in polymyositis. In dermatomyositis the cells are predominantly perivascular and perimysial, although some may be endomysial, and there is a higher proportion of B-cells and $CD4^+$ cells, some of which are T-cells, but many are dendritic cells.

In both adult and juvenile dermatomyositis an early feature is depletion of capillaries: this can be seen with immunolabeling of endothelial cell markers, MHC-I, laminin α5, or lectins such as that from *Ulex europaeus*. Blood vessels in dermatomyositis often have thickened walls, and may be enlarged and show deposits of immune complexes and the terminal component of the complement pathway, the membrane attack complex C5b-9 (MAC). With electron microscopy endothelial cells show tubuloreticular inclusions.

In IBM in addition to variation in fiber size and inflammation, rimmed vacuoles and inclusions are typical but the number variable (see Figure 5.13). The inclusions are congophilic, and several of the same proteins seen in myofibrillar myopathies are associated with the vacuoles (see above) [47]. Cytoplasmic bodies and disruption of the myofibrillar pattern with core-like areas lacking NADH-TR activity may be seen, and there is often a higher number of fibers for age devoid of cytochrome oxidase. Electron microscopy reveals the presence of 15- to 20-nm filamentous inclusions in the cytoplasm and nuclei, but absence of these does not exclude a diagnosis of IBM.

Connective tissue disorders, such as scleroderma, systemic lupus erythematosus (SLE), rheumatoid arthritis, and sarcoidosis, may show fiber necrosis and inflammatory cells, often with a vasculitis. In SLE the blood vessels walls may be thickened and can also show the tubuloreticular inclusions seen in dermatomyositis. In sarcoidosis granulomatous inflammatory infiltrates, with giant cells, lymphocytes, and macrophages, frequently occur. Nonspecific myopathic changes such as type 2 fiber atrophy are also common in connective tissue disorders. Viruses can also induce a myositis.

Other disorders

A variety of abnormalities are associated with ion channel disorders, myasthenic syndromes, and endocrine disturbances. In addition, changes can be induced by drugs and toxins. The abnormalities are nonspecific and relate mainly to changes in fiber size and fiber proportions, and the presence of necrosis and vacuolation [3].

Conclusion

Morphological studies of muscle make a major contribution to the diagnosis of neuromuscular disease. Immunoanalysis of both primary and secondary protein defects has broadened the understanding of the pathological changes, and can help to direct molecular analysis. Overlapping clinicopathological spectra, however, have created diagnostic difficulties and challenge traditional classifications. They highlight the importance of a multidisciplinary approach to diagnosis.

References

1. S. Pillen, N. van Alfen, M. J. Zwarts, Muscle ultrasound: a grown-up technique for children with neuromuscular disorders. *Muscle Nerve* **38**:3 (2008), 1213–1214.
2. E. Mercuri, A. Pichiecchio, J. Allsop, S. Messina, M. Pane, F. Muntoni, Muscle MRI in inherited neuromuscular disorders: past, present, and future. *J. Magn. Reson. Imaging* **25**:2 (2007), 433–440.
3. V. Dubowitz, C. A. Sewry, *Muscle Biopsy: A Practical Approach*, 3rd edn. (Philadelphia, PA: Saunders/Elsevier, 2007.)
4. K. G. Henriksson, [Muscle biopsy techniques.] *Scand. J. Rheumatol. Suppl.* **30** (1979), 74–79.
5. S. T. Cooper, H. P. Lo, K. N. North, Single section Western blot: improving the molecular diagnosis of the muscular dystrophies. *Neurology* **61**:1 (2003), 93–97.
6. T. G. Overton, R. P. Smith, C. A. Sewry, S. E. Holder, N. M. Fisk, Maternal contamination at fetal muscle biopsy. *Fetal Diagn. Ther.* **15**:2 (2000), 118–121.
7. A. Clerk, P. N. Strong, C. A. Sewry, Characterisation of dystrophin during development of human skeletal muscle. *Development* **114**:2 (1992), 395–402.
8. A. Clerk, C. A. Sewry, V. Dubowitz, P. N. Strong, Characterisation of dystrophin in fetuses at risk for Duchenne muscular dystrophy. *J. Neurol. Sci.* **111**:1 (1992), 82–91.
9. C. A. Sewry, J. Philpot, L. M. Sorokin, *et al.*, Diagnosis of merosin (laminin-2) deficient congenital muscular dystrophy by skin biopsy. *Lancet* **347**:9001 (1996), 582–584.
10. S. Manilal, C. A. Sewry, N. Man, F. Muntoni, G. E. Morris, Diagnosis of X-linked Emery-Dreifuss muscular dystrophy by

protein analysis of leucocytes and skin with monoclonal antibodies. *Neuromuscul. Disord.* **7**:1 (1997), 63–66.

11. E. Mercuri, Y. Yuva, S. C. Brown, *et al.*, Collagen VI involvement in Ullrich syndrome: a clinical, genetic, and immunohistochemical study. *Neurology* **58**:9 (2002), 1354–1359.
12. H. Shimizu, T. Masunaga, Y. Kurihara *et al.*, Expression of plectin and HD1 epitopes in patients with epidermolysis bullosa simplex associated with muscular dystrophy. *Arch. Dermatol. Res.* **291**:10 (1999), 531–537.
13. P. Sabatelli, S. Squarzoni, S. Petrini, *et al.*, Oral exfoliative cytology for the non-invasive diagnosis in X-linked Emery-Dreifuss muscular dystrophy patients and carriers. *Neuromuscul. Disord.* **8**:2 (1998), 67–71.
14. F. Muntoni, C. Sewry, L. Wilson, *et al.*, Prenatal diagnosis in congenital muscular dystrophy. *Lancet* **345**:8949 (1995), 591.
15. M. Brockington, S. C. Brown, A. Lampe *et al.*, Prenatal diagnosis of Ullrich congenital muscular dystrophy using haplotype analysis and collagen VI immunocytochemistry. *Prenat. Diagn.* **24**:6 (2004), 440–444.
16. P. Sabatelli, P. Bonaldo, G. Lattanzi, *et al.*, Collagen VI deficiency affects the organization of fibronectin in the extracellular matrix of cultured fibroblasts. *Matrix Biol.* **20**:7 (2001), 475–486.
17. C. Jimenez-Mallebrera, M. A. Maioli, J. Kim, *et al.*, A comparative analysis of collagen VI production in muscle, skin and fibroblasts from 14 Ullrich congenital muscular dystrophy patients with dominant and recessive COL6A mutations. *Neuromuscul. Disord.* **16**:9–10 (2006), 571–582.
18. D. Hicks, A. K. Lampe, R. Barresi, *et al.*, A refined diagnostic algorithm for Bethlem myopathy. *Neurology* **70**:14 (2008), 1192–1199.
19. C. A. Sewry, C. Jimenez-Mallebrera, S. C. Brown, F. Muntoni, Diseases of muscle. In *Greenfield's Neuropathology*, eds. S. Love, D. Louis, D. Ellison. (London: Hodder-Arnold, 2008), pp. 1725–1820.
20. M. Bitoun, S. Maugenre, P. Y. Jeannet, *et al.*, Mutations in dynamin 2 cause dominant centronuclear myopathy. *Nat. Genet.* **37**:11 (2005), 1207–1209.
21. W. M. Behan, D. W. Cossar, H. A. Madden, I. C. McKay, Validation of a simple, rapid, and economical technique for distinguishing type 1 and 2 fibres in fixed and frozen skeletal muscle. *J. Clin. Pathol.* **55**:5 (2002), 375–380.
22. G. Kollberg, M. Tulinius, T. Gilljam, *et al.*, Cardiomyopathy and exercise intolerance in muscle glycogen storage disease 0. *N. Engl. J. Med.* **357**:15 (2007), 1507–1514.
23. J. Schessl, Y. Zou, M. J. McGrath, *et al.*, Proteomic identification of FHL1 as the protein mutated in human reducing body myopathy. *J. Clin. Invest.* **118**:3 (2008), 904–912.
24. C. Windpassinger, B. Schoser, V. Straub, *et al.*, An X-linked myopathy with postural muscle atrophy and generalized hypertrophy, termed XMPMA, is caused by mutations in FHL1. *Am. J. Hum. Genet.* **82**:1 (2008), 88–99.
25. C. M. Quinzii, T. H. Vu, K. C. Min, *et al.*, X-linked dominant scapuloperoneal myopathy is due to a mutation in the gene encoding four-and-a-half-LIM protein 1. *Am. J. Hum. Genet.* **82**:1 (2008), 208–213.
26. H. Kalimo, M. L. Savontaus, H. Lang, *et al.*, X-linked myopathy with excessive autophagy: a new hereditary muscle disease. *Ann. Neurol.* **23**:3 (1988), 258–265.
27. I. Nishino, J. Fu, K. Tanji, *et al.*, Primary LAMP-2 deficiency causes X-linked vacuolar cardiomyopathy and myopathy (Danon disease). *Nature* **406**:6798 (2000), 906–910.
28. C. A. Sewry, Immunocytochemical analysis of human muscular dystrophy. *Microsc. Res. Tech.* **48**:3–4 (2000), 142–154.
29. B. Ilkovski, S. Clement, C. Sewry, K. N. North, S. T. Cooper, Defining alpha-skeletal and alpha-cardiac actin expression in human heart and skeletal muscle explains the absence of cardiac involvement in ACTA1 nemaline myopathy. *Neuromuscul. Disord.* **15**:12 (2005), 829–835.
30. I. Carbone, C. Bruno, F. Sotgia, *et al.*, Mutation in the CAV3 gene causes partial caveolin-3 deficiency and hyperCKemia. *Neurology* **54**:6 (2000), 1373–1376.
31. C. Minetti, F. Sotgia, C. Bruno, *et al.*, Mutations in the caveolin-3 gene cause autosomal dominant limb-girdle muscular dystrophy. *Nat. Genet.* **18**:4 (1998), 365–368.
32. C. G. Bonnemann, R. Modi, S. Noguchi, *et al.*, Beta-sarcoglycan (A3b) mutations cause autosomal recessive muscular dystrophy with loss of the sarcoglycan complex. *Nat. Genet.* **11**:3 (1995), 266–273.
33. M. Vainzof, M. R. Passos-Bueno, M. Canovas, *et al.*, The sarcoglycan complex in the six autosomal recessive limb-girdle muscular dystrophies. *Hum. Mol. Genet.* **5**:12 (1996), 1963–1969.
34. G. Gosztonyi, U. Naschold, Z. Grozdanovic, G. Stoltenburg-Didinger, R. Gossrau, Expression of Leu-19 (CD56, N-CAM) and nitric oxide synthase (NOS) I in denervated and reinnervated human skeletal muscle. *Microsc. Res. Tech.* **55**:3 (2001), 187–197.
35. V. Straub, A. J. Ettinger, M. Durbeej, *et al.*, Epsilon-sarcoglycan replaces alpha-sarcoglycan in smooth muscle to form a unique dystrophin-glycoprotein complex. *J. Biol. Chem.* **274**:39 (1999), 27989–27996.
36. E. Ozawa, Y. Mizuno, Y. Hagiwara, T. Sasaoka, M. Yoshida, Molecular and cell biology of the sarcoglycan complex. *Muscle Nerve* **32**:5 (2005), 563–576.
37. M. T. Wheeler, M. J. Allikian, A. Heydemann, E. M. McNally, The sarcoglycan complex in striated and vascular smooth muscle. *Cold Spring Harb. Symp. Quant. Biol.* **67** (2002), 389–397.
38. A. Zimprich, M. Grabowski, F. Asmus, *et al.*, Mutations in the gene encoding epsilon-sarcoglycan cause myoclonus-dystonia syndrome. *Nat. Genet.* **29**:1 (2001), 66–69.
39. F. Muntoni, M. Brockington, S. Torelli, S. C. Brown, Defective glycosylation in congenital muscular dystrophies. *Curr. Opin. Neurol.* **17**:2 (2004), 205–209.
40. F. Muntoni, M. Brockington, C. Godfrey, *et al.*, Muscular dystrophies due to defective glycosylation of dystroglycan. *Acta Myol.* **26**:3 (2007), 129–135.
41. S. C. Brown, S. Torelli, C. Jimenez, F. Muntoni, C. A. Sewry, Immunopathology and molecular genetics of dystrophinopathies. *Suppl. Clin. Neurophysiol.* **57** (2004), 313–321.

42. S. C. Brown, F. Muntoni, C. A. Sewry, Non-sarcolemmal muscular dystrophies. *Brain Pathol.* **11**:2 (2001), 193–205.

43. H. Topaloglu, F. Muntoni, V. Dubowitz, C. Sewry, Expression of HLA class I antigens in skeletal muscle is a diagnostic marker in juvenile dermatomyositis. *J. Child. Neurol.* **12**:1 (1997), 60–63.

44. M. Fanin, C Angelini, Muscle pathology in dysferlin deficiency. *Neuropathol. Appl. Neurobiol.* **28**:6 (2002), 461–470.

45. H. H. Goebel, I. A. Warlo, Surplus protein myopathies. *Neuromuscul. Disord.* **11**:1 (2001), 3–6.

46. D. Selcen, K. Ohno, A. G. Engel, Myofibrillar myopathy: clinical, morphological and genetic studies in 63 patients. *Brain* **127**:Pt 2 (2004), 439–451.

47. V. Askanas, W. K. Engel, Inclusion-body myositis: a myodegenerative conformational disorder associated with Abeta, protein misfolding, and proteasome inhibition. *Neurology* **66**:2 Suppl. 1 (2006), S39–S48.

48. R. Schroder, J. Reimann, P. Salmikangas, *et al.*, Beyond LGMD1A: myotilin is a component of central core lesions and nemaline rods. *Neuromuscul. Disord.* **13**:6 (2003), 451–455.

49. A. Oldfors, Hereditary myosin myopathies. *Neuromuscul. Disord.* **17**:5 (2007), 355–367.

50. L. V. Anderson, K. Davison, Multiplex Western blotting system for the analysis of muscular dystrophy proteins. *Am. J. Pathol.* **154**:4 (1999), 1017–1022.

51. H. K. Kolski, C. Hawkins, M. Zatz, *et al.*, Diagnosis of limb-girdle muscular dystrophy 2A by immunohistochemical techniques. *Neuropathology* **28**:3 (2008), 264–268.

52. R. Charlton, M. Henderson, J. Richards, *et al.*, Immunohistochemical analysis of calpain 3: advantages and limitations in diagnosing LGMD2A. *Neuromuscul. Disord.* **19**:7 (2009), 449–457.

53. L. V. Anderson, R. M. Harrison, R. Pogue, *et al.*, Secondary reduction in calpain 3 expression in patients with limb girdle muscular dystrophy type 2B and Miyoshi myopathy (primary dysferlinopathies). *Neuromuscul. Disord.* **10**:8 (2000), 553–559.

54. C. Matsuda, Y. K. Hayashi, M. Ogawa, *et al.*, The sarcolemmal proteins dysferlin and caveolin-3 interact in skeletal muscle. *Hum. Mol. Genet.* **10**:17 (2001), 1761–1766.

55. B. Udd, A. Vihola, J. Sarparanta, I. Richard, P. Hackman, Titinopathies and extension of the M-line mutation phenotype beyond distal myopathy and LGMD2J. *Neurology* **64**:4 (2005), 636–642.

56. L. V. Anderson, K. Davison, J. A. Moss, *et al.*, Characterization of monoclonal antibodies to calpain 3 and protein expression in muscle from patients with limb-girdle muscular dystrophy type 2A. *Am. J. Pathol.* **153**:4 (1998), 1169–1179.

57. R. Griggs, A. Vihola, P. Hackman, *et al.*, Zaspopathy in a large classic late-onset distal myopathy family. *Brain* **130**:Pt 6 (2007), 1477–1484.

58. C. Jimenez-Mallebrera, S. Torelli, L. Feng, *et al.*, A comparative study of alpha-dystroglycan glycosylation in dystroglycanopathies suggests that the hypoglycosylation of alpha-dystroglycan does not consistently correlate with clinical severity. *Brain Pathol.* **19**:4 (2009), 596–611.

59. K. Bushby, L. V. Anderson, C. Pollitt, I. Naom, F. Muntoni, L. Bindoff, Abnormal merosin in adults. A new form of late onset muscular dystrophy not linked to chromosome 6q2. *Brain* **121**:Pt 4 (1998), 581–588.

60. A. E. Emery, The muscular dystrophies. *Lancet* **359**:9307 (2002), 687–695.

61. M. S. Anderson, L. M. Kunkel, The molecular and biochemical basis of Duchenne muscular dystrophy. *Trends. Biochem. Sci.* **17**:8 (1992), 289–292.

62. F. Muntoni, P. Gobbi, C. Sewry, *et al.*, Deletions in the 5′ region of dystrophin and resulting phenotypes. *J. Med. Genet.* **31**:11 (1994), 843–847.

63. F. Muntoni, Is a muscle biopsy in Duchenne dystrophy really necessary? *Neurology* **57**:4 (2001), 574–575.

64. S. C. Brown, S. Torelli, M. Brockington, *et al.*, Abnormalities in alpha-dystroglycan expression in MDC1C and LGMD2I muscular dystrophies. *Am. J. Pathol.* **164**:2 (2004), 727–737.

65. A. Ferlini, C. Sewry, M. A. Melis, A. Mateddu, F. Muntoni, X-linked dilated cardiomyopathy and the dystrophin gene. *Neuromuscul. Disord.* **9**:5 (1999), 339–346.

66. K. Bushby, F. Norwood, V. Straub, The limb-girdle muscular dystrophies – diagnostic strategies. *Biochim. Biophys. Acta* **1772**:2 (2007), 238–242.

67. M. Olive, L. G. Goldfarb, A. Shatunov, D. Fischer, I. Ferrer, Myotilinopathy: refining the clinical and myopathological phenotype. *Brain* **128**:Pt 10 (2005), 2315–2326.

68. W. J. Schulte-Mattler, R. A. Kley, E. Rothenfusser-Korber, *et al.*, Immune-mediated rippling muscle disease. *Neurology* **64**:2 (2005), 364–367.

69. C. Matsuda, M. Aoki, Y. K. Hayashi, M. F. Ho, K. Arahata, R. H. Brown, Jr., Dysferlin is a surface membrane-associated protein that is absent in Miyoshi myopathy. *Neurology* **53**:5 (1999), 1119–1122.

70. M. Vainzof, L. V. Anderson, E. M. McNally, *et al.*, Dysferlin protein analysis in limb–girdle muscular dystrophies. *J. Mol. Neurosci.* **17**:1 (2001), 71–80.

71. F. Piccolo, S. A. Moore, G. C. Ford, K. P. Campbell, Intracellular accumulation and reduced sarcolemmal expression of dysferlin in limb–girdle muscular dystrophies. *Ann. Neurol.* **48**:6 (2000), 902–912.

72. E. S. Moreira, T. J. Wiltshire, G. Faulkner, *et al.*, Limb-girdle muscular dystrophy type 2G is caused by mutations in the gene encoding the sarcomeric protein telethonin. *Nat. Genet.* **24**:2 (2000), 163–166.

73. T. Weiler, C. R. Greenberg, T. Zelinski, *et al.*, A gene for autosomal recessive limb-girdle muscular dystrophy in Manitoba Hutterites maps to chromosome region 9q31–q33: evidence for another limb-girdle muscular dystrophy locus. *Am. J. Hum. Genet.* **63**:1 (1998), 140–147.

74. B. G. Schoser, P. Frosk, A. G. Engel, U. Klutzny, H. Lochmuller, K. Wrogemann, Commonality of TRIM32 mutation in causing sarcotubular myopathy and LGMD2H. *Ann. Neurol.* **57**:4 (2005), 591–595.

75. M. Brockington, D. J. Blake, P. Prandini, *et al.*, Mutations in the fukutin-related protein gene (FKRP) cause a form of congenital muscular dystrophy with secondary laminin alpha2 deficiency and abnormal glycosylation of alpha-dystroglycan. *Am. J. Hum. Genet.* **69**:6 (2001), 1198–1209.

76. C. Sewry, C. Jimenez-Mallebrera, L. Feng, R. Quinlivan, F. Muntoni, Over-expression of sarcolemmal utrophin in

patients with limb-girdle muscular dystrophies [Abstract]. *Neuromuscul. Disord.* **15**:9–10 (2005), 717.

77. P. Hackman, A. Vihola, H. Haravuori, *et al.*, Tibial muscular dystrophy is a titinopathy caused by mutations in TTN, the gene encoding the giant skeletal-muscle protein titin. *Am. J. Hum. Genet.* **71**:3 (2002), 492–500.
78. J. P. Hackman, A. K. Vihola, A. B. Udd, The role of titin in muscular disorders. *Ann. Med.* **35**:6 (2003), 434–441.
79. R. J. Barohn, A. A. Amato, Distal myopathies. *Semin. Neurol.* **19**:1 (1999), 45–58.
80. I. Nonaka, S. Noguchi, I. Nishino, Distal myopathy with rimmed vacuoles and hereditary inclusion body myopathy. *Curr. Neurol. Neurosci. Rep.* **5**:1 (2005), 61–65.
81. H. Haravuori, A. Vihola, V. Straub, *et al.*, Secondary calpain3 deficiency in 2q-linked muscular dystrophy: titin is the candidate gene. *Neurology* **56**:7 (2001), 869–877.
82. F. Muntoni, T. Voit, The congenital muscular dystrophies in 2004: a century of exciting progress. *Neuromuscul. Disord.* **14**:10 (2004), 635–649.
83. V. Dubowitz, 22nd ENMC sponsored workshop on congenital muscular dystrophy held in Baarn, The Netherlands, 14–16 May 1993. *Neuromuscul. Disord.* **4**:1 (1994), 75–81.
84. V. Dubowitz, M. Fardeau, Proceedings of the 27th ENMC sponsored workshop on congenital muscular dystrophy. 22–24 April 1994, The Netherlands. *Neuromuscul. Disord.* **5**:3 (1995), 253–258.
85. V. Dubowitz, 41st ENMC International Workshop on Congenital Muscular Dystrophy 8–10 March 1996, Naarden, The Netherlands. *Neuromuscul. Disord.* **6**:4 (1996), 295–306.
86. V. Dubowitz, 50th ENMC International Workshop: congenital muscular dystrophy. 28 February 1997 to 2 March 1997, Naarden, The Netherlands. *Neuromuscul. Disord.* **7**:8 (1997), 539–547.
87. V. Dubowitz, 68th ENMC international workshop (5th international workshop): on congenital muscular dystrophy, 9–11 April 1999, Naarden, The Netherlands. *Neuromuscul. Disord.* **9**:6–7 (1999), 446–454.
88. F. Muntoni, T. Voit, 133rd ENMC International Workshop on Congenital Muscular Dystrophy (IXth International CMD Workshop) 21–23 January 2005, Naarden, The Netherlands congenital muscular dystrophies in 2004: a century of exciting progress. *Neuromuscul. Disord.* **1514**:1110 (2005), 794635–801649.
89. C. A. Sewry, I. Naom, M. D'alessandro, *et al.*, Variable clinical phenotype in merosin-deficient congenital muscular dystrophy associated with differential immunolabelling of two fragments of the laminin alpha 2 chain. *Neuromuscul. Disord.* **7**:3 (1997), 169–175.
90. M. Vainzof, P. Richard, R. Herrmann, *et al.*, Prenatal diagnosis in laminin alpha2 chain (merosin)-deficient congenital muscular dystrophy: a collective experience of five international centers. *Neuromuscul. Disord.* **15**:9–10 (2005), 588–594.
91. Y. K. Hayashi, F. L. Chou, E. Engvall, *et al.*, Mutations in the integrin alpha7 gene cause congenital myopathy. *Nat. Genet.* **19**:1 (1998), 94–97.
92. A. K. Lampe, K. M. Bushby, Collagen VI related muscle disorders. *J. Med. Genet.* **42**:9 (2005), 673–685.
93. J. Vajsar, W. Zhang, W. B. Dobyns, *et al.*, Carriers and patients with muscle-eye-brain disease can be rapidly diagnosed by enzymatic analysis of fibroblasts and lymphoblasts. *Neuromuscul. Disord.* **16**:2 (2006), 132–136.
94. V. Allamand, P. Richard, A. Lescure, *et al.*, A single homozygous point mutation in a 3′ untranslated region motif of selenoprotein N mRNA causes SEPN1-related myopathy. *EMBO. Rep.* **7**:4 (2006), 450–454.
95. M. R. Taylor, D. Slavov, A. Gajewski, *et al.*, Thymopoietin (lamina-associated polypeptide 2) gene mutation associated with dilated cardiomyopathy. *Hum. Mutat.* **26**:6 (2005), 566–574.
96. B. G. Schoser, C. Schneider-Gold, W. Kress, *et al.*, Muscle pathology in 57 patients with myotonic dystrophy type 2. *Muscle Nerve* **29**:2 (2004), 275–281.
97. R. Cardani, E. Mancinelli, G. Rotondo, V. Sansone, G, Meola, Muscleblind-like protein 1 nuclear sequestration is a molecular pathology marker of DM1 and DM2. *Eur. J. Histochem.* **50**:3 (2006), 177–182.
98. A. Calado, F. M. Tome, B. Brais, *et al.*, Nuclear inclusions in oculopharyngeal muscular dystrophy consist of poly(A) binding protein 2 aggregates which sequester poly(A) RNA. *Hum. Mol. Genet.* **9**:15 (2000), 2321–2328.
99. V. Askanas, P. Serdaroglu, W. K. Engel, R. B. Alvarez, Immunolocalization of ubiquitin in muscle biopsies of patients with inclusion body myositis and oculopharyngeal muscular dystrophy. *Neurosci. Lett.* **130**:1 (1991), 73–76.
100. C. A. Sewry, C. Jimenez-Mallebrera, F. Muntoni, Congenital myopathies. *Curr. Opin. Neurol.* **21**:5 (2008), 569–575.
101. J. Vockley, D. A. Whiteman, Defects of mitochondrial beta-oxidation: a growing group of disorders. *Neuromuscul. Disord.* **12**:3 (2002), 235–246.
102. S. DiMauro, M. Hirano, Mitochondrial encephalomyopathies: an update. *Neuromuscul. Disord.* **15**:4 (2005), 276–286.
103. G. D. Watts, J. Wymer, M. J. Kovach, *et al.*, Inclusion body myopathy associated with Paget disease of bone and frontotemporal dementia is caused by mutant valosin-containing protein. *Nat. Genet.* **36**:4 (2004), 377–381.
104. M. C. Dalakas, The molecular pathophysiology in inflammatory myopathies. *Rev. Med. Interne* **25** Suppl 1 (2004), S14–S16.

Chapter 6

Ultrastructural study of muscle

Anders Oldfors

Introduction

Recent developments in immunohistochemistry, molecular biology, and genetics have diminished the role of electron microscopy in reaching a correct diagnosis, but it still has a place in diagnostic work-up in many cases. Supplementing light microscopy on frozen sections, electron microscopy can also be of great help in distinguishing artifacts from real pathology. Semi-thin (1 μm) resin sections, usually prepared to select regions for ultrathin sections, are also valuable for characterizing morphological alterations. In this chapter the emphasis is on structural alterations that are important in diagnostic work-up, and both semi-thin resin sections and electron micrographs are discussed.

Myofibrils

Myofibrils are composed of sarcomeres that constitute the contractile units of the muscle fiber. The sarcomeres are approximately 2 μm long and bordered at their ends by dark narrow lines (0.1 μm), Z-lines or Z-bands. Between the Z-bands are bundles of myofilaments. The thin myofilaments are attached to the Z-bands with which they form the I-band. Between I-bands, in the middle of the sarcomeres, is the A-band, which is composed of thick filaments. At each end of the A-band these thick filaments are partially overlapped by thin filaments. The myofibrils are surrounded by the intermyofibrillar network, which contains mitochondria, glycogen, sarcoplasmic reticulum, and T-tubules as well as cytoskeletal proteins such as desmin.

The major constituent of the thick (15 nm) filament is myosin. Myosin is a molecular motor that converts chemical energy into mechanical force [1]. It is a hexameric protein composed of two myosin heavy chain (MyHC) subunits, each with a molecular weight of approximately 220 kDa, and two pairs of nonidentical myosin light chain subunits (essential light chains and regulatory light chains) of approximately 20 kDa molecular weight. The MyHC has two functional domains: the globular, N-terminal head domain to which the light chains bind exhibits the motor function, and the elongated alpha-helical coiled-coil C-terminal rod domain has filament-forming properties. The globular head contains the binding sites for actin and ATP [2]. The rod domain lies along the thick filament axis. Accessory proteins, such as myomesin, M-protein, titin, desmin, and myosin-binding proteins (MyBP) C and H are necessary for the precise alignment of the thick filaments [3].

The major constituents of the thin (10 nm) filament are skeletal α-actin, tropomyosin (Tm), and the troponin (Tn) complex. The giant protein nebulin is thought to be essential for the length of the thin filament, with which it is associated. Filamentous actin (F-actin) is a polar molecule composed of a double helix of two strands of polymerized globular actin monomers. By binding to the myosin head F-actin plays a central role in muscle contraction [4]. Tm is an integral part of the thin filament of the sarcomere [5]. It is composed of two α-helical chains, forming a rod-shaped coiled-coil dimer. By overlap of a few residues at the C- and N-terminals, Tm dimers form a continuous polymer lying in each of the two grooves in F-actin in the thin filament. Tm plays an important role in the regulation of muscle contraction by controlling Ca^{2+} sensitivity and by modulating actin–myosin cross-bridge cycle kinetics [6]. The Tn complex consists of TnI, TnT, and TnC and is important for the Ca^{2+}-regulatory system. TnT is the component that binds to actin [7].

The Z-bands are composed of several proteins, the major component being α-actinin. Several thin filament proteins such as actin and nebulin and also titin are anchored to the Z-bands. Intermediate filaments, mainly desmin, form transverse links between the sarcomeres keeping them in register.

Structural changes in myofibrils are frequently seen in muscle diseases, but in most instances these alterations are unspecific and secondary. In some diseases it is the sarcomeres that are primarily affected.

Diseases of thin filament proteins

Mutations in genes encoding for the thin filament proteins actin (*ACTA1*), Tm (*TPM2* and *TPM3*), TnT (*TNNT1*), and nebulin (*NEB*) are associated with nemaline myopathy [8].

Disorders of Voluntary Muscle, 8th edn., eds. George Karpati, David Hilton-Jones, Kate Bushby and Robert C. Griggs. Published by Cambridge University Press.

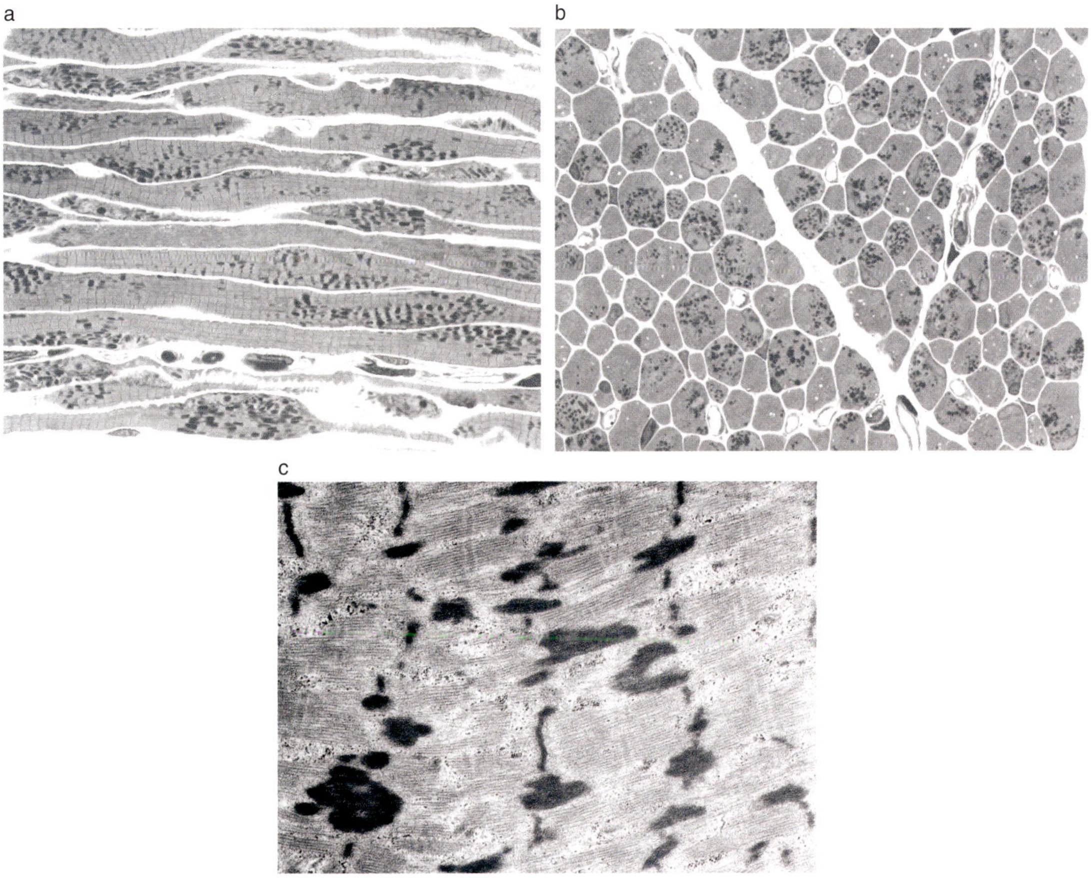

Figure 6.1a–c. (a, b) Nemaline myopathy. Longitudinal (a) and transverse (b) semi-thin resin sections in a case of nemaline myopathy caused by an *ACTA1* mutation. (a) The apparent association of nemaline rods with Z-lines and their orientation parallel to the long axis of the muscle fibers are seen. (b) In transverse sections the rods appear as dark round inclusions (x1000). (c) Electron micrograph demonstrating the similar electron density of nemaline rods as Z-line material and their localization to the Z-line region (x21 000).

Nemaline rods can be identified by light microscopy but electron microscopy is helpful if they are scarce; the latter is also valuable for verifying that inclusions are nemaline rods. They comprise an extension of the lattice of the Z-lines, from which it can be clearly seen in longitudinal sections that they originate (Figure 6.1). They measure approximately 1–7 μm in length and 0.5–1.5 μm in width. They frequently accumulate beneath the sarcolemma, exhibiting both longitudinal and transverse periodicity (Figure 6.2) [9]. Intranuclear rods can sometimes be observed in large amounts [10] and have been identified in relation to some specific *ACTA1* mutations [11]. Mutations in *ACTA1* may also be expressed as actin myopathy with accumulation of actin thin filaments beneath the sarcolemma [12, 13]. Nemaline rods are not specific and can occur in various primary hereditary and acquired muscle diseases and interestingly also in monoclonal gammopathy [14, 15].

Cap disease, described in 1981 [16], is a rare congenital myopathy with abnormal accumulation of proteins forming cap-like structures in the periphery of the muscle fibers under the sarcolemma, with reduced myosin ATPase activity and increased nicotinamide adenine dinucleotide dehydrogenase tetrazolium reductase (NADH-TR) activity. The clinical features resemble those of nemaline myopathy with infantile onset of hypotonia and muscle weakness, predominantly involving the proximal muscles, neck flexors, and the facial muscles [17, 18]. Cap disease was recently associated with a

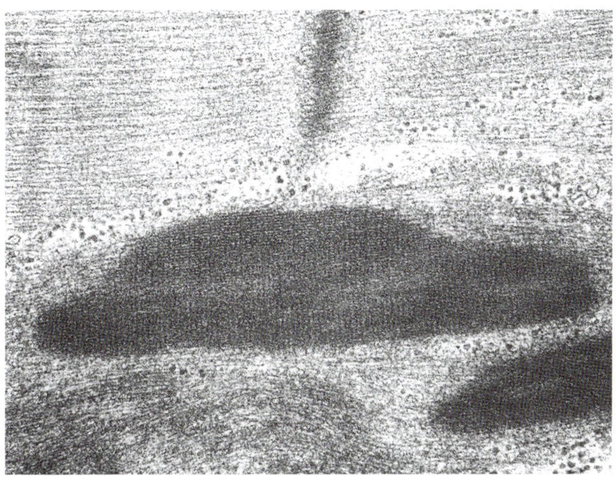

Figure 6.2. Nemaline myopathy. Nemaline rod demonstrating typical longitudinal and transverse periodicity (x50 000).

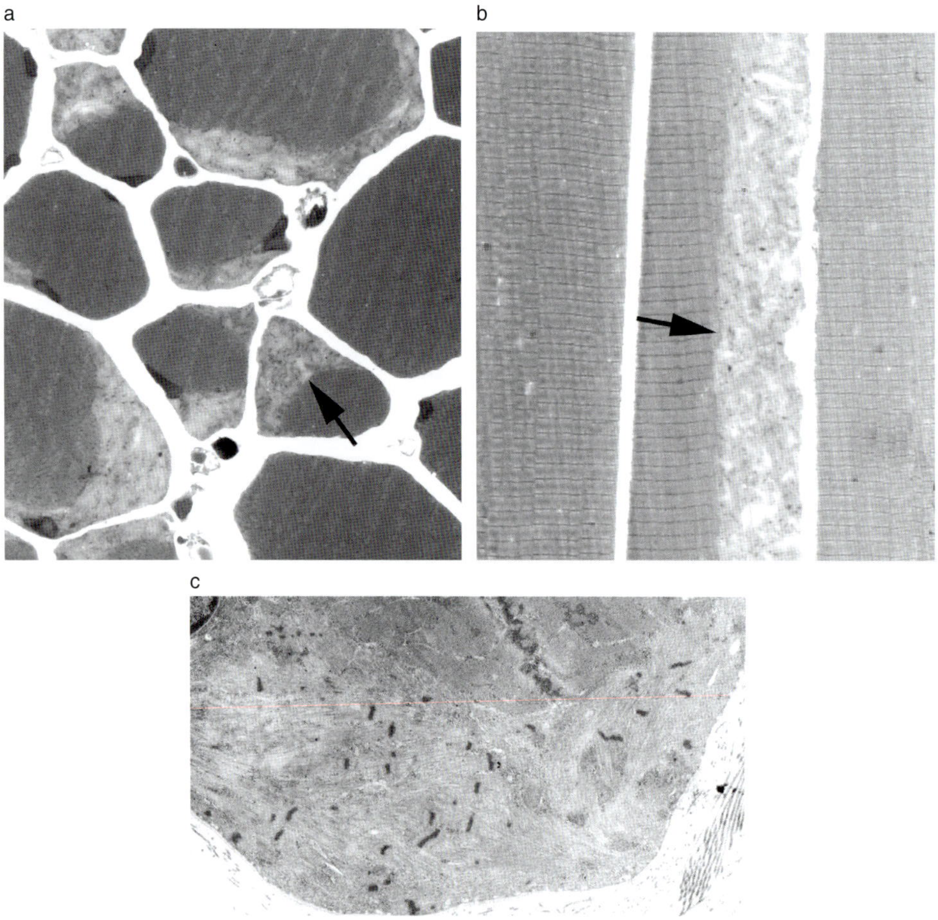

Figure 6.3a–c. (a, b) Cap disease. Transverse (a) and longitudinal (b) semi-thin resin sections in a case of cap disease caused by a *TPM2* mutation. The caps (arrows) are sharply demarcated structures with disorganization of myofibrils beneath the plasma membrane (a: x1000; b: x1000). (c) Electron micrograph of a cap structure demonstrating irregular myofibrils with partial paucity of thick filaments (x15 000).

mutation in the gene encoding for β-tropomyosin (*TPM2*) [19]. Electron microscopy of the cap structures reveals disorganization of myofibrils, partial loss of thick filaments, and thickened fragments of Z-bands without nemaline rod formation (Figure 6.3).

Diseases of thick filament proteins

Diseases that primarily or mainly affect thick filaments include hereditary myosin myopathies and acute quadriplegic myopathy. Hereditary myosin myopathies have emerged as a new group of muscle diseases with highly variable clinical features and onset during fetal development, childhood or adulthood [20]. They are caused by mutations in skeletal muscle MyHC genes. Mutations have been reported in two of the three MyHC isoforms expressed in adult limb skeletal muscle: type I (slow/β-cardiac MyHC; *MYH7*) and type IIa (*MYH2*). Laing early-onset distal myopathy and myosin storage myopathy (MSM) are associated with mutations in *MYH7*. MSM is morphologically characterized by subsarcolemmal accumulation of myosin in type 1 fibers, which appears as granular or filamentous material at the ultrastructural level (Figure 6.4), whereas Laing distal myopathy is associated with variable and unspecific muscle pathology. A myopathy associated with a specific mutation in *MYH2* is associated with congenital joint contractures and external ophthalmoplegia. Numerous rimmed vacuoles with 15- to 20-nm tubulofilamentous inclusions identical to those seen in sporadic inclusion body myositis (sIBM) (see below) occur in some individuals with this disease [21].

In acute quadriplegic myopathy (AQM), also called critical illness myopathy, there is selective loss of thick filaments [22]. AQM is typically seen in patients with severe asthma treated with high doses of steroids and neuromuscular blockade to facilitate assisted respiration. Clinical recovery proceeds for weeks or months following cessation of treatment. The selective loss of thick filaments is however not specific for AQM since it can also occur in ischemia and cancer cachexia [23].

Myofibrillar myopathy

Myofibrillar or desmin-related myopathy comprises a group of diseases with a wide spectrum of clinical findings despite morphological similarities involving alterations of the myofibrils and accumulation of various proteins, e.g., desmin, myotilin, αB-crystallin, dystrophin, and neural cell adhesion molecule (NCAM) [24]. The genes thus far associated with myofibrillar myopathy include *DES*, *CRYAB*, *ZASP*, *SEPN1*, *MYOT*, and *FLNC*. At the ultrastructural level many different

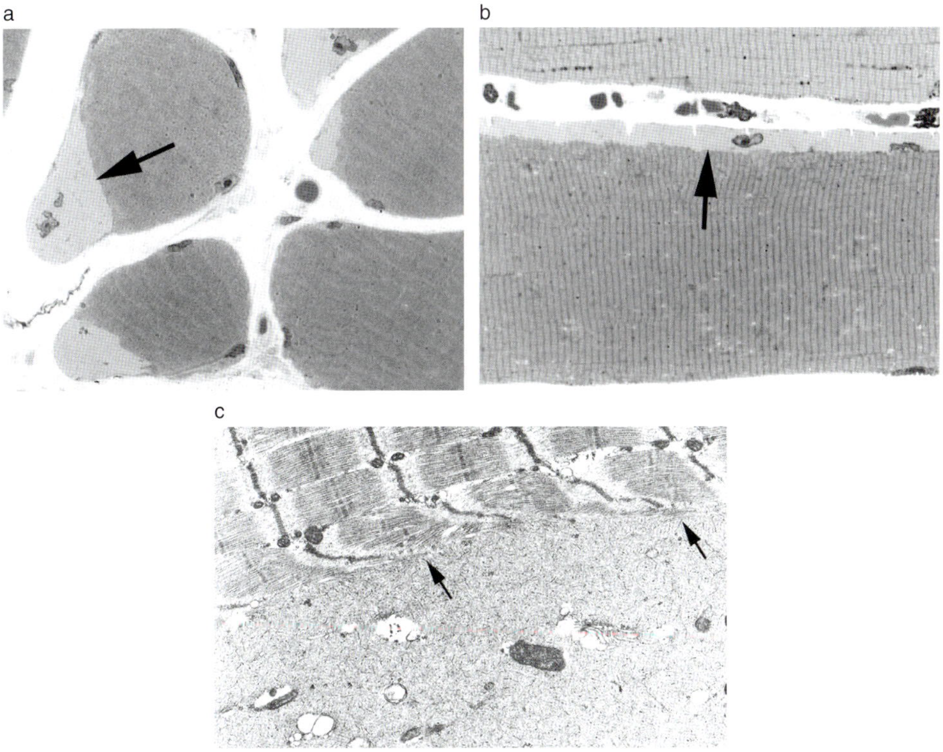

Figure 6.4a–c. (a, b) Myosin storage disease. Transverse (a) and longitudinal (b) semi-thin resin sections in a case of myosin storage disease caused by a *MYH7* mutation. There are sharply demarcated subsarcolemmal regions with accumulation of unstructured material and occasional myonuclei and cell organelles (arrows) (x1000). (c) Electron micrograph of subsarcolemmal regions with accumulation of granular or slightly filamentous material mixed with occasional cell organelles. Thick filaments of the sarcomeres (arrows) seem to disintegrate into the accumulated material (x21 000).

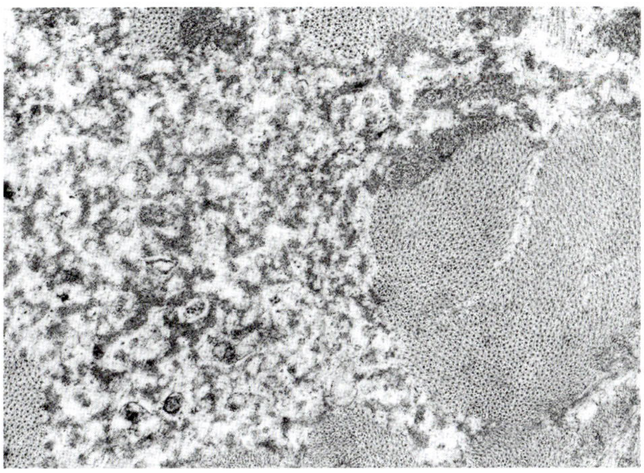

Figure 6.5. Myofibrillar myopathy. Electron micrograph illustrating granulofilamentous material (left part) accumulated between and partly engaging the myofibrils in a case of myofibrillar myopathy (x30 000).

changes involving the myofibrils can be observed: the accumulation of granulofilamentous material (also described as bands of electron-dense material or dappled dense bodies) is one such typical alteration (Figure 6.5). Some cases of myofibrillar myopathy are characterized by desmin plaques or Mallory-body-like inclusions [25, 26].

Multi-minicore and central core myopathies

In multi-mini core myopathy caused by mutations in selenoprotein N1 (*SEPN1*) and the ryanodine receptor (*RYR1*) the major structural alteration is focal disorganization of the myofibrils [27, 28] (Figure 6.6). These are unspecific changes seen in many muscle diseases but multi-minicore disease is diagnosed when they are abundant. Within the cores there is depletion of mitochondria, sarcoplasmic reticulum, and T-tubules as well as myofibrillar disorganization. *RYR1* mutations are also associated with central core disease [29] in which the core structure is a cylinder extending throughout the entire fiber (Figure 6.7). In central core disease the myofibrillar disorganization is sometimes minimal. The cores can be centrally placed but are more often located peripherally. There can be one or more cores in a fiber. The target formations seen in neurogenic muscle diseases are similar to the cores in central core disease, but the zone of mitochondrial depletion and myofibrillar disorganization is limited in length in the target formations.

Other myofibrillar changes

Organized aberrant myofibrils as seen in lobulated muscle fibers and annular myofibrils (ringbinden) are other unspecific myofibrillar changes. Annular myofibrils (Figure 6.8) are typically present in myotonic dystrophy but occur in various other myopathies as well as in denervation. The annular myofibrils encircle the peripheral part of the muscle fiber in a plane perpendicular to the long axis. Z-band streaming (Figure 6.9a) and cytoplasmic bodies (Figure 6.9b) are additional structural alterations of the sarcomeres and can be seen in numerous different neuromuscular disorders.

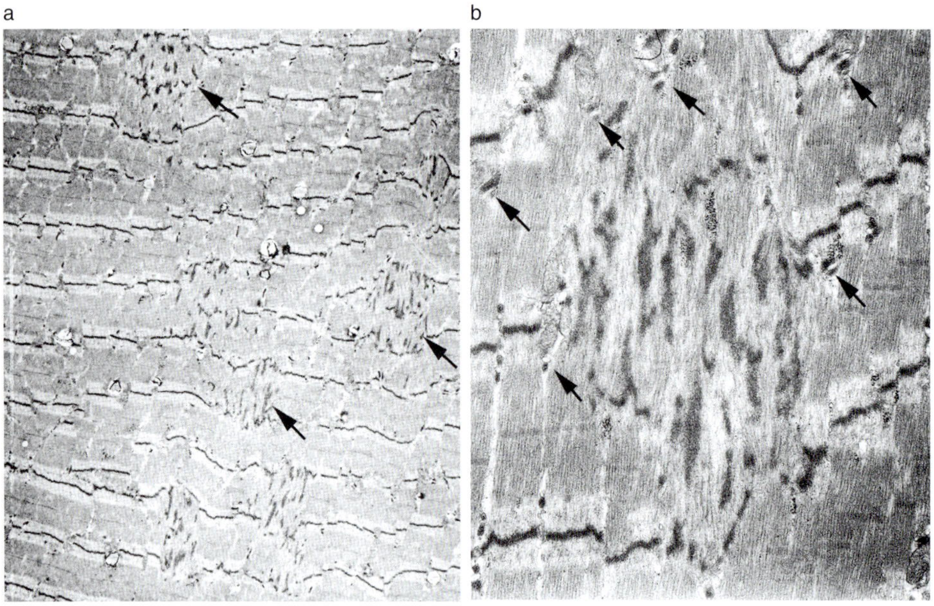

Figure 6.6a, b. Multi-minicore disease. Electron micrograph illustrating minicores (arrows) in a longitudinal section from a case with multi-minicore disease. (b) Within the minicores (center) there are no mitochondria and no sarcoplasmic reticulum. Numerous triads of T-tubules and sarcoplasmic reticulum are seen around the minicore structure (arrows) (a: x7000; b: x20 000).

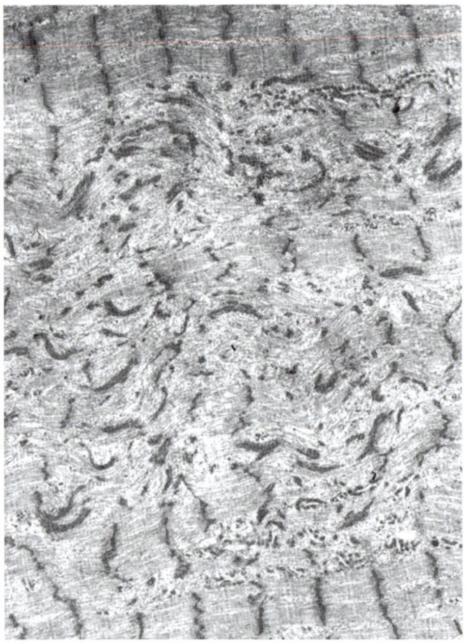

Figure 6.7. Central core disease. Electron micrograph showing longitudinal section of a muscle fiber in a patient with central core disease. Within the core, which extends along the center of the fiber, there is myofibrillar disorganization and lack of mitochondria (x7000).

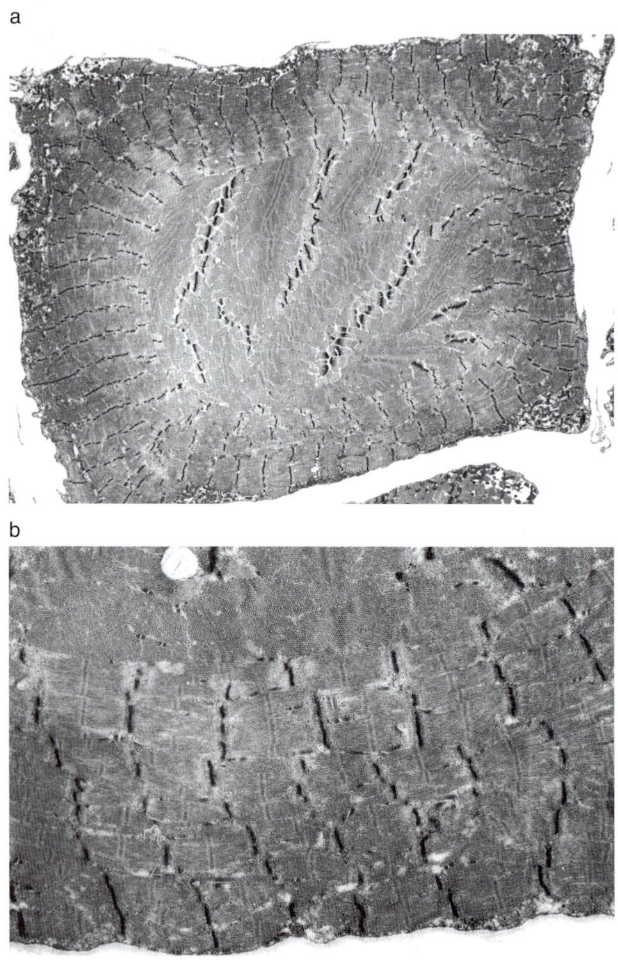

Figure 6.8a, b. Annular myofibrils. Electron micrograph of annular myofibrils in cross-section demonstrating the orientation of peripheral myofibrils perpendicular to the long axis of the fiber (a: x4500; b: x14 000).

Nuclei

In normal adult muscle, myonuclei are apposed to the sarcolemma with no intervening myofibrils. Areas within the nucleus where chromatin is being actively transcribed are pale (euchromatin), while transcriptionally inactive areas are dark (heterochromatin). Communication between cytoplasm and nucleus takes place through the nuclear pores. On the inner side of the inner nuclear membrane is a relatively uniform granular band known as the nuclear lamina. Fibrillar proteins

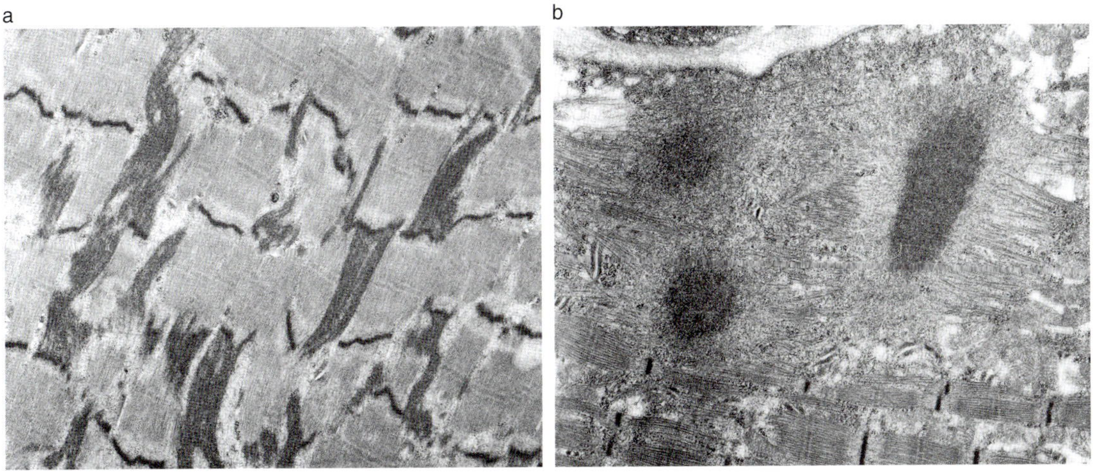

Figure 6.9a, b. Z-band streaming and cytoplasmic bodies. (a) Electron micrograph demonstrating Z-band streaming (x15 000). (b) Electron micrograph demonstrating three cytoplasmic bodies (x16 000).

called lamins, which may bind the ends of chromosomes to the lamina, are found in this region. The lamina is interrupted beneath the nuclear pores.

Displacement of nuclei from their normal subsarcolemmal position is the most common abnormality involving nuclei and is an unspecific finding in many neuromuscular diseases. Such nuclei tend to be scattered randomly in the interior of fibers. By contrast, in X-linked myotubular myopathy caused by mutations in myotubularin 1 (*MTM1*) [30] the nuclei are in the precise geometric center of the fiber, although some subsarcolemmal nuclei are also present [31]. In autosomal dominant centronuclear myopathy (CNM) caused by mutations in dynamin 2 (*DNM2*) [32] and autosomal recessive CNM caused by mutations in amphiphysin 2 (*BIN1*) [33] tight clusters of nuclei occur in the center of the fibers [34] (Figure 6.10).

Accumulation of fine tubular filaments, 8.5 nm in external diameter and up to 0.25 μm in length, within myonuclei are pathognomonic of oculopharyngeal muscular dystrophy (OPMD) [35, 36]. The filaments frequently form tangles or palisades (Figure 6.11). OPMD is caused by mutations (expansion of a short GCG triplet repeat) in the gene encoding for the nuclear poly(A)-binding protein 7 (*PABPN1*) [37]. This protein normally resides in nuclei and binds the polyadenylate tail of mRNA. GCG codes for alanine and the tubular filaments may possibly be formed by polymerized polyalanine tracts in β-pleated form.

A variety of nuclear abnormalities can be seen in sporadic inclusion body myositis, including bizarre shapes, excess heterochromatin, accumulation of tubular filaments 12–15 nm in diameter and loss of nuclear membranes (Figure 6.12). There is some evidence that the filaments reach the cytoplasm through nuclear breakdown [38, 39]. The cytoplasmic filaments tend to have a slightly larger external diameter than the nuclear ones.

The mutation that causes Emery–Dreifuss muscular dystrophy results in loss of a protein normally localized on the

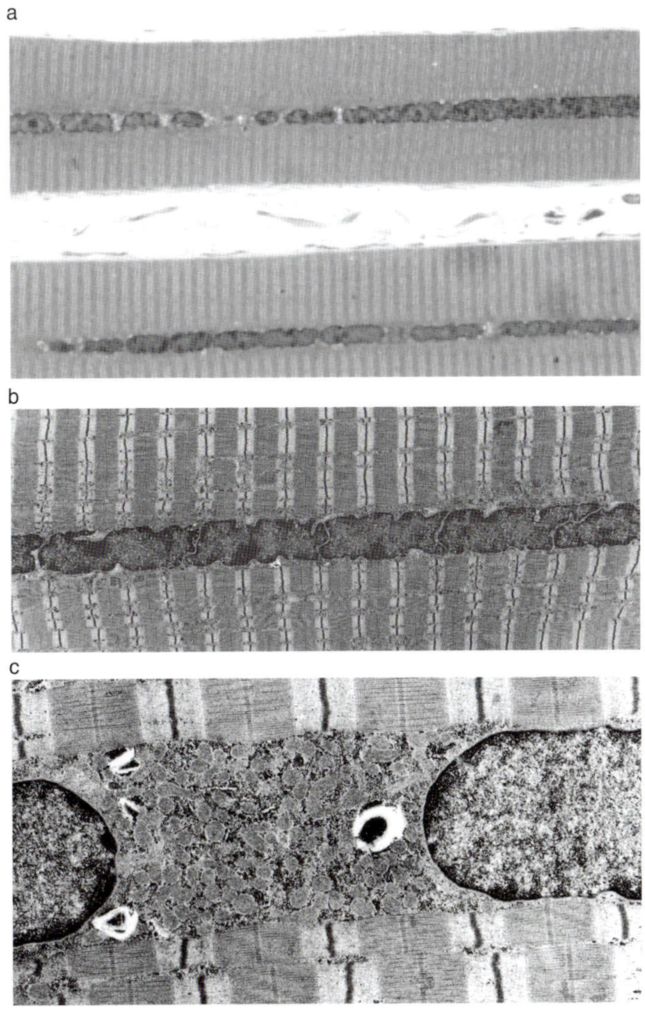

Figure 6.10a–c. Centronuclear myopathy. (a) Longitudinal semi-thin resin sections in a case of centronuclear myopathy caused by a *BIN1* mutation. There are rows of exactly centrally located nuclei and paucity of peripherally located nuclei (x1200). (b) Electron micrograph demonstrating a row of closely apposed centrally located nuclei (x4000). (c) Electron micrograph demonstrating that there is lack of myofibrils and accumulation of mitochondria in segments where the central nuclei are not completely apposed to each other (x15 000).

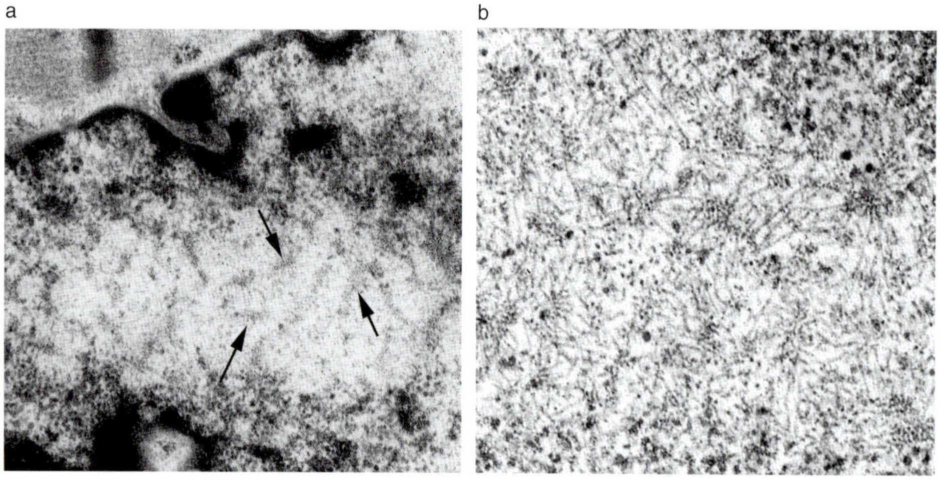

Figure 6.11a, b. Oculopharyngeal muscular dystrophy. Electron micrographs demonstrating the pathognomonic palisading intranuclear filaments (arrows) that appear tubular at high magnification (a. x30 000; b: x80 000).

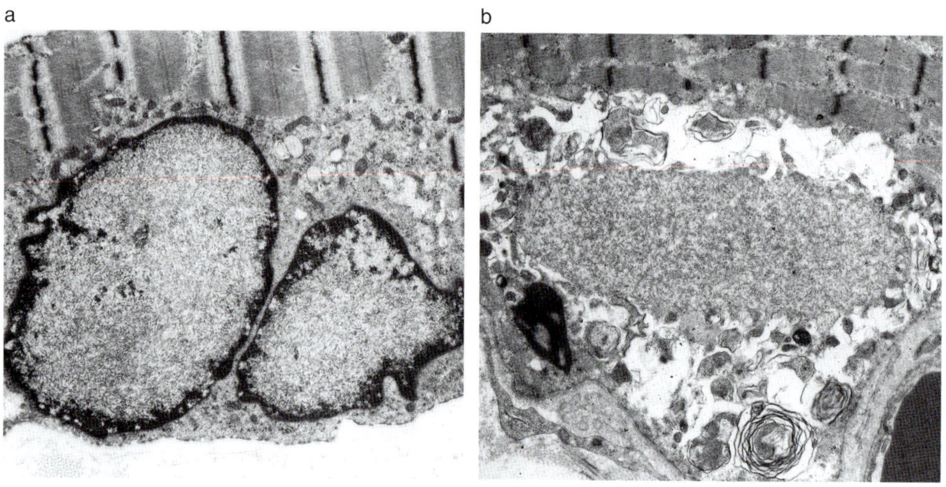

Figure 6.12a, b. Nuclear filaments in inclusion body myositis. Electron micrographs demonstrating intranuclear filaments (a) and a collection of cytoplasmic filaments (b). These images suggest that the cytoplasmic collections of filaments may be formed in nuclei and then become cytoplasmic after breaking down of the nuclear membranes (x9000).

inner nuclear membrane. Electron microscopic abnormalities of nuclei have been reported, becoming more frequent with increasing age, including formation of regular tubules 300–350 nm in diameter, nuclear pyknosis, and focal breakdown of the nuclear membranes [40].

In Marinesco–Sjögren syndrome, nuclei become surrounded by a thick membrane, which may be derived from the outer nuclear membrane and the presence of TUNEL-positive nuclei indicates that apoptosis may occur [41].

Accumulation in nuclei of masses of fine, parallel 8-nm filaments, presumably representing actin, is a nonspecific reaction. In human muscle, it is seen most often in damaged fibers in dermatomyositis. Excess globular actin can apparently diffuse into nuclei, where it can be trapped if conditions favor its polymerization into filamentous actin. Nemaline bodies can also be encountered in nuclei in some cases of nemaline myopathy caused by mutations in alpha-skeletal actin (*ACTA1*) [11]. In vitro studies have demonstrated that transfection of cultured myoblasts with a mutant actin gene construct as well as cell stress by ATP depletion will result in accumulation and polymerization of intranuclear actin [42].

Lysosomes

Together with the ubiquitin-proteasomal system, lysosomes are essential for the normal turnover of proteins and the degradation of waste material. After autophagocytosis of intracellular material and fusion of the autophagosome with the lysosome, hydrolytic enzymes will degrade the material.

Lipofuscin is a brown, autofluorescent and periodic-acid-Schiff- (PAS-) positive substance seen as granules in normal muscle, which increase with age. It is found in increased amounts in many neuromuscular disorders and represents residual bodies remaining after lysosomal degradation. Ultrastructurally the lipofuscin granules contain a mixture of different components that may exhibit very high electron density as well as components with low electron density resembling that of normal lipid droplets. Other parts may appear to be granular with moderate electron density and may be found with other more specific structures in certain lysosomal diseases such as Fabry disease or Batten disease.

Myopathies demonstrated to be primary lysosomal diseases include Pompe disease and Danon disease. X-linked myopathy

a

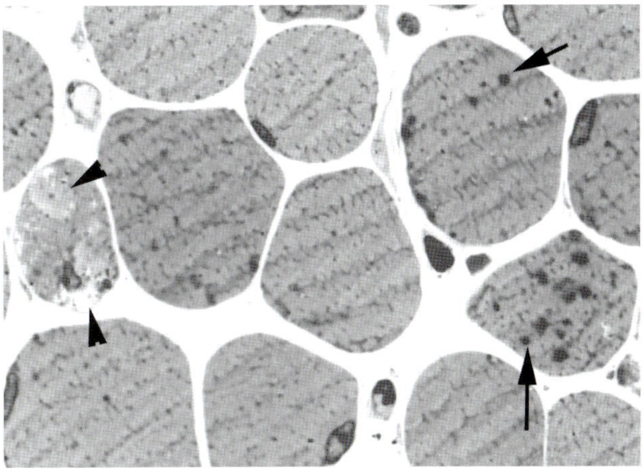

b

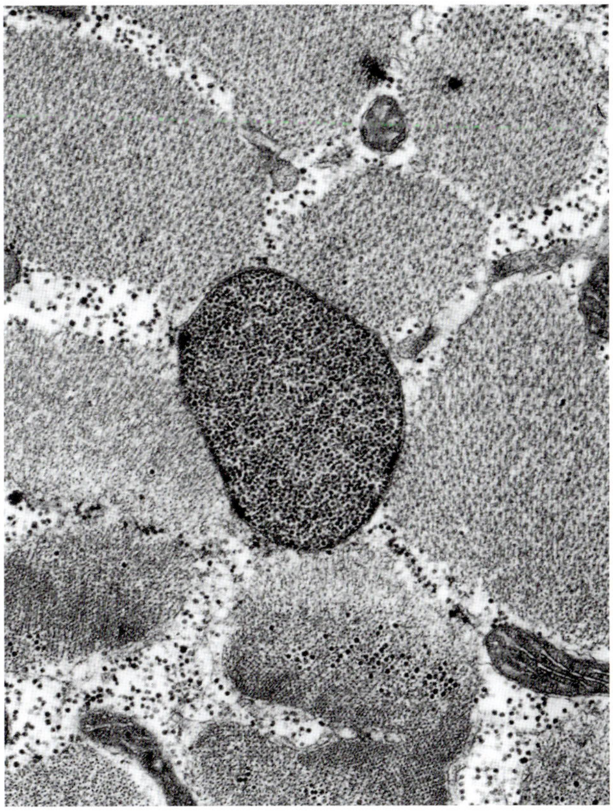

Figure 6.13a, b. Acid maltase deficiency (Pompe disease). (a) Transverse semi-thin resin sections in a case of α-glucosidase deficiency with adult onset. Some fibers show small inclusions (arrows) and occasional fibers show large inclusions (arrowheads) (x500). (b) Electron micrograph demonstrating a collection of glycogen in a single-membrane-bound space indicating lysosomal glycogen storage (x25 000).

with excessive autophagy (XMEA), infantile autophagic vacuolar myopathy, adult-onset autophagic vacuolar myopathy with multi-organ involvement, and X-linked congenital autophagic vacuolar myopathy are additional myopathies with suspected primary lysosomal etiology [43]. "Rimmed vacuoles," which can be seen in various muscle diseases, probably represent a secondary lysosomal abnormality.

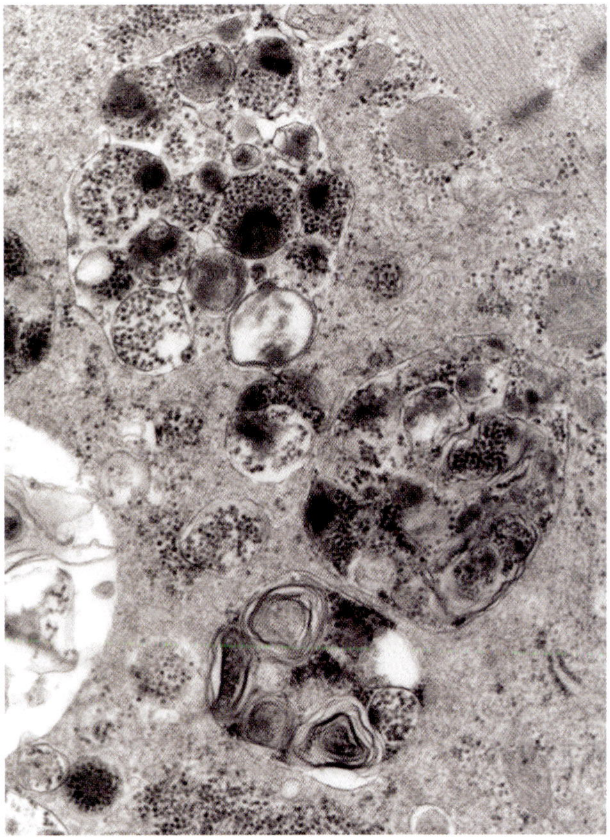

Figure 6.14. Danon disease. Electron micrograph demonstrating glycogen storage and myeloid bodies in lysosomes in a case of Danon disease due to a *LAMP2* mutation (x30 000). Courtesy of Inger Nennesmo.

Pompe disease is caused by mutations in *GAA* which encodes for lysosomal α-1,4 and α-1,6 glucosidase (acid maltase). The infantile and juvenile forms are easily recognized by the extensive accumulation of glycogen in muscle fibers [44]. The glycogen is present within as well as outside lysosomes and the increase in lysosomes can be identified by acid phosphatase staining. In some cases of the adult form there may be minimal lysosomal increase and glycogen storage, for which acid phosphatase staining and electron microscopy may be helpful. Ultrastructural examination can reveal accumulation of glycogen in lysosomes, identified as structures bound by a single membrane and filled with glycogen granules of otherwise normal appearance (Figure 6.13).

Danon disease is caused by mutations in *LAMP2*, encoding for lysosome-associated membrane protein-2 (LAMP-2) [45]. It is an X-linked disease associated with myopathy, cardiomyopathy, and mental retardation. It was originally described as "lysosomal glycogen storage disease with normal acid maltase," because of some clinical and pathological similarities to Pompe disease [46]. However, unlike acid maltase, LAMP-2 is a lysosomal structural protein. The vacuoles in Danon disease are generally small and may contain glycogen in addition to cytoplasmic debris, as well as dense and myeloid bodies (Figure 6.14). The vacuoles sometimes exhibit a basal lamina

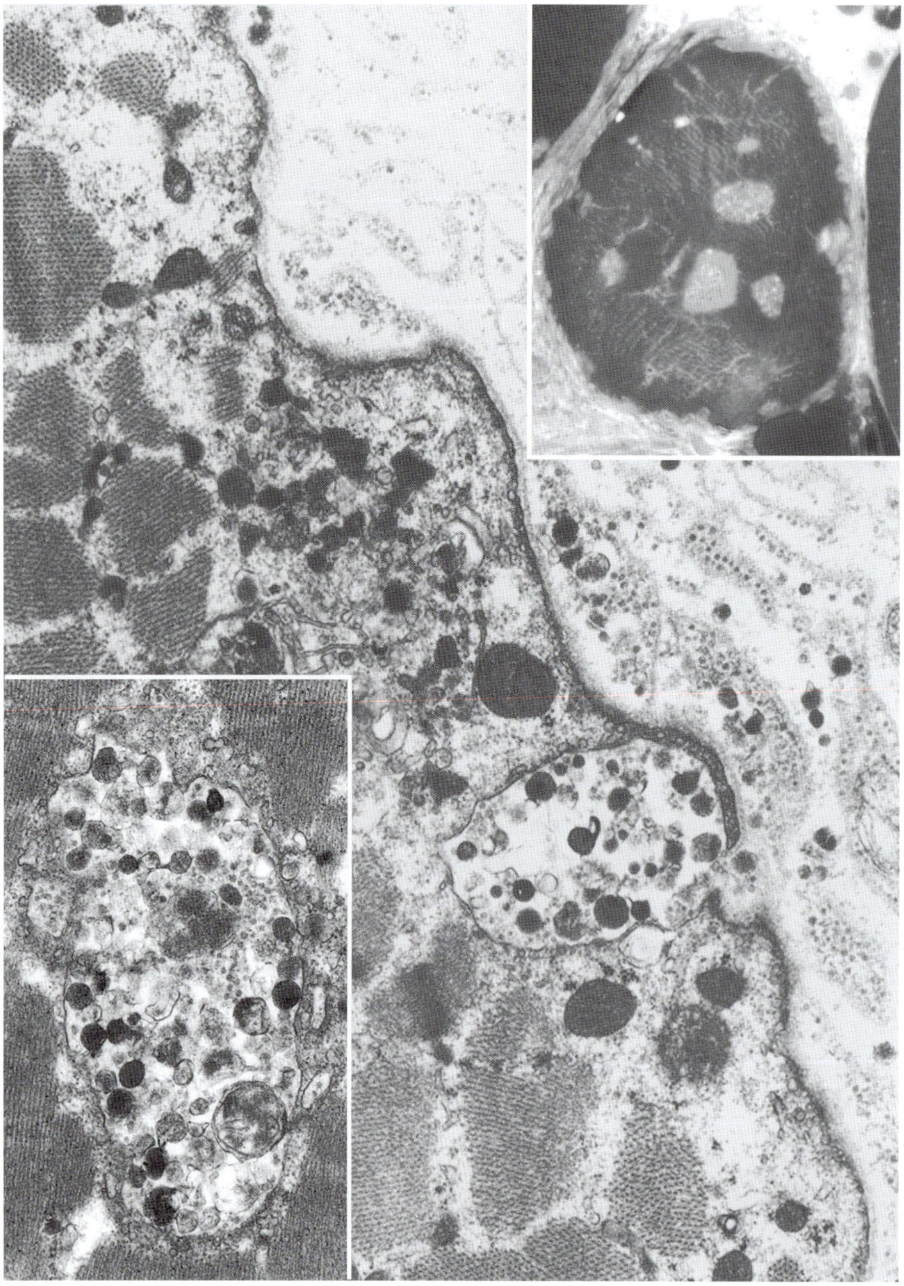

Figure 6.15. X-linked myopathy with excessive autophagy (XMEA). The upper inset illustrates a vacuolated muscle fiber with irregular plasma membrane in a case of XMEA (semi-thin resin section; x4000). The electron micrograph in the main panel illustrates an autophagic vacuole which appears to discharge the content to the extracellular space. There are several layers of basal lamina mixed with granular and osmiophilic debris (x25 000). The lower inset demonstrates an autophagic vacuole bound by a single membrane and containing cytoplasmic debris and dense bodies (x25 000). Courtesy of Hannu Kalimo.

along the luminal side of the vacuolar membrane and stain positive for dystrophin.

X-linked myopathy with excessive autophagy (XMEA) is an autophagic vacuolar myopathy without cardiomyopathy; as in the vacuoles in Danon disease, the vacuolar membrane characteristics frequently resemble those of plasma membrane [47]. Autophagic vacuoles are seen in the cytoplasm, exocytosis of the phagocytosed material occurs and the basal lamina of the muscle fibers is often multilayered (Figure 6.15).

Chloroquine myopathy causing muscle weakness occurs as a dose-dependent side-effect of treatment with chloroquine and hydroxychloroquine by inhibiting lysosomal degradation [48]. The morphological changes include upregulation of lysosomes with increased acid phosphatase activity. At the ultrastructural level there are numerous dispersed osmiophilic concentric lamellar bodies (Figure 6.16). Curvilinear bodies as seen in neuronal ceroid lipofuscinosis may also occur [49].

Rimmed vacuoles are muscle fiber vacuoles lined by granular material, with features resembling those of autophagic vacuoles and having frequent myeloid bodies at the ultrastructural level. They are typically observed in sporadic inclusion body myositis (s-IBM) and in various hereditary distal myopathies. Light microscopy of semi-thin resin sections and electron microscopy demonstrate that the rimmed vacuoles

a

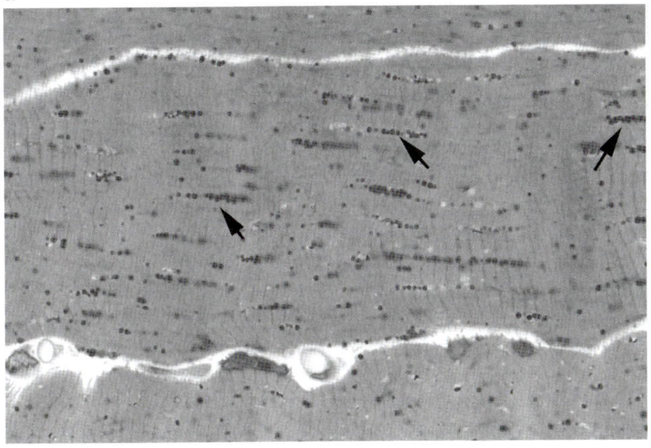

b

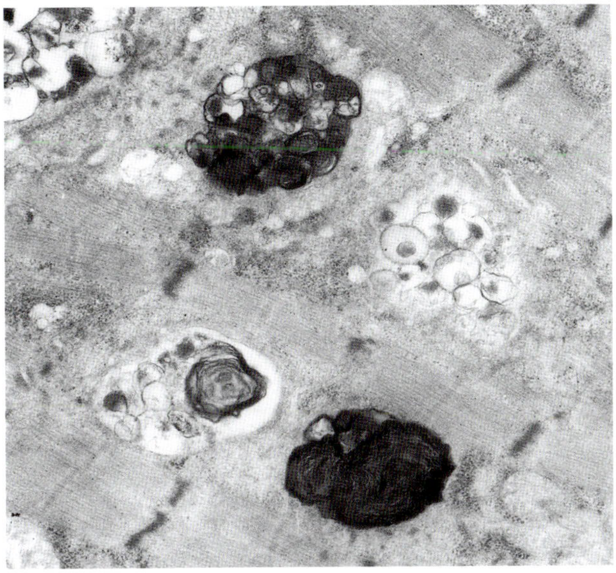

Figure 6.16a, b. Chloroquine myopathy. (a) Longitudinal semi-thin section of muscle fibers in a case of chloroquine myopathy. There are conspicuous dense small inclusions (arrows) frequently lining up in rows (x1200). (b) At the ultrastructural level the inclusions correspond to collections of concentric lamellated myeloid bodies (x18 000).

are filled with degraded organelles, myeloid structures, and membrane-bound spaces (Figure 6.17). The collections of 15- to 21-nm filaments associated with s-IBM are frequently found in association with the rimmed vacuoles (Figure 6.17). The filaments are usually referred to as tubulofilaments or paired helical filaments (PHF). They are several micrometers in length and are straight or lightly curved. They are arranged in an interlacing meshwork or form parallel bundles. In longitudinal sections they may show periodicity but are tubular in structure [50]. When the muscle tissue has been frozen and then fixed and embedded in resin the filamentous inclusions may appear as PHFs [51]. In most cases they can be identified in nuclei as well as in cytoplasm (Figure 6.17) and disintegration of such nuclei indicates the nuclear origin of filamentous inclusions (Figure 6.12).

The rimmed vacuoles in distal myopathy with rimmed vacuoles (DMRV) [52], which is allelic to hereditary inclusion body myopathy (HIBM) [53] are not due to a primary lysosomal defect since the gene defect affects GNE (UDP-GlcNAc 2-epimerase/ManNAc kinase), a cytoplasmic enzyme involved in sialic acid biosynthesis [54]. The lysosomal abnormalities associated with rimmed vacuoles are thus probably secondary to production of abnormal proteins. In some cases of myosin myopathy associated with a mutation in myosin heavy chain IIa, rimmed vacuoles are a frequent pathological alteration. This supports the concept that production of pathological proteins may trigger their formation.

Glycogen

At rest muscle mainly utilizes fatty acids as fuel whereas the energy derives from glycolysis at intense exercise. Glycogen is the most important source of the energy provided by glycolysis in muscle. Glycolysis ends with pyruvate, which enters the mitochondria for further degradation in aerobic metabolism or is converted to lactate in the case of anaerobic metabolism. Muscle glycogen synthesis accounts for disposal of up to 90% of ingested glucose. Diseases of glycogen metabolism and glycolysis therefore affect muscle energy supply and frequently cause exercise intolerance and/or episodes of myalgia, muscle cramps and rhabdomyolysis. Some of the disorders of carbohydrate metabolism are associated with fixed, slowly progressive muscle weakness. Numerous enzymes are involved in glycogen synthesis, glycogenolysis, and glycolysis. When these enzymes are defective in muscle they cause muscle glycogen storage diseases, several of which are associated with abnormal accumulation of glycogen. An exception is glycogen storage disease 0, in which there is deficiency of glycogen in muscle due to deficiency of glycogen synthase (*GYS1*) [55]. In glycogen storage diseases with abnormal accumulation of glycogen ultrastructural investigation can provide some information aiding in diagnostic work-up. In diseases due to myophosphorylase deficiency (*PYGM*; McArdle disease) [56] and other disorders of glycolysis, there is an abnormal increase of glycogen in the cytoplasm, mainly in the subsarcolemmal region. The glycogen usually has a normal ultrastructure appearing as 20- to 25-nm β-glycogen granules. In glycogen storage disease due to lysosomal α-1,4 and α-1,6 glucosidase (acid maltase, *GAA*) deficiency (Pompe disease) there is abnormal accumulation of normal-appearing glycogen in the cytoplasm as well as in lysosomes [44] (Figure 6.13). In branching enzyme deficiency (*GBE1*) and also some other forms of glycogenosis there is storage of abnormal glycogen composed of poorly branched polymeric glucose with long peripheral glucose chains [57] (Figure 6.18).

Mitochondria

Mitochondria are believed to have originated from the fusion of a eukaryotic cell with a prokaryotic cell capable of oxidative phosphorylation some 1.5 billion years ago (endosymbiotic hypothesis). Relics of this endosymbiotic event include: the double membrane structure; the circular genome with specific

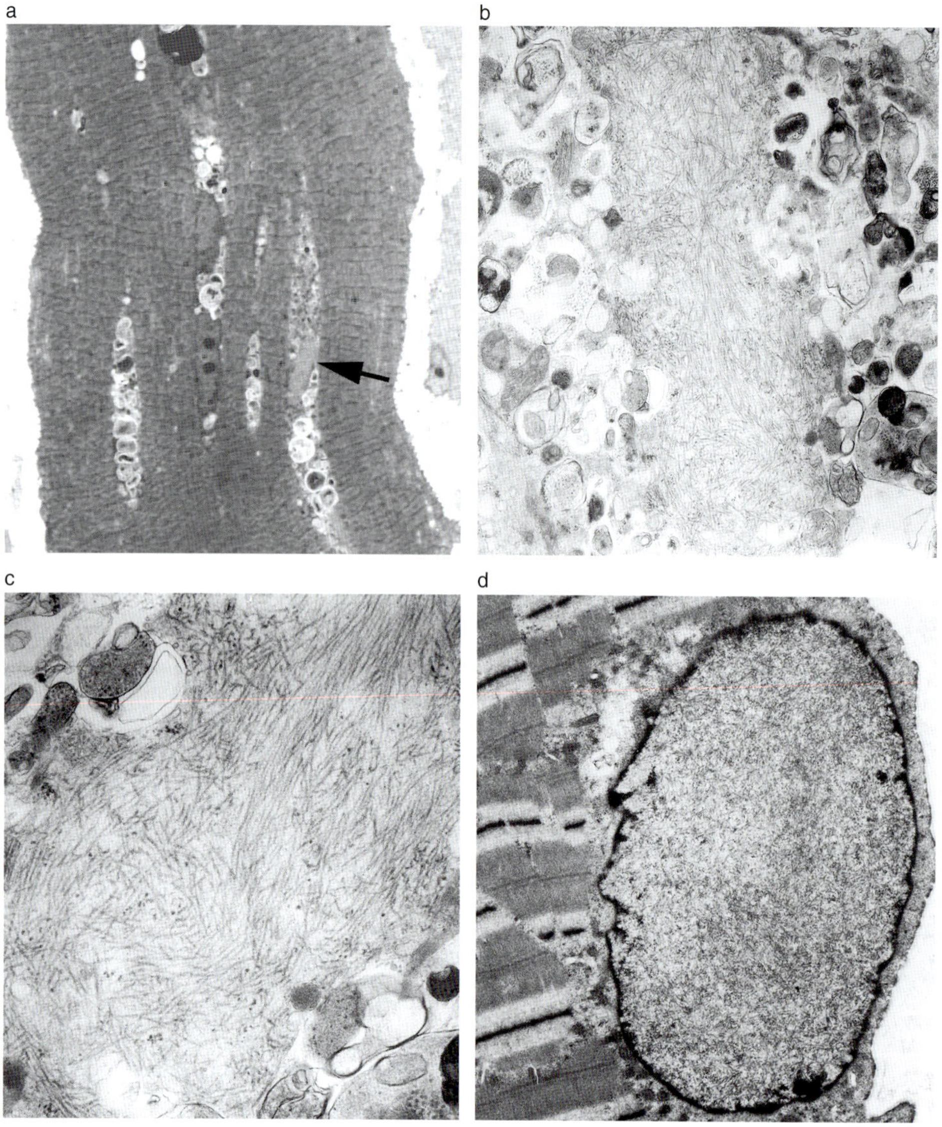

Figure 6.17a–d. Rimmed vacuoles in inclusion body myositis (IBM). (a) Longitudinal semi-thin resin section of a muscle fiber with rimmed vacuoles in a case of sporadic IBM (s-IBM). The longitudinally oriented spaces are associated with cytoplasmic debris and nuclei. Some of the material corresponds to inclusions (arrows) of 15- to 21-nm tubulofilaments as illustrated in (b) and (c) (x1200). (b, c) Electron micrographs of cytoplasmic tubulofilaments, partly membrane-bound cytoplasmic debris and myeloid bodies typical of rimmed vacuoles in s-IBM. (b; x16 000; c: x36 000). (d) Nuclear filaments in s-IBM (x11 000).

transcription, translation, and protein assembly systems; the presence of mitochondrial proteins enabling organelle dynamics and movement; the presence of specific transmembrane carrier systems for ions, metabolites, and proteins; and the numerous and diverse degradative and biosynthetic reactions carried out in addition to oxidative phosphorylation (OXPHOS).

OXPHOS – i.e., the oxidation of substrates (mainly pyruvate and fatty acids) to H_2O and CO_2, generating the bulk of ATP produced by the cell – is a main function of mitochondria. A double membrane surrounds the mitochondrion. The OXPHOS system, consisting of five enzyme complexes, is embedded in the inner membrane.

Mitochondrial disorders are usually, but not consistently, associated with myopathy, which may lead to moderate muscle wasting, exercise intolerance, muscle pain, cramps, fatigue, and episodic rhabdomyolysis. There are often no symptoms of muscle involvement despite morphological evidence of mitochondrial myopathy, which makes muscle biopsy useful for diagnosing mitochondrial disorders including in the absence of muscle symptoms. In diseases due to mitochondrial DNA (mtDNA) rearrangements or tRNA point mutations, mitochondrial myopathy with ragged red fibers (RRF) is a typical finding (Figure 6.19). The RRF usually exhibit enzyme histochemical cytochrome c oxidase deficiency and accumulation of abnormal mitochondria (Figure 6.20). These structural alterations consist of enlargement of the mitochondria, various inclusions, and abnormal arrangement of the cristae (Figure 6.21).

In some cases electron microscopy may reveal morphological changes in the mitochondria indicative of a mitochondrial disease despite normal light microscopy and enzyme histochemistry findings. However, morphological changes alone are not sufficient for a definite diagnosis of a

a

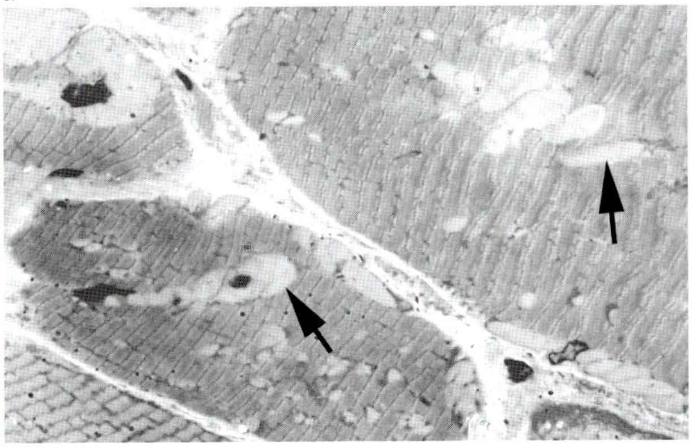

b

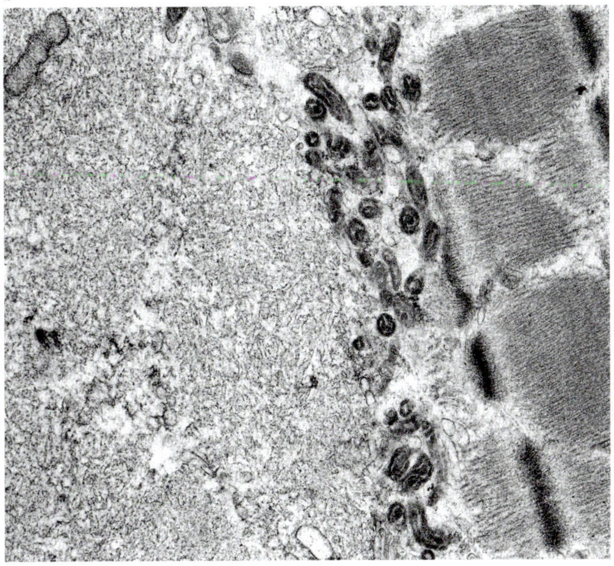

Figure 6.18a, b. Branching enzyme deficiency. (a) Semi-thin resin section in a case of branching enzyme deficiency demonstrating large sharply demarcated pale inclusions (arrows) (x1200). (b) Electron micrograph illustrating the filamentous nature of the storage material (x24 000).

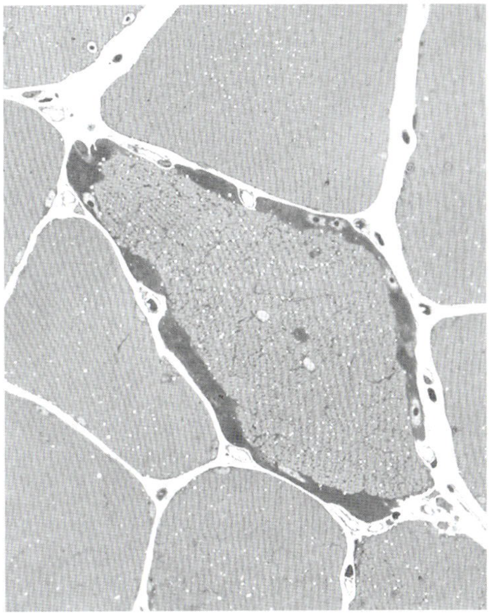

Figure 6.19. Mitochondrial myopathy. Semi-thin resin section of a ragged red fiber (RRF) in a case of mitochondrial myopathy associated with a mtDNA deletion mutation. There are large accumulations of darkly stained mitochondria in the subsarcolemmal region, an increase in cytoplasmic fat droplets and an increase in capillaries adjacent to the RRF (x900).

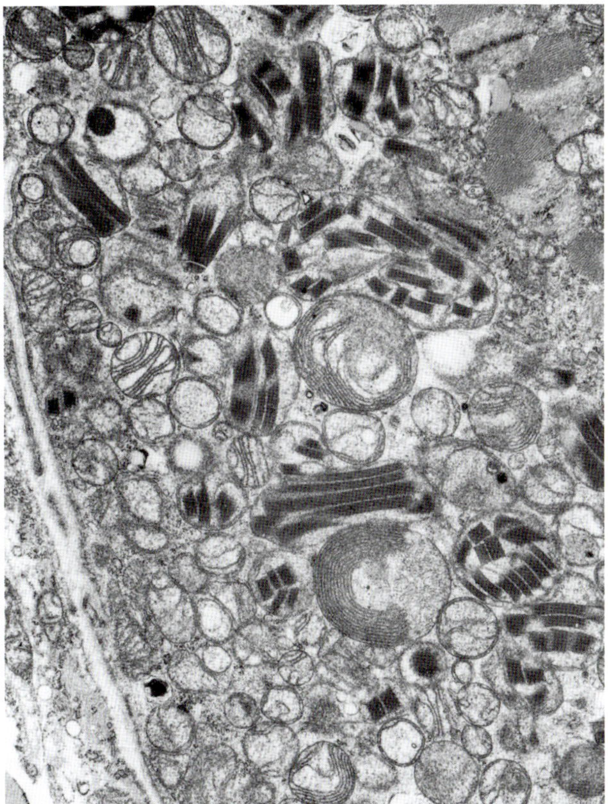

Figure 6.20. Mitochondrial myopathy. Electron micrograph illustrating the typical appearance of mitochondria in ragged red fibers. There is abnormal accumulation of mitochondria with abnormal cristae and various inclusions (x20 000).

mitochondrial disease, and there are apparently no specific ultrastructural changes associated with any of the described mtDNA mutations. Genetic and/or biochemical findings are usually necessary to support a definite diagnosis.

Only some of the mutations of protein-encoding genes of mtDNA are associated with mitochondrial myopathy. For example, the 8993T>G/C mutation in the ATPase6 gene, which is associated with Leigh syndrome (LS), and the different mutations in NADH-dehydrogenase (ND) genes associated with Leber hereditary optic neuropathy (LHON), do not present with typical mitochondrial myopathy. On the other hand, mutations in the genes encoding cytochrome *b* and cytochrome c oxidase I–III result in mitochondrial myopathy with RRF [58, 59, 60].

Mutations of nuclear genes causing OXPHOS deficiency by secondary mtDNA alterations are, in some instances, associated with mitochondrial myopathy with RRF, as seen in adPEO and mtDNA depletion disorders [61]. On the other

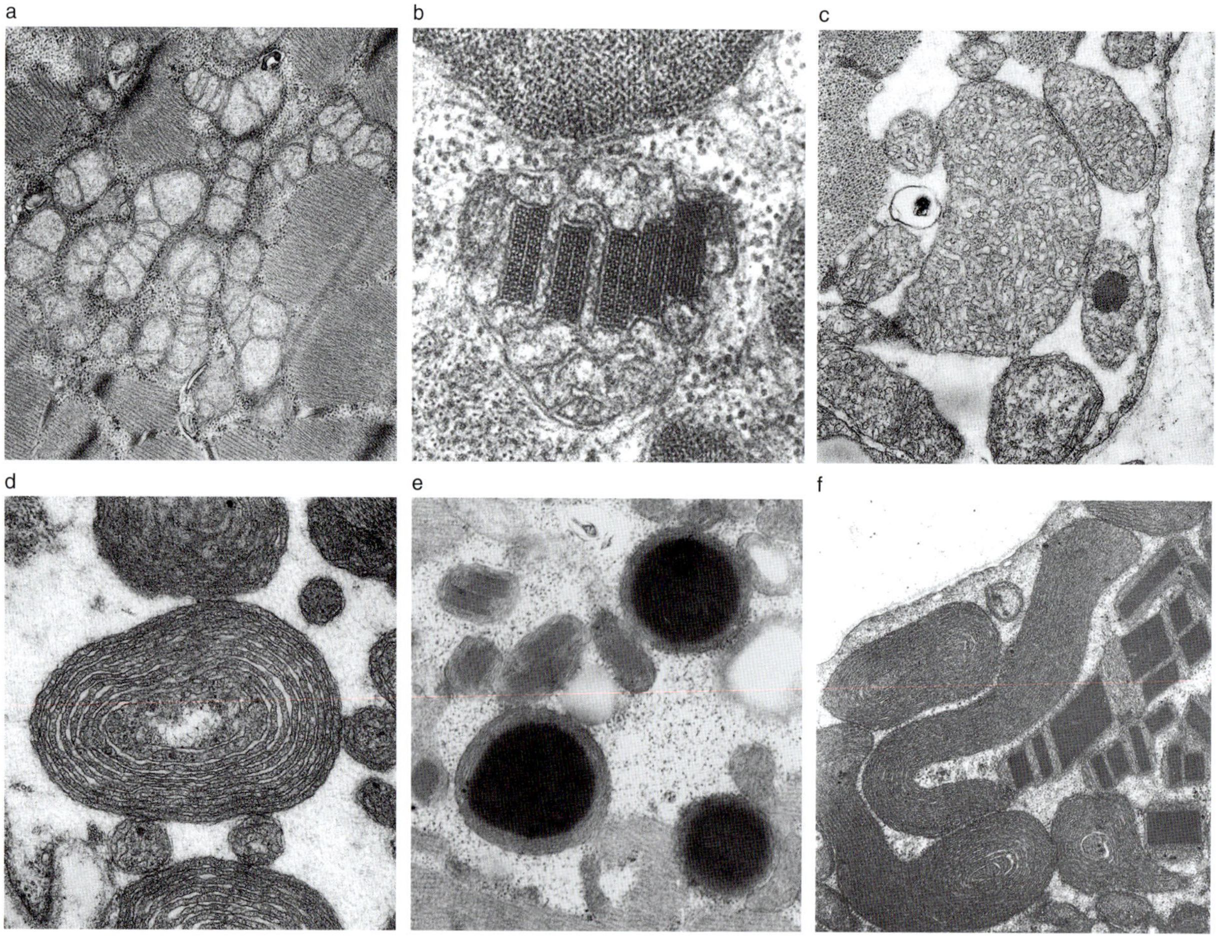

Figure 6.21. Various ultrastructural abnormalities of mitochondria (a): Sparse cristae (x22 000) (b): Paracrystalline inclusions (x75 000) (c): Tubular cristae (x30 000) (d): Circular cristae (x30 000) (e): Osmiophilic inclusions (x25 000) (f); Elongated mitochondria with densly packed circular cristae and paracrystalline inclusions (x14 000).

hand, mutations in nuclear-encoded complex I and II subunits, which are most often associated with LS, do not usually result in typical mitochondrial myopathy. *SURF1* mutations are associated with generalized cytochrome c oxidase deficiency in muscle but not with RRF [62, 63, 64].

One obstacle to diagnostic work on mitochondrial myopathies is the frequent presence of age-related mitochondrial changes [65] and mitochondrial alterations that occur secondary to other disease processes, e.g., in inclusion body myositis [66]. A special disease entity called "late-onset mitochondrial myopathy" has emerged as a differential diagnosis in these cases [67]. These aging-associated mitochondrial changes are due to somatic mutations of mtDNA, with clonal expansion of mutated mtDNA molecules causing segmental cytochrome c oxidase deficiency.

Intracellular lipid storage

Free fatty acids are normally taken up by muscle fibers from the blood and then further metabolized by the mitochondria. Lipids can be stored in muscle fibers in the form of triglycerides, forming lipid droplets usually in close association with mitochondria in the intermyofibrillar region. Abnormal lipid storage can be observed in diseases compromising lipid metabolism in muscle. However, excessive lipid storage is not a consistent finding in all these diseases. Lipid dysmetabolism in muscle presents as two major clinical syndromes: chronic progressive proximal muscle weakness and acute recurrent muscle weakness with myalgia and rhabdomyolysis.

Fatty acyl-CoA esters are imported into the mitochondria by means of carnitine and the carnitine palmitoyl-transferase (CPT-I and CPT-II) system. In primary carnitine deficiency (CDSP) due to mutations in the carnitine transporter gene (*SLC22A5*) [68] muscle frequently exhibits abnormal lipid storage that can be identified by lipid histochemistry and electron microscopy (Figure 6.22). This lipid storage is reversible by carnitine supplementation. In CPT-II deficiency, on the other hand, lipid storage does not usually occur and muscle pathology is dominated by the changes associated with acute rhabdomyolysis and the ensuing regeneration.

Within mitochondria, fatty acyl-CoA is metabolized by β-oxidation to acetyl-CoA which enters the Krebs cycle. This system involves several enzymes that can be associated with disease if defective, but pathological lipid accumulation is not a consistent finding. Each β-oxidation cycle produces reduced flavine adenine dinucleotide ($FADH_2$) and NADH. Electrons from $FADH_2$ are transferred to coenzyme Q (CoQ) in the respiratory chain by electron transferring flavoprotein (ETF) and ETF:oxidoreductase (EFT:QO). Mutations in the gene encoding EFT:QO (*ETFDH*) underlie riboflavin-responsive multiple acyl-CoA dehydrogenase deficiency (RR-MADD) [69]. This disease is associated with chronic myopathy and abnormal lipid storage in most instances (Figure 6.23). However, myopathies with extreme lipid accumulation are usually disorders of oxidative phosphorylation (respiratory chain disorders) (Figure 6.23). Ultrastructural alterations of mitochondria can be seen in lipid storage myopathies of various etiologies, including CDSP and RR-MADD, but are usually more marked in the primary respiratory chain diseases.

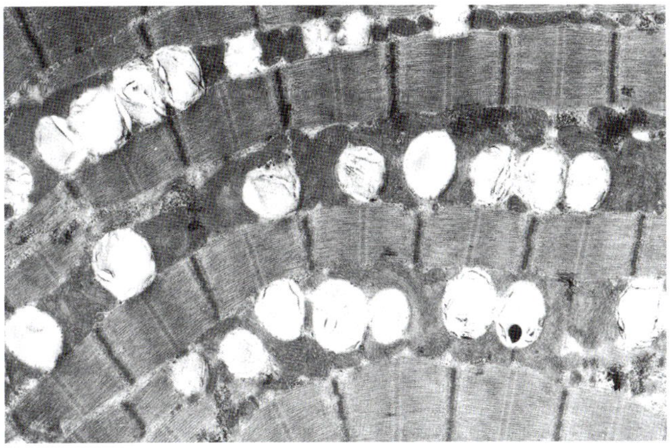

Figure 6.22. Primary carnitine deficiency. Electron micrograph illustrating abnormal amounts of lipid droplets and mitochondria, which are located between myofibrils (x11 000).

Sarcoplasmic reticulum and T-tubules

The sarcoplasmic reticulum takes up and stores calcium ions and releases them when activated by the voltage-gated calcium

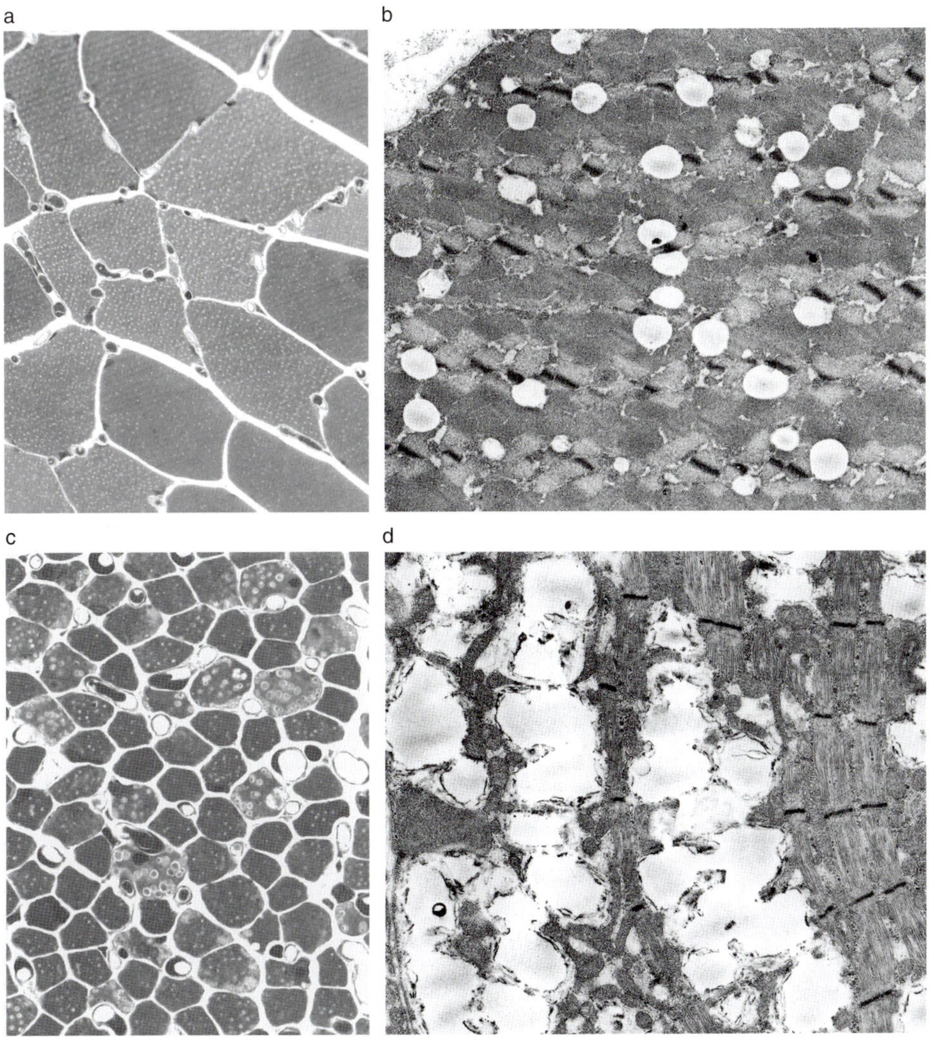

Figure 6.23a–d. Lipid storage myopathies. (a, b) Lipid storage myopathy caused by multiple acyl CoA dehydrogenase deficiency associated with a mutation in *ETFDH*. (c, d): Lipid storage myopathy in a child associated with a respiratory chain disease. (a, c) Semi-thin resin sections (a: x450; c: x450). (b, d) Electron micrographs (b: x6000; d: x8000). In both disorders there is abnormal lipid accumulation. In (c) and (d) the lipid storage is extreme.

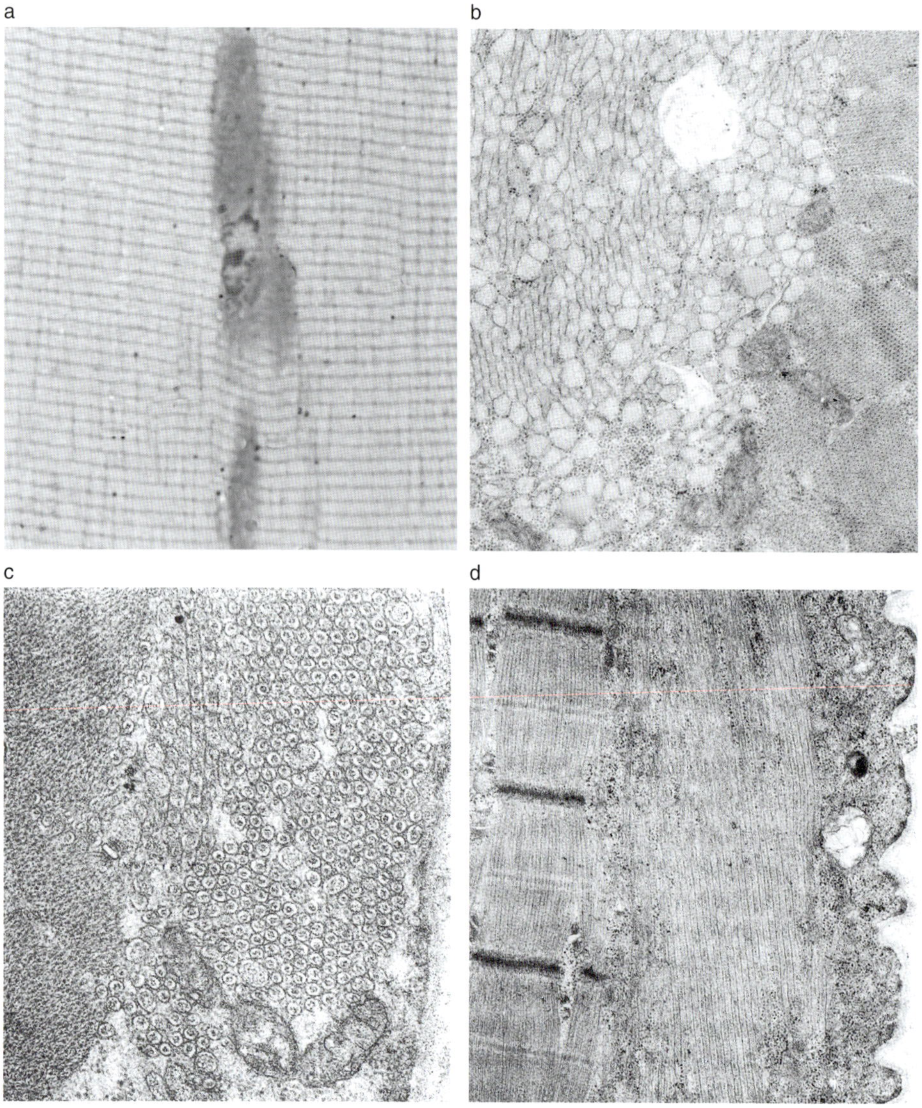

Figure 6.24a–d. Myopathy with tubular aggregates. (a, b) Congenital myopathy with tubular aggregates in type 1 and type 2 fibers. (a) Longitudinal semi-thin resin section demonstrating a collection of centrally located tubular aggregates close to a nucleus (x 1200). (b) Electron micrograph demonstrating the tubular aggregates in cross-section (x20 000). (c, d) Myopathy with tubular aggregates in type 2 fibers associated with cramps and muscle pain. (c) Ultrastructure of subsarcolemmal tubular aggregates in cross-section. Many of them appear to have inner tubules (x32 000). (d) Ultrastructure of subsarcolemmal tubular aggregates in longitudinal section (x16 000).

channel in the T-tubule membrane. Calcium uptake is dependent on the calcium-activated ATPase in the tubular component of the sarcoplasmic reticulum. Calcium release takes place through the ryanodine receptor, a large tetrameric molecule interposed between the terminal cisternae and the T-tubule membrane. The conjuncture of T-tubule and two flanking cisternae is known as a triad. The lateral cisternae tend to have finely granular contents of low to medium density. The T-tubular lumen is in continuity with the extracellular space, and the T-tubular membrane is in continuity with the plasmalemma, although the two membranes differ in their protein composition.

Tubular aggregates are formed from masses of parallel tubules (Figure 6.24). Their continuity with membranes of the sarcoplasmic reticulum has been demonstrated. An appearance of double-walled tubules is often encountered, but the inner tubules are probably not formed from true membranes. Abundance of tubular aggregates can be found in type 2 fibers in males, in association with a cramp and myalgia syndrome [70]. They can also occur in a congenital myopathy with autosomal recessive or dominant inheritance and then affecting both type 1 and type 2 fibers [71] (Figure 6.24). Furthermore, they are seen in periodic paralysis syndromes and other conditions [70].

T-system networks due to proliferation of T-tubules are a common reaction in chronically injured muscle fibers, for example in muscular dystrophy or inflammatory myopathy [72, 73] (Figure 6.25).

Sarcolemma

The sarcolemma is composed of the basal lamina and the plasma membrane. The plasma membrane is a lipid bilayer in which numerous proteins, the presence and distribution of

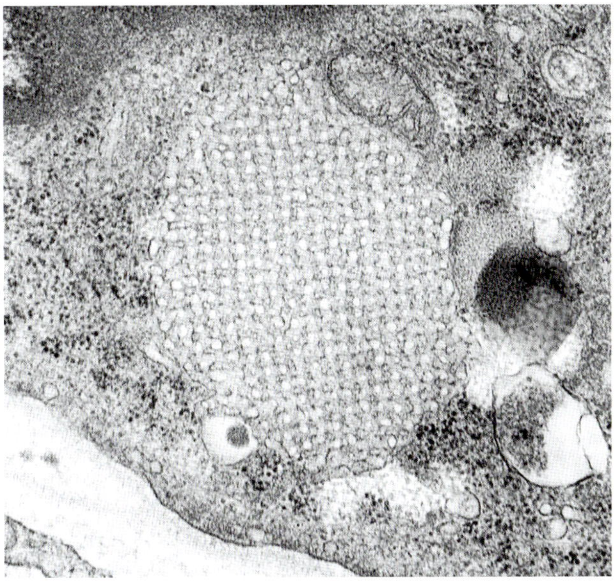

Figure 6.25. T-system network. Ultrastructure of T-system network in a case of myositis (x35 000).

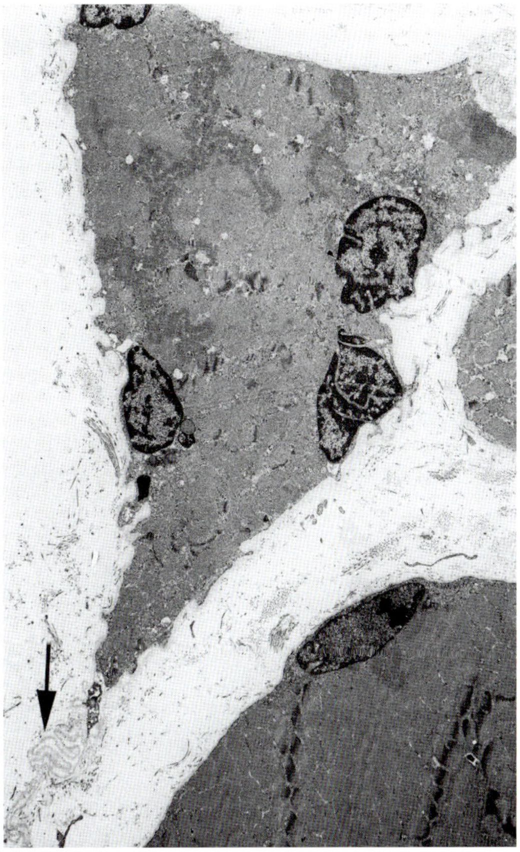

Figure 6.26. Neurogenic atrophy. Ultrastructure of an atrophic muscle fiber with folds of redundant basal lamina (arrow) in a case of neurogenic muscular atrophy (x5000).

which can only be determined by immunostaining, are embedded. The basal lamina has two visible components with electron microscopy: the lamina lucida, which borders the plasmalemma, and the lamina densa. The pallor of the lamina lucida is crossed by vaguely discernible strands, and it contrasts with the darkness of the lamina densa. Proteins in the lamina densa include type IV collagen and laminin-2 (merosin). Links between the basal lamina and the plasmalemma are normally formed by interaction of merosin with sarcoglycans and α-dystroglycan. The sarcoglycans and dystroglycans, in turn, are linked to dystrophin in the submembranous cytoskeleton, which is linked to cytoskeletal actin.

In Duchenne muscular dystrophy, deficiency of dystrophin leads to paucity of sarcoglycans and dystroglycans. This is reflected by reduplication of many segments of basal lamina and occasional segments of plasma membrane denuded of basal lamina [74]. In some cases of Duchenne muscular dystrophy, fibers can be found in which segments of plasma membrane are absent. These fibers do not show the usual signs of necrosis, although they contain some vacuoles formed from T-tubules. Their myofibrils may be contracted or relaxed. This condition may be an initial stage of necrosis in Duchenne muscular dystrophy.

Basal lamina abnormalities are characteristically seen in denervation atrophy, as well as in other types of muscle fiber atrophy, in which sleeves of redundant basal lamina form long prolongations of the angular corners of fibers (Figure 6.26). Reduplication of basal lamina can be seen in various conditions, e.g., XMEA (Figure 6.15).

Inflammatory cell infiltration

Inflammatory myopathies are acquired diseases in which the inflammatory reaction is of major importance for pathogenesis. These diseases may be autoimmune or related to an infection. The major autoimmune idiopathic inflammatory myopathies are dermatomyositis, polymyositis (PM) and s-IBM. Macrophagic myofasciitis is an acquired apparently iatrogenic form of myositis. The diagnosis in these disorders rests on a combination of clinical findings, laboratory data, and muscle biopsy [75].

In PM and s-IBM, inflammatory cells (T-cells and macrophages) typically surround and invade non-necrotic muscle fibers. However, these cells do not invade the muscle cells. With electron microscopy this is seen as the presence of inflammatory cells inside the muscle fiber beneath the basal lamina but the plasma membrane of the muscle cell remains intact and separates the muscle cell from the invading inflammatory cells (Figures 6.27 and 6.28).

Macrophagic myofasciitis was first reported in 1998 [76]. Muscle biopsy reveals infiltration by large macrophages with finely granular PAS-positive content. The pathophysiology of this disease has been traced to the presence of an aluminum adjuvant used in hepatitis A and B and tetanus vaccines; the adjuvant aggregates at the site of injection [77]. Electron microscopy shows macrophage infiltrates with crystalline inclusions appearing as aggregates of needle-shaped dense structures (Figure 6.29).

Vessels

In normal adult muscle, the lumen of a capillary is seen in most intersections of the interstitial space among muscle fibers. Roughly 1.5 capillary lumina accompany each muscle cell, and there are about 400–500 lumina per square millimeter of transverse muscle fiber area. In newborn infants, the number of capillaries per muscle fiber is far lower than in adults.

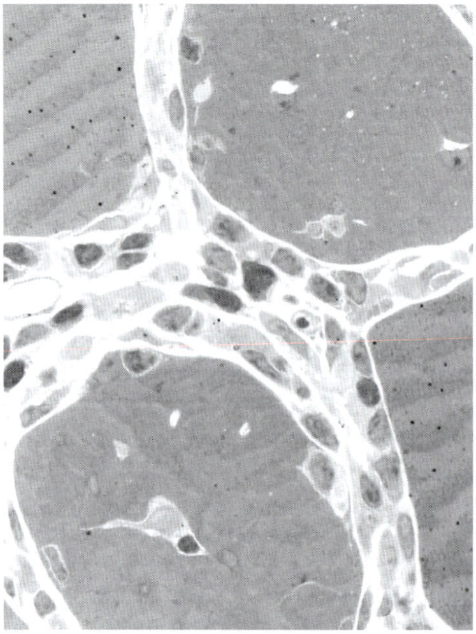

Figure 6.27. Inflammatory cell infiltration in sporadic inclusion body myositis (s-IBM). Semi-thin resin section in a case of s-IBM demonstrating inflammatory cells, which surround and invade muscle fibers (x1100).

There is some lability in the capillary network. In denervation atrophy, as muscle fibers shrink, the capillaries surrounding them come closer together, causing an increase in the number of capillaries per unit of transverse muscle fiber area. The muscle appears overvascularized. At the same time, the endothelial cells of certain capillary lines undergo cell death [78]. In denervated muscle, one can often see an occasional capillary that is represented only by a basal lamina circle without endothelium.

Destruction and loss of capillaries is a characteristic finding in dermatomyositis. It is a cause rather than a result of atrophy [79]. The number of capillaries per unit of transverse muscle fiber area drops. At the ultrastructural level, the vessels exhibit hyperplasia of endothelial cells, obliteration and necrosis of capillaries, and tubuloreticular inclusions (Figures 6.30 and 6.31). These inclusions can be generated in lymphocytes in vitro by interferon treatment. They are seen in endothelial cells, lymphocytes, and monocytes in viral infections and in collagen vascular disease. In intramuscular capillaries, they are rare outside of dermatomyositis, lupus myositis, and HIV infection. They are thus diagnostically useful, especially as they are virtually never seen in polymyositis. Perifascicular areas are most often involved. Proliferation of thin-walled venules is sometimes present next to an area of capillary loss. Necrosis of larger vessels is seen in a few cases, where it is often associated with infarcts. Capillary death leaves the basal lamina behind as a marker of where the capillary had been.

Thickening of the basal lamina of capillaries, appearing as a pale gray ground-glass density, is seen most commonly in diabetic patients (Figure 6.32). It occasionally occurs without any obvious cause. In an extreme form ("pipe-stem capillaries") it has been reported in connection with connective tissue disease [80].

a b

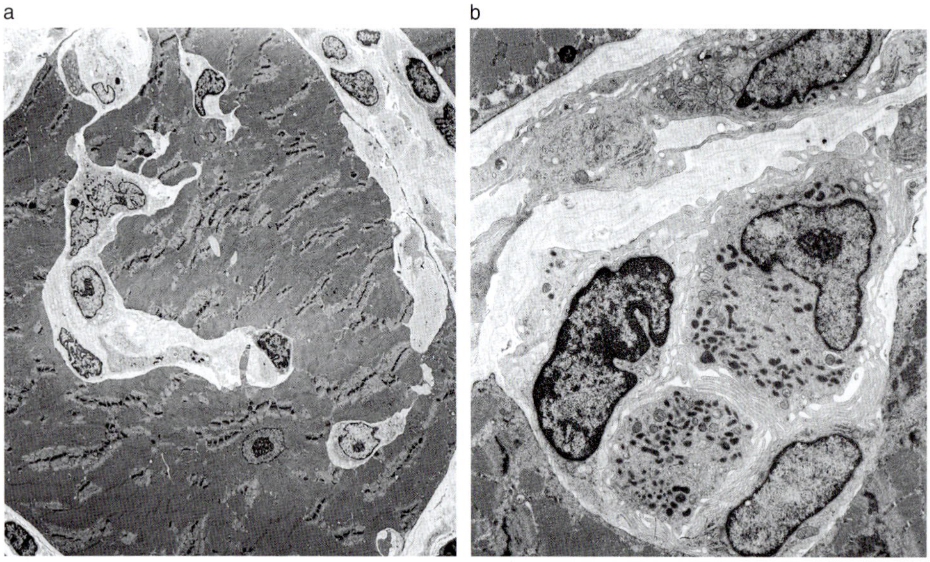

Figure 6.28a, b. Inflammatory cell infiltration in sporadic inclusion body myositis (s-IBM). (a, b) Electron micrograph demonstrating invasion of inflammatory cells in a muscle fiber. The inflammatory cells are lymphocytes and macrophages invading across the basal lamina but not through the plasma membrane (a: x2500; b: x10 000).

a

b c

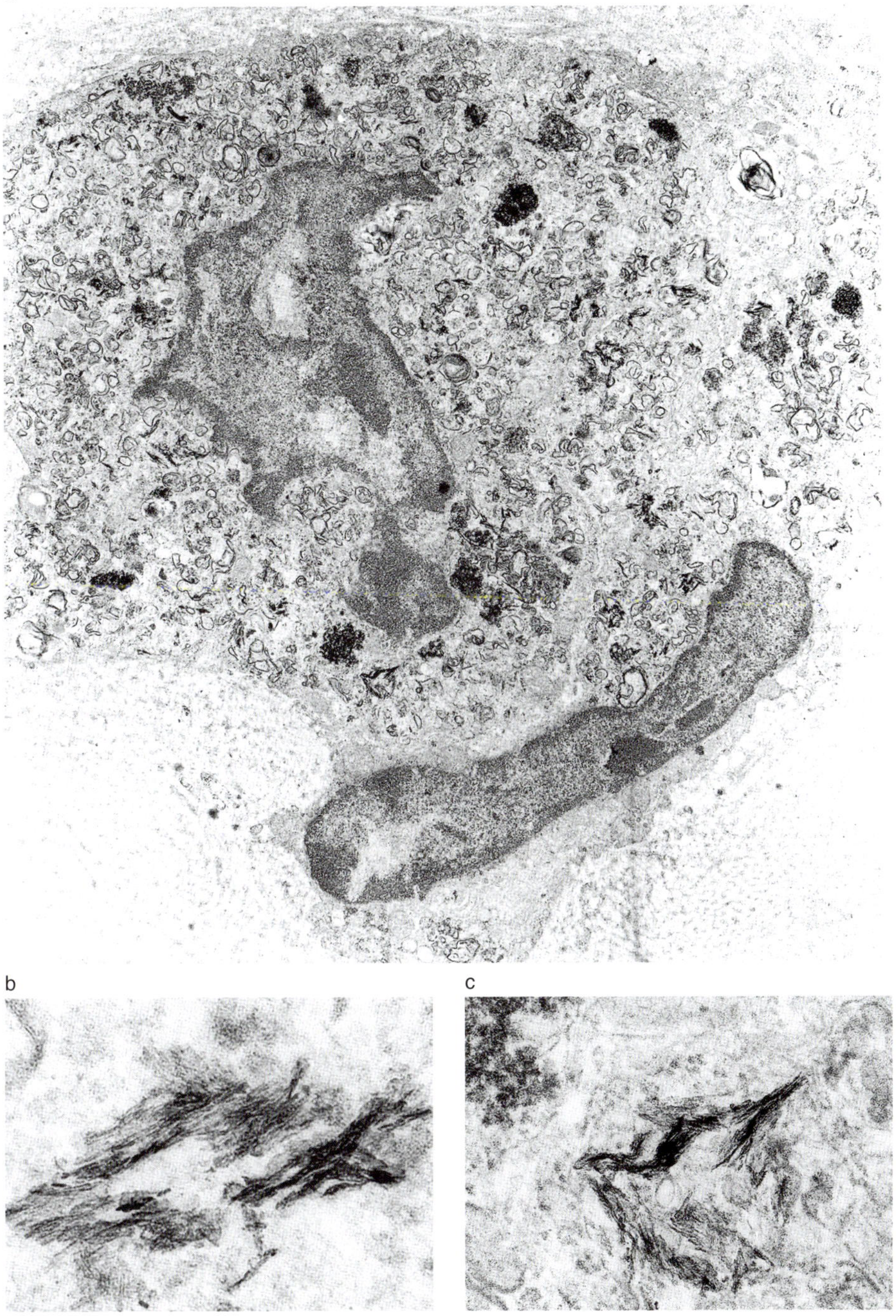

Figure 6.29a–c. Macrophagic myofasciitis. (a) Electron micrograph of a macrophage with numerous electron-dense intracytoplasmic inclusions (x13 000) in a case of macrophage myofasciitis. (b, c) At high magnification the inclusions frequently exhibit a spicular structure (x60 000).

An excess of capillaries is seen in some patients with inclusion body myositis and in those with marked histochemical type 1 fiber predominance. RRF are often surrounded, and even indented, by an excess number of capillary lumina (Figure 6.19).

Extracellular matrix

Normally very little collagen is present between muscle fibers. An exception is in the neighborhood of neuromuscular junctions, where a small amount of collagen tends to encircle muscle fibers. Muscle that has been severely damaged from a variety of causes tends to contain increased endomysial connective tissue, usually in the form of rather loose, randomly oriented collagen. In muscular dystrophies such as Duchenne and Becker muscular dystrophy, the connective tissue proliferation, which begins to occur early, is distinctive, consisting of discrete dense bundles of collagen laid parallel to the muscle fibers. Fibrosis in other conditions, such as polymyositis and inclusion body myositis, is less discrete, less organized, and

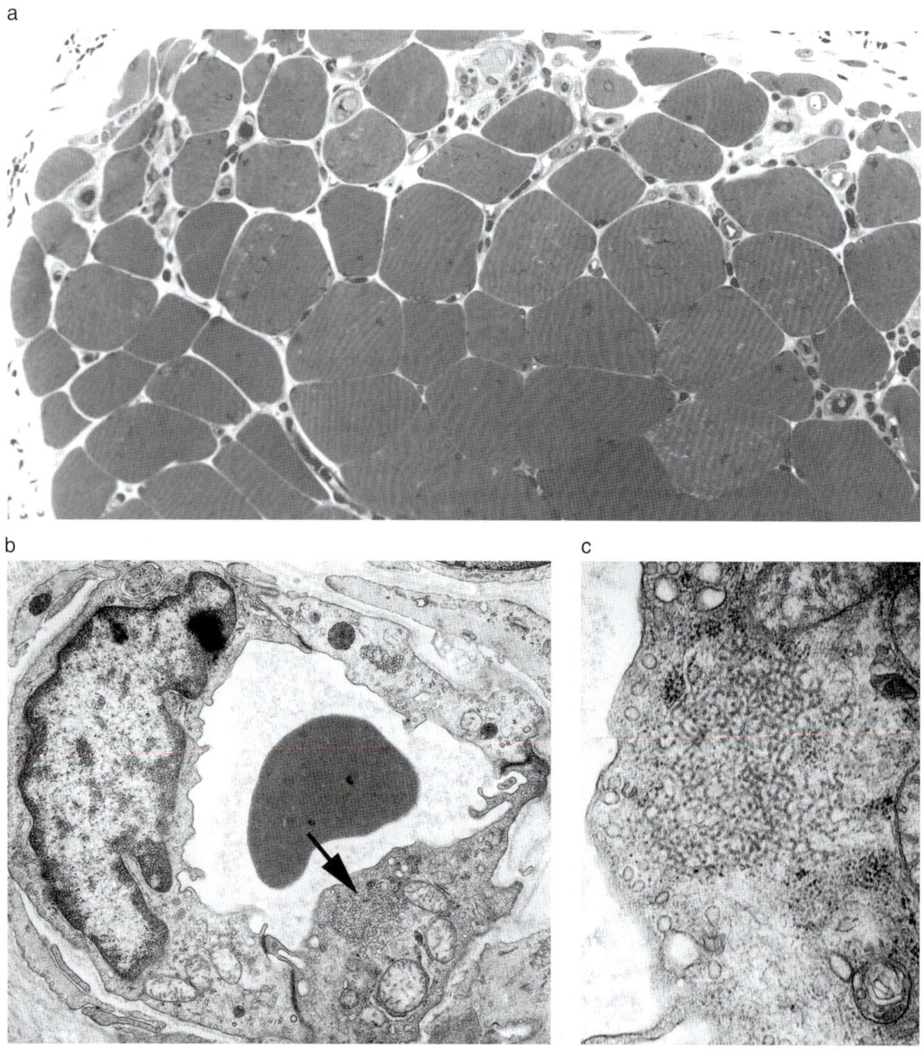

Figure 6.30a–c. Dermatomyositis. (a) Semi-thin resin section in a case of dermatomyositis demonstrating perifascicular atrophy (x400). (b, c) Electron micrographs illustrating a microtubular aggregate in an endothelial cell (b: x20 000; c: x40 000).

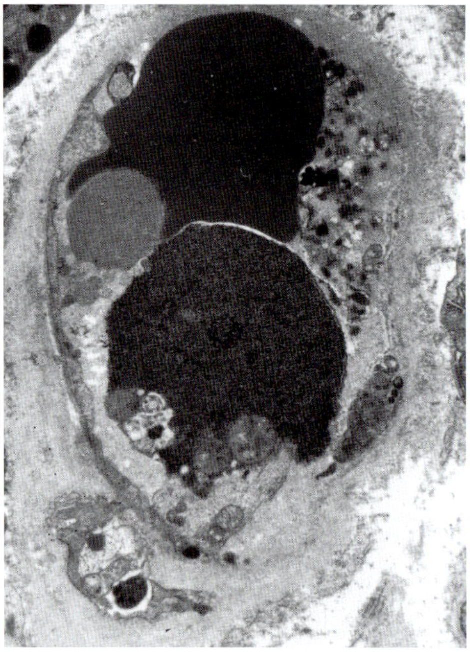

Figure 6.31. Dermatomyositis. Electron micrograph illustrating a capillary with degenerated endothelial cells in a region of perifascicular atrophy (x18 000).

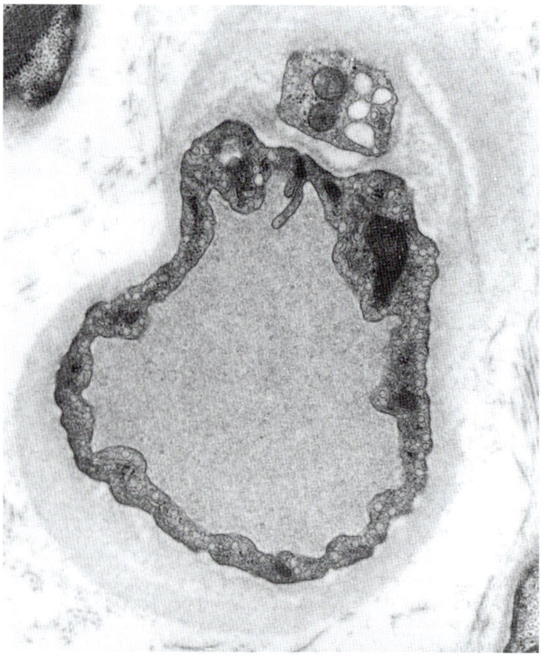

Figure 6.32. Diabetes angiopathy. Electron micrograph demonstrating a capillary with thickened basal lamina in diabetes (x18 000).

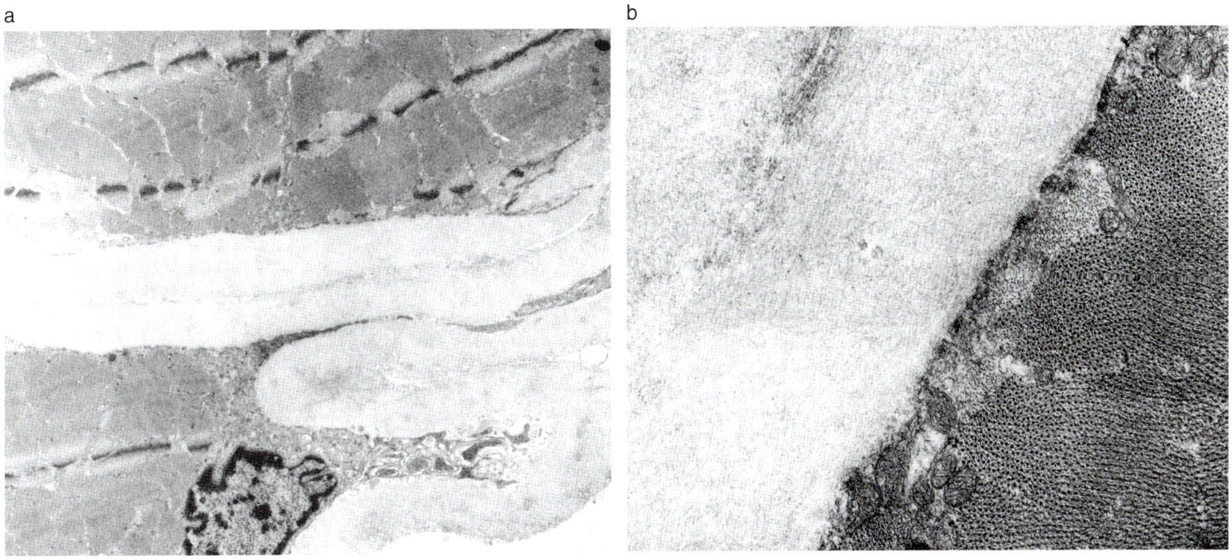

Figure 6.33a, b. Amyloid myopathy. (a, b) Electron micrographs illustrating deposition of fibrillar material surrounding the muscle fibers. The basal lamina of the sarcolemma is partly not visible (b). The amyloid in this case is of AL type (a: x7000; b: x30 000).

more obviously related to cell loss. When muscle cells have been lost and replaced by fat cells, collagen also tends to be lost.

Extracellular amyloid deposition may occur in different sporadic and hereditary types of amyloidosis, and does not usually cause clinical symptoms. Some patients may develop generalized muscle weakness sometimes associated with pseudohypertrophy of muscles and macroglossia. These cases are usually associated with plasma cell dyscrasia and monoclonal immunoglobulin light chain production (systemic AL amyloidosis) [81, 82, 83]. Electron microscopy reveals a deposition of nonbranching filaments, about 10 nm wide, around blood vessels and between muscle fibers (Figure 6.33).

Necrosis and regeneration

Necrosis entails the death of a cell, its inability to maintain homeostasis, and its inevitable transition to debris. Since muscle cells are multinucleated and elongated, necrosis in them is usually segmental because a demarcation membrane is formed, limiting the extension of the necrosis during focal muscle fiber injury [84]. Although several reports suggest that apoptosis can occur in skeletal muscle fibers, this issue is not totally clear at present. At least in the case of the cytoplasmic changes accompanying segmental death of a mature skeletal muscle cell, no distinction can be made between apoptosis and necrosis.

Necrosis occurs in many, but by no means all, muscle diseases. Many reactions of muscle cells do not promote necrosis, and in many diseases necrosis occurs at such a low rate that it is rarely seen in biopsies. In Duchenne muscular dystrophy, it is usually prominent until late in the disease, when few fibers are left. Necrotic fibers often appear to be clustered in Duchenne muscular dystrophy; in contrast, necrotic fibers appear to be single and random in polymyositis. Necrosis is less commonly seen in dermatomyositis, in which it may follow one of two patterns: occasional fibers at the periphery of fascicles or many adjacent fibers comprising the larger part of a fascicle (i.e., an infarct).

Marked hypercontraction and tearing of myofibrils may be seen in early stages of experimental necrosis. Mitochondria lose their laterally elongated shape and become round and dark, often forming chains. While hypercontraction can cause the myofibrillar material of necrotic fibers to appear darker than normal, within hours they lose density until they are paler than normal. This happens without phagocytosis. In some instances remnants of sarcomeres can be seen within macrophages (Figure 6.34). The nuclei of necrotic fibers disappear rapidly; the nuclei seen within necrotic fibers are those of phagocytes or regenerative cells. Invasion of necrotic fibers by mononuclear phagocytes is probably rare before 10 hours have passed. In Duchenne muscular dystrophy, where monocytes are already present in the interstitial tissue, it may occur more rapidly. Invasion of necrotic muscle fibers by monocytes is dependent on blood supply. In the center of infarcts, necrotic fibers can persist for some time with neither phagocytosis nor regeneration occurring.

Regeneration comes from the migration and proliferation of satellite cells, which appear first as thin cells on the periphery of the old fiber. During one stage of the necrosis–regeneration process, a mixture of proliferating satellite cells and macrophages fills the empty basal lamina tube (Figure 6.34). After proliferation the satellite cells grow and then fuse. The numerous ribosomes make their cytoplasm bluish when the cells are stained with hematoxylin and eosin. After

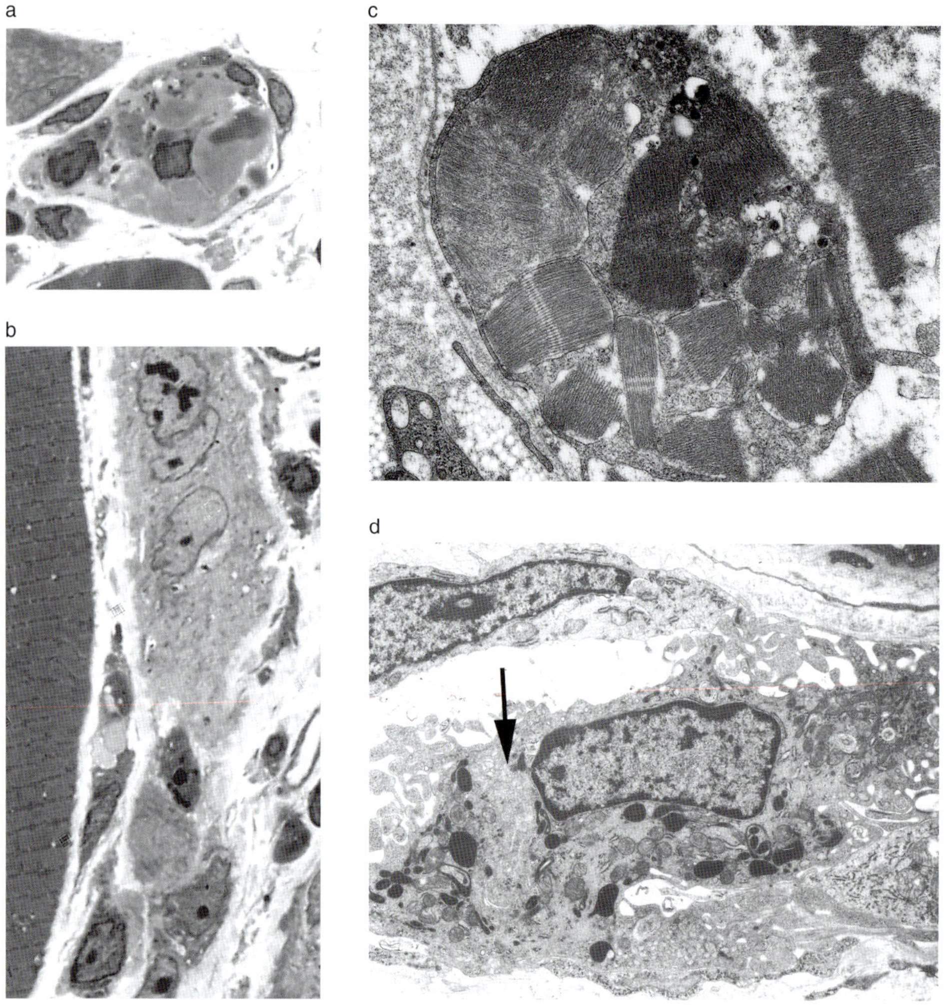

Figure 6.34a–d. Muscle fiber necrosis and regeneration. Illustrations from a case of congenital muscular dystrophy. (a) Transverse semi-thin resin section of a necrotic muscle fiber invaded by macrophages (x1000). (b) Longitudinal semi-thin resin section showing a muscle fiber after necrosis at a stage when the basal lamina tube contains macrophages and proliferating myoblasts (x1600). (c) Electron micrograph demonstrating a macrophage that has phagocytosed sarcomeres (x14 000). (d) Electron microscopy of the same fiber demonstrated in (b) illustrating myoblasts and a macrophage with numerous lysosomes (arrow) within the basal lamina tube (x3200).

they have fused, myofibrils develop, at first separated by considerable cytoplasmic space. Nuclei are large and pale with large nucleoli and are often located at a distance from the sarcolemma.

References

1. K. M. Ruppel, J. A. Spudich, Structure-function analysis of the motor domain of myosin. *Annu. Rev. Cell Dev. Biol.* **12** (1996), 543–573.
2. I. Rayment, H. M. Holden, M. Whittaker, *et al.*, Structure of the actin-myosin complex and its implications for muscle contraction. *Science* **261** (1993), 58–65.
3. K. A. Clark, A. S. McElhinny, M. C. Beckerle, C. C. Gregorio, Striated muscle cytoarchitecture: an intricate web of form and function. *Annu. Rev. Cell Dev. Biol.* **18** (2002), 637–706.
4. T. D. Pollard, Actin. *Curr. Opin. Cell Biol.* **2** (1990), 33–40.
5. P. W. Gunning, G. Schevzov, A. J. Kee, E. C. Hardeman, Tropomyosin isoforms: divining rods for actin cytoskeleton function. *Trends. Cell. Biol.* **15** (2005), 333–341.
6. S. V. Perry, Vertebrate tropomyosin: distribution, properties and function. *J. Muscle Res. Cell Motil.* **22** (2001), 5–49.
7. S. V. Perry, Troponin T: genetics, properties and function. *J. Muscle Res. Cell Motil.* **19** (1998), 575–602.
8. N. G. Laing, Congenital myopathies. *Curr. Opin. Neurol.* **20** (2007), 583–589.
9. E. P. Morris, G. Nneji, J. M. Squire, The three-dimensional structure of the nemaline rod Z-band. *J. Cell Biol.* **111** (1990), 2961–2978.
10. R. J. Barohn, C. E. Jackson, K. S. Kagan-Hallet, Neonatal nemaline myopathy with abundant intranuclear rods. *Neuromuscul. Disord.* **4** (1994), 513–520.
11. K. J. Nowak, D. Wattanasirichaigoon, H. H. Goebel, *et al.*, Mutations in the skeletal muscle alpha-actin gene in patients with actin myopathy and nemaline myopathy. *Nat. Genet.* **23** (1999), 208–212.
12. H. H. Goebel, J. R. Anderson, C. Hubner, *et al.*, Congenital myopathy with excess of thin myofilaments. *Neuromuscul. Disord.* **7** (1997), 160–168.
13. J. C. Sparrow, K. J. Nowak, H. J. Durling, *et al.*, Muscle disease caused by mutations in the skeletal muscle alpha-actin gene (ACTA1). *Neuromuscul. Disord.* **13** (2003), 519–531.
14. B. Eymard, J. C. Brouet, H. Collin, *et al.*, Late-onset rod myopathy associated with monoclonal gammopathy. *Neuromuscul. Disord.* **3** (1993), 557–560.
15. C. E. Keller, A. P. Hays, L. P. Rowland, *et al.*, Adult-onset nemaline myopathy and monoclonal gammopathy. *Arch. Neurol.* **63** (2006), 132–134.

16. A. Fidzianska, B. Badurska, B. Ryniewicz, I. Dembek, "Cap disease": new congenital myopathy. *Neurology* **31** (1981), 1113–1120.
17. A. Fidzianska, "Cap disease" – a failure in the correct muscle fibre formation. *J. Neurol. Sci.* **201** (2002), 27–31.
18. J. M. Cuisset, C. A. Maurage, J. F. Pellissier, *et al.*, "Cap myopathy": case report of a family. *Neuromuscul. Disord.* **16** (2006), 277–281.
19. H. Tajsharghi, M. Ohlsson, C. Lindberg, A. Oldfors, Congenital myopathy with nemaline rods and cap structures caused by a mutation in the beta-tropomyosin gene (TPM2). *Arch. Neurol.* **64** (2007), 1334–1338.
20. A. Oldfors, Hereditary myosin myopathies. *Neuromuscul. Disord.* **17** (2007), 355–367.
21. T. Martinsson, A. Oldfors, N. Darin, *et al.*, Autosomal dominant myopathy: missense mutation (Glu-706 to Lys) in the myosin heavy chain IIa gene. *Proc. Natl. Acad. Sci. U. S. A.* **97** (2000), 14614–14619.
22. M. J. Danon, S. Carpenter, Myopathy with thick filament (myosin) loss following prolonged paralysis with vecuronium during steroid treatment. *Muscle Nerve* **14** (1991), 1131–1139.
23. S. Carpenter, G. Karpati, S. Rothman, G. Watters, The childhood type of dermatomyositis. *Neurology* **26** (1976), 952–962.
24. D. Selcen, K. Ohno, A. G. Engel, Myofibrillar myopathy: clinical, morphological and genetic studies in 63 patients. *Brain* **127** (2004), 439–451.
25. A. Ferreiro, C. Ceuterick-de Groote, J. J. Marks, *et al.*, Desmin-related myopathy with Mallory body-like inclusions is caused by mutations of the selenoprotein N gene. *Ann. Neurol.* **55** (2004), 676–686.
26. A. Kostera-Pruszczyk, B. Goudeau, A. Ferreiro, *et al.*, Myofibrillar myopathy with congenital cataract and skeletal anomalies without mutations in the desmin, alphaB-crystallin, myotilin, LMNA or SEPN1 genes. *Neuromuscul. Disord.* **16** (2006), 759–762.
27. A. Ferreiro, S. Quijano-Roy, C. Pichereau, *et al.*, Mutations of the selenoprotein N gene, which is implicated in rigid spine muscular dystrophy, cause the classical phenotype of multiminicore disease: reassessing the nosology of early-onset myopathies. *Am. J. Hum. Genet.* **71** (2002), 739–749.
28. H. Jungbluth, C. R. Muller, B. Halliger-Keller, *et al.*, Autosomal recessive inheritance of RYR1 mutations in a congenital myopathy with cores. *Neurology* **59** (2002), 284–287.
29. Y. Zhang, H. S. Chen, V. K. Khanna, *et al.*, A mutation in the human ryanodine receptor gene associated with central core disease. *Nat. Genet.* **5** (1993), 46–50.
30. J. Laporte, L. J. Hu, C. Kretz, *et al.*, A gene mutated in X-linked myotubular myopathy defines a new putative tyrosine phosphatase family conserved in yeast. *Nat. Genet.* **13** (1996), 175–182.
31. A. Oldfors, M. Kyllerman, J. Wahlstrom, *et al.*, X-linked myotubular myopathy: clinical and pathological findings in a family. *Clin. Genet.* **36** (1989), 5–14.
32. M. Bitoun, S. Maugenre, P. Y. Jeannet, *et al.*, Mutations in dynamin 2 cause dominant centronuclear myopathy. *Nat. Genet.* **37** (2005), 1207–1209.
33. A. S. Nicot, A. Toussaint, V. Tosch, *et al.*, Mutations in amphiphysin 2 (BIN1) disrupt interaction with dynamin 2 and cause autosomal recessive centronuclear myopathy. *Nat. Genet.* **39** (2007), 1134–1139.
34. P. Y. Jeannet, G. Bassez, B. Eymard, *et al.*, Clinical and histologic findings in autosomal centronuclear myopathy. *Neurology* **62** (2004), 1484–1490.
35. F. M. Tome, M. Fardeau, Nuclear inclusions in oculopharyngeal dystrophy. *Acta Neuropathol.* **49** (1980), 85–87.
36. F. M. Tome, D. Chateau, A. Helbling-Leclerc, M. Fardeau, Morphological changes in muscle fibers in oculopharyngeal muscular dystrophy. *Neuromuscul. Disord.* **7** Suppl 1 (1997), S63–S69.
37. B. Brais, J. P. Bouchard, Y. G. Xie, *et al.*, Short GCG expansions in the PABP2 gene cause oculopharyngeal muscular dystrophy. *Nat. Genet.* **18** (1998), 164–167.
38. S. Carpenter, Inclusion body myositis, a review. *J. Neuropathol. Exp. Neurol.* **55** (1996), 1105–1114.
39. S. A. Greenberg, J. L. Pinkus, A. A. Amato, Nuclear membrane proteins are present within rimmed vacuoles in inclusion-body myositis. *Muscle Nerve* **34** (2006), 406–416.
40. A. Fidzianska, D. Toniolo, I. Hausmanowa-Petrusewicz, Ultrastructural abnormality of sarcolemmal nuclei in Emery-Dreifuss muscular dystrophy (EDMD). *J. Neurol. Sci.* **159** (1998), 88–93.
41. Y. Suzuki, N. Murakami, Y. Goto, *et al.*, Apoptotic nuclear degeneration in Marinesco-Sjogren syndrome. *Acta Neuropathol.* **94** (1997), 410–415.
42. A. Domazetovska, B. Ilkovski, S. T. Cooper, *et al.*, Mechanisms underlying intranuclear rod formation. *Brain* **130** (2007), 13275–13284.
43. I. Nishino, Lysosomal myopathies. In: F. L. Mastaglia, D. Hilton Jones, eds., *Handbook of Clinical Neurology.* (Edinburgh: Elsevier, 2007), pp. 205–214.
44. P. S. Kishnani, R. R. Howell, Pompe disease in infants and children. *J. Pediatr.* **144** (2004), S35–S43.
45. I. Nishino, J. Fu, K. Tanji, *et al.*, Primary LAMP-2 deficiency causes X-linked vacuolar cardiomyopathy and myopathy (Danon disease). *Nature* **406** (2000), 906–910.
46. M. J. Danon, S. J. Oh, S. DiMauro, *et al.*, Lysosomal glycogen storage disease with normal acid maltase. *Neurology* **31** (1981), 51–57.
47. H. Kalimo, M. L. Savontaus, H. Lang, *et al.*, X-linked myopathy with excessive autophagy: a new hereditary muscle disease. *Ann. Neurol.* **23** (1988), 258–265.
48. T. Masuda, H. Ueyama, K. Nakamura, *et al.*, Skeletal muscle expression of clathrin and mannose 6-phosphate receptor in experimental chloroquine-induced myopathy. *Muscle Nerve* **31** (2005), 495–502.
49. H. E. Neville, C. A. Maunder-Sewry, J. McDougall, *et al.*, Chloroquine-induced cytosomes with curvilinear profiles in muscle. *Muscle Nerve* **2** (1979), 376–381.
50. J. Mikol, P. A. Felten, F. Ferchal, *et al.*, Inclusion-body myositis: clinicopathological studies and isolation of an adenovirus type 2 from muscle biopsy specimen. *Ann. Neurol.* **11** (1982), 576–581.

51. V. Askanas, W. K. Engel, M. Bilak, *et al.*, Twisted tubulofilaments of inclusion body myositis muscle resemble paired helical filaments of Alzheimer brain and contain hyperphosphorylated tau. *Am. J. Pathol.* **144** (1994), 177–187.

52. I. Nonaka, N. Sunohara, S. Ishiura, E. Satoyoshi, Familial distal myopathy with rimmed vacuole and lamellar (myeloid) body formation. *J. Neurol. Sci.* **51** (1981), 141–155.

53. Z. Argov, R. Yarom, "Rimmed vacuole myopathy" sparing the quadriceps. A unique disorder in Iranian Jews. *J. Neurol. Sci.* **64** (1984), 33–43.

54. I. Eisenberg, N. Avidan, T. Potikha, *et al.*, The UDP-N-acetylglucosamine 2-epimerase/N-acetylmannosamine kinase gene is mutated in recessive hereditary inclusion body myopathy. *Nat. Genet.* **29** (2001), 83–87.

55. G. Kollberg, M. Tulinius, T. Gilljam, *et al.*, Cardiomyopathy and exercise intolerance in muscle glycogen storage disease 0. *N. Engl. J. Med.* **357** (2007), 1507–1514.

56. S. DiMauro, A. L. Andreu, C. Bruno, G. M. Hadjigeorgiou, Myophosphorylase deficiency (glycogenosis type V; McArdle disease). *Curr. Mol. Med.* **2** (2002), 189–196.

57. C. Bruno, D. Cassandrini, S. Assereto, *et al.*, Neuromuscular forms of glycogen branching enzyme deficiency. *Acta Myol.* **26** (2007), 75–78.

58. A. L. Andreu, M. G. Hanna, H. Reichmann, *et al.*, Exercise intolerance due to mutations in the cytochrome b gene of mitochondrial DNA. *N. Engl. J. Med.* **341** (1999), 1037–1044.

59. A. L. Andreu, K. Tanji, C. Bruno, *et al.*, Exercise intolerance due to a nonsense mutation in the mtDNA ND4 gene. *Ann. Neurol.* **45** (1999), 820–823.

60. G. Kollberg, A. R. Moslemi, C. Lindberg, *et al.*, Mitochondrial myopathy and rhabdomyolysis associated with a novel nonsense mutation in the gene encoding cytochrome c oxidase subunit I. *J. Neuropathol. Exp. Neurol.* **64** (2005), 123–128.

61. G. Kollberg, A. R. Moslemi, N. Darin, *et al.*, POLG1 mutations associated with progressive encephalopathy in childhood. *J. Neuropathol. Exp. Neurol.* **65** (2006), 758–768.

62. Z. Zhu, J. Yao, T. Johns, *et al.*, SURF1, encoding a factor involved in the biogenesis of cytochrome c oxidase, is mutated in Leigh syndrome. *Nat. Genet.* **20** (1998), 337–343.

63. M. O. Pequignot, R. Dey, M. Zeviani, *et al.*, Mutations in the SURF1 gene associated with Leigh syndrome and cytochrome C oxidase deficiency. *Hum. Mutat.* **17** (2001), 374–381.

64. A. R. Moslemi, M. Tulinius, N. Darin, *et al.*, SURF1 gene mutations in three cases with Leigh syndrome and cytochrome c oxidase deficiency. *Neurology* **61** (2003), 991–993.

65. G. Fayet, M. Jansson, D. Sternberg, *et al.*, Ageing muscle: clonal expansions of mitochondrial DNA point mutations and deletions cause focal impairment of mitochondrial function. *Neuromuscul. Disord.* **12** (2002), 484–493.

66. A. Oldfors, A. R. Moslemi, L. Jonasson, *et al.*, Mitochondrial abnormalities in inclusion-body myositis. *Neurology* **66** (2006), S49–S55.

67. W. Johnston, G. Karpati, S. Carpenter, *et al.*, Late-onset mitochondrial myopathy. *Ann. Neurol.* **37** (1995), 16–23.

68. J. Nezu, I. Tamai, A. Oku, *et al.*, Primary systemic carnitine deficiency is caused by mutations in a gene encoding sodium ion-dependent carnitine transporter. *Nat. Genet.* **21** (1999), 91–94.

69. R. K. Olsen, S. E. Olpin, B. S. Andresen, *et al.*, ETFDH mutations as a major cause of riboflavin-responsive multiple acyl-CoA dehydrogenation deficiency. *Brain* **130** (2007), 2045–2054.

70. N. L. Rosenberg, H. E. Neville, S. P. Ringel, Tubular aggregates. Their association with neuromuscular diseases, including the syndrome of myalgias/cramps. *Arch. Neurol.* **42** (1985), 973–976.

71. M. H. Tulinius, A. Lundberg, A. Oldfors, Early-onset myopathy with tubular aggregates. *Pediat. Neurol.* **15** (1996), 68–71.

72. S. M. Chou, T. Miike, Ultrastructural abnormalities and perifascicular atrophy in childhood dermatomyositis with special reference to transverse tubular system-sarcoplasmic reticulum junctions. *Arch. Pathol. Lab. Med.* **105** (1981), 76–85.

73. T. Miike, Y. Ohtani, H. Tamari, *et al.*, An electron microscopical study of the T-system in biopsied muscles from Fukuyama type congenital muscular dystrophy. *Muscle Nerve* **7** (1984), 629–635.

74. S. Carpenter, G. Karpati, Duchenne muscular dystrophy: plasma membrane loss initiates muscle cell necrosis unless it is repaired. *Brain* **102** (1979), 147–161.

75. M. C. Dalakas, Inflammatory disorders of muscle: progress in polymyositis, dermatomyositis and inclusion body myositis. *Curr. Opin. Neurol.* **17** (2004), 561–567.

76. R. K. Gherardi, M. Coquet, P. Cherin, *et al.*, Macrophagic myofasciitis: an emerging entity. Groupe d'Etudes et Recherche sur les Maladies Musculaires Acquises et Dysimmunitaires (GERMMAD) de l'Association Francaise contre les Myopathies (AFM). *Lancet* **352** (1998), 347–352.

77. R. K. Gherardi, F. J. Authier, Aluminum inclusion macrophagic myofasciitis: a recently identified condition. *Immunol. Allergy Clin. North Am.* **23** (2003), 699–712.

78. S. Carpenter, G. Karpati, Necrosis of capillaries in denervation atrophy of human skeletal muscle. *Muscle Nerve* **5** (1982), 250–254.

79. A. M. Emslie-Smith, A. G. Engel, Microvascular changes in early and advanced dermatomyositis: a quantitative study. *Ann. Neurol.* **27** (1990), 343–356.

80. A. M. Emslie-Smith, A. G. Engel, J. Duffy, C. A. Bowles, Eosinophilia myalgia syndrome: I. Immunocytochemical evidence for a T-cell-mediated immune effector response. *Ann. Neurol.* **29** (1991), 524–528.

81. S. Spuler, A. Emslie-Smith, A. G. Engel, Amyloid myopathy: an underdiagnosed entity. *Ann. Neurol.* **43** (1998), 719–728.

82. J. E. Chapin, M. Kornfeld, A. Harris, Amyloid myopathy: characteristic features of a still underdiagnosed disease. *Muscle Nerve* **31** (2005), 266–272.

83. A. Windhagen, J. Bufler, S. Neudecker, Gross muscle pseudohypertrophy in myeloma-associated light chain amyloidosis. *Neurology* **65** (2005), 1670.

84. T. Hurme, H. Kalimo, M. Lehto, M. Jarvinen, Healing of skeletal muscle injury: an ultrastructural and immunohistochemical study. *Med. Sci. Sports Exerc.* **23** (1991), 801–810.

Chapter 7

Diagnostic imaging of muscle

Eugenio Mercuri and Marianne de Visser

From the pioneering work of O'Doherty *et al.* [1] and of Heckmatt *et al.* [2], increasing attention has been devoted to the usefulness of muscle imaging in the diagnosis of neuromuscular disorders. Ultrasonography (US) and computed tomography (CT) have been used for many years to identify the extent and distribution of muscle changes in neuromuscular disorders but more recently magnetic resonance imaging (MRI) has become the "gold standard" for imaging muscle involvement in inherited and acquired muscle disorders. Using different sequences muscle MRI can not only accurately identify the extent of replacement of skeletal muscle by fat or fibrotic tissue but also recognize specific patterns of involvement in genetically different muscle disorders. Muscle MRI has proven to be a valuable adjunct to the clinical examination in the differential diagnosis of muscle disorders sharing a clinical overlap and it is becoming increasingly used in clinical settings to tailor subsequent genetic investigations. More recently a possible role of muscle MRI as a research tool is suggested to better understand the pathophysiology of various muscle diseases and possible changes over time and in response to treatment.

In this chapter we will discuss pros and cons of the different imaging techniques providing an update of the clinical application of muscle MRI in neuromuscular disorders.

Technical aspects

A full review of the different types of muscle imaging is beyond the scope of this chapter. However, some basic information will help to better understand the pros and cons of each of the available techniques. Many radiologists have limited experience with muscle imaging in chronic muscle diseases and it is important for the referring clinician to have a clear idea of some of the general technical aspects in order to select the most appropriate protocol.

The great advantages of muscle ultrasound are that it is easily accessible, is portable, easy to perform in clinical settings, and can be easily used in children. US has proven to be a valuable screening tool to identify the presence of muscle involvement and to guide muscle biopsies [3, 4, 5]. Furthermore, because US scans are also inexpensive and do not use ionizing radiation, they can be easily repeated to document the progression of muscle involvement. The possibility of recording dynamically also allows the visualization of fasciculations in neurogenic disorders, and in particular in motor neuron disorders. However, these diseases will not be addressed in this chapter.

The interpretation of the scans however is highly operator-dependent and its use in identifying specific patterns of muscle involvement is limited by the difficulties in detecting muscle changes in deep-seated muscles when the muscles closer to the probe are severely affected.

In contrast, CT provides a better view of the overall pattern of muscle involvement but, because of the use of ionizing radiation, and the bone artifacts which hamper interpretation, its use has progressively been replaced by muscle MRI. Nevertheless, it can still be applied in adults with chronic muscle disorders for guidance of a muscle biopsy and for recognition of patterns of muscle involvement if access to MRI and costs are an issue.

Magnetic resonance imaging has obvious advantages related not only to the absence of ionizing radiation but also to the possibility of using multiplanar imaging that is highly important in patients affected by muscle disorders. Patients with chronic inherited disorders often have severe contractures of their limbs and cannot be easily adjusted into conventional positions as requested for CT scanning. Another major advantage is that MRI also provides different sequences, demonstrating different pathological changes. Comparative studies using both CT and MR techniques have shown that MRI T_1-weighted images have a higher sensitivity than CT [6, 7] for identifying fatty replacement in muscles. Another advantage of muscle MRI is that it is much more accurate in estimating "nonmuscular tissues" such as subcutaneous and connective tissue. The possibility of using additional sequences, such as T_2 sequences with fat suppression or short time inversion recovery (STIR) enhances the detection of water content and edema within the muscle.

Disorders of Voluntary Muscle, 8th edn., eds. George Karpati, David Hilton-Jones, Kate Bushby and Robert C. Griggs. Published by Cambridge University Press.

The most commonly used protocols for muscle MRI include T_1-weighed (T_1W), T_2-weighted (T_2W) images, and STIR sequences. T_1-weighted images show differences in T_1 relaxation times between tissues with different structure and density and are very sensitive in differentiating healthy muscle, which has a long T_1 relaxation time, from fat, which has a relatively low T_1 relaxation time. T_1-weighted images are therefore very sensitive in detecting chronic changes such as those observed in muscular dystrophies and more generally in chronic myopathies but are less sensitive at detecting acute changes due to increased water in muscle or to inflammation. Due to its long T_2 relaxation, muscle edema is better seen on T_2-weighted images as high signal intensity. T_2-weighted images, therefore, can provide better information on acute changes secondary to increased water content but as both fat and water are associated with increased signal on T_2-weighted imaging, edema cannot always be distinguished from fat [8, 9]. In those cases other techniques such as STIR or proton density with fat suppression will remove the signal originating from fat, allowing visualization of edema and water. These sequences are most important in patients with a suspected diagnosis of inflammatory myopathy. True edema or edema-like changes can also be found as a nonspecific finding in various neuromuscular conditions and diseases such as facioscapulohumeral muscular dystrophy or Duchenne muscular dystrophy [10].

One limitation of this detailed protocol is however the duration of the scan, which is not tolerated by unsedated pediatric patients or by patients with contractures or abnormal postures. A recently proposed shorter protocol has been found to be suitable for the pediatric population. This includes transverse T_1-weighted spin echo sequence images through two different regions of the lower limbs, one for hips and thighs and one for calves, for a total scanning time of less than 30 minutes [11].

In the last few years increasing attention has been devoted to the possible use of MRI as an aid to understanding the mechanisms of skeletal muscle damage in muscular dystrophy by using contrast-agent-enhanced MRI [12].

The disadvantages of MRI are mainly related to its costs and to practical aspects such as that this tool cannot be used in patients carrying pacemakers or other indwelling metallic objects.

Another technique that has gained much interest over recent years is magnetic resonance spectroscopy (MRS). Muscle phosphorus (P) MRS can be used as a diagnostic tool in patients suspected of metabolic myopathies and mitochondrial disorders (see [13] for review) but has also been used in various forms of muscular dystrophies. Its application in patients with Duchenne and Becker muscular dystrophies and with limb-girdle muscular dystrophies suggests that different forms of dystrophies have different mechanisms of impairment of energy metabolism [14]. Proton nuclear magnetic resonance spectroscopy (^{1}H-MRS) can also be used to study skeletal muscle metabolism, e.g., changes in fatty acid chains, membrane lipid fluidity, and amino acid residues [15].

Muscular dystrophies

Several studies have recently highlighted how different forms of genetically distinct muscular dystrophies have different patterns of muscle involvement even when there is a significant overlap between the clinical phenotypes. We will briefly describe MRI findings in the most common forms of muscular dystrophies.

Duchenne and Becker muscular dystrophies

Standard T_1-weighted MRI scans may be normal in boys with Duchenne muscular dystrophy (DMD) in the early stages [16] or only show hypertrophy of the muscle bulk in the calves without any marked signal abnormalities (E.M., personal observation). With progression of clinical signs there is progressive muscle involvement with a well-defined pattern evolving over time [16, 17, 18].

T_1 sequences in young children with DMD show abnormal signal in the more proximal muscles, involving gluteus maximus and adductor magnus muscles, followed by rectus femoris, and biceps femoris muscles. Sartorius, gracilis, semitendinosus, and semimembranosus muscles appear to be selectively preserved [19] (Figure 7.1a–d).

At calf level, gastrocnemius muscles are affected earlier and more severely than other muscle groups. The use of T_2 and STIR imaging shows additional signs of edema in relatively spared muscles suggesting that an inflammatory component may also play a role in this progressive condition. This finding is of particular interest as a better understanding of the mechanism underlying muscle damage and the recognition of early signs may help when exploring mechanisms of action of candidate drugs for therapeutic trials.

In individuals with Becker muscular dystrophy there is a milder but similar pattern of selective muscle involvement that evolves over longer periods of observation [16, 20].

In the 1980s MRI studies were also conducted in DMD carriers showing significantly higher T_1 values in the proximal muscles as compared to normal females, caused by degenerative muscular changes accompanied by interstitial edema [21, 22].

Limb-girdle muscular dystrophies

The term "limb-girdle muscular dystrophies" includes a quite wide and heterogeneous group of genetically distinct forms of muscular dystrophies. The two most frequent forms of LGMD are the autosomal recessive form due to mutations in the calpain-3 gene (calpain-deficient LGMD, LGMD2A) and another autosomal recessive form with reduction of α-dystroglycan due to mutations in the FKRP gene (LGMD2I).

LGMD2A is generally associated with marked and progressive involvement of the posterior thigh muscles [23]. The

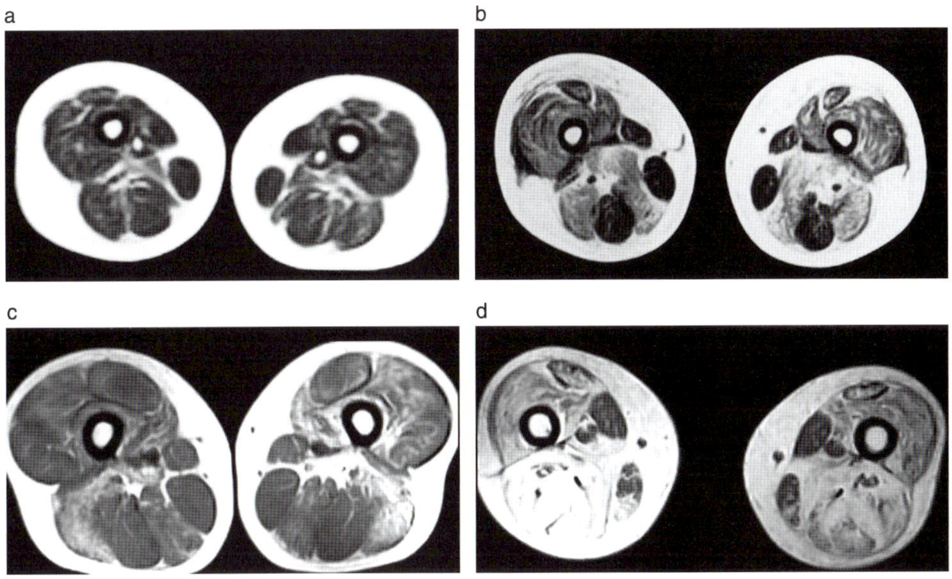

Figure 7.1a–d. Transverse T_1-weighted images through thigh muscles in four patients with Duchenne muscular dystrophy. Note the progressive involvement of the biceps femoris, adductor magnus and vastus muscles with selective sparing of the anteromedial muscles and of the semitendinosus (a, b, c) that remain relatively spared even in the nonambulant patient with more severe clinical involvement (d).

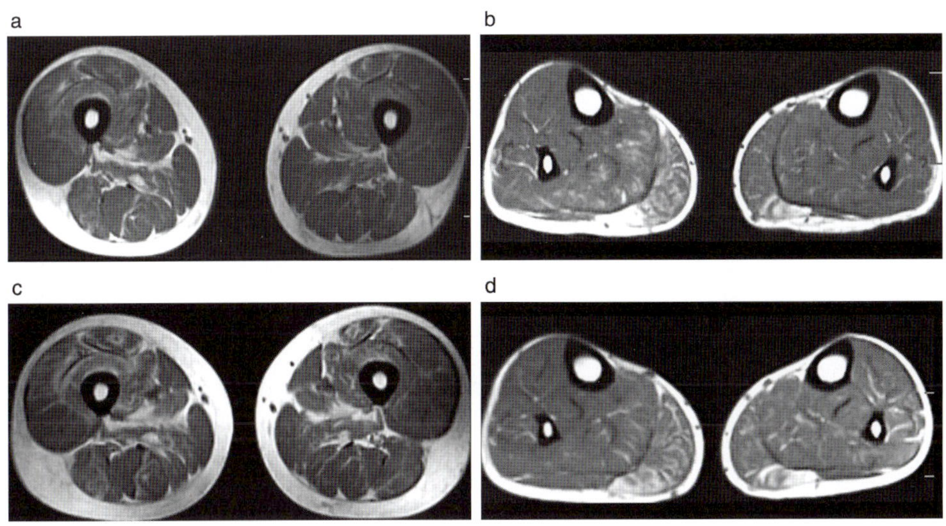

Figure 7.2a–d. Transverse T_1-weighted images through thigh (a, c) and calf (b, d) muscles in two patients with LGMD2A. Note the selective involvement of the adductor magnus in the initial phases and the initial involvement of the vastus medialis and rectus femoris muscles in two patients with mild clinical involvement (c). At calf level there is a selective involvement of the medial head of the gastrocnemius muscle (b, d).

severity of the changes observed on MRI is related to the severity of clinical involvement. Patients with a mild phenotype and minimal weakness show predominant changes in the adductors (Figure 7.2a and c) and semimembranosus muscles while patients with restricted ambulation have a more diffuse involvement of the posterolateral muscles of the thigh and of the vastus intermedius with relative sparing of the vastus lateralis, sartorius, and gracilis muscles (Figure 7.3).

At calf level all patients showed involvement of the medial head of the gastrocnemius (Figures 7.2b, d, 7.3) and of the soleus muscle (Figure 7.3b), with relative sparing of the lateral head of the gastrocnemius muscle.

The pattern observed in patients with LGMD2A shows some overlap but also some differences with that observed in patients affected by the form of LGMD secondary to FKRP mutations (LGMD2I) [24]. While at thigh level there is predominant involvement of the adductor magnus and of the posterior thigh muscles in both LGMD2A and LGMD2I patients, there is less sparing of the anterior muscles in LGMD2I, and a significant hypertrophy of sartorius and gracilis muscles (Figure 7.4).

At calf level patients with LGMD2I also have a predominant involvement of the posterior muscles but without the striking differential involvement between the medial and the lateral head of the gastrocnemius observed in LGMD2A (Figure 7.4).

Less has been reported about other forms of LGMDs. In a study describing MRI and MRS findings in calf muscles in patients with sarcoglycan deficiency on muscle biopsy, T_1- and T_2-weighted images showed marked changes in the soleus muscles with only minimal changes in the gastrocnemius muscles. At variance with the other forms of LGMD recently

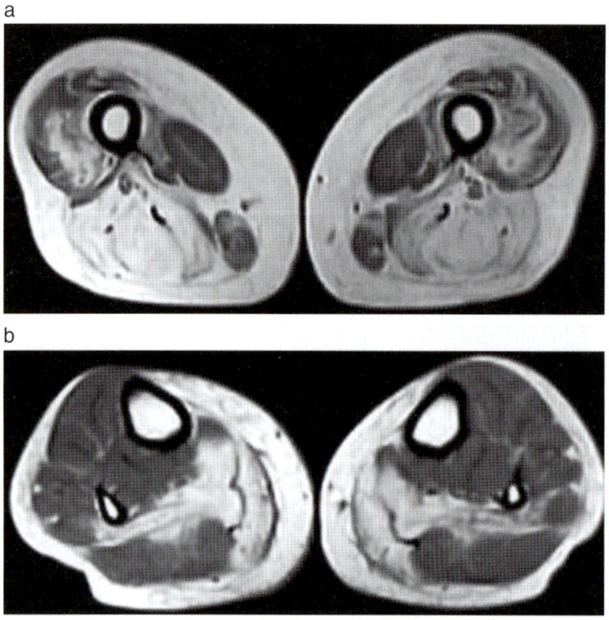

Figure 7.3a,b. Transverse T_1-weighted images through thigh and calf muscles in a severely affected patient with LGMD2A. Note that although the pattern of involvement is more severe than in the patients in Figure 7.2, there is still selective involvement of the posterior muscles of the thigh (a) at calf level of the medial head of the gastrocnemius and the soleus muscles (b).

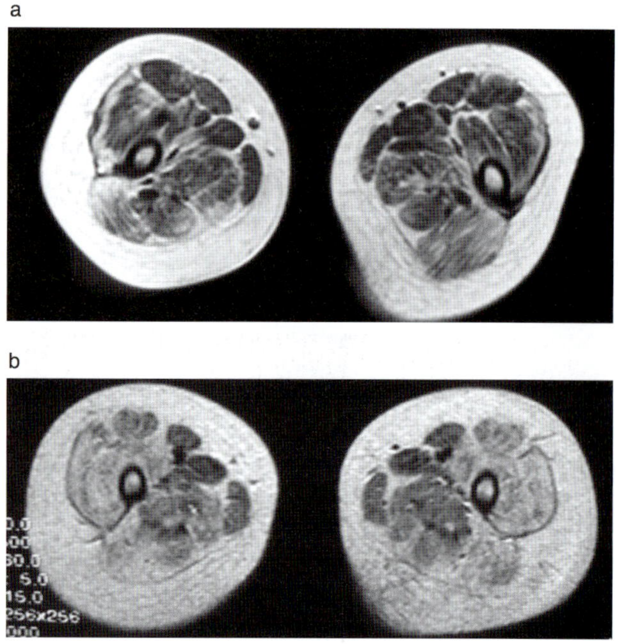

Figure 7.5a,b. Transverse T_1-weighted images through thigh muscles in non-ambulant patients with Ullrich congenital muscular dystrophy. Note the diffuse involvement with relative selected sparing of all the anteromedial muscles.

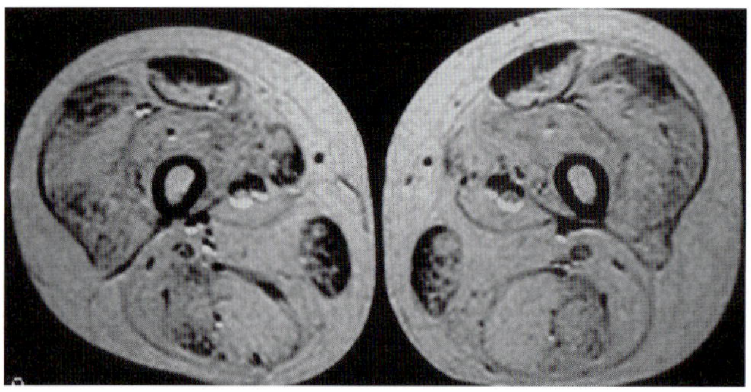

Figure 7.4. Transverse T_1-weighted images through thigh muscles in a non-ambulant patient with the form of LGMD associated with FKRP mutations (LGMD2I). Note the diffuse predominant involvement of the adductor muscles and relative sparing of rectus and gracilis muscles.

described, patients with sarcoglycan deficiency had more involvement of the anterior muscles with abnormal signal in both tibialis anterior and peroneal muscles [14].

LGMD2B, which is caused by mutations in the dysferlin gene, manifests with proximal muscle weakness. In the early stages, weakness is detected only in the posterior compartment muscles of the lower limbs (hamstrings and adductors), which is confirmed by muscle imaging. Although the first localization of muscle weakness was pelvifemoral, there was often early and subclinical involvement of the soleus muscles [25].

Congenital muscular dystrophies

In the last few years, several genes responsible for individual forms of congenital muscular dystrophies (CMD) have been identified. There are no systematic studies evaluating muscle MRI in all the genetically recognized forms of CMD but a few recent studies have reported muscle MRI findings in the forms with a predominantly "rigid" phenotype, namely Ullrich congenital muscular dystrophy (UCMD) and rigid spine muscular dystrophy type 1 (RSMD1), two genetically distinct forms of CMD with overlapping clinical features such as rigidity of the spine and early respiratory involvement, and normal or only mildly elevated creatine kinase (CK).

Ullrich CMD is due to mutations in one of the three collagen VI genes and is characterized by a combination of marked distal laxity and contractures. Muscle MRI at thigh level shows selective sparing of sartorius, gracilis, adductor longus, and often of the rectus femoris [26, 27] with involvement of the posterior and lateral muscles. The rectus femoris muscle often shows an "internal shadow" that can also be appreciated on US while the quadriceps muscles have a peculiar pattern of signal increase typically pronounced at the periphery of the muscles with relative preservation of the muscle belly (Figure 7.5). A similar appearance of peripheral involvement of the muscle is observed at calf level with a typical appearance of the gastrocnemius and soleus muscles.

In contrast, patients with RSMD1, a condition secondary to deficiency in selenoprotein N 1, have a variable involvement of the thigh muscles depending on the severity of motor impairment but, at variance with UCMD, they all show involvement of the sartorius muscle that is often severely affected and associated with selective preservation of rectus femoris and gracilis muscles [28, 29] (Figure 7.6).

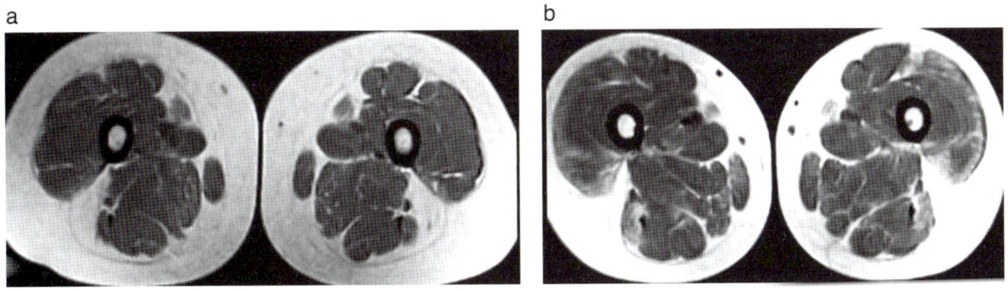

Figure 7.6a,b. Transverse T_1-weighted images through thigh muscles in two patients with RSMD 1 with *SEPN1* mutations. Note the selective involvement of the sartorius and the sparing of the other anteromedial muscles.

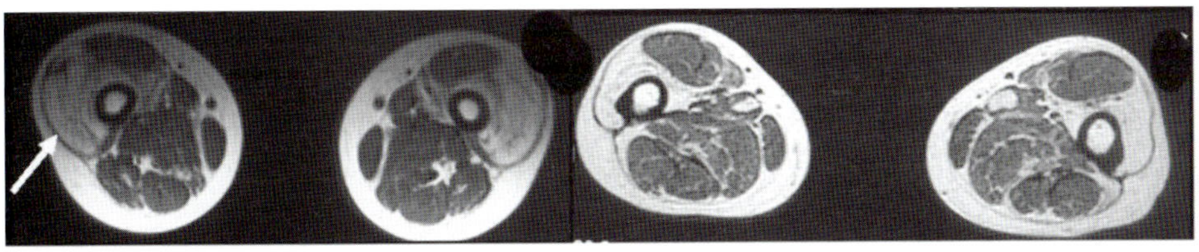

Figure 7.7. Transverse T_1-weighted images through thigh muscles in two patients with autosomal dominant Emery–Dreifuss muscular dystrophy with *LMNA* mutations. Note the striking selective involvement of the vastus muscles with sparing of the rectus femoris that shows remarkable hypertrophy.

Emery–Dreifuss muscular dystrophy

The autosomal dominant form (*EDMD2*) is the most common form of Emery–Dreifuss muscular dystrophy and is due to mutations in *LMNA*, which encodes for the nuclear envelope proteins lamins A and C, while the X-linked variant (EDMD) is due to a defect of emerin, a nuclear membrane protein encoded by the *STA* gene. The two forms share some clinical signs but have a different pattern of muscle involvement on muscle MRI [30].

At thigh level patients with the dominant form often have a selective involvement of the vastus lateralis and intermedius muscles (Figure 7.7), although this pattern is less clear in patients with more severe weakness who have lost ambulation. These patients show more diffuse involvement of thigh muscles. Patients with the X-linked form in contrast have minimal involvement of the thigh muscles.

At calf level patients with the dominant form have a differential involvement of the medial and lateral head of the gastrocnemius with the medial head always predominantly involved and relative sparing of the lateral one. This pattern is more obvious in mildly affected patients but can also be recognized in patients with more severe clinical impairment and more diffuse changes on MRI. Patients with the X-linked form in contrast have preferential involvement of the soleus muscle.

In patients with the dominant form muscle MRI can provide additional information. As mutations in the *LMNA* gene are also responsible for a dominantly inherited partial lipodystrophy of the Dunningan type, patients with the dominant form may also present abnormalities of fat distribution that are often minor [31], but an association with a full-blown picture of LGMD does occur [32]. These patients, especially after the first decades or if severely affected, tend to accumulate fat in the neck and the abdomen, while they have very little fat in the subcutaneous tissue of the limbs.

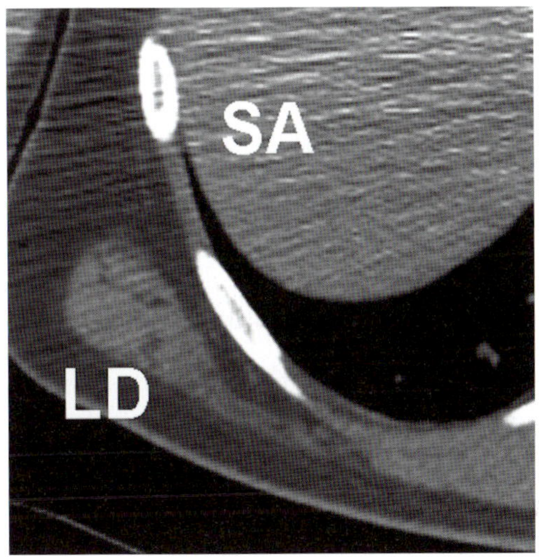

Figure 7.8. CT scan of patient with facioscapulohumeral dystrophy showing fatty replacement of the serratus anterior muscle (SA) whereas the latissimus dorsi (LD) muscle is preserved.

Facioscapulohumeral dystrophy

Facioscapulohumeral muscular dystrophy (FSHD), an autosomal dominant myopathy associated with a deletion on chromosome 4q35, has a variable age of onset and a wide range of clinical expression even within families. Weakness of facial and/or shoulder girdle muscles, often asymmetrical, is usually the presenting symptom in the second decade. Therefore, the most evident abnormalities on muscle imaging are to be found in the biceps and triceps brachii and in the periscapular muscles (Figure 7.8). However, in FSHD lower extremity involvement is rather common and sometimes the presenting manifestation of the disease [33] (Figure 7.9a, b). A systematic MRI study on the pattern of leg muscle involvement revealed asymmetrical involvement in 15% of the cases [34]. The semimembranosus muscle appeared to be the most affected muscle (Figure 7.9c) followed by the tibialis anterior

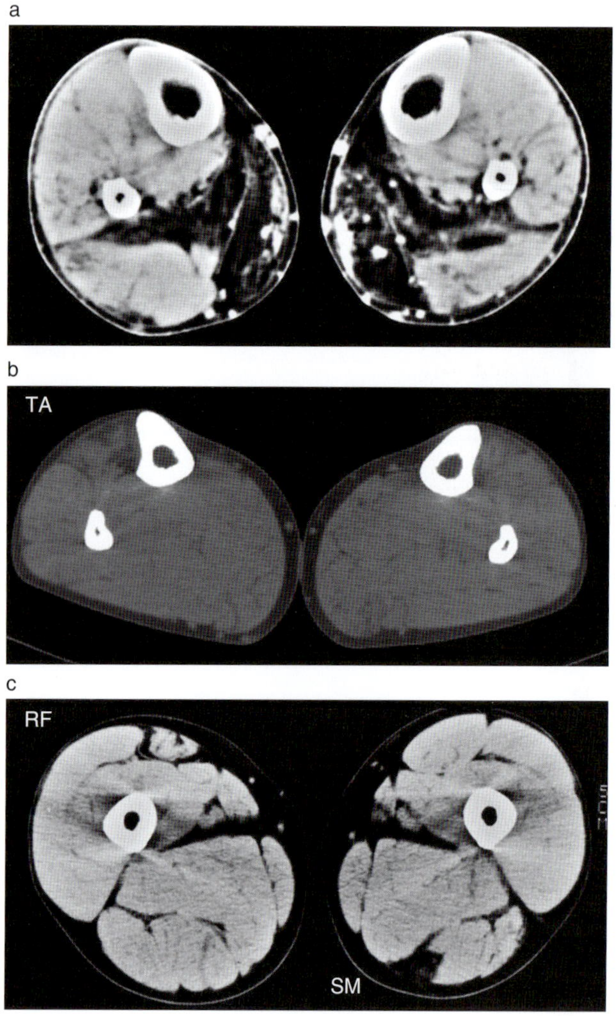

Figure 7.9a–c. CT scan of patient with facioscapulohumeral dystrophy showing bilateral fatty replacement of the medial head of the gastrocnemius muscles and the soleus muscles at the lower leg level (a) in one patient, whereas another patient has asymmetrical involvement of the tibialis anterior (TA) muscle (b). At thigh level (c) there is involvement of the right-sided rectus femoris (RF) and the left-sided semimembranosus muscle (SM).

compartment (Figure 7.9b), the biceps femoris, the semitendinosus, the medial head of the gastrocnemius muscle (Figure 7.9a), and the adductor group. The vastus, gluteal, and peroneal muscles were mostly unaffected and the psoas muscle did not show evidence of involvement in any of the investigated subjects. Muscle imaging enables us to show subclinical involvement of one or more constituent parts of compound muscles such as the quadriceps femoris (Figure 7.9c), hamstrings (Figure 7.9c), hip adductors, and gastrocnemius muscles (Figure 7.9a).

Congenital myopathies

Congenital myopathies are another genetically heterogeneous group of inherited muscle disorders. Two studies have systematically correlated muscle MRI and genetic findings in a large

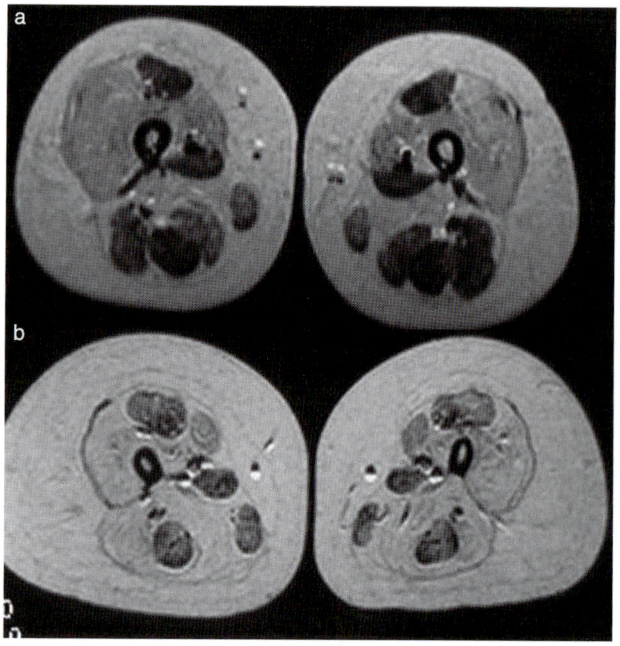

Figure 7.10a,b. Transverse T_1-weighted images through thigh muscles in two patients with central core myopathy and *RYR1* mutations. Note the marked signal increase in the vastus, sartorius, and adductor magnus muscles with relative sparing of rectus femoris, adductor longus, gracilis, and semitendinosus muscles.

cohort of patients with different forms of congenital myopathies [35, 36].

Central core disease

Patients with central core disease and *RYR1* mutation show a pattern of selective involvement of the vastus, sartorius, and adductor magnus and relative sparing of rectus femoris, adductor longus, and hamstring muscles [35] (Figure 7.10).

At calf level there is marked involvement of the soleus, the lateral head of the gastrocnemius, and the peroneal group with relative sparing of tibialis anterior and other anterior compartment muscles.

Minicore myopathy

In patients with minicore myopathy due to mutations in the selenoprotein N 1 gene, muscle MRI changes in the lower limb may be normal with the exception of isolated sartorius involvement (E.M., personal observation), with a similar pattern to that observed in the forms of CMD with rigid spine also due to mutations in the same gene.

Patients with mutations in *RYR1* have a pattern of selectivity similar to that found in central core disease.

Nemaline myopathy

Less has been reported for patients with nemaline myopathy and the findings appear to be more heterogeneous reflecting the number of genes involved and the wide range of clinical

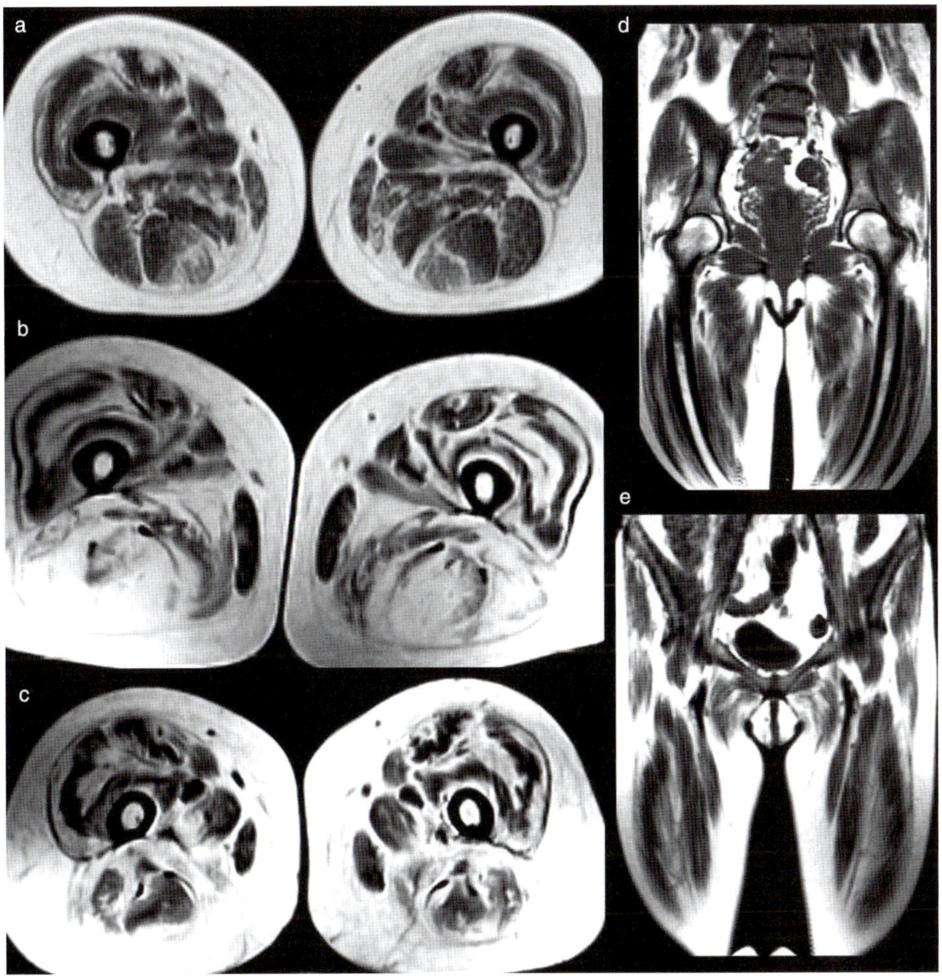

Figure 7.11a–e. Transverse T_1-weighted images through thigh muscles in three patients with Bethlem myopathy (a, b, c). Note the peripheral involvement of the vastus lateralis with sparing of the internal part of the muscles that can be observed even in the nonambulant patient (c). All three patients also have the typical "internal shadow" in the rectus femoris. Coronal images (d, e) also highlight the peripheral involvement of the vastus and the sparing of the central part of these muscles.

phenotypes described even in association with mutations in a single gene, such as reported for *ACTA1* [36, 37].

Bethlem myopathy

Bethlem myopathy is an autosomal dominant myopathy caused by mutations in collagen VI genes. Muscle MRI findings are similar to those observed in UCMD, the form of CMD also due to mutations in the collagen VI genes. Although the changes in Bethlem myopathy are generally milder there is a significant overlap between the milder cases of UCMD and the older or more severe patients with Bethlem myopathy. In patients with Bethlem myopathy the vastus muscles are the most frequently affected thigh muscles, with a rim of abnormal signal at the periphery of the muscle and relative sparing of the central part [26, 38] (Figure 7.11a–c) and relative sparing of the rectus femoris that however shows a central area of abnormal signal within the muscle (central shadow) (Figure 7.11a, b) that can also be observed on muscle ultrasound [39]. The peripheral involvement of the vastus muscles with sparing of the central part can also be well appreciated on coronal images (Figure 7.11d, e). This pattern is better appreciated in patients with mild involvement but can still be recognized even in patients with more severe or advanced involvement.

At calf level the involvement is less severe with a rim of abnormal signal at the periphery of soleus and gastrocnemius muscles (Figure 7.12a, b).

Distal myopathies

As in limb-girdle muscular dystrophies there is a wide range of distal myopathies with considerable clinical and genetic heterogeneity.

Muscle imaging can be helpful in showing involvement of clinically unaffected muscles, e.g., in recessively inherited Miyoshi myopathy, another phenotype of dysferlinopathy. The disease usually affects individuals in early adulthood who present with the inability to walk on tiptoe. Markedly elevated serum CK activity is a hallmark of the disease. Subsequent to calf muscle involvement (Figure 7.13a) the disease process spreads to the gluteus minimus (Figure 7.13b) muscles and the thigh muscles, hamstrings more than quadriceps (Figure 7.13c), but this may initially escape the attention of the clinician unless the strength of each of these muscles is specifically assessed [40, 41].

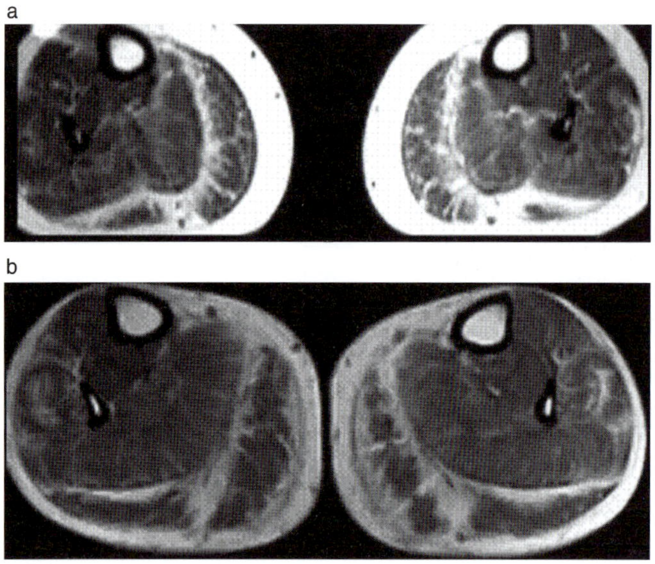

Figure 7.12a,b. Transverse T_1-weighted images through calf muscles in two patients with Bethlem myopathy: note the rim of increased signal between soleus and gastrocnemius muscles.

Laing myopathy is an autosomal dominantly inherited early-onset distal myopathy caused by mutations in the slow skeletal muscle fiber myosin heavy chain gene in which foot and great toe extensor involvement is the initial symptom and sign both clinically and on muscle imaging [42] (Figure 7.14).

Tibial muscular dystrophy (TMD) was first reported in Finland. Mutations in the titin gene have been shown to be responsible for TMD. Usually, the onset of this disease occurs in late adult life and there is a relatively benign course, as is also the case in Welander myopathy, first reported in Sweden and subsequently in Finland. Welander disease is linked to a locus on 2p13. Both diseases have an autosomal dominant inheritance pattern. In TMD the first symptoms and signs appear in the anterior tibial and extensor digitorum muscles, whereas in Welander myopathy these muscles become affected some 10 years after involvement of the extensors of the fingers [43]. In both diseases other muscles including the calf muscles and posterior thigh muscles are gradually replaced by fatty tissue.

A recessively inherited distal myopathy due to mutations in the nebulin gene which usually gives rise to a nemaline myopathy was described in Finland. The patients present with foot drop followed by finger extensor and neck flexor involvement and eventually also the proximal limb muscles become affected. Muscle imaging shows preferential anterior tibial muscle involvement in the early stages as in tibial muscular dystrophy [44].

Mutations in the caveolin-3 gene (autosomal dominant caveolinopathy) give rise to a wide range of clinical manifestations including a limb-girdle syndrome, distal myopathy, calf hypertrophy, rippling muscle disease, and hyperCKemia, sometimes occurring within the same kinship [45]. In the distal phenotype the anterior tibial muscle is preferentially affected on clinical examination. In addition to atrophy and fatty degeneration in the anterior leg compartment MRI may

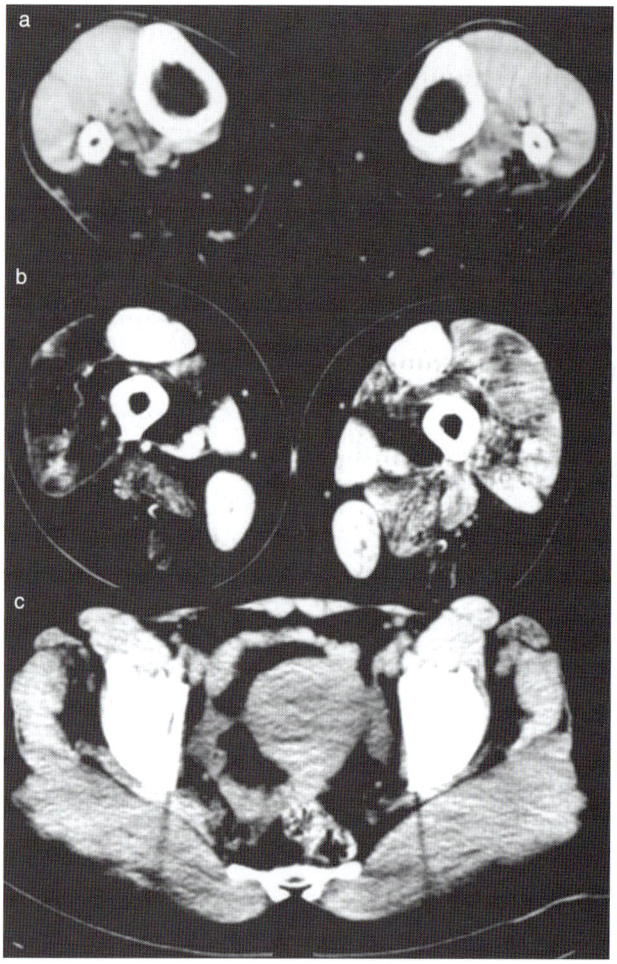

Figure 7.13a–c. CT scan of patient with dysferlin-negative Miyoshi myopathy showing fatty replacement at calf level of the soleus and the gastrocnemius muscles, medial and lateral head (a), at the pelvic girdle level of the gluteus minimus muscles (b), and of the thigh muscles including the quadriceps muscles, adductors, and hamstrings, right more than left with preservation of the rectus femoris and of sartorius and gracilis muscles (c).

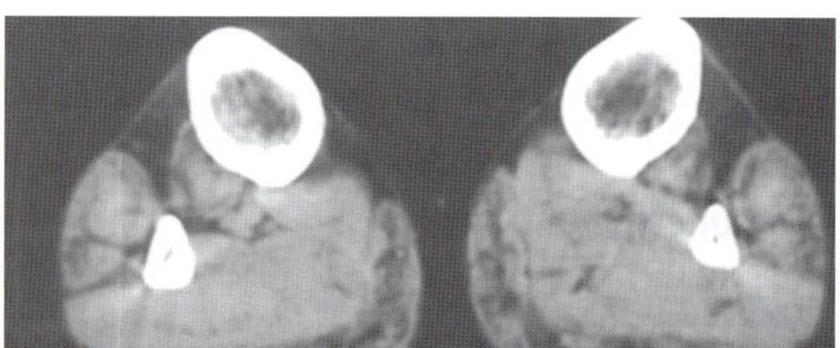

Figure 7.14. CT scan of patient with Laing myopathy showing fatty replacement of both anterior tibialis muscles. The gastrocnemius muscles are slightly affected.

also show involvement of the hypertrophic medial gastrocnemius muscles on T_2-weighted images which is then designated as pseudohypertrophy [45].

Quadriceps-sparing inclusion body myopathy is an autosomal recessive disorder that manifests after the age of 20 with foot drop and ascending weakness and wasting gradually involving

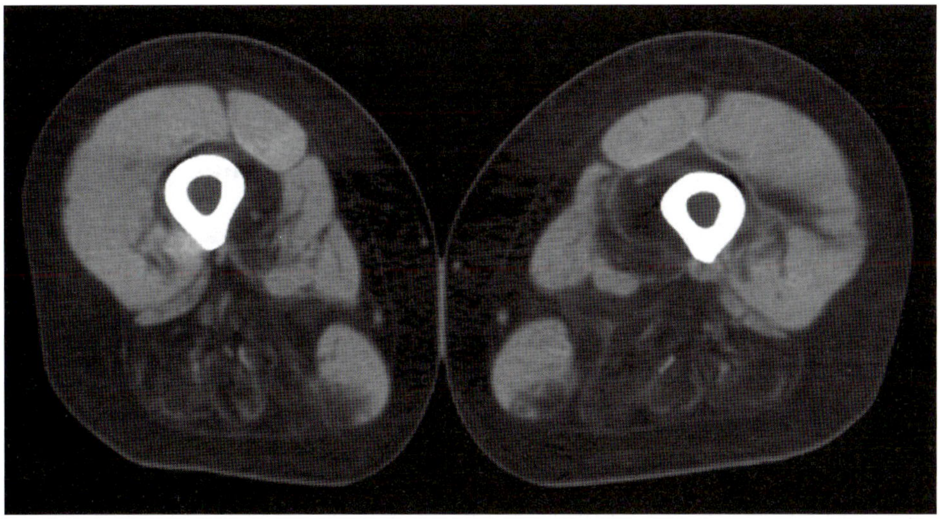

Figure 7.15. CT scan of adult patient with Pompe disease showing fatty replacement of the hamstrings, the adductor magnus, and vastus intermedius muscles.

all limb muscles, but sparing the quadriceps. The disease is caused by mutations in the *GNE* gene UDP-GlcNAc-2-epimerase, the complex enzyme responsible for *N*-acetylneuraminic acid (sialic acid) biosynthesis. In spite of preserved strength and size even the quadriceps muscle becomes subclinically affected as is shown by MRI, especially late in the disease [46].

Other distal myopathies in which muscle imaging findings have been described in order to delineate the phenotype include myofibrillar myopathies, e.g., myotilinopathy, zaspopathy, and desminopathy [47, 48, 49]. In myotilinopathy in all four compartments of the lower leg the skeletal muscle was replaced by fatty tissue, whereas in asymptomatic gene carriers only the soleus muscle was affected [47]. In zaspopathy muscle imaging studies show a pattern of early involvement of posterior calf muscles, particular the gastrocnemius and soleus muscles, and late involvement of all lower leg muscles [48]. In desminopathy there is concomitant involvement of the muscles of the thigh (semitendinosus, followed by the sartorius and gracilis muscles) and of the peroneal and anterior tibial muscles albeit that clinically the disease initially presented with toe walking due to ankle contractures and distal muscle weakness [49].

Metabolic myopathies

Pompe disease or glycogen storage disease type II, is an autosomal recessive disorder caused by deficiency of the lysosomal enzyme acid α-glucosidase resulting in lysosomal accumulation of glycogen in most tissues. Infantile, juvenile, and adult variants of Pompe disease are classified according to the age at onset, rate of progression, and extent of tissue involvement. Patients with the adult-onset form present after the age of 20 with slowly progressive lower limb weakness, frequently associated with severe diaphragm weakness in one-third of the cases. Muscle imaging studies show that the paraspinal muscles at lumbar level, the psoas, and among the thigh muscles the adductor magnus and hamstrings (Figure 7.15), are initially affected. Gradually the vastus muscles, and in particular the

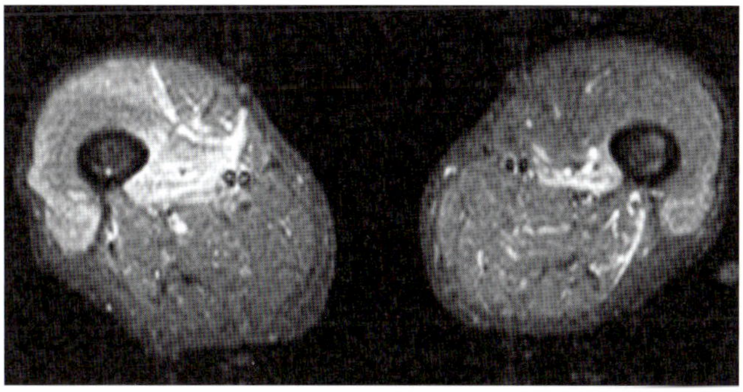

Figure 7.16. Short T_1 inversion recovery (STIR) MRI image of upper legs of adult patient with dermatomyositis showing hyperintensity of the vastus medialis muscles, predominantly on the right.

vastus intermedius (Figure 7.15) and medialis, become progressively involved [50, 51].

Disorders which clinically manifest with rhabdomyolysis such as McArdle disease and glycolytic diseases usually reveal normal muscle imaging findings between the attacks. However, during the exacerbation, the muscles shows focal edematous changes [52].

Results of muscle imaging in mitochondrial disorders are inconsistent. Often few abnormalities are observed which may indicate that the myopathy in mitochondrial myopathies is caused by energy failure rather than structural abnormalities in the skeletal muscles [52].

Inflammatory myopathies

Idiopathic inflammatory diseases such as dermatomyositis and polymyositis manifest with muscle edema, whereas sporadic inclusion body myositis (sIBM), which is a chronic myodegenerative disease associated with inflammation, shows fatty infiltration of the skeletal muscle by fat. MRI can readily assess a change in subacute muscle inflammation which is visible as a high signal intensity on fat-suppressed T_2-weighted and STIR MRI images [53] (Figure 7.16). In contrast, in sIBM there is

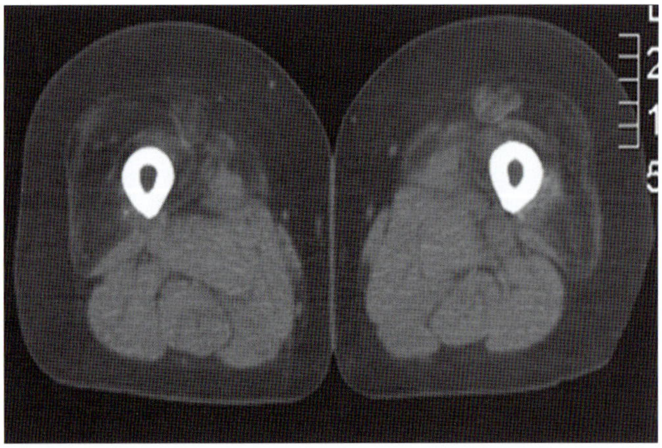

Figure 7.17. Patient with sporadic inclusion body myositis showing fatty replacement of the quadriceps femoris muscles.

replacement of skeletal muscle by fat [54]. Another important difference between dermatomyositis/polymyositis and sIBM is the distribution of muscle changes. In the former, there is predominantly proximal and symmetrical involvement, whereas in sIBM muscle changes are often asymmetrical and often located in distal muscles of the limbs (anterior tibial muscles and deep finger flexors), also at an early stage, although involvement of the quadriceps muscle is also an early and characteristic feature [54] (Figure 7.17).

A MRI-guided muscle biopsy might reduce the number of false-negative biopsies although the sensitivity of MRI to detect abnormalities is 80% [55].

Another application of MRI in inflammatory myopathies is the evaluation of treatment by monitoring the signal intensities [56].

References

1. D. S. O'Doherty, D. Schellinger, V. Raptopoulos, Computed tomographic patterns of pseudohypertrophic muscular dystrophy: preliminary results. *J. Comput. Assist. Tomogr.* **1** (1977), 482–486.
2. J. Z. Heckmatt, V. Dubowitz, S. Leeman, Detection of pathological change in dystrophic muscle with B-scan ultrasound imaging. *Lancet* **1** (1980), 1389–1390.
3. J. Z. Heckmatt, S. Leeman, V. Dubowitz, Ultrasound imaging in the diagnosis of muscle disease. *J. Pediatr.* **101** (1992), 656–660.
4. J. Z. Heckmatt, V. Dubowitz, Diagnostic advantage of needle muscle biopsy and ultrasound imaging in the detection of focal pathology in a girl with limb girdle dystrophy. *Muscle Nerve* **8** (1985), 705–709.
5. S. M. Zuberi, N. Matta, S. Nawaz, *et al.*, Muscle ultrasound in the assessment of suspected neuromuscular disease in childhood. *Neuromuscul. Disord.* **9** (1999), 203–207.
6. H. Schedel, C. D. Reimers, M. Nägele, *et al.*, Imaging techniques in myotonic dystrophy. A comparative study of ultrasound, computed tomography and magnetic resonance imaging of skeletal muscles. *Eur. J. Radiol.* **15** (1992), 230–238.
7. O. Ozsarlak, E. Schepens, P. M. Parizel, *et al.*, Hereditary neuromuscular diseases. *Eur. J. Radiol.* **40** (2001), 184–197.
8. C. D. Reimers, P. Fisher, D. E. Pongratz, Histopathological basis of muscle imaging. In *Muscle Imaging in Health and Disease*, eds. J. L. Fleckenstein, J. V. Crues III, C. D. Reimers. (New York: Springer, 1996), pp. 183–192.
9. J. L. Fleckenstein, MRI of neuromuscular disease: the basics. *Semin. Musculoskelet. Radiol.* **4** (2000), 393–419.
10. H. Schedel, C. D. Reimers, T. Vogl, *et al.*, Muscle edema in MR imaging of neuromuscular diseases. *Acta Radiol.* **36** (1995), 228–232.
11. E. Mercuri, A. Pichiecchio, S. Counsell, *et al.*, A short protocol for muscle MRI in children with muscular dystrophies. *Eur. J. Paediatr. Neurol.* **6** (2002), 305–307.
12. V. Straub, K. M. Donahue, V. Allamand, *et al.*, Contrast agent-enhanced magnetic resonance imaging of skeletal muscle damage in animal models of muscular dystrophy. *Magn. Reson. Med.* **44** (2000), 655–659.
13. Z. Argov, M. Lofberg, D. L. Arnold, Insights into muscle diseases gained by phosphorus magnetic resonance spectroscopy. *Muscle Nerve* **23** (2000), 13–16.
14. R. Lodi, F. Muntoni, J. Taylor, *et al.*, Correlative MR imaging and 31P-MR spectroscopy study in sarcoglycan deficient limb girdle muscular dystrophy. *Neuromuscul. Disord.* **7** (1997), 505–511.
15. P. A. Narayana, E. F. Jackson, I. J. Butler, 1H-MRS of muscle physiology and pathophysiology. In *Muscle Imaging in Health and Disease*, eds. J. L. Fleckenstein, J. V. Crues III, C. D. Reimers. (New York: Springer, 1996), pp. 133–148.
16. A. E. Lamminen, Magnetic resonance imaging of primary skeletal muscle disease: patterns of distribution and severity of involvement. *Br. J. Radiol.* **63** (1990), 946–950.
17. H. Nagao, T. Morimoto, N. Sano, *et al.*, Magnetic resonance imaging of skeletal muscle in patients with Duchenne muscular dystrophy – serial axial and sagittal section studies. *No To Hattatsu* **23** (1991), 39–43.
18. K. Matsumura, I. Nakano, N. Fukuda, *et al.*, Proton spin-lattice relaxation time of Duchenne dystrophy skeletal muscle by magnetic resonance imaging. *Muscle Nerve* **11** (1988), 97–102.
19. M. Liu, H. Chino, T. Ishihara, Muscle damage progression in Duchenne muscular dystrophy evaluated by a new quantitative computed tomographic method. *Arch. Phys. Med. Rehabil.* **73** (1993), 507–514.
20. M. de Visser, B. Verbeeten Jr, Computed tomography of the skeletal musculature in Becker-type muscular dystrophy and benign infantile spinal muscular atrophy. *Muscle Nerve* **8** (1985), 435–444.
21. H.-D. Rott, M. Santellani, W. Rödl, G. Nebel, Duchenne muscular dystrophy: carrier detection by ultrasound and computerised tomography. *Lancet* **2** (1983), 1199–2000.
22. K. Matsumura, I. Nakano, N. Fukuda, *et al.*, Duchenne muscular dystrophy carriers. Proton spin-lattice relaxation times of skeletal muscles on magnetic resonance imaging. *Neuroradiology* **31** (1989), 373–376.
23. E. Mercuri, K. Bushby, E. Ricci, *et al.*, Muscle MRI findings in patients with limb girdle muscular dystrophy with calpain 3

deficiency (LGMD2A), and early contractures. *Neuromuscul. Disord.* **15** (2005), 164–171.

24. D. Fischer, M. C. Walter, K. Kesper, *et al.*, Diagnostic value of muscle MRI in differentiating LGMD2I from other LGMDs. *J. Neurol.* **252** (2005), 538–547.
25. I. Majhneh, G. Marconi, K. Bushby, *et al.*, Dysferlinopathy (LGMD2B): a 23-year follow-up study of 10 patients homozygous for the same frameshifting dysferlin mutations. *Neuromusc. Disord.* **11** (2001), 20–26.
26. E. Mercuri, A. Lampe, J. Allsopp, *et al.*, Muscle MRI in Ullrich congenital muscular dystrophy and Bethlem myopathy. *Neuromusc. Disord.* **15** (2005), 303–310.
27. E. Mercuri, C. Cini, A. Pichiecchio, *et al.*, Muscle magnetic resonance imaging in patients with Ullrich congenital muscular dystrophy. *Neuromusc. Disord.* **13** (2003), 554–557.
28. E. Mercuri, B. Talim, B. Moghdaszadeh, *et al.*, Clinical and imaging findings in six cases of congenital muscular dystrophy with rigid spine syndrome linked to chromosome 1p (RSMD1). *Neuromusc. Disord.* **12** (2002), 631–638.
29. K. M. Flanigan, L. Kerr, M. B. Bromberg, *et al.*, Congenital muscular dystrophy with rigid spine syndrome: a clinical, pathological, radiological, and genetic study. *Ann. Neurol.* **47** (2000), 152–161.
30. E. Mercuri, S. Counsell, J. Allsop, *et al.*, Selective muscle involvement on magnetic resonance imaging in autosomal-dominant Emery-Dreifuss muscular dystrophy. *Neuropediatrics* **33** (2002), 10–14.
31. M. C. Vantyghem, P. Pigny, C. A. Maurage, *et al.*, Patients with familial partial lipodystrophy of the Dunnigan type due to a LMNA R482W mutation show muscular and cardiac abnormalities. *J. Clin. Endocrinol. Metab.* **89** (2004), 5337–5346.
32. A. J. Van der Kooi, G. Bonne, B. Eymard, *et al.*, Lamin A/C mutations with lipodystrophy, cardiac abnormalities, and muscular dystrophy. *Neurology* **27** (2002), 620–623.
33. A. J. Van der Kooi, M. C. Visser, N. Rosenberg, *et al.*, Extension of the clinical range of facioscapulohumeral dystrophy: report of six cases. *J. Neurol. Neurosurg. Psychiatry* **69** (2000), 114–116.
34. D. B. Olsen, P. Gideon, T. D. Jeppesen, J. Vissing, Leg muscle involvement in facioscapulohumeral muscular dystrophy assessed by MRI. *J. Neurol.* **253** (2006), 1437–1441.
35. H. Jungbluth, M. R. Davis, C. Muller, *et al.*, Magnetic resonance imaging of muscle in congenital myopathies associated with RYR1 mutations. *Neuromusc. Disord.* **14** (2004), 785–790.
36. H. Jungbluth, C. A. Sewry, S. Councell, *et al.*, Magnetic resonance imaging of muscle in nemaline myopathy. *Neuromusc. Disord.* **14** (2004), 779–784.
37. H. Jungbluth, C. A. Sewry, S. C. Brown, *et al.*, Mild phenotype of nemaline myopathy with sleep hypoventilation due to a mutation in the skeletal muscle alpha-actin (ACTA1), gene. *Neuromusc. Disord.* **11** (2001), 35–41.
38. E. Mercuri, C. Cini, S. Counsell, *et al.*, Muscle MRI findings in a three-generation family affected by Bethlem myopathy. *Eur. J. Paediatr. Neurol.* **6** (2002), 309–314.
39. C. G. Bonnemann, K. Brockmann, F. Hanefeld, Muscle ultrasound in Bethlem myopathy. *Neuropediatrics* **34** (2003), 335–336.
40. W. H. Linssen, N. C. Notermans, Y. Van der Graaf, *et al.*, Miyoshi-type distal muscular dystrophy. Clinical spectrum in 24 Dutch patients. *Brain* **120** (1997), 1989–1996.
41. L.-S. Ro, G.-J. Lee-Chen, T.-C. Lin, *et al.*, Phenotypic features and genetic findings in 2 Chinese families with Miyoshi distal myopathy. *Arch. Neurol.* **61** (2004), 1594–1599.
42. T. Voit, P. Kutz, B. Leube, *et al.*, Autosomal dominant distal myopathy: further evidence of a chromosome 14 locus. *Neuromusc. Disord.* **11** (2001), 11–19.
43. I. Mahjneh, A. E. Lamminen, B. Udd, *et al.*, Muscle magnetic resonance imaging shows distinct diagnostic patterns in Welander and tibial muscular dystrophy. *Acta Neurol. Scand.* **110** (2004), 87–93.
44. C. Wallgren-Pettersson, V.-L. Lehtokari, H. Kalimo, *et al.*, Distal myopathy caused by homozygous missense mutations in the nebulin gene. *Brain* **130** (2007), 1465–1476.
45. D. Fischer, A. Schroers, I. Blümcke, *et al.*, Consequences of a novel caveolin-3 mutation in a large German family. *Ann. Neurol.* **53** (2003), 233–241.
46. O. M. Vasconcelos, R. Raju, M. C. Dalakas, GNE mutations in an American family with quadriceps-sparing IBM and lack of mutations in s-IBM. *Neurology* **59** (2002), 1776–1779.
47. J. Berciano, E. Gallardo, R. Domínguez-Perles, *et al.*, Autosomal-dominant distal myopathy with a myotilin S55F mutation: sorting out the phenotype. *J. Neurol. Neurosurg. Psychiatry* **79** (2008), 205–208.
48. R. Griggs, A. Vihola, P. Hackman, *et al.*, Zaspopathy in a large classic late-onset distal myopathy family. *Brain* **130** (2007), 1477–1484.
49. M. Olivé, J. Armstrong, F. Miralles, *et al.*, Phenotypic patterns of desminopathy associated with three novel mutations in the desmin gene. *Neuromuscul. Disord.* **17** (2007), 443–450.
50. A. E. J. De Jager, T. M. van der Vliet, T. C. van der Ree, *et al.*, Muscle computed tomography in adult-onset acid maltase deficiency. *Muscle Nerve* **21** (1998), 398–400.
51. A. Pichiecchio, C. Uggetti, S. Ravaglia, *et al.*, Muscle MRI in adult-onset acid maltase deficiency. *Neuromusc. Disord.* **14** (2004), 51–55.
52. Z. Argov, D. L. Arnold, MR spectroscopy and MR imaging in metabolic myopathies. *Neurol. Clin.* **18** (2000), 35–52.
53. S. M. Maillard, R. Jones, C. Owens, *et al.*, Quantitative assessment of MRI T2 relaxation time of thigh muscles in juvenile dermatomyositis. *Rheumatology* **43** (2004), 603–608.
54. B. A. Phillips, L. A. Cala, G. W. Thickbroom, *et al.*, Patterns of muscle involvement in inclusion body myositis: clinical and magnetic resonance imaging study. *Muscle Nerve* **24** (2001), 1526–1534.
55. C. D. Reimers, H. Schedel, J. L. Fleckenstein, *et al.*, Magnetic resonance imaging of skeletal muscles in idiopathic inflammatory myopathies of adults. *J. Neurol.* **241** (1994), 306–314.
56. J. T. Studýnková, F. Charvát, K. Jarosová, J. Vencovský, MRI in the assessment of polymyositis and dermatomyositis. *Rheumatology* **46** (2007), 1174–1179.

Section 3A
Chapter

8

Description of muscle disease – general aspects

The clinical assessment and a guide to classification of the myopathies

David Hilton-Jones and John T. Kissel

Introduction

The molecular genetics revolution has resulted in a wealth of new information on the pathogenesis of most myopathies, and a resulting fundamental change in the way these disorders are diagnosed and classified [1]. Whereas traditionally it was a rare patient who avoided muscle biopsy, largely because there were few other practical methods to investigate muscle structure and function, current advances in laboratory medicine (Table 8.1), especially in the field of molecular genetics, have drastically reduced the indications for biopsy, especially for those with many types of muscular dystrophy. For example, a boy with suspected Duchenne dystrophy should now be evaluated through a serum creatine kinase (CK) assay and direct genetic analysis for an Xp21 mutation before electrodiagnostic testing and muscle biopsy are even considered.

It is ironic, however, that this increase in the number and sophistication of diagnostic tests has, if anything, *increased* the crucial role of the bedside history and examination in the diagnostic process. It is still chiefly through the history and examination that the clinician makes the initial determination that a disorder is likely to be myopathic, and no amount of laboratory testing, including genetic testing, can compensate for an erroneous impression based on an incomplete, hastily performed history and examination. Moreover, some muscle disorders have findings so characteristic that they can be diagnosed with relative certainty at the bedside (Table 8.2). More frequently, the data gathered from the history and examination permit the generation of diagnostic hypotheses, which can then be assessed through appropriate diagnostic studies. Equally important is the fact that the process of history taking and performing the examination through the "laying on of hands" represents the first and most important interaction between physician and patient. It is during this initial contact that the patient develops trust in the clinician and the rapport necessary for a successful therapeutic relationship is established. This chapter will begin with a discussion of the neuromuscular history and examination as a prelude to discussing other aspects of the evaluation of patients with suspected muscle disease. In the course of each discussion, various classification schemes that may be helpful in approaching these patients, both diagnostically and conceptually, will be presented, followed by some thoughts on a global classification scheme for muscle disorders. The aim throughout is to provide practical advice that will be of benefit to the clinician.

History

Although the basic elements of the history (presenting complaint, history of the present illness, past medical history, drug history, family history, social history, and review of symptoms) are the same for neuromuscular complaints as for other medical problems, certain features are unique to the patient with suspected myopathy. One of the most notable differences is that some of the more common muscle symptoms, such as pain and fatigue, are not amenable to direct observation or quantification by the examiner, and they often occur in patients with no definable muscle disease. Conversely, other symptoms, such as weakness, may develop so slowly that patients may not realize it and not complain of it during the history.

Presenting complaint

Skeletal muscle has a limited repertoire of responses to insults so that the chief complaint in most myopathy patients is usually limited to one or more of the following: weakness, resting or exercise-induced muscle pain, muscle enlargement or atrophy, muscle "overactivity" or delayed relaxation (e.g., cramps, myotonia), fatigue, or (rarely) myoglobinuria.

Weakness

Weakness is by far the most common presenting symptom of patients with a definable muscle disease. Patients may use the term "weakness" to refer to any of a number of symptoms, including fatigue, restricted movement owing to orthopedic or mechanical problems, reduced exercise capacity, or occasionally even sensory disturbances. Conversely, patients frequently use words such as deadness, heaviness, aching or even

Disorders of Voluntary Muscle, 8th edn., eds. George Karpati, David Hilton-Jones, Kate Bushby and Robert C. Griggs. Published by Cambridge University Press.

Table 8.1. Diagnostic testing useful in patients with suspected muscle disease

Clinical history and examination
Computerized quantitative muscle testing[a]
Biochemical tests
Blood and urine analyses (e.g., serum creatine kinase)
Exercise tests (forearm exercise test, treadmill or bicycle ergometry)
Enzyme assay
Neurophysiological studies
Nerve conduction studies
Electromyography
Single fiber electromyography
Repetitive stimulation studies
Muscle imaging[a]
Muscle biopsy
Routine histology and histochemistry
Immunocytochemistry
Specific enzyme assays
Genetic tests (e.g., mitochondrial DNA)
Molecular genetic testing
Specific gene tests for disease (e.g., Xp21 deletion in Duchenne dystrophy)
Genetic tests associated with disease (e.g., 4q5 deletion in FSH dystrophy)
Linkage analysis

Note: [a]These are not essential and indeed are not available in many specialist departments. However, they are often used in research and imaging can be of great value in determining the pattern of muscle involvement, which may help direct further investigation.

Table 8.2. Myopathies that can often be diagnosed (or strongly suspected) at the bedside

- Duchenne muscular dystrophy
- Emery–Dreifuss syndrome
- Facioscapulohumeral muscular dystrophy
- Oculopharyngeal muscular dystrophy
- Rigid spine syndrome
- Myotonic dystrophy
- Myotonia congenita
- Dermatomyositis
- Inclusion body myositis
- Some endocrine myopathies
- Some mitochondrial cytopathies
- Acid maltase deficiency (if there is diaphragmatic involvement)

numbness to describe what is actually muscle weakness. It is obviously crucial for the examiner to pin down precisely the nature of the presenting complaint, and what the patient means by "weakness." Questions detailing functional limitations induced by the weakness are usually required to make this determination.

Accurate delineation of the duration of weakness, rate of progression, distribution of involved muscles and whether the weakness is persistent or intermittent are also crucial. Making these determinations by history alone can be difficult, particularly in slowly progressive disorders that have their onset years or decades prior to the patient's initial presentation. Weakness may be relatively static, as in some congenital myopathies; progressive, as in most dystrophies; fluctuating, as in the myasthenic disorders; intermittent, as in the periodic paralyses and some myotonic disorders; or exercise related, as in many metabolic disorders.

The distribution of weakness is in many respects the most important aspect to be elucidated, as it provides important clues to the diagnosis; it is determined from both the history and examination. Although there are many exceptions to any rule concerning distribution of involved muscles, most patients with myopathy can be grouped into one of several patterns of involvement. One classification scheme that has found widespread clinical use is based on recognizing one of six predominant patterns of weakness [2, 3] (Table 8.3). Taking a goal-directed history aimed at placing the patient conceptually into one of these six groups can go a long way towards arriving at an accurate diagnosis.

The most common distribution of weakness by far is that of exclusively or predominantly proximal extremity and axial muscles (including neck flexors) or *limb-girdle* involvement (Figure 8.1; video clip 1). This pattern is seen in many hereditary and acquired myopathies and therefore the pattern probably *least* helpful in arriving at a specific diagnosis. This pattern results in difficulty getting out of chairs or car seats, going up and down steps, arising from a squat or getting off the floor. Proximal arm weakness manifests historically as difficulty reaching to get things from shelves, or difficulty with self-care activities such as shaving, combing or setting hair, brushing teeth or even raising the arms enough to put on a shirt or sweater.

Less frequently, and for reasons that are entirely unknown, disorders such as myotonic dystrophy, distal myopathies, and inclusion body myositis (IBM) can cause a *predominantly distal pattern* of weakness (Figure 8.2, video clip 2). This distribution produces leg complaints such as tripping over curbs and difficulty walking in fields or over uneven ground or thick carpeting. Patients may notice difficulty standing on their toes while reaching for objects or during exercise classes. Patients may notice "slapping" feet caused by foot drop, and they may begin wearing high-topped shoes or boots to stabilize

Table 8.3. Classification of muscle disease based on pattern of muscle involvement

- I. Limb-girdle pattern
  - Inflammatory myopathies (polymyositis and dermatomyositis)
  - Multiple types of muscular dystrophy
    - Duchenne and Becker dystrophies
    - Limb-girdle muscular dystrophies
    - Emery–Dreifuss humeroperoneal dystrophy[a]
    - Congenital muscular dystrophies
  - Congenital myopathy
    - Nemaline myopathy[a]
    - Central core myopathy[a]
    - Centronuclear myopathy
- II. Predominantly distal weakness pattern
  - Distal myopathies
    - Late adult-onset distal myopathy (Welander)
    - Late adult-onset distal myopathy (Markesbery/Griggs)
    - Early adult-onset distal myopathy (Nonaka)
    - Early adult-onset distal myopathy (Miyoshi)
    - Early adult-onset distal myopathy (Laing)
  - Myofibrillar myopathy
  - Childhood-onset distal myopathy
  - Myotonic dystrophy
  - Facioscapulohumeral dystrophy[a]
  - Scapuloperoneal myopathy[a]
  - Inflammatory myopathies – inclusion body myositis
  - Sarcoidosis
  - Metabolic myopathies
    - Debrancher deficiency
- III. Scapuloperoneal pattern
  - Facioscapulohumeral muscular dystrophy
  - Scapuloperoneal dystrophy
  - Emery–Dreifuss dystrophy
  - Limb-girdle muscular dystrophies (especially types 1B, 2A, 2C–F, 2I)
  - Phosphorylase deficiency
  - Acid maltase deficiency
- IV. Distal upper-extremity/proximal lower-extremity pattern
  - Inclusion body myositis
- V. Ocular pattern causing ptosis or ophthalmoplegia
  - Ptosis usually without ophthalmoplegia
    - Myotonic dystrophy
  - Congenital myopathies
    - Centronuclear myopathy
    - Nemaline myopathy
    - Central core myopathy
  - Desmin storage myopathy (rarely)
  - Ptosis with ophthalmoplegia
    - Oculopharyngeal muscular dystrophy
    - Oculopharyngodistal myopathy
    - Mitochondrial chronic progressive external ophthalmoplegia
- VI. Prominent neck extensor pattern of weakness
  - Disorders with isolated or predominant neck extensor weakness
    - "Dropped head syndrome" [isolated neck extensor myopathy (INEM)]
    - Myasthenia gravis
    - Myopathy with hyperparathyroidism
    - Hyperthyroid myopathy
  - Disorders with neck extensor weakness in advanced stages and concurrent neck flexor weakness
    - Polymyositis
    - Dermatomyositis
    - Inclusion body myositis
    - Carnitine deficiency
    - Facioscapulohumeral dystrophy
    - Myotonic dystrophy
    - Congenital myopathy

Note: [a]Foot-drop can be an early/presenting feature.

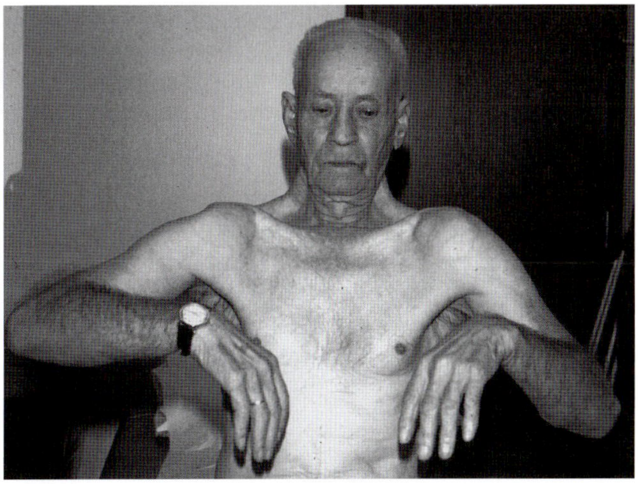

Figure 8.1. Patient with proximal weakness in predominantly limb-girdle pattern (polymyositis). The patient is trying to abduct his shoulders to 90°.

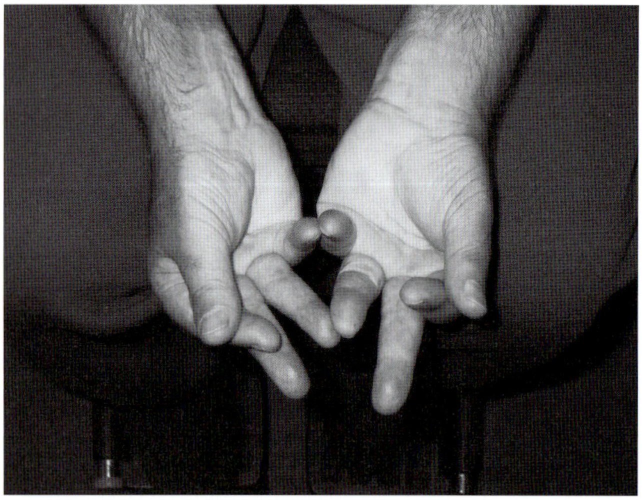

Figure 8.2. Patient with predominantly distal weakness (inclusion body myositis). The patient is attempting to make a fist bilaterally.

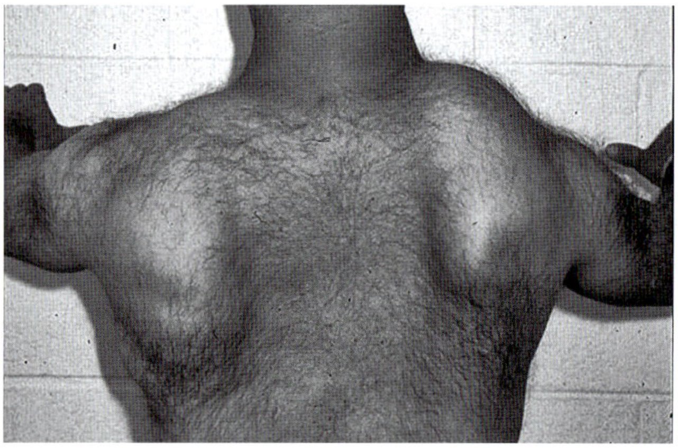

Figure 8.3. Facioscapulohumeral dystrophy. Note the scapular winging and elevation of the right scapula.

the ankle. Distal arm weakness produces difficulty opening car doors, turning keys, opening jars, wringing-out a cloth, picking up objects while shopping, and buttoning clothes.

An even less common pattern of weakness occurs when the proximal upper-extremity peri-scapular muscles and distal lower-extremity weakness of the anterior compartment are affected resulting in a *scapuloperoneal pattern* of involvement (video clip 3). This pattern is most frequently encountered in conjunction with facial weakness in the setting of facioscapulohumeral dystrophy. These patients often relate a history of prominent scapulae and "sloped-shoulders" noticed by classmates during gym class or sporting events at school (Figure 8.3). Some are criticized for their "poor posture." Others are noticed to have these features while trying on clothes or during a medical examination. Frequently, children or teenagers note difficulty doing activities involving the shoulders that are performed easily by peers, such as climbing trees or a rope, throwing a ball or swinging a golf club. The facial weakness in these patients is usually bilateral and

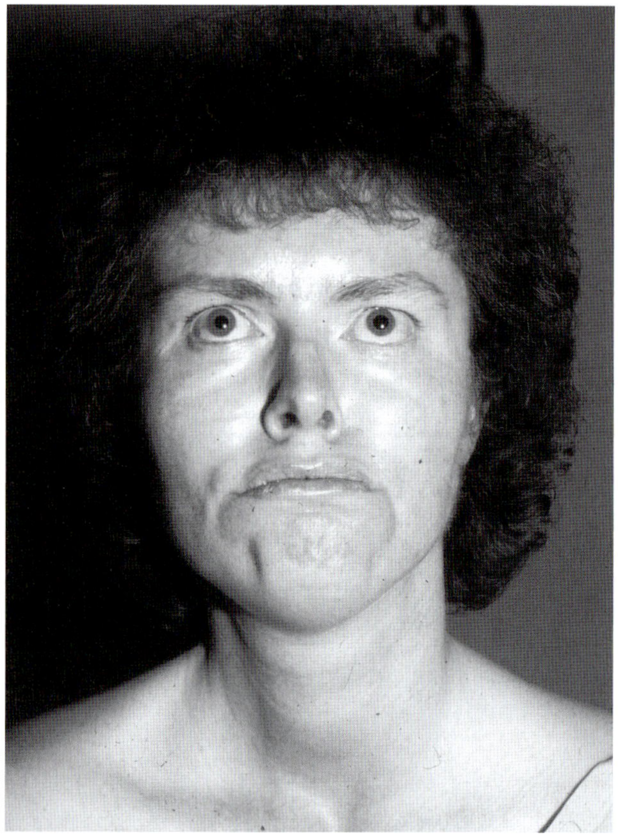

Figure 8.4. Facial appearance in facioscapulohumeral dystrophy. Note the prominence of the lips and mild lower lid ectropion.

relatively symmetrical; consequently, subtle facial weakness is often overlooked by the patient and naive examiner until it becomes severe. Frequently, patients are asymptomatic even with marked objective weakness. Questioning may elicit a history of having a "funny smile" (Figure 8.4), or difficulty blowing-up balloons, whistling, drinking through a straw, and clearing food caught between the lips and gums. One of our patients was even arrested when they were unable to blow into a police breath-alcohol analyzer! Severe facial weakness may also cause dysarthria.

Arguably, the most characteristic pattern of involvement is that of a combination of distal forearm wrist and finger flexor muscles, and quadriceps weakness. This *distal upper-extremity and proximal lower-extremity pattern* may be asymmetrical and is essentially pathognomonic for inclusion body myositis [4, 5] (video clip 4). These patients complain of difficulty lifting objects and doing fine manipulations, such as picking up coins, winding their wrist-watch, or doing crafts and hobbies. Such patients also complain of frequent falls caused by their "knees giving out," and difficulties going down stairs.

Predominant involvement of the *ocular muscles* produces a distinctive picture that results from a relatively restricted group of muscle disorders (Figure 8.5; video clip 5). Patients may complain of ptosis because of the cosmetic appearance noticed while shaving or putting on make-up, or because it is

a

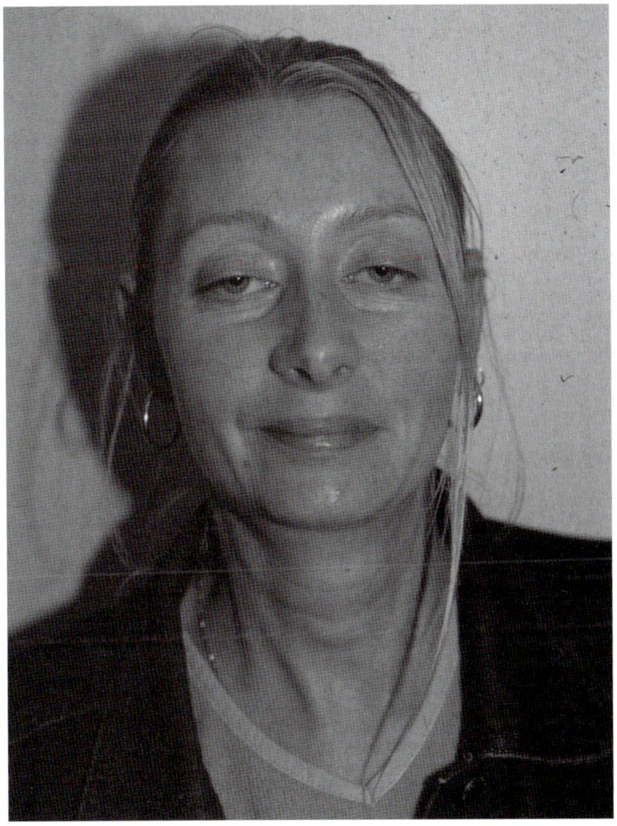

b

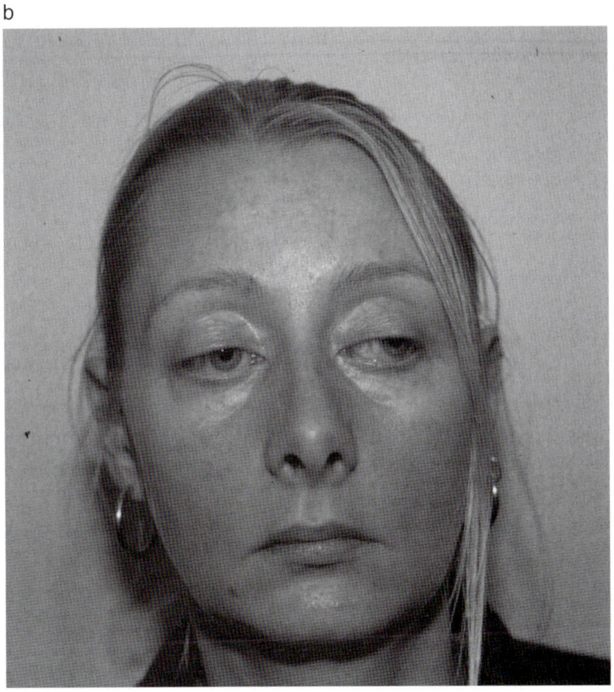

Figure 8.5a, b. Ophthalmoplegia/ptosis pattern. Note the ptosis (a) and external ophthalmoplegia (b). (b) The patient is trying to look to the extreme left but movement of each eye is incomplete.

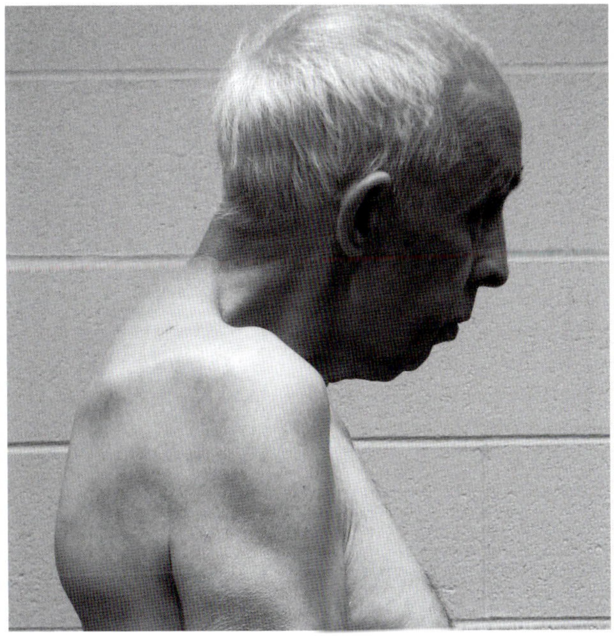

Figure 8.6. Neck extensor weakness (idiopathic neck extensor myopathy).

severe enough to cover the pupil and obscure vision. With mild or chronic ptosis, the lid droop is often first noticed by an acquaintance. When the onset of ptosis is uncertain, the examiner should request old pictures of the patient, which frequently will reveal mild ptosis long before it was noticed by the patient. Constant ptosis occurs in myotonic dystrophy, mitochondrial cytopathies, oculopharyngeal dystrophy, and several congenital muscle syndromes. Weakness of extraocular muscles may result in a history of diplopia, although in mitochondrial disorders diplopia is uncommon despite restricted eye movements because of the chronicity of the symptoms [6]. Diplopia rarely occurs in oculopharyngeal dystrophy and myotonic dystrophy. Variable ptosis and diplopia are pathognomonic of myasthenia gravis. Thyroid ophthalmopathy can produce ptosis, although it more commonly causes lid retraction and a history of staring; diplopia may be constant or fluctuating in this case.

A final, unusual but distinctive, pattern of muscle involvement occurs in those conditions that can present with a dramatic degree of weakness of the neck extensor muscles, often with relative sparing of the neck flexors. Patients with this *neck extensor pattern* (Figure 8.6; video clip 6) complain of difficulty looking forward, such as when watching television, and also of significant neck pain. Frequently the patient has to support the head with the hand when conversing with acquaintances. This pattern usually occurs superimposed on one of the previously described patterns, most commonly the limb-girdle syndromes. Predominant or isolated neck extensor weakness, although most commonly seen in association with amyotrophic lateral sclerosis and myasthenia gravis, can also occur as a distinct muscle disorder, a disorder sometimes referred to as "dropped head syndrome" or *isolated neck extensor myopathy* (INEM). When also associated with forward flexion of the whole spine, the term camptocormia is sometimes used [7], or axial myopathy [8].

Respiratory muscle involvement

Mild respiratory muscle weakness is usually asymptomatic. The earliest symptoms of respiratory failure are typically caused not by hypoxia directly but rather by fragmentation of sleep and retention of carbon dioxide. Typical symptoms include nightmares, frequent needs to be turned at night, early morning headache or confusion, and excessive daytime sleepiness. Other symptoms, the significance of which may easily be missed, include fear of going to bed and anorexia (you can't swallow and breathe at the same time). With increased severity, patients complain of shortness of breath on exertion and orthopnea. Respiratory insufficiency typically occurs in the later stages of disorders causing progressive weakness, such as Duchenne dystrophy, long after the patient has become wheelchair-dependent. Certain disorders, however, such as acid maltase deficiency, myasthenia gravis (rarely), critical illness myopathy, and carnitine palmitoyl-transferase deficiency may present with respiratory failure, or respiratory failure develops when the patient is still ambulant. Other conditions in which respiratory failure can develop while the patient is still ambulant include limb-girdle muscular dystrophy type 2I, Emery–Dreifuss syndrome, rigid spine muscular dystrophy, and various congenital myopathies (e.g., nemaline myopathy) [9]. Recognizing ventilatory failure [10] is of crucial importance because it is readily treatable, with marked symptomatic improvement, by noninvasive positive pressure ventilation techniques.

Pain

Muscle pain is by far the most common muscle complaint encountered by clinicians. In some population studies, up to 10% of individuals complained of diffuse muscle discomfort. Muscle pain is a nonspecific symptom that can arise from a variety of general medical, rheumatological, orthopedic, neurological, and psychiatric conditions. Even intense muscle pain may be unrelated to primary muscle disease. In fact, evaluation of patients with muscle pain alone (i.e., without accompanying weakness) usually does not reveal a muscle disease in the usual sense [11, 12, 13]; many of these patients are diagnosed with fibromyalgia [14]. Muscle pain is also often a major feature of the chronic fatigue syndrome, in which in the majority of patients there is no evidence of muscle pathology [15, 16]. Part of the difficulty in evaluating muscle pain relates to confusion in the patients' descriptions of their symptoms. Patients frequently use the word "pain" to refer to a number of abnormal sensations, including aching, stiffness, numbness, burning, restlessness, and swelling. Patients with cramping and contractures (see below) will also usually complain of muscle pain.

The most common muscle pain is a deep discomfort, often described as "burning" or "dull ache." This pain can be either focal and localized to an individual muscle or group of muscles (Table 8.4) or widespread and generalized (Table 8.5). Muscle conditions that cause focal pain usually involve local trauma, an infiltrating process (such as tumor or sarcoidosis), vascular disorders (either arterial ischemia or venous thrombophlebitis), local bacterial or parasitic infections, glycolytic metabolic disorders, and occasionally toxins (especially the statin agents). Diffuse myalgia is most common after viral infection but also occurs in polymyositis and dermatomyositis (but usually only when the onset is acute or subacute), toxic or infectious myopathies, and a few rare metabolic or endocrine myopathies. In most of these disorders, pain is accompanied by weakness, which can be mild to devastating. Diffuse myalgia without weakness is seen in polymyalgia rheumatica and fibromyalgia.

Table 8.4. Disorders causing localized muscle pain[a]

Trauma (including compartment syndromes)
Ischemia
Infection
• Bacterial
• Parasitic
Metabolic and toxic myopathies
• Acute alcoholic myopathy
• Some glycogenoses
• Statin myopathy
Inflammation
• Sarcoidosis
• Eosinophilic fasciitis
Neuralgic amyotrophy
Focal (compressive and ischemic) peripheral nerve lesions

Note: [a]But not necessarily primary myopathic disorders.

It is also useful to distinguish between pain present at rest (most of the conditions listed in Table 8.5) and that which comes on only during exercise, which usually suggests one of the metabolic myopathies (Table 8.6). Numerous drugs may also cause a painful myopathy (Table 8.7) and over the past decade, so-called "cholesterol lowering agent myopathy" (CLAM) or statin myopathy has become an increasingly common cause of diffuse muscle pain, with or without weakness [17, 18, 19, 20]. The origin of muscle pain in most conditions unfortunately remains uncertain even after extensive evaluations [13].

Contractures

The term contracture is used to refer to two different phenomena. In many chronic neuromuscular disorders, there is shortening of muscles and an inability to stretch the muscle passively to its proper length because of fibrosis. Such fixed contractures, which are in themselves painless, are rarely the

Table 8.5. Disorders causing generalized muscle pain[a]

Dermatomyositis and polymyositis (if acute/subacute)
Infections
• Viral (e.g., coxsackie, poliomyelitis)
• Toxoplasmosis
Drug-induced myopathies (see Table 8.7)
Steroid withdrawal
Metabolic myopathies
• Metabolic bone disease
• Hypothyroid myopathy
• CPT[b] deficiency
• Acute alcoholic myopathy
Polymyalgia rheumatica
Eosinophilia-myalgia syndrome
Connective tissue disorders
Guillain–Barré syndrome
Porphyria
Amyotrophic lateral sclerosis
Parkinson disease
In association with fever

Notes: [a]But not necessarily primary myopathic disorders. [b]CPT = carnitine palmitoyl-transferase.

Table 8.6. Disorders associated with exercise-induced muscle pain

Ischemia (claudication)
Muscular dystrophies
• Duchenne
• Becker
Metabolic myopathies
• Glycogenoses
• Mitochondrial cytopathies
• CPT[a] deficiency
• Brody syndrome
Tubular aggregate myopathy
Dermatomyositis

Note: [a]CPT = carnitine palmitoyl-transferase.

presenting complaint in patients with muscle disease since they are usually a late feature of most diseases. In a few disorders, such as Emery–Dreifuss dystrophy (Figure 8.7), Bethlem myopathy, LGMD type 1B (lamin A/C deficiency), and the rigid spine syndrome, contractures may be an early and striking feature affecting both limbs and spine.

Table 8.7. Drugs causing painful myopathy[a]

Amiodarone	Labetalol
Cimetidine	Statin lipid-lowering agents
Clofibrate	Nifedipine
Ciclosporin	D-Penicillamine
EACA[b]	Procainamide
Emetine	Salbutamol
Gemfibrozil	L-Tryptophan
Gold	Vincristine
Heroin	Zidovudine

Notes: [a]This list is incomplete and lists only the more commonly used drugs associated with painful myopathy. For more detailed discussion see Argov and Mastaglia, Chapter 24. [b]EACA = epsilon-aminocaproic acid.

The term contracture is also used to describe sustained, electrically silent, muscle contractions that produce hard nodules in the muscle and may persist for hours, in severe cases leading to myoglobinuria. Such contractures are painful, usually occur with exercise and are the hallmark of the glycolytic metabolic myopathies and a few other muscle disorders (Table 8.8). The pathogenesis of contractures in these conditions is poorly understood, although they probably result from a disturbance of high-energy metabolic pathways.

Cramps

Cramping is also accompanied by intense muscle pain and can produce a palpable mass in the muscle. Unlike contractures, cramps may occur at rest, are explosive in onset and short in duration, and may be relieved by passive stretching of the muscle. Electromyographic (EMG) study of a cramp reveals high-frequency motor unit discharges similar to a maximal contraction [21]. Cramps, particularly those in the gastrocnemius muscle, occur in all normal individuals. Although the etiology of cramps is uncertain, evidence suggests they originate in the intramuscular motor nerve terminals [22, 23]. As such, widespread cramps usually indicate neurogenic disease (e.g., amyotrophic lateral sclerosis, peripheral neuropathy) or metabolic disorders that alter the nerve microenvironment (e.g., hypothyroidism, dehydration, and uremia).

Stiffness and other muscle hyperactivity states

"Stiffness" is another word often used by patients to describe a number of different phenomena, some of which may be painful. Most commonly, the term is used to describe muscle that feels tight, is resistant to passive stretch, and does not relax normally. Stiffness can arise from a wide range of neurological disorders affecting every part of the neuraxis, as well as medical conditions that cause metabolic derangements which disrupt muscle relaxation [22]. Although stiffness and pain frequently overlap, many patients with excessive stiffness

a b

c

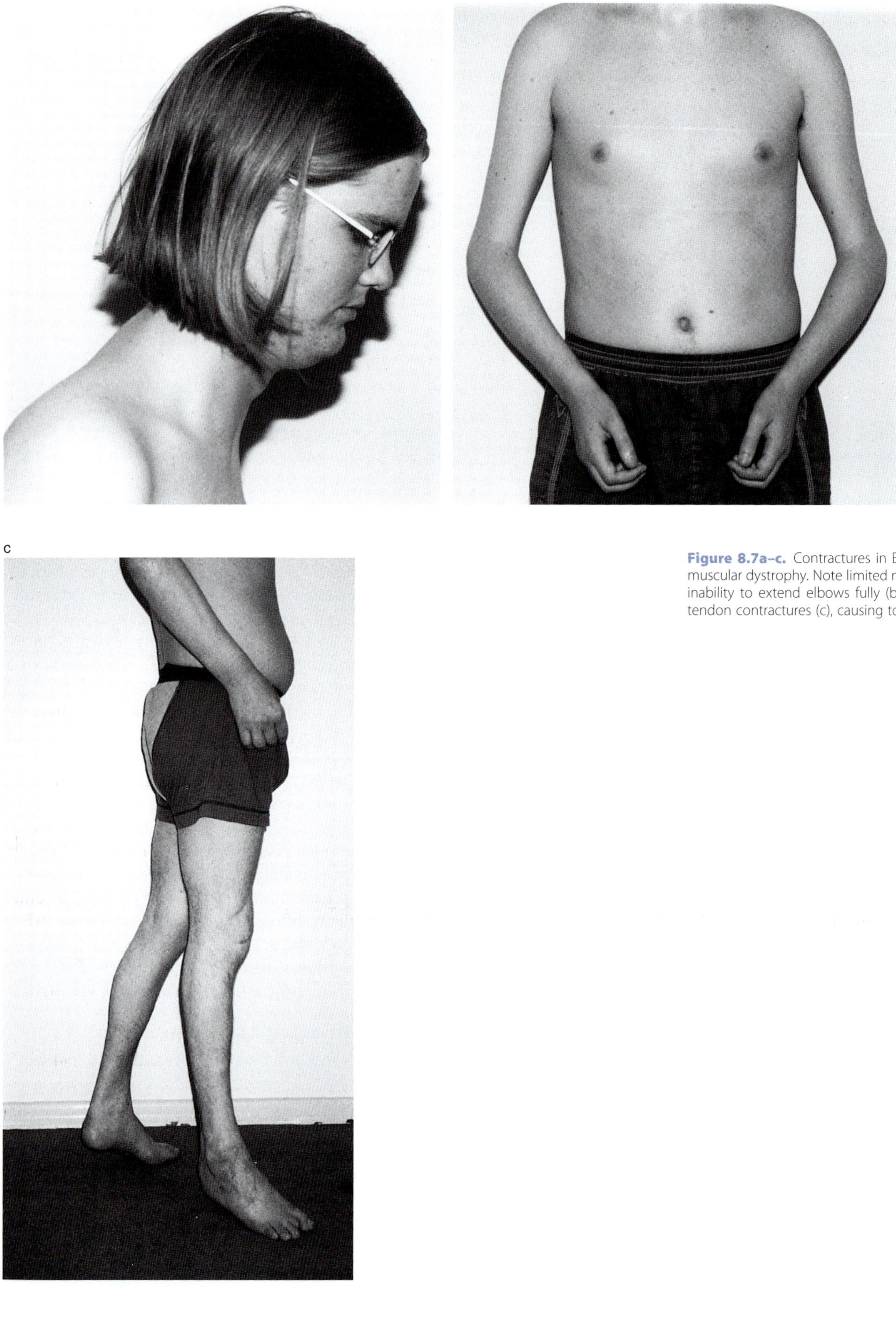

Figure 8.7a–c. Contractures in Emery–Dreifuss muscular dystrophy. Note limited neck flexion (a), inability to extend elbows fully (b), and Achilles tendon contractures (c), causing toe walking.

Table 8.8. Muscle disorders associated with contractures

Myopathies associated with glycolytic/glycogenolytic enzyme defects
Phosphorylase deficiency (McArdle disease)
Phosphofructokinase deficiency
Phosphoglycerate kinase deficiency
Phosphoglycerate mutase deficiency
Lactate dehydrogenase deficiency
Debrancher enzyme deficiency
Paramyotonia congenita
Hypothyroid myopathy with myoedema
Rippling muscle syndrome
Brody disease

related to central mechanisms (e.g., spasticity or rigidity) do not have significant pain.

Myotonia is the most common muscle phenomenon that results in stiffness. It is caused by recurrent depolarization of the muscle membrane, characterized on electrophysiological studies by waxing and waning rhythmical discharges (video clip 7). Patients experience stiffness and slowed relaxation, most evident after voluntary contraction and percussion of the muscle. Myotonia is seen in four main conditions. In myotonic dystrophy type 1, by far the most common condition associated with myotonia, patients complain of difficulty releasing objects after a firm grasp, or of stiffness in the hands and forearms [24]. Myotonia may also affect tongue movements and chewing, and some patients notice dysphagia because of myotonia in the upper esophagus. Patients usually complain more of weakness than myotonia. Patients with myotonic dystrophy may be asymptomatic, even when myotonia is evident on examination. Myotonic dystrophy type 2, formerly referred to as proximal myotonic myopathy (or PROMM), is characterized, as the name suggests, by predominantly proximal weakness and myotonia [25]. In these patients, the myotonia is frequently subclinical, and often detectable only with EMG, although patients frequently complain of stiffness and aching in affected muscles. In myotonia congenita, a chloride channelopathy, there is severe generalized myotonia, which is usually worse after rest and on initiation of movement [26, 27]. A severe episode of myotonia may be followed by transient weakness of the affected muscles. Facial muscles can be involved, resulting in a blepharospasm-like appearance after forceful eye closure. In the sodium channelopathies (paramyotonia congenita and hyperkalemic periodic paralysis), myotonia may be exacerbated by continued activity (paradoxical myotonia), whereas in the other conditions myotonia lessens with sustained action [27]. It may also be markedly exacerbated by cold. The facial, forearm, and hand muscles tend to be the most affected [26].

Some rare muscle disorders can also be associated with muscle stiffness. Brody syndrome is caused by a deficiency of sarcoplasmic reticulum calcium-ATPase, which causes exercised-induced stiffness and cramping, and slowed muscle relaxation [28]. Rippling muscle syndrome is either acquired (associated with myasthenia gravis) [29] or inherited (associated with mutations affecting caveolin-3) [30]. Patients complain of stiffness; on examination, stretching or percussion of muscle sets off waves of rippling [31].

Two neurogenic disorders with prominent muscle overactivity are neuromyotonia and stiff-person syndrome. Neuromyotonia, characterized by stiffness, cramps, myokymia, increased sweating and occasionally sensory symptoms, may be associated with a variety of inherited and acquired disorders. Autoimmunity is involved in at least some acquired disease [32, 33, 34]. In stiff-person syndrome, the axial and then limb muscles develop severe painful spasms and stiffness giving rise to spinal deformity and gait disturbance. Most cases are associated with antibodies to glutamic acid decarboxylase, an enzyme crucial in inhibitory GABAergic pathways [35, 36].

Fatigue

Fatigue refers to a sense of tiredness, lack of energy, and a tendency to avoid physical (and often mental) activities because of exhaustion [37]. Fatigue is a multifactorial phenomenon, depending upon the individual's emotional state, sleep habits, cardiopulmonary status, conditioning, and overall medical status [21, 37]. Although some myopathies (most notably mitochondrial disorders, some metabolic myopathies, and myotonic dystrophy), and neuromuscular junction disorders can be associated with significant fatigue, fatigue in isolation almost never indicates a primary myopathy. However, many patients with muscle disease and weakness complain of fatigue and decreased endurance, since they must perform routine activities with less muscle (the so-called overuse syndrome).

In patients complaining of fatigue and decreased endurance, it is important to determine exactly why certain activities cannot be performed, particularly in relation to other complaints. Patients often use the term weakness when trying to describe fatigue. For example, many fatigued patients will complain of inability to perform some routine activity, such as going up a flight of stairs or walking one block, because of weakness, when in reality they are simply too fatigued and exhausted and could accomplish the activity if strength alone were the issue. Motivation and emotional status are also important in this regard, as many patients with clinical depression will complain of weakness and fatigue.

Muscle wasting and enlargement

Patients with myopathic disorders rarely complain of muscle wasting as their primary complaint. Unlike neurogenic disease, where the degree of wasting often parallels weakness, wasting

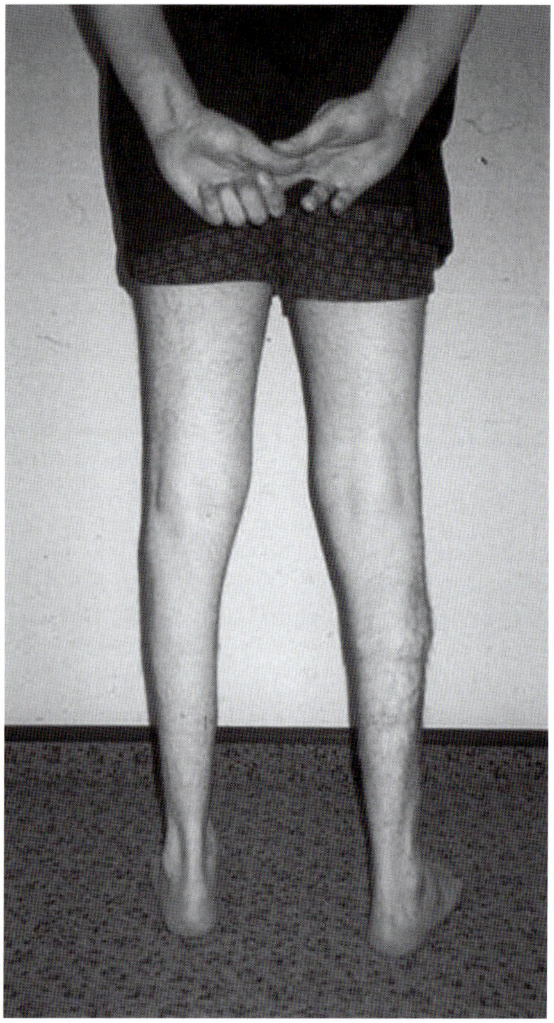

Figure 8.8. Distal pattern. Gastrocnemius atrophy in Miyoshi myopathy.

may be slight or absent in myopathies, even with severe weakness. Early wasting is often difficult for the patient (or examiner) to see, particularly if the patient is obese. In some diseases, wasting may be focal and affect only certain muscles. This can result in an unusual appearance that may bring the patient to medical attention; the marked gastrocnemius atrophy seen in some of the distal myopathies (Figure 8.8) (e.g., Miyoshi myopathy) is an example. In other disorders, wasting is evident only as the disease progresses and weakness becomes severe.

Muscle enlargement, either focal or generalized, is seen in a number of disorders (Table 8.9). True hypertrophy, which involves enlargement of muscle fibers as a result of repetitive activity, is seen in some cases of myotonia congenita (Figure 8.9) and neuromyotonia. In other instances, enlargement is better termed pseudohypertrophy and results from replacement of damaged muscle by fat and connective tissue. The pattern of muscle enlargement can help to suggest the diagnosis, the calf enlargement seen in boys with dystrophin-related dystrophies being the best example.

Table 8.9. Neuromuscular disorders associated with muscle hypertrophy or pseudohypertrophy

Muscular dystrophies
Duchenne/Becker
Manifesting carriers of Duchenne
Limb-girdle dystrophies
Myotonia congenita
Neuromyotonia
Spinal muscular atrophy
Spinal nerve root compression (e.g., S1 root irritation and calf hypertrophy)
Debrancher enzyme deficiency
Cysticercosis

Myoglobinuria

Any disorder that disrupts muscle membranes may allow release of myoglobin into the blood (myoglobinemia) and then excretion in urine (myoglobinuria) [38]. Patients typically notice discoloration of the urine ranging from light-brown to dark brown-black; they describe the urine as dark, smoky, rusty or like Coca-Cola or whisky. Such discoloration must be distinguished from other causes of pigmenturia, including drugs, hemolysis, and porphyria. Myoglobinuria, which may cause renal failure from acute tubular necrosis, is always paralleled by markedly increased serum CK. Some common causes of myoglobinuria are listed in Table 8.10.

Systemic symptoms

The review of systems, while too often neglected in the history taking, is nevertheless an extremely important part of the evaluation in neuromuscular disorders. Patients with myopathic complaints frequently will have symptoms related to other organ systems that can be very helpful in suggesting the type of muscle disease present. Other patients may present with chief complaints unrelated to skeletal muscle per se. Although frequently tedious, an accurate review of systems allows for the early identification of symptoms that suggest a myopathy and yet may have been overlooked by the patient, or that point towards a disease that involves systems other than muscle. Significant symptoms must be pursued by a review of old records or by discussions with the patient's primary care physician or other involved specialists. The following symptoms are discussed according to organ-system involvement.

Heart

Cardiac involvement in myopathies is common (Table 8.11) and may cause significant morbidity and mortality. It can assume many forms and involve either the contractile or

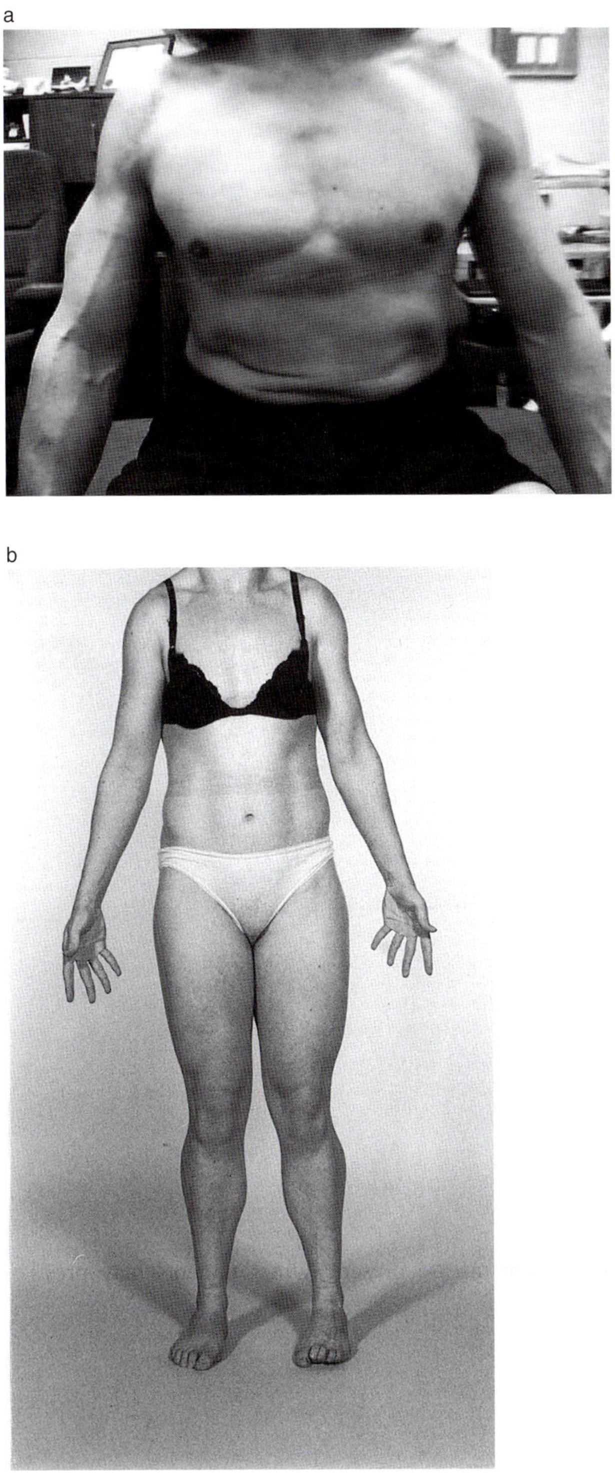

Figure 8.9a, b. Muscle enlargement in myotonia congenita.

Table 8.10. Causes of myoglobinuria

Intensive exercise in normal individuals

Inherited myopathies

- Metabolic
  - Glycogenoses (e.g., myophosphorylase deficiency)
  - Lipid disorders (e.g., carnitine palmitoyl-transferase deficiency)
  - Malignant hyperthermia
- Dystrophic
  - Duchenne and Becker

Acquired myopathies

- Dermatomyositis and polymyositis
- Infections
  - Viral
  - Bacterial

Ischemia and trauma

- Crush injury
- Status epilepticus
- Electric shock
- Arterial insufficiency

Drugs and toxins

- Alcohol
- Opiates
- Clofibrate
- Statins
- Snake venom
- Bacterial toxins
- Carbon monoxide

Others

- Neuroleptic malignant syndrome
- Severe metabolic disturbances
- Fever and heat stroke
- Idiopathic

conduction systems, producing symptoms of cardiac failure or arrhythmias, respectively. It can occasionally be difficult to distinguish respiratory symptoms caused by cardiac failure from those resulting from primary respiratory failure, and consultation with medical specialists is often indicated. It is crucial to identify cardiac involvement early since it may be amenable to therapy.

Liver

In both childhood and adult debranching enzyme deficiency, hepatomegaly may cause symptomatic protrusion of the abdomen. In branching enzyme deficiency, hepatomegaly is associated with ascites; without liver transplantation death ensues from hepatic failure. Neonatal and childhood liver

Table 8.11. Myopathies associated with cardiac involvement

Cardiomyopathy

- Duchenne and Becker muscular dystrophy
- Limb-girdle muscular dystrophy (rarely)
- Emery–Dreifuss syndrome (late)
- Dermatomyositis
- Infantile acid maltase deficiency
- Disorders of lipid metabolism
- Debranching enzyme deficiency
- Mitochondrial cytopathies
- Alcoholic cardiomyopathy
- Endocrine myopathies

Arrhythmias

- Myotonic dystrophy
- Emery–Dreifuss syndrome
- Mitochondrial cytopathies
- Periodic paralysis (particularly Andersen syndrome)

Table 8.12. CNS and eye symptoms and signs in mitochondrial disorders

- Stroke-like episodes
- Deafness
- Epilepsy
- Headache
- Ataxia
- Movement disorders
- Myoclonus
- Encephalopathy
- Dementia
- Dysphagia
- Pigmentary retinopathy
- Optic atrophy
- Progressive external ophthalmoplegia

involvement is common in disorders of carnitine metabolism and fatty acid β-oxidation and may be seen in the mitochondrial cytopathies.

Central nervous system

Mitochondrial cytopathies are frequently associated with central nervous system (CNS) symptoms and signs. CNS involvement, including ocular symptoms, may even be the presenting feature of these disorders (Table 8.12). Some CNS involvement also occurs in dystrophinopathies, where the intelligence quotient (IQ) of patients averages lower than controls. This difference is often not apparent in individual patients and seldom helps in making a diagnosis. In contrast, the lower IQ and personality differences seen in myotonic dystrophy are usually more apparent; patients with congenital myotonic dystrophy invariably require special-needs schooling. A lower than average IQ is also a feature of some congenital myopathies. An interesting example of asymptomatic CNS involvement with muscle disease occurs in congenital muscular dystrophy with laminin-α2 chain (merosin) deficiency, where white matter hypomyelination is seen by magnetic resonance imaging (MRI), but patients rarely have intellectual impairment [39, 40]. In contrast, severe CNS, and sometimes eye, involvement is seen in the congenital muscular dystrophies relating to abnormality of α-dystroglycan glycosylation, such as Walker–Warburg syndrome and muscle–eye–brain disease [41].

Table 8.13. Disorders that can affect both skeletal muscle and peripheral nerves

- Alcohol
- Amyloidosis
- Chronic renal failure
- Collagen vascular disorders
  - Rheumatoid arthritis
  - Systemic lupus erythematosus
  - Systemic vasculitides
- Drugs
  - Gold
  - Vincristine
- Endocrinopathies
  - Acromegaly
  - Hypothyroidism
- Malnutrition
- Mitochondrial cytopathies
- Paraneoplastic syndromes
- Sarcoidosis

Peripheral nervous system

As already discussed, patients often use words like deadness or numbness to describe muscle weakness. Occasionally, patients may even say that touching the affected extremity does not "feel" normal. There are, however, many disorders that may involve both muscle and peripheral nerve and, therefore, produce symptoms referable to both systems (Table 8.13). In these patients, it is important not to misinterpret the sensory complaints as indicating involvement of only the peripheral nervous system.

Table 8.14. Endocrine disorders that can cause a myopathy

- Hypothyroidism
- Hyperthyroidism
- Graves ophthalmopathy
- Cushing syndrome
- Addison disease
- Hyperparathyroidism
- Hypoparathyroidism
- Acromegaly
- Hypopituitarism
- Primary hyperaldosteronism
- Phaeochromocytoma

Eyes

Ptosis and altered ocular motility are the most common ocular symptoms related to muscle disease (as discussed above). Other ocular problems, however, may also be associated with myopathies. Pigmentary retinopathy, optic atrophy or both may occur with mitochondrial disorders, but symptomatic visual impairment is unusual [42]. Eye involvement with severe visual failure may be seen in some congenital muscular dystrophies, as noted above.

Endocrine system

Although most endocrinopathies can, if severe enough, produce a myopathy (Table 8.14), the almost universal availability of rapid biochemical screening for most hormones has rendered clinically significant endocrine myopathies very uncommon [43]. It is still important, however, to question patients about symptoms that may be related to an underlying endocrinological disorder. Myasthenia gravis is associated with an increased incidence of thyroid dysfunction (and vice versa), which may exacerbate the myasthenia. Mitochondrial cytopathies have been linked with several endocrine disorders, including diabetes mellitus. A specific form of periodic paralysis, thyrotoxic periodic paralysis, is linked to hyperthyroidism.

Kidneys

Myoglobinuria as a cause of renal damage has already been discussed. Chronic renal failure from any cause, along with dialysis and subsequent renal tubular acidosis, can cause myopathy through several mechanisms [43].

Gastrointestinal system

Many neuromuscular disorders affect the gastrointestinal tract; conversely, a number of bowel disorders cause myopathy. The most common gastrointestinal-related symptom in myopathic patients is dysphagia, which usually relates to weakness of the pharyngeal muscles and upper third of the esophagus. Dysphagia is particularly prominent in myotonic dystrophy, oculopharyngeal dystrophy, inclusion body myositis, and myasthenia gravis. Gastric stasis and intestinal dysmotility causing bowel pseudo-obstruction, and constipation may result from involvement of smooth muscle, as in myotonic dystrophy. More frequently, constipation can arise from simple immobility resulting from generalized weakness. In myotonic dystrophy, symptoms similar to irritable bowel syndrome, and fecal soiling in childhood, are common. In the rare MNGIE syndrome (mitochondrial myopathy, peripheral neuropathy, gastrointestinal disease, and encephalopathy), nausea, vomiting, and diarrhea are caused by gut dysmotility [44, 45].

Skin

The muscle disease most commonly associated with skin involvement is dermatomyositis. The "classic" heliotrope discoloration of the eyelids is much less frequent than erythema of the face and upper chest (sun-exposed areas) and of the hands, particularly over the knuckles (Figure 8.10). Raynaud phenomenon can also occur in this disorder. Various types of skin rash can result from underlying vasculitis, which may also involve muscle. Such rashes occasionally bring patients to medical attention before weakness is symptomatic. Other rare cutaneous manifestations of myopathy include lipomatosis, a feature of some mitochondrial disorders (Figure 8.11), and jaundice, which is seen in approximately 25% of those with phosphofructokinase deficiency. Collagen VI disorders (e.g., Ullrich myopathy) are often associated with cutaneous features including abnormal scarring and hyperkeratosis pilaris (sandpaper-like skin).

Past medical history

The past medical history should focus predominantly on four key areas. Firstly and most importantly, the presence of any underlying illnesses associated with muscle involvement needs to be identified. These disorders include the various connective tissue disorders, endocrine disturbances, and renal or hepatic failure. Secondly, any disorder associated with peripheral neuropathy or other symptoms that may be confused with a myopathy must be identified (e.g., diabetes mellitus). Similarly, it is crucial to recognize prior surgeries (such as cervical or lumbar laminectomies, thoracic outlet surgery, carpal tunnel release) that may affect the neurological history or examination and the patient's functional status. A third key area concerns anesthetic exposure. Many myopathies cause subclinical respiratory muscle involvement that is asymptomatic until the patient is stressed with general anesthesia. A history of being "difficult to wake up" or needing prolonged assisted ventilation after general anesthesia can be important clues to the presence of an underlying muscle disorder. Such a history is often obtained from patients with myotonic dystrophy, who also may give a history of peri- or postoperative cardiac arrhythmias. Patients with subclinical myasthenia gravis also may present with acute

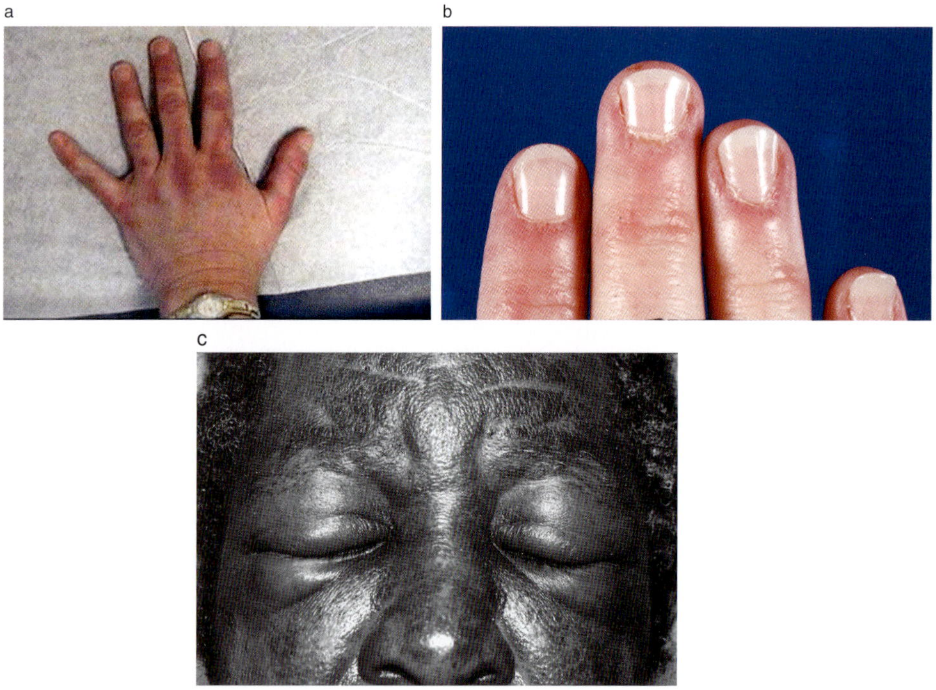

Figure 8.10a–c. Skin rash in dermatomyositis. Erythema over the knuckles (a) and dilatation of nail-bed capillaries (b). (c) The facial rash in an African-American.

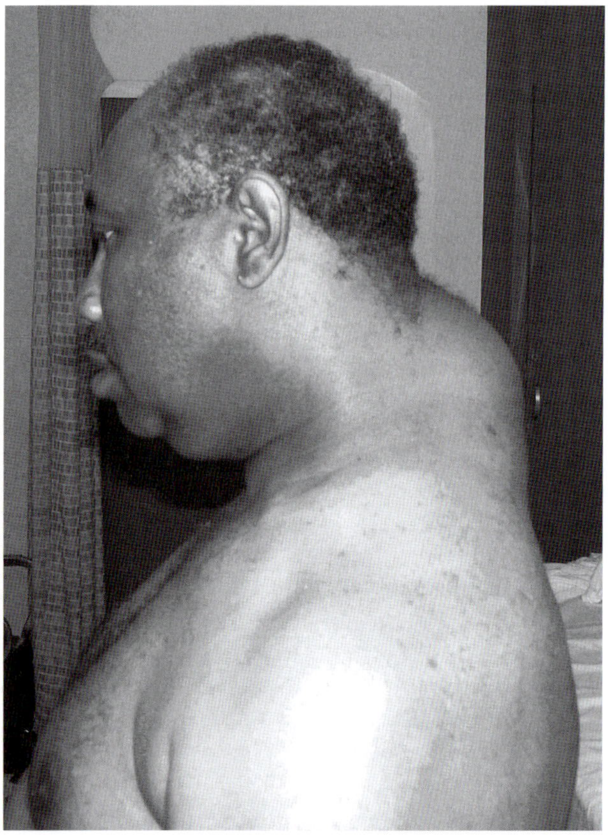

Figure 8.11. Lipomatosis in mitochondrial cytopathy.

deterioration following either anesthetic agents or neuromuscular blockers. A history of malignant hyperthermia with general anesthesia is also a "red flag" for an occult myopathy. Although malignant hyperthermia frequently occurs in isolation or in association with central core disease, anesthesia-induced hyperthermic reactions may also occur in patients with Duchenne or Becker muscular dystrophy [46].

Table 8.15. Drugs causing painless myopathy[a]

- Amiodarone
- Chloroquine
- Colchicine
- Corticosteroids
- Heroin
- Hypokalemia-inducing drugs (e.g., diuretics)
- Perhexiline

Note: [a]This list is incomplete and lists only the more commonly used drugs associated with painless myopathy. For more detailed references see Chapter 24.

A final important area in the history relates to past and current medication use and toxin exposure. The examiner must identify all legal or illicit medications the patient is taking, over-the-counter products as well as all nutritional or vitamin supplements and even homeopathic remedies. In this context, a history of hypercholesterolemia or hyperlipidemia may be a clue that a statin agent has been used at some time in the past. The common pharmacological agents associated with myopathy are listed in Table 8.7 and 8.15; these agents are discussed more extensively in Chapter 24.

Family history

The family history is of obvious importance in patients with suspected muscle disease, but obtaining an accurate family history can sometimes require a great deal of effort by the examiner. A common mistake is asking vague general questions concerning whether any family members have a similar disease as the patient, an approach that is often unproductive. Rather, it is essential to ask specifically about the health, functional status, and associated medical conditions of each family member in the nuclear group (parents, siblings, and children). Questions addressed to specific issues, such as the need for canes, braces or wheelchairs, functional limitations and postural or skeletal deformities, are often more rewarding than questions about muscle diseases. Frequently, family members have been diagnosed with "arthritis" or various orthopedic disorders when a muscle disorder was actually present. The examiner also must address the fact that family members may be very reluctant to discuss the possibility of a genetic disorder and even try to deceive family members and physicians. In some families, particularly those with certain autosomal dominant disorders (e.g., facioscapulohumeral dystrophy), phenotypic variability may be such that even those carrying the abnormal gene can be asymptomatic. This phenomenon is typical in conditions such as myotonic dystrophy, which show true genetic anticipation, and facioscapulohumeral dystrophy in which females tend to be less severely affected. If an inherited disorder is being considered and the parents are living, consideration should be given to their assessment, even if asymptomatic, but with due thought and discussion – there are numerous potential ethical and practical issues relating to possibly unwanted diagnosis in an asymptomatic individual. An important point in this regard, however, is that because of possible spontaneous mutations or genetic heterogeneity, even a negative evaluation of parents and other family members does not necessarily rule out an inherited myopathy.

Social history

Relatively few aspects of the social history are pertinent to the diagnosis of the patient with suspected myopathy. Information about alcohol consumption and tobacco use is of obvious importance, although "alcoholic myopathy" is an uncommon and controversial entity. Information on recreational drug exposure and sexual preference are important clues to possible muscle disease related to human immunodeficiency virus (HIV). Even initial denial of such risk factors should not be accepted without question in the appropriate clinical situation. Conversely, but not discussed further here, the consequences of a muscle disorder on the patient's social functioning are often dramatic and should be explored in this part of the history.

Physical examination

The examination of the patient with a suspected muscle disorder flows naturally from, and is directed by, information gleaned from the history. Given the associations between myopathies and general medical disorders, the examination cannot be confined to assessment of the muscles alone but rather must encompass a general examination. Systems suspected to be involved because of information obtained in the history of the present illness or review of systems must receive special attention. Examination of the cardiovascular and pulmonary systems is always indicated. The goal is to identify a systemic disorder that may be associated with myopathy.

A neurological examination to exclude possible central or peripheral nervous system disorders that might explain the patient's symptoms should be performed in all patients. A more detailed CNS examination is essential in patients suspected of having a mitochondrial cytopathy (Table 8.12). The retinopathy in these disorders is mainly peripheral and, therefore, it may be necessary to dilate the pupils to detect it. Hearing loss may be mild and easily overlooked. Examination of the peripheral nervous system, including sensory examination, is also vital, not only to exclude neurogenic disorders from the differential diagnosis but also because a number of conditions can involve both nerves and muscle (Table 8.13). The following section will focus on the muscle examination but will not review basic techniques, which should be familiar to all clinicians. Of course, the examination really begins as soon as the patient enters the consulting room and continues during the history taking, before being formalized in the standard examination.

Muscle examination

All too often, the muscle assessment is restricted to "pushing and pulling" on muscles to assess strength, with little attention paid to other aspects of the examination. A complete skeletal muscle examination includes the classic components of inspection, palpation, and percussion.

Inspection and palpation

The muscle examination should always begin with an adequate inspection of the undressed but appropriately gowned patient. The muscles under inspection should be completely relaxed, so that a patient's efforts to support the limb do not result in subtle voluntary contractions that may be misinterpreted as fasciculations. Any wasting or hypertrophy and any involuntary movements (e.g., fasciculation, rippling, myokymia) should be noted, in addition to any skeletal abnormalities, such as pectus excavatum, kyphoscoliosis or scapular winging. Inspection is best performed by region, including the individual limbs and the entire back and trunk. Such an approach helps to identify patterns of muscle and orthopedic findings that can be useful diagnostically, such as the shoulder and pectoral findings in facioscapulohumeral dystrophy (Figure 8.3). Palpating the muscles is appropriate during this phase of the examination. Palpation may help to detect subtle atrophy not readily apparent on inspection. Rarely, a mass or nodule can be palpated, as with an abscess or diabetic muscle infarction. Palpation also permits assessment of muscle texture; for example, the doughy feel of the gastrocnemius in

Table 8.16. Muscles/actions that should be assessed in patients with suspected neuromuscular disease

- Cranial nerve innervated muscles
  - Eyelid elevation
  - Eye movement
  - Facial muscles
  - Palatal movements
  - Neck flexion/extension
  - Shoulder shrugging
  - Tongue movements
- Limbs and trunk
  - Scapula – fixation
  - Shoulder – abduction and adduction
  - Elbow – flexion and extension
  - Wrist – flexion and extension
  - Finger – flexion, extension, and abduction
  - Hip – flexion and extension
  - Knee – flexion and extension
  - Ankle – dorsiflexion and plantar flexion
  - Trunk – sitting from lying
  - Gait – assess walking, running, walking on heels and tip-toe
- Respiratory muscles
  - Diaphragm – movement on inspiration

patients with Duchenne dystrophy or the fibrotic, ropey feel of muscles replaced by connective tissue and fat in patients with various dystrophies can be appreciated.

Strength assessment

Strength assessment is clearly the most important aspect of the muscle examination. In general, groups of muscles having specific actions on a joint should be tested rather than individual muscles (Table 8.16). With rare exceptions, it is important that a standard group of muscles be tested in every patient, with more specific testing performed as indicated by the presenting symptoms. For example, in patients with mainly proximal involvement, the examiner should assess other shoulder muscles, such as the supra- and infraspinatus, as well as other muscles around the hips, such as the hip abductors, adductors, and internal and external rotators. If there is evidence of mainly distal weakness, other distal functions should be examined, such as the long finger flexors and extensors, intrinsic hand muscles, ankle eversion and inversion, and the small muscles of the feet. Selective involvement of specific muscles in the same anatomical area is typical for many muscular dystrophies. In facioscapulohumeral dystrophy, for example,

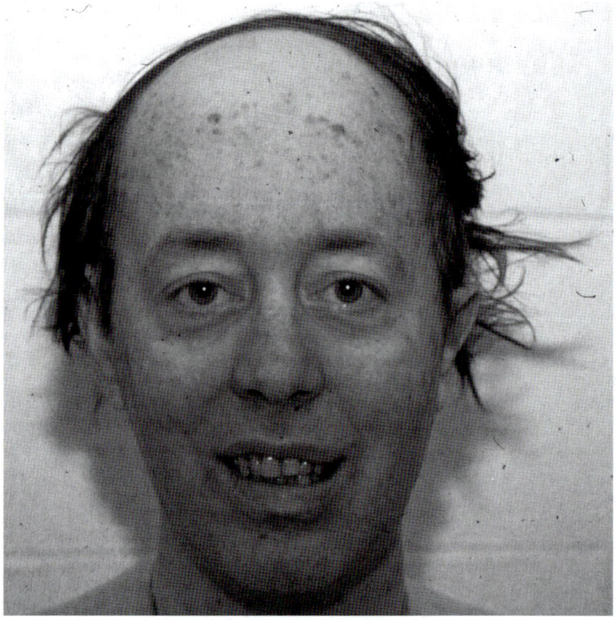

Figure 8.12. Temporal wasting in myotonic dystrophy.

the biceps and triceps are significantly affected but the deltoids are usually relatively spared.

No aspect of the muscle examination is more important in providing clues to the diagnosis than the pattern of muscle weakness. The common patterns of weakness encountered in myopathy patients have already been discussed above in relation to the history (video clips 1–6). From the examination perspective, it is convenient to consider separately muscles innervated by the cranial nerves, limb and trunk muscles, and the respiratory muscles, since different methods are involved in testing these areas.

Cranial nerve innervated muscle

Mild ptosis and ophthalmoplegia may be subtle and difficult to detect on examination. Patients with significant ptosis may tilt their head backwards, raise their eyebrows or wrinkle their foreheads in an attempt to look out from under ptotic lids (referred to as "overactivity of frontalis"). When assessing ptosis and eye movement, it is crucial to check for fatigability in addition to weakness and restriction of movement. Wasting and atrophy of the temporalis muscles may produce the "hatchet face" appearance characteristic of myotonic dystrophy (Figure 8.12), although it may occur in other disorders. The masseters are best tested by having the patient clench their teeth and move the jaw from side to side while the masseter is palpated. The most common disorder resulting in masseter weakness is myasthenia gravis.

Mild symmetrical facial weakness can also be difficult to detect. Although patients often have a somewhat blank, drooped, "myopathic" expression, this may easily be overlooked on cursory examination, particularly if it is the examiner's first encounter with the patient. Asking the patient to smile broadly, show their teeth, wrinkle their forehead, blow a

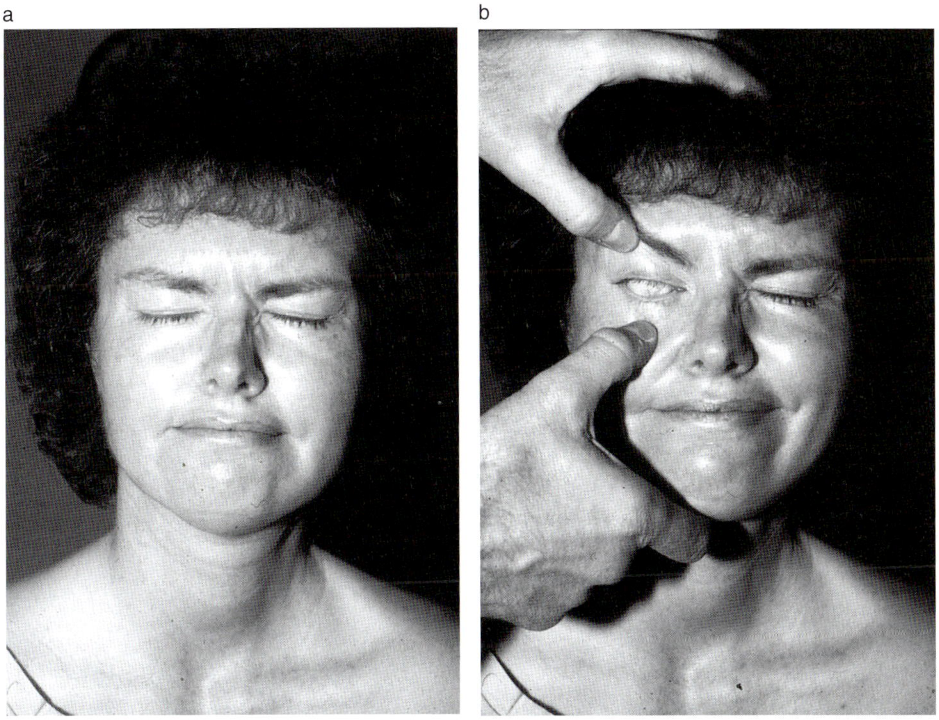

Figure 8.13a, b. Failure to bury eyelashes with eye closure (a) and demonstration of weak eye closure (b) (perform with great care!).

kiss, and whistle may bring out the abnormalities. One sensitive test is to ask the patient to close their eyes tightly: failure to bury the eyelashes completely indicates weakness (Figure 8.13). Another method is to try to force the eyelids open with the thumbs, although this is sometimes poorly tolerated by the patient. Pursing the lips can be helpful in patients with facioscapulohumeral dystrophy, where involvement is often asymmetrical, particularly in the orbicularis oris muscle, resulting in an odd, twisted smile with dimpling at the corner of the mouth and a depressed and "flat" appearance to the patient's face. When asked to whistle or blow a kiss, the lips frequently form a characteristic transverse or horizontal configuration (Figure 8.14). Significant facial weakness also results in hollow sounding speech, and, if the lips are affected, difficulty pronouncing consonants such as b, f, m, and p.

Speech is an excellent method for assessing tongue and palate strength. Palatal weakness produces speech that is nasal and "airy," with difficulty pronouncing sounds such as k and the hard g. In contrast, tongue weakness produces thick, slurred speech and difficulty with sounds such as d, l, n, and t. Having the patient protrude the tongue and push forward and sideways against a tongue-blade is another way to assess tongue strength. Swallowing can be assessed by observing the patient eat and drink. The time taken to swallow a certain fluid volume, or the number of swallows taken, may be recorded as an objective measure of swallowing.

Many muscle disorders cause weakness of the neck flexors and extensors. These muscles can be tested in the supine and prone positions, respectively, so that their actions against gravity can be determined. Neck flexor weakness with relatively

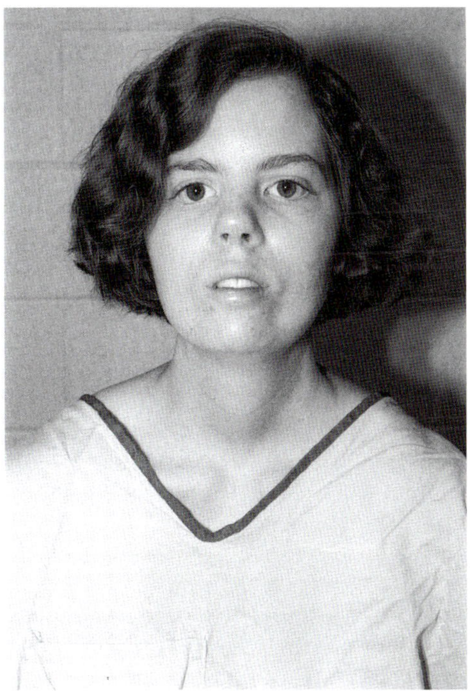

Figure 8.14. Transverse smile in facioscapulohumeral dystrophy.

preserved extensor strength can be seen in many conditions and is common in disorders such as myotonic dystrophy, myasthenia gravis, and the inflammatory myopathies. Preferential involvement of the neck extensors is much less common and, as discussed above, it may be seen in myasthenia gravis,

Table 8.17. MRC scale of muscle strength

Grade 0	No contraction
Grade 1	Flicker of contraction
Grade 2	Active movement, with gravity eliminated
Grade 3	Active movement against gravity
Grade 4–	Active movement against slight resistance
Grade 4	Active movement against moderate resistance
Grade 4+	Active movement against strong resistance
Grade 5	Normal power

poly- or dermatomyositis, myotonic dystrophy, and the so-called dropped head syndrome or isolated neck extensor myopathy [7, 47].

Limb and trunk muscles

Table 8.16 lists muscle groups that should be tested in all patients presenting with a suspected muscle problem. The findings on this basic screening, as well as the patient's specific symptoms, will indicate if other limb muscles should be tested. Although the basic procedure of manual muscle testing is familiar to all clinicians, several aspects deserve comment. The first point when assessing strength is that it is crucial to have the patient in the appropriate position for testing each muscle, both to assess function against gravity and to provide the optimum opportunity to detect subtle weakness. Hip abductors, for example, should never be tested in the seated position; rather the patient should be placed on their side. It is also crucial to test muscle groups on both sides of the body, as the degree of symmetry or asymmetry of involvement may also help guide the diagnosis.

Most clinicians employ the positions, methods, and 5-point grading scale outlined in *Aids to the Examination of the Peripheral Nervous System* [48] (Table 8.17). Although there may be considerable inter- and intraobserver variability with this grading scale, clinical trials have shown that manual testing can be accurate and reproducible if performed by experienced evaluators [49]. Clinicians familiar with this scheme who use it routinely find it invaluable in documenting the status of their patients. Various computerized systems have been developed, most of which employ strain gauge tensiometers or hand-held dynamometers that record the maximal force a muscle can generate and then compare the values with those of age- and sex-matched controls [50, 51]. These systems are widely used in clinical trials but are not available to most clinicians for routine clinical use.

A second major point concerning muscle testing is that accurate strength determinations cannot be made in patients who do not give a maximal effort or who are in significant pain. Frequently, joint pain results in a rapid collapse of the extremity during manual muscle testing that is misinterpreted as weakness. Patients with psychogenic or functional

Table 8.18. Simple bedside tests of muscle function

- Lying supine on examining table and lifting head
- Lying supine on examining table and lifting lower limb straight up. Measure heel–couch distance
- Sitting up from lying
- Standing up from "standard" chair – with or without use of upper limbs
- Stepping onto a standard stool, beginning with each leg
- Rising from a squat
- Time to walk a specific distance
- Distance walked in a specific time (e.g., the 6-min walk test)
- Ability to run and hop
- Ability to walk on heels and on tip-toe
- Ability to climb steps in "child" or "adult" fashion[a]
- Raising arms over the head

Note: [a]For example, one at a time or one after another.

"weakness" may also give-way suddenly when tested. These patients often adjust the resistance they offer to match the force applied by the examiner. Patients with genuine weakness rarely "give-way" in this fashion; rather, they offer resistance that, although not normal, is uniform through the range of motion.

The final, and perhaps most important, point concerning manual muscle testing is that it represents only part of the strength assessment and should never be interpreted in isolation. Rather, the results of manual muscle testing must always be assessed in conjunction with simple bedside functional tests, which, although not truly quantitative, nevertheless give a clearer picture of the patient's abilities and how they are compromised by weakness. Such functional analyses are also informative in younger children, where detailed manual muscle testing is usually not feasible. Table 8.18 lists the most useful functional tests performed in the clinic. Many experienced clinicians feel that this type of functional testing is superior to manual muscle testing in determining whether a patient's weakness is improving or worsening and is less subject to interobserver variability [52]. A patient with mild lower limb weakness, for example, may be able to walk normally and get up from a chair without pushing with the arms but may not be able to rise from a squat. The subsequent ability to rise from a squat provides convincing evidence that improvement has occurred. Conversely, an inability to rise from a chair as well as rise from a squat would indicate that there has likely been deterioration.

Functional testing is also the best way to assess axial strength and muscle fatigability. Weakness of truncal muscles may be evident when the patient tries to sit up from lying. With greater weakness there may be spinal deformity in the form of scoliosis or kyphosis, a common finding in Duchenne dystrophy, many of the congenital and limb-girdle dystrophies, and several congenital myopathies. Fatigue, a pronounced feature in myasthenia gravis and some metabolic myopathies, may be assessed by timing the number of seconds a patient can stand with outstretched arms, or by counting the number of squats the patient can perform in a row.

Respiratory muscles

Patients may have advanced respiratory muscle insufficiency before they develop symptoms of respiratory failure and signs at the bedside become obvious. It is imperative to assess respiratory function, particularly in patients with muscle disorders associated with diaphragmatic weakness, such as Duchenne dystrophy, acid maltase deficiency, myotonic dystrophy, and some congenital myopathies. At the bedside, respiratory reserve can be estimated by having the patient take a deep breath and count slowly while exhaling. The availability of hand-held spirometers permits easy and more accurate testing of forced vital capacity [53]. As respiratory weakness progresses, paradoxical movement of the abdominal wall may be observed. Normally, on inspiration, the upper abdomen moves outward as the diaphragm descends. If the diaphragm is weak it is drawn up on inspiration by negative intrathoracic pressure, and the abdominal wall moves inwards. The use of accessory muscles, including the sternocleidomastoid and other cervical muscles, may also be observed (video clip 8).

Percussion of muscle and abnormal relaxation phenomena

Although usually not a major part of the muscle examination, muscle percussion can elicit several reactions helpful in suggesting diagnoses. By far the most common of these phenomena is percussion myotonia, best elicited by sharply tapping the thenar eminence with a reflex hammer (Figure 8.15; video clip 9). Percussion myotonia is most commonly seen in myotonic dystrophy but is more widespread and severe in myotonia congenita (Figure 8.16). Patients with one of the sodium channelopathies or proximal myotonic myopathy may also have percussion myotonia. Most of these disorders also cause grip myotonia, demonstrated by asking the patient to grip the examiner's fingers tightly for several seconds and then release rapidly (Figure 8.17; video clip 10). Muscle percussion can also elicit myoedema, or mounding-phenomenon, which manifests as a muscle ridge or lump that may persist for many seconds. This rare phenomenon is usually seen in the setting of myxedema or severe malnutrition. Percussion, or relaxation after contraction, may trigger the phenomenon of muscle rippling (video clip 11), the causes of which were noted above.

Reflex testing

As in all neurological disease, reflex testing is an important part of the examination of patients with suspected muscle disease. As a rule, tendon reflexes are normal in myopathies until late in the course, when wasting and weakness are advanced. There are, however, several important exceptions

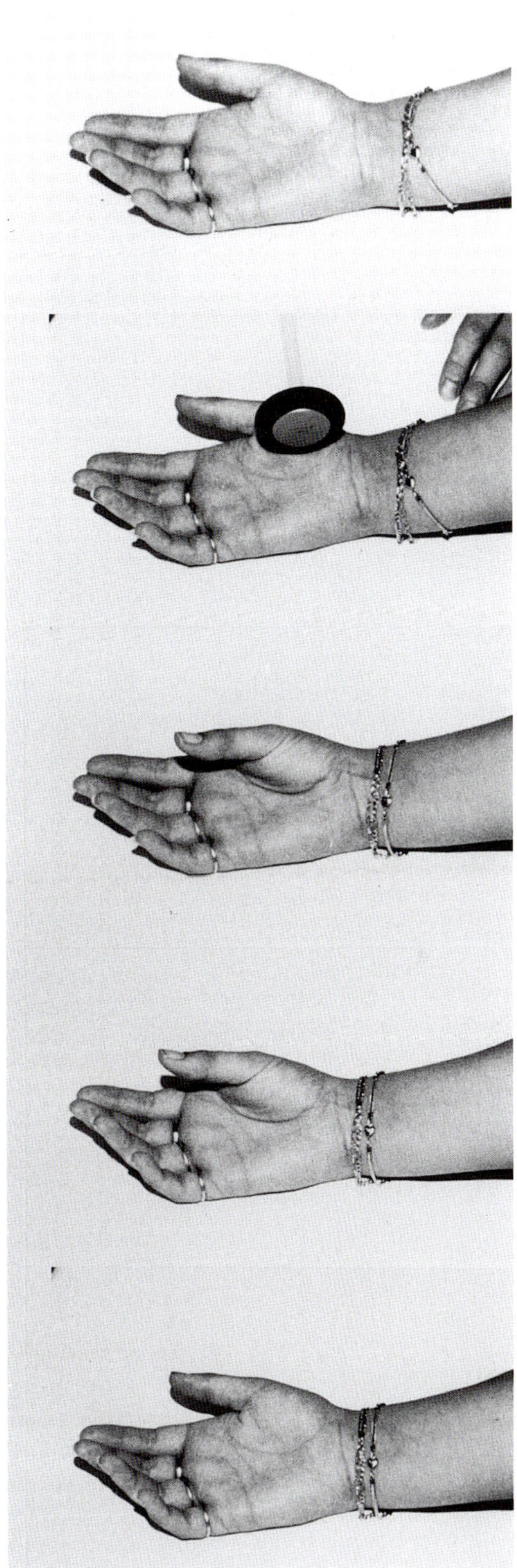

Figure 8.15. Percussion myotonia in myotonic dystrophy. The thenar eminence is given a sharp tap with the tendon hammer – subsequent pictures taken at 2-second intervals.

a

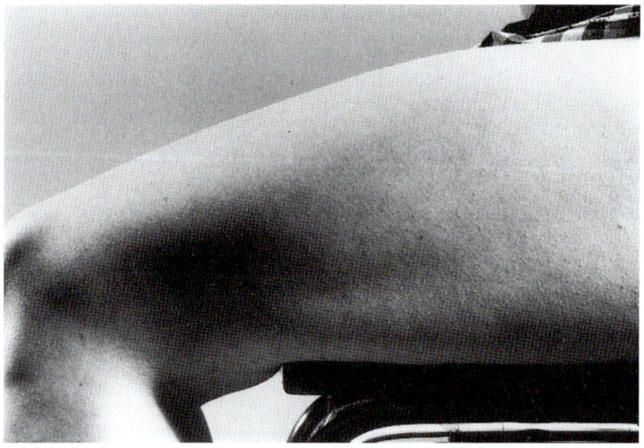

b

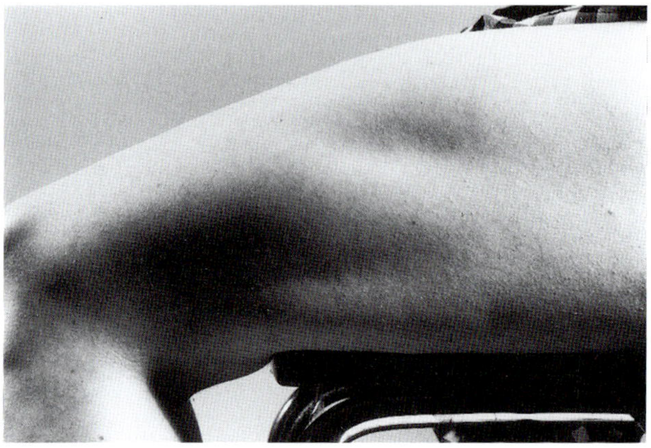

Figure 8.16a, b. Percussion myotonia in myotonia congenita. Following a sharp tap with a tendon hammer, there is a sustained localized depression that lasted about 5 seconds.

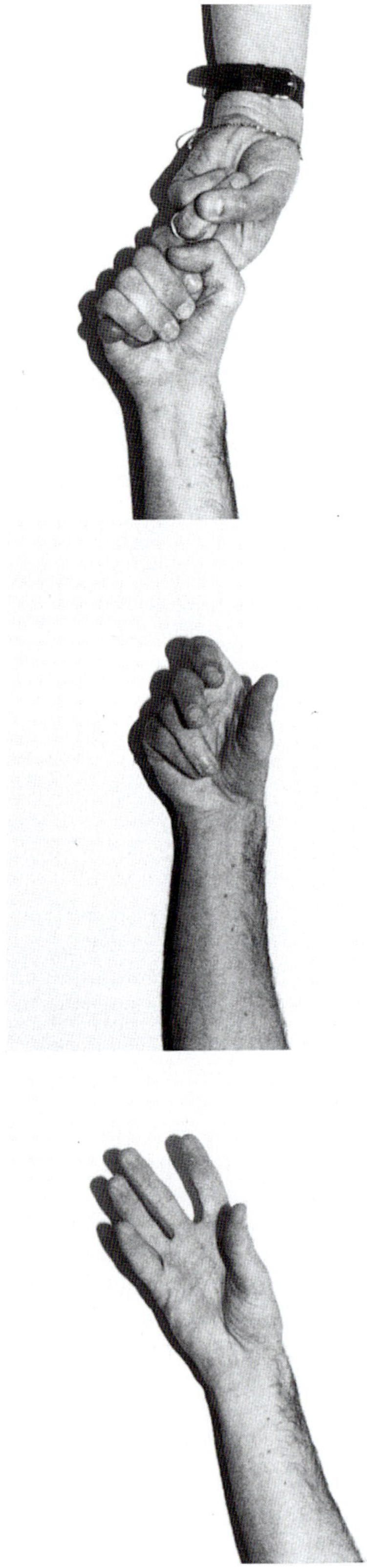

Figure 8.17. Grip myotonia in myotonic dystrophy. The patient was asked to grip the examiner's fingers for 3 seconds, and then to release and open their hand fully as quickly as possible. The following two pictures were taken at 3-second intervals.

to this rule. In the Lambert–Eaton syndrome, absent tendon reflexes may reappear after sustained contraction of the appropriate muscle (i.e., reflex potentiation). In contrast, the reflexes in myasthenia gravis are often relatively brisk. Delayed or slowed relaxation of the reflexes is typical of hypothyroidism, although this can be difficult to detect in an individual patient unless the relaxation is quite abnormal. This is perhaps most often elicited in the ankle jerks but is sometimes better seen with the supinator reflex.

Muscle examination in children

Disorders beginning in early infancy and childhood cause particular problems for the clinician, since the patient cannot present their own history and the standard adult neurological examination is in many respects not appropriate or applicable (or even possible!) in infants or very young children. An excellent review of the approach to neuromuscular problems in childhood is Dubowitz's classic monograph [54]. Areas unique to the childhood assessment include details of the pregnancy, labor and delivery, and early motor and intellectual milestones.

Weakness in young children usually manifests initially as delayed motor milestones, although in some congenital myopathies the mother may notice reduced fetal movements during pregnancy. Perinatal features of note include hypotonia (floppy baby) and feeding and breathing difficulties. In older children, it is crucial, but often difficult, to determine the age of onset and whether the weakness is static, improving or progressive. Children with muscle diseases are frequently thought to be simply "a little slow" or "kind of clumsy" by their parents, siblings, and pediatricians, and the seriousness of the problem may be overlooked until the weakness is advanced. It may take many years of observation before one can determine with any certainty the rate of progression of the disorder, an important feature in determining prognosis. The family may be able to comment on muscle atrophy or hypertrophy, and even in very young children it may be evident that exercise induces pain. The parents' description of the child's problems, watching the child play in the examining room, and performing functional tests as discussed above usually reveal more compared with a rigid, structured interview and formal examination.

Initial differential diagnosis

Based on findings gleaned from the history and examination, the clinician should usually be able place the patient into one of the six patterns of weakness listed in Table 8.3, and then formulate a differential diagnosis that can be refined by subsequent laboratory investigations. A discussion of the differential diagnosis for each set of symptoms and signs that patients may manifest is beyond the scope of this chapter; much of this material is covered in subsequent chapters on specific disorders. Two fundamental issues, however, need to be addressed in all patients and deserve discussion here. The first issue concerns making the initial distinction between whether the patient is likely to have a primary muscle disorder, as opposed to a disease of the neuromuscular junction, anterior horn cells, peripheral nerves, central nervous system, or even a non-neurological process. While this may seem straightforward, the distinction between these entities can often be difficult on clinical grounds alone. Features favoring a peripheral nerve disorder are sensory symptoms and signs; however, not all neuropathies (e.g., demyelinating polyneuropathies) cause demonstrable sensory involvement. Distal myopathies can simulate the Charcot–Marie–Tooth syndromes (in which sensory features can be slight or absent) as well as the distal spinal muscular atrophies. A possible additional source of confusion is that most myopathies causing severe disability and immobility may result in sensory symptoms because of secondary compressive neuropathies.

Once the determination is made that the disorder is likely to be myopathic, the second fundamental issue concerns identification of the specific myopathy present. For this determination, many clinicians try to classify patients into one of two broad groups according to whether the disorder is likely to be genetic/hereditary or acquired (Table 8.19). Obviously, a family history of similar difficulties is strong evidence that the condition is inherited, but coincidental disorders in other family members may be unrelated and can be very misleading. Age of onset is often a powerful discriminator (Table 8.20). Duchenne dystrophy, for example, does not present at age 15 years, and the primary periodic paralyses do not present in old age. In contrast, oculopharyngeal muscular dystrophy rarely presents in early adult life, but mitochondrial external ophthalmoplegia can present at any age.

Table 8.19. Major categories of primary muscle disease

- I. Hereditary disorders
  - Muscular dystrophies
  - Congenital myopathies
  - Myotonic dystrophies
  - Channelopathies
  - Primary metabolic myopathies
    - Disorders of carbohydrate metabolism
    - Disorders of lipid metabolism
  - Mitochondrial cytopathies
- II. Acquired myopathies
  - Inflammatory myopathies
  - Endocrine myopathies
  - Toxic and drug-induced myopathies
  - Myopathies associated with systemic illness

Rate of progression may also be informative. Many congenital disorders are nonprogressive or change only slowly with time. Inflammatory myopathies, but not dystrophies, may have a very acute onset with severe weakness developing within days. Metabolic disorders and channelopathies may cause slowly progressive weakness, over many decades, but with superimposed acute exacerbations. The pattern of weakness may also be highly informative. Dystrophies tend to "pick out" certain muscles, whereas inflammatory myopathies are less selective. Cardiac involvement occurs in only certain myopathies, and the mitochondrial cytopathies have many nonmyopathic features. By the end of the interview and examination, therefore, a relatively short list of possible diagnoses should be under consideration. This list can then be refined further through judicious testing, as discussed in the next section.

Approach to laboratory investigation

With few exceptions (e.g., typical myotonic dystrophy), all patients suspected of having a muscle disorder should have a serum creatine kinase (CK) determination. Although many patients should also undergo neurophysiological studies, these are certainly not necessary in all patients, since other tests may

Table 8.20. Clinical classification of myopathies based on age at onset

Myopathies presenting at birth
Congenital myopathies
Congenital myotonic dystrophy
Congenital muscular dystrophies
Glycogen storage diseases (acid maltase and, rarely, phosphorylase deficiencies)
Lipid storage diseases (carnitine deficiency)
Myopathies presenting in childhood
Congenital myopathies
Endocrine-metabolic disorders – hypokalemia, hypocalcemia, hypercalcemia
Glycogen storage disease (acid maltase deficiency)
Dermatomyositis (polymyositis only rarely)
Disorders of fatty acid transport and metabolism
Mitochondrial myopathies
Muscular dystrophies
Duchenne dystrophy
Becker dystrophy
Multiple types of LGMD
FSH dystrophy
Myopathies presenting in adulthood
Distal myopathies
Congenital myopathies (especially centronuclear and nemaline myopathies)
Endocrine myopathies – thyroid, parathyroid, adrenal, pituitary disorders
Inflammatory myopathies
Polymyositis
Dermatomyositis
Inclusion body myositis
Viral (HIV, HTLV-1)
Metabolic myopathies – acid maltase deficiency, disorders of lipid transport and metabolism, debrancher deficiency, phosphorylase b kinase deficiency
Muscular dystrophies
LGMD
FSH dystrophy
Becker dystrophy
Emery–Dreifuss dystrophy
Myotonic dystrophies
Mitochondrial myopathies
Toxic myopathies – especially alcohol myopathy and statin myopathy

be more specific (e.g., genetic testing in myotonic dystrophy). If these evaluations indicate a myopathy, and there is no evidence for an endocrinopathy, systemic disorder (e.g., sepsis/critical illness), or drug or toxin exposure (especially in relation to statin use), then the patient's condition is likely to fall into one of the other broad categories of myopathy listed in Table 8.21, which also lists the investigations most useful in reaching a diagnosis. It is important to remember that testing in the muscle diseases may serve different purposes depending on the type of test and the nature of the problem. Some tests, such as enzyme assays in metabolic disorders and DNA analyses in genetic disorders, provide a specific diagnosis. Other tests, such as the forearm exercise test, suggest the type of problem but not an exact diagnosis. Still other studies, such as electrocardiography, reveal abnormalities that are a consequence of the primary myopathy but provide few clues to the underlying disorder. Finally, there are investigations, such as magnetic resonance spectroscopy, which are currently mainly of research value.

In some muscular dystrophies (e.g., facioscapulohumeral dystrophy), the diagnosis can often be strongly suspected on the basis of clinical features and family history. Gene studies are becoming increasingly important for most of the muscular dystrophies (and especially the myotonic dystrophies, facioscapulohumeral dystrophy, oculopharyngeal dystrophy, and Duchenne and Becker dystrophies) and have made muscle biopsy unnecessary. This is an important concept, especially since routine histochemical and electron microscopy studies in the dystrophies are rarely unique or diagnostic anyway, an exception being the characteristic intranuclear inclusions seen in oculopharyngeal muscular dystrophy [55]. Immunochemistry and immunoblotting are major tools in the study of many limb-girdle and congenital dystrophies, and in those patients with dystrophin disorders with no identifiable Xp21 mutation; at present, the identification of a protein abnormality by such methods often helps direct appropriate DNA analysis. For inflammatory myopathies, muscle biopsy remains the sine qua non of diagnosis [56, 57]. Electromyography may be suggestive but is never diagnostic and serum CK may be normal. Inflammatory changes within muscle may be patchy, however, and result in a noninformative biopsy. Routine histology may be diagnostic but electron microscopy (for filaments in inclusion body myositis) and immunocytochemistry (for complement membrane attack complex in dermatomyositis, and MHCI expression in various forms of myositis) may provide additional information.

The metabolic myopathies are rare but among the most complicated and difficult of the myopathies to investigate [58]. Exercise tests, if performed correctly by experienced personnel, may help to determine the site of metabolic dysfunction as a prelude to specific biochemical investigations or muscle biopsy [59, 60]. Histochemical staining of biopsy material may sometimes demonstrate directly the enzyme deficiency or show accumulated products (e.g., glycogen, lipid) resulting from the blocked metabolic pathway. Enzyme assay may also be

Table 8.21. Diagnostic testing for major categories of primary muscle disease

I. Hereditary disorders

Muscular dystrophies
- Muscle biopsy
- Histology
- Immunocytochemistry
- Immunoblotting
- DNA studies

Congenital myopathies
- Muscle biopsy
- Histology
- Immunocytochemistry
- Immunoblotting
- DNA studies

Myotonic dystrophies
- DNA studies

Channelopathies
- Neurophysiological studies
- Serum potassium changes during attacks (for periodic paralysis)
- Provocation tests (for periodic paralysis)
- DNA studies

Mitochondrial myopathies
- Muscle biopsy
- Histology
- Histochemistry
- DNA studies

Primary metabolic myopathies – disorders of carbohydrate metabolism
- Forearm exercise test (assay lactate and ammonia)
- Magnetic resonance spectroscopy
- Muscle biopsy
- Histochemistry
- Enzyme assay
- Muscle biochemistry
- Blood cells
- Fibroblasts
- Leukocyte glycogen storage
- DNA studies

Primary metabolic myopathies – disorders of lipid metabolism
- Urinalysis
- Organic acids
- Acylcarnitines
- Prolonged fasting (assay free fatty acids, lactate, pyruvate, uric acid, ammonia, ketone bodies, glucose, creatine kinase)
- Aerobic exercise (assay as above)
- Carnitine assay
- Blood
- Muscle
- Enzyme assay
- Muscle
- Fibroblasts
- Liver
- DNA studies

Mitochondrial cytopathies
- Resting blood lactate and pyruvate
- Aerobic exercise (assay lactate, pyruvate, ammonia, glucose)
- Muscle biopsy
- Histochemistry
- Mitochondrial DNA studies
- Magnetic resonance spectroscopy

II. Acquired myopathies

Inflammatory myopathies
- Muscle biopsy
- Histology
- Immunocytochemistry
- Electron microscopy
- Skin biopsy

performed on a biopsy sample. For disorders where the genetic defect is known, DNA analysis can often be performed on a blood sample, but at a research level mRNA studies on muscle may be useful. An important exception is mitochondrial DNA deletion/duplication syndromes in which the genetic defect is best detected in muscle, not lymphocytes. For the channelopathies, electromyography is useful, particularly if myotonia is present [27]. In the periodic paralyses, monitoring potassium levels during spontaneous attacks may be diagnostic and obviate the need for more risky provocative tests. Direct gene analysis is rapidly becoming the investigation of choice for these disorders [61].

Neurophysiology

It is frustrating but all too true that even after the most thorough assessment it may be impossible at the bedside to make even the fundamental determination of whether the patient has a myopathy or a disorder affecting some other part of the neuraxis. Neurophysiological studies are the most valuable method to make this distinction. Although many techniques are now available in clinical neurophysiology departments, those most pertinent to the assessment of possible muscle disorders include nerve conduction studies, electromyography, and studies of neuromuscular transmission. These are all discussed in more detail elsewhere in this volume (see Section 2), and only two points will be stressed here. The first is that although these techniques will usually clearly indicate whether the patient has a neurogenic or myopathic disorder, this is not invariably true. For example, there are some diseases that mainly produce a myopathy but that may also be associated with a subclinical neuropathy (e.g., mitochondrial disorders, myotonic dystrophy, and inclusion body myositis). The second point is that the neurophysiological studies, like any test in medicine, cannot be interpreted in isolation but must always be analyzed in light of the clinical findings and the results of other testing.

Biochemical studies

The biochemical tests available to evaluate patients with muscle disease range from the simple and inexpensive serum CK assay to complex and time-consuming exercise protocols and phosphorus magnetic resonance spectroscopy. Other biochemical studies are useful for diagnosing various endocrinological or metabolic disorders (such as thyroid disease) that may be associated with muscle disease. The CK is by far the most common, and useful, serum test obtained in the muscle clinic.

Creatine kinase assay

Creatine kinase is an enzyme that catalyzes the reversible reaction by which adenosine diphosphate (ADP) and phosphocreatine form adenosine triphosphate (ATP) and creatine, but knowledge of this reaction is not important in understanding the significance of the assay in clinical practice. Elevation of the serum CK is a nonspecific marker of muscle damage and occurs in a wide variety of muscle diseases. Simply put, damaged muscle allows the enzyme to leak out into the circulation. It is important to remember that CK elevation can occur in diseases not of muscle origin, including neuropathies and anterior horn cell disorders; conversely, many muscle diseases do not cause an increase in CK. For example, CK is often normal in the two common forms of adult muscular dystrophy, namely myotonic dystrophy and facioscapulohumeral dystrophy. It is also crucial to remember that CK levels vary among normal individuals on the basis of gender, race, age, and physical activity. Black males, for example, may have CK values two or three times higher than standard laboratory grouped control values [62]. Many normal individuals have levels higher than the upper reference limit quoted by most laboratories and commercial kit manufacturers [63, 64].

Table 8.22. Causes of elevated creatine kinase (CK) in apparently normal individuals

- Hypothyroidism
- Becker muscular dystrophy
- Female carriers of the Duchenne/Becker muscular dystrophy gene
- Susceptibility to malignant hyperthermia
- Drugs causing subclinical myopathy (e.g., statins for treating hypercholesterolemia)
- High level of physical exercise

Fractionating the CK isoforms is not helpful in assessing muscle disease.

The highest CK elevations are seen with rhabdomyolysis from any cause. In Duchenne and Becker dystrophies, some of the sarcoglycanopathies, and disorders such as Miyoshi myopathy, the serum CK is markedly elevated in the early stages but declines later on as muscle mass is reduced. In the inflammatory myopathies, serum CK is usually, but not always, elevated, more so in dermatomyositis and polymyositis than in inclusion body myositis. Although it is tempting in these disorders to use the CK level to monitor progress, there is an imprecise relationship between serum CK and strength. For example, serum CK typically falls to normal within weeks of starting steroids but weakness may take much longer to improve. Serum CK elevation may also result from muscle injury that does not involve a muscle disease in the usual sense, such as muscle trauma (e.g., intramuscular injections, electric shock), sepsis, hypothermia, vigorous exercise, cardiac injury, and severe dyskinesias. More common is the patient with elevated serum CK without obvious cause or weakness. Common causes of elevated CK in an otherwise asymptomatic individual are shown in Table 8.22. It is unusual to make a specific diagnosis in a patient with no weakness or pain and a modest elevation in CK (up to three to five times normal). Many of these patients have idiopathic, sometimes hereditary, hyperCKemia and do not develop serious muscle disease, even on long-term follow-up [65].

Other serum and urine tests

Although other muscle enzymes and proteins can be assayed (e.g., myoglobin, aldolase, carbonic anhydrase III, aspartate transaminase (AST), alanine transaminase (ALT)), none offers an advantage over the CK test. A relatively common situation in this regard concerns patients found on routine blood testing to have an elevated ALT and/or AST level. Since ALT and AST are markers of hepatic function, these patients are often suspected of having liver disease, even though other liver function tests are normal. Some patients undergo liver biopsy before a CK value is obtained and it is realized that the transaminase is of muscle origin. In mitochondrial disorders, serum (and spinal fluid) lactate may be elevated at rest, a finding that can be a useful screening test. In the rare disorders of lipid metabolism, blood and urine carnitine and acylcarnitine assays are helpful. Tandem mass spectrometry is a recently developed method to study disorders of fatty acid β-oxidation [66]. Myoglobin levels are elevated in patients with rhabdomyolysis, although a more obvious manifestation of this disorder is myoglobinuria, which causes a positive dip-stick reaction that may be confused with the presence of blood.

Enzyme assays

In many metabolic myopathies, the diagnosis is secured only after enzyme assay on a muscle biopsy specimen frozen immediately in liquid nitrogen and stored at −70°C. In some disorders, assays can be performed on blood, urine, fibroblast cultures, and liver biopsy specimens.

Exercise tests

Exercise tests are used chiefly in the investigation of metabolic myopathies but they may also be beneficial in some channelopathies. Forearm exercise testing can be performed at the bedside, while aerobic bicycle exercise is more complex and requires specialized equipment; both should be performed at neuromuscular referral centers by experienced staff. Phosphorus magnetic resonance spectroscopy has proven useful in the research setting but is available in few centers and is not yet practical for routine diagnosis. These tests are discussed in more detail elsewhere in this book and in other reviews [58].

Forearm exercise test

The forearm exercise test is a simple screen for defects of glycogenolysis and glycolysis. The test is not without risk, and compartment syndromes or rhabdomyolysis with secondary renal compromise can occur, especially if the test is done under ischemic conditions (i.e., forearm ischemic exercise test). Because of these concerns, and the fact that oxidative metabolism contributes little in early intense exercise, most muscle centers perform the test under nonischemic conditions [67]. In this test, an intravenous line is placed in an antecubital vein and kept patent with heparin. After baseline blood samples are obtained, the patient exercises by squeezing a sphygmomanometer bulb to exhaustion (usually over 1–2 min). After exercise stops, further blood samples are taken at 1, 2, 3, 5, 10, and 15 min. Samples are assayed for lactate and ammonia, which requires pre-iced sample tubes and rapid processing. The normal response is a three- to fivefold increase over baseline for both lactate and ammonia (Figure 8.18). In disorders of glycogenolysis and glycolysis, the lactate response curve is reduced (or absent) and the rise in ammonia excessive. Conversely, myoadenylate deaminase deficiency results in a normal lactate rise but little or no increase in ammonia (Figure 8.19). With submaximal effort, neither lactate nor ammonia increases [68, 69]. A variation on the forearm exercise test which examines oxygen extraction from the samples has also shown promise as a screen for mitochondrial disorders [70].

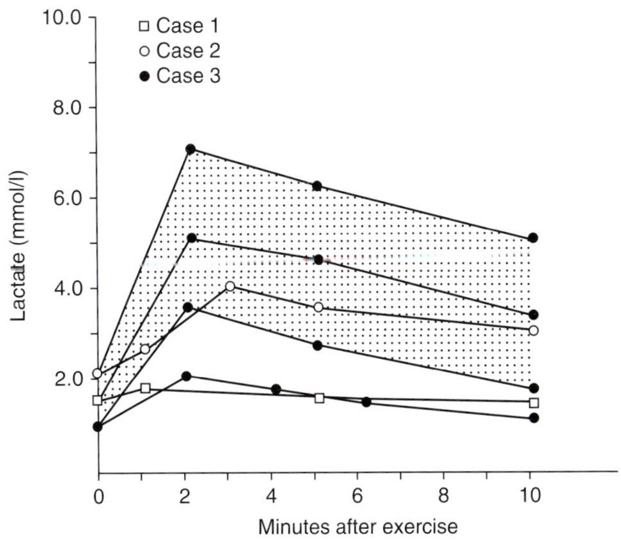

Figure 8.18. Venous lactate response to 1 minute of forearm exercise in three patients with phosphoglycerate mutase deficiency. The shaded area represents the mean and range of normal control responses to the same exercise protocol. None of the patients shows even a twofold rise in lactate above baseline. (Reproduced with permission from Kissel, J. T, Beam, W., Bresolin, N. *et al.*, (1985). Physiologic assessment of phosphoglycerate mutase deficiency: Incremental exercise tests. *Neurology* **35**, 828–833.)

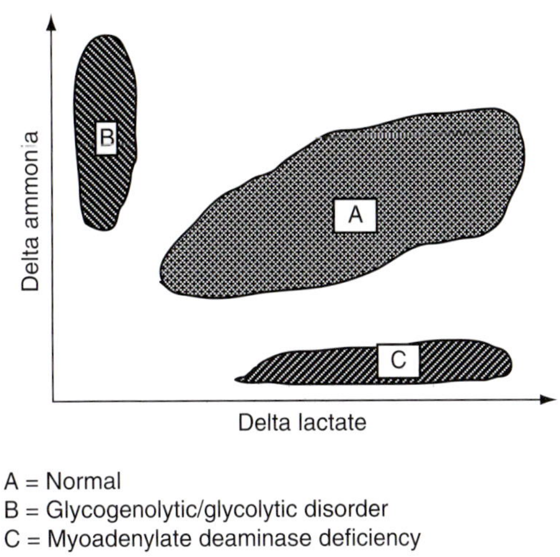

Figure 8.19. An alternative method of presenting the results of a forearm exercise study. The change from baseline for ammonia and lactate are presented on the vertical and horizontal axes respectively. Normally both rise following exercise. In glycogenoses there is a failure of increase in lactate, but a somewhat greater than normal rise in ammonia. In myoadenylate deaminase deficiency, there is a failure of increase in ammonia, but a normal rise in lactate.

Aerobic bicycle exercise test

The main clinical value of aerobic exercise testing is in the investigation of patients suspected of having disorders of oxidative metabolism, such as the mitochondrial disorders. In the test, the patient typically exercises for 15 minutes, and lactate and pyruvate are measured during exercise and recovery. Many protocols are used; one of the most satisfactory being the subanaerobic threshold exercise test [60, 71]. A defect in

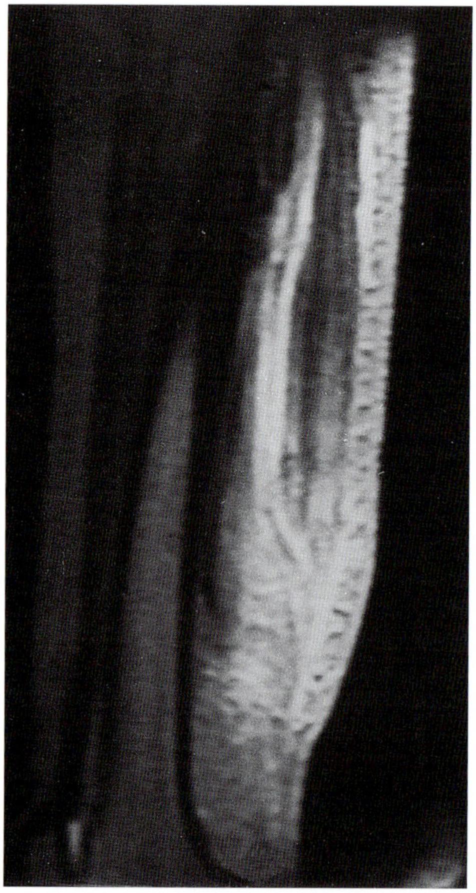

Figure 8.20. A T_2-weighted MRI of the thigh from a patient with diabetic thigh muscle infarction. There is diffuse high signal in the posterior muscles, including the biceps femoris, semimembranosus, and semitendinosus muscles. The bone and quadriceps muscles (on the left of the figure) appear normal. (From Barohn, R. J. and Kissel, J. T. Case of the month-painful thigh mass in a young woman: diabetic muscle infarction. *Muscle Nerve* **15**, 850–855. ©1992 John Wiley. Reprinted with permission.)

the Krebs' cycle or respiratory chain results in the pyruvate formed during glycolysis being reduced to lactate. In disorders of oxidative metabolism, there is an abnormal increase in serum lactate and also an abnormal lactate/pyruvate ratio.

Phosphorus magnetic resonance spectroscopy

Although phosphorus magnetic resonance spectroscopy is available routinely in relatively few muscle centers, it has already contributed significantly to the understanding of a number of disorders, principally the metabolic myopathies [58, 72].

Muscle imaging

Although muscle imaging can prove invaluable in selected patients, such as those with diabetic thigh muscle infarction (Figure 8.20), it is a rare patient in whom imaging is an indispensable part of the diagnostic process. The standard imaging modalities, ultrasound, computed tomography (CT) scanning, and MRI, can all be used and each provides somewhat different information. Imaging may demonstrate early and selective muscle involvement not evident to even the most experienced clinical eye. For example, forearm flexor muscle involvement may be detected by MRI scanning in patients with inclusion body myositis prior to the onset of the characteristic finger flexor weakness [5]. Imaging may also be used to evaluate the severity of the disease process in a given area, assess disease progression or regression, demonstrate fatty replacement in degenerating muscles or help to localize inflammatory deposits in disorders such as sarcoidosis. These issues and the use of imaging in evaluating patients with muscle disease are covered in more detail in Chapter 7.

Muscle biopsy

Despite advances in genetics and molecular biology, muscle biopsy remains an important diagnostic tool in evaluating many types of muscle disorder. The material obtained through biopsy can be studied through histological, histochemical, immunocytochemical, biochemical, electron microscopic or genetic techniques; these methodologies, along with interpretive aspects related to muscle biopsies, are reviewed in Chapters 5 and 6. Like neurophysiological studies, biopsy results must always be interpreted in the light of the clinical presentation and other laboratory studies. It is also important to remember that pathological changes may be very focal, both between muscles and within a given muscle. This is particularly common in the inflammatory myopathies, where an initial biopsy may show no abnormality while a second specimen from an adjacent area shows striking pathology. It is often helpful in such cases to sample multiple levels through the specimen. Biopsy appearances in specific disorders are considered throughout this volume, and there are also several excellent monographs on muscle biopsy [73, 74].

Molecular genetics diagnosis

The impact of molecular genetics on the description, classification, and understanding of the hereditary muscle disorders cannot be overstated. Over the past two decades, the field has advanced so rapidly that genetic testing has become a routine part of the evaluation of many muscle diseases, and it is crucial for all clinicians to have at least some understanding of the main methodologies involved. These are discussed in the chapters relating to specific disorders and will not be considered further here, except in terms of their impact on diagnosis. The single most important technique leading to the identification of disease-associated genes has been that of positional cloning (also called reverse genetics), which allows the defective gene responsible for a disease to be isolated so that the protein product of the gene can be identified. This is accomplished by studying large informative families with a clearly defined disorder using polymorphic markers to identify the approximate chromosomal location of the gene. The exact position of the gene is then determined using finer mapping techniques. Expressed transcripts of candidate genes from the area are

Table 8.23. Types of gene mutation seen in the commoner neuromuscular disorders

Large deletions	Duchenne/Becker muscular dystrophy (most patients)
Small deletions and point mutations	Duchenne/Becker muscular dystrophy (up to 30%)
Deletion	Spinal muscular atrophy
	Mitochondrial cytopathies (especially chronic external ophthalmoplegia) – in mitochondrial DNA
	Hereditary liability to pressure palsies
Duplication	Hereditary motor and sensory neuropathy Ia
Point mutations	Sarcoglycanopathies
	Limb girdle dystrophy 2A (calpain-deficient)
	Congenital muscular dystrophy (merosin deficient)
	Many metabolic disorders
	Channelopathies
	Myotonia congenita
	Emery–Dreifuss X-linked muscular dystrophy
	Hereditary motor and sensory neuropathy (several)
	Mitochondrial cytopathies (in mitochondrial DNA)
	Congenital myasthenic syndromes
Nucleotide repeat expansion	Myotonic dystrophies
	Kennedy syndrome
Deletion of repeat units	Facioscapulohumeral muscular dystrophy

assessed until the responsible gene is identified. The protein product can then be deduced from the nucleotide sequence. Another approach is to study candidate genes likely to be responsible for a given disorder, based on specific pathophysiological or biochemical features of that disease.

Several different types of mutation have been identified in muscle disorders, as summarized in Table 8.23. The disorders for which commercial tests were available at the time this chapter was written are also indicated. The identification of the gene defect responsible for a given disease may have immediate clinical import from a number of perspectives. Most obviously, such an identification is likely to be a major prerequisite to the development of effective therapy, whether by gene therapy or by some pharmacological or biochemical means (see Chapter 9). There are also immediate practical benefits to the patient and their family of having a specific genetic marker:

- Provides precise diagnosis and information about disease pathogenesis
- Usually limits need for additional testing
- Often permits carrier detection
- Allows identification of presymptomatic or at-risk individuals
- In some instances, may permit prenatal diagnosis and accurate genetic counseling
- Provides diagnostic homogeneity for patients participating in clinical trials
- May eventually be useful in identifying patients for gene therapy trials
- Occasionally may suggest phenotypic expression and severity of disease (but should never replace clinical determinations of disease severity or be used only rarely to provide detailed prognostic information to patient or family).

Although most of these benefits are self-evident they are considered further in Chapter 9 and in the discussions of each disorder.

Guide to classification

This section will conclude that there is not, and probably never can be, a single, universally applicable system for classifying muscle disorders. When considering how to classify, one first has to answer the question "why bother to try?", which then immediately leads to a second question, "what approach or system should be used?" The most important of the many possible answers to these questions include:

- To provide a clinically based framework that helps the clinician to categorize the nature of the problem that they are seeing at the bedside, and that will help with the diagnostic approach, management, and possible therapy
- To classify on the basis of the known molecular defect, which might be in terms of either the specific protein involved, or the organelle or functional component (such as the contractile apparatus, excitation–contraction coupling mechanism) that is defective
- To classify on the basis of the underlying DNA abnormality and the affected gene, e.g., mutation leading to a premature stop codon, gene duplication, nucleotide repeat expansion disorder affecting RNA metabolism, repeat contraction disorder, or other process

Each of these systems has its merits and attractions, but several problems are immediately apparent. The last approach is only applicable to inherited myopathies, as opposed to acquired, and requires that the specific DNA abnormality has been identified; which, of course, is currently not always the case. Nevertheless, such an approach to classification will undoubtedly be of great value in the future, when specific

Table 8.24. Proposed system for classifying muscle disease

Group	Associated with
Structural/linking proteins	Nucleus: membrane or other
	Mitochondria
	Contractile apparatus
	Sarcolemmal membrane
	Other
Contractile proteins	
Ion channel proteins	
Associated with enzyme activity	Energy-related processes: glycolysis, lipid oxidation, mitochondrial enzymes, adenylate deaminase
	Non-energy-related processes: proteases, protein kinases, phosphatases
Other proteins	Nucleus
	Mitochondria
	Contractile apparatus
	Membranes
	Other
Protein storage	
Secondary diseases	Inflammation and autoimmunity
	Immunological disease
	Infectious disease
	Systemic disease
	Toxins

therapeutic approaches based on particular DNA mutations, have been developed – for example, a recent newspaper headline stated that the development of a particular drug that would "read-through" a premature stop codon could cure [sic] 3000 genetic diseases!

In the last edition of this book, Michael Brooke proposed a system for classifying muscle disease on the basis of the protein defect and the associated disruption of normal muscle function (Table 8.24) and provided a correlation between older terminology and the underlying molecular defect (Table 8.25) [75]. Although the protein defect is known for most inherited disorders, it certainly is not for many (if not most) acquired disorders. Furthermore, there may be considerable uncertainty and even controversy concerning the exact role of a particular protein, or how absence of that protein, or its presence in mutated form, leads to loss of normal muscle function. For example, even now, over 20 years after its discovery, there remains debate as to all of the functions of dystrophin in relation to Duchenne dystrophy – although its structural

Table 8.25. Correlation of the older terminology for muscle diseases with the underlying molecular defects, where known

Older terminology	"New" terminology
Emery–Dreifuss dystrophy	Emerin deficiency, lamin A deficiency
Nemaline myopathy	Nebulin deficiency, α-tropomyosin deficiency
Duchenne/Becker dystrophies	Dystrophin deficiency
"Limb-girdle" dystrophies	Deficiencies of α-, β-, γ-, and δ-sarcoglycan, laminin α_2- and β_1-chains, dysferlin, caveolin, calpain-3
Epidermolysis bullosa muscular dystrophy	Plectin deficiency
Bethlem myopathy	Collagen VI deficiency
Fukuyama dystrophy	Fukutin deficiency
Hypokalemic periodic paralysis (autosomal dominant)	Calcium channel
Hyperkalemic periodic paralysis (autosomal dominant)	Sodium channel
Myotonia cogenita	Chloride channel
Malignant hyperthermia	Ryanodine receptor
Central core disease	Ryanodine receptor
Congenital muscular dystrophy	Deficiencies of laminin α_2-chain and γ-sarcoglycan
Myoshi myopathy	Dysferlin deficiency
Myotonic dystrophy	Myotonin protein kinase deficiency
Myotubular myopathy	Myotubularin deficiency
Oculopharyngeal dystrophy	Poly-A-binding protein

function is universally accepted, additional disease mechanisms may relate, for example, to a role in membrane signal processing.

When considering the inherited myopathies, what has proved particularly difficult for those desirous of a simple classification system has been the increasing realization of the extent of phenotypic and genotypic heterogeneity. Many years ago it was presumed that mutation of a specific gene would affect the protein product of that gene, and that that would lead to a *specific* phenotype. In the field of neuromuscular disorders the concept of genotypic heterogeneity has long been recognized. Perhaps the best example is Charcot–Marie–Tooth syndrome, which was originally described as a specific clinical entity, but for which we now know that there are over 30 different genes that may be causatively involved.

Table 8.26. Different phenotypes caused by different mutations within the same gene

Lamin A/C
Autosomal dominant Emery–Dreifuss syndrome
Autosomal recessive Emery–Dreifuss syndrome
Limb-girdle muscular dystrophy type 1B
Partial lipodystrophy syndromes
Progeria
Restrictive dermopathy
Mandibuloacral dysplasia
Autosomal recessive Charcot–Marie–Tooth syndrome type 2B1
Dystrophin
Duchenne muscular dystrophy
Becker muscular dystrophy
X-linked cramp-myalgia syndrome
Isolated hyperCKemia
Isolated cardiomyopathy

This is a relatively easy concept to understand in the sense that whichever genes are involved, the outcome is the same; that is, distal nerve disruption which causes a uniform clinical picture. Similarly, in the field of muscle diseases, mutations in numerous genes can produce a limb-girdle dystrophy picture, and Emery–Dreifuss syndrome can be caused by mutations affecting either lamin A/C or emerin (both nuclear envelope proteins).

More unexpected has been the discovery that mutations affecting one gene can lead to more than one phenotype. The first observation to be made in this regard was not very surprising; namely, that mutations affecting different parts of the same gene may give rise to very different phenotypes. This can readily be understood in terms of differing critical functions for different parts of the encoded protein, the effects of altered splicing patterns, involvement of specific promoters, and a host of other variables that help determine genotype/phenotype correlations. As examples, the different phenotypes that can be associated with lamin A/C and dystrophin mutations are shown in Table 8.26.

The second observation was more surprising, but perhaps should not have been that unexpected; the same mutation in different individuals, even different members of the same family, can lead to a different phenotype. Examples relating to caveolin, dysferlin and lamin A/C are shown in Table 8.27. The principle of penetrance has long been recognized; lack of penetrance means that an individual carrying an abnormal dominant gene may not show features of the condition at the same age as do other affected family members. In a family tree it can appear that a dominant disorder has jumped a generation. This has been observed frequently in facioscapulohumeral dystrophy, where it has also been noted that females, in general, tend to be less severely affected than males. The cause of phenotypic variability from either the same mutation within a gene, or from variable penetrance, presumably relates to the modifying effect of other genes; it is extremely difficult to take such phenomena into account when trying to develop a system of classification.

Table 8.27. The same mutation leading to different phenotypes

Caveolin
Autosomal dominant limb-girdle muscular dystrophy type 1C
Rippling-muscle disease
Distal myopathy
HyperCKemia
Dysferlin
Miyoshi distal myopathy
Autosomal recessive limb-girdle muscular dystrophy type 2B
Lamin A/C
Autosomal dominant limb-girdle muscular dystrophy type 1B
Dilated cardiomyopathy

The distinction between inherited and acquired disorders is a fundamental one, but one that it may not be possible to make when the patient first presents. At the time of writing, it is a general observation that most acquired myopathies (with the notable exception of inclusion body myositis) can improve or resolve, either by removing or treating the cause (e.g., drug-induced myopathy, endocrinopathy) or by drug therapy (e.g., immunosuppression for myositis). In contrast, aside from enzyme replacement therapy for Pompe disease [76], there are as yet no other specific DNA-based or molecular treatments for the inherited myopathies, although symptomatic drug therapy is available for some (e.g., mexiletine for treating myotonia, acetazolamide for periodic paralysis, corticosteroids in Duchenne dystrophy, and various drugs for cardiomyopathy). But the identification of an inherited myopathy has obvious implications with respect to genetic counseling issues.

At the beginning of this chapter we stated that "The molecular genetics revolution has resulted in a wealth of new information on the pathogenesis of most myopathies, and a resulting fundamental change in the way these disorders are diagnosed and classified." We should perhaps have changed the last part of that sentence to read "... are diagnosed and *might be* classified." Although some myologists might like to think that we can now create a rational classification scheme for myopathies that does *not* rely solely on clinical features and distribution of weakness, it can be seen that we are still some distance from that goal, and may never achieve it. To use the terms Xp21 dystrophy or dystrophinopathy might suggest clever insight or molecular wisdom, but to the clinician the term Duchenne muscular dystrophy has a precision in

Table 8.28. Partial classification of the more common muscular dystrophies based on inheritance and genetic defect

Disease	Chromosome	Affected protein	Testing[a]		
X-linked recessive			**IC**	**IB**	**DNA**
Duchenne/Becker	Xp21	Dystrophin	√	√	√
Emery–Dreifuss	Xq28	Emerin	√	√	√
Autosomal dominant limb-girdle dystrophies (LGMD 1)					
LGMD 1A	5q22.3–31.3	Myotilin			√
LGMD 1B	1q11–21	Lamin A & C			√
LGMD 1C	3p25	Caveolin-3	√	√	√
LGMD 1D	7q	?	NA		
LGMD 1E	6q23	?	NA		
LGMD 1F	7q32.1	?	NA		
LGMD 1G	4p21	?			
Autosomal recessive limb-girdle dystrophies (LGMD 2)					
LGMD 2A	15q15.1–21.1	Calpain 3		√	√
LGMD 2B[b]	2p13	Dysferlin	√	√	√
LGMD 2C	13q12	γ-sarcoglycan		√	√
LGMD 2D	17q12–21.3	α-sarcoglycan		√	√
LGMD 2E	4q12	β-sarcoglycan		√	√
LGMD 2F	5q33–34	δ-sarcoglycan		√	√
LGMD 2G	17q11–12	Telethonin			√
LGMD 2H	9q31–33	E3-ubiquitin-ligase (TRIM 32)			√
LGMD 2I	19q13	Fukutin-related protein (FKRP)			√
LGMD 2J	2q31	ZASP			√
LGMD 2K	9q34	POMT1			√
LGMD 2L	11q13	Fukutin			√
Congenital muscular dystrophies (CMD) – all autosomal recessive					
Laminin-α-2 CMD	6q22–23	Laminin-α-2 chain	√	√	√
α-7 Integrin CMD	12q13	α-7 Integrin			√
CMD with normal CNS	19q13	Fukutin-related protein (FKRP)			√
Fukuyama CMD	9q31–33	Fukutin			√
Walker–Warburg CMD	9q31	POMT1			√
Muscle–eye–brain CMD	1p32	POMGnT1			√
Rigid spine syndrome	1p35–36	Selenoprotein N1			√
Autosomal dominant distal dystrophies/myopathies					
Late adult-onset (Welander)	2p13	?	NA		
Late adult-onset (Markesbery)	2q31	ZASP			√
Early adult-onset (Laing)	14q11	MYH7			√
Autosomal recessive distal dystrophies/myopathies					
Early adult-onset[c] (Nonaka)	9p1–q1	GNE			√
Early adult-onset[b] (Miyoshi)	10q22.3–q23.2	Dysferlin	√	√	√

Table 8.28. (cont.)

Disease	Chromosome	Affected protein	Testing[a]		
X-linked recessive			IC	IB	DNA
Quadriceps-sparing myopathy[c]	9p1–q1	GNE			√
Other dystrophies (all autosomal dominant)					
Facioscapulohumeral	4q35	?			√
Scapuloperoneal dystrophy	12	?	NA		
Oculopharyngeal	14q11.2–13	PABP2			√
Myotonic dystrophy (DM1)	19q13.3	DMPK			√
Myotonic dystrophy (DM2)	3q21	ZNF9			√

Notes: [a]Testing – IC = immunocytochemistry, IB = immunoblotting (western blotting), DNA = mutation testing. [b]LGMD 2B and Miyoshi distal dystrophy are allelic conditions. [c]Nonaka myopathy and quadriceps-sparing myopathy are allelic conditions.

summarizing the highly characteristic clinical features of this specific condition that will never be bettered by molecular terminology. Recent advances have been largely in the area of inherited myopathies, and the causes and mechanisms in most acquired myopathies remain elusive.

Despite the foregoing discussion, it would be quite wrong to conclude that there are no classification systems that are of use to the clinician; far from it. But what are available and what are of value are rather simple classifications that are of particular use in the clinical setting. In practice, it is helpful to use more than one system. We have discussed these in the earlier section on the clinical approach to the patient with muscle disease, when virtually all patients are able to be placed in one of six categories, depending solely on the pattern of muscle involvement (Table 8.3). Subclassification within each category can then be made by noting additional clinical features such as age of onset (Table 8.20), presence or absence of contractures (Table 8.8), presence and type of cardiac involvement (Table 8.11), and presence and pattern of pain (Tables 8.4, 8.5, 8.6).

A very simple, but all embracing, classification of myopathies is shown in Table 8.19. Each category encompasses numerous different disorders which present their own challenges for more detailed classification and this is discussed in detail in the relevant chapters covering each disorder. If we consider the muscular dystrophies, it is possible to provide a more comprehensive classification (Table 8.28) including details of inheritance patterns (highly useful in clinical practice) and molecular information (essential in aiding appropriate laboratory assessment). Entries in this table emphasize phenotypic and genetic heterogeneity – thus there are numerous molecular causes of limb-girdle muscular dystrophy, and mutations in some genes can cause more than one phenotype, as discussed above. It can readily be seen that if a comprehensive classification such as used in Table 8.28 were applied to each of the entries in the simple classification of Table 8.19, then many pages of text would be required, producing a listing that would be unwieldy and largely unhelpful in everyday practice.

It is fitting to conclude by returning to some of Brooke's observations [75]. In moving from the era of clinical description to the molecular era he bemoaned, "the disappearance into the genetic laboratory of every aspiring fellow, together with much of the funding." The molecular scientists do not yet have all of the answers, and may never do so, at least in terms of clinical applicability. Now more than ever, we really *are* "between two eras," with "a danger inherent in trying to establish a permanent foundation during a time of transition." Watch this space for future developments!

References

1. G. Karpati, M. Sinnreich, The molecular era of myology. *J. Neuropathol. Exp. Neurol.* **62**:12 (2003), 1203–1210.
2. R. Lane, G. Fuller, Clinical presentation: symptoms and signs of muscle disease and their interpretation. In *Handbook of Muscle Disease*, First Edition, ed. R. Lane. (New York: Marcel Dekker, 1996), pp. 1–17.
3. R. J. Barohn, General approach to muscle diseases. In *Cecil Textbook of Medicine*, eds. L. Golman, D. Ausiello. (Philadelphia, PA: W. B. Saunders, 2004), pp. 2370–2379.
4. A. A. Amato, G. S. Gronseth, C. E. Jackson, *et al.*, Inclusion body myositis: clinical and pathological boundaries. *Ann. Neurol.* **40**:4 (1996), 581–586.
5. E. A. Sekul, C. Chow, M. C. Dalakas, Magnetic resonance imaging of the forearm as a diagnostic aid in patients with sporadic inclusion body myositis. *Neurology* **48**:4 (1997), 863–866.
6. R. K. H. Petty, A. E. Harding, J. A. Morgan-Hughes, The clinical features of mitochondrial myopathy. *Brain* **109** (1986), 915–938.
7. J. S. Katz, G. I. Wolfe, D. K. Burns, W. W. Bryan, J. L. Fleckenstein, R. J. Barohn, Isolated neck extensor myopathy: a common cause of dropped head syndrome. *Neurology* **46**:4 (1996), 917–921.

8. I. Mahjneh, G. Marconi, A. Paetau, A. Saarinen, T. Salmi, H. Somer, Axial myopathy – an unrecognised entity. *J. Neurol.* **249**:6 (2002), 730–734.
9. N. Shahrizaila, W. J. Kinnear, A. J. Wills, Respiratory involvement in inherited primary muscle conditions. *J. Neurol. Neurosurg. Psychiatry* **77**:10 (2006), 1108–1115.
10. T. Shahrizaila, W. Kinnear, Recommendations for respiratory care of adults with muscle disorders. *Neuromuscul. Disord.* **17**:1 (2007), 13–15.
11. K. R. Mills, R. H. T. Edwards, Investigative strategies for muscle pain. *J. Neurol. Sci.* **58** (1983), 73–88.
12. M. Filosto, P. Tonin, G. Vattemi, *et al.*, The role of muscle biopsy in investigating isolated muscle pain. *Neurology* **68**:3 (2007), 181–186.
13. J. T. Kissel, Muscle biopsy in patients with myalgia: still a painful decision. *Neurology* **68**:3 (2007), 170–171.
14. J. T. Kissel, The problem of fibromyalgia. *Muscle Nerve* **25**:4 (2002), 473–476.
15. D. Hilton-Jones, The clinical features of some miscellaneous neuromuscular disorders. In *Disorders of Voluntary Muscle*, Sixth Edition, eds. J. Walton, G. Karpati, D. Hilton-Jones. (Edinburgh: Churchill Livingstone, 1994), pp. 967–987.
16. J. Kissel, R. G. Miller, Muscle pain and fatigue. In *Muscle Diseases*, eds. A. H. Schapira, R. C. Griggs. (Woburn: Butterwort-Heinemann, 1999), pp. 33–58.
17. Z. Argov, F. L. Mastaglia, Drug-induced neuromuscular disorders in man. In *Disorders of Voluntary Muscle*, Sixth Edition, eds. J. Walton, G. Karpati, D. Hilton-Jones. (Edinburgh: Churchill Livingstone, 1994), pp. 989–1029.
18. S. Franc, S. Dejager, E. Bruckert, M. Chauvenet, P. Giral, G. Turpin, A comprehensive description of muscle symptoms associated with lipid-lowering drugs. *Cardiovasc. Drugs Ther.* **17**:5–6 (2003), 459–465.
19. S. K. Baker, Molecular clues into the pathogenesis of statin-mediated muscle toxicity. *Muscle Nerve* **31**(5) (2005), 572–580.
20. W. W. Campbell, Statin myopathy: the iceberg or its tip? *Muscle Nerve* **34**:4 (2006), 387–390.
21. R. Layzer, Muscle pain, cramps and fatigue. In *Myology*, Second Edition, eds. A. Engel, C. Franzini-Armstrong. (New York: McGraw-Hill, 1994), pp. 1754–1768.
22. R. G. Auger, AAEM minimonograph #44: diseases associated with excess motor unit activity. *Muscle Nerve* **17**:11 (1994), 1250–1263.
23. T. M. Miller, R. B. Layzer, Muscle cramps. *Muscle Nerve* **32**:4 (2005), 431–442.
24. P. S. Harper, *Myotonic Dystrophy*, Third Edition. (London: W. B. Saunders, 2001.)
25. J. W. Day, K. Ricker, J. F. Jacobsen, *et al.*, Myotonic dystrophy type 2: molecular, diagnostic and clinical spectrum. *Neurology* **60**:4 (2003), 657–664.
26. A. J. Hudson, G. C. Ebers, D. E. Bulman, The skeletal muscle sodium and chloride channel diseases. *Brain* **118**: (1995), 547–563.
27. E. Fournier, K. Viala, H. Gervais, *et al.*, Cold extends electromyography distinction between ion channel mutations causing myotonia. *Ann. Neurol.* **60**:3 (2006), 356–365.
28. J. A. P. Hiel, P. J. H. Jongen, P. J. E. Poels, *et al.*, Sarcoplasmic reticulum Ca^{2+}-adenosine triphosphate deficiency (Brody's disease). In *Handbook of Muscle Disease*, ed. R. J. M. Lane. (New York: Marcel Dekker, 1996), pp. 473–478.
29. S. A. Greenberg, Acquired rippling muscle disease with myasthenia gravis. *Muscle Nerve* **29**:1 (2004), 143–146.
30. R. C. Betz, B. G. Schoser, D. Kasper, *et al.*, Mutations in CAV3 cause mechanical hyperirritability of skeletal muscle in rippling muscle disease. *Nat. Genet.* **28**:3 (2001), 218–219.
31. K. Ricker, R. T. Moxley, R. Rohkamm, Rippling muscle disease. *Arch. Neurol.* **46** (1989), 405–408.
32. P. Shillito, P. C. Molenaar, A. Vincent, *et al.*, Acquired neuromyotonia: evidence for autoantibodies directed against K^{+} channels of peripheral nerves. *Ann. Neurol.* **38**:5 (1995), 714–722.
33. I. K. Hart, J. Newsom-Davis, Neuromyotonia. In *Handbook of Muscle Disease*, ed. R. J. M. Lane. (New York: Marcel Dekker, 1996), pp. 355–363.
34. J. Newsom-Davis, The emerging diversity of neuromuscular junction disorders. *Acta Myol.* **26**:1 (2007), 5–10.
35. J. T. Kissel, R. J. Elble, Stiff-person syndrome: stiff opposition to a simple explanation. *Neurology* **51**:1 (1998), 11–14.
36. M. C. Dalakas, Advances in the pathogenesis and treatment of patients with stiff person syndrome. *Curr. Neurol. Neurosci. Rep.* **8**:1 (2008), 48–55.
37. L. B. Krupp, D. A. Pollina, Mechanisms and management of fatigue in progressive neurological disorders. *Curr. Opin. Neurol.* **9**:6 (1996), 456–460.
38. J. Sieb, A. Penn, Myoglobinuria. In *Myology*, Third Edition, eds. A. Engel, C. Franzini-Armstrong. (New York: McGraw-Hill, 2004), pp. 1677–1692.
39. C. Y. Tsao, J. R. Mendell, J. Rusin, M. Luquette, Congenital muscular dystrophy with complete laminin-alpha2-deficiency, cortical dysplasia, and cerebral white-matter changes in children. *J. Child Neurol.* **13**:6 (1998), 253–256.
40. C. Y. Tsao, J. R. Mendell, The childhood muscular dystrophies: making order out of chaos. *Semin. Neurol.* **19**:1 (1999), 9–23.
41. C. Godfrey, E. Clement, R. Mein, *et al.*, Refining genotype phenotype correlations in muscular dystrophies with defective glycosylation of dystroglycan. *Brain* **130**:Pt 10 (2007), 2725–2735.
42. M. A. Mullie, A. E. Harding, R. K. Petty, H. Ikeda, J. A. Morgan-Hughes, M. D. Sanders, The retinal manifestations of mitochondrial myopathy. A study of 22 cases. *Arch Ophthalmol.* **103**:12 (1985), 1825–1830.
43. J. Kissel, J. R. Mendell, Endocrine myopathies. In *Handbook of Clinical Neurology*, eds. L. P. Rowland, S. DiMauro. (New York: Elsevier Science, 1992), pp. 527–551.
44. M. Hirano, G. Silvestri, D. M. Blake, *et al.*, Mitochondrial neurogastrointestinal encephalomyopathy (MNGIE): clinical, biochemical, and genetic features of an autosomal recessive mitochondrial disorder. *Neurology* **44**:4 (1994), 721–727.
45. M. C. Lara, M. L. Valentino, J. Torres-Torronteras, M. Hirano, R. Marti, Mitochondrial neurogastrointestinal encephalomyopathy (MNGIE): biochemical features and therapeutic approaches. *Biosci. Rep.* **27**:1–3 (2007), 151–163.

46. J. Hayes, F. Veyckemans, B. Bissonnette, Duchenne muscular dystrophy: an old anesthesia problem revisited. *Paediatr. Anaesth.* **18**:2 (2008), 100–106.

47. G. A. Suarez, J. J. Kelly, The dropped head syndrome. *Neurology* **42** (1992), 1625–1627.

48. *Aids to the Examination of the Peripheral Nervous System*, Fourth Edition. (Oxford: Saunders, 2000.)

49. R. Tawil, M. P. McDermott, J. R. Mendell, J. Kissel, R. C. Griggs, Facioscapulohumeral muscular dystrophy (FSHD): design of natural history study and results of baseline testing. FSH-DY Group. *Neurology* **44**:3 Pt 1 (1994), 442–446.

50. T. Munsat, *Quantification of Neurologic Deficit*. (Stoneham: Butterworth, 1989.)

51. K. E. Personius, S. Pandya, W. M. King, R. Tawil, M. P. McDermott, Facioscapulohumeral dystrophy natural history study: standardization of testing procedures and reliability of measurements. The FSH DY Group. *Phys. Ther.* **74**:3 (1994), 253–263.

52. M. Brooke, *A Clinician's View of Neuromuscular Diseases*. (Baltimore, MD: Williams and Wilkins, 1986.)

53. R. A. C. Hughes, D. Bihari, Acute neuromuscular respiratory paralysis. *J. Neurol. Neurosurg. Psychiatry* **56** (1993), 334–343.

54. V. Dubowitz, *Muscle Disorders in Childhood*, Second Edition. (London: Saunders, 1995.)

55. F. M. S. Tome, D. Chateau, A. Helbling-Leclerc, M. Fardeau, Morphological changes in muscle fibers in oculopharyngeal muscular dystrophy. *Neuromuscul. Disord.* **7**:Suppl 1 (1997), S63–S69.

56. N. Chahin, A. G. Engel, Correlation of muscle biopsy, clinical course, and outcome in PM and sporadic IBM. *Neurology* **70**:6 (2008), 418–424.

57. J. T. Kissel, Polymyositis: not a unicorn or mythological beast. . . but maybe a duck? *Neurology* **70**:6 (2008), 414–415.

58. D. Hilton-Jones, M. Squier, D. J. Taylor P. Matthews, *Metabolic Myopathies*, First Edition. (London: W. B. Saunders, 1995.)

59. R. G. Haller, L. A. Bertocci, Exercise evaluation of metabolic myopathies. In *Myology*, Second Edition, eds. A. G. Engel, C. Franzini-Armstrong. (New York: McGraw-Hill, 1994), pp. 807–821.

60. R. Lane, Exercise tests. In *Handbook of Muscle Disease*, ed. R. Lane. (New York: Marcel Dekker, 1996.)

61. S. L. Venance, S. C. Cannon, D. Fialho, *et al.*, The primary periodic paralyses: diagnosis, pathogenesis and treatment. *Brain* **129**:Pt 1 (2006), 8–17.

62. E. T. Wong, C. Cobb, M. K. Umehara, *et al.*, Heterogeneity of serum creatine kinase activity among racial and gender groups of the population. *Am. J. Clin. Pathol.* **79**:5 (1983), 582–586.

63. E. I. Lev, I. Tur-Kaspa, I. Ashkenazy, *et al.*, Distribution of serum creatine kinase activity in young healthy persons. *Clin. Chim. Acta* **279**:1–2 (1999), 107–115.

64. L. M. Brewster, G. Mairuhu, A. Sturk, G. A. van Montfrans, Distribution of creatine kinase in the general population: implications for statin therapy. *Am. Heart J.* **154**:4 (2007), 655–661.

65. E. D'Adda, M. Sciacco, M. E. Fruguglietti, *et al.*, Follow-up of a large population of asymptomatic/oligosymptomatic hyperCKemic subjects. *J. Neurol.* **253**:11 (2006), 1399–1403.

66. K. G. Sim, J. Hammond, B. Wilcken, Strategies for the diagnosis of mitochondrial fatty acid beta-oxidation disorders. *Clin. Chim. Acta* **323**:1–2 (2002), 37–58.

67. P. Kazemi-Esfarjani, E. Skomorowska, T. D. Jensen, R. G. Haller, J. Vissing, A nonischemic forearm exercise test for McArdle disease. *Ann. Neurol.* **52**:2 (2002), 153–159.

68. R. A. Coleman, J. M. Stajich, V. W. Pact, M. A. Pericak-Vance, The ischemic exercise test in normal adults and in patients with weakness and cramps. *Muscle Nerve* **9** (1986), 216–221.

69. S. P. Sinkeler, R. A. Wevers, E. M. Joosten, *et al.*, Improvement of screening in exertional myalgia with a standardized ischemic forearm test. *Muscle Nerve* **9** (1986), 731–737.

70. T. D. Jensen, P. Kazemi-Esfarjani, E. Skomorowska, J. Vissing, A forearm exercise screening test for mitochondrial myopathy. *Neurology* **58**:10 (2002), 1533–1538.

71. L. Nashef, R. J. M. Lane, Screening for mitochondrial cytopathies: the sub-anaerobic threshold exercise test (SATET). *J. Neurol. Neurosurg. Psychiatry* **52**: (1989), 1090–1094.

72. P. Laforet, C. Wary, S. Duteil, *et al.*, [Exploration of exercise intolerance by ^{31}P NMR spectroscopy of calf muscles coupled with MRI and ergometry.] *Rev. Neurol. (Paris)* **159**:1 (2003), 56–67.

73. V. Dubowitz, C. Sewry, *Muscle Biopsy. A Practical Approach*. (China: Saunders, 2007.)

74. S. Carpenter, G. Karpati, *Pathology of Skeletal Muscle*. (Oxford: Oxford University Press, 2001.)

75. M. Brooke, The classification of muscle diseases. In *Disorders of Voluntary Muscle*, eds. G. Karpati, D. Hilton-Jones, R. C. Griggs. (Cambridge: Cambridge University Press, 2001), pp. 374–384.

76. T. M. Geel, P. M. McLaughlin, L. F. de Leij, M. H. Ruiters, K. E. Niezen-Koning, Pompe disease: current state of treatment modalities and animal models. *Mol. Genet. Metab.* **92**:4 (2007), 299–307.

Tentative Video Clips

Clip 1. Limb-girdle pattern of weakness

Clip 2. Patient with predominantly distal weakness

Clip 3. Scapuloperoneal pattern of weakness

Clip 4. Patient with IBM, distal upper extremity/proximal lower extremity

Clip 5. Ocular weakness pattern (mitochondrial)

Clip 6. Isolated neck extensor weakness

Clip 7. EMG of myotonia

Clip 8. Accessory muscle use with breathing

Clip 9. Percussion myotonia

Clip 10. Grip myotonia

Clip 11. Muscle rippling

Chapter 9

The principles of molecular therapies for muscle diseases

George Karpati and Rénald Gilbert

Background

The application of molecular science and technology to medicine since the 1990s has had a major impact on the understanding of the pathogenesis, pursuit of investigation, and planning of high-tech therapy of human diseases. In that sense, myology has been an outstanding beneficiary of the advent of molecular science and in this chapter the prospects of molecular therapies for muscle diseases will be highlighted.

It is important to realize that this chapter is restricted only to the discussion of the *principles* of the subject. For detailed discussion, the reader is referred to up-to-date relevant papers and reviews. The other important point to emphasize is that the field is an exceptionally rapidly moving one and that some items discussed may have become outdated by the time the reader consults this chapter.

Definitions

Molecular therapies are defined as those treatment modalities that are based on the negation or at least partial correction of important molecular defects that have major disease-causing effect(s) on the structure and/or function of cells in a given tissue(s). This definition entails the need for a precise knowledge and understanding of the basic molecular defects and the pathogenesis of the disease in question. Molecular therapies are also termed "gene therapy" since in many instances the target of the therapeutic intervention is a particular gene mutated in that disease. However, in this chapter, therapeutic approaches for treating the defects of mitochondrial genes are not included.

Molecular therapies may be curative or at least substantially beneficial. In contrast to molecular therapies, conventional treatments are usually, but not invariably, based on empirical principles and consist mainly of the treatment of symptoms.

Types of molecular therapies in myology

Most muscle diseases for which molecular therapies are currently planned or contemplated are genetically determined but there is no reason why in some nongenetic diseases molecular therapies could not be applied. For example, in some dysimmune myopathies, such as inflammatory muscle diseases, where the molecular background of the fundamental deleterious immunopathological features is known, appropriate corrections of such phenomena by molecular intervention could have therapeutic effect.

In genetic diseases, the target of the therapy is either directly a mutated gene itself or a mechanism (transcription or translation) related to the expression of that gene. It is important to emphasize that effective molecular therapeutic modalities are different in recessive versus dominant diseases (see below).

Cell therapy for muscle (i.e., transplantation of myogenic precursor or progenitor cells) may also be considered a cell-mediated gene therapy although one of its more important roles is tissue replacement (see below).

The most extensive efforts in developing effective molecular therapies in myology have been directed to Duchenne muscular dystrophy (DMD) and therefore, in this chapter, DMD will be used as the main prototype for recessive muscle disease. For dominant diseases, myotonic dystrophy type 1 will be used as a convenient prototype.

Indications for molecular therapies

Since most forms of molecular therapies are complex, expensive, and potentially risky, indications for their application require precise practical and ethical considerations. The key point is the assessment of the risk/benefit ratio. If a disease is prematurely fatal or entails severe downgrading of the quality of life, even a relatively risky procedure is justifiable. From the economic point of view, cost-effectiveness is also an important factor.

From the practical standpoint, the critical technical and scientific issues must be optimized in preclinical models before human trials are contemplated. For DMD, the mdx mouse [1] or the Golden Retriever Dystrophic (GRD) dog [2] models are very useful for such purposes.

Disorders of Voluntary Muscle, 8th edn., eds. George Karpati, David Hilton-Jones, Kate Bushby and Robert C. Griggs. Published by Cambridge University Press.

Specific modalities of molecular therapies for recessive diseases

The main types of molecular therapy applicable to *recessive diseases* using DMD as the prototype include the following:
Directly applied approaches

- Gene replacement
- Direct correction of genomic defect
- Correction of the deleterious effect(s) of the gene defect on the primary transcript
- Translational interference
- Upregulation of analog molecules

Indirect approaches

- Stimulation of muscle fiber regeneration
- Induction of muscle fiber hypertrophy
- Limiting fibrosis

Gene replacement

This approach consists of introduction into muscle fibers of a normal or at least functionally adequate version of the mutated gene which can produce a normal or near-normal protein product of the gene in question, which in the case of DMD is the one that encodes dystrophin. This gene is mutated in DMD and as a result muscle fibers are devoid of dystrophin protein; thus, they become highly susceptible to necrosis.

For gene replacement, there are a set of operational items that need to be optimized in preclinical models before human trials are initiated. These include the identification of the optimal transferable gene or at least the coding sequence thereof (cDNA), the use of a strong and preferably muscle-specific promoter, the use of a safe and efficient vector that can deliver a substantial number of expression cassettes to the myonuclei (transduction), and the determination of an efficient and safe route of administration of the vector/gene construct (reviewed in [3, 4, 5, 6]).

In terms of the *transferable gene*, because of the huge size of the entire dystrophin gene, only the coding sequence of the gene (cDNA) has been used. This has included the full-length cDNA (13.5 kb) [7, 8, 9], or a truncated "minigene" (6.5 kb) [10, 11, 12], or a really short microdystrophin cDNA (3.5–4.0 kb) [13, 14, 15]. The latter has been designed to fit the limited insert capacity of the adeno-associated viral vector (see below). Concerning the *promoters*, an ideal promoter is one that has a strong activity but at the same time is muscle specific to avoid production of dystrophin in cells where it is not needed and, in fact, where it may be deleterious. According to these criteria, several strong constitutive (viral) promoters (CMV, RSV and CAG or CB) are not ideal, but the most promising muscle-specific promoter, the one that controls the creatine kinase gene, is weaker than the viral promoter [16, 17]. Nevertheless, recent modifications of this promoter have shown promising results [18].

As far as the gene *vectors* are concerned, they are required because there are no natural molecules at the eukaryotic cell surface that can serve as a receptor or transporter of genetic material. The most favored vectors for in vivo use have been either plasmids (mediating "naked" gene transfer) or viral vectors. Unfortunately, plasmid-based gene transfer to muscle fibers is of low efficiency even when using enhancing procedures (electroporation or sonoporation, or intravascular delivery) that have been developed to improve the transduction efficiency of plasmid DNA [19, 20, 21, 22, 23]. Of the viral vectors, the most widely tested ones are the variably modified adenovirus (AV) vectors or the adeno-associated virus (AAV) vector. The most advanced AV is the one from which all early viral genes are removed ("gutted virus"), resulting in a very large insert capacity (35 kb) and a much reduced unwanted immunogenicity [24, 25]. However, AV vector fails to integrate, even partially, into the host genome, which is a negative feature for the treatment of a disease such as DMD; this is most likely because of a compromise in the longevity of transgene expression. Another negative feature of the AV vector is the fact that the specific primary receptors necessary for its intracellular entry (CAR) are scarce in mature muscle fibers. Long-term (up to 1 year), efficient and safe microdystrophin gene transfer has been demonstrated after treatment of mdx mice using AAV vectors [26, 27]. It was originally thought that AAV vectors integrated into the cell chromosomes. Recent studies however indicated that integration is a relatively rare event [28]. Hence, re-administration of AAV vectors will probably be necessary to provide sustained dystrophin expression in muscle. Importantly, the small AAV vector insert capacity for the gene payload is limited to about 4.5 kb, requiring drastic truncation of the dystrophin cDNA.

With regard to the *route of administration*, intramuscular injection is the simplest, but it is not practical because of the widespread distribution of muscle tissue. Obviously, intravascular (intra-arterial or retrograde intravenous) dissemination of the gene construct (containing the expression cassette that consists of the promoter plus the cDNA and the polyA tail) is the route of choice.

None of the numerous tested combinations of the cited options has yet proved absolutely ideal in preclinical experiments, as various setbacks have compromised the efficiency and safety of the procedures and protocols. These include poor transduction of mature muscle fibers, a limited period of effective transgene expression, and deleterious immune reactions against the vector and/or transgene protein. However, some paradigms appeared to be more promising than others. For example, the intravascular administration of an AAV vector of a choice serotype carrying a dystrophin microgene controlled by an abridged creatine kinase (CK) promoter had sufficiently promising results in preclinical models [15, 29] that human trials have been initiated (see below). Furthermore, in other gene replacement experiments of more limited preclinical success, meticulous dissection of the causes of the suboptimal results will enable investigators to improve the attractiveness of some of these paradigms.

Direct correction of the genomic defect

Theoretically, direct correction of the DNA abnormality (mutation) would be an attractive therapeutic approach [30], but in diseases such as DMD where a large percentage of mutations consist of variable deletions or duplications, such undertaking in vivo is not feasible. Even in less extensive types of mutations, such as a single base change causing a premature stop codon, it is simpler to bring about a therapeutic effect by manipulations of the primary transcript or mRNA (see below).

Therapeutic manipulations of the primary transcript

The effect of deletion mutations upon the functionality of the dystrophin gene depends on whether the deleted exons leave the mRNA configuration in-frame or out-of-frame. In the former scenario, the resulting mRNA is capable of generating at least a truncated dystrophin with some functional value and a less severe clinical phenotype. However, if the deletion causes an out-of-frame configuration, the primary RNA transcript and the mRNA will contain a premature stop codon downstream from the deletion and translation beyond that point is obviated. The resulting highly truncated dystrophin protein is not viable and complete dystrophin deficiency ensues with resulting necrosis of the muscle fibers and a full-blown DMD phenotype. This second scenario, however, can be modified if the out-of-frame mutation in the primary RNA transcript is transformed into an in-frame mutation. This is possible by manipulating the splicing mechanism using a process in which one or more additional exons downstream are spliced out to transform the deletion profile into the in-frame configuration (reviewed in [31, 32]). This will permit the generation of a variably truncated dystrophin with some functional value. Thus, the clinical phenotype is transformed from severe DMD to a less severe Becker muscular dystrophy (BMD) phenotype. The manipulation of the splicing to bring about the cited effects can be made with use of custom-designed oligonucleotides, or morpholinos or small RNA that can block the splicing at a specific exon–intron junction resulting in the loss of one or more additional exon(s) ("exon skipping") [33]. The blockage of the splicing at a specific donor or receptor site is brought about by preventing access of the active moiety of the relevant spliceosome to that site. For example, a deletion that involves exons 45–54 inclusively causes an out-of-frame configuration of the primary transcript since in the resulting mRNA the adjacent exons 44–55 are not in-frame and a premature stop codon forms downstream within exon 55. If the normal splicing at the junction of exon and intron 44 is obviated, exon 44 is also spliced out (along with intron 44) and the configuration of the adjacent exons 43–55 of the mRNA is now in-frame.

The exon skipping approach can also be used to remove a primary stop codon [34, 35, 36 37]. For example, in the mdx mouse a primary stop codon in exon 23 causes complete dystrophin deficiency. Removal of exon 23, including the stop codon, leaves an in-frame configuration with the juxtaposition of exons 22–24 in the transcript and mRNA. While the principle of the selective exon removal approach is attractive and proved to work in some experimental models in vivo, it must be realized that it has considerable drawbacks. This includes the fact that it only mitigates the phenotype and for every case custom-designed nucleotides must be designed. Thus the cost-efficiency of the procedure is not really great. Nevertheless, limited human trials are underway [33, 38].

Translational interference

This approach is applicable to cases in which the mutation consists of a primary premature stop codon due to a single missense base change. The gene defect causes premature translational arrest and the truncated protein is unstable causing total dystrophin deficiency and a DMD phenotype. The procedure is based on modification of the normal translational process by which the premature stop codon is ignored by the ribosomes. Thus, premature translational arrest does not occur and a near-normal dystrophin can be produced. The phenomenon has been dubbed as translational "read-through." Initially, gentamicin [39] was proposed for such a role but in subtoxic doses it did not work in four DMD patients [40]. More recently, a synthetic orally administered small molecule, dubbed PTC124, has been found to be encouraging in preclinical experiments [41].

Presently the apparently nontoxic PTC124 drug is undergoing phase I/II trials in properly selected muscular dystrophy patients. Regretfully, the chemical structure and the molecular mechanism of its action have not been revealed by the manufacturer and the reason why it apparently does not have a "read-through" action on normal stop codons has not been explained satisfactorily. Furthermore, the percentage of read-through events/non-read-through translation per unit time, which would determine its efficiency, remain unknown.

Upregulation of a normally occurring functional analog of the missing or abnormal protein

It has been realized for some time that immature isoproteins are functionally similar to their mature versions and that the immature isoform may functionally substitute for the absence of the mature version. This phenomenon was first identified in the genetic deficiency of glycogen phosphorylase (causing McArdle disease), where the temporary emergence of the immature isoforms of glycogen phosphorylase in regenerating muscle fibers, encoded at a different locus, could compensate for the deficiency of the mature enzyme [42]. In fact, this approach is being explored as a molecular therapy for McArdle disease, which creates major functional disturbance of the use of skeletal muscles [43].

An even more exciting situation of this type is applicable to DMD where dystrophin has a close functional and structural paralogue but that is normally only expressed in the neuromuscular or myotendinous junctions [44]. This molecule, utrophin, is encoded at a locus on chromosome 6. There is ample experimental evidence to show that, if in animal models of dystrophin deficiency the expression of utrophin is made to substantially increase such that it is abundantly expressed on the surface of muscle fibers ("extrasynaptic expression"), most features of the dystrophy are mitigated or negated. Such marked extrasynaptic utrophin expression has been induced in mdx/utrophin transgenic mice [45, 46, 47]. In postnatal dystrophin-deficient models, a marked increase of extrasynaptic utrophin can be achieved by utrophin gene transfer, in which the promoter of the transgenic utrophin ensures extrasynaptic localization of the neutrophin [48, 49, 50, 51], or by enhancing the transcription or translation of the endogenous utrophin [52], or by inhibiting the proteolytic turnover of the very small amount of utrophin normally generated in the extrasynaptic location. This latter scenario was achieved to a remarkable degree by creating a low-grade inflammation in the mdx muscle [53]. In such a situation it appeared that certain inflammatory cytokines inhibited the activity of calpain-1/2, a known proteolytic enzyme of utrophin [54]. A major search is underway to find a nontoxic molecule whose administration produces a mild to moderate inhibition of calpain-1/2 and thus augments, for the long-term, the extrasynaptic utrophin level. The strategy of relying therapeutically on large amounts of extrasynaptic utrophin appears to be superior to achieving dystrophin expression by gene replacement since utrophin is an immunologically inoffensive molecule in dystrophin-deficient hosts, whereas neodystrophin is an immunostimulant.

Indirect approaches

Stimulation of muscle fiber regeneration [55]

As indicated above, the fundamental defect in DMD is deficiency of dystrophin which predisposes muscle fibers to segmental necrosis usually triggered by lengthening contractions. Regeneration of necrotic muscle fiber segments after a single or few a cycles of necrosis is usually strong and based on the mitotic activation of the normally dormant myogenic precursor or progenitor cells, also called "satellite cells." However, these cells do not have an unlimited capacity to divide, and after about 50–60 mitotic divisions they become senescent and then unable to contribute to regeneration. Since in DMD, and in some other dystrophies, regenerated fibers also undergo unlimited cycles of necrosis, most muscle fibers eventually reach the stage of regeneration failure. This leads to muscle fiber loss with adipose and fibrous tissue replacement, which is the basis of progressive muscle atrophy and weakness of the dystrophic muscles. From the above discussion it would follow that if this regeneration failure could be reduced or obviated, the catastrophic dystrophic phenotype could be averted. However, it appears that this mitotic constraint (also called Hayflick constraint) is based on a genetic program insinuated in the cell cycle program that cannot be eradicated or overcome. An artificially induced increase of the myogenic transcription factors (myoD, myogenin, myf 5, etc.) cannot overcome this mitotic constraint [56].The inhibition of the myostatin system (see below) might attain a degree of myogenic cell stimulation, but not necessarily an override of the Hayflick constraint.

One possible approach to deal with the cited regeneration failure based on senescence of the myogenic progenitor cells is the introduction of quasi stem cells with a myogenic differentiating potential as well as immortality. Such cells were identified as mesoangioblasts, which are believed to derive from pericytes of blood vessels [57, 58, 59]. If such cells are introduced into dystrophic muscles, some may fuse into the host muscle fibers endowing them with quasi infinite regenerating potential. In addition, if they derive from a normal source, they could also function as agents of cell-mediated transfer of the dystrophin gene, thus even preventing necrosis. Other mesangioblasts may fuse with each other and create new muscle fibers, which, if innervated, could amount to cell and tissue replacement of lost muscle fibers.

Induction of muscle fiber hypertrophy [60]

A novel molecule, called myostatin, was recently discovered which is a negative regulator of muscle fiber growth and mass and it also acts as a suppressor of the proliferation and differentiation of myogenic precursor cells. In this capacity, inhibition of its action could lead to muscle fiber hypertrophy and stimulation of muscle fiber growth and possibly enhancement of regeneration. In fact, ample experimental evidence is available to prove the validity of the above-cited points. It was hypothesized that the muscle fiber hypertrophy that could be induced by myostatin inhibition might have therapeutic effects in various muscular dystrophies. In fact, in mdx mice myostatin inhibition has improved various dystrophic indices [61, 62, 63]. However, it is not clear if this was due to the creation of muscle fiber hypertrophy or stimulation of muscle fiber regeneration or perhaps both. In fact, in DMD, it has been established that having a small caliber actually protects muscle fibers from necrosis, which would imply that muscle fiber hypertrophy, by itself, might be counterproductive for the long-term [64]. However, no precise study has been performed to determine if by myostatin inhibition the mitotic constraint of the myogenic progenitor cells has been lifted. Since there are many convenient means of inhibiting the myostatin system [i.e., inhibition of the binding of myostatin to its receptor (activin type IIB) at the muscle fiber surface by the application of follistatin or inactivation of the circulating activated myostatin by specific antibodies, etc.], therapeutic trials in DMD and in other dystrophies are likely to follow [60].

Limiting intramuscular fibrosis [65]

As indicated earlier, in dystrophic muscles in general, but in DMD in particular, endomysial connective tissue is abnormally increased. While the stimulus and source of the endomysial collagen overproduction remain unclear, it is certain that, in addition to the loss of muscle fibers, the excess fibrous tissue compromises muscle function. Thus, limiting fibrosis could have therapeutic value. One theory maintains that endomysial fibrosis is a reaction to the loss of muscle fibers, while another holds that it is a byproduct of the basic dystrophic process [65]. For example, the phagocytic macrophages that are mobilized in response to muscle fiber necrosis may generate soluble fibrogenic cytokines that enhance collagen production by interstitial fibroblasts. This may be analogous to excess fibrous tissue production in interstitial pulmonary fibrosis, in scleroderma, or in chronic graft versus host reaction. Monoclonal antibodies are available to inactivate fibrogenic cytokines but they tend to activate intramuscular inflammation [65].

Specific modalities of molecular therapies for dominant diseases

In dominant diseases the source of molecular pathogenicity is the mutant allele, which is characterized as *dominant negative effect*. The activity of the normal allele is not capable of negating or even mitigating the dominant negative effect of the mutant allele. In fact, a reduction of the amount of the protein product of the affected gene is not pathogenic and therefore gene replacement does not make sense. In light of these facts, the molecular therapeutic strategies for dominant diseases differ from those discussed above for recessive diseases. The dominant negative effect related to the dominant allele may be mediated by an abnormal primary transcript/mRNA or the abnormal relevant protein. The best example of the former is the abnormal primary RNA transcript that is produced by the mutant allele in myotonic dystrophy type 1 (MyD1) as a result of the expansion of a CTG trinucleotide repeat in the 5′ untranslated region of the *DMPK* gene (reviewed in [66, 67, 68]). The abnormal RNA transcript originating from the mutant allele accumulates in the myonuclei and sequesters important molecules, such as Muscleblind 1, that have an important role in the splicing of primary transcripts [69, 70]. This, in turn, will give rise to several "misspliced" abnormal proteins, such as the chloride channel and the insulin receptor, etc., thus producing a multisystem disease. In other words, MyD1 is a classical Mendelian single gene mutation scenario masquerading as a multigenic disease. Thus, the pathogenic role is that of the RNA and not the protein. Accordingly, the molecular therapeutic approaches include selective silencing of the mutant gene by RNAi or introducing genes that encode extra amounts of splicing factors that are "soaked up" by the abnormal primary transcript [71, 72]. In another situation exemplified by Huntington disease caused by an expansion of CAG trinucleotide in the coding sequence of the Huntingtin gene, the pathogenic culprit is the mutant protein containing variable but abnormal lengths of polylysine tracts, which binds to different cellular proteins corrupting their function [73]. In such a situation, the protein related to the mutant allele has the pathogenic role. Molecular therapeutic interventions in this scenario include silencing the mutant allele or inhibiting the formation of, or inactivating, the mutant Huntingtin.

Conclusions

From the foregoing discussion it is clear that by utilizing the molecular scientific background of a disease and employing molecular techniques, it is possible to design and explore the usefulness of diverse molecular therapies for genetic muscle diseases. However, it is also clear that molecular therapies are still in their infancy. Certainly, they lag behind the development of molecular diagnostics. However, increasing preclinical and clinical studies are underway in several laboratories (not detailed for logistic reasons) which will surely lead to practicable, safe, effective, and cost-effective therapeutic modalities [74].

The key issues to consider at this stage are:

- Of the several available and sometimes competitive strategies discussed earlier, which one is the most suitable for a given case?
- At what stage of a disease is it practical and ethical to intervene? Common sense would indicate that earlier is better.
- Proper education of the public and of individual patients and their families concerning molecular therapies is of utmost importance to dispel some misconceptions and false presumptions concerning molecular science in general and molecular therapies in particular.
- Continue research efforts to develop molecular approaches for the treatment of nongenetic muscle diseases.

References

1. P. Sicinski, Y. Geng, A. S. Ryder-Cook, E. A. Barnard, M. G. Darlison, P. J. Barnard, The molecular basis of muscular dystrophy in the mdx mouse: a point mutation. *Science* **30** (1989), 1578–1580.
2. B. A. Valentine, B. J. Cooper, A. De Lahunta, R. O. Quinn, J. T. Blue, Canine X-linked muscular dystrophy. An animal model of Duchenne muscular dystrophy: clinical studies. *J. Neurol. Sci.* **88** (1988), 69–81.
3. J. S. Chamberlain, Gene therapy of muscular dystrophy. *Hum. Mol. Genet.* **11** (2002), 2355–2362.
4. K. J. Nowak, K. E.Davies, Duchenne muscular dystrophy and dystrophin: pathogenesis and opportunities for treatment. *EMBO Rep.* **5** (2004), 872–876.
5. J. V. Chakkalakal, J. Thompson, R. J. Parks, B. J. Jasmin, Molecular, cellular, and pharmacological therapies for Duchenne/Becker muscular dystrophies. *FASEB J.* **19** (2005), 880–891.

6. K. Foster, H. Foster, J. G. Dickson, Gene therapy progress and prospects: Duchenne muscular dystrophy. *Gene Ther.* **13** (2006), 1677–1685.
7. S. E. Haecker, H. H. Stedman, R. J. Balice-Gordon, *et al.*, In vivo expression of full-length human dystrophin from adenoviral vectors deleted of all viral genes. *Hum. Gene Ther.* **7** (1996), 1907–1914.
8. C. DelloRusso, J. M. Scott, D. Hartigan-O'Connor, *et al.*, Functional correction of adult mdx mouse muscle using gutted adenoviral vectors expressing full-length dystrophin. *Proc. Natl. Acad. Sci. U. S. A.* **99** (2002), 12979–12984.
9. R. Gilbert, R. W. Dudley, A. B. Liu, B. J. Petrof, J. Nalbantoglu, G. Karpati, Prolonged dystrophin expression and functional correction of mdx mouse muscle following gene transfer with a helper-dependent (gutted) adenovirus-encoding murine dystrophin. *Hum. Mol. Genet.* **12** (2003), 1287–1299.
10. N. Vincent, T. Ragot, H. Gilgenkrantz, *et al.*, Long-term correction of mouse dystrophic degeneration by adenovirus-mediated transfer of a minidystrophin gene. *Nat. Genet.* **5** (1993), 130–134.
11. N. Deconinck, T. Ragot, G. Marechal, M. Perricaudet, J. M. Gillis, Functional protection of dystrophic mouse (mdx) muscles after adenovirus-mediated transfer of a dystrophin minigene. *Proc. Natl. Acad. Sci. U. S. A.* **93** (1996), 3570–3574.
12. G. Acsadi, H. Lochmuller, A. Jani, *et al.*, Dystrophin expression in muscles of mdx mice after adenovirus-mediated in vivo gene transfer. *Hum. Gene Ther.* **7** (1996), 129–140.
13. B. Wang, J. Li, X. Xiao, Adeno-associated virus vector carrying human minidystrophin genes effectively ameliorates muscular dystrophy in mdx mouse model. *Proc. Natl. Acad. Sci. U. S. A.* **97** (2000), 13714–13719.
14. S. Q. Harper, M. A. Hauser, C. DelloRusso, *et al.*, Modular flexibility of dystrophin: implications for gene therapy of Duchenne muscular dystrophy. *Nat. Med.* **8** (2002), 253–261.
15. P. Gregorevic, M. J. Blankinship, J. M. Allen, *et al.*, Systemic delivery of genes to striated muscles using adeno-associated viral vectors. *Nat. Med.* **10** (2004), 828–834.
16. N. Larochelle, W. Oualikene, P. Dunant, *et al.*, The short MCK1350 promoter/enhancer allows for sufficient dystrophin expression in skeletal muscles of mdx mice. *Biochem. Biophys. Res. Commun.* **292** (2002), 626–631.
17. M. A. Hauser, A. Robinson, D. Hartigan-O'Connor, *et al.*, Analysis of muscle creatine kinase regulatory elements in recombinant adenoviral vectors. *Mol. Ther.* **2** (2000), 16–25.
18. M. Z. Salva, C. L. Himeda, P. W. Tai, *et al.*, Design of tissue-specific regulatory cassettes for high-level rAAV-mediated expression in skeletal and cardiac muscle. *Mol. Ther.* **15** (2007), 320–329.
19. Q. L. Lu, G. Bou-Gharios, T. A. Partridge, Non-viral gene delivery in skeletal muscle: a protein factory. *Gene Ther.* **10** (2003), 131–142.
20. M. J. Molnar, R. Gilbert, Y. Lu, *et al.*, Factors influencing the efficacy, longevity, and safety of electroporation-assisted plasmid-based gene transfer into mouse muscles. *Mol. Ther.* **10** (2004), 447–455.
21. G. Danialou, A. S. Comtois, R. W. Dudley, *et al.*, Ultrasound increases plasmid-mediated gene transfer to dystrophic muscles without collateral damage. *Mol. Ther.* **6** (2002), 687–693.
22. H. Herweijer, J. A. Wolff, Progress and prospects: naked DNA gene transfer and therapy. *Gene Ther.* **10** (2003), 453–458.
23. G. Zhang, V. Budker, P. Williams, V. Subbotin, J. A. Wolff, Efficient expression of naked DNA delivered intraarterially to limb muscles of nonhuman primates. *Hum. Gene Ther.* **12** (2001), 427–438.
24. S. Kochanek, High-capacity adenoviral vectors for gene transfer and somatic gene therapy. *Hum. Gene Ther.* **10** (1999), 2451–2459.
25. R. Alba, A. Bosch, M. Chillon, Gutless adenovirus: last-generation adenovirus for gene therapy. *Gene Ther.* **12**:Suppl 1 (2005), S18–S27.
26. T. Athanasopoulos, I. R. Graham, H. Foster, G. Dickson, Recombinant adeno-associated viral (rAAV) vectors as therapeutic tools for Duchenne muscular dystrophy (DMD). *Gene Ther.* **11**:Suppl 1 (2004), S109–S121.
27. M. J. Blankinship, P. Gregorevic, J. S. Chamberlain, Gene therapy strategies for Duchenne muscular dystrophy utilizing recombinant adeno-associated virus vectors. *Mol. Ther.* **13** (2006), 241–249.
28. B. C. Schnepp, K. R. Clark, D. L. Klemanski, C. A. Pacak, P. R. Johnson, Genetic fate of recombinant adeno-associated virus vector genomes in muscle. *J. Virol.* **77** (2003), 3495–3504.
29. P. Gregorevic, J. M. Allen, E. Minami, *et al.*, rAAV6-microdystrophin preserves muscle function and extends lifespan in severely dystrophic mice. *Nat. Med.* **12** (2006), 787–789.
30. T. A. Rando, M. H. Disatnik, L. Z. Zhou, Rescue of dystrophin expression in mdx mouse muscle by RNA/DNA oligonucleotides. *Proc. Natl. Acad. Sci. U. S. A.* **97** (2000), 5363–5368.
31. G. McClorey, S. Fletcher, S. Wilton, Splicing intervention for Duchenne muscular dystrophy. *Curr. Opin. Pharmacol.* **5** (2005), 529–534.
32. A. Artsma-Rus, G. J. vanOmmen, Antisense-mediated exon skipping: a versatile tool with therapeutic and research applications. *RNA* **13** (2007), 1609–1624.
33. J. C. van Deutekom, A. A. Janson, I. B. Ginjaar, *et al.*, Local dystrophin restoration with antisense oligonucleotide PRO051. *N. Engl. J. Med.* **357** (2007), 2677–2686.
34. Q. L. Lu, C. J. Mann, F. Lou, *et al.*, Functional amounts of dystrophin produced by skipping the mutated exon in the mdx dystrophic mouse. *Nat. Med.* **9** (2003), 1009–1014.
35. C. J. Mann, K. Honeyman, A. J. Cheng, *et al.*, Antisense-induced exon skipping and synthesis of dystrophin in the mdx mouse. *Proc. Natl. Acad. Sci. U. S. A.* **98** (2001), 42–47.
36. M. A. Denti, A. Rosa, G. D'Antona, *et al.*, Body-wide gene therapy of Duchenne muscular dystrophy in the mdx mouse model. *Proc. Natl. Acad. Sci. U. S. A.* **103** (2006), 3758–3763.
37. A. Goyenvalle, A. Vulin, F. Fougerousse, *et al.*, Rescue of dystrophic muscle through U7 snRNA-mediated exon skipping. *Science* **306** (2004), 1796–1799.
38. C. Bertoni, Clinical approaches in the treatment of Duchenne muscular dystrophy (DMD) using oligonucleotides. *Front. Biosci.* **13** (2008), 517–527.

39. E. R. Barton-Davis, L. Cordier, D. I. Shoturma, S. E. Leland, H. L. Sweeney, Aminoglycoside antibiotics restore dystrophin function to skeletal muscles of mdx mice. *J. Clin. Invest.* **104** (1999), 375–381.

40. P. Dunant, M. C. Walter, G. Karpati, H. Lochmuller, Gentamicin fails to increase dystrophin expression in dystrophin-deficient muscle. *Muscle Nerve* **27** (2003), 624–627.

41. E. M. Welch, E. R. Barton, J. Zhuo, *et al.*, PTC124 targets genetic disorders caused by nonsense mutations. *Nature* **447** (2007), 87–91.

42. G. Karpati, Mitigation of deleterious effects of certain abnormal genes in immature skeletal muscle cells. *Trends Neurosci.* **7** (1985), 524–525.

43. J. Howell, K. R. Walker, L. Davies, *et al.*, Adenovirus and adeno-associated virus-mediated delivery of human myophosphorylase cDNA and LacZ cDNA to muscle in the ovine model of McArdle's disease: expression and re-expression of glycogen phosphorylase. *Neuromuscul. Disord.* **18** (2008), 248–268.

44. G. Karpati, Utrophin muscles in on the action. *Nat. Med.* **3** (1997), 22–23.

45. J. A. Rafael, J. M. Tinsley, A. C. Potter, A. E. Deconinck, K. E. Davies, Skeletal muscle-specific expression of a utrophin transgene rescues utrophin-dystrophin deficient mice. *Nat. Genet.* **19** (1998), 79–82.

46. J. Tinsley, N. Deconinck, R. Fisher, *et al.*, Expression of full-length utrophin prevents muscular dystrophy in mdx mice. *Nat. Med.* **4** (1998), 1441–1444.

47. J. M. Tinsley, A. C. Potter, S. R. Phelps, R. Fisher, J. I. Trickett, K. E. Davies, Amelioration of the dystrophic phenotype of mdx mice using a truncated utrophin transgene. *Nature* **384** (1996), 349–353.

48. J. R. Deol, G. Danialou, N. Larochelle, *et al.*, Successful compensation for dystrophin deficiency by a Helper-dependent adenovirus expressing full-length utrophin. *Mol. Ther.* **15** (2007), 1767–1774.

49. M. Cerletti, T. Negri, F. Cozzi, *et al.*, Dystrophic phenotype of canine X-linked muscular dystrophy is mitigated by adenovirus-mediated utrophin gene transfer. *Gene Ther.* **10** (2003), 750–757.

50. P. M. Wakefield, J. M. Tinsley, M. J. Wood, R. Gilbert, G. Karpati, K. E. Davies, Prevention of the dystrophic phenotype in dystrophin/utrophin-deficient muscle following adenovirus-mediated transfer of a utrophin minigene. *Gene Ther.* **7** (2000), 201–204.

51. R. Gilbert, J. Nalbantoglu, B. J. Petrof, *et al.*, Adenovirus-mediated utrophin gene transfer mitigates the dystrophic phenotype of mdx mouse muscles. *Hum. Gene Ther.* **10** (1999), 1299–1310.

52. E. Mattei, N. Corbi, M. G. Di Certo, *et al.*, Utrophin up-regulation by an artificial transcription factor in transgenic mice. *PLoS ONE* **2** (2007), e774.

53. I. Waheed, R. Gilbert, J. Nalbantoglu, G. H. Guibinga, B. J. Petrof, G. Karpati, Factors associated with induced chronic inflammation in mdx skeletal muscle cause posttranslational stabilization and augmentation of extrasynaptic sarcolemmal utrophin. *Hum. Gene Ther.* **16** (2005), 489–501.

54. I. Courdier-Fruh, A. Briguet, Utrophin is a calpain substrate in muscle cells. *Muscle Nerve* **33** (2006), 753–759.

55. G. Karpati, M. Molnar, Muscle fiber regeneration in human skeletal muscle diseases. In *Skeletal Muscle Regeneration and Repair*, eds. S. Schiaffino, T. Partridge. (New York: Springer, 2008), pp. 199–215.

56. T. Nastasi, N. Rosenthal, Boosting muscle regeneration. In *Skeletal Muscle Regeneration and Repair*, eds. S. Schiaffino, T. Partridge. (New York: Springer, 2008), pp. 335–355.

57. A. Dellavalle, M. Sampaolesi, R. Tonlorenzi, *et al.*, Pericytes of human skeletal muscle are myogenic precursors distinct from satellite cells. *Nat. Cell Biol.* **9** (2007), 255–267.

58. M. Sampaolesi, S. Blot, G. D'Antona, *et al.*, Mesoangioblast stem cells ameliorate muscle function in dystrophic dogs. *Nature* **444** (2006), 574–579.

59. B. Peault, M. Rudnicki, Y. Torrente, *et al.*, Stem and progenitor cells in skeletal muscle development, maintenance, and therapy. *Mol. Ther.* **15** (2007), 867–877.

60. A. Nadeau, G. Karpati, Are big muscles necessarily good muscles? *Ann. Neurol.* **63** (2008), 543–545.

61. K. R. Wagner, A. C. McPherron, N. Winik, S. J. Lee, Loss of myostatin attenuates severity of muscular dystrophy in mdx mice. *Ann. Neurol.* **52** (2002), 832–836.

62. S. Bogdanovich, K. J. Perkins, T. O. Krag, L. A. Whittemore, T. S. Khurana, Myostatin propeptide-mediated amelioration of dystrophic pathophysiology. *FASEB J.* **19** (2005), 543–549.

63. S. Bogdanovich, T. O. Krag, E. R. Barton, *et al.*, Functional improvement of dystrophic muscle by myostatin blockade. *Nature* **420** (2002), 418–421.

64. G. Karpati, S. Carpenter, S. Prescott, Small-caliber skeletal muscle fibers do not suffer necrosis in mdx mouse dystrophy. *Muscle Nerve* **11** (1988), 795–803.

65. L. Passerini, P. Bernasconi, F. Baggi, *et al.*, Fibrogenic cytokines and extent of fibrosis in muscle of dogs with x-linked golden retriever muscular dystrophy. *Neuromuscul. Disord.* **12** (2002), 828–835.

65. F. Andreetta, P. Bernasconi, F. Baggi, *et al.*, Immunomodulation of TGF-beta1 in mdx mouse inhibits connective tissue proliferation in diaphragm but increases inflammatory response: Implications for antifibrotic therapy. *J. Neuroimmunol.* **175** (2006), 77–86.

66. L. P. Ranum, J. W. Day, Myotonic dystrophy: RNA pathogenesis comes into focus. *Am. J. Hum. Genet.* **74** (2004), 793–804.

67. L. P. Ranum, T. A. Cooper, RNA-mediated neuromuscular disorders. *Annu. Rev. Neurosci.* **29** (2006), 259–277.

68. R. J. Osborne, C. A. Thornton, RNA-dominant diseases. *Hum. Mol. Genet.* **15**: Spec No 2 (2006), R162–R169.

69. H. Jiang, A. Mankodi, M. S. Swanson, R. T. Moxley, C. A. Thornton, Myotonic dystrophy type 1 is associated with nuclear foci of mutant RNA, sequestration of muscleblind proteins and deregulated alternative splicing in neurons. *Hum. Mol. Genet.* **13** (2004), 3079–3088.

70. R. N. Kanadia, K. A. Johnstone, A. Mankodi, *et al.*, A muscleblind knockout model for myotonic dystrophy. *Science* **302** (2003), 1978–1980.

71. R. N. Kanadia, J. Shin, Y. Yuan, *et al.*, Reversal of RNA missplicing and myotonia after muscleblind overexpression in a mouse poly(CUG) model for myotonic dystrophy. *Proc. Natl. Acad. Sci. U. S. A.* **103** (2006), 11748–11753.

72. E. M. Ovan-Wright, B. L. Davidson, RNAi: a potential therapy for the dominantly inherited nucleotide repeat diseases. *Gene Ther.* **13** (2006), 525–531.

73. J. Shao, M. I. Diamond, Polyglutamine diseases: emerging concepts in pathogenesis and therapy. *Hum. Mol. Genet.* **16**: Spec No 2 (2007), R115–R123.

74. D. J. Wells, Treatments for muscular dystrophy: increased treatment options for Duchenne and related muscular dystrophies. *Gene Ther.* **15**:5 (2008), 1077–1078.

Section 3B Chapter 10

Description of muscle disease – specific diseases

Dystrophinopathies

Michael Sinnreich

History

An excellent and exhaustive summary of the history of Duchenne muscular dystrophy is provided by Eric. P. Hoffman in the previous edition of this book [1]. The disease that would later carry his name appears to have been described before the renowned Duchenne de Boulogne published on the disorder in 1868 [2].

Phenotypes

Duchenne muscular dystrophy

Duchenne muscular dystrophy (DMD) affects about 1 in 3500 live male births, which makes it the most common inherited disease of childhood. Although some infants may be floppy, the most common earliest clinical presentation is delay in walking, sometimes exceeding 18 months of age, and Duchenne boys tend to appear clumsy. Later, affected boys develop difficulty running or climbing stairs, and often use the Gower maneuver to arise from the floor, appreciated by the families at around 3–5 years of age. DMD is a multisystem disease with clinical involvement of skeletal muscles, heart, and the central nervous system.

Wasting and weakness affect muscles of the shoulder and pelvic girdles, with lower extremities being predominantly involved causing a waddling gait. Other muscle groups may show an increased contour, (often called hypertrophy or pseudohypertrophy), most prominently seen in the calves. Due to imbalance of muscle strength in most large joints, the stronger muscles permanently shorten and contractures ensue. The majority of DMD patients will have lost independent ambulation at around age 12 years and wheelchair dependency will further aggravate the contractures. Although some DMD patients lose ambulation later (so-called outliers), patients who remain ambulatory beyond age 16 are considered to suffer from the Becker type of dystrophinopathy. Respiratory compromise due to thoracic scoliosis and ventilatory muscle weakness may lead to pneumonia or respiratory failure, which is the most common cause of death in the late teens or early twenties. However, intensive cardiorespiratory care may delay the fatal outcome [3], in some cases into the fourth decade.

Cardiac involvement is present in about 90% of DMD boys, and is the cause of death in about 20% [4, 5, 6]. Cardiac disease manifests as dilated cardiomyopathy and/or arrhythmia usually in the second decade of life, although the actual disease process in the heart starts much earlier [7]. Therefore, abnormalities on investigation are more frequent than symptomatic presentation. Signs of heart failure may go unrecognized for a long period of time because of the reduced physical activity level due to skeletal muscle weakness.

The mean intelligence coefficient for Duchenne boys is about one standard deviation below the population mean [8]. The cognitive impairment in DMD is nonprogressive and does not correlate with muscle weakness. Many studies suggest that verbal intelligence and verbal skills are more affected than performance intelligence.

Dystrophinopathy patients have abnormal electroretinograms with reduction or absence of the b-wave in the dark adapted state [9]. The b-wave of the electroretinogram represents response to photoreceptor-mediated light stimulation by the middle and inner retinal neurons.

Becker muscular dystrophy (BMD)

Becker muscular dystrophy is a milder form of dystrophinopathy, with later disease onset, presenting usually in the teenage years. The incidence of this disease is about 1 in 17 000 live male births [10]. The disease has a slower progression than in patients with DMD but involves essentially the same muscle groups [11]. The disease can be so mild as to become symptomatic only in adult life, and cases presenting with muscle weakness in the sixth decade have been reported [12]. Such cases require differentiation from other forms of limb-girdle muscular dystrophy. Calf pain during exercise that is relieved by rest has been described as a typical, and often presenting, symptom in a large proportion of Becker patients [13]. Ninety percent of Becker patients develop a cardiomyopathy, which is the cause of death in about 50% [14, 15, 16, 17, 18]. As BMD patients are more active than DMD patients, their hearts have a higher

Disorders of Voluntary Muscle, 8th edn., eds. George Karpati, David Hilton-Jones, Kate Bushby and Robert C. Griggs. Published by Cambridge University Press.

workload. Some BMD patients may become symptomatic from cardiomyopathy prior to developing significant skeletal muscle weakness [19]. Intellectual impairment is less marked than in DMD. Reproductive fitness is lower in BMD than in limb-girdle muscular dystrophy patients with comparable disability [20].

X-linked cardiomyopathy

X-linked dilated cardiomyopathy is one end of the large clinical spectrum of dystrophinopathies presenting with predominant involvement of heart muscle. Although clinically skeletal muscles appear relatively spared, serum creatine kinase (CK) levels are elevated and skeletal muscle biopsy shows myopathic changes [21]. The disease typically affects males in their second decade, and can be fatal within 12–24 months if patients do not receive a heart transplant.

Carrier women can be affected later in life in a similar manner and while disease progression is less rapid it can nevertheless be likewise fatal.

Carrier women

There are several possibilities for how a woman can be carrier for a dystrophin mutation. The woman may have inherited an X-chromosome containing a dystrophin mutation from one of her parents. In this case, all her cells will contain an X-chromosome that carries the mutation. Placental female mammals inactivate one of their X-chromosomes randomly (in contrast to marsupials where always the paternal X-chromosome is inactivated). Therefore, only one X-chromosome will be transcriptionally active [22]. X-inactivation (or lyonization) occurs very early in embryonic development, and descendants of a given cell retain the same inactivation pattern. Depending on the degree of skewed inactivation and clonal propagation, a female carrier can manifest symptoms of the disease, ranging from mild asymmetrical weakness [23] to expression of the full disease. Rarely monozygotic twin girls can show varied phenotypes due to differently skewed X-inactivation [24, 25]. Muscle biopsy usually shows a mosaic dystrophin expression which can differ depending on the sample site.

As a large proportion of dystrophin mutations are spontaneous, a mutation can arise in the sperm or in the oozyte prior to conception. In such instances, all the cells of the body will carry the mutation, and disease severity will depend on the degree and distribution of skewed X-inactivation.

If, however, the spontaneous mutation occurs after conception, the patient will be a mosaic with some cells containing two normal X-chromosomes, and other cells containing an X-chromosome with the dystrophin mutation. The clinical phenotype of these carrier women depends on the extent of mosaicism, which can be restricted to the germline, to the somatic cells or involve both the germline and somatic cells.

In Turner syndrome (45, XO) there is monosomy for the X-chromosome. If the X-chromosome carries a dystrophin gene mutation, the patient will express the dystrophinopathy phenotype [26].

In female embryos with X-chromosomal-autosomal translocation, the nonaffected X-chromosome is preferentially inactivated. Therefore, an X-chromosomal translocation that would disrupt the dystrophin locus could lead to a Duchenne phenotype in a girl. Such translocations led to the identification of the dystrophin gene [27] (see below).

The majority of carrier women do not complain of clinical symptoms of neuromuscular impairment. Symptoms are present in only about 20% of obligate carriers. However, a proportion of these women may have considerable muscle weakness. Weakness in BMD carriers is more rare than in DMD carriers. Signs of dilated cardiomyopathy are found in between 7% and 11% of carrier women [28, 29, 30]. Skeletal muscle weakness and cardiomyopathy do not have to occur in the same patient. Several reports have commented that carrier woman with skeletal muscle involvement do not necessarily have cardiomyopathy and vice versa.

Duchenne muscular dystrophy mimics and atypical phenotypes

Before dystrophin gene and protein analysis became routinely available, some patients suffering from spinal muscular atrophy, limb-girdle muscular dystrophies with distal weakness [31], congenital muscular dystrophy [32], metabolic myopathies [13], and nonprogressive myalgia and cramps [33] could not be differentiated reliably from dystrophinopathies. Furthermore, dystrophinopathies may present with unusual phenotypes such as quadriceps myopathy [34], or asymmetrical calf involvement in carrier women [23], as well as asymptomatic elevation of serum CK activity [35].

Molecular background

The discovery of the molecular defect of DMD in 1987 was the first triumph of "reverse genetics." This discovery was based on the molecular analysis of a patient who had a chromosomal gene deletion leading to DMD, retinitis pigmentosa, chronic granulomatous disease, and the McLeod red blood cell phenotype [36]. These studies led to the eventual cloning of the DMD gene [37, 38]. Leading up to this discovery were genetic linkage studies that confirmed the localization of the DMD gene to chromosome Xp21 [39]. Using the same genetic markers, it was found that BMD was allelic to DMD [40].

Genetic analysis of manifesting female carriers who had an X-autosomal translocation made a more precise localization of the culprit gene possible [41]. The specific autosome involved in each translocation was different, but the X-chromosomal breakpoint was always the same on the short arm of the X-chromosome, Xp21 [27, 42, 43] and X-chromosomal sequences flanking the breakpoint were identified, which were lacking in boys with DMD [41, 44] (Figure 10.1).

The gene encoding dystrophin is the largest known to date, covering up to 3 Mb of DNA, and its 79 exons are interspersed with some enormous introns [38]. Its large size may render it more vulnerable to mutations. The transcribed mRNA of the full-length isoform is 14 kb in length and the full-length protein is 427 kDa in molecular mass [45]. It takes about 16 hours to transcribe the mRNA which is cotranscriptionally spliced [46].

The dystrophin family contains the autosomal homologue, utrophin, and several small dystrophin-related proteins called dystrobrevins.

The muscle isoform of dystrophin consists of 3685 amino acids and is primarily expressed in skeletal muscle, smooth muscle, and cardiac muscle cells. The protein can be divided into four domains [47]:

1. An N-terminal globular domain of 240 amino acids that is similar in sequence to α-actinin and β-spectrin, containing two calponin homology domains that bind to F-actin [48]. This region is encoded by exons 1–8.

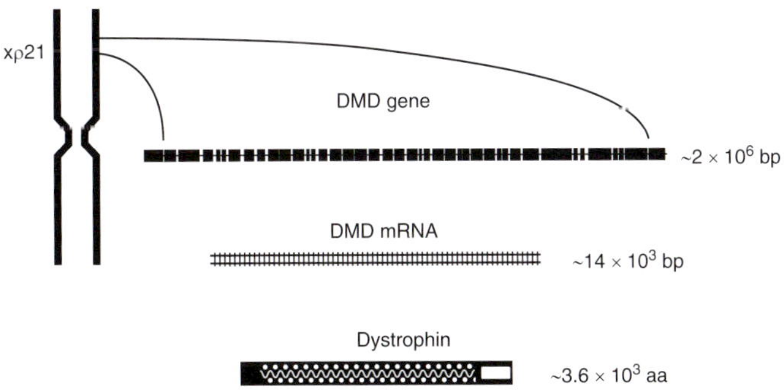

Figure 10.1. A schematic diagram of the dystrophin gene, mRNA, and protein. (Taken from Hoffman, E. P., *Disorders of Voluntary Muscle*, 7th edition, with permission [1]).

2. A rod-shaped domain, encoded by exons 9–62, and containing 2400 residues [49]. It consists of 24 spectrin-like repeats, which are interrupted by four flexible hinge regions, two of which are located at either end of the rod domain while the other two are located within the rod domain between repeats 3 and 4, as well as between repeats 19 and 20. The function of the rod domain is primarily to link the N-terminal actin-binding domain to the cysteine-rich domain, and thus it provides a link between the cytoskeleton and the dystrophin-associated glycoprotein complex (DGC). It also has some weak inherent actin-binding capabilities which are located around spectrin repeats 11–13.
3. A cysteine-rich domain that contains the crucial binding sites to β-dystroglycan, a WW domain [50], 2EF hand domains, and a ZZ domain [51]. It is encoded by exons 63–69.
4. A C-terminal domain which includes two alpha helical coiled-coil domains that bind dystrobrevin [52]. The C-terminal domain is 420 amino acids long and is encoded by exons 70–79. The C-terminal domain is subject to various sorts of alternative splicing.

In addition to various splice variants predominantly involving the C-terminus, a number of dystrophin isoforms are generated by several promoters which are controlled in a tissue-specific manner (Figure 10.2).

The muscle promoter controls transcription in skeletal muscle, heart, and smooth muscle as well as in the retina. Tissue expression of muscle dystrophin is developmentally regulated [53]. In the human fetus, muscle dystrophin is detectable as early as at 9 weeks of gestation. In cell culture

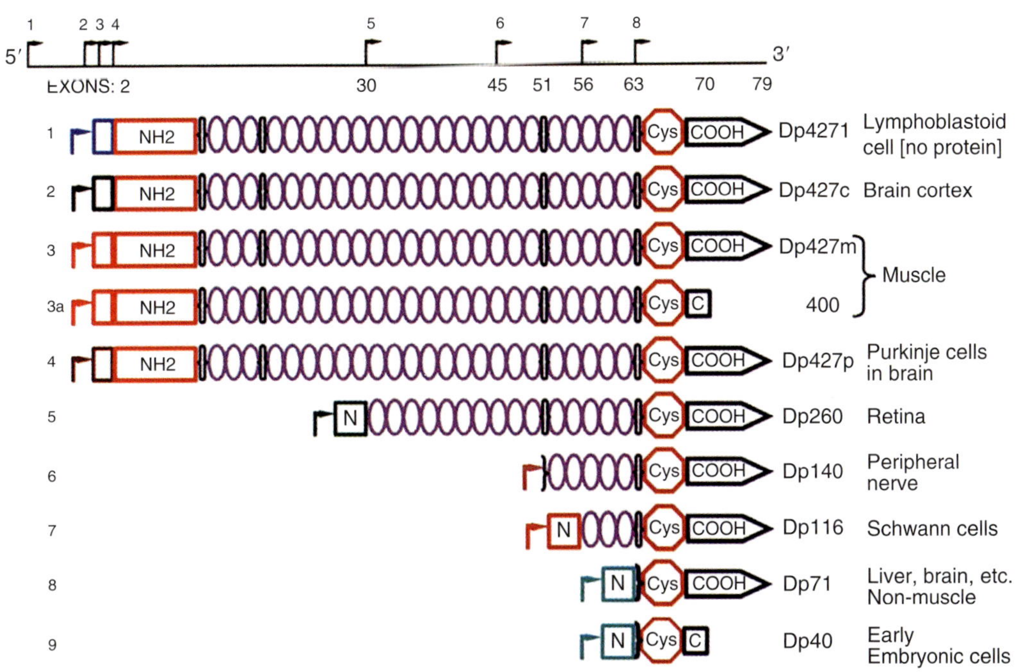

Figure 10.2. Schematic diagram of dystrophin isoforms and tissue distribution. For details see text. (Taken from Anderson, L. V. B., *Structural and Molecular Basis of Skeletal Muscle Diseases*, World Federation of Neurology, with permission from the volume editor, G. Karpati).

myoblasts express muscle dystrophin when they begin to differentiate into myotubes [54, 55].

The promoter, which is active in cortical neurons, is located upstream of the muscle promoter [56]. It drives transcription starting at its own first exon. This exon is spliced to the common exon 2 of the dystrophin gene [57]. Cortical dystrophin can be transcribed in skeletal muscle in case the muscle promoter is deleted. Such a scenario is seen in X-linked dilated cardiomyopathy, where deletions of the muscle promoter lead to cardiac disease and skeletal muscle is relatively spared [58].

Dystrophin in Purkinje cells of the cerebellum is driven by a promoter located between the muscle promoter and the common exon 2 [59]. It drives transcription starting with its own short exon which is spliced to the common exon 2 of dystrophin.

In lymphoblastoid cells an additional promoter sequence was identified 500 kb upstream of the cortical promoter. It drives transcription from its own first short exon, which is spliced to the common exon 3 of the dystrophin gene [60].

Shorter dystrophin isoforms have their initiation of transcription within the dystrophin gene by a variety of promoters that are interspersed within the intronic regions. The nomenclature for these dystrophin proteins (Dp) is based on their molecular weight.

Dp260 is expressed in retina, brain, and heart. Transcription starts with a unique exon that is spliced to the common exon 30 of the dystrophin gene [61].

Dp140 is found throughout the central nervous system and kidney, but not in skeletal or cardiac muscle. Its promoter lies in the large intron between exons 44 and 45, which is a hotspot for mutations. Transcription starts from a unique exon, which, however, is not translated. This exon is spliced to exon 51, which is the first translated exon of this isoform [62]. Lack of this isoform has been associated with cognitive impairment in dystrophinopathies [63].

Dp116 is expressed in Schwann cells of the peripheral nervous system where it is concentrated in the nodes of Ranvier. The promoter for this isoform lies in intron 55 and transcription is initiated from a unique exon which splices to exon 56 [64].

Dp71 is the major isoform in brain [65, 66], where it is predominantly expressed in the dentate gyrus. It is also found in heart and gut, but not in skeletal muscle. Dp71 has been associated with synaptic plasticity and its absence due to mutation in its gene has been linked to intellectual impairment [67]. The promoter for this isoform lies in intron 62, and the transcription initiation site lies upstream of exon 63. The last 13 hydrophilic amino acids of dystrophin are replaced in this isoform by a stretch of 31 amino acids, which confer hydrophobicity to this region [68].

Dp40 is ubiquitously expressed. The N-terminal part of the protein is identical to Dp71, but the C-terminus is markedly shortened, containing only 48 amino acids from the C-terminus of the full-length isoform. It is the only dystrophin isoform expressed in early embryonic stem cells [69].

Utrophin

Utrophin is an autosomal homologue of dystrophin; its gene is located on chromosome 6q24 in humans and it is transcribed by two promoters (A and B) [70] which are active in many tissues [71]. Similar to dystrophin, the utrophin gene also encodes several short isoforms [72, 73]. Whereas under normal conditions, dystrophin is expressed throughout the sarcolemmal membrane in adult skeletal muscle fibers, utrophin expression is restricted to the neuromuscular and to the myotendinous junctions [74, 75]. Utrophin is expressed in regenerating skeletal muscle fibers [74, 76], and as such can be used as an immunohistochemical marker of muscle regeneration. In tissue culture utrophin is expressed in myoblasts. In the absence of dystrophin, utrophin expression is post-transcriptionally upregulated and utrophin will be expressed in the extrasynaptic sarcolemmal membrane [74]. Utrophin has a molecular weight of 395 kDa and has similar domains to dystrophin [77]. Its N-terminal actin-binding domain has a high homology with the corresponding domain of dystrophin and binds to filamentous actin [78]. The utrophin rod domain lacks certain sequences present in dystrophin's rod domain and, contrary to dystrophin, does not bind actin [79]. The cysteine-rich domain and the C-terminal domain again share a high homology with dystrophin [80]. Overexpression of utrophin can rescue the dystrophic phenotype of dystrophin-deficient mice [81, 82]. Further evidence that utrophin can partially compensate for dystrophin comes from the observation that double-knock-out mice for dystrophin and utrophin have a much more severe phenotype than mice deficient for dystrophin alone [83]. In those double-knock-out animals even extraocular muscles are not spared [84]. Also, a boy defcient for both dystrophin and utrophin showed a very severe phenotype [85]. Thus therapeutic strategies are being developed that include upregulation of endogenous utrophin or vector-based delivery of the utrophin gene to combat dystrophin deficiency [86, 87, 88].

Dystrophin protein and its functional partners

The function and maintenance of skeletal muscle cell integrity depend upon interactions of the muscle with the surrounding basement membrane and underlying cytoskeleton [89]. Trans-sarcolemmal receptor complexes provide critical mechanical links between the basement membrane and the cytoskeleton and are involved in signaling functions. The two most important of these receptor complexes in skeletal muscle cells are the dystrophin–glycoprotein complex [90] and the α7–β1 integrin complex [91].

These receptor complexes have a costameric distribution along the sarcolemma. Costameres are striated-muscle-specific variations of focal adhesions that are usually present in non-muscle cells [92]. These subsarcolemmal protein assemblies serve to physically couple the force-generating sarcomeres with the sarcolemma. They include, like focal adhesion in nonmuscle cells, the proteins vinculin, α-actinin and β1-integrin [93].

Through the intermediate filament desmin, costameres establish a link to the Z-disk of the sarcomeres around which they align in register [93].

The normal functions of dystrophin even in skeletal muscle fibers are still not fully elucidated but it appears that it has at least three major functions probably in synergy with the cited dystrophin-associated molecules:

1. The most important function is mechanical reinforcement of the surface membrane so that muscle fibers can withstand the contraction or stretch-induced mechanical stresses without becoming necrotic [94]. In normal states, lengthening contractions occurring in everyday physical activity in certain muscles are examples of where the presence of dystrophin is necessary for minimizing the prevalence of muscle fiber necrosis.
2. Molecular signaling from the extracellular domain to the interior of muscle fibers. This is more presumed that actually proven. For example, the putative intracellular chemical mediators and the target functions have not been identified although homeostasis of muscle fiber volume and the function of certain types of sarcolemmal/T-tubular calcium channels were suspected target parameters [95].
3. Control of the microcirculation of muscle by ensuring the normal localization of neuronal nitric oxide synthase (nNOS) [96].

The dystrophin-associated glycoprotein complex (DGC) consists of three distinct subgroups referred to as the dystroglycans [97], sarcoglycans [98], and the syntrophin complex [99] (Figure 10.3).

The dystroglycans form the core of the DGC. Through binding to the cysteine-rich domain of dystrophin, they provide the link between the intracellular actin cytoskeleton and the extracellular matrix. The dystroglycans (DG) are transcribed from one gene (*DAG1*) and are post-translationally modified to yield a transmembrane β-subunit and a heavily glycosylated extracellular α-subunit [100]. Glycosylation of α-dystroglycan occurs in a tissue-specific manner; thus, the molecular weight for α-dystroglycan differs according to its tissue distribution [101]. While β-dystroglycan interacts with proteins located at the internal sarcolemmal surface, α-dystroglycan interacts with components of the specialized extracellular matrix, or basement membrane [100].

α-Dystroglycan binds to laminins via their LG domains, and interacts with other LG-domain-containing proteins such as agrin, perlecan, and neurexins, which are located in the basement membrane [102].

Thus a continuous link is established between the actin cytoskeleton and the extracellular matrix via dystrophin, β-dystroglycan, α-dystroglycan, and laminin. Mutations in the dystroglycan gene itself have not yet been reported, and are probably not compatible with life. In the mouse, targeted deletion of the dystroglycan gene is embryonically lethal as the basal lamina (Reichert's membrane) which separates the embryonic yolk sac cavity from the maternal circulation cannot form [103].

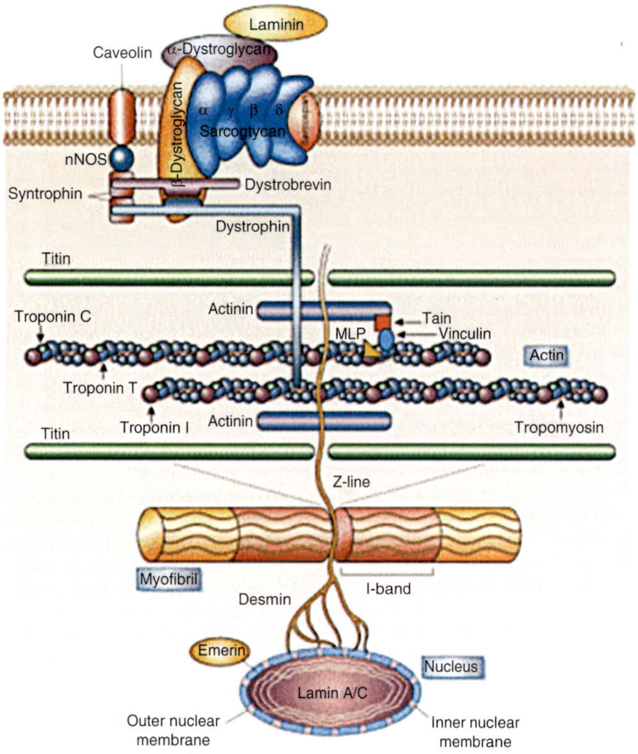

Figure 10.3. Schematic representation of the dystrophin–glycoprotein complex. (With permission for reproduction given by G. Karpati.)

However, a wide spectrum of diseases has been observed with glycosylation defects of α-dystroglycan, as this modification is essential for the interaction of α-dystroglycan with the extracellular matrix. In brain, hypoglycosylation of α-dystroglycan leads to neuronal migration defects [104], and in skeletal muscle, hypoglycosylation of α-dystroglycan leads to muscular dystrophy [105]. Thus, glycosylation disorders of α-dystroglycan have a wide clinical spectrum ranging from severe congenital muscular dystrophies with prominent structural brain abnormalities to milder forms of muscular dystrophies with a limb-girdle phenotype. These disorders are reviewed in Chapter 3.

The absence of the structural continuity between the cytoskeleton and the extracellular matrix leads to muscle cell damage [94]. Several lines of evidence suggest that dystrophin provides mechanical support to the sarcolemma. The rod domain of dystrophin is structurally similar to spectrin, the absence of which leads to increased erythrocyte membrane instability in hereditary spherocytosis [106]. Dystrophin-deficient myotubes show reduced membrane stiffness and cultured myofibers from dystrophin-deficient mdx mice demonstrate increased susceptibility for rupture from osmotic shock [107]. It has been shown that dystrophin-deficient muscles suffer greater than normal levels of membrane rupture during muscle contraction [108]. Isolated diaphragm and extensor digitorum muscles from dystrophin-deficient mdx and control mice were subjected to a range of contraction

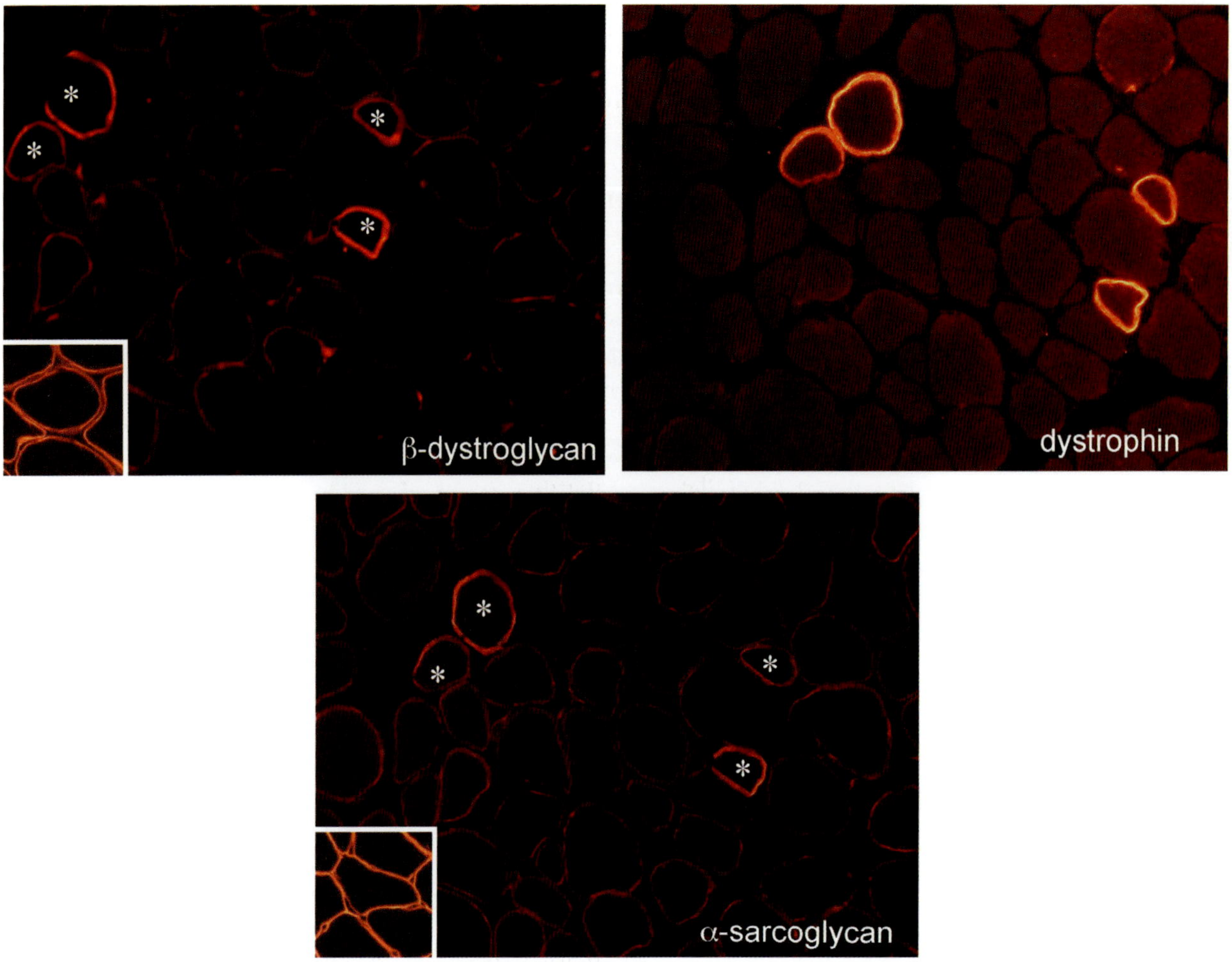

Figure 10.4. Absence of dystrophin leads to secondary reduction of components of the dystrophin–glycoprotein complex (DGC), as shown here for β-dystroglycan and α-sarcoglycan. Note that the dystrophin in revertant fibers can recruit the DGC to the sarcolemma. These fibers however are too few to compensate for the dystrophin loss throughout the muscle. Small inserts show control staining. Original magnification 350×.

conditions in vitro to produce various levels of membrane stress. The experiments were performed in the presence of a membrane-impermeable dye to identify muscle fibers with disrupted membranes. Mdx muscle fibers demonstrated significantly higher susceptibility to membrane rupture. Interestingly, in vitro, the diaphragm was less susceptible to such injury than the limb muscles tested. Because in vivo, in the mdx mouse, the diaphragm shows the most marked myopathological alterations, these findings would suggest that the preferential degeneration of the diaphragm in the mdx mouse is a reflection of its higher workload rather than an intrinsic vulnerability of this muscle to contraction-induced injury.

The sarcoglycans are a family of six transmembrane proteins (alpha, beta, gamma, delta, epsilon, and zeta) [99]. Sarcoglycanopathies are reviewed in detail in Chapter 11. They form hetero-tetrameric complexes which are composed in a tissue-specific manner, and are thought to stabilize the DGC together with sarcospan. In skeletal and heart muscle the complex consists of an alpha, beta, gamma, and delta subunit. Mutations of any of those sarcoglycans lead to a specific subtype of recessively inherited limb-girdle muscular dystrophies (LGMD2D, 2E, 2C, and 2F) [98]. As the sarcoglycans associate early with each other in the cell sorting compartment to form a tetrameric complex, the absence of one sarcoglycan will lead to a secondary reduction of the other three. Despite the fact that the sarcoglycans are secondarily reduced in the case of dystrophin deficiency (Figure 10.4), dystrophin and the dystroglycans are not typically reduced in cases of primary sarcoglycan deficiencies (Figure 10.5.)

The above-mentioned observations suggest an important structural function for dystrophin and the DGC, specifically in establishing a physical link for force transduction between the actin cytoskeleton and the extracellular matrix. However, there is also evidence to suggest that dystrophin and the DGC are involved in cell signaling. The structural and signaling functions of the DCG are not mutually exclusive.

Dystrophin binds indirectly via syntrophin to nNOS, which is thereby recruited to the sarcolemma. In the absence

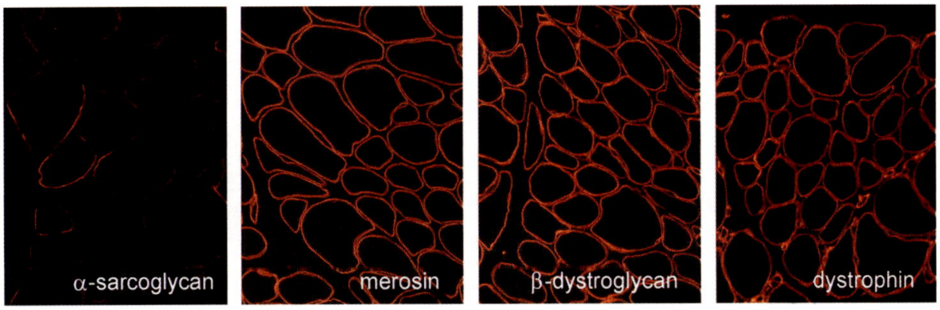

Figure 10.5. Whereas dystrophin deficiency leads to a secondary reduction of members of the DGC, primary deficiency of any of the sarcoglycans does not lead to the reciprocal deficiency of dystrophin, shown here for a patient with primary α-sarcoglycanopathy. Original magnification 140×.

of dystrophin the concentration of nNOS at the cell membrane [109] and in the cytoplasm diminishes [110] and the mRNA levels of nNOS are reduced [110]. nNOS produces the freely diffusible signaling molecule nitric oxide (NO). NO can act as a vasodilator in exercising muscle where it can blunt the vasoconstrictor response to reflex sympathetic activation [111]. nNOS is present predominantly in fast-twitch fibers, where it is thought to be responsible for maintaining an adequate blood supply during exercise. Such modulation was shown to be defective during contraction of nNOS-deficient skeletal muscles both of mdx mice and nNOS-deficient mice [96]. Moreover, this mechanism is defective in children with DMD, but not in children with muscle diseases that have no influence on nNOS sarcolemmal localization [112]. NO mediates its effects in part via cyclic GMP (cGMP). A drug that inhibits cGMP breakdown, such as the phosphodiesterase-5 inhibitor sildenafil, has recently been shown to prevent cardiomyopathic changes that are associated with dystrophin deficiency [113]. This is one example suggesting that the DGC has also signaling functions in addition to its structural role.

Caveolin-3 also associates with the DGC by binding to β-dystroglycan where it competes for the same binding site as dystrophin, and caveolin-3 is increased in dystrophin-deficient muscle [114]. Caveolin-3 is the muscle-specific family member of caveolins, which is the principal component of caveolar membranes [115]. Caveolae are vesicular invaginations of the plasma membrane measuring 50–100 nm in diameter [116]. Caveolins participate in vesicular trafficking events and signal transduction processes by acting as scaffolding proteins to organize and concentrate specific lipids and lipid-modified signaling molecules within caveolar membranes. Mutations in caveolin are usually missense with a dominant negative effect, as mutant caveolin proteins aggregate in the Golgi apparatus and are not expressed at the cell surface. Clinical phenotypes associated with caveolinopathies are limb-girdle muscular dystrophy type 1C, distal myopathy, and rippling muscle disease [117]. These different phenotypes can occur in different patients who have identical mutations, and can also be overlapping within the same individual [118]. Overexpression of caveolin-3 in transgenic mice leads to a muscular dystrophy phenotype and a downregulation of dystrophin expression [119]. Caveolin-3 is also implicated in T-tubule biogenesis and caveolin-3 knock-out mice develop mild myopathic changes with T-tubule abnormalities [120]. The DGC is excluded from lipid raft domains in caveolin-deficient mice [120].

Through α-actinin the C-terminal part of dystrophin can associate with the integrin system [121].

Integrins form a large family of cell surface receptors that mediate cell–extracellular matrix interactions and provide a similar link between the cytoskeleton and the extracellular matrix as the DGC. α7β1-integrin is the major integrin form found in adult skeletal muscle [91]. Mutations in the α7-integrin gene cause a congenital myopathy [122], which despite its clinical severity shows only mild histopathological features on muscle biopsy, which consist of mild fiber size variation. It is thought that the α7β1-integrin system is primarily responsible for the stability of the myotendinous junction, whereas the DGC is essential for the lateral integrity of the myofiber [91]. The presence of either complex is essential, as double-knock-out mice lacking dystrophin and α7β1-integrin develop a severe dystrophy and die within 4 weeks after birth [123].

Much information has been gained concerning dystrophin's function and the function of the DGC from complementation studies in dystrophin-deficient mice.

A commonly used mouse model is the mdx mouse which has a point mutation in exon 23 (3185C > T) that introduces a stop codon into the open reading frame which abolishes the dystrophin expression [124].

Phenotypically the mice are unaffected until age 2–4 weeks when prominent necrosis occurs. This is followed by regeneration and the mice survive. Regenerated fibers keep as a mark internally situated myonuclei, and in older mice up to 80% of fibers show central nucleation. The diaphragm is the muscle to have the most distinct dystrophic myopathology, which is scarce in other muscles; therefore, the diaphragm of the mdx mouse is generally used to assess the therapeutic effect of a given regimen.

A better animal model for the human disease is the Golden Retriever Dog [125]. The dog has a mutation in the splice acceptor site of exon 7, which leads to skipping of exon 7 and to the disruption of the open reading frame further downstream in exon 8. These dogs develop signs of muscle weakness at age 8–10 weeks and display a dystrophic muscle pathology. Because of their large size and pathology, which is closer to the human condition, these dogs are a better study model for therapeutic approaches than the mdx mouse.

In mouse transgenic experiments truncated dystrophin constructs were introduced into a dystrophin-deficient background. The information gained has helped to elucidate the effects that human mutations in the dystrophin gene can have on muscle pathology. More importantly, it has led to the development of therapeutic strategies, some of which have already advanced to the clinical trial stage. Numerous transgenic mice with different dystrophin constructs were generated, and only a few of those are briefly described here.

As the dystrophin-associated glycoproteins were characterized, it was observed that many of those proteins showed secondary deficiency in dystrophin-deficient muscle [126]. One circulating hypothesis was that it might be the deficiency of these proteins rather than the absence of dystrophin per se that led to muscle fiber damage [127]. Further strengthening such hypothesis was the fact that mutations in DGC proteins could lead to muscular dystrophy without affecting dystrophin expression, such as seen in sarcoglycanopathies [99]. However, overexpression of the short isoform Dp71 in a dystrophin-deficient mdx mouse could restore the dystrophin glycoprotein complex at the sarcolemma, but was unable to alleviate the muscular dystrophy phenotype [128, 129]. Dp71 contains the cysteine-rich domain as well as the C-terminal domain of dystrophin but lacks the rod domain and the actin-binding domain. These studies demonstrated that the fragment containing the cysteine-rich domain and the C-terminus of dystrophin was sufficient to restore the DGC at the sarcolemma, but was unable to counteract the muscle degeneration. It demonstrated a critical role for the dystrophin protein domains not included in this short isoform, and pointed towards the importance of the physical link between the actin cytoskeleton and the extracellular matrix which is provided by the full-length dystrophin.

Dp116 was able to restore the DGC at the sarcolemma of mdx mice but was likewise unable to alleviate the dystrophic phenotype [130]. Dp116 contains the C-terminal domain, the cysteine-rich domain and only two complete spectrin-like repeats. However, overexpression of Dp260 in an mdx background could partially alleviate the muscular dystrophy phenotype [131]. This is likely due to the actin-binding capabilities of the rod domain fragment contained in this isoform.

To further map the binding properties of the C-terminal part of dystrophin, deletion mutants of dystrophin were introduced as transgenes into dystrophin-deficient mdx mice [132]. Constructs lacking protein sequences encoded by exons 71–78 were able to assemble all the components of the DGC at the sarcolemma and were able to mitigate the dystrophic phenotype, indicating that the C-terminus of dystrophin is dispensable in the mdx mouse. As the omitted fragment also includes the binding sites for dystrobrevin (exons 74/75) and syntrophin (exons 73/74), the experiment demonstrated that these two proteins can functionally associate with the DGC in the absence of a direct link with dystrophin.

Led by clinical observations in patients with large deletions in the rod domain who exhibited a mild clinical phenotype, a detailed functional analysis was made of dystrophin deletion mutants, which were introduced as transgenes into mdx mice [133]. Dystrophin transgenes lacking extensive parts of the rod domain were able to prevent a wide variety of functional characteristics of the muscular dystrophy and protected the muscles against damage caused by muscle activity [133]. By deleting also the C-terminal domain, a mini-dystrophin molecule small enough to be incorporated into an adeno-associated viral (AAV) vector was generated [133]. AAV vectors are currently the vector of choice for somatic gene therapy directed towards muscle, as they have a high muscle tropism, low immunogenicity, and no pathogenicity [134]. Muscles of mdx mice injected with this construct showed reversal of the histopathological features of the disease. The same group administered such microdystrophin AAV particles systemically to dystrophin-utrophin double-knock-out animals and could preserve muscle function and prolong the life span of these severely dystrophic mice [135].

Mutations of the dystrophin gene

The functional effects of the mutations are determined by both the nature of the mutation and its location in the dystrophin gene. The nature of the mutations includes deletions or duplications (in-frame and out-of-frame) as well as small or single nucleotide changes. Deletions have two "hot spots" (Figure 10.6).

Mutations are determined by the effect they have on the reading frame for protein translation and by their localization along the gene. Large intragenic deletions involving single or multiple exons are the most common mutations, which are present in around 60% in DMD and 80% in BMD [136]. About 10% of mutations are duplications and the remainder are small or single nucleotide substitutions. When these mutations lead to premature termination of translation, or if they are located in a critical area of the dystrophin protein, they lead to the DMD phenotype. If the open reading frame is preserved or if missense mutations are located in less crucial protein domains, then a BMD phenotype may result [137].

Patients with an intermediate DMD/Becker phenotype have either missense mutations that are located in a functionally important domain, or they have frame-shifting deletions that can undergo somatic restoration through exon skipping [138, 139, 140].

Whereas small gene alterations are mostly individually distinct and are randomly distributed throughout the gene, deletions in the dystrophin gene are located at two hotspots [38, 141]. About 30% of deletions occur at the proximal hotspot and many are located in the large intron after exon 2. Two-thirds of deletions occur at the distal hotspot, particularly in intron 44, leading in many instances to in-frame deletions of exons 45–47, 45–48, 45–49, giving rise to a BMD phenotype.

Mutations in X-linked dilated cardiomyopathy are located at two hotspots of the dystrophin gene; one hotspot is in the region of the skeletal muscle promoter and exon 1–7, while the other is around exon 48–51. It is thought that skeletal muscle

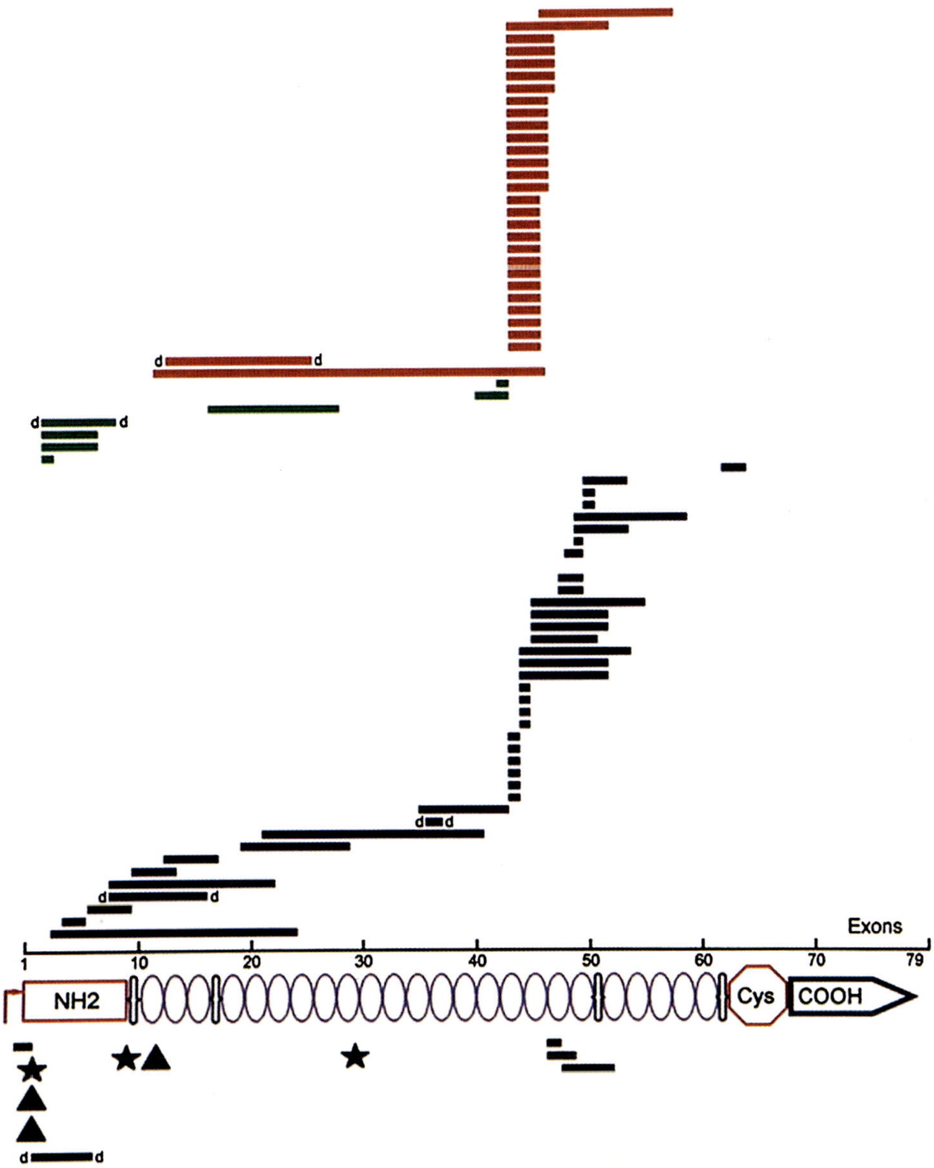

Figure 10.6. Diagram to illustrate the distribution and extent of deletions in patients with BMD (red bars), intermediate D/BMD (green bars), DMD (blue bars) and X-linked dilated cardiomyopathy (black). d = duplication, stars = point mutations, arrow heads = insertions. (Taken from Anderson, L. V. B., *Structural and Molecular Basis of Skeletal Muscle Diseases*, World Federation of Neurology, with permission from the volume editor, G. Karpati).

tissue can escape the deleterious effect of dystrophin absence by alternative splicing, which may not be possible in the heart.

X-linked dilated myopathy cases have been reported where a region of the dystrophin gene was deleted that included the muscle promoter as well as the first muscle exon. Because patients had high levels of dystrophin in their skeletal muscle, it must be assumed that transcription in those cases was driven by the brain or Purkinje cell promoter. This explains the preferential cardiac involvement in patients with these deletions, where the brain or Purkinje promoters are inactive, but transcription from these promoters is possible in skeletal muscle [58].

Exceptions to the reading frame hypothesis exist. It has been observed that certain out-of-frame deletions, in particular of exons 3–7, are associated with a Becker phenotype [142, 143]. These deletions lead, contrary to expectations, to the generation of a partially functional dystrophin protein, likely through exon skipping.

In-frame deletions that cause DMD are rare, and they involve crucial domains of the dystrophin protein [144]. A very rare missense mutation (Asp3335His) associated with a DMD phenotype has been reported, with normal size dystrophin, near-normal dystrophin protein levels, and the presence of the DGC at the sarcolemma [145].

Pathogenesis of muscle fiber damage in dystrophinopathies

The study of the microscopic pathology of muscle in dystrophinopathies has been of great help in the formulation of ideas about the pathogenesis of muscle fiber damage. The following pathogenic events appear to cause muscle fiber necrosis, which is often segmental.

The dystrophin deficiency leads to structural weakness and to tears in the sarcolemma. When the membrane repair process fails, calcium-rich extracellular fluid enters through the sarcolemmal gaps [146]. Calcium overload is initially buffered by the sarcoplasmic reticulum, the mitochondria, and intracellular calcium-binding proteins such as parvalbumin and calmodulin. Once the calcium buffering capacity is reached, calcium-dependent proteases (calpains) are activated which lead to digestion of cytoskeletal and myofibrillar proteins. Calcium-mediated activation of phospholipases leads to further membrane damage [147, 148]. To test a causal relationship between calpain activation and muscle cell death in dystrophin deficiency, mdx mice were generated that overexpress a calpastatin transgene in muscle [149]. Calpastatin is a specific, endogenous inhibitor of m- and u-calpains. Transgenic mice crossed with mdx mice had fewer as well as smaller lesions, and fewer regenerating fibers, indicating reduced necrosis. The extent of improvement correlated with the level of calapastatin expression. Membrane damage, as assessed by procion orange and creatine kinase assays, was unchanged, supporting the idea that calpains act downstream of the primary muscle defect.

Interestingly, calcium levels are elevated in dystrophin-deficient muscles even when the plasmalemma is intact, as has been shown in cultured myotubes of Duchenne human or mdx mouse origin [95, 150]. This elevation of intracellular free calcium concentration was associated with increased open probability of calcium leak channels, suggesting an inherent defect in calcium regulation of the dystrophin-deficient cell.

In response to the increased intracellular calcium concentration, mitochondria form a large pore complex, leading to loss of matrix and intermembrane contents, and to swelling of the mitochondria [151]. If not reversed, the mitochondrion can rupture and lead to cell necrosis and apoptosis. The process of mitochondrial pore formation is regulated by cyclophilin D, a mitochondrial matrix prolyl cis-trans isomerase. Mice deleted for the gene encoding cyclophilin D show protection from necrotic cell death in the brain and heart after ischemic injury [152, 153]. Crossing cyclophilin-D-deficient mice with δ-sarcoglycan-deficient mice showed markedly less dystrophic disease in heart and skeletal muscle in the double-knock-out animals [154]. Furthermore, treatment of mdx mice with a cyclophilin D inhibitor reduced mitochondrial swelling and necrotic disease manifestations [154]. These experiments suggest that mitochondrial-mediated necrosis represents an additional disease mechanism that could be therapeutically influenced by inhibition of cyclophilin D.

The role of apoptosis in DMD is unclear. Some workers have found evidence to suggest that apoptosis may contribute to the pathogenesis of dystrophinopathies in mdx mice [155, 156] and Duchenne patients [157, 158], but other studies could not demonstrate signs of apoptosis in human dystrophinopathies [159, 160, 161]. One study [158] suggested that chromatin fragmentation in necrotic and regenerating areas of the dystrophic muscle is part of the normal regulating events during muscle regeneration, as a similar degree of apoptosis can be seen in embryonal myogenesis. This, and another study [158, 161] found that macrophages are also affected by apoptosis after successful removal of necrotic fibers.

Oxidative stress has been implicated in the pathophysiology of myofiber degeneration [162]. Myofibers from mdx mice are more easily killed when exposed to oxidants [163] than when exposed to other metabolic stresses [163]. Furthermore, myoblast cultures derived from mdx mice that were transgenic for different truncated forms of dystrophin showed a positive correlation between the susceptibility to oxidative damage and myopathology of the respective transgenic lines [164].

Muscles collected from mdx mice before the onset of myopathology show increased levels of antioxidant enzymes suggesting that oxidative stress may be an early event in dystrophinopathies [165]. However, sampling of muscles from mdx mice after necrosis had occurred showed that levels of antioxidant enzymes and products of lipid peroxidation were consistently higher than in control mice, regardless of whether the muscle was affected or spared [166], suggesting that increased oxidative stress alone is insufficient to cause the dystrophic phenotype. Along these lines, further experiments demonstrated that oxidative stress has the potential to promote pathology but would require an additional insult to the cell homeostasis, such as physical membrane damage [167]. In this regard, the dystrophin-deficient muscle membrane is particularly susceptible to lengthening contractions [168]. The different reasons for a weakened sarcolemma are discussed above, but greatly attributable to the disrupted physical link between the actin cytoskeleton and the extracellular matrix. The low level of extrasynaptic utrophin is insufficient to rescue the dystrophin-deficient muscle fiber, but likely mitigates the pathology to a certain degree. The additional absence of utrophin in double-knock-out dystrophin–utrophin mice leads to a much more severe phenotype compared to the dystrophin-deficient mdx mouse. In the double-knock-out mice, even extraocular muscles are involved which are spared in dystrophin deficiency [84]. Sparing of extraocular muscles was attributed to several mechanisms: a better calcium handling capability [169]; a utrophin level which is three times as elevated as in limb muscles [84]; and muscle fiber smallness, as the higher surface to volume ratio will reduce the tension exerted on the plasma membrane, according to the Law of Laplace [170].

In addition to calcium derangements, influx of extracellular fluid through the plasmalemmal gaps leads to intracellular activation of complement and thereby to further damage of intracellular membranous organelles and recruitment of macrophages [171]. Macrophages and T-cells are the most common leukocytic populations in dystrophic muscle [172] and macrophages derived from mdx mice can be cytolytic to cultured myotubes [173]. The contribution of the inflammatory infiltrate seen in biopsies of Duchenne patients however is uncertain, even if in experimental mouse models depletion of T-cells reduces the extent of myopathology [174] and their passive transfer to healthy murine recipients results in pathology [174]. In Duchenne patients both prednisone and azathioprine decrease the number of inflammatory cells [175], but only prednisone had a beneficial effect on the disease, and its mode of action is likely not explained by its anti-inflammatory effect (see below).

As muscle fibers degenerate, satellite cells become activated. It is thought that the replication cycles available to the satellite cells are limited [176], and once this regenerative capacity is exhausted, no new muscle fibers can form and fibrosis ensues. This hypothesis is supported by the observation that the telomere length in Duchenne boys is shorter than in control subjects [177]. However, elegant experiments showed that aged satellite cells could effectively regenerate when they were transplanted into young animals [178]. Regeneration of aged satellite cells was as effective as regeneration from young satellite cells. This would suggest that environmental factors contribute to the apparent senescence of satellite cells. Such a hypothesis is strengthened by the observation that aged muscle stem cells that were exposed to a youthful systemic milieu through parabiotic pairings of aged and young mice repair muscle nearly as well as young satellite cells [179]. This would suggest that the diminished regenerative potential of aged muscle is not primarily due to intrinsic aging of satellite cells, but rather to the effects of the aged environment on satellite-cell function. In this context, increased Wnt signaling during aging has been implicated, and has been shown to alter the satellite cell fate and to increase fibrosis [180].

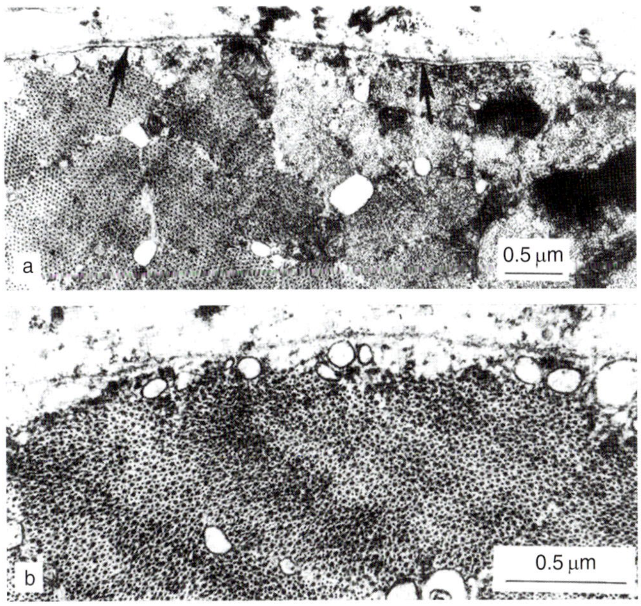

Figure 10.7. Electron microscopic picture of a non-necrotic myofiber of a DMD patient showing the earliest abnormalities: plasmalemmal defects. (a) Arrows point to the region of plasmalemmal loss. (b) Plasmalemma is missing along the entire segment of the cell surface. However basement membrane is preserved above the plasmalemmal defect. Cysterns of sarcotubular or T-tubular origin align at the periphery in an apparent attempt to reseal the membrane defect. (Permission for reproduction given by S. Carpenter and G. Karpati).

Diagnosis

When the diagnosis of dystrophinopathy is suspected on the basis of clinical phenotype and X-linked inheritance, patients will undergo laboratory testing to verify the diagnosis.

Serum creatine kinase (CK)

Serum CK levels are elevated as this cytosolic enzyme will leak out through the plasma membrane gaps of the affected muscle fibers or from necrotic fibers.

In DMD and BMD, 100% of affected individuals will show an elevation of serum CK activity levels as early as after birth. It is usually in the range of 40–60 times above the normal level in DMD patients, while in BMD patients it is usually less, at about 5–20 times above normal. Serum CK levels often show daily variability due to a variety of factors, mainly physical activity. Therefore using serum CK levels as an endpoint in therapeutic evaluation requires caution. As the disease progresses and muscle tissue becomes replaced with adipose and fibrous tissue, serum CK levels usually decline [181].

Patients presenting with dilated X-linked cardiomyopathy may also show an increase in serum CK levels, indicating that the disease is not solely restricted to cardiac muscle but involves skeletal muscle as well. Xp21-linked cardiomyopathy without serum CK elevation has been reported as well [182].

Women who are carriers of DMD or BMD mutations will show a relatively mild increase in serum CK activity (2–10 times the normal level) [183, 184].

Microscopic study of muscle biopsies

Myopathology in DMD, including classical pathology as well as specific cytochemistry, is quite typical. The earliest myopathology is discernible by electron microscopy in the form of focal gaps of the plasma membrane and the apposition of flat cisterns to these gaps (Figure 10.7 [185, 186]). The plasma membrane gaps are responsible for the massive influx of the calcium-rich extracellular fluid, triggering necrosis (Figure 10.8). However, these gaps are assumed to be sealed frequently by the flat cisterns' membranes.

The cardinal classical myopathological features revealed by light microscopy are segmental necrosis and phagocytosis of small clusters (four to ten) of muscle fibers as well as regenerating fibers in a similar distribution (Figure 10.9). Early light microscopic features of muscle fiber necrosis are pale staining and a rounded appearance. The intermyofibrillar network becomes indistinct, giving the fibers a ground glass appearance. Prenecrotic fibers may be recognizable by the presence of stainable precipitated calcium salts, particularly in the periphery of the fiber (Figure 10.8). An unusual plethora of hypercontracted fibers is also present. Macrophages invade necrotic fibers within a few hours after the plasmalemma is lost. They can be visualized by their strong reactivity to acid phosphatase and are also abundant in the interstitial space. Regeneration is recognized by small caliber muscle fibers with basophilic cytoplasm and prominent myonuclei with large nucleoli (Figure 10.9). Other cytochemical indices of regenerating muscle fibers include positive diffuse cytoplasmic desmin immunostaining, as well as immunoreactivity to immature myosin heavy chain isoforms, N-CAM, myoD and class I major histocompatibility complex (MHC). Regeneration, however, is not perfect and consequences of aberrant regeneration are recognizable as small-caliber fibers, forked fibers, and myopathic type grouping (Figure 10.10) [187]. However, the worst outcome of imperfect regeneration is the complete failure of regeneration leading to progressive loss of muscle fibers. This is best recognized by empty skeins of basal lamina on electron microscopy (Figure 10.11). As muscle fiber loss continues, progressive increase of endomysial connective tissue becomes evident (Figure 10.9).

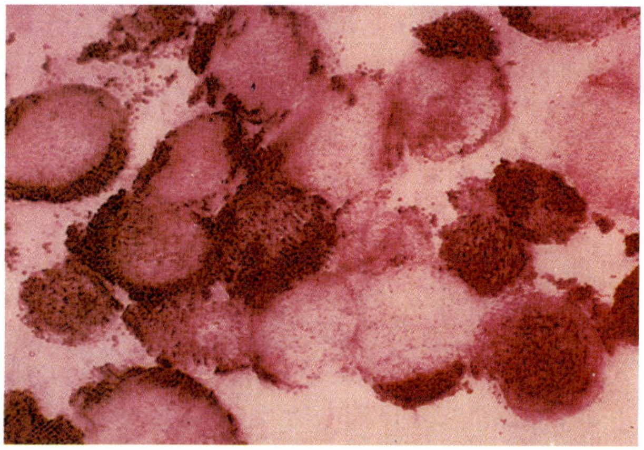

Figure 10.8. Calcium staining in non-necrotic and necrotic muscle fibers of DMD stained with glyoxal-bis-(2-hydroxyanil), GBHA. See the predominantly subsarcolemmal distribution of calcium depositis in many fibers. Original magnification 350×. (Permission for reproduction given by G. Karpati).

Histochemistry and cytochemistry

Reliable and affordable antibodies are available to demonstrate the most informative abnormalities on cryostat sections of the muscle biopsies. The deficiency of dystrophin is best demonstrated by using the three antibodies marketed by Novocastra Laboratories, Newcastle, UK (Figure 10.12). Each of these antibodies recognizes an epitope at three different regions of the dystrophin protein (N-terminus, mid-rod region, and C-terminus). This permits demonstration of the possible presence of specifically truncated dystrophin molecules in BMD (Figure 10.13). Sarcolemmal immunostaining can be continuous if large amounts of the truncated Becker protein are made. Otherwise the sarcolemmal staining pattern may be interrupted. In DMD there is total deficiency of dystrophin in all muscle fibers. However, in usually less than 1% of the fibers, full or partial circumferential dystrophin immunostaining is present. These fibers are called "revertant" fibers (Figures 10.4, 10.12). These are believed to be due to somatic mosaicism with reverse mutations leading to the repair of the translational frame [188, 189]. Significantly decreased sarcolemmal staining for the sarcoglycans and the dystroglycans can also be demonstrated by appropriate antibodies (Figure 10.4). This is an asymmetrical relationship, as in primary sarcoglycan deficiency, dystrophin and dystroglycans are not usually reduced (Figure 10.5). An additional interesting feature is the presence of extrasynaptic

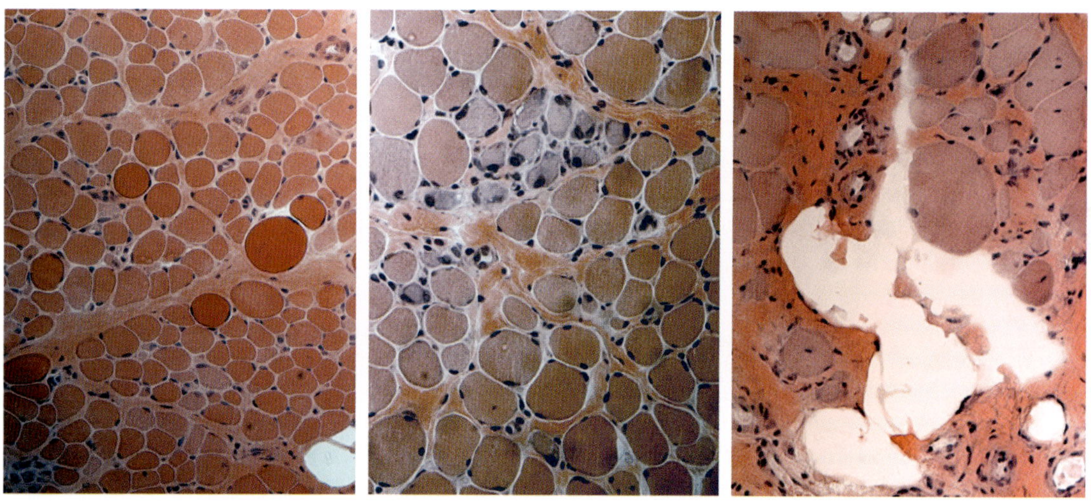

Figure 10.9. Hematoxylin & eosin staining of skeletal muscle biopsies from Duchenne boys at different ages. The figure on the left is from a 2-year-old boy, the middle figure from a 6-year-old boy and the figure on the right from an 11-year-old boy. See on the left marked variation in fiber size and hypercontracted eosinophilic fibers, typical of dystrophinopathies. In the middle panel there is a cluster of regenerating fibers with basophilic cytoplasm and large nuclei with prominent nucleoli. Necrosis of muscle fibers often occurs in clusters in DMD. When the regeneration fails, muscle tissue is replaced by adipose and fibrous tissue, as seen in the left panel. Original magnification 140×.

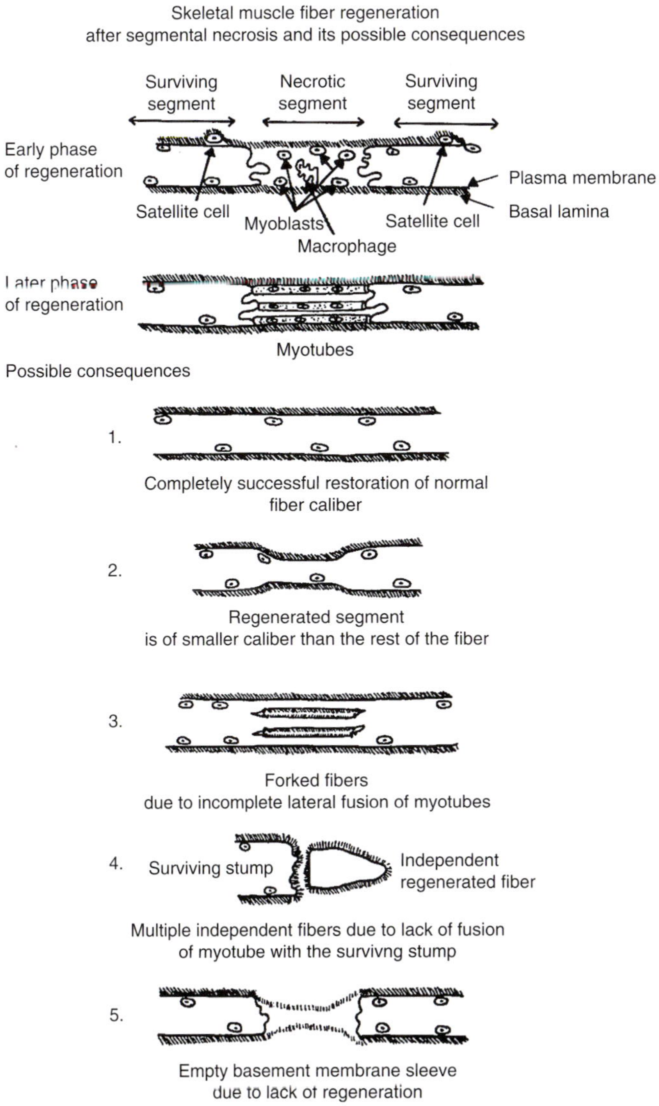

Figure 10.10. Schematic representation of skeletal muscle fiber regeneration after segmental necrosis and its possible consequences. (Permission for reproduction given by G. Karpati.)

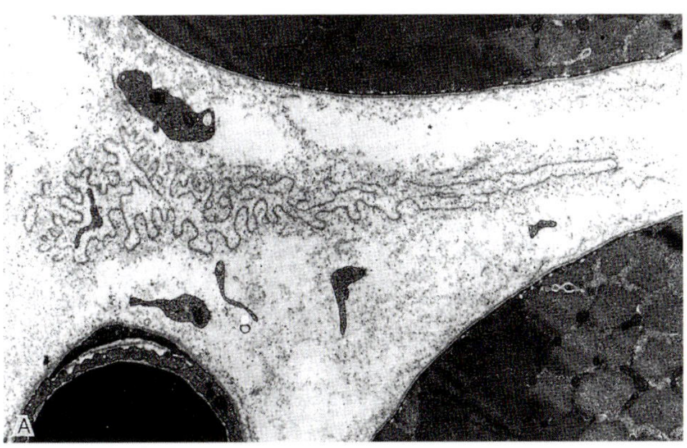

Figure 10.11. Failed regeneration of a muscle fiber. The only residual is a skein of basement membrane. (Permission for reproduction given by G. Karpati.)

utrophin immunostaining in many muscle fibers, particularly, but not exclusively, in regenerating ones (Figure 10.14). Despite the fact that in experimental paradigms transgenically supplied utrophin can mitigate the deleterious effects of dystrophin deficiency [86, 87, 88], correlation between the number of extrasynaptically utrophin-positive muscle fibers and the severity of the clinical phenotype is difficult to make.

In female carriers, dystrophin immunohistochemistry may show a mosaic of dystrophin-positive and -negative fiber segments as explained earlier (Figure 10.15).

Western blot

In DMD, immunoblot analysis shows the total absence of dystrophin, as can be expected from the negative dystrophin immunohistochemistry. In contrast, in BMD, a smaller than normal amount of variably truncated dystrophin is well demonstrable by the appropriate antibody on Western blot and it provides diagnostically useful information.

DMD: as most mutations in DMD are out-of-frame, no full-length dystrophin product is produced, and thus Western blots with antibodies directed against the C-terminus will show no detectable protein. N-terminal, rod-domain or polyclonal antibodies can detect, at times, multiple bands in cases of DMD on Western blots, representing truncated forms of the protein or protein products produced by exon skipping [190] (Figure 10.12).

BMD: polyclonal antibodies and/or antibodies directed against multiple epitopes of the dystrophin protein should be used, as deletion mutations may lead to internal truncation of the dystrophin protein. Thus absent immunostaining with antibodies directed against only one epitope may lead to the erroneous diagnosis of DMD. Bands of abnormal size on Western blot can help guide the molecular diagnosis and can suggest the size of the gene deletion or duplication [191] (Figure 10.13).

Cytogenetic analysis

Males

Duchenne muscular dystrophy patients with Xp21 gene deletion may have additional disorders as part of a contiguous gene deletion syndrome, including retinitis pigmentosa, chronic granulomatous disease, and McLeod red cell phenotype [36] or glycerol kinase deficiency and adrenal hypoplasia [192]. Patients with these large genomic deletions led to the identification of the dystrophin locus (see above). Deletions or rearrangements involving chromosome Xp21 should be excluded through morphological analysis and *in situ* hybridization techniques in such patients.

Females

Girls may develop classical DMD as a result of either skewed X-inactivation, or if they carry only one X-chromosome such

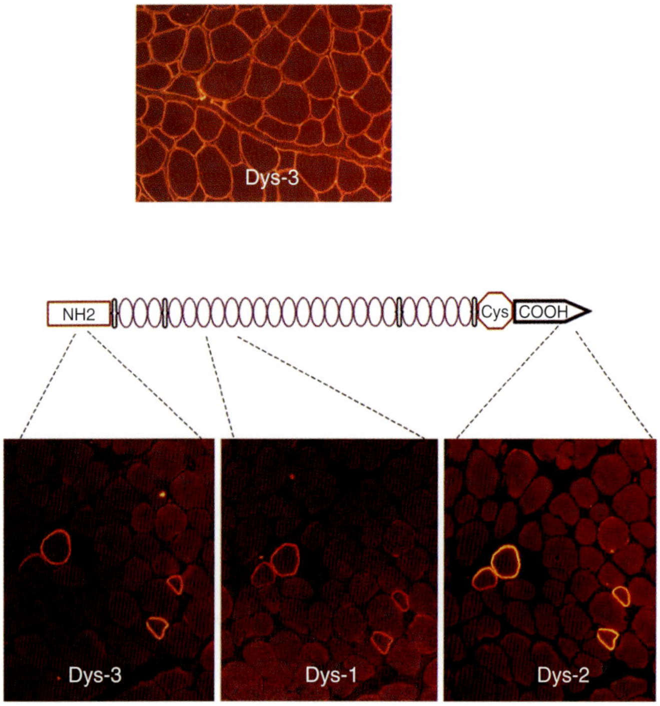

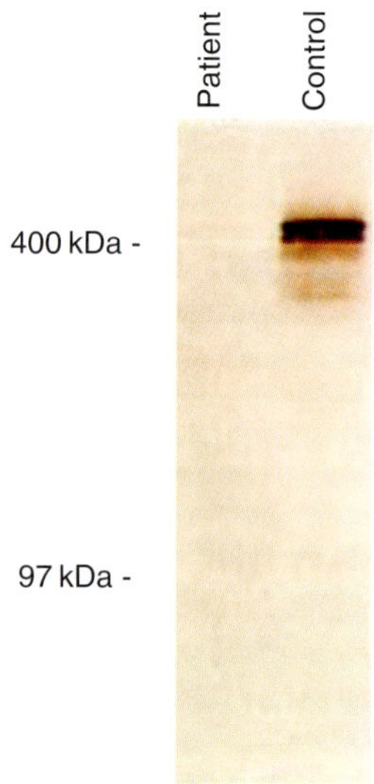

Figure 10.12. Dystrophin immunohistochemistry of skeletal muscle from a 5-year-old Duchenne boy stained with antibodies that recognize the N-terminal dystrophin domain (Dys-3, Novocastra), the rod domain (Dys-1, Novocastra), and the C-terminal domain (Dys-2, Novocastra). Absent dystrophin staining is seen with all antibodies, except for a few "revertant" fibers in which the open reading frame has been reconstituted. The upper panel shows a normal control for dystrophin staining with Dys-3. Western blot analysis with polyclonal antibodies shows complete absence of dystrophin staining in the patient's lane, whereas dystrophin staining is seen in the control lane. The double dystrophin band in the control lane is due to differential splicing at the C-terminus of dystrophin. Original magnification 140×.

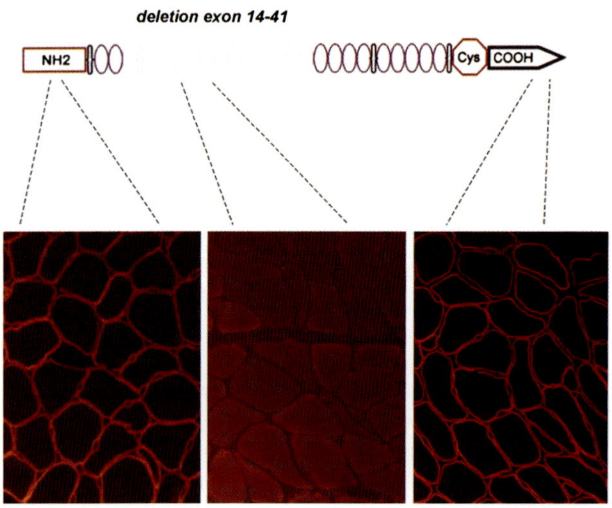

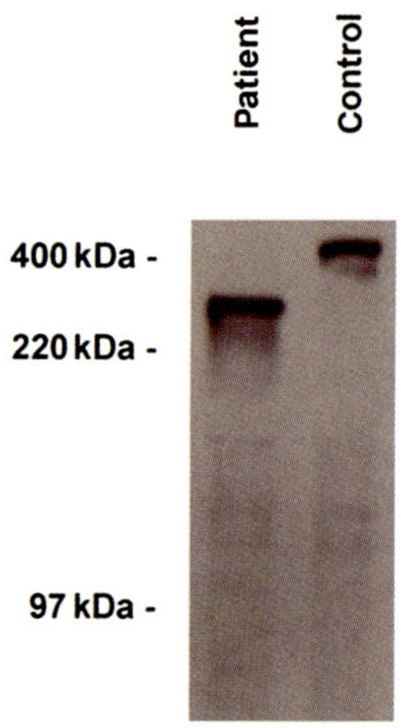

Figure 10.13. Immunohistochemistry of skeletal muscle of a patient with late-onset Becker muscular dystrophy. Antibody labeling is as in Figure 10.12. Note the absence of labeling to the rod domain, but the high-intensity labeling with the N-terminal and C-terminal antibody, suggesting an internal deletion with preservation of the reading frame. This was confirmed by subsequent molecular analysis which showed a large deletion spanning exon 14 to exon 41, which equates to about 40% of the entire protein. This is demonstrated in the Western blot, which shows large amounts of a dystrophin molecule with significantly reduced molecular weight. This truncated dystrophin molecule must retain significant biological activity, as the patient became symptomatic only at age 47, and was still ambulatory at age 64. Original magnification 350×.

as in Turner syndrome, or they inherit two copies of a mutated X-chromosome from one parent (uniparental disomy). Therefore, cytogenetic analysis should be performed in girls with classical Duchenne phenotype.

Molecular testing

Southern blotting has been the most conventional technique used for the detection of deletions and duplications [193]. This technique was subsequently replaced by multiplex polymerase chain reaction (PCR) [194]. In this approach multiple exons that are most frequently deleted are co-amplified; common protocols use up to 18 exons located around mutation hot spots and can detect between 90% and 98% of deletions [195, 196].

Real-time PCR has been used to detect deletions and duplications in female carriers [197, 198].

New molecular methods combining hybridization and PCR amplification of DNA fragments were adapted to efficiently detect exon deletions and duplications in the DMD gene, namely multiplex amplifiable probe hybridization (MAPH) [199] and multiplex ligation-dependent probe amplification (MLPA) [200].

In MAPH, exon-specific DNA probes are used that differ in length but which all have an identical flanking sequence at

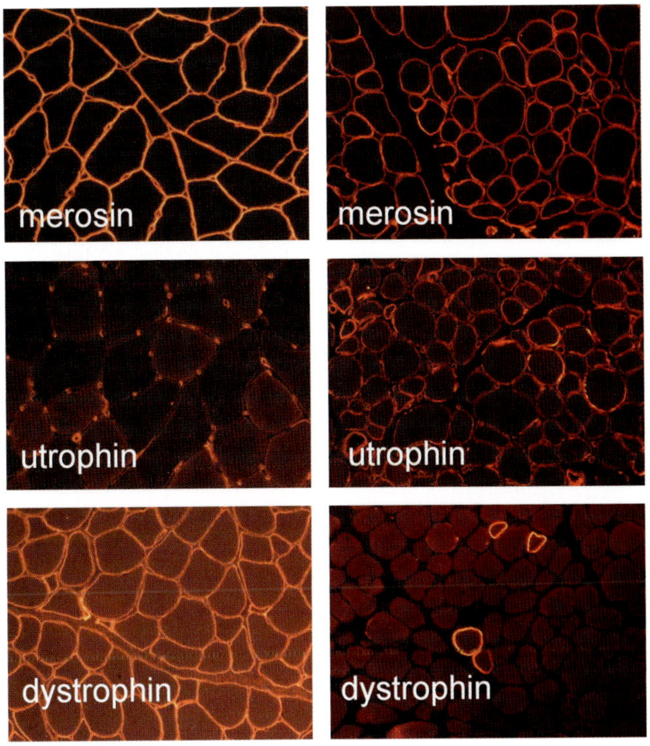

Figure 10.14. Upregulation of extrasynaptic utrophin. Under normal conditions utrophin B expression in skeletal muscle is restricted to the neuromuscular junction and utrophin A is seen around blood vessels (left panel). In dystrophin deficiency, utrophin expression is increased, as seen in extrasynaptic areas of the sarcolemma. This is thought to be a compensatory reaction; however, expression levels are not high enough to mitigate the dystrophic phenotype. Original magnification 140×.

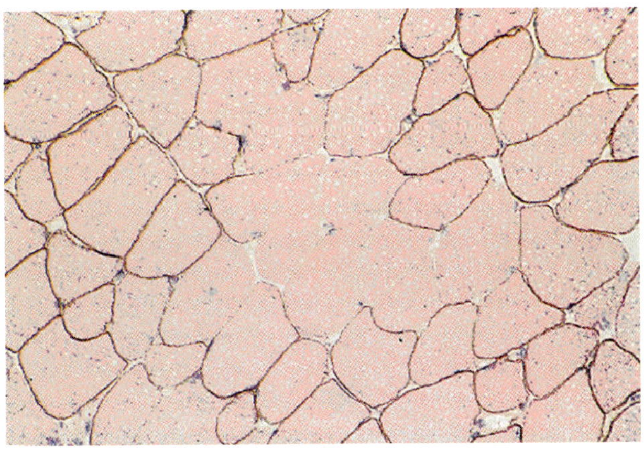

Figure 10.15. This is a non-manifesting but obligate DMD carrier's biopsy; peroxidase-labeled dystrophin immunostaining with polyclonal antibodies. A small group of muscle fibers lack dystrophin immunostaining presumably corresponding to a segment of fibers with skewed inactivation of the normal X-chromosome. Original magnification 350×. (Permission for reproduction given by G. Karpati.)

their 3′ end as well as another identical sequence at their 5′ end. These probes are hybridized with the genomic DNA. Subsequent washing will eliminate any unbound probe. Genomic DNA and probe hybrids are then denatured and the probes are subjected to PCR amplification.

Since all the probes can be amplified with the same primer pair, one reaction can be performed to amplify up to 40 probes. As each probe was designed to have a distinct size which can be correlated to the probed exon, the amplified probes can be separated by electrophoresis. The intensity of the bands can be correlated to internal standards and thus duplications or deletions of any specific gene fragment can be assessed. Advantages of MAPH are that probe generation is simple and because the probes are usually long, single base polymorphisms will not interfere with hybridization. However, MAPH probes are inherently amplifiable as each probe contains the necessary primer sequences. This carries a contamination risk, as any nonhybridized probe that is not removed will amplify, with the potential risk of yielding false-negative results.

Multiplex ligation-dependent probe amplification also uses the hybridization technique followed by PCR amplification. In MLPA each probe set is composed of two halves, which are specifically designed to hybridize to adjacent DNA sequences of a given exon. The exon-specific sequence of one half is flanked by a universal primer sequence. The exon-specific sequence of the other half also has a universal primer sequence at its end; however, it contains a spacer fragment of a defined length in between, such that the length of each spacer fragment can be attributed to a specific exon. Genomic DNA is hybridized with both halves of all probes. As each half of a probe will be located directly adjacent to its other half after hybridization, a ligation step unites both halves to one continuous probe. This newly generated "full probe" now becomes amplifiable by PCR as it is flanked by universal primers on either side. Probe halves that do not hybridize because of lack of an exon will not be ligated and will not amplify. Amplification products are then separated by electrophoresis according to size, and depending on the intensities of each band, duplication or deletion of any probed exon can be assessed. MLPA has the advantage that nonhybridized probes will not be amplified, thus reducing the risk of missing an exonic deletion. However, the short length of the specific probe region carries the risk that polymorphisms may interfere with hybridization and may lead to overcalling of exonic deletions.

The above-mentioned methods detect deletions and duplications but not point mutations or small rearrangements. Detection of such mutations requires direct sequencing of all exons, exon–intron boundaries and promoters, as these mutations are not localized to any specific hotspot. Several strategies have been developed to increase mutation detection rates and cost-effectiveness. Most of these strategies are PCR based and include a screening strategy to narrow down the amplicon that will most likely harbor the mutation. Various techniques have been developed to attain this aim each with its advantages and disadvantages. Such techniques include single-strand conformational polymorphism analysis (SSCP), which takes advantage of the altered electrophoretic mobility of single-stranded DNA molecules that harbor nucleotide polymorphisms. An improvement of this method has been called "detection of virtually all mutations-SSCP" (DOVAM-S) [201]. Other methods of screening for small mutations include denaturing high-performance liquid chromatography (DHPLC) [202], single condition amplification/internal primer analysis (SCAIP) [203] and denaturing gradient gel electrophoresis (DGGE) [204] amongst others.

Given the current technical advances in and ready availability of molecular diagnosis through gene analysis, many authors advocate first performing genetic testing in a patient with clinical findings suggestive of a dystrophinopathy before performing a muscle biopsy, as the latter carries a potential but low risk of complications, and can be psychologically traumatizing for a child.

Therapy

Most current therapies for DMD are palliative and include physiotherapy, orthopedic intervention, mainly stretching, bracing, surgical procedures for contractures and thoracic scoliosis, medications for osteopenia, cardiorespiratory intervention, psychological support, and dietary measures [205].

Physiotherapy should be offered to encourage activity and promote muscle function. Exercises are best performed in the hydrotherapy pool and exercise against resistance should be avoided as it could accelerate muscle fiber damage [206]. After an ambulant child loses ankle dorsiflexion he should be offered night splints. Once children become nonambulant, sitting ankle–foot orthoses should be prescribed to avoid painful contractures. If ankle contractures develop then they may need to be surgically addressed, and after surgery ankle–foot orthoses should be worn to delay re-occurrence. Knee–ankle–foot orthoses may prolong ambulation and thus delay contractures. In nonambulant children, standing frames or walkers can be used to delay contractures. Wheelchairs should have supportive seating to avoid postural contractures.

Scoliosis surgery should be performed when the Cobb angle is greater than 20° [207]. Preferably, surgery is performed when the spine is still relatively mobile and boys still have the cardiorespiratory fitness for the operation. Spinal bracing can be offered to children whose cardiorespiratory function does not allow surgery.

Respiratory management in DMD should include serial measurements of forced vital capacity [208]. Once this parameter falls below 40% of the predicted value, then overnight oximetry should be installed to detect nocturnal respiratory compromise. Nocturnal hypoventilation should be treated by noninvasive nocturnal ventilation [209]. Children with respiratory compromise are prone to chest infections and should be vaccinated against flu and pneumococcus pneumonia. Antibiotics should be provided promptly in cases of infection along with cough augmentation techniques.

Clinical signs of cardiomyopathy become evident only in very late stages of heart disease, because of inactivity due to skeletal muscle weakness. Once cardiomyopathy is clinically apparent, the left ventricular ejection fraction is markedly reduced to about 10% of normal, leading then to death within 12 months. Cardiac investigations should be performed every 2 years until age 10 years, and yearly thereafter [14]. Angiotensin converting enzyme (ACE) inhibitors and beta-blockers should be initiated when cardiac abnormalities are detected, although a recent study suggests that ACE inhibitors are beneficial if introduced prior to any detectable cardiac abnormalities [210].

Before any surgical intervention patients should undergo cardiac evaluation. During surgery depolarizing muscle relaxants should be avoided because of risk of hyperkalemia [211]. Because of inactivity, bone mineral density is reduced in DMD boys. After long bone fractures, patients should be mobilized early to avoid contractures. The use of long-term steroid treatment further precipitates osteoporosis. This should be counteracted with vitamin D, calcium, sunshine, and physical activity. Bisphosphonate administration had a positive effect on bone mineral density in Duchenne boys who received deflazacort treatment [212].

Several randomized, placebo-controlled clinical trials, many open label clinical trials, and large case series of glucocorticoid corticosteroids suggest that there is a significant increase in strength, timed function tests, and cardiorespiratory function in patients with DMD. These studies have recently been summarized [213, 214, 215]. A commonly accepted dosing regimen consists of daily prednisone 0.75 mg/kg or deflazacort 0.9 mg/kg per day, which is tapered as the child grows older. Treatment response can be observed as early as 10 days after initiation of treatment and reaches a plateau after 3 months. The treatment response can be sustained for approximately 3 years. Because of significant side-effects of steroid treatment such as weight gain, hypertension, cushingoid appearance, behavioral changes, growth retardation, and cataracts, intermittent dosing has been suggested [216] and a recent study demonstrated efficacy against placebo of an intermittent dosing regimen [217]. Currently clinical trials are in the planning stages to compare long-term daily versus intermittent glucocorticoid corticosteroid treatment [218]. Most Duchenne patients receive steroid treatment at around age 5 until they lose ambulation. Some authors suggest that long-term glucocorticoid corticosteroid treatment may be beneficial even beyond the age of loss of ambulation [219], but this has not yet been assessed in a controlled randomized clinical trial. Also, the question remains open as to at what age would be the best time to initiate glucocorticoid corticosteroid treatment.

The biological effect of glucocorticoid corticosteroid treatment is unclear, and several hypothesis have been put forward [214]:

- Altering the mRNA levels of structural, signaling, and immune response genes [220]
- Reducing cytotoxic T-lymphocytes [221]
- Lowering calcium influx and concentration [222]
- Increasing laminin expression and myogenic repair [223]
- Retarding muscle apoptosis and cellular infiltration [224]

- Enhancing dystrophin expression [225]
- Affecting neuromuscular transmission [226]
- Protecting against mechanically induced fiber damage [227]
- Slowing the rate of skeletal muscle breakdown [228]

Cell therapies

Cell therapies consist of the introduction of normal myogenic progenitors and precursor cells or even stem cells into affected muscles [229, 230]. The main purpose of these procedures is to either use the cells as vectors for dystrophin gene transfer or to provide replacement for lost muscle fibers. In the former case, the injected normal myogenic cells fuse with the dystrophin-deficient host fibers, providing them with nuclei that contain a normal dystrophin gene. In the latter case, the transplanted myogenic cells fuse with each other and if they become innervated they could function as replaced tissue to compensate for the dystrophic loss of fibers. Experimental cell replacement therapy approaches for muscular dystrophy have been pursued for a long time and include experiments whereby normal muscle is transplanted into a dystrophic animal [231, 232]. Ethical issues, in particular availability of newborn muscle that would be more easily reinnervated and re-vascularized, made it difficult to pursue this avenue further. A different experimental procedure consists of injecting donor muscle precursor cells (myoblasts) into a dystrophic host [233], thereby hoping for fusion of donor myoblasts, which express dystrophin, with the dystrophin-deficient host myotubes. Obstacles that have to be overcome with this experimental technique are: (1) reduced survival of injected myoblasts; (2) limited distribution and fusion of donor myoblasts with host muscle; (3) immune response to donor myoblasts. Human clinical trials involving myoblast transfer were not successful in improving muscle strength, despite multiple injections of a large number of donor myoblasts [234, 235, 236]. Other experimental strategies involved the genetic manipulation of donor myoblasts ex vivo, through introduction of a dystrophin transgene, followed by injection of the manipulated myoblasts into a recipient host [237, 238].

Additional cell-based experiments included systemic delivery of muscle precursor cells, which can be isolated from bone marrow [239], muscle [240] or the perivascular bed (so-called mesangioblasts) [241], into a host recipient. Recently, improved muscle function has been reported in dystrophic Golden Retriever dogs treated with intra-arterial delivery of such mesangioblasts [242].

Molecular therapies

An entire chapter (Chapter 9) is devoted to the subject of molecular therapies and the reader is referred to this chapter for details. Briefly, the following types of molecular therapies are being developed in preclinical models of DMD and in some cases clinical trials have already been initiated: dystrophin gene replacement, correction of the genomic gene defect, removing specific and selected exons from the transcribed primary constructs (exon skipping), prevention of the recognition of stop codons by ribosomes during the translational process (stop codon read-through), upregulation of functional analogs of dystrophin, such as extrasynaptic utrophin, as well as producing muscle hypertrophy by inhibition of the myostatin pathway.

The appropriateness of these various techniques and strategies will have to be adapted to individual circumstances.

Genetic counseling

Accurate genetic counseling requires meticulous documentation of the phenotype of the entire pedigree of the patient's family. It is important to emphasize that the ultimate advice to the family is made only in terms of statistical probability. The ultimate decision about procreative plans is made by the parents.

The basic principles are based on the fundamental facts that the inheritance of the dystrophinopathies are X-linked and that the pathogenic mutation in the mother may be inherited or develop de novo in her germ cells. The following practical examples are useful to consider [243]:

Because dystrophinopathies are inherited in an X-linked mode, a father of an affected male cannot be a carrier.

A woman with one affected son and no other affected family members may be one of the following:

- A carrier
- A somatic mosaic including the germline
- A germline mosaic
- Not a carrier, the mutation arose in the ovum, and the mutation is present in all cells of her son
- Not a carrier, the mutation arose after conception and her son is a mosaic

Sisters of a boy with an apparent de novo mutation are at risk of being carriers, because their mother could be a germline mosaic and subsequent siblings have a risk in the order of 5% to 10% of being affected (in the case of a male) or a carrier (in the case of a female).

The same holds true for sister of a woman who is a carrier due to a new mutation.

A woman with more than one affected son and no family history can be:

- A full carrier
- A somatic mosaic including her germline
- A germline mosaic

If a woman has an affected son and also an affected family member in her maternal lineage, such as a brother or maternal uncle, she is a definite carrier

A woman with at least one affected brother but no affected offspring is a possible carrier

A woman can be a carrier because:

- She inherited the mutation from her mother who is a carrier
- Either of her parents is a mosaic including the germline

- Either of her parents is a germline mosaic
- The ovum or sperm from which she arose contained the mutation
- The mutation arose after conception and she is a somatic mosaic including her germline

Offspring of a non-mosaic male proband:

- In the case of DMD, patients usually do not have the reproductive fitness, or may die before they reproduce
- In the case of BMD, or X-linked dilated cardiomyopathy, all female offspring will be obligate carriers

Prenatal testing

Identification of the X-chromosome carrying the mutation is a prerequisite for prenatal diagnosis. This can be done either by identifying the mutation or by establishing linkage to polymorphic markers in cases where there is a family history. Cells for DNA analysis are obtained from chorionic villus biopsies at 10–12 weeks of gestational age, or from amniocentesis at 15–18 weeks of gestational age.

Preimplantation diagnosis

As for prenatal diagnosis, preimplantation diagnosis requires knowledge about the affected X-chromosome, either through linkage or through identification of the disease-causing mutation.

Future perspectives

So far the application of molecular science to the dystrophinopathies has resulted in several major benefits. These include a good understanding of the pathogenesis, availability of precise diagnostic tests that allow accurate diagnosis, and genetic counseling. This knowledge has opened the way to designing and eventually employing effective and safe new therapeutic strategies. In this category a great deal of further progress is expected and in the next edition of this volume the reader should expect to be informed about such progress.

References

1. E. P. Hoffman, Dystrophinopathies. In *Disorders of Voluntary Muscle*. Seventh Edition, eds. G. Karpati, D. Hilton-Jones, R. C. Griggs. (Cambridge, UK: Cambridge University Press, 2001), pp. 385–432.
2. G. B. A. Duchenne, Recherche sur la paralysie musculaire pseudo-hypertrophique ou paralysie myo-sclerotique. *Arch. Gen. Med.* **11** (1868), 5–25, 179–209, 305–321, 421–443, 552–588.
3. M. Eagle, J. Bourke, R. Bullock, *et al.*, Managing Duchenne muscular dystrophy – the additive effect of spinal surgery and home nocturnal ventilation in improving survival. *Neuromuscul. Disord.* **17**:6 (2007), 470–475.
4. J. Finsterer, C. Stollberger, The heart in human dystrophinopathies. *Cardiology* **99**:1 (2003), 1–19.
5. J. M. de Kermadec, H. M. Becane, A. Chenard, F. Tertrain, Y. Weiss, Prevalence of left ventricular systolic dysfunction in Duchenne muscular dystrophy: an echocardiographic study. *Am. Heart. J.* **127**:3 (1994), 618–623.
6. G. Corrado, A. Lissoni, S. Beretta, *et al.*, Prognostic value of electrocardiograms, ventricular late potentials, ventricular arrhythmias, and left ventricular systolic dysfunction in patients with Duchenne muscular dystrophy. *Am. J. Cardiol.* **89**:7 (2002), 838–841.
7. American Academy of Pediatrics Section on Cardiology and Cardiac Surgery, Cardiovascular health supervision for individuals affected by Duchenne or Becker muscular dystrophy. *Pediatrics* **116**:6 (2005), 1569–1573.
8. S. Cotton, N. J. Voudouris, K. M. Greenwood, Intelligence and Duchenne muscular dystrophy: full-scale, verbal, and performance intelligence quotients. *Dev. Med. Child. Neurol.* **43**:7 (2001), 497–501.
9. D. A. Pillers, D. E. Bulman, R. G. Weleber, *et al.*, Dystrophin expression in the human retina is required for normal function as defined by electroretinography. *Nat. Genet.* **4**:1 (1993), 82–86.
10. A. E. Emery, Population frequencies of inherited neuromuscular diseases – a world survey. *Neuromuscul. Disord.* **1**:1 (1991), 19–29.
11. A. E. Emery, R. Skinner, Clinical studies in benign (Becker type) X-linked muscular dystrophy. *Clin. Genet.* **10**:4 (1976), 189–201.
12. M. Yazaki, K. Yoshida, A. Nakamura, *et al.*, Clinical characteristics of aged Becker muscular dystrophy patients with onset after 30 years. *Eur. Neurol.* **42**:3 (1999), 145–149.
13. K. M. Bushby, D. Gardner-Medwin, The clinical, genetic and dystrophin characteristics of Becker muscular dystrophy. I. Natural history. *J. Neurol.* **240**:2 (1993), 98–104.
14. K. Bushby, F. Muntoni, J. P. Bourke, 107th ENMC International Workshop: the management of cardiac involvement in muscular dystrophy and myotonic dystrophy 7th–9th June 2002, Naarden, the Netherlands. *Neuromuscul. Disord.* **13**:2 (2003), 166–172.
15. E. M. Hoogerwaard, W. G. de Voogt, A. A. Wilde, *et al.*, Evolution of cardiac abnormalities in Becker muscular dystrophy over a 13-year period. *J. Neurol.* **244**:10 (1997), 657–663.
16. M. Saito, H. Kawai, M. Akaike, K. Adachi, Y. Nishida, S. Saito, Cardiac dysfunction with Becker muscular dystrophy. *Am. Heart. J.* **132**:3 (1996), 642–647.
17. P. Melacini, M. Fanin, G. A. Danieli, *et al.*, Cardiac involvement in Becker muscular dystrophy. *J. Am. Coll. Cardiol.* **22**:7 (1993), 1927–1934.
18. G. Nigro, L. I. Comi, L. Politano, *et al.*, Evaluation of the cardiomyopathy in Becker muscular dystrophy. *Muscle Nerve* **18**:3 (1995), 283–291.
19. E. Kuhn, W. Fiehn, J. M. Schroder, H. Assmus, A. Wagner, Early myocardial disease and cramping myalgia in Becker-type muscular dystrophy: a kindred. *Neurology* **29**:8 (1979), 1144–1149.
20. S. Eggers, V. Lauriano, M. Melo, *et al.*, Why is the reproductive performance lower in Becker (BMD) as compared to limb girdle (LGMD) muscular dystrophy male patients? *Am. J. Med. Genet.* **60**:1 (1995), 27–32.

21. L. Mestroni, M. Giacca, Molecular genetics of dilated cardiomyopathy. *Curr. Opin. Cardiol.* **12**:3 (1997), 303–309.

22. P. Avner, E. Heard, X-chromosome inactivation: counting, choice and initiation. *Nat. Rev. Genet.* **2**:1 (2001), 59–67.

23. L. Merlini, Calf myopathy with a twist. *Neuromuscul. Disord.* **4**:1 (1994), 13–15.

24. S. D. Pena, G. Karpati, S. Carpenter, F. C. Fraser, The clinical consequences of X-chromosome inactivation: Duchenne muscular dystrophy in one of monozygotic twins. *J. Neurol. Sci.* **79**:3 (1987), 337–344.

25. J. R. Lupski, C. A. Garcia, H. Y. Zoghbi, E. P. Hoffman, R. G. Fenwick, Discordance of muscular dystrophy in monozygotic female twins: evidence supporting asymmetric splitting of the inner cell mass in a manifesting carrier of Duchenne dystrophy. *Am. J. Med. Genet.* **40**:3 (1991), 354–364.

26. P. Ferrier, F. Bamatter, D. Klein, Muscular dystrophy (Duchenne) in a girl with Turner's Syndrome. *J. Med. Genet.* **42** (1965), 38–46.

27. M. Zatz, A. M. Vianna-Morgante, P. Campos, A. J. Diament, Translocation (X;6) in a female with Duchenne muscular dystrophy: implications for the localisation of the DMD locus. *J. Med. Genet.* **18**:6 (1981), 442–447.

28. E. M. Hoogerwaard, P. A. van der Wouw, A. A. Wilde, *et al.*, Cardiac involvement in carriers of Duchenne and Becker muscular dystrophy. *Neuromuscul. Disord.* **9**:5 (1999), 347–351.

29. L. Grain, M. Cortina-Borja, C. Forfar, D. Hilton-Jones, J. Hopkin, M. Burch, Cardiac abnormalities and skeletal muscle weakness in carriers of Duchenne and Becker muscular dystrophies and controls. *Neuromuscul. Disord.* **11**:2 (2001), 186–191.

30. L. Politano, V. Nigro, G. Nigro, *et al.*, Development of cardiomyopathy in female carriers of Duchenne and Becker muscular dystrophies. *J. Am. Med. Assoc.* **275**:17 (1996), 1335–1338.

31. K. J. Felice, Distal weakness in dystrophin-deficient muscular dystrophy. *Muscle Nerve* **19**:12 (1996), 1608–1610.

32. A. Prelle, R. Medori, M. Moggio, *et al.*, Dystrophin deficiency in a case of congenital myopathy. *J. Neurol.* **239**:2 (1992), 76–78.

33. F. J. Samaha, J. G. Quinlan, Myalgia and cramps: dystrophinopathy with wide-ranging laboratory findings. *J. Child. Neurol.* **11**:1 (1996), 21–24.

34. N. Sunohara, K. Arahata, E. P. Hoffman, *et al.*, Quadriceps myopathy: forme fruste of Becker muscular dystrophy. *Ann. Neurol.* **28**:5 (1990), 634–639.

35. A. Morrone, E. Zammarchi, P. C. Scacheri, *et al.*, Asymptomatic dystrophinopathy. *Am. J. Med. Genet.* **69**:3 (1997), 261–267.

36. U. Francke, H. D. Ochs, B. de Martinville, *et al.*, Minor Xp21 chromosome deletion in a male associated with expression of Duchenne muscular dystrophy, chronic granulomatous disease, retinitis pigmentosa, and McLeod syndrome. *Am. J. Hum. Genet.* **37**:2 (1985), 250–267.

37. L. M. Kunkel, A. P. Monaco, W. Middlesworth, H. D. Ochs, S. A. Latt, Specific cloning of DNA fragments absent from the DNA of a male patient with an X chromosome deletion. *Proc. Natl. Acad. Sci. U. S. A.* **82**:14 (1985), 4778–4782.

38. M. Koenig, E. P. Hoffman, C. J. Bertelson, A. P. Monaco, C. Feener, L. M. Kunkel, Complete cloning of the Duchenne muscular dystrophy (DMD) cDNA and preliminary genomic organization of the DMD gene in normal and affected individuals. *Cell* **50**:3 (1987), 509–517.

39. J. M. Murray, K. E. Davies, P. S. Harper, L. Meredith, C. R. Mueller, R. Williamson, Linkage relationship of a cloned DNA sequence on the short arm of the X chromosome to Duchenne muscular dystrophy. *Nature* **300**:5887 (1982), 69–71.

40. H. M. Kingston, M. Sarfarazi, N. S. Thomas, P. S. Harper, Localisation of the Becker muscular dystrophy gene on the short arm of the X chromosome by linkage to cloned DNA sequences. *Hum. Genet.* **67**:1 (1984), 6–17.

41. R. G. Worton, C. Duff, J. E. Sylvester, R. D. Schmickel, H. F. Willard, Duchenne muscular dystrophy involving translocation of the dmd gene next to ribosomal RNA genes. *Science* **224**:4656 (1984), 1447–1449.

42. R. M. Greenstein, M. P. Reardon, T. S. Chan, *et al.*, An (X;11) translocation in a girl with Duchenne muscular dystrophy Repository identification No GM1695. *Cytogenet. Cell. Genet.* **27**:4 (1980), 268.

43. C. Verellen-Dumoulin, M. Freund, R. De Meyer, *et al.*, Expression of an X-linked muscular dystrophy in a female due to translocation involving Xp21 and non-random inactivation of the normal X chromosome. *Hum. Genet.* **67**:1 (1984), 115–119.

44. P. N. Ray, B. Belfall, C. Duff, *et al.*, Cloning of the breakpoint of an X;21 translocation associated with Duchenne muscular dystrophy. *Nature* **318**:6047 (1985), 672–675.

45. E. P. Hoffman, R. H. Brown Jr., L. M. Kunkel, Dystrophin: the protein product of the Duchenne muscular dystrophy locus. *Cell* **51**:6 (1987), 919–928.

46. C. N. Tennyson, H. J. Klamut, R. G. Worton, The human dystrophin gene requires 16 hours to be transcribed and is cotranscriptionally spliced. *Nat. Genet.* **9**:2 (1995), 184–190.

47. M. Koenig, A. P. Monaco, L. M. Kunkel, The complete sequence of dystrophin predicts a rod-shaped cytoskeletal protein. *Cell* **53**:2 (1988), 219–228.

48. R. G. Hammonds, Jr., Protein sequence of DMD gene is related to actin-binding domain of alpha-actinin. *Cell* **51**:1 (1987), 1.

49. R. A. Cross, M. Stewart, J. Kendrick-Jones, Structural predictions for the central domain of dystrophin. *FEBS Lett.* **262**:1 (1990), 87–92.

50. X. Huang, F. Poy, R. Zhang, A. Joachimiak, M. Sudol, M. J. Eck, Structure of a WW domain containing fragment of dystrophin in complex with beta-dystroglycan. *Nat. Struct. Biol.* **7**:8 (2000), 634–638.

51. C. P. Ponting, D. J. Blake, K. E. Davies, J. Kendrick-Jones, S. J. Winder, ZZ and TAZ: new putative zinc fingers in dystrophin and other proteins. *Trends. Biochem. Sci.* **21**:1 (1996), 11–13.

52. D. J. Blake, J. M. Tinsley, K. E. Davies, A. E. Knight, S. J. Winder, J. Kendrick-Jones, Coiled-coil regions in the carboxy-terminal domains of dystrophin and related proteins: potentials for protein-protein interactions. *Trends. Biochem. Sci.* **20**:4 (1995), 133–135.

53. A. Clerk, P. N. Strong, C. A. Sewry, Characterisation of dystrophin during development of human skeletal muscle. *Development* **114**:2 (1992), 395–402.

54. A. A. Lev, C. C. Feener, L. M. Kunkel, R. H.Brown Jr., Expression of the Duchenne's muscular dystrophy gene in cultured muscle cells. *J. Biol. Chem.* **262**:33 (1987), 15817–15820.

55. U. Nudel, K. Robzyk, D. Yaffe, Expression of the putative Duchenne muscular dystrophy gene in differentiated myogenic cell cultures and in the brain. *Nature* **331**:6157 (1988), 635–638.

56. U. Nudel, D. Zuk, P. Einat, *et al.*, Duchenne muscular dystrophy gene product is not identical in muscle and brain. *Nature* **337**:6202 (1989), 76–78.

57. F. M. Boyce, A. H. Beggs, C. Feener, L. M. Kunkel, Dystrophin is transcribed in brain from a distant upstream promoter. *Proc. Natl. Acad. Sci. U. S. A.* **88**:4 (1991), 1276–1280.

58. F. Muntoni, M. Cau, A. Ganau, *et al.*, Brief report: deletion of the dystrophin muscle-promoter region associated with X-linked dilated cardiomyopathy. *N. Engl. J. Med.* **329**:13 (1993), 921–925.

59. D. C. Gorecki, A. P. Monaco, J. M. Derry, A. P. Walker, E. A. Barnard, P. J. Barnard, Expression of four alternative dystrophin transcripts in brain regions regulated by different promoters. *Hum. Mol. Genet.* **1**:7 (1992), 505–510.

60. H. Nishio, Y. Takeshima, N. Narita, *et al.*, Identification of a novel first exon in the human dystrophin gene and of a new promoter located more than 500 kb upstream of the nearest known promoter. *J. Clin. Invest.* **94**:3 (1994), 1037–1042.

61. V. N. D'souza, T. M. Nguyen, G. E. Morris, W. Karges, D. A. Pillers, P. N. Ray, A novel dystrophin isoform is required for normal retinal electrophysiology. *Hum. Mol. Genet.* **4**:5 (1995), 837–842.

62. H. G. Lidov, S. Selig, L. M. Kunkel, Dp140: a novel 140 kDa CNS transcript from the dystrophin locus. *Hum. Mol. Genet.* **4**:3 (1995), 329–335.

63. A. Bardoni, G. Felisari, M. Sironi, *et al.*, Loss of Dp140 regulatory sequences is associated with cognitive impairment in dystrophinopathies. *Neuromuscul. Disord.* **10**:3 (2000), 194–199.

64. T. J. Byers, H. G. Lidov, L. M. Kunkel, An alternative dystrophin transcript specific to peripheral nerve. *Nat. Genet.* **4**:1 (1993), 77–81.

65. D. Rapaport, D. Lederfein, J. T. den Dunnen, *et al.*, Characterization and cell type distribution of a novel, major transcript of the Duchenne muscular dystrophy gene. *Differentiation* **49**:3 (1992), 187–193.

66. S. Bar, E. Barnea, Z. Levy, S. Neuman, D. Yaffe, U. Nudel, A novel product of the Duchenne muscular dystrophy gene which greatly differs from the known isoforms in its structure and tissue distribution. *Biochem. J.* **272**:2 (1990), 557–560.

67. M. P. Moizard, A. Toutain, D. Fournier, *et al.*, Severe cognitive impairment in DMD: obvious clinical indication for Dp71 isoform point mutation screening. *Eur. J. Hum. Genet.* **8**:7 (2000), 552–556.

68. D. Lederfein, Z. Levy, N. Augier, *et al.*, A 71-kilodalton protein is a major product of the Duchenne muscular dystrophy gene in brain and other nonmuscle tissues. *Proc. Natl. Acad. Sci. U. S. A.* **89**:12 (1992), 5346–5350.

69. J. M. Tinsley, D. J. Blake, K. E. Davies, Apo-dystrophin-3: a 2.2kb transcript from the DMD locus encoding the dystrophin glycoprotein binding site. *Hum. Mol. Genet.* **2**:5 (1993), 521–524.

70. E. A. Burton, J. M. Tinsley, P. J. Holzfeind, N. R. Rodrigues, K. E. Davies, A second promoter provides an alternative target for therapeutic up-regulation of utrophin in Duchenne muscular dystrophy. *Proc. Natl. Acad. Sci. U. S. A.* **96**:24 (1999), 14025–14030.

71. D. R. Love, D. F. Hill, G. Dickson, *et al.*, An autosomal transcript in skeletal muscle with homology to dystrophin. *Nature* **339**:6219 (1989), 55–58.

72. J. Wilson, W. Putt, C. Jimenez, Y. H. Edwards, Up71 and up140, two novel transcripts of utrophin that are homologues of short forms of dystrophin. *Hum. Mol. Genet.* **8**:7 (1999), 1271–1278.

73. D. J. Blake, J. N. Schofield, R. A. Zuellig, *et al.*, G-utrophin, the autosomal homologue of dystrophin Dp116, is expressed in sensory ganglia and brain. *Proc. Natl. Acad. Sci. U. S. A.* **92**:9 (1995), 3697–3701.

74. G. Karpati, S. Carpenter, G. E. Morris, K. E. Davies, C. Guerin, P. Holland, Localization and quantitation of the chromosome 6-encoded dystrophin-related protein in normal and pathological human muscle. *J. Neuropathol. Exp. Neurol.* **52**:2 (1993), 119–128.

75. A. O. Gramolini, J. Wu, B. J. Jasmin, Regulation and functional significance of utrophin expression at the mammalian neuromuscular synapse. *Microsc. Res. Tech.* **49**:1 (2000), 90–100.

76. F. Galvagni, M. Cantini, S. Oliviero, The utrophin gene is transcriptionally up-regulated in regenerating muscle. *J. Biol. Chem.* **277**:21 (2002), 19106–19113.

77. M. Pearce, D. J. Blake, J. M. Tinsley, *et al.*, The utrophin and dystrophin genes share similarities in genomic structure. *Hum. Mol. Genet.* **2**:11 (1993), 1765–1772.

78. S. J. Winder, L. Hemmings, S. K. Maciver, *et al.*, Utrophin actin binding domain: analysis of actin binding and cellular targeting. *J. Cell. Sci.* **108**:Pt 1 (1995), 63–71.

79. K. J. Amann, A. W. Guo, J. M. Ervasti, Utrophin lacks the rod domain actin binding activity of dystrophin. *J. Biol. Chem.* **274**:50 (1999), 35375–35380.

80. S. J. Winder, T. J. Gibson, J. Kendrick-Jones, Dystrophin and utrophin: the missing links! *FEBS Lett.* **369**:1 (1995), 27–33.

81. J. A. Rafael, J. M. Tinsley, A. C. Potter, A. E. Deconinck, K. E. Davies, Skeletal muscle-specific expression of a utrophin transgene rescues utrophin-dystrophin deficient mice. *Nat. Genet.* **19**:1 (1998), 79–82.

82. J. R. Deol, G. Danialou, N. Larochelle, *et al.*, Successful compensation for dystrophin deficiency by a helper-dependent adenovirus expressing full-length utrophin. *Mol. Ther.* **15**:10 (2007), 1767–1774.

83. A. E. Deconinck, J. A. Rafael, J. A. Skinner, *et al.*, Utrophin-dystrophin-deficient mice as a model for Duchenne muscular dystrophy. *Cell* **90**:4 (1997), 717–727.

84. J. D. Porter, J. A. Rafael, R. J. Ragusa, J. K. Brueckner, J. I. Trickett, K. E. Davies, The sparing of extraocular muscle in dystrophinopathy is lost in mice lacking utrophin and dystrophin. *J. Cell. Sci.* **111**:Pt 13 (1998), 1801–1811.

85. M. P. Chevron, B. Echenne, J. Demaille, Absence of dystrophin and utrophin in a boy with severe muscular dystrophy. *N. Engl. J. Med.* **331**:17 (1994), 1162–1163.

86. G. Karpati, R. Gilbert, B. J. Petrof, J. Nalbantoglu, Gene therapy research for Duchenne and Becker muscular dystrophies. *Curr. Opin. Neurol.* **10**:5 (1997), 430–435.

87. P. Miura, B. J. Jasmin, Utrophin upregulation for treating Duchenne or Becker muscular dystrophy: how close are we? *Trends Mol. Med.* **12**:3 (2006), 122–129.

88. R. C. Hirst, K. J. McCullagh, K. E. Davies, Utrophin upregulation in Duchenne muscular dystrophy. *Acta. Myol.* **24**:3 (2005), 209–216.

89. K. P. Campbell, J. T. Stull, Skeletal muscle basement membrane-sarcolemma-cytoskeleton interaction minireview series. *J. Biol. Chem.* **278**:15 (2003), 12599–12600.

90. V. Straub, K. P. Campbell, Muscular dystrophies and the dystrophin-glycoprotein complex. *Curr. Opin. Neurol.* **10**:2 (1997), 168–175.

91. U. Mayer, Integrins: redundant or important players in skeletal muscle? *J. Biol. Chem.* **278**:17 (2003), 14587–14590.

92. J. M. Ervasti, Costameres: the Achilles' heel of Herculean muscle. *J. Biol. Chem.* **278**:16 (2003), 13591–13594.

93. T. J. Patel, R. L. Lieber, Force transmission in skeletal muscle: from actomyosin to external tendons. *Exerc. Sport. Sci. Rev.* **25** (1997), 321–363.

94. B. J. Petrof, The molecular basis of activity-induced muscle injury in Duchenne muscular dystrophy. *Mol. Cell. Biochem.* **179**:1–2 (1998), 111–123.

95. P. Y. Fong, P. R. Turner, W. F. Denetclaw, R. A. Steinhardt, Increased activity of calcium leak channels in myotubes of Duchenne human and mdx mouse origin. *Science* **250**:4981 (1990), 673–676.

96. G. D. Thomas, M. Sander, K. S. Lau, P. L. Huang, J. T. Stull, R. G. Victor, Impaired metabolic modulation of alpha-adrenergic vasoconstriction in dystrophin-deficient skeletal muscle. *Proc. Natl. Acad. Sci. U. S. A.* **95**:25 (1998), 15090–15095.

97. R. Barresi, K. P. Campbell, Dystroglycan: from biosynthesis to pathogenesis of human disease. *J. Cell. Sci.* **119** Pt 2 (2006), 199–207.

98. E. Ozawa, Y. Mizuno, Y. Hagiwara, T. Sasaoka, M. Yoshida, Molecular and cell biology of the sarcoglycan complex. *Muscle Nerve* **32**:5 (2005), 563–576.

99. M. J. Allikian, E. M. McNally, Processing and assembly of the dystrophin glycoprotein complex. *Traffic* **8**:3 (2007), 177–183.

100. D. E. Michele, K. P. Campbell, Dystrophin-glycoprotein complex: post-translational processing and dystroglycan function. *J. Biol. Chem.* **278**:18 (2003), 15457–15460.

101. O. Ibraghimov-Beskrovnaya, A. Milatovich, T. Ozcelik, *et al.*, Human dystroglycan: skeletal muscle cDNA, genomic structure, origin of tissue specific isoforms and chromosomal localization. *Hum. Mol. Genet.* **2**:10 (1993), 1651–1657.

102. R. Timpl, D. Tisi, J. F. Talts, Z. Andac, T. Sasaki, E. Hohenester, Structure and function of laminin LG modules. *Matrix Biol.* **19**:4 (2000), 309–317.

103. R. A. Williamson, M. D. Henry, K. J. Daniels, *et al.*, Dystroglycan is essential for early embryonic development: disruption of Reichert's membrane in Dag1-null mice. *Hum. Mol. Genet.* **6**:6 (1997), 831–841.

104. E. C. Olson, C. A. Walsh, Smooth, rough and upside-down neocortical development. *Curr. Opin. Genet. Dev.* **12**:3 (2002), 320–327.

105. F. Muntoni, M. Brockington, D. J. Blake, S. Torelli, S. C. Brown, Defective glycosylation in muscular dystrophy. *Lancet.* **360**:9343 (2002), 1419–1421.

106. J. A. Chasis, P. Agre, N. Mohandas, Decreased membrane mechanical stability and in vivo loss of surface area reflect spectrin deficiencies in hereditary spherocytosis. *J. Clin. Invest.* **82**:2 (1988), 617–623.

107. A. Menke, H. Jockusch, Decreased osmotic stability of dystrophin-less muscle cells from the mdx mouse. *Nature* **349**:6304 (1991), 69–71.

108. B. J. Petrof, J. B. Shrager, H. H. Stedman, A. M. Kelly, H. L. Sweeney, Dystrophin protects the sarcolemma from stresses developed during muscle contraction. *Proc. Natl. Acad. Sci. U. S. A.* **90**:8 (1993), 3710–3714.

109. J. E. Brenman, D. S. Chao, H. Xia, K. Aldape, D. S. Bredt, Nitric oxide synthase complexed with dystrophin and absent from skeletal muscle sarcolemma in Duchenne muscular dystrophy. *Cell* **82**:5 (1995), 743–752.

110. W. J. Chang, S. T. Iannaccone, K. S. Lau, *et al.*, Neuronal nitric oxide synthase and dystrophin-deficient muscular dystrophy. *Proc. Natl. Acad. Sci. U. S. A.* **93**:17 (1996), 9142–9147.

111. K. S. Lau, R. W. Grange, W. J. Chang, K. E. Kamm, I. Sarelius, J. T. Stull, Skeletal muscle contractions stimulate cGMP formation and attenuate vascular smooth muscle myosin phosphorylation via nitric oxide. *FEBS Lett.* **431**:1 (1998), 71–74.

112. M. Sander, B. Chavoshan, S. A. Harris, *et al.*, Functional muscle ischemia in neuronal nitric oxide synthase-deficient skeletal muscle of children with Duchenne muscular dystrophy. *Proc. Natl. Acad. Sci. U. S. A.* **97**:25 (2000), 13818–13823.

113. M. Khairallah, R. J. Khairallah, M. E. Young, *et al.*, Sildenafil and cardiomyocyte-specific cGMP signaling prevent cardiomyopathic changes associated with dystrophin deficiency. *Proc. Natl. Acad. Sci. U. S. A.* **105**:19 (2008), 7028–7033.

114. S. Repetto, M. Bado, P. Broda, *et al.*, Increased number of caveolae and caveolin-3 overexpression in Duchenne muscular dystrophy. *Biochem. Biophys. Res. Commun.* **261**:3 (1999), 547–550.

115. J. R. Glenney, D. Soppet, Jr. Sequence and expression of caveolin, a protein component of caveolae plasma membrane domains phosphorylated on tyrosine in Rous sarcoma virus-transformed fibroblasts. *Proc. Natl. Acad. Sci. U. S. A.* **89**:21 (1992), 10517–10521.

116. E. J. Smart, G. A. Graf, M. A. McNiven, *et al.*, Caveolins, liquid-ordered domains, and signal transduction. *Mol. Cell. Biol.* **19**:11 (1999), 7289–7304.

117. S. E. Woodman, F. Sotgia, F. Galbiati, C. Minetti, M. P. Lisanti, Caveolinopathies: mutations in caveolin-3 cause four distinct autosomal dominant muscle diseases. *Neurology* **62**:4 (2004), 538–543.

118. D. Fischer, A. Schroers, I. Blumcke, *et al.*, Consequences of a novel caveolin-3 mutation in a large German family. *Ann. Neurol.* **53**:2 (2003), 233–241.

119. F. Galbiati, D. Volonte, J. B. Chu, *et al.*, Transgenic overexpression of caveolin-3 in skeletal muscle fibers induces a Duchenne-like muscular dystrophy phenotype. *Proc. Natl. Acad. Sci. U. S. A.* **97**:17 (2000), 9689–9694.

120. F. Galbiati, J. A. Engelman, D. Volonte, *et al.*, Caveolin-3 null mice show a loss of caveolae, changes in the microdomain

distribution of the dystrophin-glycoprotein complex, and t-tubule abnormalities. *J. Biol. Chem.* **276**:24 (2001), 21425–21433.

121. J. E. Hance, S. Y. Fu, S. C. Watkins, A. H. Beggs, M. Michalak, Alpha-actinin-2 is a new component of the dystrophin-glycoprotein complex. *Arch. Biochem. Biophys.* **365**:2 (1999), 216–222.
122. Y. K. Hayashi, F. L. Chou, E. Engvall, *et al.*, Mutations in the integrin alpha 7 gene cause congenital myopathy. *Nat. Genet.* **19**:1 (1998), 94–97.
123. C. Guo, M. Willem, A. Werner, *et al.*, Absence of alpha 7 integrin in dystrophin-deficient mice causes a myopathy similar to Duchenne muscular dystrophy. *Hum. Mol. Genet.* **15**:6 (2006), 989–998.
124. P. Sicinski, Y. Geng, A. S. Ryder-Cook, E. A. Barnard, M. G. Darlison, P. J. Barnard, The molecular basis of muscular dystrophy in the mdx mouse: a point mutation. *Science* **244**:4912 (1989), 1578–1580.
125. B. A. Valentine, N. J. Winand, D. Pradhan, *et al.*, Canine X-linked muscular dystrophy as an animal model of Duchenne muscular dystrophy: a review. *Am. J. Med. Genet.* **42**:3 (1992), 352–356.
126. K. Ohlendieck, K. P. Campbell, Dystrophin-associated proteins are greatly reduced in skeletal muscle from mdx mice. *J. Cell. Biol.* **115**:6 (1991), 1685–1694.
127. E. P. Hoffman, Dystrophin associated proteins fail in filling dystrophin's shoes. *Nat. Genet.* **8**:4 (1994), 311–312.
128. D. S. Greenberg, Y. Sunada, K. P. Campbell, D. Yaffe, U. Nudel, Exogenous Dp71 restores the levels of dystrophin associated proteins but does not alleviate muscle damage in mdx mice. *Nat. Genet.* **8**:4 (1994), 340–344.
129. G. A. Cox, Y. Sunada, K. P. Campbell, J. S. Chamberlain, Dp71 can restore the dystrophin-associated glycoprotein complex in muscle but fails to prevent dystrophy. *Nat. Genet.* **8**:4 (1994), 333–339.
130. L. M. Judge, M. Haraguchiln, J. S. Chamberlain, Dissecting the signaling and mechanical functions of the dystrophin-glycoprotein complex. *J. Cell. Sci.* **119**:Pt 8 (2006), 1537–1546.
131. L. E. Warner, C. Dello Russo, R. W. Crawford, *et al.*, Expression of Dp260 in muscle tethers the actin cytoskeleton to the dystrophin-glycoprotein complex and partially prevents dystrophy. *Hum. Mol. Genet.* **11**:9 (2002), 1095–1105.
132. G. E. Crawford, J. A. Faulkner, R. H. Crosbie, K. P. Campbell, S. C. Froehner, J. S. Chamberlain, Assembly of the dystrophin-associated protein complex does not require the dystrophin COOH-terminal domain. *J. Cell. Biol.* **150**:6 (2000), 1399–1410.
133. S. Q. Harper, M. A. Hauser, C. Dello Russo, *et al.*, Modular flexibility of dystrophin: implications for gene therapy of Duchenne muscular dystrophy. *Nat. Med.* **8**:3 (2002), 253–261.
134. M. J. Blankinship, P. Gregorevic, J. S. Chamberlain, Gene therapy strategies for Duchenne muscular dystrophy utilizing recombinant adeno-associated virus vectors. *Mol. Ther.* **13**:2 (2006), 241–249.
135. P. Gregorevic, J. M. Allen, E. Minami, *et al.*, rAAV6-microdystrophin preserves muscle function and extends lifespan in severely dystrophic mice. *Nat. Med.* **12**:7 (2006), 787–789.
136. M. Koenig, A. H. Beggs, M. Moyer, *et al.*, The molecular basis for Duchenne versus Becker muscular dystrophy: correlation of severity with type of deletion. *Am. J. Hum. Genet.* **45**:4 (1989), 498–506.
137. A. P. Monaco, C. J. Bertelson, S. Liechti-Gallati, H. Moser, L. M. Kunkel, An explanation for the phenotypic differences between patients bearing partial deletions of the DMD locus. *Genomics* **2**:1 (1988), 90–95.
138. L. V. Nicholson, M. A. Johnson, K. M. Bushby, *et al.*, Integrated study of 100 patients with Xp21 linked muscular dystrophy using clinical, genetic, immunochemical, and histopathological data. Part 1. Trends across the clinical groups. *J. Med. Genet.* **30**:9 (1993), 728–736.
139. L. V. Nicholson, M. A. Johnson, K. M. Bushby, *et al.*, Integrated study of 100 patients with Xp21 linked muscular dystrophy using clinical, genetic, immunochemical, and histopathological data. Part 2. Correlations within individual patients. *J. Med. Genet.* **30**:9 (1993), 737–744.
140. L. V. Nicholson, M. A. Johnson, K. M. Bushby, *et al.*, Integrated study of 100 patients with Xp21 linked muscular dystrophy using clinical, genetic, immunochemical, and histopathological data. Part 3. Differential diagnosis and prognosis. *J. Med. Genet.* **30**:9 (1993), 745–751.
141. M. C. Wapenaar, T. Kievits, K. A. Hart, *et al.*, A deletion hot spot in the Duchenne muscular dystrophy gene. *Genomics* **2**:2 (1988), 101–108.
142. S. B. Malhotra, K. A. Hart, H. J. Klamut, *et al.*, Frame-shift deletions in patients with Duchenne and Becker muscular dystrophy. *Science* **242**:4879 (1988), 755–759.
143. S. B. Gangopadhyay, T. G. Sherratt, J. Z. Heckmatt, *et al.*, Dystrophin in frameshift deletion patients with Becker muscular dystrophy. *Am. J. Hum. Genet.* **51**:3 (1992), 562–570.
144. L. V. Nicholson, K. M. Bushby, M. A. Johnson, D. Gardner-Medwin, I. B. Ginjaar, Dystrophin expression in Duchenne patients with "in-frame" gene deletions. *Neuropediatrics* **24**:2 (1993), 93–97.
145. L. R. Goldberg, I. Hausmanowa-Petrusewicz, A. Fidzianska, D. J. Duggan, L. S. Steinberg, E. P. Hoffman, A dystrophin missense mutation showing persistence of dystrophin and dystrophin-associated proteins yet a severe phenotype. *Ann. Neurol.* **44**:6 (1998), 971–976.
146. P. R. Turner, T. Westwood, C. M. Regen, R. A. Steinhardt, Increased protein degradation results from elevated free calcium levels found in muscle from mdx mice. *Nature* **335**:6192 (1988), 735–738.
147. D. A. Jones, M. J. Jackson, G. McPhail, R. H. Edwards, Experimental mouse muscle damage: the importance of external calcium. *Clin. Sci. (Lond)*, **66**:3 (1984), 317–322.
148. M. J. Jackson, D. A. Jones, R. H. Edwards, Experimental skeletal muscle damage: the nature of the calcium-activated degenerative processes. *Eur. J. Clin. Invest.* **14**:5 (1984), 369–374.
149. M. J. Spencer, R. L. Mellgren, Overexpression of a calpastatin transgene in mdx muscle reduces dystrophic pathology. *Hum. Mol. Genet.* **11**:21 (2002), 2645–2655.
150. J. M. Alderton, R. A. Steinhardt, How calcium influx through calcium leak channels is responsible for the elevated levels of calcium-dependent proteolysis in dystrophic myotubes. *Trends. Cardiovasc. Med.* **10**:6 (2000), 268–272.

151. N. Zamzami, G. Kroemer, The mitochondrion in apoptosis: how Pandora's box opens. *Nat. Rev. Mol. Cell. Biol.* **2**:1 (2001), 67–71.

152. C. P. Baines, R. A. Kaiser, N. H. Purcell, *et al.*, Loss of cyclophilin D reveals a critical role for mitochondrial permeability transition in cell death. *Nature* **434**:7033 (2005), 658–662.

153. A. C. Schinzel, O. Takeuchi, Z. Huang, *et al.*, Cyclophilin D is a component of mitochondrial permeability transition and mediates neuronal cell death after focal cerebral ischemia. *Proc. Natl. Acad. Sci. U. S. A.* **102**:34 (2005), 12005–12010.

154. D. P. Millay, M. A. Sargent, H. Osinska, *et al.*, Genetic and pharmacologic inhibition of mitochondrial-dependent necrosis attenuates muscular dystrophy. *Nat. Med.* **14**:4 (2008), 442–447.

155. M. Sandri, U. Carraro, M. Podhorska-Okolov, *et al.*, Apoptosis, DNA damage and ubiquitin expression in normal and mdx muscle fibers after exercise. *FEBS Lett.* **373**:3 (1995), 291–295.

156. J. G. Tidball, D. E. Albrecht, B. E. Lokensgard, M. J. Spencer, Apoptosis precedes necrosis of dystrophin-deficient muscle. *J. Cell. Sci.* **108**:Pt 6 (1995), 2197–2204.

157. M. Sandri, C. Minetti, M. Pedemonte, U. Carraro, Apoptotic myonuclei in human Duchenne muscular dystrophy. *Lab. Invest.* **78**:8 (1998), 1005–1016.

158. D. S. Tews, H. H. Goebel, DNA-fragmentation and expression of apoptosis-related proteins in muscular dystrophies. *Neuropathol. Appl. Neurobiol.* **23**:4 (1997), 331–338.

159. A. Migheli, T. Mongini, C. Doriguzzi, *et al.*, Muscle apoptosis in humans occurs in normal and denervated muscle, but not in myotonic dystrophy, dystrophinopathies or inflammatory disease. *Neurogenetics* **1**:2 (1997), 81–87.

160. A. Inukai, Y. Kobayashi, K. Ito, *et al.*, Expression of Fas antigen is not associated with apoptosis in human myopathies. *Muscle Nerve* **20**:6 (1997), 702–709.

161. M. Olive, J. A. Martinez-Matos, J. Montero, I. Ferrer, Apoptosis is not the mechanism of cell death of muscle fibers in human muscular dystrophies and inflammatory myopathies. *Muscle Nerve* **20**:10 (1997), 1328–1330.

162. J. G. Tidball, M. Wehling-Henricks, The role of free radicals in the pathophysiology of muscular dystrophy. *J. Appl. Physiol.* **102**:4 (2007), 1677–1686.

163. T. A. Rando, M. H. Disatnik, Y. Yu, A. Franco, Muscle cells from mdx mice have an increased susceptibility to oxidative stress. *Neuromuscul. Disord.* **8**:1 (1998), 14–21.

164. M. H. Disatnik, J. S. Chamberlain, T. A. Rando, Dystrophin mutations predict cellular susceptibility to oxidative stress. *Muscle Nerve* **23**:5 (2000), 784–792.

165. M. H. Disatnik, J. Dhawan, Y. Yu, *et al.*, Evidence of oxidative stress in mdx mouse muscle: studies of the pre-necrotic state. *J. Neurol. Sci.* **161**:1 (1998), 77–84.

166. R. J. Ragusa, C. K. Chow, J. D. Porter, Oxidative stress as a potential pathogenic mechanism in an animal model of Duchenne muscular dystrophy. *Neuromuscul. Disord.* **7**:6–7 (1997), 379–386.

167. R. W. Dudley, G. Danialou, K. Govindaraju, L. Lands, D. E. Eidelman, B. J. Petrof, Sarcolemmal damage in dystrophin deficiency is modulated by synergistic interactions between mechanical and oxidative/nitrosative stresses. *Am. J. Pathol.* **168**:4 (2006), 1276–1287, quiz 1404–1405.

168. B. Weller, G. Karpati, S. Carpenter, Dystrophin-deficient mdx muscle fibers are preferentially vulnerable to necrosis induced by experimental lengthening contractions. *J. Neurol. Sci.* **100**:1–2 (1990), 9–13.

169. T. S. Khurana, R. A. Prendergast, H. S. Alameddine, *et al.*, Absence of extraocular muscle pathology in Duchenne's muscular dystrophy: role for calcium homeostasis in extraocular muscle sparing. *J. Exp. Med.* **182**:2 (1995), 467–475.

170. G. Karpati, S. Carpenter, Small-caliber skeletal muscle fibers do not suffer deleterious consequences of dystrophic gene expression. *Am. J. Med. Genet.* **25**:4 (1986), 653–658.

171. A. G. Engel, G. Biesecker, Complement activation in muscle fiber necrosis: demonstration of the membrane attack complex of complement in necrotic fibers. *Ann. Neurol.* **12**:3 (1982), 289–296.

172. K. Arahata, A. G. Engel, Monoclonal antibody analysis of mononuclear cells in myopathies. IV: Cell-mediated cytotoxicity and muscle fiber necrosis. *Ann. Neurol.* **23**:2 (1988), 168–173.

173. M. Wehling, M. J. Spencer, J. G. Tidball, A nitric oxide synthase transgene ameliorates muscular dystrophy in mdx mice. *J. Cell. Biol.* **155**:1 (2001), 123–131.

174. M. J. Spencer, E. Montecino-Rodriguez, K. Dorshkind, J. G. Tidball, Helper (CD4(+)) and cytotoxic (CD8(+)) T cells promote the pathology of dystrophin-deficient muscle. *Clin. Immunol.* **98**:2 (2001), 235–243.

175. R. C. Griggs, R. T. Moxley, J. R. Mendell 3rd, *et al.*, Duchenne dystrophy: randomized, controlled trial of prednisone (18 months) and azathioprine (12 months). *Neurology* **43**:3 Pt 1 (1993), 520–527.

176. H. M. Blau, C. Webster, G. K. Pavlath, Defective myoblasts identified in Duchenne muscular dystrophy. *Proc. Natl. Acad. Sci. U. S. A.* **80**:15 (1983), 4856–4860.

177. S. Decary, C. B. Hamida, V. Mouly, J. P. Barbet, F. Hentati, G. S. Butler-Browne, Shorter telomeres in dystrophic muscle consistent with extensive regeneration in young children. *Neuromuscul. Disord.* **10**:2 (2000), 113–120.

178. B. M. Carlson, J. A. Faulkner, Muscle transplantation between young and old rats: age of host determines recovery. *Am. J. Physiol.* **256:6** Pt 1 (1989), C1262–C1266.

179. I. M. Conboy, M. J. Conboy, A. J. Wagers, E. R. Girma, I. L. Weissman, T. A. Rando, Rejuvenation of aged progenitor cells by exposure to a young systemic environment. *Nature* **433**:7027 (2005), 760–764.

180. A. S. Brack, M. J. Conboy, S. Roy, *et al.*, Increased Wnt signaling during aging alters muscle stem cell fate and increases fibrosis. *Science* **317**:5839 (2007), 807–810.

181. M. Zatz, D. Rapaport, M. Vainzof, *et al.*, Serum creatine-kinase (CK) and pyruvate-kinase (PK) activities in Duchenne (DMD) as compared with Becker (BMD) muscular dystrophy. *J. Neurol. Sci.* **102**:2 (1991), 190–196.

182. L. Mestroni, C. Rocco, D. Gregori, G. Sinagra, A. Di Lenarda, S. Miocic, *et al.*, Familial dilated cardiomyopathy: evidence for genetic and phenotypic heterogeneity. Heart Muscle Disease Study Group. *J. Am. Coll. Cardiol.* **34**:1 (1999), 181–190.

183. E. M. Hoogerwaard, E. Bakker, P. F. Ippel, *et al.*, Signs and symptoms of Duchenne muscular dystrophy and Becker

muscular dystrophy among carriers in The Netherlands: a cohort study. *Lancet* **353**:9170 (1999), 2116–2119.

184. D. R. Sumita, M. Vainzof, S. Campiotto, *et al.*, Absence of correlation between skewed X inactivation in blood and serum creatine-kinase levels in Duchenne/Becker female carriers. *Am. J. Med. Genet.* **80**:4 (1998), 356–361.

185. B. Mokri, A. G. Engel, Duchenne dystrophy: electron microscopic findings pointing to a basic or early abnormality in the plasma membrane of the muscle fiber. *Neurology* **25**:12 (1975), 1111–1120.

186. S. Carpenter, G. Karpati, Duchenne muscular dystrophy: plasma membrane loss initiates muscle cell necrosis unless it is repaired. *Brain* **102**:1 (1979), 147–161.

187. H. Schmalbruch, Regenerated muscle fibers in Duchenne muscular dystrophy: a serial section study. *Neurology* **34**:1 (1984), 60–65.

188. M. Uchino, M. Tokunaga, S. Mita, *et al.*, PCR and immunocytochemical analyses of dystrophin-positive fibers in Duchenne muscular dystrophy. *J. Neurol. Sci.* **129**:1 (1995), 44–50.

189. K. L. Burrow, D. D. Coovert, C. J. Klein, *et al.*, Dystrophin expression and somatic reversion in prednisone-treated and untreated Duchenne dystrophy CIDD Study Group. *Neurology* **41**:5 (1991), 661–666.

190. D. E. Bulman, S. B. Gangopadhyay, K. G. Bebchuck, R. G. Worton, P. N. Ray, Point mutation in the human dystrophin gene: identification through western blot analysis. *Genomics* **10**:2 (1991), 457–460.

191. A. Bornemann, L. V. Anderson, Diagnostic protein expression in human muscle biopsies. *Brain Pathol.* **10**:2 (2000), 193–214.

192. B. T. Darras, U. Francke, Myopathy in complex glycerol kinase deficiency patients is due to 3′ deletions of the dystrophin gene. *Am. J. Hum. Genet.* **43**:2 (1988), 126–130.

193. B. T. Darras, M. Koenig, L. M. Kunkel, U. Francke, Direct method for prenatal diagnosis and carrier detection in Duchenne/Becker muscular dystrophy using the entire dystrophin cDNA. *Am. J. Med. Genet.* **29**:3 (1988), 713–726.

194. J. S. Chamberlain, R A. Gibbs, J E. Ranier, P N. Nguyen, C T. Caskey, Deletion screening of the Duchenne muscular dystrophy locus via multiplex DNA amplification. *Nucleic Acids Res.* **16**:23 (1988), 11141–11156.

195. A. H. Beggs, M. Koenig, F. M. Boyce, L. M. Kunkel, Detection of 98% of DMD/BMD gene deletions by polymerase chain reaction. *Hum. Genet.* **86**:1 (1990), 45–48.

196. S. Abbs, S. C. Yau, S. Clark, C. G. Mathew, M. Bobrow, A convenient multiplex PCR system for the detection of dystrophin gene deletions: a comparative analysis with cDNA hybridisation shows mistypings by both methods. *J. Med. Genet.* **28**:5 (1991), 304–311.

197. S. C. Yau, M. Bobrow, C. G. Mathew, S. J. Abbs, Accurate diagnosis of carriers of deletions and duplications in Duchenne/Becker muscular dystrophy by fluorescent dosage analysis. *J. Med. Genet.* **33**:7 (1996), 550–558.

198. F. Joncourt, B. Neuhaus, K. Jostarndt-Foegen, S. Kleinle, B. Steiner, S. Gallati, Rapid identification of female carriers of DMD/BMD by quantitative real-time PCR. *Hum. Mutat.* **23**:4 (2004), 385–391.

199. S. White, M. Kalf, Q. Liu, *et al.*, Comprehensive detection of genomic duplications and deletions in the DMD gene, by use of multiplex amplifiable probe hybridization. *Am. J. Hum. Genet.* **71**:2 (2002), 365–374.

200. V. Gatta, O. Scarciolla, A. R. Gaspari, *et al.*, Identification of deletions and duplications of the DMD gene in affected males and carrier females by multiple ligation probe amplification (MLPA). *Hum. Genet.* **117**:1 (2005), 92–98.

201. J. R. Mendell, C. H. Buzin, J. Feng, *et al.*, Diagnosis of Duchenne dystrophy by enhanced detection of small mutations. *Neurology* **57**:4 (2001), 645–650.

202. R. R. Bennett, J. den Dunnen, K. F. O'Brien, B. T. Darras, L. M. Kunkel, Detection of mutations in the dystrophin gene via automated DHPLC screening and direct sequencing. *BMC Genet.* **2** (2001), 17.

203. K. M. Flanigan, A. von Niederhausern, D. M. Dunn, J. Alder, J. R. Mendell, R. B. Weiss, Rapid direct sequence analysis of the dystrophin gene. *Am. J. Hum. Genet.* **72**:4 (2003), 931–939.

204. R. M. Hofstra, I. M. Mulder, R. Vossen, *et al.*, DGGE-based whole-gene mutation scanning of the dystrophin gene in Duchenne and Becker muscular dystrophy patients. *Hum. Mutat.* **23**:1 (2004), 57–66.

205. K. Bushby, V. Straub, Nonmolecular treatment for muscular dystrophies. *Curr. Opin. Neurol.* **18**:5 (2005), 511–518.

206. M. Eagle, Report on the muscular dystrophy campaign workshop: exercise in neuromuscular diseases Newcastle, January 2002. *Neuromuscul. Disord.* **12**:10 (2002), 975–983.

207. S. Cervellati, N. Bettini, M. Moscato, A. Gusella, E. Dema, R. Maresi, Surgical treatment of spinal deformities in Duchenne muscular dystrophy: a long term follow-up study. *Eur. Spine J.* **13**:5 (2004), 441–448.

208. J. D. Finder, D. Birnkrant, J. Carl, *et al.*, Respiratory care of the patient with Duchenne muscular dystrophy: ATS consensus statement. *Am. J. Respir. Crit. Care Med.* **170**:4 (2004), 456–465.

209. M. Eagle, S. V. Baudouin, C. Chandler, D. R. Giddings, R. Bullock, K. Bushby, Survival in Duchenne muscular dystrophy: improvements in life expectancy since 1967 and the impact of home nocturnal ventilation. *Neuromuscul. Disord.* **12**:10 (2002), 926–929.

210. D. Duboc, C. Meune, G. Lerebours, J. Y. Devaux, G. Vaksmann, H. M. Becane, Effect of perindopril on the onset and progression of left ventricular dysfunction in Duchenne muscular dystrophy. *J. Am. Coll. Cardiol.* **45**:6 (2005), 855–857.

211. W. Klingler, F. Lehmann-Horn, K. Jurkat-Rott, Complications of anaesthesia in neuromuscular disorders. *Neuromuscul. Disord.* **15**:3 (2005), 195–206.

212. G. A. Hawker, R. Ridout, V. A. Harris, C. C. Chase, L. J. Fielding, W. D. Biggar, Alendronate in the treatment of low bone mass in steroid-treated boys with Duchennes muscular dystrophy. *Arch. Phys. Med. Rehabil.* **86**:2 (2005), 284–288.

213. A. Y. Manzur, T. Kuntzer, M. Pike, A. Swan, Glucocorticoid corticosteroids for Duchenne muscular dystrophy. *Cochrane Database Syst. Rev.* **2** (2004), CD003725.

214. R. T. Moxley 3rd, S. Ashwal, S. Pandya, *et al.*, Practice parameter: corticosteroid treatment of Duchenne dystrophy: report of the Quality Standards Subcommittee of the American Academy of

Neurology and the Practice Committee of the Child Neurology Society. *Neurology* **64**:1 (2005), 13–20.

215. C. K. Silversides, G. D. Webb, V. A. Harris, D. W. Biggar, Effects of deflazacort on left ventricular function in patients with Duchenne muscular dystrophy. *Am. J. Cardiol.* **91**:6 (2003), 769–772.

216. V. Dubowitz, Prednisone in Duchenne dystrophy. *Neuromuscul. Disord.* **1**:3 (1991), 161–163.

217. E. A. Beenakker, J. M. Fock, M. J. Van Tol, *et al.*, Intermittent prednisone therapy in Duchenne muscular dystrophy: a randomized controlled trial. *Arch. Neurol.* **62**:1 (2005), 128–132.

218. K. Bushby, R. Griggs, 145th ENMC International Workshop: planning for an International Trial of Steroid Dosage Regimes in DMD (FOR DMD), 22–24th October 2006, Naarden, The Netherlands. *Neuromuscul. Disord.* **17**:5 (2007), 423–428.

219. W. D. Biggar, V. A. Harris, L. Eliasoph, B. Alman, Long-term benefits of deflazacort treatment for boys with Duchenne muscular dystrophy in their second decade. *Neuromuscul. Disord.* **16**:4 (2006), 249–255.

220. F. Muntoni, I. Fisher, J. E. Morgan, D. Abraham, Steroids in Duchenne muscular dystrophy: from clinical trials to genomic research. *Neuromuscul. Disord.* **12**:Suppl 1 (2002), S162–S165.

221. J. T. Kissel, K. L. Burrow, K. W. Rammohan, J. R. Mendell, Mononuclear cell analysis of muscle biopsies in prednisone-treated and untreated Duchenne muscular dystrophy CIDD Study Group. *Neurology* **41**:5 (1991), 667–672.

222. L. Metzinger, A. C. Passaquin, W. J. Leijendekker, P. Poindron, U. T. Ruegg, Modulation by prednisolone of calcium handling in skeletal muscle cells. *Br. J. Pharmacol.* **116**:7 (1995), 2811–2816.

223. J. E. Anderson, M. Weber, C. Vargas, Deflazacort increases laminin expression and myogenic repair, and induces early persistent functional gain in mdx mouse muscular dystrophy. *Cell Transplant.* **9**:4 (2000), 551–564.

224. S. Kojima, A. Takagi, T. Watanabe, [Effect of prednisolone on apoptosis and cellular infiltration in mdx mouse muscle]. *Rinsho. Shinkeigaku.* **39**:11 (1999), 1109–1113.

225. O. Hardiman, R. M. Sklar, R. H. Brown, Jr., Methylprednisolone selectively affects dystrophin expression in human muscle cultures. *Neurology* **43**:2 (1993), 342–345.

226. T. Fukudome, N. Shibuya, T. Yoshimura, K. Eguchi, Short-term effects of prednisolone on neuromuscular transmission in the isolated mdx mouse diaphragm. *Tohoku J. Exp. Med.* **192**:3 (2000), 211–217.

227. S. C. Jacobs, A. L. Bootsma, P. W. Willems, P. R. Bar, J. H. Wokke, Prednisone can protect against exercise-induced muscle damage. *J. Neurol.* **243**:5 (1996), 410–416.

228. Z. Rifai, S. Welle, R. T. Moxley 3rd, M. Lorenson, R. C. Griggs, Effect of prednisone on protein metabolism in Duchenne dystrophy. *Am. J. Physiol.* **268**:1 Pt 1 (1995), E67–E74.

229. B. Peault, M. Rudnicki, Y. Torrente, *et al.*, Stem and progenitor cells in skeletal muscle development, maintenance, and therapy. *Mol. Ther.* **15**:5 (2007), 867–877.

230. J. V. Chakkalakal, J. Thompson, R. J. Parks, B. J. Jasmin, Molecular, cellular, and pharmacological therapies for Duchenne/Becker muscular dystrophies. *FASEB J.* **19**:8 (2005), 880–891.

231. T. A. Partridge, M. Grounds, J. C. Sloper, Evidence of fusion between host and donor myoblasts in skeletal muscle grafts. *Nature* **273**:5660 (1978), 306–308.

232. P. K. Law, J. L. Yap, New muscle transplant method produces normal twitch tension in dystrophic muscle. *Muscle Nerve* **2**:5 (1979), 356–363.

233. T. Partridge, Myoblast transplantation. *Neuromuscul. Disord.* **12**: Suppl 1 (2002), S3–S6.

234. G. Karpati, D. Ajdukovic, D. Arnold, *et al.*, Myoblast transfer in Duchenne muscular dystrophy. *Ann. Neurol.* **34**:1 (1993), 8–17.

235. E. Gussoni, G. K. Pavlath, A. M. Lanctot, *et al.*, Normal dystrophin transcripts detected in Duchenne muscular dystrophy patients after myoblast transplantation. *Nature* **356**:6368 (1992), 435–438.

236. J. R. Mendell, J. T. Kissel, A. A. Amato, *et al.*, Myoblast transfer in the treatment of Duchenne's muscular dystrophy. *N. Engl. J. Med.* **333**:13 (1995), 832–838.

237. P. A. Moisset, D. Skuk, I. Asselin, *et al.*, Successful transplantation of genetically corrected DMD myoblasts following ex vivo transduction with the dystrophin minigene. *Biochem. Biophys. Res. Commun.* **247**:1 (1998), 94–99.

238. P. A. Moisset, Y. Gagnon, G. Karpati, J. P. Tremblay, Expression of human dystrophin following the transplantation of genetically modified mdx myoblasts. *Gene. Ther.* **5**:10 (1998), 1340–1346.

239. G. Ferrari, G. Cusella-DeAngelis, M. Coletta, *et al.*, Muscle regeneration by bone marrow-derived myogenic progenitors. *Science* **279**:5356 (1998), 1528–1530.

240. Z. Qu, L. Balkir, J. C. van Deutekom, P. D. Robbins, R. Pruchnic, J. Huard, Development of approaches to improve cell survival in myoblast transfer therapy. *J. Cell. Biol.* **142**:5 (1998), 1257–1267.

241. M. Sampaolesi, Y. Torrente, A. Innocenzi, *et al.*, Cell therapy of alpha-sarcoglycan null dystrophic mice through intra-arterial delivery of mesoangioblasts. *Science* **301**:5632 (2003), 487–492.

242. M. Sampaolesi, S. Blot, G. D'Antona, *et al.*, Mesoangioblast stem cells ameliorate muscle function in dystrophic dogs. *Nature* **444**:7119 (2006), 574–579.

243. A. J. van Essen, A. L. Kneppers, A. H. van der Hout, *et al.*, The clinical and molecular genetic approach to Duchenne and Becker muscular dystrophy: an updated protocol. *J. Med. Genet.* **34**:10 (1997), 805–812.

Chapter 11

Muscular dystrophies presenting with proximal muscle weakness

Mariz Vainzof and Kate Bushby

A general introduction to the "limb-girdle muscular dystrophies": definition of the entities and basis for their classification

Proximal muscle weakness is a primary problem in a large number of patients with very variable underlying disease entities. For the purpose of this chapter, the emphasis will be on the recognized inherited diseases within the "limb-girdle" muscular dystrophy (LGMD) classification [1]. From original clinical descriptions dating back to the 1950s, the LGMD group has been controversial. Its original designation was to allow distinction from the more commonly recognized Duchenne and Becker phenotypes, and facioscapulohumeral muscular dystrophy [2]. For a period it was argued that "LGMD" patients actually all had alternative diagnoses, and the term fell from favor [3, 4]. With the advent of molecular genetic techniques able to identify the cause of novel disease entities, it soon became clear that amongst patients with inherited disease causing a proximal muscular dystrophy a variety of different diseases with different underlying genetic causes could be identified. From this concept arose the group of diseases that is now recognized under the "LGMD" classification, which is remarkably heterogeneous [5, 6, 7, 8]. For many of the genes involved in LGMD, it has emerged that there may be marked phenotypic heterogeneity as well, with several different phenotypes associated with mutations in particular genes. So the shared minimum features between the disorders in this classification are the presence of an inherited progressive muscle weakness and wasting affecting at least in a proportion of cases predominantly the proximal musculature.

Amongst the recognized types of LGMD, severity ranges from severe forms with onset in the first decade of life and rapid progression, to milder forms of later onset and slower progression (for reviews, see [5, 6, 7, 8]. Inheritance may be autosomal dominant (LGMD1) or recessive (LGMD2). From 1998 to the time of writing, 21 LGMD genes, 7 autosomal dominant (AD) and 14 autosomal recessive (AR), have been mapped. The AD forms are relatively rare and probably represent less than 10% of all LGMD. The seven AD-LGMD forms are: LGMD1A at 5q31, coding for the protein myotilin [9, 10]; LGMD1B at 1q11, coding for lamin A/C [11, 12]; LGMD1C at 3p25, coding for caveolin-3 [13, 14, 15]; LGMD1D at 7q [16]; LGMD1E at 6q23 [17]; LGMD1F at 7q32 [18]; and LGMD1G at 4p21, mapped in a Brazilian family [19].

The protein products of 13 out of the 14 AR forms have been identified. Four genes, localized at 17q21, 4q12, 13q12, and 5q33, respectively code for α-sarcoglycan (α-SG), β-SG, γ-SG, and δ-SG, which are glycoproteins of the sarcoglycan subcomplex of the dystrophin-associated glycoprotein complex (DGC) [20, 21, 22, 23, 24, 25, 26, 27, 28, 29, 30, 31, 32]. Mutations in these genes cause LGMD2D, 2E, 2C, and 2F respectively, and constitute a distinct subgroup of LGMD, i.e., the sarcoglycanopathies. Among the clinically milder forms, LGMD2A, at 15q15.1, codes for calpain-3 [33, 34]; LGMD2B, at 2p13, codes for dysferlin [35, 36]; and LGMD2G, at 17q12, codes for the sarcomeric telethonin [37]. The fukutin-related protein gene (FKRP), mapped at 19q13.3, was identified as the gene responsible for the LGMD2I form, as well as the severe form of congenital muscular dystrophy (MDC1C) [38, 39]. Other gene-encoding proteins responsible for the glycosylation of α-dystroglycan may cause a limb-girdle phenotype as well as a congenital muscular dystrophy and these forms of LGMD have been defined as LGMD2K, 2M and 2N [40]. The protein TRIM32 has been identified as the gene product of the LGMD2H form at 9q31–34 [41, 42]. LGMD2J was recently described in the Finnish population as the result of autosomal recessive mutations in the titin gene while dominant mutations cause tibial muscular dystrophy [43, 44].

Table 11.1 lists the different entities recognized within this classification and shows that for many of these the underlying genetic defect has been identified, allowing precise molecular diagnosis and an understanding of shared and discrete pathological mechanisms. Figure 11.1 shows a diagrammatic representation of the localization of the various proteins involved within the muscle fiber. There are distinct geographical variations in the proportions of different diseases reported in different populations. Where founder mutations for some of

Disorders of Voluntary Muscle, 8th edn., eds. George Karpati, David Hilton-Jones, Kate Bushby and Robert C. Griggs. Published by Cambridge University Press.

Table 11.1. Classification of the limb-girdle muscular dystrophies. AD, autosomal dominant; AD EDMD, autosomal dominant Emery–Dreifuss muscular dystrophy; AR autosomal recessive; LGMD, limb-girdle muscular dystrophy; SG, sarcoglycan

LGMD forms		Chromosome	Protein	OMIM number	Other diseases associated with this gene	Relative prevalence/founder mutations
AD	LGMD1A	5q31	Myotilin	159000	Myofibrillar myopathies, spheroid body myopathy (see Chapter 25)	Common mutation in all populations
	LGMD1B	1q11–q21	Lamin A/C	159001	Many including AD EDMD and dilated cardiomyopathy (see Chapter 14)	Present worldwide: private mutations usual
	LGMD1C	3p25	Caveolin-3	607780	Rippling muscle disease, hyperCKemia, myalgia, hypertrophic cardiomyopathy	Present worldwide at low frequency: private mutations usual
	LGMD1D	7q	?	603511		Few reported cases
	LGMD1E	6q23	?	602067	Cardiomyopathy and conduction defect: CMD1F	Few reported cases
	LGMD1F	7q32	?	608423		Few reported cases
	LGMD1G	4p21	?	609115		Few reported cases
AR	LGMD2A	15q15.1	Calpain-3	253600		Founder mutations in several populations. One of the most common forms of AR LGMD worldwide
	LGMD2B	2p13	Dysferlin	253601	Miyoshi myopathy (see Chapter 16)	Founder populations in Libyan Jewish and Canadian populations. More common in southern than northern Europe
	LGMD2C	13q12	γ-sarcoglycan	253700		Present worldwide. Founder mutation del521T in Tunisia and North Africa
	LGMD2D	17q12–q21.33	α-sarcoglycan	608099		Present worldwide. Frequent SG form in all populations. Common Arg77Cys mutation. Independent of ethnicity
	LGMD2E	4q12	β-sarcoglycan	604286		Common in Northern and Southern Indiana Amish; Bern, Switzerland
	LGMD2F	5q33	δ-sarcoglycan	601287		All over the world. A common African–Brazilian ancestry mutation (del656C)
	LGMD2G	17q12	Telethonin	601954		Rarely reported outside Brazil
	LGMD2H	9q31–q34	TRIM32	254110	Sarcotubular myopathy	Rarely reported outside Hutterite population of Canada
	LGMD2I	19q13.3	FKRP	607155	MDC1C (see Chapter 12)	Common Northern European founder mutation
	LGMD2J	2q31	Titin	608807	Heterozygous mutations cause AD tibial muscular dystrophy (see Chapter 16)	Reported only in Finland
	LGMD2K	9q34	POMT1	609308	Walker–Warburg syndrome See Chapter 12)	Few reported cases
	LGMD2L	11p14.3?	?	611307		Reported in French Canadian families
	LGMD2M	9q31	Fukutin	611588	Fukuyama muscular dystrophy (see Chapter 12)	Prevalent mutation in Japan
	LGMD2N	14q24	POMT2	607439	Walker–Warburg syndrome (see Chapter 12)	Few reported cases

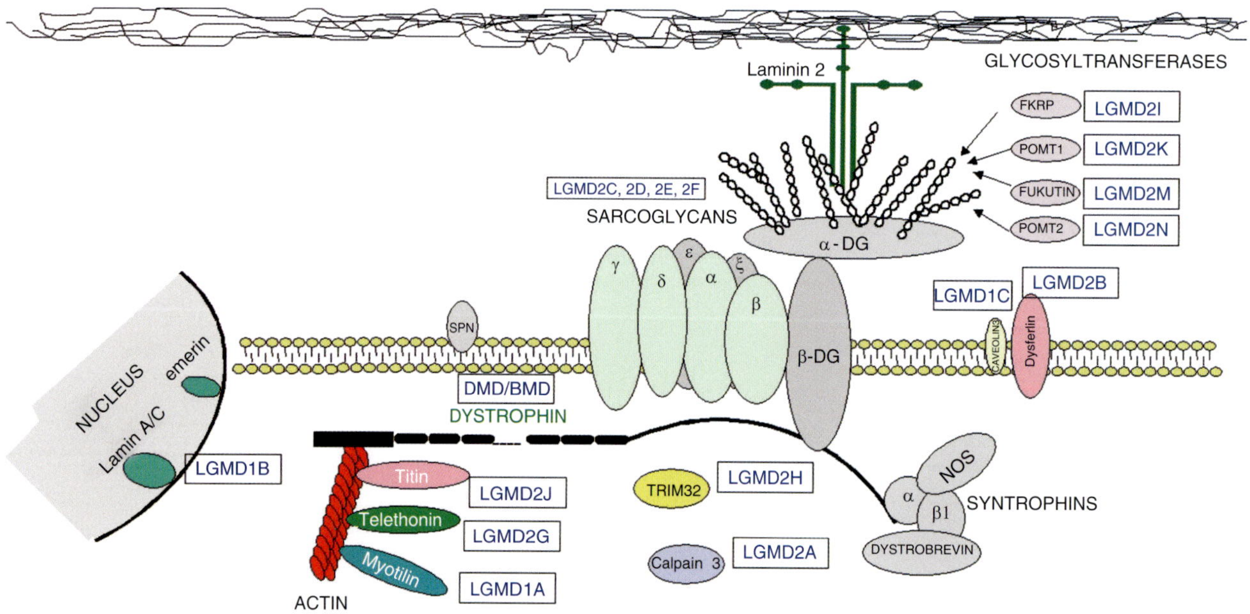

Figure 11.1. Diagrammatic representation of the localization of the various proteins involved within the muscle fiber.

the genes are reported in specific population groups this can be a useful tool for diagnosis in these populations.

For many of these conditions the gold standard diagnostic test now is detection of the responsible mutation [45, 46, 47, 48]. Frequently, taking a muscle biopsy and using a range of antibodies to different muscle proteins may help in pinpointing the underlying protein defect (Figures 11.2 and 11.3) and thereby directing mutation detection to the appropriate gene. Precise diagnosis is necessary to allow genetic counseling as well as to direct management towards associated complications particularly in the respiratory and cardiac systems. As targeted therapeutics become a reality in the future, precise diagnosis will become imperative.

Prevalence

There are some problems in comparing the prevalence of the different types of LGMD as the ways used to define the different entities as well as the denominators for the different studies are not uniform. In Brazil the relative proportion of the different forms among classified patients with AR LGMD (through DNA and/or muscle protein analysis) from 120 families was found to be 32% for LGMD2A, 22% for LGMD2B, 32% for the sarcoglycanopathy group, 3% for LGMD2G, and 11% for LGMD2I [49]. In the Italian population, looking at both dominant and recessive diagnoses LGMD2A was the most common with 28.4%, dysferlinopathy 18.7%, sarcoglycanopathy 18.1%, LGMD2I 6.4%, LGMD1C 1.3% and undetermined diagnosis 27.1% [50]. In the North of England population, LGMD2A represented 26.5% of the whole LGMD group, LGMD2I 19.1%, sarcoglycanopathy 11.7%, LGMD2B 5.9%, and unclassified LGMD 27.9% [51]. In this population group the limb-girdle muscular dystrophies as a whole represented 6.15% of the total clinic population (when the most common diagnoses were myotonic dystrophy and dystrophinopathies). In Australia, calpainopathy represented 8% of a total muscular dystrophy population and dysferlinopathy 5%, while LGMD2I was less frequent (3%) [52]. By contrast, LGMD2I represents a common type of LGMD in the German and Scandinavian populations [53, 54]. The most common LGMDs in the United States are calpainopathies, dysferlinopathies, sarcoglycanopathies, and dystroglycanopathies [55] with a distribution of immunophenotypes of 12% calpainopathy, 18% dysferlinopathy, 15% sarcoglycanopathy, 15% dystroglycanopathy and 1.5% caveolinopathy. In the Netherlands, LGMD2A is the most common LGMD form, consisting of 21% of the classified families. LGMD2B is rare, while sarcoglycanopathies and LGMD2I account for 16% and 8% of the classified families, respectively [56].

The overall approach to diagnosis and management

In a case of suspected LGMD, an important starting point remains the exclusion of other possible diagnosis. Given that dystrophinopathy is more common than LGMD in all populations, it should be excluded by protein and molecular genetic testing if the phenotype is suspicious. Other diagnoses which may present in an "LGMD" manner include facioscapulohumeral muscular dystrophy when the facial weakness may be very mild, Bethlem myopathy if the typical contractures are overlooked or mild, myotonic dystrophy type 2, Pompe disease, spinal muscular atrophy especially types 3 and 4, and congenital myopathies including nemaline myopathy and central core disease. Mitochondrial and myasthenic syndromes may both at times also present with a phenotype of a proximal myopathy [57, 58, 59].

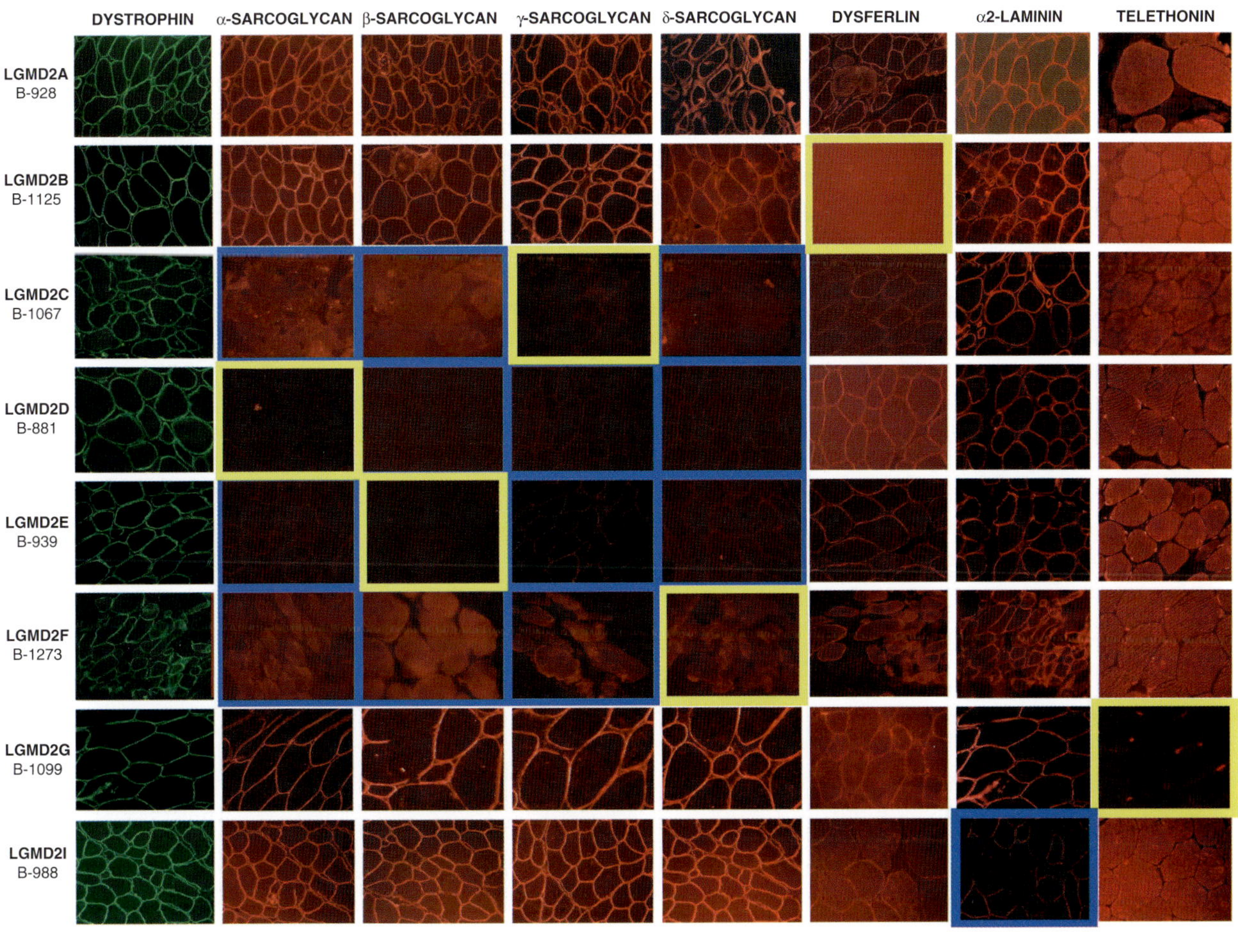

Figure 11.2. Immunohistochemical analysis for muscle proteins in patients with AR forms of LGMDs. Yellow square, primary deficient protein; blue square, secondary deficient proteins.

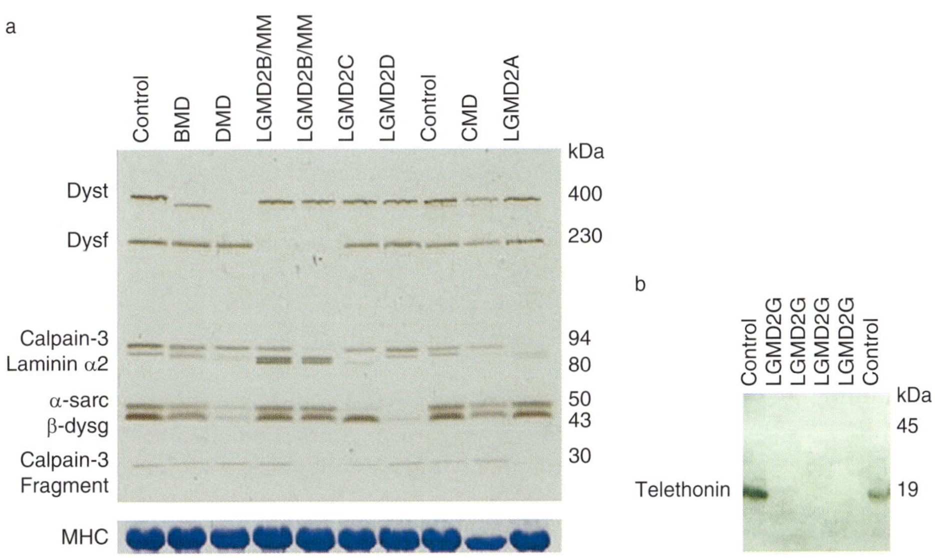

Figure 11.3a, b. (a) Example of multiplex Western blotting for several muscle proteins; (b) for telethonin.

As will be apparent from the text of this chapter, in many situations clinical clues to the diagnosis may be very useful; these frequently can be confirmed or developed by the findings from protein testing using a range of specific antibodies though increasingly the demonstration of the underlying mutation is the gold standard for diagnosis. As this is such a heterogeneous group, basing the request for genetic analysis on the findings from clinical examination, creatine kinase levels, and the results of protein immunoanalysis is crucial for targeting resources appropriately. Basic histology and electromyography is not likely to be of value in discriminating between the different diseases but will provide important information on differential diagnoses. As no specific treatments yet exist for any of the limb-girdle muscular dystrophies, the basic principles of management include the recognition of the risk of complications, such as arrhythmias, cardiomyopathy or respiratory impairment, and appropriate proactive surveillance and management. These actions in themselves can be responsible for an increase in quality of life and longevity [45, 46, 47].

Genetic counseling

Key to the management of patients with any inherited disease, an early diagnosis allows precise genetic counseling, provides the potential to prevent and treat complications, and is frequently of psychological importance to the patient. Once the precise definition of the type of LGMD has been achieved, genetic counseling follows the basic principles of autosomal recessive or dominant inheritance. In autosomal recessive conditions, the parents are typically heterozygous carriers of one of the mutations. When there is consanguinity, both parents will have inherited the same mutation from one common ancestor. Therefore, for the parents of a child with a proven autosomal recessive muscular dystrophy, there is a recurrence risk of 25% for a future child of this couple being affected by the same disease (and mutations). Brothers and sisters of the affected person will have a two-thirds chance of being carriers, and other family members may also be carriers. However, as most of these mutations are very rare, the probability of a carrier having a child with another carrier in the general population is low, and the risk is considered very small. The risks of having another affected child are increased within populations with founder mutations and where there is consanguinity: careful counseling to explain the risks in these situations is required.

In the autosomal dominant diseases it can be more difficult to determine the definitive diagnosis, because protein-based diagnosis may be less specific and indeed for many of the recognized forms of autosomal dominant LGMD, the causative gene has not yet been identified. When a large family with an obvious autosomal dominant transmission is diagnosed, genetic counseling is clearer and of course again the definition of the causative mutation allows predictive testing for the inheritance of the disease from an affected parent (the risk being 50:50). There are various situations though where counseling can be complex. Dominant mutations can in some cases be nonpenetrant, and late onset of disease can also cause problems. In many dominant diseases missense sequence changes are often private so that determination of the pathogenicity may be difficult. It may also be difficult to provide clear guidance about prognosis in predictive situations. A further pitfall in the recognition of, and genetic counseling for, dominant diseases, and one which may take a degree of explanation, is that new dominant mutations are increasingly recognized in this group. For most of the diseases in this group, the possibility and importance of a preclinical diagnosis must also be carefully analyzed. A preclinical diagnosis is generally only recommended when some clinical prevention of complication is possible, or if this information is important for reproductive decisions. In these cases, the patient must be very well supported psychologically and medically. With the definition of the causative mutation prenatal diagnosis is also possible and the options for prenatal or even preimplantation diagnosis can be discussed according to local availability.

Dominant diseases within the LGMD classification

Amongst patients with a suspected diagnosis of LGMD, the autosomal dominant diagnoses are much less frequent than autosomal recessive disease, accounting for around 10% of cases [60, 61]. Specific features of the different diagnoses might lead to suspicion of these diseases: of course with dominant disease a key feature may be the presence of affected family members in other generations, but as it is now known that new dominant mutations and germline mosaicism may be relatively common, the absence of a positive family history should not detract from thinking of these diseases if the clinical features are suggestive. All of the dominant diseases present with a high degree of phenotypic variability and require a high index of suspicion in order to achieve the diagnosis. Different affected family members may also show different manifestations of disease.

LGMD1A

Definition

LGMD1A per se remains a rare diagnosis, established in only two large pedigrees with a proximal muscle weakness and variable dysarthria where the disease could be linked to chromosome 5q [9, 10, 62]. Definition of the involvement of the myotilin gene in these patients provides evidence of an overlap with the myofibrillar myopathies [62] (see Chapter 25). Therefore, a careful search for features more commonly described in myofibrillar myopathy patients (accumulation of desmin and myotilin on the muscle biopsy for example, or the presence of cardiac disease or respiratory impairment) is indicated in suspected cases.

Clinical features

In the original descriptions of LGMD1A, the age of onset was in young adulthood, with proximal muscle weakness present alongside, in around 50% of patients, nasal speech. Creatine kinase (CK) levels were raised to 1.5–9 times normal. Contractures were frequently present in the Achilles tendons [9, 10]. As myotilin mutations are much more commonly reported in patients with a distal myopathy, and even patients with an initial proximal presentation may have distal weakness later in the disease [63] (see discussion in Chapter 25) the diagnosis would have to be suspected in patients presenting with distal muscle weakness predominantly.

Molecular genetics and pathogenesis

Several point mutations in myotilin have been described in patients with LGMD1A, myofibrillar myopathy, and sphenoid body myopathy. A mouse with the first reported LGMD1A mutation develops myofibrillar pathology, suggesting a shared pathomechanism across the diseases and that strict genotype–phenotype correlations between these different groups are unlikely [64].

Diagnosis

While the gold standard for diagnosis is the definition of a mutation in the myotilin gene, the diagnosis can be suggested in a number of ways. From a clinical perspective, patients with myotilinopathy frequently present with distal rather than proximal muscle weakness, so a careful search for distal weakness in the index case and/or their family is indicated. Dysarthria was reported in the first LGMD1A family, but is also seen in the other forms of myofibrillar myopathy. Magnetic resonance imaging may prove to be a useful tool for defining the pattern of muscle involvement in detail. Examination of the muscle biopsy with antibodies to myotilin and desmin may reveal the presence of accumulation of these proteins within the muscle fiber. Electron microscopy provides a useful adjunct to diagnosis in specialized hands (Goebbels *et al.*, in preparation).

Management

In general, patients with myofibrillar myopathy are at risk of cardiac complications in the form of cardiomyopathy and arrhythmia [63]. As genotype–phenotype correlations within the different types of myofibrillar myopathy become clearer, there is some indication that myotilin mutations are less likely to be associated with these complications than, for example, mutations in desmin. However, at our current state of knowledge, given the generally overlapping phenotypes it is wise to suggest that patients with myotilin mutations should be offered cardiac screening both by echocardiogram and electrocardiography, and also should be monitored for respiratory muscle weakness, including assessment in the supine position which will detect involvement of the diaphragm. Standard management modalities are appropriate for detected abnormalities, such as use of a pacemaker or implantable defibrillator for progressive arrhythmia, cardioactive drugs in cardiomyopathy, and home nocturnal ventilation for respiratory failure. Management of Achilles tendon contractures with physiotherapy, splinting and if necessary surgery is indicated as with any neuromuscular patient, especially if the contractures are interfering with ambulation.

LGMD1B

Definition

This form of LGMD is allelic with autosomal dominant Emery–Dreifuss muscular dystrophy (EDMD) and both are caused by lamin A/C mutations. This condition is discussed in detail in Chapter 14. Other phenotypes with mutations in the lamin A/C gene include autosomal dominant dilated cardiomyopathy with conduction system disease, pure autosomal dominant dilated cardiomyopathy (with conduction system disease in some cases), 217 focal lipidystrophy of the Dunnigan type, autosomal recessive axonal polyneuropathy (CMT2A), and mandibuloacral dysplasia, as well as Hutchinson–Gilford progeria [12, 65, 66, 67, 68, 69, 70, 71, 72, 73, 74, 75, 76, 77, 78, 79, 80]. Around 60% of patients with laminopathy have involvement of skeletal and/or cardiac muscle. Combinations of phenotypes also are beginning to emerge and there can be considerable phenotypic variability even within the same family. An LGMD phenotype with cardiac involvement is probably less common than the presentation as autosomal dominant EDMD characterized by a more humeroperoneal pattern of weakness and prominent contractures. Here the discussion is restricted to the LGMD phenotype.

Clinical features

In the LGMD presentation of laminopathy the age of onset falls within a wide range from 4 to 38 years with occasional earlier onset in childhood with more rapid progression also possible [81]. The disease appears to be fully penetrant by age 45 in all the obligatory mutation carriers in the original Dutch pedigrees. The progression of weakness is generally slow, with upper-extremity involvement setting in only around 40 years of age in the original report. Later in the course of the disease contractures may develop at the elbow and Achilles tendon, but usually not in the neck extensors or the paraspinal muscles, where they typically manifest in the Emery–Dreifuss presentation (Figure 11.4). CK values may be normal or moderately elevated, around 1.5- to 3-fold. Of great importance are diagnosis and adequate follow-up of the cardiac status. Cardiac involvement starts insidiously and may first manifest in the third to fourth decades as a first-degree atrioventricular (AV) block, followed in the fourth to fifth decade by second-degree heart block, and eventually progressing to a complete AV block. However, significant left ventricular disease can develop as well. Normal cardiac studies at a younger age do not rule out a laminopathy as presentation may be delayed into middle adult life. Early sudden cardiac death has occurred in

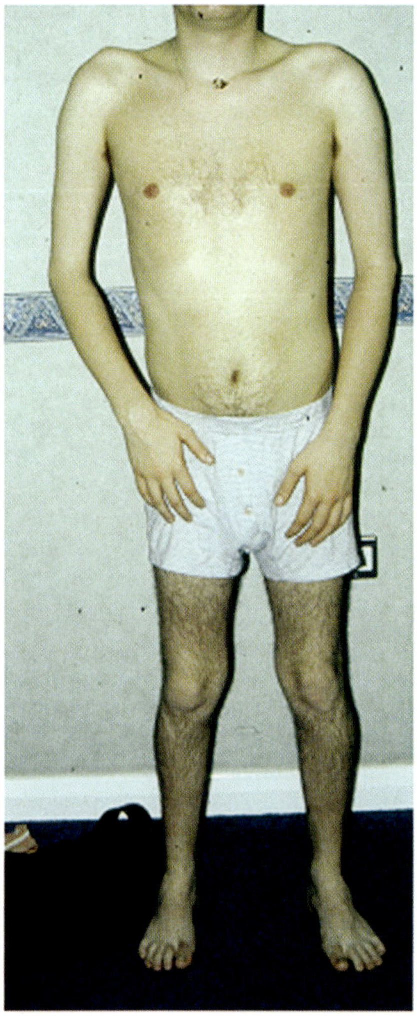

Figure 11.4. LGMD1B. Note overlap with AD EDMD (elbow contractures).

laminopathy in general and in very rare cases may even be the presenting feature [66]. It can occur even with a pacemaker in place [82, 83, 84]. In the original families with autosomal dominant Emery–Dreifuss phenotype several members presented with cardiac disease only, whereas in all the members of the original LGMD1B pedigrees there was some muscle weakness in the presence of cardiac involvement, although sometimes only noted in hindsight. Rarely, there may also be frank dilated cardiomyopathy in addition to the conduction system disease.

Although an LGMD core phenotype within laminopathy can be recognized, there is definite clinical overlap with a more classic Emery–Dreifuss phenotype on the one hand and a pure cardiac phenotype with conduction system disease on the other. These different manifestations are best regarded as a continuum, because distinct genotype–phenotype correlations explaining these different phenotypes have not emerged as yet. A rare case of a child born to parents both affected with LGMD1B has been reported [85]. There was fetal akinesia and the child died at birth with severe congenital muscular dystrophy; there were lamin A/C mutations on both alleles.

Molecular genetics

Mutations in LMNA underlying the LGMD presentation are summarized on the Leiden muscular dystrophy website and the UMD database (www.dmd.nl/md.html). A significant proportion of LMNA mutations arise de novo. No clear genotype–phenotype correlation has emerged to distinguish LGMD1B from autosomal dominant EDMD and familial dilated cardiomyopathy with conduction system disease, as the different presentations can occur within the same family on the basis of identical mutation. It appears that the mutations causing the partial lipodystrophy (Dunnigan type) phenotype are largely restricted to codon 482 in exon 8 [86]. However, a mutation directly adjacent to this codon (Tyr481His) has been described in a 67-year-old patient with LGMD without contractures, while there was cardiac disease only in other family members. Other patients had both lipodystrophy and cardiac disease (Arg28Trp;Arg62Gly) [87]. Mutations in additional genes have also been reported to exacerbate the phenotype [79].

Diagnosis

Mutation detection is the gold standard for diagnosis in laminopathy. The severe and frequent cardiac complications together with the pleiotropic clinical presentations associated with these mutations mean that a high level of suspicion of the diagnosis is necessary. Antibody studies for lamin A/C on muscle biopsy sections will appear normal, as the heterozygous mutations presumably act in a functionally dominant-negative way on the intermediate filament network of the inner nuclear membrane, thereby not affecting the immunoreactivity for lamin A/C to a measurable degree. Thus, direct mutation analysis in the lamin A/C gene must be initiated to prove or rule out the diagnosis in suggestive patients, even if the family history is negative. As the majority of mutations are missense and often private, careful attention to the likely pathogenicity of any change found is essential.

Management

No curative treatment is available, but placement of an implantable defibrillator will prevent potentially fatal cardiac arrhythmia [82, 83, 84, 88]. Careful cardiac monitoring of patients is mandatory throughout the course of the disease, as ventricular arrhythmias may become a problem only as the disease progresses. It is important to consider a device with an integrated cardioverter/defibrillator, as sudden ventricular tachyarrhythmias can be a cause of sudden cardiac death that would not be treated merely by pacing. It is therefore very important to make a timely diagnosis. The progression to clinically significant dilated cardiomyopathy is more important in the lamin A/C-related than in the X-linked form of EDMD. Patients with laminopathy may also develop significant nocturnal respiratory impairment as the condition progresses, so surveillance for this complication, as well as intervention with nocturnal respiratory support when necessary, is also indicated. Physiotherapy with or without orthopedic intervention is indicated for contractures.

With the major implications of laminopathy and the need for cardiac surveillance even in cases with minor skeletal muscle disease, presymptomatic testing is often requested. Due to the high number of missense lamin A/C changes, which may be of unknown pathogenicity, it is very important indeed that putative mutations are checked rigorously against mutation databases and protein prediction programs and that caution is taken in offering presymptomatic testing while the nature of a change in the lamin A/C gene is not fully secure. This should only be done in conjunction with experienced genetic counseling.

LGMD1C, caveolinopathy

Definition

LGMD1C is a manifestation of mutations in the caveolin-3 gene, which may also present with other phenotypes including rippling muscle disease, distal myopathy, and hyperCKemia. It appears in most series to be a rare cause of LGMD.

Clinical features

Mutations in the caveolin-3 gene define caveolinopathy, one presentation of which may be with a limb-girdle muscular dystrophy. However, there are several alternative presentations of caveolin mutations, with the possibility for phenotypic heterogeneity within individual families [13, 14, 15, 50, 89, 90]. The mildest presentation is with hyperCKemia and in fact patients with caveolinopathy may be very strong and athletic. HyperCKemia may also be seen with muscle cramping. In a recent Newcastle series, 50% of the patients presented with myalgia in some cases associated with myoglobinuria, so caveolinopathy should be amongst the differential diagnoses for patients presenting with muscle pain (Aboumousa *et al.* in preparation). Muscle pain has also been reported associated with the LGMD form of caveolinopathy where the more prominent complaint however was of proximal muscle weakness which was in most cases mild to moderate, and might be accompanied by hypertrophy of the calf or other muscles (Figure 11.5). Rippling muscle disease due to caveolinopathy has been reported in patients with or without associated muscle weakness and may be found in childhood and young adulthood before weakness is present. The major findings in rippling muscle disease are muscle stiffness, together with electrically silent rippling, and percussion- or pressure-induced rapid muscle contractions (PIRCS). Patients may report muscle rippling, which may be stimulated mechanically or by activity, or they may be unaware of this phenomenon which may be induced by percussion. Distal myopathy has also been reported in caveolinopathy: overlap in the range of phenotypes seen with a single mutation or within single families indicates that genotype–phenotype correlations are not straightforward [91]. The clinical features associated with caveolinopathy are therefore variable and indeed may vary within families and within patients over time. For example a patient may be detected with hyperCKemia when he or she is very strong and athletic and at that stage may have rippling inducible on investigation: subsequently proximal and/or distal muscle weakness with or without myalgia may become the predominant symptom. Muscle hypertrophy may be observed especially in the calves and CK levels may be elevated from 4 to 24 times normal levels.

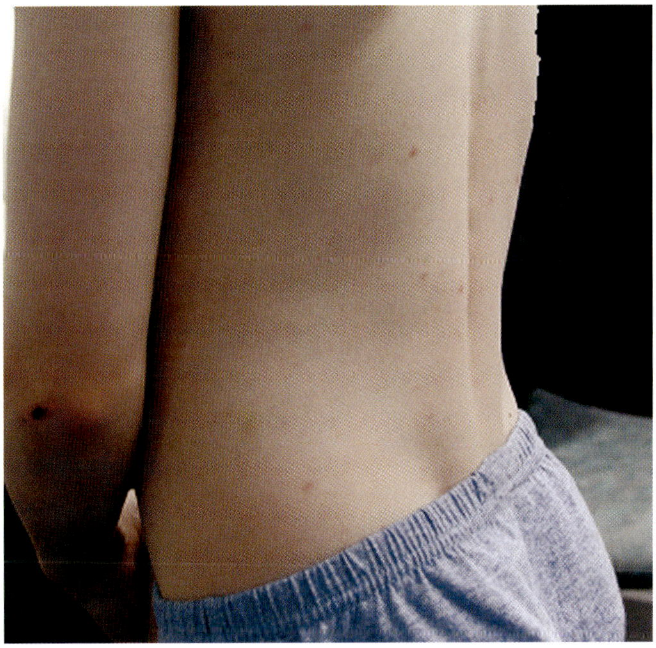

Figure 11.5. LGMD1C. Note paraspinal muscle hypertrophy.

Although one family has been reported with hypertrophic cardiomyopathy associated with caveolin-3 mutation, cardiomyopathy is not to date a recognized complication of muscular dystrophy associated with caveolin-3 mutations [92].

Diagnosis

Demonstration of a heterozygous pathogenic mutation in the caveolin-3 gene is the definitive diagnostic test and allows distinction from other causes of these presentations: rippling muscle disease has a number of different causes including as a manifestation of autoimmune disease and in these patients there may also be a secondary reduction in caveolin-3 labeling in muscle. Patients with CAV3 mutations usually show complete absence of caveolin-3 expression in muscle and this can be used to direct mutation testing in patients with one of the suggestive phenotypes. The deficiency of the protein is due to a dominant negative effect of heterozygous mutations, suggesting that mutant caveolin-3 proteins might interfere with the formation of normal homo-oligomers, which, in turn, leads to an accelerated degradation of the misfolded caveolin-3 proteins [14, 93]. A secondary reduction of caveolin-3 protein may sometimes be observed in patients with an autoimmune rippling muscle disease as well as in some patients with dysferlinopathy [94, 95].

LGMD1D

The two families described as linked to the LGMD1D locus on 7q had progressive proximal leg weakness with or without proximal arm weakness, absent ankle deep-tendon reflexes, occasional family members with dysphagia and elevated CK values [16]. The diagnostic evaluation of at least one affected member per family documented a myopathic process. Neither electromyography nor muscle biopsy demonstrated any pathognomonic features of other disorders. Clinically, they did not show any of the additional features reported in other types of ADLGMD such as the dysarthria reported in LGMD1A or cardiac defects in LGMD1B.

LGMD1E

LGMD type 1E has prominent cardiac involvement, although the primary genetic defect is not yet known. This type has been defined in a single large North American family with more than 25 affected members in which genetic linkage to chromosome 6q23 has been established [17].

In the original large family, the age of onset in males was in the late teens, whereas it was about a decade later in females. Weakness was predominantly proximal and only very slowly progressive, so that loss of ambulation was the exception. Contractures were not a prominent feature and occurred only late in the course of the disease. Much as in the case of LGMD1B (laminopathy), the cardiac manifestations mainly presented as arrhythmias in the form of AV conduction disturbances. Sudden cardiac death occurred in this family also. As in laminopathy, dilated cardiomyopathy and/or arrhythmias may be present at onset or develop later in the course of the disease. There were no patients with cardiac disease in the absence of skeletal muscle weakness. The serum CK level was elevated up to fourfold, but it was normal in other affected members of the family. Calf hypertrophy was reported.

A genetic diagnosis can only be made in a family large enough for meaningful linkage analysis. It seems impossible to differentiate this disorder from laminopathy (LGMD1B) on clinical grounds alone. It is imperative that lamin A/C mutations are excluded in all cases.

LGMD1F

LGMD1F was described in a large Spanish kindred in which 32 members spanning 5 generations were affected with autosomal dominant limb-girdle muscular dystrophy and subsequently linkage was described to chromosome 7q32 [18, 96]. Two forms were delineated based on age at onset: a juvenile form with onset before age 15 years (66%), and an adult-onset form starting around the third or fourth decade (28%). All affected patients showed characteristic pelvic and shoulder girdle proximal weakness, and patients affected earlier showed a faster progression. Pelvic girdle impairment was more severe and occurred earlier than shoulder girdle weakness, and distal weakness often occurred later. In some patients with early onset there was also mild facial weakness and scapular winging, making facioscapulohumeral muscular dystrophy an important differential diagnosis. Respiratory muscles were clinically affected in four patients with juvenile onset. Muscle biopsies of five patients showed myopathic or dystrophic changes, including abnormal fiber size and variation, increased connective tissue, degenerative fibers, occasional central nuclei, and, in three cases, rimmed vacuoles. There was no cardiac involvement, dysarthria, calf hypertrophy, or contractures.

Linkage to a 3.68-Mb region on chromosome 7q32.1–q32.2 has been described, termed LGMD1F (maximum 2-point Lod score of 7.56 at marker D7S2544). All affected members had a common disease haplotype. No mutation was identified in the filamin C gene which mapped to the candidate interval.

LGMD1G

This form of autosomal dominant LGMD was identified in a Caucasian Brazilian family in which 12 members had a mild adult-onset form of muscular dystrophy [19]. Age at onset ranged from 30 to 47 years with proximal lower limb weakness in most patients, muscle cramps in one patient, and upper limb weakness in one patient. Clinical phenotype was quite stereotyped but some variability was also recognized, mostly regarding age at onset. Lower limbs were affected in all patients. Typical features of LGMD, such as marked proximal amyotrophy and abolished myotatic reflexes, were constantly present in affected muscles. With the exception of distal stiffness of toes and fingers, the clinical phenotype of this new form of muscular dystrophy is similar to that of other AD LGMD. Nine of ten patients eventually had upper limb weakness. With the exception of the youngest patient, all patients developed progressive and permanent restriction of finger and toe flexion and reduced range of movement in the interphalangeal joints. Normal strength was retained in the intrinsic hand muscles. Serum creatine kinase was increased in all but two patients up to 10 times the normal level. Muscle biopsy showed fiber size variation with very discrete perimysial fibrosis, and several necrotic fibers with rimmed vacuoles. Scattered groups of small atrophic angulated fibers were also observed. However, a mosaic of type I/II fibers was detected in the ATPase reactions, with no clear evidence of fiber type grouping. The NADH reaction showed a conserved myofibrillar network. All five patients and three unaffected family members older than 45 years had type II diabetes mellitus.

A genome-wide linkage search mapped the disease locus to a 7-Mb region at 4q21. In silico analysis of this region showed the presence of a large number of genes. From the 40 genes found in this region so far, 11 coded for hypothetical proteins. Among the 29 known genes, 8 are expressed in muscle and might be good candidates for LGMD1G.

Muscle protein immunohistochemical and Western blot analyses revealed a normal pattern for the following proteins: dystrophin, sarcoglycans, calpain-3, dysferlin, and telethonin. Some of the vacuoles were clearly labeled with antibodies for

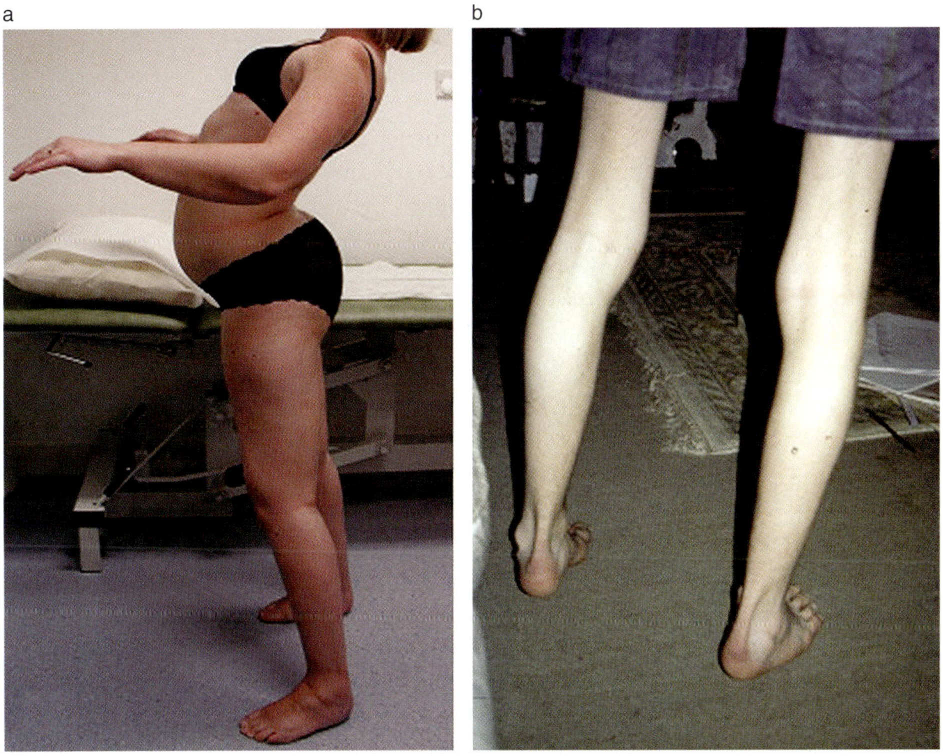

Figure 11.6a, b. LGMD2A. Extreme hyperlordosis (a) may be a feature, as may early Achilles tendon contractures and atrophic calves (b).

sarcolemmal proteins, such as dystrophin and α-sarcoglycan, confirming the presence of sarcolemmal membrane in the vacuoles.

Autosomal recessive forms of LGMD

LGMD2A – calpainopathy

Definition

LGMD2A is the most frequent form of LGMD in many populations, accounting for about 25%–30% of the identified forms [50, 51]. However, there are pockets of particularly high frequency especially in the Basque region and Ile de Reunion [33, 97, 98]. A common mutation is reported in Russia and Eastern Europe [99, 100, 101].

Clinical features

LGMD2A can present at any age from infancy (toe walking can be seen as an early presentation) to late adulthood when it is most likely to be seen as a relatively indolent proximal muscle weakness (Figure 11.6). The majority of cases though present between 8 and 15 years with difficulties climbing stairs or running [30, 33, 50, 102, 103, 104, 105, 106, 107, 108]. Initial complaints therefore tend to localize to the pelvic girdle, and this is reflected on examination with typically a very clear and almost stereotypic pattern of muscle weakness involving the posterior thigh and hip muscles especially, with relative preservation of the quadriceps and hip abductors. Calf hypertrophy may be present, alternatively there may be a markedly atrophic phenotype. Despite there often being few complaints at this stage about upper girdle involvement, scapular winging is typically present even at presentation and a prominent lumbar lordosis is also frequently seen. Contractures are present in a subset of patients and typically involve predominantly the Achilles tendon, elbow, and neck. Clinical delineation from Emery–Dreifuss muscular dystrophy may be difficult in these cases, but may be helped by MRI [109]. As with almost any of the LGMDs, rarely patients may present with muscle stiffness and pain [98, 110]. In determining the key clinical determinants which can distinguish calpainopathy from other forms of LGMD, the presence of preserved respiratory function, contractures, especially of the Achilles tendons, and scapular winging have been shown to be particularly discriminatory [108] as is the absence of cardiac involvement and a posterior pattern of muscle involvement.

Evolution in LGMD2A is variable but always progressive. Typically, patients lose independent ambulation between 11 and 28 years after onset of the disease. Complications with Achilles tendon contractures may require surgery, but cardiac and respiratory complications are rare. Life expectancy in most cases will be normal. Some unexpected results were also observed in calpainopathy, suggesting that the spectrum of phenotypic variability may be broader than suspected. This includes the confirmation of LGMD2A in a family with clinical characteristics of neurogenic spinal muscular atrophy, or patients with normal serum CK levels [111].

Molecular genetics and pathogenesis

LGMD2A is caused by mutations in the calpain-3 gene at 15q15.1 [34]. The human calpain-3 gene comprises 24 exons, covers a genomic region of ~40 kb, is expressed predominantly in the skeletal muscle as a 3.5-kb transcript, and encodes a protein of 94 kDa [34, 112, 113]. LGMD2A patients present a wide range of distinct pathogenic mutations distributed along the entire length of the calpain-3 gene. Over 100 distinct pathogenic mutations have been identified, including nonsense, missense, deletions/insertions, splice-site mutations (Leiden database at www.dmd.nl/capn3_home.html, accessed 27 April 2009). About 70% are private variant mutations, 60%–70% are single base pair alterations, most being (~80%) missense mutations, a few stop codons, and about 15% are splicing defects. However, some recurrent mutations are found more frequently in some populations such as the Basque, Amish, Japanese, Brazilians, Eastern Europeans, and Italians [97, 99, 100, 105, 114].

Calpain-3 is a muscle-specific calcium-activated neutral protease 3 which binds to titin and plays a role in the disassembly of sarcomeric protein, though it may also have a regulatory role in the modulation of transcription factors and in the regulation of apoptotic factors [115, 116, 117]. The calpains, or calcium-activated neutral proteases, are a family of proteins including two ubiquitous forms (calpain-1 and -2), two stomach-specific forms, and the muscle-specific form CAPN3 (calpain-3). All are heterodimers with distinct large catalytic subunits (~80 kDa) and a common regulatory small subunit of 30 kDa. The large calpain subunits can be subdivided into four domains: The N-terminal region of domain I is autocatalytically processed during activation by Ca^{2+} ions, suggesting that domain I is involved in the regulation of activity. Domain II is considered to be the cysteine protease module. Domain IV contains structures for calcium binding and thus this domain may be involved in the calcium activation of the calpains. No function has yet been assigned to domain III. The muscle-specific calpain-3 form differs in structure from the ubiquitous forms by having three unique insertions, which increase its molecular weight to 94 kDa: NS at the beginning of domain I, IS1 in protease domain II, and IS2 in domain III [112, 118, 119, 120].

Genotype–phenotype correlations

Although there is a marked inter- and intra-familial heterogeneity in the severity of the clinical course in LGMD2A it has been suggested that on average missense mutations are usually associated with a milder phenotype than null mutations. The analysis of Brazilian LGMD2A patients showed that on average the ages at onset and ascertainment were significantly higher in groups of patients with missense mutations on both alleles or one missense and one in-frame deletion than in the groups of patients who were compound heterozygous for missense/null mutations or patients carrying null mutations (frameshift or stop codon mutations) or splicing site changes on both alleles. However, the mean ages of onset and ascertainment did not differ between the two last groups which suggests that one null mutation is enough to determine a more severe phenotype [105, 111]. Similar broad relationships between the presence of null mutations and severity have been reported in other groups [108, 113, 118, 121].

Diagnosis

The recognition of the characteristic clinical features in calpainopathy, alongside a typically elevated serum CK (usually elevated at least 10× normal, though rare outliers are described), can be a very useful adjunct to diagnosis as neither protein nor mutation testing in LGMD2A is infallible.

Muscle histological analysis shows a mainly dystrophic pattern, with muscle fibers with necrosis and regeneration, variable size of muscle fibers, lobulated fibers, split fibers, an internal nucleus, and increased endomysial and perimysial fibrosis. Analysis of muscle biopsies from some asymptomatic and early-stage patients with LGMD2A showed a consistent but unusual pattern with isolated fascicles of degenerating fibers in an almost normal muscle. These findings suggest that a peculiar pattern of focal degeneration occurs in calpainopathy, independent of the type of mutation or the amount of calpain-3 in the muscle [8]. This has also been confirmed in calpain-3 knockout mice, which presented similar atrophic features, small foci of muscular necrosis, and abnormal sarcomere formation [122]. There have been reports of eosinophilic myositis as an early histological manifestation of calpainopathy, but this does not appear to be specific or sensitive as a marker of the diagnosis [108, 123].

The use of calpain-3 antibodies is a very useful adjunct to diagnosis, though the antibodies currently available are not reliable for immunolabeling of sections in the diagnostic setting such that testing has to rely on Western blotting [108, 124, 125] (Figure 11.3). In a recent study of 85 UK patients, it was shown that the interpretation of protein expression obtained by Western blot is complex and involves the analysis of a number of bands detected by two antibodies for calpain-3 [108]. Loss of all three calpain bands was 100% specific for LGMD2A, but this pattern was found in only 23% of cases of proven mutation. Absence or reduction of the 60-kDa bands was also highly specific for LGMD2A, while increased abundance was highly predictive of no mutations being found even where other bands were reduced, suggesting that this is the most sensitive marker of artifactual protein degradation.

Although careful evaluation of the pattern of calpain-3 in muscle on immunoblotting can be very helpful in directing the diagnosis, the finding of normal levels of calpain-3 in muscle in association with calpain-3 mutations is a consistent finding in around 20%–30% of recent mutation series, leading to the suggestion that additional analysis of autoproteolytic function or a proteolytic function of calpain-3 could be usefully added to the diagnostic process. Many of the mutations found in these cases could be consistent with the alteration of one of the proteolytic functions of the protein [50, 108, 126, 127, 128]. On the other hand, a secondary reduction in calpain-3 levels has been reported in dysferlinopathy [129, 130] and LGMD2J [131] and other muscular dystrophies. Protein analysis in calpainopathy is therefore complex and requires the input of

a b

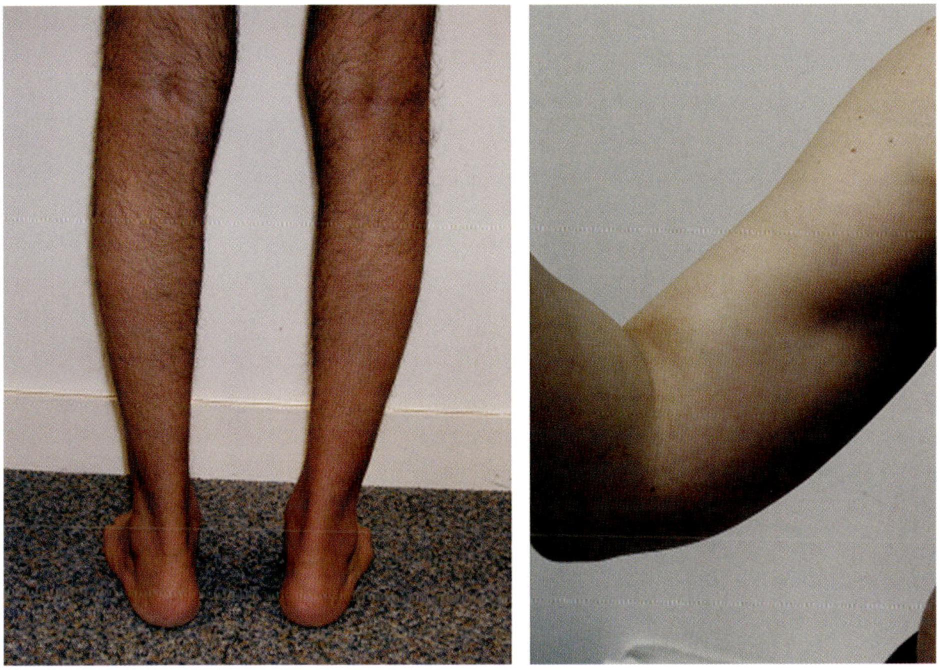

Figure 11.7a, b. LGMD2B. Note loss of medial gastrocnemius (a) and focal loss of biceps (b).

specialized laboratories together with careful interpretation in the light of clinical data.

There is a further complexity in diagnosis of LGMD2A at the level of gene analysis. Although of course screening for mutations in the 24 exons of the CAP3 gene can be performed using several different methodologies, such as direct sequencing, single-strand conformation polymorphism (SSCP) or denaturing high-performance liquid chromatography (DHPLC), and many mutation series are published, most confirm a problem in locating the second expected mutation in around 20%–25% of cases. Furthermore, most mutations represent private variants limiting the usefulness of targeted mutation testing except in specific population groups [50, 106, 107, 108, 110, 113, 118, 132, 133, 134]. Nonetheless, genetic analysis in LGMD2A has become the gold standard for diagnosis.

Management

The contractures, which relatively frequently present in LGMD2A at the Achilles tendons, require physiotherapy input and may need surgery depending on how they respond to stretching and splinting. Respiratory and cardiac problems are not common.

LGMD2B – dysferlinopathies

Definition

Two distinct phenotypes were initially associated with mutations in this gene: Miyoshi myopathy, with predominantly distal muscle wasting, and LGMD2B, with a proximal weakness. Other variant presentations such as with calf pain and swelling, anterior tibial onset or a (probably relatively frequent) proximo-distal distribution are also increasingly recognized [35, 36, 56, 135, 136, 137, 138].

Mutations causing LGMD2B are present in low frequency in many populations, being about 1% of the recessive LGMD forms, and 33% of the distal myopathies. On the other hand LGMD2B may be the most prevalent form (35%–45%) in some populations such as in the Cajun/Arcadian population of North America and founder mutations are present in the Libyan Jewish population and the Jews of the Caucasus [139, 140]. In the Brazilian population and Italian populations it is the second most prevalent form of AR-LGMD [49, 50] while it appears to be less common in the UK [51].

Clinical features

There are a number of clinical features of dysferlinopathy which are almost pathognomonic of the diagnosis. For the vast majority of patients, onset of symptoms is in the late teens or early twenties, often with normal or even outstanding sporting ability before that. The initial symptoms may be difficulty standing on tiptoe (Miyoshi distal myopathy presentation), foot drop (distal myopathy with anterior tibial presentation), proximal muscle weakness ("LGMD2B" presentation), or a mixture of proximal and distal weakness. Involvement of the shoulder girdle is a much later event, though asymptomatic local atrophy of the biceps may be seen before that (Figure 11.7). At diagnosis, serum CK levels are markedly elevated (frequently 100× normal or higher). A history of calf pain and/or swelling preceding the development of weakness even by several years can frequently be elicited. Otherwise, calf hypertrophy is very rare; indeed dysferlinopathy is typically an atrophic disease. Misdiagnosis as polymyositis is common due to the apparently sudden nature of the onset (and frequent presence of inflammatory cells in the muscle biopsy). However the weakness does not respond to steroid medication. The presence of different patterns of clinical muscle involvement in the presence of the same homozygous mutation in the same family or population group indicates that genotype–phenotype relations are not simple and that other genes may be involved in determining the pattern of muscle involvement in these patients. Progression of the disease is somewhat variable. For some patients there appears to be relatively rapid progression of disease and early confinement to a wheelchair. In others the disease may be much more slowly progressive. Complications of cardiac and respiratory impairment are not reported as frequent clinical complications, though suggestions of cardiomyopathy in animal models of dysferlinopathy have prompted the reporting of occasional cases of dysferlinopathy with cardiac disease, of uncertain significance. From published series it does not appear that life expectancy is significantly reduced in these patients with respiratory complications coming at a late stage with severe muscle involvement if at all, and indeed a very mild presentation in the seventies has recently been reported indicating that dysferlin mutations may be compatible with very mild disease [30, 49, 138, 139, 141, 142, 143, 144].

Molecular genetics and pathogenesis

LGMD2B is caused by mutations in the dysferlin gene, which spans a region of 150 kb, contains over 55 exons and is transcribed as a 8.5 major mRNA expressed strongly in skeletal muscle, heart and placenta [36, 37]. Dysferlin is a ubiquitously expressed 230-kDa molecule localized predominantly at the sarcolemma [145] and expressed at early stages of development. A specific loss of dysferlin labeling is observed in muscle biopsies from patients with mutations in the LGMD2B/MM gene [130, 145] (Figures 11.2 and 11.3). It appears however that the sarcolemmal localization of dysferlin can be altered during regeneration, in muscular dystrophies, and in the presence of membrane damage [52, 146, 147, 148]. This may relate to the putative role of dysferlin in membrane repair [149].

Dysferlin mutations have been described affecting all regions of this large gene. The variations in phenotype are not well explained by the mutation type and a variety of mutations are reported with occasional founder mutations such as in the Libyan Jewish population [139].

Diagnosis

The combination of age and type of onset, together with very marked CK elevation, can be highly indicative of a diagnosis of dysferlinopathy. Muscle biopsies from LGMD2B patients typically show rather milder dystrophic features than might be expected from the degree of CK elevation. However, the presence of inflammatory cells is common.

Protein analysis in dysferlinopathy is useful (Figures 11.2 and 11.3). Combining immunoanalysis of muscle sections with immunoblotting is the most informative, as currently available diagnostic antibodies may work relatively poorly on muscle sections and there is variability of dysferlin localization which can lead to confusion in interpretation. On the other hand, a total deficiency of dysferlin on Western blotting appears to be specific to dysferlinopathy, and a secondary deficiency of calpain-3 can also be seen [130, 145] (Figure 11.3). The Miyoshi phenotype is genetically heterogeneous, with another locus on chromosome 10 and others are also likely to exist due to the presence of further families not linked either to dysferlin or the chromosome 10 locus [150].

An alternative route to the diagnosis of dysferlinopathy has been suggested via the examination of monocytes, in which dysferlin is highly expressed [137, 151].

Mutation detection in the large dysferlin gene will confirm the diagnosis but does not provide useful information on phenotypic correlations, with many families showing discordant phenotypes despite sharing the same homozygous mutations.

Management

There are few complications of dysferlinopathy aside from the progressive decrease in muscle strength, which, regardless of the initial mode of presentation, eventually affects both the proximal and distal musculature. Foot drop may be managed with the provision of ankle–foot orthoses. Contractures are rare until later stages and respiratory muscle strength appears to be well maintained. There is not yet good evidence for clinically relevant cardiac disease despite some reports of problems in mouse models and a few older patients in whom the relevance of any cardiac involvement could not be fully assessed [152, 153]. Where long-term follow-up has been reported in dysferlinopathy, the disease appears to be compatible with a normal life expectancy.

Sarcoglycanopathies

Definition

The sarcoglycanopathies may in some cases be amongst the most severe forms of LGMD though once again there is variation in severity. Nonetheless, the first clinical descriptions of what later turned out to be sarcoglycanopathy designated the disease as severe childhood autosomal recessive muscular dystrophy and commented on its phenotypic similarity to Duchenne muscular dystrophy. The frequency of sarcoglycanopathies varies between different populations, and it has been estimated at 15% in the American population, ~25% in Italian patients [50, 55], and accounts for about 32% of classified LGMD-affected Brazilian patients [50]. It is less frequent in the UK.

As to the relative proportion of each of the sarcoglycanopathies, while in Europe and North America the great majority of the patients deficient for the SG proteins are affected by LGMD2D [154, 155, 156], LGMD2C corresponds to almost 100% of the sarcoglycanopathies in Northern Africa [157]. From the same studies LGMD2F seems to be very rare all over

a b

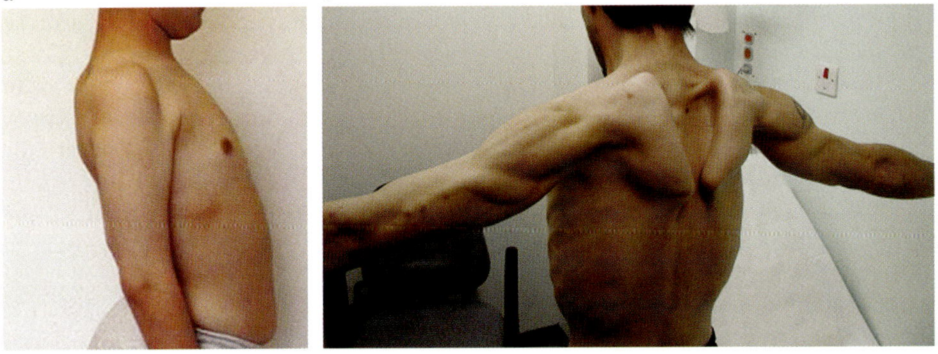

Figure 11.8a, b. Sarcoglycanopathy. (a) Severe weakness with hyperlordosis. (b) Prominent scapular winging and localized hypertrophy.

the world. The four subtypes are well represented in Brazil, with a relative frequency of 23% for LGMD2C, 40% for LGMD2D, 23% for LGMD2E, and 14% for LGMD2F [50, 158].

Clinical features

Given that the sarcoglycans belong to the same protein complex as dystrophin, it is probably not a surprise that their phenotypes overlap with dystrophinopathy and that the spectrum of severity seen in sarcoglycanopathy reflects the spectrum of dystrophinopathy as well, with the more severe end of the spectrum being equivalent to Duchenne muscular dystrophy and the milder to the Becker phenotypes (Figure 11.8). It does not appear that there are significant clinical distinguishing features between the different sarcoglycanopathies. An important distinguishing factor from dystrophinopathy however is the absence of any intellectual involvement; rather more subtle pointers to the diagnosis in distinction from dystrophinopathy are the relatively greater degree of scapular winging that may be seen in sarcoglycanopathy patients. There is a bias towards childhood rather than adult onset, though both may be seen: most patients with sarcoglycanopathy will present between 6 and 8 years of age. Calf and other muscle hypertrophy including the tongue is frequent, CK levels are usually elevated to 10–100 times normal at least in active disease. The disease course is always progressive and respiratory and cardiac involvement may be seen with increasing severity of disease; however, they are only infrequently seen early in the disease course. Cardiac involvement may be more prevalent with δ- and β-sarcoglycanopathy but has been reported in association with mutations in α- and γ-sarcoglycanopathy as well [49, 154, 155, 159, 160, 161, 162, 163, 164, 165, 166, 167].

Molecular genetics and pathogenesis

The four components of the SG complex known to be involved in muscular dystrophy include α-SG, β-SG, γ-SG, and δ-SG; these are transmembrane glycoproteins which, together with sarcospan, dystrophin, dystroglycans, syntrophins, and α-dystrobrevin, constitute the dystrophin–glycoprotein complex (DGC). The DGC acts as a linker between the cytoskeleton of the muscle cell and the extracellular matrix, providing mechanical support to the plasma membrane during myofiber contraction. Besides this structural function, there is now increasing evidence that the DGC might play a role in cellular communication, as highlighted by its interaction with signaling molecules [168, 169].

Mutations in the genes for α-SG, β-SG, γ-SG, and δ-SG cause LGMD2D, 2E, 2C, and 2F respectively. Many different mutations have already been identified in all the sarcoglycan genes, including missense, splicing, nonsense, small and large gene deletions (listed at www.dmd.nl, accessed 28 April 2009).

Two additional SG proteins which are not directly involved in the diagnosis of LGMD are epsilon-sarcoglycan (ε-SG) and zeta-sarcoglycan (ζ-SG). The structure of the ε-SG gene is similar to that of α-SG, and is expressed in a wide variety of tissues [170, 171]. In the smooth muscle ε-SG is an integral part of the DGC, replacing α-SG [172]. Mutations in the ε-SG gene have been identified in patients with myoclonus-dystonia syndrome, an autosomal dominant nondegenerative central nervous system disorder [173]. Pedigree analysis showed reduced penetrance of the phenotype upon maternal inheritance of the mutated allele, indicating genomic imprinting.

Zeta-sarcoglycan (ζ-SG), identified due to its similarity to γ-SG and the human ζ-SG gene, shares the same intron–exon organization as the γ-SG and δ-SG genes [174]. The protein is localized in the plasma membrane of skeletal and cardiac muscle, and has been found to be associated with the SG complex. No specific disease was associated with mutations in the ζ-SG gene.

Diagnosis

As dystrophinopathy is far more common than sarcoglycanopathy in most populations, the most important initial test outside those populations where sarcoglycanopathy is particularly frequent is exclusion of dystrophinopathy by searching for a causative mutation [deletion/duplication by multiplex ligation-dependent probe amplification (MLPA) and point mutation detection by sequencing]. Dystrophinopathy would also be detected on muscle biopsy. Biopsy analysis is also very useful in the diagnosis of sarcoglycanopathy. Given the multimeric nature of the dystrophin-associated complex, loss of one of the complex members usually causes a secondary loss or at least reduction of the other complex members as well (Figures 11.2 and 11.3). The patterns of abnormalities seen in association with primary defects in one or other of the sarcoglycan genes are not always predictable. A secondary loss of dystrophin may also be seen mainly in patients with primary γ-SG deficiency. This is a particularly important point in the distinction between sarcoglycanopathy and milder cases of dystrophinopathy, for example Becker muscular dystrophy and manifesting carriers of dystrophinopathy. Despite preliminary surveys suggesting that the pattern of protein loss might act as a useful pointer to the primary gene involved, in most muscle biopsies from patients with a sarcoglycanopathy, the primary loss or deficiency of any one of the four sarcoglycans, β-SG and δ-SG in particular, leads to a secondary deficiency of the whole subcomplex [175, 176] (Figure 11.2). A recent review of primary sarcoglycanopathy in the Newcastle UK Diagnostic Centre for LGMD indicated that prediction of the primary protein involvement can be difficult even with use of the whole range of sarcoglycan antibodies (Klinge *et al.* submitted).

Genotype–phenotype correlations

Severe Duchenne-like presentations tend to be relatively common among these patients, with onset occurring early in childhood and confinement to a wheelchair before the age of 16 years. Patients harboring null mutations in both alleles of one of the SG genes as well as a drastic decrease of the entire SG complex usually but not always show a severe phenotype. In the Brazilian population, the majority of the severely affected LGMD patients have a sarcoglycanopathy [177]. Nevertheless, milder courses have also been described in LGMD2C, 2D, and 2E patients, and intrafamilial variability in clinical course is frequently described.

Most patients with missense changes in both alleles also show a dramatic reduction of the primary protein together with variable deficiency of the secondary SGs. This pattern has usually been associated with a severe clinical course in LGMD2E and 2F but with both mild and severe presentations in LGMD2D. Within this last subgroup, clinical variability among patients homozygous for the same mutation seems to correlate with the residual amount of γ-SG in the muscle, despite the absence of the other three SGs in all of them. However, normal or almost normal levels of the primarily involved SG in the muscle have been found in some rare LGMD2C and LGMD2D patients [175, 178].

Management

The management principles for sarcoglycanopathies mirror those for dystrophinopathy. Attention to strength and joint range of movement necessitates physiotherapy input and if necessary orthopedic intervention. Assessment of respiratory function will identify the correct timing for nocturnal ventilatory support and cardiac evaluation is necessary to identify patients requiring treatment for cardiomyopathy. Scoliosis may be a problem in the more severely affected patients, and necessitate spinal surgery. Although glucocorticoid corticosteroid medication is now accepted as a gold standard for improving strength in Duchenne muscular dystrophy, reaching clear evidence that it is also of benefit in sarcoglycanopathy is difficult due to the small patient numbers and the heterogeneity of the condition. Anecdotal stories of benefit in individual patients suggest that a trial of steroids in patients fully informed about the possibility of side-effects and the uncertainty of benefit might be indicated in controlled conditions.

LGMD2G – telethoninopathy

Definition

LGMD2G is a relatively mild form of autosomal recessive muscular dystrophy with a wide spectrum of inter- and intra-familial clinical variability, identified and described in Brazilian families and now also in a group of ethnic Chinese [179]. LGMD2G is relatively rare even in Brazil, accounting for about 4% of the classified AR-LGMD forms [37, 180].

The age of onset ranges from 9 to 15 years and loss of ambulation may occur after the fourth decade. Cardiac involvement is frequent. Serum CK is 3- to 30-fold increased. Muscle biopsy shows a dystrophic pattern, including rimmed vacuoles.

Clinical features

In the nine initially described LGMD2G patients from three families, the age at onset ranged from 9 to 15 years, with marked weakness in the distal muscles of the legs and proximal involvement. Of these patients, five lost the ability to walk within their third or fourth decade, whereas the remaining four remained ambulant at age 22–44 years [38] (Figure 11.9). Cardiac involvement was observed in three of six affected members from one of the families, while in the second family clinical features of the three affected members resemble those observed in LGMD2A and 2B, with the involvement of some distal muscles. Age at onset, typically characterized by difficulty in walking and climbing stairs, ranged from 2 to 15 years. All of these patients have pronounced calf hypertrophy (one asymmetrical) [37, 180].

Molecular genetics and pathogenesis

LGMD2G is caused by mutations in the telethonin gene or TCAP [37, 180], mapped to 17q12, and the coding region is formed by only two exons. Telethonin is a sarcomeric protein of 19 kDa present in the Z-disk of the sarcomere of striated and cardiac muscle [181]. Telethonin is one of the substrates of the serine kinase domain of titin. The specific function of telethonin and its interaction with other muscle proteins is still unknown.

Two different pathogenic changes have first been identified in three Brazilian LGMD2G families: c.157C > T (Q53X) and c.639–640delGG. Both changes lead to premature stop codons. In a screening of 200 patients with a clinical diagnosis of LGMD, previously excluded through DNA and/or muscle

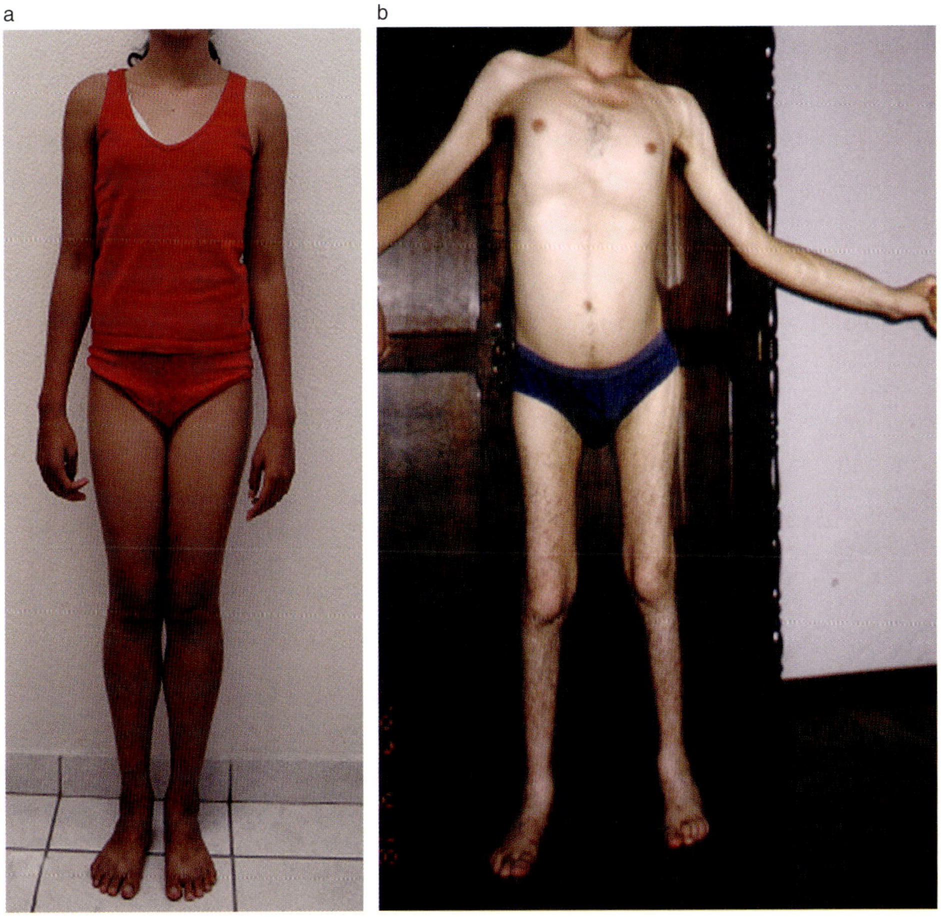

Figure 11.9a, b. LGMD2G. (a) Mild clinical course in a 13-year-old patient. (b) A severe course in a 35-year-old patient.

protein analysis for known autosomal recessive LGMD forms, we have identified the same 157C > T mutation in homozygosity, in four additional patients from three new families, and the 1229A > C polymorphism in six patients (two heterozygotes and four homozygotes). These results confirm that the 157C > T mutation is prevalent in Brazilian LGMD2G [180]. A third mutation causing LGMD2G, a homozygous eight base pair duplication (c.26–33 dup-AGGTGTCG), was found in three affected individuals of ethnic Chinese background [179].

Genotype–phenotype correlations

As already observed in the majority of LGMD forms, no direct clinical correlation is observed in patients with LGMD2G carrying the same c.157C > T (Q53X) mutation. The duplication mutation in Chinese patients also results in a total deficiency of the protein in the muscle. Clinical features were shared among these patients, including late childhood or adolescent onset and distal as well as proximal muscle weakness, with striking selective muscle involvement and signs, including scapula winging, finger and foot drop, and calf hypertrophy. One identification of one relatively asymptomatic individual suggests a high variation in clinical severity. The mutation was also found in the heterozygous state in a screening of normal controls of the same ethnic background. This suggests that LGMD2G may not be too rare among this population.

A mutation in the telethonin/TCAP gene (R87Q) was also identified in one patient with dilated cardiomyopathy [182]. Additionally, two mutations in the telethonin/TCAP gene, T137I and R153H, were found in two patients, in a screening of 346 patients with hypertrophic cardiomyopathy (HCM) and one additional mutation, E132Q, was found in one among 136 patients with dilated cardiomyopathy (DCM). It was demonstrated by a qualitative assay that the HCM-associated mutations augment the ability of telethonin to interact with titin and calsarcin-1, whereas the DCM-associated mutations impair the interaction of telethonin with muscle LIM protein (MLP), titin, and calsarcin-1. It was concluded that the difference in clinical phenotype (HCM or DCM) may be correlated with the property of altered binding among the Z-disk components [183].

Diagnosis

Immunohistochemical and Western blot analysis using an antibody against the whole protein showed total absence of telethonin in patients from all families, suggesting that protein analysis can be used to direct patients for mutation screening

(Figures 11.2 and 11.3). No intermediate protein products of the mutated gene were identified, using additional antibodies against the N-terminal domain of telethonin. Histological analysis showed a dystrophic pattern of muscle degeneration in all studied patients, including fiber size variation, slight degree of connective tissue infiltration, presence of a high number of internally localized nuclei, splitting, and a variable degree of rimmed vacuoles. Only one patient showed the presence of spread ghost fibers. Histochemical analysis revealed the presence of a mosaic pattern of type I/II fibers, with a type I predominance in two patients and type II predominance in a third patient. Small groups of fibers from the same type were observed in three patients, a type I fiber atrophy in five patients, while one patient showed type II atrophy [184].

Additional protein studies on LGMD2G patients have shown normal expression of dystrophin, sarcoglycans, dysferlin, calpain-3, and titin. However, a reduction in the amount of the recently identified sarcomeric protein myopalladin was observed in muscle fibers from the LGMD2G patients, suggesting an interaction between telethonin and myopalladin [184]. Furthermore, immunofluorescence analysis for α-actinin-2 and myotilin showed a normal cross-striation pattern, suggesting that at least part of the Z-line of the sarcomere is preserved. Telethonin was clearly present in the rods in muscle fibers from patients with nemaline myopathy, confirming its localization in the Z-line of the sarcomere.

Ultrastructural analysis confirmed the maintenance of the integrity of the sarcomeric architecture. Therefore, mutations in the telethonin gene do not seem to alter sarcomere integrity [184].

LGMD2H (TRIM32-related dystrophy)

This muscular dystrophy was identified among the Hutterites of Canada, in whom genetic linkage was established to chromosome 9q31–34. A homozygous missense mutation in the putative E3 ubiquitin ligase TRIM32 was demonstrated in affected patients within these families, thus introducing a novel pathogenic concept for the muscular dystrophies. The mutation (Asp487Asn) occurs in the first of three NHL domains presumably responsible for protein–protein interactions. Mutations in TRIM32 are also described in patients diagnosed with sarcotubular myopathy [41, 42, 185].

The age of onset is usually in the mid 20s, but may be as early as 8 years of age. The presenting complaint is proximal weakness with a waddling gait, sometimes associated with fatigue and back pain. Progression tends to be somewhat slower than in other autosomal recessive LGMDs. Later in the disease, there is weakness in the upper extremity with involvement of the deltoid and trapezius muscles as well as some distal weakness in the anterior peroneal group and the brachioradialis, and possibly some mild facial involvement. By ECG there is also evidence for some degree of cardiac involvement that remains subclinical. Loss of ambulation may occur in some patients in their 40s. Serum CK levels are elevated 5- to 50-fold.

The muscle biopsy specimens show changes consistent with muscular dystrophy. Even though the presumed function of TRIM32 is in tagging proteins for degradation, no conspicuous protein accumulations or inclusions have been detected in the muscle fibers so far.

Limb-girdle muscular dystrophy associated with abnormalities of-dystroglycan

Definition

In recent years the identification of a group of muscular dystrophies characterized by a shared feature of abnormal glycosylation of α-dystroglycan has highlighted a new pathogenic mechanism in muscular dystrophy. A hallmark of mutations in the genes encoding proteins important in the glycosylation of α-dystroglycan is huge clinical variability with a spectrum of disease severity from severe congenital muscular dystrophy with or without structural brain and eye defects (discussed in more detail in Chapter 12) to limb-girdle muscular dystrophies presenting with much milder disease and without CNS complications. The most common form of limb-girdle muscular dystrophy where the underlying pathomechanism is likely to be abnormal glycosylation of α-dystroglycan is LGMD2I, due to FKRP mutations [38, 39]. Here the LGMD phenotype is more common than the congenital muscular dystrophy phenotype and indeed the majority of cases with milder disease share a common mutation (C826A).

LGMD2I occurs worldwide and the common mutation has been shown to share a common haplotype [186]. The frequency of LGMD2I shows some regional variations with an apparent north–south gradient of frequency in Europe. Therefore it is as frequent as or more frequent than LGMD2A in most of Northern Europe (with the exception of the Netherlands) and less common in the south of Europe and Australia than LGMD2A and LGMD2B [52, 54, 56, 114]. In the areas with higher prevalence of the disease, the ready testing for the common mutation can be a useful route to the diagnosis.

Clinical features

LGMD2I is characterized by a high variability in clinical course, with a spectrum of phenotypes ranging from a Duchenne-like disease course to milder phenotypes with a slow progression, though even the milder cases may show complications of cardiomyopathy and respiratory impairment. Its allelic form MDC1C is characterized by onset of symptoms within the first few months of life, and in the MDC1C form there is inability to walk. Within the spectrum of patients with MDC1C there are some who have major structural brain defects, though this is less common than with some of the other α-dystroglycanopathies. Patients usually show elevated

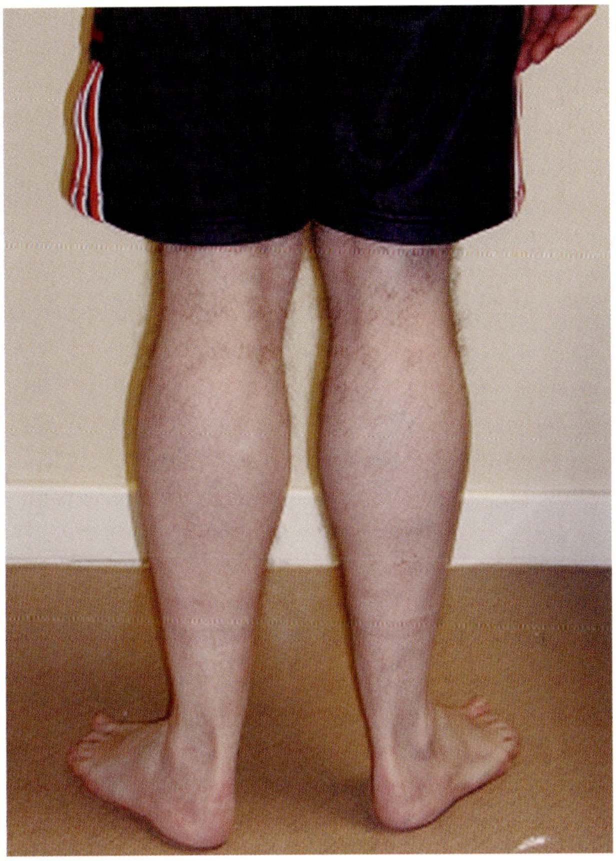

Figure 11.10. LGMD2I Calf hypertrophy is a common feature.

serum CK, and histological changes are characteristic of a muscular dystrophy.

The LGMD phenotype of FKRP mutations is quite variable in severity and at its most severe can present as a disorder of at least Duchenne-like severity with early loss of ambulation at the end of the first decade or at the beginning of the second decade. In these early-onset cases there may be delayed motor milestones or hypotonia during the first year of life. The spectrum extends to milder phenotypes with even late adult onset essentially resembling Becker muscular dystrophy. This is typically the most common presentation of LGMD2I especially when patients are homozygous for the common C826A mutation. The muscle weakness has a pronounced predilection for axial muscles, neck flexors, and the proximal limb muscles. There may also be mild facial weakness, in particular in the very early onset cases. Muscles of the shoulder girdle may be weaker than those of the pelvic girdle, with atrophy of the pectoralis major and deltoid muscles. In contrast, there can be prominent hypertrophy of the tongue, the brachioradialis, the calves, and possibly other leg muscles (Figure 11.10). There is often prominent lordosis. Exercise-induced muscle cramping is not uncommon and rhabdomyolysis precipitated by anesthesia has been reported. Clinically significant dilated cardiomyopathy develops in about half of patients and is independent of the severity of the skeletal muscle weakness [187, 188]. There is also an important respiratory involvement in patients with FKRP mutations, manifesting initially as a drop in forced vital capacity followed by nocturnal hypoventilation on the basis of diaphragmatic weakness. In contrast to Duchenne and Becker muscular dystrophies, it is important to note that the respiratory failure can occur while the patient is still ambulatory. Intelligence is not affected. CK levels are typically high, ranging from 10 to 100 times higher than normal [54, 187, 189, 190, 191].

Molecular genetics and pathogenesis

The FKRP protein is probably required for the post-translational modification of dystroglycan since a variable reduction of α-dystroglycan expression is observed in the skeletal muscle biopsy of affected individuals [40, 192, 193]. In addition, several cases show a deficiency of laminin-α2 either by immunocytochemistry or, more often, by Western blotting [194] (Figures 11.2 and 11.3).

The 12-kb FKRP gene is composed of three noncoding exons and a single large exon that contains part of the 5′ untranslated region, the entire open reading frame and the 3′ untranslated region [39]. The FKRP gene encodes a 495-amino-acid protein and has a 1488-bp open reading frame. Sequence analysis of FKRP predicts the presence of a hydrophobic transmembrane-spanning region (amino acids 4–28) followed by a "stem region" and the putative catalytic c domain. A similar molecular organization is found in several Golgi-resident glycosyltransferases.

Although the function of FKRP is still unknown, it has been suggested that it might be involved in the glycosylation of α-DG in muscle membrane. The DG complex is important in muscle formation and maintenance, and cell adhesion, and it also plays an important role in the function of other tissues, such as brain, kidneys, and peripheral nerves. A single gene *DAG1* encodes a polypeptide that is post-translationally modified to yield the two glycoproteins referred to as α- and β-DG [195, 196]. α-DG is a heavily glycosylated peripheral membrane component of the dystrophin-associated glycoprotein complex (DGC), whilst β-DG is a transmembrane protein that links to dystrophin intracellularly. The disruption of this linkage underlies several forms of muscular dystrophy, underscoring its importance in striated muscle, which contributes to the structural integrity of the sarcolemma [189, 192, 196, 197].

Genotype–phenotype correlations

In a group of British patients, the results of the molecular genetic studies were correlated with the clinical and pathological findings and allowed the recognition of three groups of patients: (1) MDC1C, who were either compound heterozygotes for one nonsense and one missense or homozygotes for missense mutations; (2) LGMD21 severe (DMD-like) who had the leu276Ile mutation plus one other mutation (not exclusively null); and (3) LGMD2I mild, who almost invariably were homozygotes for the common Leu276Ileu mutation. This latter mutation appears to be a mild mutation as the patients homozygous for it had the mildest phenotype and better preserved α-DG staining, while it was never observed in patients with MDC1C [193]. The possibility of variability of phenotype even in patients homozygous for the common mutation must be borne in mind [198].

Among 13 Brazilian LGMD genealogies, including 20 individuals with mutations in the FKRP gene, the commonest Leu276Ileu "European" mutation was found in 35% (9/26) out of the mutated LGMD2I alleles [199]. In two unrelated LGMD2I families, homozygous for novel missense mutations, four asymptomatic individuals were identified, all older than 20 years. At the more severe end of the spectrum, Schwartz *et al.* [200] found that 13 of 102 sporadic patients with a phenotype resembling Duchenne or Becker muscular dystrophy but without mutations in the dystrophin gene had mutations in the FKRP gene, consistent with a diagnosis of LGMD2I [200]. Four of seven patients showed reduced or irregular immunostaining for dystrophin on muscle biopsy. In two cases, a diagnosis of Becker muscular dystrophy had been made based on muscle biopsy and clinical findings, and prenatal diagnoses had been performed in their families based on that erroneous assumption. This finding underlines the importance of comprehensive genetic testing before assumptions of neuromuscular diseases are made and genetic counseling provided based on these assumptions.

An interesting explanation for a clinical variability in LGMD2I was found in a study of three affected sisters and a highly variable clinical course. FKRP gene sequencing showed that all three sisters carried a nonsense paternal mutation (W225X). The two oldest sisters with a severe phenotype carried two maternal mutations V79M and P89A. However, the youngest sister with a milder course carried the paternal and only the V79M maternal mutation, due to an intragenic recombination [201].

Diagnosis

Serum CK levels are increased 4- to 100-fold in most affected individuals. On muscle biopsy, a variation in muscle fiber size, necrotic and regenerating fibers, type I predominance, and mildly increased connective tissue replacement are observed.

Secondary protein abnormalities are common in this group of diseases, including a reduction of laminin-α2 labeling, mainly on immunoblots (Figure 11.3), and reduced Western blot labeling for laminin-β_1. A variable reduction of α-DG expression was also observed in skeletal muscle biopsies from affected individuals, with a reduction in molecular weight observed by immunoblotting, which could indicate an association with a glycosylation defect. The analysis of 10 proteins in 13 molecularly classified Brazilian LGMD2I patients showed a significant reduction of laminin-α2 in almost all, with no direct correlation with the secondary reduction of α-DG or the type of mutation [202] (Figure 11.2).

Although a variable finding, in the majority of patients there will be a secondary reduction of α-DG and laminin-α2 immunoreactivity which is more commonly seen on immunoblotting. Other secondary protein abnormalities have been observed as well, including a reduction of calpain-3. α-Dystroglycan on immunohistochemical analysis using antibodies raised against glycosylated epitopes may be much more prominently reduced, providing an important diagnostic clue for the presence of this type of disorder. It should be noted that the protein abnormalities may be quite diverse, and none in itself is specific for LGMD2I. However, in the appropriate clinical context, any of these abnormalities should prompt mutation analysis in the FKRP gene. Genetic analysis is relatively simple, as a single missense mutation predominates in the milder cases, and the entire open reading frame coding for the protein is contained on exon 4 of the gene. In some of the populations where the prevalence of LGMD2I is high, this in itself offers a straightforward screening test for a patient with a suspected LGMD and a high CK.

Management

The early recognition of dilated cardiomyopathy and early respiratory failure is of great importance. Cardiac disease may be detected preclinically to allow early introduction of prophylactic treatment: "routine" management of cardiomyopathy is indicated and in some cases even cardiac transplantation may be necessary [187, 188]. Respiratory impairment may manifest first as diaphragmatic weakness so investigation of respiratory muscle strength when lying as well as sitting is mandatory. Night-time ventilatory assistance should be able to be introduced in a timely manner. In this type of recessive LGMD, serious and life-threatening complications that are amenable to treatment may supervene at a stage when the patient is still ambulant; therefore, it is very important to establish the correct diagnosis. The phenotypic overlap with dystrophinopathy can lead to problems with genetic counseling. That the genetic implications of the two disorders are so different provides a further practical reason for determining the correct diagnosis by mutation analysis. Although no trials have been conducted of corticosteroid treatment in LGMD2I, there is a report of benefit [203] which has also been seen in LGMD2K [204].

Other forms of LGMD with abnormal glycosylation of α-dystroglycan

As the detection of abnormal glycosylation of α-dystroglycan on muscle biopsy has been more widely applied, the spectrum of disease associated with mutations classically involved in forms of congenital muscular dystrophies and specifically muscle eye brain disease and Walker–Warburg syndrome has expanded. The designations LGMD2K, 2M, and 2N have all been used to define forms of LGMD associated with mutations in one of the genes which much more frequently are seen with congenital muscular dystrophy presentations (Table 11.1 and see Chapter 12).

LGMD2K was defined in seven patients from six consanguineous Turkish families with autosomal recessive muscular dystrophy and mental retardation [205]. An eighth British patient, who was not from a consanguineous family, had a similar phenotype. All patients acquired early motor milestones, excluding a congenital muscular dystrophy. Age at onset ranged from 1 to 6 years, with difficulty in walking and climbing stairs. Other features included slow progression, proximal muscle weakness, mild muscle hypertrophy, increased serum CK, microcephaly, and mental retardation (IQ range 50–76). Brain imaging was normal in all cases, with no structural abnormalities or white matter changes. Skeletal muscle biopsy showed dystrophic changes, including mild fibrosis with many regenerating and few necrotic fibers, increased fiber size variability, and multiple central nuclei. Immunohistochemical staining showed severe hypoglycosylation of α-dystroglycan. The Turkish patients subsequently were shown to have a homozygous mutation in the POMT1 gene [206] which is more commonly associated with Walker–Warburg syndrome.

In a similar story LGMD2K was defined in three children from two unrelated families with autosomal recessive LGMD [204]. All developed hypotonia and muscle weakness in infancy between ages 4 and 10 months. Two patients presented with severe acute motor deterioration after febrile viral illnesses; the third patient already had motor symptoms but also showed deterioration after a febrile illness at age 3 years. The patients showed mainly proximal muscle weakness with delayed motor development, decreased endurance, frequent falls, proximal muscle weakness, hypertrophy of lower limb muscles, and increased serum CK. All three patients eventually achieved independent ambulation. Skeletal muscle biopsies showed virtually absent glycosylation of α-dystroglycan and dystrophic features with mild macrophage infiltration. All patients had normal intellectual development, normal brain structure, and, interestingly for the perspective of therapy, responded very well to steroid treatment. These patients were compound heterozygotes for mutations in the fukutin gene, already known to cause Fukuyama congenital muscular dystrophy, a common form of muscular dystrophy in Japan where it typically causes early-onset disease with mental retardation. In the Japanese population there is a common retrotransposon mutation, which is not seen in the patients with milder disease. Other genes involved in congenital muscular dystrophy phenotypes (POMT2: LGMD2N [207] and LARGE) have a similarly broad spectrum of severity. At the moment though it would appear that relative to the large number of patients with LGMD due to FKRP mutations, for all the other α-dystroglycan-altering genes, the congenital muscular dystrophy phenotype is much more common [40]. It is also clear that other genes remain to be identified which can cause a secondary reduction in α-dystroglycan labeling in muscle.

LGMD2J

LGMD2J is a rare autosomal recessive muscular dystrophy, so far described only in a large consanguineous Finnish family [208, 209, 210] and caused by a homozygous mutation in the titin gene. Relatives of these patients, heterozygous for the same titin gene mutation, were affected by a milder form of distal tibial myopathy (TMD) [211]. LGMD2J is therefore a homozygous manifestation of the dominantly inherited titin gene mutation which is the cause of TMD. Clinically, LGMD2J patients described so far show severe progressive proximal weakness with onset ranging from the first to the third decade. Late-onset distal weakness has also been observed. Loss of ambulation can occur between third and sixth decades. Facial muscle weakness, joint contractures, and cardiac involvement have not been reported [208, 209]. CK levels were greatly elevated in all patients.

The titin gene (TTN) maps to chromosome 2q24.3 [212] and encodes the biggest single peptide found in humans. Titin is a central sarcomeric myofilament, expressed in heart and skeletal muscle, localized beside myosin and actin filaments and spanning half of the sarcomere from the Z-line to the M-line. It plays a mechanical role, keeping the contractile element of skeletal muscle centrally in the sarcomere during cycles of contraction and extension, and is responsible for muscle elasticity. Titin binds different proteins including calpain-3 and seems to play a role in stabilizing calpain-3 from autolytic degradation. All affected individuals characterized to date have a homozygous 11-bp deletion/insertion in the last TTN exon that affects the C-terminus of protein, close to the calpain-3 binding site. TTN mutations which involve residues located in the cardiac-specific N2-B region cause dilated cardiomyopathy type 1G (CMD1G) and hypertrophic cardiomyopathy [211]. Reported muscle biopsies in LGMD2J patients show typical dystrophic changes. Severe reduction or absence of calpain-3 has been observed by Western blot analysis, suggesting a possible effect of the mutation on the calpain-3 binding sites in titin [131].

LGMD2L

The locus on chromosome 11p defined as LGMD2L was described in 14 French Canadian patients from 8 different families with LGMD with quadriceps atrophy [213]. Age at onset ranged from 11 to 50 years. The majority of patients reported muscle pain. Although the severity of the phenotype was variable, all affected individuals had prominent weakness and atrophy of the quadriceps femoris muscles, often with asymmetrical involvement. Serum CK was normal or significantly increased. EMG studies showed myopathic changes, and muscle biopsies showed dystrophic changes with increased connective tissue and fiber splitting. Two patients with more advanced disease showed neurogenic changes on EMG. MRI studies on four patients showed atrophy of the biceps brachii and quadriceps femoris muscles with fatty infiltration. Four patients were wheelchair-bound after an average disease duration of 12 years. Less common findings included facial weakness in two patients and calf hypertrophy in four. Inheritance was consistent with autosomal recessive disease and linkage analysis identified a candidate region on chromosome 11p14.3. Further families remain to be defined.

Future perspectives

The potential to reach a definitive diagnosis based on the identification of the causative mutation in patients presenting with a proximal muscular dystrophy is now very impressive. Series of patients from different parts of the world are consistently showing that a diagnosis can be reached in 50%–75% of these patients and these figures are constantly improving as new genes and proteins are identified. The diagnostic process relies on a careful evaluation of the clinical and family history, the pattern of muscle involvement, level of elevation of CK, and the results of specific muscle biopsy and DNA analyses [45, 48]. The benefits to families of precise genetic counseling are clear: management implications are also better recognized and a proactive approach to cardiac and respiratory management in particular has a positive impact on quality of life and longevity [47]. Therapies based on the underlying genetic defect for many of these conditions are under development, and strategies such as gene replacement, stem cell transplantation, replacing the defective or absent gene with an alternative, increasing muscle mass or using pharmacological agents to alter the mutation or its downstream effects are at various stages of preclinical or even clinical development [214]. This in itself leads to new challenges. Identification of patient cohorts to be able to participate in trials amongst these rare disorders will necessitate international collaboration. Methods appropriate for measuring outcomes will need to be developed and validated in groups for whom generally long-term natural history studies are not available. Collaboration on these issues has already become a priority while the development of these therapies is still ongoing, and this is an issue which unites patient organizations, funding organizations and industry, together with the clinicians caring for these patients. These efforts will be essential for the expedited developments of treatments within this patient group.

Acknowledgments

The collaboration of the following people is gratefully acknowledged: Mayana Zatz, Lydia Yamamoto, Rita C. M. Pavanello, Ivo Pavanello, Helga C. A. Silva, Maria Rita Passos-Bueno, Marta Canovas, Volker Straub, Hanns Lochmuller, Rita Barresi, Fiona Norwood, and Michela Guglieri. M. V. is supported by grants from FAPESP- CEPID, CNPq FINEP, and ABDIM-Petrobras. K. B. is supported by grants from the EU (TREAT-NMD), the MRC, the AFM, and the MDC. Support from the National Specialist Commissioning Group in the UK for the LGMD national diagnostic and advisory service is also gratefully acknowledged.

References

1. K. M. Bushby, J. S. Beckmann, The limb-girdle muscular dystrophies – proposal for a new nomenclature. *Neuromuscul. Disord.* **5** (1995), 337–343.
2. J. N. Walton, F. J. Nattrass, On the classification, natural history and treatment of the myopathies. *Brain* **77** (1954), 169–231.
3. J. N. Walton, *Disorders of Voluntary Muscles.* Third Edition. (Edinburgh: Churchill Livingstone, 1974.)
4. J. N. Walton, D. Gardner-Medwin, The clinical examination of the voluntary muscles. In *Disorders of Voluntary Muscles.* Third Edition, ed. J. N. Walton. (Edinburgh: Churchill Livingstone, 1974), pp. 517–560.
5. K. M. Bushby, Making sense of the limb-girdle muscular dystrophies. *Brain* **122**:Pt 8 (1999), 1403–1420.
6. M. Zatz, M. Vainzof, M. R. Passos-Bueno, Limb-girdle muscular dystrophy: one gene with different phenotypes, one phenotype with different genes. *Curr. Opin. Neurol.* **13** (2000), 511–517.
7. S. H. Laval, K. M. Bushby, Limb-girdle muscular dystrophies – from genetics to molecular pathology. *Neuropathol. Appl. Neurobiol.* **30** (2004), 91–105.
8. M. Vainzof, M, Zatz, Protein defects in neuromuscular diseases. *Braz. J. Med. Biol. Res.* **36** (2003), 543–555.
9. M. A. Hauser, S. K. Horrigan, P. Salmikangas, *et al.*, Myotilin is mutated in limb girdle muscular dystrophy 1A. *Hum. Mol. Genet.* **9** (2000), 2141–2147.
10. M. A. Hauser, C. B. Conde, V. Kowaljow, *et al.*, Myotilin mutation found in second pedigree with LGMD1A. *Am. J. Hum. Genet.* **71** (2002), 1428–1432.
11. A. J. van der Kooi, M. van Meegen, T. M. Ledderhof, E. M. McNally, M. de Visser, P. A, Bolhuis, Genetic localization of a newly recognized autosomal dominant limb-girdle muscular dystrophy with cardiac involvement (LGMD1B), to chromosome 1q11–21. *Am. J. Hum. Genet.* **60** (1997), 891–895.
12. A. Muchir, G. Bonne, A. J. van der Kooi, *et al.*, Identification of mutations in the gene encoding lamins A/C in autosomal dominant limb girdle muscular dystrophy with atrioventricular conduction disturbances (LGMD1B). *Hum. Mol. Genet.* **9** (2000), 1453–1459.
13. I. Carbone, C. Bruno, F. Sotgia, *et al.*, Mutation in the CAV3 gene causes partial caveolin-3 deficiency and hyperCKemia. *Neurology* **54** (2000), 1373–1376.
14. C. Minetti, F. Sotgia, C. Bruno, *et al.*, Mutations in the caveolin-3 gene cause autosomal dominant limb-girdle muscular dystrophy. *Nat. Genet.* **18** (1998), 365–368.
15. E. M. McNally, E. de Sa Moreira, D. J. Duggan, *et al.*, Caveolin-3 in muscular dystrophy. *Hum. Mol. Genet.* **7** (1998), 871–877.
16. M. C. Speer, J. M. Vance, J. M. Grubber, *et al.*, Identification of a new autosomal dominant limb-girdle muscular dystrophy locus on chromosome 7. *Am. J. Hum. Genet.* **64** (1999), 556–562.
17. D. N. Messina, M. C. Speer, M. A. Pericak-Vance, E. M. McNally, Linkage of familial dilated cardiomyopathy with conduction defect and muscular dystrophy to chromosome 6q23. *Am. J. Hum. Genet.* **61** (1997), 909–917.
18. L. Palenzuela, A. L. Andreu, J. Gamez, *et al.*, A novel autosomal dominant limb-girdle muscular dystrophy (LGMD 1F), maps to 7q32.1–32.2. *Neurology* **61** (2003), 404–406.
19. A. Starling, F. Kok, M. R. Passos-Bueno, M. Vainzof, M. Zatz, A new form of autosomal dominant limb-girdle muscular dystrophy (LGMD1G), with progressive fingers and toes flexion limitation maps to chromosome 4p21. *Eur. J. Hum. Genet.* **12** (2004), 1033–1040.

20. K. Matsumura, K. P. Campbell, Dystrophin-glycoprotein complex: its role in the molecular pathogenesis of muscular dystrophies. *Muscle Nerve* **17** (1994), 2–15.

21. S. L. Roberds, F. Leturcq, V. Allamand, *et al.*, Missense mutations in the adhalin gene linked to autosomal recessive muscular dystrophy. *Cell* **78** (1994), 625–633.

22. L. E. Lim, F. Duclos, O. Broux, *et al.*, Beta-sarcoglycan: characterization and role in limb-girdle muscular dystrophy linked to 4q12. *Nat. Genet.* **11** (1995), 257–265.

23. S. Noguchi, E. M. McNally, K. Ben Othmane, *et al.*, Mutations in the dystrophin-associated protein gamma-sarcoglycan in chromosome 13 muscular dystrophy. *Science* **270** (1995), 819–822.

24. Y. Sunada, K. P. Campbell, Dystrophin-glycoprotein complex: molecular organization and critical roles in skeletal muscle. *Curr. Opin. Neurol.* **8** (1995), 379–384.

25. D. Jung, F. Duclos, B. Apostol, *et al.*, Characterization of delta-sarcoglycan, a novel component of the oligomeric sarcoglycan complex involved in limb-girdle muscular dystrophy. *J. Biol. Chem.* **271** (1996), 32321–32329.

26. E. M. McNally, M. R. Passos-Bueno, C. G. Bonnemann, *et al.*, Mild and severe muscular dystrophy caused by a single gamma-sarcoglycan mutation. *Am. J. Hum. Genet.* **59** (1996), 1040–1047.

27. V. Nigro, G. Piluso, A. Belsito, *et al.*, Identification of a novel sarcoglycan gene at 5q33 encoding a sarcolemmal 35 kDa glycoprotein. *Hum. Mol. Genet.* **5** (1996), 1179–1186.

28. T. Yoshida, H. Hanada, Y. Iwata, Y. Pan, M. Sigekawa, Expression of a dystrophin-sarcoglycan complex in serum-deprived BC3H1 cells and involvement of alpha-sarcoglycan in substrate attachment. *Biochem. Biophys. Res. Commun.* **225** (1996), 11–15.

29. D. J. Duggan, D. Manchester, K. P. Stears, D. J. Mathews, C. Hart, E. P. Hoffman, Mutations in the delta-sarcoglycan gene are a rare cause of autosomal recessive limb-girdle muscular dystrophy (LGMD2). *Neurogenetics* **1** (1997), 49–58.

30. M. R. Passos-Bueno, M. Vainzof, E. S. Moreira, M. Zatz, Seven autosomal recessive limb-girdle muscular dystrophies in the Brazilian population: from LGMD2A to LGMD2G. *Am. J. Med. Genet.* **82** (1999), 392–398.

31. R. Barresi, C. Di Blasi, T. Negri, *et al.*, Disruption of heart sarcoglycan complex and severe cardiomyopathy caused by beta sarcoglycan mutations. *J. Med. Genet.* **37** (2000), 102–107.

32. T. L. Gouveia, J. F. Paim, R. C. Pavanello, M. Zatz, M. Vainzof, Sarcoglycanopathies: a multiplex molecular analysis for the most common mutations. *Diagn. Mol. Pathol.* **15** (2006), 95–100.

33. M. Fardeau, B. Eymard, C. Mignard, F. M. Tome, I. Richard, J. S. Beckmann, Chromosome 15-linked limb-girdle muscular dystrophy: clinical phenotypes in Reunion Island and French metropolitan communities. *Neuromuscul. Disord.* **6** (1996), 447–453.

34. I. Richard, O. Broux, V. Allamand, *et al.*, Mutations in the proteolytic enzyme calpain 3 cause limb-girdle muscular dystrophy type 2A. *Cell* **81** (1995), 27–40.

35. R. Bashir, S. Britton, T. Strachan, *et al.*, A gene related to *Caenorhabditis elegans* spermatogenesis factor fer-1 is mutated in limb-girdle muscular dystrophy type 2B. *Nat. Genet.* **20** (1998), 37–42.

36. J. Liu, M. Aoki, I. Illa, *et al.*, Dysferlin, a novel skeletal muscle gene, is mutated in Miyoshi myopathy and limb girdle muscular dystrophy. *Nat. Genet.* **20** (1998), 31–36.

37. E. S. Moreira, T. J. Wiltshire, G. Faulkner, *et al.*, Limb-girdle muscular dystrophy type 2G is caused by mutations in the gene encoding the sarcomeric protein telethonin. *Nat. Genet.* **24** (2000), 163–166.

38. M. Brockington, D. J. Blake, P. Prandini, *et al.*, Mutations in the fukutin-related protein gene (FKRP), cause a form of congenital muscular dystrophy with secondary laminin alpha2 deficiency and abnormal glycosylation of alpha-dystroglycan. *Am. J. Hum. Genet.* **69** (2001), 1198–1209.

39. M. Brockington, Y. Yuva, P. Prandini, *et al.*, Mutations in the fukutin-related protein gene (FKRP), identify limb girdle muscular dystrophy 2I as a milder allelic variant of congenital muscular dystrophy MDC1C. *Hum. Mol. Genet.* **10** (2001), 2851–2859.

40. C. Godfrey, E. Clement, R. Mein, *et al.*, Refining genotype phenotype correlations in muscular dystrophies with defective glycosylation of dystroglycan. *Brain* **130** (2007), 2725–2735.

41. T. Weiler, C. R. Greenberg, T. Zelinski, *et al.*, A gene for autosomal recessive limb-girdle muscular dystrophy in Manitoba Hutterites maps to chromosome region 9q31-q33: evidence for another limb-girdle muscular dystrophy locus. *Am. J. Hum. Genet.* **63** (1998), 140–147.

42. P. Frosk, T. Weiler, E. Nylen, *et al.*, Limb-girdle muscular dystrophy type 2H associated with mutation in TRIM32, a putative E3-ubiquitin-ligase gene. *Am. J. Hum. Genet.* **70** (2002), 663–672.

43. D. Selcen, K. Bushby, Titinopathies: what happens when a big gene mutates in a big family? *Neurology* **64** (2005), 596–597.

44. P. Hackman, A. Vihola, H. Haravuori, *et al.*, Tibial muscular dystrophy is a titinopathy caused by mutations in TTN, the gene encoding the giant skeletal-muscle protein titin. *Am. J. Hum. Genet.* **71** (2002), 492–500.

45. K. Bushby, F. Norwood, V. Straub, The limb-girdle muscular dystrophies - diagnostic strategies. *Biochim. Biophys. Acta* **1772** (2007), 238–242.

46. V. Straub, K. Bushby, The childhood limb-girdle muscular dystrophies. *Semin. Pediatr. Neurol.* **13** (2006), 104–114.

47. K. Bushby, V. Straub, Nonmolecular treatment for muscular dystrophies. *Curr. Opin. Neurol.* **18** (2005), 511–518.

48. F. Norwood, M. de Visser, B. Eymard, H. Lochmuller, K. Bushby, EFNS guideline on diagnosis and management of limb girdle muscular dystrophies. *Eur. J. Neurol.* **14** (2007), 1305–1312.

49. M. Zatz, F. de Paula, A. Starling, M. Vainzof, The 10 autosomal recessive limb-girdle muscular dystrophies. *Neuromuscul. Disord.* **13** (2003), 532–544.

50. M. Guglieri, F. Magri, M. G. D'Angelo, *et al.*, Clinical, molecular, and protein correlations in a large sample of genetically diagnosed Italian limb girdle muscular dystrophy patients. *Hum. Mutat.* **29**:2 (2008), 258–266.

51. F. Norwood, C. Harling, P. Chinnery, *et al.*, Prevalence of gentic muscle clinic population. *Brain* (in press).

52. H. P. Lo, S. T. Cooper, F. J. Evesson, *et al.*, Limb-girdle muscular dystrophy: diagnostic evaluation, frequency and clues to pathogenesis. *Neuromuscul. Disord.* **18**:1 (2007), 34–44.

53. M. C. Walter, J. A. Petersen, R. Stucka, *et al.*, FKRP (826C > A), frequently causes limb-girdle muscular dystrophy in German patients. *J. Med. Genet.* **41** (2004), e50.

54. M. L. Sveen, M. Schwartz, J. Vissing, High prevalence and phenotype-genotype correlations of limb girdle muscular dystrophy type 2I in Denmark. *Ann. Neurol.* **59** (2006), 808–815.

55. S. A. Moore, C. J. Shilling, S. Westra, *et al.*, Limb-girdle muscular dystrophy in the United States. *J. Neuropathol. Exp. Neurol.* **65** (2006), 995–1003.

56. A. J. van der Kooi, W. S. Frankhuizen, P. G. Barth, *et al.*, Limb-girdle muscular dystrophy in the Netherlands: gene defect identified in half the families. *Neurology* **68** (2007), 2125–2128.

57. R. McFarland, H. Swalwell, E. L. Blakely, *et al.*, The m.5650G > A mitochondrial tRNA(Ala), mutation is pathogenic and causes a phenotype of pure myopathy. *Neuromuscul. Disord.* **18**:1 (2008), 63–67.

58. J. Palace, D. Lashley, J. Newsom-Davis, *et al.*, Clinical features of the DOK7 neuromuscular junction synaptopathy. *Brain* **130** (2007), 1507–1515.

59. J. S. Muller, A. Herczegfalvi, J. J. Vilchez, *et al.*, Phenotypical spectrum of DOK7 mutations in congenital myasthenic syndromes. *Brain* **130** (2007), 1497–1506.

60. A. J. van der Kooi, H. B. Ginjaar, H. F. Busch, J. H. Wokke, P. G. Barth, M. de Visser, Limb girdle muscular dystrophy: a pathological and immunohistochemical reevaluation. *Muscle Nerve* **21** (1998), 584–590.

61. K. Bushby, Report on the 12th ENMC sponsored international workshop – the "limb-girdle" muscular dystrophies. *Neuromuscul. Disord.* **2** (1992), 3–5.

62. L. H. Yamaoka, C. A. Westbrook, M. C. Speer, *et al.*, Development of a microsatellite genetic map spanning 5q31-q33 and subsequent placement of the LGMD1A locus between D5S178 and IL9. *Neuromuscul. Disord.* **4** (1994), 471–475.

63. D. Selcen, A. G. Engel, Mutations in myotilin cause myofibrillar myopathy. *Neurology* **62** (2004), 1363–1371.

64. S. M. Garvey, S. E. Miller, D. R. Claflin, J. A. Faulkner, M. A. Hauser, Transgenic mice expressing the myotilin T57I mutation unite the pathology associated with LGMD1A and MFM. *Hum. Mol. Genet.* **15** (2006), 2348–2362.

65. G. Bonne, M. R. Di Barletta, S. Varnous, *et al.*, Mutations in the gene encoding lamin A/C cause autosomal dominant Emery-Dreifuss muscular dystrophy. *Nat. Genet.* **21** (1999), 285–288.

66. H. M. Becane, G. Bonne, S. Varnous, *et al.*, High incidence of sudden death with conduction system and myocardial disease due to lamins A and C gene mutation. *Pacing Clin. Electrophysiol.* **23** (2000), 1661–1666.

67. M. Raffaele Di Barletta, E. Ricci, G. Galluzzi, *et al.*, Different mutations in the LMNA gene cause autosomal dominant and autosomal recessive Emery-Dreifuss muscular dystrophy. *Am. J. Hum. Genet.* **66** (2000), 1407–1412.

68. S. Shackleton, D. J. Lloyd, S. N. Jackson, *et al.*, LMNA, encoding lamin A/C, is mutated in partial lipodystrophy. *Nat. Genet.* **24** (2000), 153–156.

69. K. L. Wilson, The nuclear envelope, muscular dystrophy and gene expression. *Trends Cell. Biol.* **10** (2000), 125–129.

70. K. L. Wilson, M. S. Zastrow, K. K. Lee, Lamins and disease: insights into nuclear infrastructure. *Cell* **104** (2001), 647–650.

71. A. De Sandre-Giovannoli, M. Chaouch, S. Kozlov, *et al.*, Homozygous defects in LMNA, encoding lamin A/C nuclear-envelope proteins, cause autosomal recessive axonal neuropathy in human (Charcot-Marie-Tooth disorder type 2), and mouse. *Am. J. Hum. Genet.* **70** (2002), 726–736.

72. G. Novelli, A. Muchir, F. Sangiuolo, *et al.*, Mandibuloacral dysplasia is caused by a mutation in LMNA-encoding lamin A/C. *Am. J. Hum. Genet.* **71** (2002), 426–431.

73. A. M. Pendas, Z. Zhou, J. Cadinanos, *et al.*, Defective prelamin A processing and muscular and adipocyte alterations in Zmpste24 metalloproteinase-deficient mice. *Nat. Genet.* **31** (2002), 94–99.

74. A. J. van der Kooi, G. Bonne, B. Eymard, *et al.*, Lamin A/C mutations with lipodystrophy, cardiac abnormalities, and muscular dystrophy. *Neurology* **59** (2002), 620–623.

75. A. De Sandre-Giovannoli, R. Bernard, P. Cau, *et al.*, Lamin a truncation in Hutchinson-Gilford progeria. *Science* **300** (2003), 2055.

76. A. Todorova, B. Halliger-Keller, M. C. Walter, M. C. Dabauvalle, H. Lochmüller, C. R. Müller, A synonymous codon change in the LMNA gene alters mRNA splicing and causes limb girdle muscular dystrophy type 1B. *J. Med. Genet.* **40** (2003), e115.

77. E. Mercuri, M. Poppe, R. Quinlivan, *et al.*, Extreme variability of phenotype in patients with an identical missense mutation in the lamin A/C gene: from congenital onset with severe phenotype to milder classic Emery-Dreifuss variant. *Arch. Neurol.* **61** (2004), 690–694.

78. M. C. Walter, T. N. Witt, B. S. Weigel, *et al.*, Deletion of the LMNA initiator codon leading to a neurogenic variant of autosomal dominant Emery-Dreifuss muscular dystrophy. *Neuromuscul. Disord.* **15** (2005), 40–44.

79. F. Muntoni, G. Bonne, L. G. Goldfarb, *et al.*, Disease severity in dominant Emery Dreifuss is increased by mutations in both emerin and desmin proteins. *Brain* **129** (2006), 1260–1268.

80. H. Lochmüller, M. Wehnert, What message does the nuclear envelope hold? *Neurology* **68** (2007), 1879–1880.

81. W. Fang, C. C. Huang, N. S. Chu, C. J. Chen, C. S. Lu, C. C. Wang, Childhood-onset autosomal-dominant limb-girdle muscular dystrophy with cardiac conduction block. *Muscle Nerve* **20** (1997), 286–292.

82. C. Meune, J. H. Van Berlo, F. Anselme, G. Bonne, Y. M. Pinto, D. Duboc, Primary prevention of sudden death in patients with lamin A/C gene mutations. *N. Engl. J. Med.* **354** (2006), 209–210.

83. J. H. van Berlo, W. G. de Voogt, A. J. van der Kooi, *et al.*, Meta-analysis of clinical characteristics of 299 carriers of LMNA gene mutations: do lamin A/C mutations portend a high risk of sudden death? *J. Mol. Med.* **83** (2005), 79–83.

84. G. Bonne, J. Capeau, M. de Visser, *et al.*, 82nd ENMC international workshop, 5th international Emery-Dreifuss muscular dystrophy (EDMD), workshop, 1st workshop of the MYO-CLUSTER project EUROMEN (European muscle envelope nucleopathies), 15–16 September 2000, Naarden, the Netherlands. *Neuromuscul. Disord.* **12** (2002), 187–194.

85. M. Lammens, A. Muchir, K. Schwartz, *et al.*, Phenotypic characterisation of a patient with a homozygous mutation of the lamin A/C gene. *Neurology* **56** Suppl 3, (2001), 438–439.

86. D. J. Lloyd, R. C. Trembath, S. Shackleton, A novel interaction between lamin A and SREBP1: implications for partial lipodystrophy and other laminopathies. *Hum. Mol. Genet.* **11** (2002), 769–777.

87. A. Garg, R. A. Speckman, A. M. Bowcock, Multisystem dystrophy syndrome due to novel missense mutations in the amino-terminal head and alpha-helical rod domains of the lamin A/C gene. *Am. J. Med.* **112** (2002), 549–555.

88. K. M. D. Bushby, F. Muntoni, J. P. Bourke, The management of cardiac complications in muscular dystrophy and myotonic dystrophy. Proceedings of 107th ENMC Workshop. *Neuromuscul. Disord.* **13** (2003), 166–172.

89. M. Vorgerd, K. Ricker, F. Ziemssen, *et al.*, A sporadic case of rippling muscle disease caused by a de novo caveolin-3 mutation. *Neurology* **57** (2001), 2273–2277.

90. C. Kubisch, B. G. Schoser, M. von Düring, *et al.*, Homozygous mutations in caveolin-3 cause a severe form of rippling muscle disease. *Ann. Neurol.* **53** (2003), 512–520.

91. D. Fischer, A. Schroers, I. Blumcke, *et al.*, Consequences of a novel caveolin-3 mutation in a large German family. *Ann. Neurol.* **53** (2003), 233–241.

92. T. Hayashi, T. Arimura, K. Ueda, *et al.*, Identification and functional analysis of a caveolin-3 mutation associated with familial hypertrophic cardiomyopathy. *Biochem. Biophys. Res. Commun.* **313** (2004), 178–184.

93. M. Ho, R. H. Brown, Caveolinopathies. In: *Structural and Molecular Basis of Skeletal muscle Diseases*, ed. G. Karpati. (Basel: ISN Neuropath Press, 2002), pp. 33–36.

94. T. C. Watkins, L. M. Zelinka, M. Kesic, C. F. Ansevin, G. R. Walker, Identification of skeletal muscle autoantigens by expression library screening using sera from autoimmune rippling muscle disease (ARMD), patients. *J. Cell. Biochem.* **99** (2006), 79 87.

95. W. J. Schulte-Mattler, R. A. Kley, E. Rothenfusser-Korber, *et al.*, Immune-mediated rippling muscle disease. *Neurology* **64** (2005), 364–267.

96. J. Gamez, C. Navarro, A. L. Andreu, *et al.*, Autosomal dominant limb-girdle muscular dystrophy: a large kindred with evidence for anticipation. *Neurology* **56** (2001), 450–454.

97. M. Urtasun, A. Saenz, C. Roudaut, *et al.*, Limb-girdle muscular dystrophy in Guipuzcoa (Basque Country, Spain). *Brain* **121**:Pt 9 (1998), 1735–1747.

98. M. Fardeau, D. Hillaire, C. Mignard, *et al.*, Juvenile limb-girdle muscular dystrophy. Clinical, histopathological and genetic data from a small community living in the Reunion Island. *Brain* **119**: Pt 1 (1996), 295–308.

99. T. V. Pogoda, I. N. Krakhmaleva, N. A. Lipatova, N. I. Shakhovskaya, S. S. Shishkin, S. A. Limborska, High incidence of 550delA mutation of CAPN3 in LGMD2 patients from Russia. *Hum. Mutat.* **15** (2000), 295.

100. B. Georgieva, A. Todorova, I. Tournev, V. Mitev, P. Plageras, I. Kremensky, 550delA mutation in the calpain 3 (CAPN3), gene: DMD/BMD, SMA, or LGMD2A–clinically misdiagnosed cases. *Am. J. Med. Genet. A.* **136** (2005), 399–400.

101. N. Canki-Klain, A. Milic, B. Kovac, *et al.*, Prevalence of the 550delA mutation in calpainopathy (LGMD 2A), in Croatia. *Am. J. Med. Genet. A.* **125** (2004), 152–156.

102. M. R. Passos-Bueno, E. S. Moreira, S. K. Marie, *et al.*, Main clinical features of the three mapped autosomal recessive limb-girdle muscular dystrophies and estimated proportion of each form in 13 Brazilian families. *J. Med. Genet.* **33** (1996), 97–102.

103. H. Kawai, M. Akaike, M. Kunishige, *et al.*, Clinical, pathological, and genetic features of limb-girdle muscular dystrophy type 2A with new calpain 3 gene mutations in seven patients from three Japanese families. *Muscle Nerve* **21** (1998), 1493–1501.

104. C. Pollitt, L. V. Anderson, R. Pogue, K. Davison, A. Pyle, K. M. Bushby, The phenotype of calpainopathy: diagnosis based on a multidisciplinary approach. *Neuromuscul. Disord.* **11** (2001), 287–296.

105. F. de Paula, M. Vainzof, M. R. Passos-Bueno, *et al.*, Clinical variability in calpainopathy: what makes the difference? *Eur. J. Hum. Genet.* **10** (2002), 825–832.

106. A. Sáenz, F. Leturcq, A. M. Cobo, *et al.*, LGMD2A: genotype-phenotype correlations based on a large mutational survey on the calpain 3 gene. *Brain* **128** (2005), 732–742.

107. B. Balci, S. Aurino, G. Haliloglu, *et al.*, Calpain-3 mutations in Turkey. *Eur. J. Pediatr.* **165** (2006), 293–298.

108. E. J. Groen, R. Charlton, R. Barresi, *et al.*, Analysis of the UK diagnostic strategy for limb girdle muscular dystrophy 2A. *Brain* **130** (2007), 3237–3249.

109. E. Mercuri, K. Bushby, E. Ricci, *et al.*, Muscle MRI findings in patients with limb girdle muscular dystrophy with calpain 3 deficiency (LGMD2A), and early contractures. *Neuromuscul. Disord.* **15** (2005), 164–171.

110. F. L. Chou, C. Angelini, D. Daentl, *et al.*, Calpain III mutation analysis of a heterogeneous limb-girdle muscular dystrophy population. *Neurology* **52** (1999), 1015–1020.

111. A. Starling, F. de Paula, H. Silva, M. Vainzof, M. Zatz, Calpainopathy: how broad is the spectrum of clinical variability? *J. Mol. Neurosci.* **21** (2003), 233–236.

112. L. V. Anderson, K. Davison, J. A. Moss, *et al.*, Characterization of monoclonal antibodies to calpain 3 and protein expression in muscle from patients with limb-girdle muscular dystrophy type 2A. *Am. J. Pathol.* **153** (1998), 1169–1179.

113. I. Richard, L. Brenguier, P. Dincer, *et al.*, Multiple independent molecular etiology for limb-girdle muscular dystrophy type 2A patients from various geographical origins. *Am. J. Hum. Genet.* **60** (1997), 1128–1138.

114. M. Fanin, A. C. Nascimbeni, L. Fulizio, C. Angelini, The frequency of limb girdle muscular dystrophy 2A in northeastern Italy. *Neuromuscul. Disord.* **15** (2005), 218–224.

115. S. Baghdiguian, M. Martin, I. Richard, *et al.*, Calpain 3 deficiency is associated with myonuclear apoptosis and profound perturbation of the IkappaB alpha/NF-kappaB pathway in limb-girdle muscular dystrophy type 2A. *Nat. Med.* **5** (1999), 503–511.

116. I. Richard, C. Roudaut, S. Marchand, *et al.*, Loss of calpain 3 proteolytic activity leads to muscular dystrophy and to apoptosis-associated IkappaBalpha/nuclear factor kappaB pathway perturbation in mice. *J. Cell. Biol.* **151** (2000), 1583–1590.

117. H. Sorimachi, S. Kimura, K. Kinbara, *et al.*, Structure and physiological functions of ubiquitous and tissue-specific calpain

species. Muscle-specific calpain, p94, interacts with connectin/titin. *Adv. Biophys.* **33** (1996), 101–122.

118. I. Richard, C. Roudaut, A. Sáenz, *et al.*, Calpainopathy – a survey of mutations and polymorphisms. *Am. J. Hum. Genet.* **64** (1999), 1524–1540.

119. H. Sorimachi, Y. Ono, K. Suzuki, Skeletal muscle-specific calpain, p94, and connectin/titin: their physiological functions and relationship to limb-girdle muscular dystrophy type 2A. *Adv. Exp. Med. Biol.* **481** (2000), 383–395.

120. L. V. Anderson, Optimized protein diagnosis in the autosomal recessive limb-girdle muscular dystrophies. *Neuromuscul. Disord.* **6** (1996), 443–446.

121. P. Dincer, F. Leturcq, I. Richard, *et al.*, A biochemical, genetic, and clinical survey of autosomal recessive limb girdle muscular dystrophies in Turkey. *Ann. Neurol.* **42** (1997), 222–229.

122. I. Kramerova, E. Kudryashova, J. G. Tidball, M. J. Spencer, Null mutation of calpain 3 (p94), in mice causes abnormal sarcomere formation in vivo and in vitro. *Hum. Mol. Genet.* **13** (2004), 1373–1388.

123. M. Krahn, A. Lopez de Munain, N. Streichenberger, *et al.*, CAPN3 mutations in patients with idiopathic eosinophilic myositis. *Ann. Neurol.* **59** (2006), 905–911.

124. M. J. Spencer, J. G. Tidball, L. V. Anderson, *et al.*, Absence of calpain 3 in a form of limb-girdle muscular dystrophy (LGMD2A). *J. Neurol. Sci.* **146** (1997), 173–178.

125 L. V. B. Anderson, Multiplex western blot analysis of the muscular dystrophy proteins. In *Muscular Dystrophy: Methods and Protocols*, eds. K. M. D. Bushby, L. V. B. Anderson. (Totowa, NJ: Humana Press, 2001), pp. 369–386.

126. A. Milic, N. Daniele, H. Lochmüller, *et al.*, A third of LGMD2A biopsies have normal calpain 3 proteolytic activity as determined by an in vitro assay. *Neuromuscul. Disord.* **17** (2007), 148–156.

127. R. Lanzillo, S. Aurino, M. Fanin, *et al.*, Early onset calpainopathy with normal non-functional calpain 3 level. *Dev. Med. Child. Neurol.* **48** (2006), 304–306.

128. M. Fanin, L. Fulizio, A. C. Nascimbeni, *et al.*, Molecular diagnosis in LGMD2A: mutation analysis or protein testing? *Hum. Mutat.* **24** (2004), 52–62.

129. L. V. Anderson, R. M. Harrison, R. Pogue, *et al.*, Secondary reduction in calpain 3 expression in patients with limb girdle muscular dystrophy type 2B and Miyoshi myopathy (primary dysferlinopathies). *Neuromuscul. Disord.* **10** (2000), 553–559.

130. M. Vainzof, L. V. Anderson, E. M. McNally, *et al.*, Dysferlin protein analysis in limb-girdle muscular dystrophies. *J. Mol. Neurosci.* **17** (2001), 71–80.

131. H. Haravuori, A. Vihola, V. Straub, *et al.*, Secondary calpain3 deficiency in 2q-linked muscular dystrophy: titin is the candidate gene. *Neurology* **56** (2001), 869–877.

132. N. Minami, I. Nishino, O. Kobayashi, K. Ikezoe, Y. Goto, I. Nonaka, Mutations of calpain 3 gene in patients with sporadic limb-girdle muscular dystrophy in Japan. *J. Neurol. Sci.* **171** (1999), 31–37.

133. J. Chae, N. Minami, Y. Jin, *et al.*, Calpain 3 gene mutations: genetic and clinico-pathologic findings in limb-girdle muscular dystrophy. *Neuromuscul. Disord.* **11** (2001), 547–555.

134. G. Piluso, L. Politano, S. Aurino, *et al.*, Extensive scanning of the calpain-3 gene broadens the spectrum of LGMD2A phenotypes. *J. Med. Genet.* **42** (2005), 686–693.

135. I. Illa, Distal myopathies. *J. Neurol.* **247** (2000), 169–174.

136. K. Nguyen, G. Bassez, M. Krahn, *et al.*, Phenotypic study in 40 patients with dysferlin gene mutations: high frequency of atypical phenotypes. *Arch. Neurol.* **64** (2007), 1176–1182.

137. I. Illa, N. de Luna, R. Dominguez-Perles, *et al.*, Symptomatic dysferlin gene mutation carriers: characterization of two cases. *Neurology* **68** (2007), 1284–1289.

138. A. Diers, M. Carl, G. Stoltenburg-Didinger, M. Vorgerd, S. Spuler, Painful enlargement of the calf muscles in limb girdle muscular dystrophy type 2B (LGMD2B), with a novel compound heterozygous mutation in DYSF. *Neuromuscul. Disord.* **17** (2007), 157–162.

139. Z. Argov, M. Sadeh, K. Mazor, *et al.*, Muscular dystrophy due to dysferlin deficiency in Libyan Jews. Clinical and genetic features. *Brain* **123**:Pt 6, (2000), 1229–1237.

140. E. Leshinsky-Silver, Z. Argov, L. Rozenboim, *et al.*, Dysferlinopathy in the Jews of the Caucasus: a frequent mutation in the dysferlin gene. *Neuromuscul. Disord.* **17** (2007), 950–954.

141. T. Weiler, R. Bashir, L. V. Anderson, *et al.*, Identical mutation in patients with limb girdle muscular dystrophy type 2B or Miyoshi myopathy suggests a role for modifier gene(s). *Hum. Mol. Genet.* **8** (1999), 871–877.

142. S. N. Illarioshkin, I. A. Ivanova-Smolenskaya, C. R. Greenberg, *et al.*, Identical dysferlin mutation in limb-girdle muscular dystrophy type 2B and distal myopathy. *Neurology* **55** (2000), 1931–1933.

143. I. Illa, C. Serrano-Munuera, E. Gallardo, *et al.*, Distal anterior compartment myopathy: a dysferlin mutation causing a new muscular dystrophy phenotype. *Ann. Neurol.* **49** (2001), 130–134.

144. I. Mahjneh, G. Marconi, K. Bushby, L. V. Anderson, H. Tolvanen-Mahjneh, H. Somer, Dysferlinopathy (LGMD2B): a 23-year follow-up study of 10 patients homozygous for the same frameshifting dysferlin mutations. *Neuromuscul. Disord.* **11** (2001), 20–26.

145. L. V. Anderson, K. Davison, J. A. Moss, *et al.*, Dysferlin is a plasma membrane protein and is expressed early in human development. *Hum. Mol. Genet.* **8** (1999), 855–861.

146. Y. Huang, S. H. Laval, A. van Remoortere, *et al.*, AHNAK, a novel component of the dysferlin protein complex, redistributes to the cytoplasm with dysferlin during skeletal muscle regeneration. *FASEB J.* **21** (2007), 732–742.

147. F. Piccolo, S. A. Moore, G. C. Ford, K. P. Campbell, Intracellular accumulation and reduced sarcolemmal expression of dysferlin in limb-girdle muscular dystrophies. *Ann. Neurol.* **48** (2000), 902–912.

148. L. Klinge, S. Laval, S. Keers, *et al.*, From T-tubule to sarcolemma: damage-induced dysferlin translocation in early myogenesis. *FASEB J.* **21** (2007), 1768–1776.

149. D. Bansal, K. Miyake, S. S. Vogel, *et al.*, Defective membrane repair in dysferlin-deficient muscular dystrophy. *Nature* **423** (2003), 168–172.

150. J. K. Jaiswal, G. Marlow, G. Summerill, *et al.*, Patients with a non-dysferlin Miyoshi myopathy have a novel membrane repair defect. *Traffic* **8** (2007), 77–88.

151. M. Ho, E. Gallardo, D. McKenna-Yasek, N. de Luna, I. Illa, R. H. Brown Jr., A novel, blood-based diagnostic assay for limb girdle muscular dystrophy 2B and Miyoshi myopathy. *Ann. Neurol.* **51** (2002), 129–133.

152. K. Wenzel, C. Geier, F. Qadri, *et al.*, Dysfunction of dysferlin-deficient hearts. *J. Mol. Med.* **85** (2007), 1203–1214.

153. R. Han, D. Bansal, K. Miyake, *et al.*, Dysferlin-mediated membrane repair protects the heart from stress-induced left ventricular injury. *J. Clin. Invest.* **117** (2007), 1805–1813.

154. C. Angelini, M. Fanin, M. P. Freda, D. J. Duggan, G. Siciliano, E. P. Hoffman, The clinical spectrum of sarcoglycanopathies. *Neurology* **52** (1999), 176–179.

155. D. J. Duggan, J. R. Gorospe, M. Fanin, E. P. Hoffman, C. Angelini, Mutations in the sarcoglycan genes in patients with myopathy. *N. Engl. J. Med.* **336** (1997), 618–624.

156. R. Fadic, A. J. Waclawik, P. J. Lewandoski, B. P. Lotz, Muscle pathology and clinical features of the sarcolemmopathies. *Pediatr. Neurol.* **16** (1997), 79–82.

157. K. B. Othmane, D. Loeb, R. Hayworth-Hodgte, *et al.*, Physical and genetic mapping of the CMT4A locus and exclusion of PMP-2 as the defect in CMT4A. *Genomics* **28** (1995), 286–290.

158. E. S. Moreira, M. Vainzof, O. T. Suzuki, R. C. Pavanello, M. Zatz, M. R. Passos-Bueno, Genotype-phenotype correlations in 35 Brazilian families with sarcoglycanopathies including the description of three novel mutations. *J. Med. Genet.* **40** (2003), E12.

159. A. K. Meena, D. Sreenivas, C. Sundaram, *et al.*, Sarcoglycanopathies: a clinico-pathological study. *Neurol. India* **55** (2007), 117–121.

160. S. J. White, S. U. de Willige, D. Verbove, *et al.*, Sarcoglycanopathies and the risk of undetected deletion alleles in diagnosis. *Hum. Mutat.* **26** (2005), 59.

161. M. C. Walter, G. Dekomien, B. Schlotter-Weigel, *et al.*, Respiratory insufficiency as a presenting symptom of LGMD2D in adulthood. *Acta Myol.* **23** (2004), 1–5.

162. L. Politano, V. Nigro, L. Passamano, *et al.*, Evaluation of cardiac and respiratory involvement in sarcoglycanopathies. *Neuromuscul. Disord.* **11** (2001), 178–185.

163. L. Merlini, J. C. Kaplan, C. Navarro, *et al.*, Homogeneous phenotype of the gypsy limb-girdle MD with the gamma-sarcoglycan C283Y mutation. *Neurology* **54** (2000), 1075–1079.

164. F. Calvo, S. Teijeira, J. M. Fernandez, *et al.*, Evaluation of heart involvement in gamma-sarcoglycanopathy (LGMD2C). A study of ten patients. *Neuromuscul. Disord.* **10** (2000), 560–566.

165 C. G. Bonnemann, Disorders of the sarcoglycan complex (sarcoglycanopathies). In *Neuromuscular Diseases: From Basic Mechanisms to Clinical Management*, ed. F. Deymeer. (Basel: Karger, 2000), pp. 26–43.

166. A. J. van der Kooi, W. G. de Voogt, P. G. Barth, *et al.*, The heart in limb girdle muscular dystrophy. *Heart* **79** (1998), 73–77.

167. A. Prelle, G. P. Comi, L. Tancredi, *et al.*, Sarcoglycan deficiency in a large Italian population of myopathic patients. *Acta Neuropathol. Berl.* **96** (1998), 509–514.

168. M. Yoshida, E. Ozawa, Glycoprotein complex anchoring dystrophin to sarcolemma. *J. Biochem. Tokyo* **108** (1990), 748–752.

169. T. Rando, The dystrophin-glycoprotein complex, cellular signalling and the regulation of cell survival in the muscular dystrophies. *Muscle Nerve* **24** (2001), 1575–1594.

170. A. J. Ettinger, G. Feng, J. R. Sanes, Epsilon-sarcoglycan, a broadly expressed homologue of the gene mutated in limb-girdle muscular dystrophy 2D. *J. Biol. Chem.* **272** (1997), 32534–32538.

171. E. M. McNally, C. T. Ly, L. M. Kunkel, Human epsilon-sarcoglycan is highly related to alpha-sarcoglycan (adhalin), the limb girdle muscular dystrophy 2D gene. *FEBS Lett.* **422** (1998), 27–32.

172. V. Straub, A. J. Ettinger, M. Durbeej, *et al.*, Epsilon-sarcoglycan replaces alpha-sarcoglycan in smooth muscle to form a unique dystrophin-glycoprotein complex. *J. Biol. Chem.* **274** (1999), 27989–27996.

173. A. Zimprich, M. Grabowski, F. Asmus, *et al.*, Mutations in the gene encoding epsilon-sarcoglycan cause myoclonus-dystonia syndrome. *Nat. Genet.* **29** (2001), 66–69.

174. M. T. Wheeler, S. Zarnegar, E. M. McNally, Zeta-sarcoglycan, a novel component of the sarcoglycan complex, is reduced in muscular dystrophy. *Hum. Mol. Genet.* **11** (2002), 2147–2154.

175. M. Vainzof, M. R. Passos-Bueno, M. Canovas, *et al.*, The sarcoglycan complex in the six autosomal recessive limb-girdle muscular dystrophies. *Hum. Mol. Genet.* **5** (1996), 1963–199.

176. C. G. Bonnemann, Limb-girdle muscular dystrophies: an overview. *J. Child. Neurol.* **14** (1999), 31–33.

177. M. Vainzof, M. R. Passos-Bueno, R. C. Pavanello, S. K. Marie, A. S. Oliveira, M. Zatz, Sarcoglycanopathies are responsible for 68% of severe autosomal recessive limb-girdle muscular dystrophy in the Brazilian population. *J. Neurol. Sci.* **164** (1999), 44–49.

178. R. H. Crosbie, C. S. Lebakken, K. H. Holt, *et al.*, Membrane targeting and stabilization of sarcospan is mediated by the sarcoglycan subcomplex. *J. Cell. Biol.* **145** (1999), 153–165.

179. W. Yee, Z. Pramono, C. Tan, P. Kathiravelu, P. Lai, Limb girdle muscular dystrophy 2G and novel TCAP mutation in ethnic chinese. *Neuromuscul. Disord.* **17**:9 (2007), 814.

180. B. L. Lima, T. L. Gouveia, R. C. Pavanello, *et al.*, LGMD2G: screening for mutations in a large sample of Brazilian patients allows the identification of new cases. *Neuromuscul. Disord.* **15** (2005), 687.

181. G. Valle, G. Faulkner, A. de Antoni, *et al.*, Telethonin, a novel sarcomeric protein of heart and skeletal muscle. *FEBS Lett.* **415** (1997), 163–168.

182. R. Knoll, M. Hoshijima, H. M. Hoffman, *et al.*, The cardiac mechanical stretch sensor machinery involves a Z disc complex that is defective in a subset of human dilated cardiomyopathy. *Cell* **111** (2002), 943–955.

183. T. Hayashi, T. Arimura, M. Itoh-Satoh, *et al.*, Tcap gene mutations in hypertrophic cardiomyopathy and dilated cardiomyopathy. *J. Am. Coll. Cardiol.* **44** (2004), 2192–2201.

184. M. Vainzof, E. S. Moreira, O. T. Suzuki, *et al.*, Telethonin protein expression in neuromuscular disorders. *Biochim. Biophys. Acta* **1588** (2002), 33–40.

185. B. G. Schoser, P. Frosk, A. G. Engel, U. Klutzny, H. Lochmüller, K. Wrogemann, Commonality of TRIM32 mutation in causing sarcotubular myopathy and LGMD2H. *Ann. Neurol.* **57** (2005), 591–595.

186. P. Frosk, C. R. Greenberg, A. A. Tennese, *et al.*, The most common mutation in FKRP causing limb girdle muscular dystrophy type 2I (LGMD2I), may have occurred only once

and is present in Hutterites and other populations. *Hum. Mutat.* **25** (2005), 38–44.

187. M. Poppe, J. Bourke, M. Eagle, *et al.*, Cardiac and respiratory failure in limb-girdle muscular dystrophy 2I. *Ann. Neurol.* **56** (2004), 738–741.
188. C. Gaul, M. Deschauer, C. Tempelmann, *et al.*, Cardiac involvement in limb-girdle muscular dystrophy 2I: conventional cardiac diagnostic and cardiovascular magnetic resonance. *J. Neurol.* **253** (2006), 1317–1322.
189. E. Mercuri, M. Brockington, V. Straub, *et al.*, Phenotypic spectrum associated with mutations in the fukutin-related protein gene. *Ann. Neurol.* **53** (2003), 537–542.
190. M. Poppe, L. Cree, J. Bourke, *et al.*, The phenotype of limb-girdle muscular dystrophy type 2I. *Neurology* **60** (2003), 1246–1251.
191. M. C. Walter, J. A. Petersen, R. Stucka, *et al.*, FKRP (826C > A), frequently causes limb-girdle muscular dystrophy in German patients. *J. Med. Genet.* **41** (2004), e50.
192. F. Muntoni, M. Brockington, D. J. Blake, S. Torelli, S. C. Brown, Defective glycosylation in muscular dystrophy. *Lancet* **360** (2002), 1419–1421.
193. S. C. Brown, S. Torelli, M. Brockington, *et al.*, Abnormalities in alpha-dystroglycan expression in MDC1C and LGMD2I muscular dystrophies. *Am. J. Pathol.* **164** (2004), 727–737.
194. K. Bushby, L. V. Anderson, C. Pollitt, I. Naom, F. Muntoni, L. Bindoff, Abnormal merosin in adults. A new form of late onset muscular dystrophy not linked to chromosome 6q2. *Brain* **121**:Pt 4, (1998), 581–588.
195. D. E. Michele, R. Barresi, M. Kanagawa, *et al.*, Post-translational disruption of dystroglycan-ligand interactions in congenital muscular dystrophies. *Nature* **418** (2002), 417–422.
196. R. D. Cohn, Dystroglycan: important player in skeletal muscle and beyond. *Neuromuscul. Disord.* **15** (2005), 207–217.
197. F. Muntoni, Journey into muscular dystrophies caused by abnormal glycosylation. *Acta Myol.* **23** (2004), 79–84.
198. P. B. Kang, C. A. Feener, E. Estrella, *et al.*, LGMD2I in a North American population. *BMC. Musculoskelet. Disord.* **8** (2007), 115.
199. F. de Paula, N. Vieira, A. Starling, *et al.*, Asymptomatic carriers for homozygous novel mutations in the FKRP gene: the other end of the spectrum. *Eur. J. Hum. Genet.* **11** (2003), 923–930.
200. M. Schwartz, J. M. Hertz, M. L. Sveen, J. Vissing, LGMD2I presenting with a characteristic Duchenne or Becker muscular dystrophy phenotype. *Neurology* **64** (2005), 1635–1637.
201. N. M. Vieira, D. Schlesinger, F. de Paula, M. Vainzof, M. Zatz, Mutation analysis in the FKRP gene provides an explanation for a rare cause of intrafamilial clinical variability in LGMD2I. *Neuromuscul. Disord.* **16** (2006), 870–873.
202. L. U. Yamamoto, M. Canovas, R. C. M. Pavanello, *et al.*, Muscle protein alterations in patients with mutations in the Fukutin Related Protein gene. In Annual Meeting of the American Society of Human Genetics, volume 73, pp. 556. *Am. J. Hum. Genet.* **556** (2003).
203. N. Darin, A. K. Kroksmark, A. C. Ahlander, A. R. Moslemi, A. Oldfors, M. Tulinius, Inflammation and response to steroid treatment in limb-girdle muscular dystrophy 2I. *Eur. J. Paediatr. Neurol.* **11** (2007), 353–357.
204. C. Godfrey, D. Escolar, M. Brockington, *et al.*, Fukutin gene mutations in steroid-responsive limb girdle muscular dystrophy. *Ann. Neurol.* **60** (2006), 603–610.
205. P. Dincer, B. Balci, Y. Yuva, *et al.*, A novel form of recessive limb girdle muscular dystrophy with mental retardation and abnormal expression of alpha-dystroglycan. *Neuromuscul. Disord.* **13** (2003), 771–778.
206. B. Balci, G. Uyanik, P. Dincer, *et al.*, An autosomal recessive limb girdle muscular dystrophy (LGMD2), with mild mental retardation is allelic to Walker-Warburg syndrome (WWS), caused by a mutation in the POMT1 gene. *Neuromuscul. Disord.* **15** (2005), 271–275.
207. R. Biancheri, A. Falace, A. Tessa, *et al.*, POMT2 gene mutation in limb-girdle muscular dystrophy with inflammatory changes. *Biochem. Biophys. Res. Commun.* **363** (2007), 1033–1037.
208. B. Udd, Limb-girdle type muscular dystrophy in a large family with distal myopathy: homozygous manifestation of a dominant gene? *J. Med. Genet.* **29** (1992), 383–389.
209. B. Udd, H. Haravuori, H. Kalimo, *et al.*, Tibial muscular dystrophy – from clinical description to linkage on chromosome 2q31. *Neuromuscul. Disord.* **8** (1998), 327–332.
210. B. Udd, J. Partanen, P. Halonen, *et al.*, Tibial muscular dystrophy. Late adult-onset distal myopathy in 66 Finnish patients. *Arch. Neurol.* **50** (1993), 604–608.
211. B. Udd, A. Vihola, J. Sarparanta, I. Richard, P. Hackman, Titinopathies and extension of the M-line mutation phenotype beyond distal myopathy and LGMD2J. *Neurology* **64** (2005), 636–642.
212. H. Haravuori, P. Makela-Bengs, B. Udd, *et al.*, Assignment of the tibial muscular dystrophy locus to chromosome 2q31. *Am. J. Hum. Genet.* **62** (1998), 620–626.
213. J. Jarry, M. F. Rioux, V. Bolduc, *et al.*, A novel autosomal recessive limb-girdle muscular dystrophy with quadriceps atrophy maps to 11p13-p12. *Brain* **130** (2007), 368–380.
214. N. Daniele, I. Richard, M. Bartoli, Ins and outs of therapy in limb girdle muscular dystrophies. *Int. J. Biochem. Cell. Biol.* **39** (2007), 1608–1624.

Chapter 12

Dystrophic myopathies of early childhood onset (congenital muscular dystrophies)

Carsten G. Bönnemann and Enrico Bertini

Introduction

Since the late 1990s, molecular genetic advances have led to a great expansion of knowledge pertaining to the classification and molecular pathogenesis of the congenital muscular dystrophies (CMDs). First recognized by Batten in his classical description of 1909 [1], the designation congenital muscular dystrophy now encompasses a heterogeneous group of genetically, clinically, and biochemically distinct entities, and in essence applies to infants presenting with muscle weakness at birth or within the first few months of life in association with a muscle biopsy showing features of a dystrophic myopathy [2]. However, the dystrophic aspects in the muscle biopsy may not be prominent early on so that a biopsy just displaying myopathic features is still compatible with a diagnosis of CMD, as long as there are no other specific histological findings suggestive of an alternative diagnosis. The CMDs can currently be classified into four major groups based on the genes involved and on the predicted function and localization of their respective protein products: (1) abnormalities of α-dystroglycan glycosylation and defects in other membrane receptors (fukutin, POMGnT1, POMT1, POMT2, FKRP, LARGE, and ITGA7), (2) abnormalities of extracellular matrix proteins (LAMA2, COL6A1, COL6A2, COL6A3), (3) abnormalities of nuclear proteins (lamin A/C and nesprin), and (4) abnormalities at the level of the endoplasmic reticulum (SEPN1). The molecular classes 1 and 2 involve the extracellular matrix and its receptors on muscle and taken together account for the majority of CMD patients.

Congenital muscular dystrophies as a group begin in the prenatal or in the perinatal period presenting with hypotonia and weakness, although symptoms and disabilities may also first become apparent somewhat later during the first year of life. There may also be associated contractures or hypermobility of various joints as well as significant central nervous system (CNS) and ocular involvement in some forms. Careful attention to such clinical clues as well as paraclinical findings such as CNS and muscle imaging is important in guiding the diagnostic work-up. Immunohistochemistry of muscle biopsy sections using a battery of antibodies is further useful in directing the clinician to the appropriate genetic testing necessary to confirm the diagnosis.

Abnormalities of α-dystroglycan glycosylation and other membrane receptors

Alpha-dystroglycanopathies (disorders of *O*-mannosyl-glycosylation)

Definition of the entity or entities; basis for their classification

The group of CMDs characterized by abnormal *O*-mannosyl-glycosylation of α-dystroglycan (α-dystroglycanopathies) include the Fukuyama-type (fukutin related) congenital muscular dystrophy (FCMD) [#253800] muscle eye brain disease (MEB) [#253280], Walker–Warburg syndrome (WWS) [#236670], congenital muscular dystrophy 1C (FKRP related or MDC1C) [#606612] which is allelic to limb-girdle muscular dystrophy (LGMD2I) [#607155], and congenital muscular dystrophy 1D (LARGE-related MDC1D) [#608840] [2, 3, 4, 5, 6, 7, 8, 9]. All the phenotypes along this spectrum are genetically heterogeneous with mutations residing in at least six genes encoding proven or putative glycosyltransferases [10]. The immunohistochemical hallmark for all of these conditions is reduced staining for glycosylated α-dystroglycan with preserved staining for the α-dystroglycan core protein by immunohistochemistry in the muscle sarcolemma [11]. Hypoglycosylation of specifically the *O*-mannosyl-glycosylated residues of α-dystroglycan in skeletal muscle is associated with abolished ligand binding activity of laminin-α2, agrin, and neurexin [11]. This diminished binding activity results in a variable secondary deficiency of laminin-α2 in tissues, particularly brain and muscle. Consistent with these observations, all identified gene products underlying disorders in this group are thought to play a role in this glycosylation process of α-dystroglycan. Mutations in the glycosyltransferase genes of protein *O*-mannose β1,2-*N*-acetylglucosaminyltransferase 1 (POMGnT1) [*606822] and protein *O*-mannosyltransferase 1 and 2 (POMT1 [*607423] and POMT2 [*607439]) were initially identified in patients with MEB and WWS, respectively [4, 7, 9]. In addition, other

Disorders of Voluntary Muscle, 8th edn., eds. George Karpati, David Hilton-Jones, Kate Bushby and Robert C. Griggs. Published by Cambridge University Press.

responsible gene products discovered in this group, including fukutin [*607440], fukutin-related protein (FKRP) [*606596], and LARGE [*603590] are also predicted to be structurally similar to glycosyltransferases and are thought to directly and indirectly cooperate in this process [12].

While initial studies suggested a tight association between mutations in each of the individual genes and specific phenotypes [3, 4, 6, 7, 9], more recently it has become increasingly clear that mutations in each gene can be associated with a wide and largely overlapping phenotypic spectrum, as is illustrated most strikingly in the case of FKRP mutations, which can cause a spectrum ranging from severe WWS to mild late-onset limb-girdle muscular dystrophy (LGMD) [13, 14, 15].

The first gene to be related to an α-dystroglycanopathy [3] was fukutin in Fukuyama-type congenital muscular dystrophy (FCMD), an autosomal recessive disorder initially described in the Japanese population [16]. Its incidence is relatively high in Japan, as most Japanese FCMD patients carry an ancestral 3-kb retrotransposonal insertion in the 3′ noncoding region of the fukutin gene. Fukutin was also the first gene in this group of disorders for which a glycosyltransferase function was suggested on the basis of the presence of a DXD motif in the amino acid sequence [17]. Fukutin-related protein gene (FKRP) was then initially characterized based upon its sequence homology with fukutin, including the presence of the DXD motif [18]. Mutations in the FKRP gene were initially detected in the two distinct phenotypes of congenital muscular dystrophy type 1C (MDC1C) and limb-girdle muscular dystrophy type 2I (LGMD 2) [10]. However, FKRP mutations at this point are associated with the widest phenotypic spectrum amongst the α-dystroglycanopathies, including patients exhibiting lissencephaly, pachygyria, and brain stem hypoplasia suggestive of the Walker–Warburg phenotype as well as patients with mental retardation and evidence of cerebellar abnormalities such as cerebellar cysts [19, 20].

Muscle eye brain disease (MEB) is an autosomal recessive disorder originally described in genetically isolated Finnish populations. It is characterized by congenital muscular dystrophy, ocular abnormalities (congenital myopia, glaucoma, and retinal hypoplasia), and significant structural brain malformations (pachygyria, cerebellar hypoplasia, and a flat brain stem) [4]. Using a positional cloning strategy, mutations in the gene coding for POMGnT1, a type II membrane protein similar to other Golgi glycosyltransferases, have now been described in the Finnish patients and in patients throughout the world [21]. However, it is now clear that the phenotype of MEB is also genetically heterogeneous and mutations in other genes along the α-dystroglycan *O*-mannosyl-glycosylation pathway may additionally underlie variations of this phenotype [13]. Walker–Warburg syndrome (WWS) is the final and most severe of the classic syndromes in this group of disorders, characterized by severe brain involvement including lissencephaly type II (cobblestone complex), posterior fossa malformations, and severe eye malformations leading to early lethality. Using positional cloning, mutations in the gene *POMT1* coding for protein-*O*-mannosyl transferase 1 were originally reported as underlying the condition [7]. However, *POMT1* mutations have also been subsequently found in considerably milder presentations, such as limb-girdle muscle dystrophies with mental retardation with or without microcephaly and normal brain MRI [22] or CMD with mental retardation and variable brain involvement on brain MRI, ranging from normal to an MEB phenotype [13, 15] consistent with the idea of a phenotypic spectrum. Mutations in the gene coding for protein-*O*-mannosyl transferase 2 (*POMT2*) were initially described in typical WWS patients [9], but two compound heterozygous missense mutations were recently reported in a child with a milder phenotype characterized by mental retardation, microcephaly, cerebellar hypoplasia, and increased cisterna magna resembling the MEB phenotype [14] and in other patients with CMD who also had some cortical atrophy [23]. The identification of altered glycosylation of α-dystroglycan due to a loss-of-function mutation of a putative glycosyltransferase named Large in the myodystrophy mouse model (Largemyd) was the first demonstration that abnormal glycosylation can cause a neuromuscular disorder in an animal model and also generated an additional candidate gene for human α-dystroglycanopathies [24]. Analysis of the human LARGE gene for the presence of mutations in 36 patients with muscular dystrophy and mental retardation, or structural brain changes or abnormal α-dystroglycan immunolabeling, which were unlinked to any other reported CMD loci, led to the identification of mutations in a 17-year-old girl with congenital weakness, profound mental retardation, abnormal electroretinogram (abnormal b wave), abnormal white matter, and subtle abnormalities of neuronal migration [8]. This condition has been referred to as MDC1D. Recently a patient with WWS was also found to carry mutations in the LARGE gene [25], again emphasizing genetic heterogeneity within the clinical conditions and pleiotropy of the individual genes.

Salient diagnostic criteria

The various forms of CMD with α-dystroglycan deficiency (including WWS, MEB, FCMD, MDC1C, and MDC1D, and overlap syndromes) form a broad clinical spectrum ranging from the most severe manifestations of WWS via various combinations of a muscular dystrophy with brain anomalies/mental retardation and eye involvement to a pure muscular dystrophy with normal brain function. The anatomical hallmarks of the central nervous system involvement include lissencephaly type II (cobblestone complex), ranging from complete lissencephaly to more focal pachygyria, polymicrogyria, pontocerebellar hypoplasia, and abnormalities of cerebellar foliation and cerebellar cysts (Figure 12.1). There may also be hydrocephalus, and occipital encephalocele in extreme cases. The white matter signal on T_2-weighted MRI is often abnormal. In its typical appearance the pattern of CNS involvement on imaging can be highly characteristic for these conditions and therefore be of great diagnostic help. Since the underlying genetic defects in this group of disorders are mutations in known or putative glycosyltransferase enzymes and cooperating proteins, which among their substrates most prominently include α-dystroglycan, α-dystroglycanopathies are characterized by an apparent deficiency of immunolabeling of α-dystroglycan using antibodies directed against glycosylated α-dystroglycan (Figure 12.2).

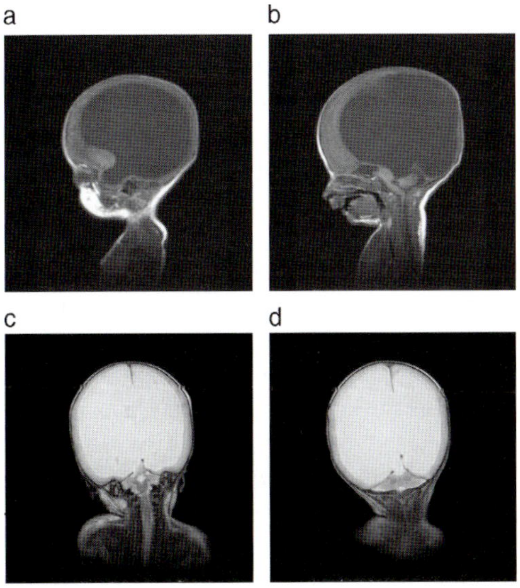

Figure 12.1a–d. MRI of a 4-month-old child with Walker–Warburg syndrome (WWS). (a, b) T_1-weighted parasagittal (a) and sagittal sections (b). (c, d) T_2-weighted coronal sections. Note severe hydrocephalus, marked ponto-cerebellar hypoplasia, and type II lissencephaly (cobblestone complex). Now at age 1 year the child has not achieved any head control but shows some antigravity movements of upper limbs and is able to suck and swallow.

Molecular genetics and pathogenesis

Perturbation of the synthesis specifically of *O*-mannosyl tetra-saccharides (a fairly rare modification in mammals) leads to hypoglycosylation of α-dystroglycan and abolishes ligand-binding activity [11, 26]. It is believed that hypoglycosylation of α-dystroglycan and subsequently diminished binding of dystroglycan to its various ligand partners, in particular to laminin-α2, leads to a disruption of the critical link between the cytoskeleton and extracellular matrix in skeletal muscle. The pathological changes in the human central nervous system are thought to be secondary to defects of the pial glia limitans that resemble the morphological findings observed in mice with a tissue-specific deletion of dystroglycan in brain [27], although there are probably additional perturbations that play a role. Phenotypic severity appears to correlate approximately with the degree of depletion of α-dystroglycan and secondary reduction in laminin-α2 [16].

Salient clinical phenotypical features

Fukuyama-type congenital muscular dystrophy (FCMD) patients manifest muscle weakness and general hypotonia usually appearing before 9 months of age. The infant appears floppy and exhibits significant motor developmental delay. Poor sucking and a mildly weak cry during the neonatal period are noticed in about half of the cases [28], while feeding difficulties and respiratory distress are rare at this early stage but may become more prominent as the disease progresses. Proximal muscles of the upper body (i.e., neck, shoulder girdle, and upper arm) and distal muscles of lower limbs (especially calf muscles) tend to be affected more significantly. Joint

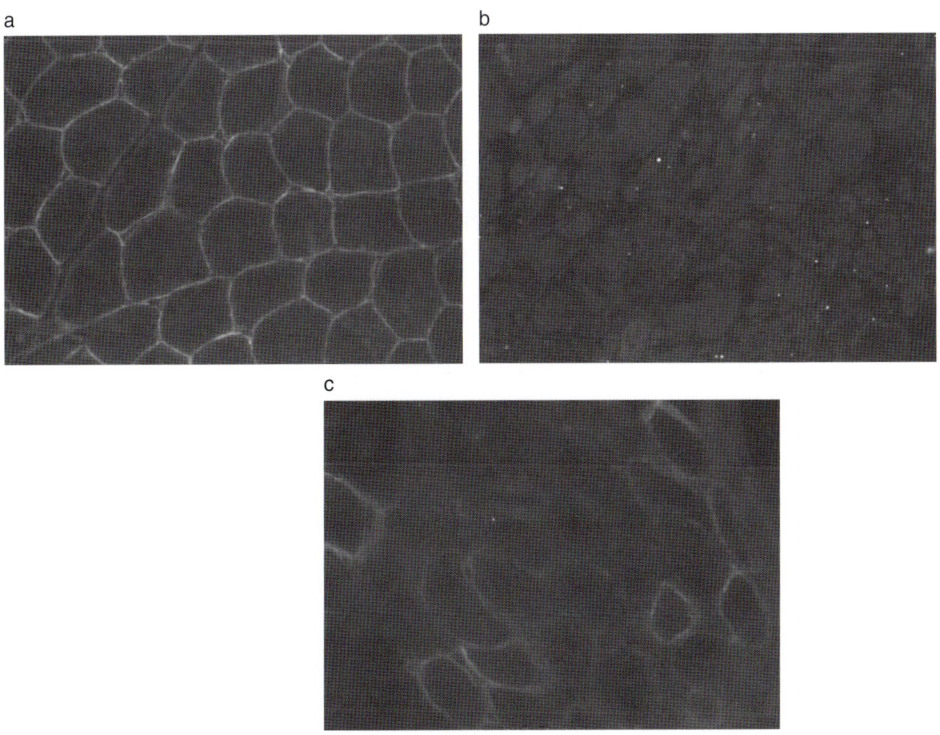

Figure 12.2a–c. Histochemical staining for glycosylated α-dystroglycan in a control subject (a), in an affected patient with markedly reduced staining (b) and in an affected patient with partial reduction of staining (c).

contractures are not prominent at birth. However, hip, knee, and ankle contractures generally start appearing before 1 year of age. In some cases, limitation of hip abduction is already apparent at 3 months of age. Muscle pseudohypertrophy may become evident in the calves and forearms by early childhood. Involvement of facial muscles tends to result in characteristic changes in appearance with aging, but the mouth remains partially open from infancy because of facial weakness. Functional disability is more severe in FCMD patients than in DMD patients; usually the maximum level of motor function achieved is sliding while sitting on the buttocks, and most FCMD patients are never able to walk. In the Japanese experience patients usually become bedridden before 10 years of age and most of them die by 20 years of age. Cardiomyopathy can occur [29]. Mental retardation is generally in the severe to moderate range (IQ scores lie between 30 and 50). Seizures manifest in about half of the cases. Possible eye involvement includes myopia, cataract, abnormal eye movement, pale optic disk, and retinal detachment, although most patients are capable of making visual contact [28]. A variety of brain malformations are the most common and characteristic changes in the central nervous system. They include polymicrogyria, pachygyria, and agyria of the cerebrum (type II lissencephaly) as well as abnormalities of cerebellar folia. In addition, focal interhemispheric fusion, fibroglial proliferation of the leptomeninges, mild to moderate ventricular dilatation, and hypoplasia of the corticospinal tracts are observed. Brain MRI most prominently shows the pachygyria in the cerebral cortex and transient high signal in the white matter on T_2-weighted images; hypoplasia of the pons and cerebellum as well as cerebellar cysts can also be seen. The high intensity of the white matter on T_2-weighted images is thought to be due to delayed myelination. It appears that patients who are homozygous for the initially described ancestral retrotransposon insertion mutation have a rather milder phenotype, while disease severity (associated eye abnormalities such as retinal detachment and microphthalmos) increases in patients who are compound heterozygous for the ancestral mutation and a more severe loss-of-function mutation [30]. Recently fukutin mutations have been related to unusual phenotypes such as steroid-responsive LGMD [31] or early-onset and prominent dilated cardiomyopathy with no muscle involvement or minimal muscle weakness [32]. It is reasonable to expect that this spectrum will broaden.

Walker–Warburg syndrome represents the most severe manifestation amongst the dystroglycanopathies, with most patients dying before the age of 3 years [33]. The disease is characterized by the presence of a congenital muscular dystrophy (14/14), in which motor development is virtually absent or severely retarded. Ocular abnormalities are frequent, such as retinal detachment and malformations (18/18), cataracts (7/20), microphthalmia (8/21), anterior and posterior chamber malformations (16/21), optic nerve hypoplasia, coloboma (3/15), and glaucoma. Structural brain abnormalities occur in the form of type II lissencephaly (cobblestone complex characterized microscopically by markedly disorganized cytoarchitecture with complete lack of lamination and numerous glial heteropias) (21/21), agenesis of the corpus callosum, cerebellar and pontine hypoplasia or Dandy–Walker malformation (20/20), ventricular dilatation with or without hydrocephalus (11/19), and rarely occipital encephalocele (5/21). Other rare associated symptoms reported are: cardiovascular abnormalities, cleft lip and palate (4/21), renal–urinary malformations (5/8), and gonadal dysplasia [34]. Motor development is virtually absent or severely retarded.

Muscle eye brain disease is characterized by the presence of a congenital muscular dystrophy, ocular abnormalities (congenital myopia, glaucoma, and retinal hypoplasia), mental retardation, and structural brain malformations (pachygyria with preferential frontoparietal involvement and polymicrogyria, cerebellar hypoplasia and hypoplastic and flat brain stem; the pachygyria represents a more restricted occurrence of the same pathology that is also seen in lissencephaly II/cobblestone complex). Pseudohypertrophy of various muscles including tongue hypertrophy is frequently seen in these patients. Some patients may show predominantly pontocerebellar involvement. Cerebellar abnormalities may include cysts or other forms of cerebellar dysplasia, which appear to be rather typical in individuals with FKRP mutations underlying the MEB phenotype, or cerebellar hypoplasia with enlarged cisterna magna as previously reported in patients with mutations in POMT1 and POMT2 [13, 14].

Other patients with mental retardation may have a structurally normal brain on MRI or may present with isolated microcephaly, as has been seen in patients harboring POMT1 mutations [15, 22]. Although structural brain involvement or mental retardation seemed to have been present in the majority of patients known to have POMT1 or POMT2 mutations, more recently exceptions have been noted including the identification of a POMT2 homozygous missense mutation in a girl with a mild LGMD phenotype together with markedly elevated serum creatine kinase (CK) levels, and absence of any brain involvement [35].

As noted before, to date FKRP gene mutations have been found to be associated with the widest clinical spectrum. The earliest recognized phenotypes are MDC1C and LGMD2I [10]. However, in a series of 13 patients presenting with CMD and FKRP mutations, only 5/13 patients had the typical phenotype originally described for MDC1C, while 3/13 had isolated cerebellar cysts and mental retardation, and 5/13 showed that cerebellar cysts were associated with structural brain changes involving the posterior fossa and the cortex, resembling MEB or mild WWS [14]. Classic severe WWS has now also been associated with mutations in FKRP. Thus, more patients with FKRP-related CMD had evidence for brain involvement than did not [14]. These observations point towards a clinical spectrum of presentation of FKRP mutations, ranging from WWS to the mildest presentations of pure muscle involvement. The main difference between the two phenotypes presenting with just isolated muscle weakness (MDC1C and LGMD2I) is that patients in the MDC1C category generally present with severe muscle weakness early in life and usually do not achieve ambulation. In contrast, in LGMD2I the age at onset of symptoms ranges between 2 and 40 years, with a clinically heterogeneous presentation ranging from asymptomatic isolated hyperCK-emia, to exertional myoglobinuria to different degrees of pelvic and shoulder muscle involvement frequently associated with dilated cardiomyopathy (DCM), which has been reported in a high proportion of LGMD2I patients. Most LGMD2I patients develop DCM in an age-dependent manner and usually the evolution of cardiomyopathy reflects the progression of skeletal muscle weakness [35]. Contractures are generally mild, lumbar lordosis without signs of spinal rigidity and hypertrophy of the calves are frequent, while tongue hypertrophy is very rare. Nonetheless, the relationship between skeletal myopathy and cardiomyopathy is complex. Recently early-onset prominent DCM with no muscle involvement or minimal muscle weakness was reported in children harboring the common homozygous Leu276Ile FKRP mutation [36] similar to what has been reported for mutations in the Fukutin gene [32], thus further increasing the clinical spectrum of dystroglycanopathies.

Genotype–phenotype correlations

Mutations in POMT1 alone accounted for about 20% of WWS patients in a recent series [13]. Analyzing all currently known genes related to the *O*-mannosyl glycosylation of α-dystroglycan in a recent series of 41 families, about 50% of WWS patients can be explained, with POMT1, POMT2, and POMGnT1 mutations found in the majority of patients ([37]; van Brokhoven, personal communication). Thus, it is likely that more genes remain to be identified in WWS. Overall it appears that, in the case of the POMT1 and POMT2 genes, mutations leading to severe functional defects (e.g., prematurely truncated protein, involvement of residues crucial for the enzymatic activity, etc.) are associated with severe MEB or WWS phenotypes, whereas missense changes that are distant from crucial protein domains or that affect amino acids that are not highly conserved result in milder phenotypes such as CMD with mental retardation and normal MRI [13, 15, 37], or even LGMD, as is the case for POMT2 [38].

Mutations in the *POMGnT1* gene have also been identified in patients outside of Finland following the first description of a disease-causing mutation in that population. The Finnish founder mutation, c.153911G4A [4], predicting an in-frame deletion of 42 amino acids (p.Leu472_513- His del), has also frequently been reported in other series of patients with severe clinical presentations consistent with the Finnish disease [37]. Interestingly, genotype–phenotype correlations reveal that patients with milder clinical presentation most often exhibit a mutation located towards the 3′ end of the *POMGnT1* gene, while patients with a more severe phenotype (including a degree of brain involvement) tend to have mutations toward the 5′ end of the gene [39].

For *fukutin* a broad correlation between genotype and phenotype in FCMD patients has been recognized. It appears that patients who are homozygous for the ancestral Japanese mutation (insertion of a retrotransposon) have a rather milder phenotype, while disease severity (including associated eye abnormalities such as retinal detachment and microphthalmos) increases in patients who are compound heterozygous for the ancestral mutation and have a more severe loss-of-function mutation on the other allele [30]. Interestingly, in contrast to fukutin-null mice, which are not viable, homozygous null mutations in the human *fukutin* gene have recently been characterized in two patients of Turkish origin, suggesting that human life is compatible with a homozygous null mutation [40]. These patients presented with a more severe, WWS-like phenotype compared to the general FCMD patient population in Japan, and had evidence for substantial depletion of α-dystroglycan as shown by immunofluorescence.

The *FKRP* gene consists of four exons, with the entire coding region confined to exon 4. Most of the CMD associated *FKRP* mutations are private while the n. 826C > A (p.Leu276Ile) mutation is particularly common in LGMD2I patients and has been reported to confer a relatively mild phenotype when present in the homozygous state, but can be associated with much more variable presentations when present in the compound heterozygous state, depending on the nature and severity of the second mutation [6]. As noted before, within the α-dystroglycanopathies, FKRP mutations are associated with the broadest clinical spectrum at this point.

Diagnostic approaches (biochemistry, pathology, histochemistry, immunocytochemistry, fine structure, immunoblot, mutational analysis, imaging)

Muscle biopsies from patients with α-dystroglycanopathy in general reveal a dystrophic pattern with myofiber necrosis, increased variability in fiber diameter, central nuclei, and an increase in connective and fatty tissue, although in some patients the findings may be much less conspicuous. Immunohistochemical staining with a monoclonal antibody recognizing glycosylated epitopes of the α-dystroglycan protein on unfixed frozen tissue sections serves as a straightforward tool in the diagnostic muscle biopsy work-up of dystroglycanopathies irrespective of the specific gene mutation (Figure 12.2). In patients presenting with the most severe clinical variants (WWB, MEB) of CMD there usually is a profound depletion of properly glycosylated α-dystroglycan, causing a secondary reduction of laminin-α2-binding activity in skeletal muscle and peripheral nerve. In the milder clinical variants, such as LGMD2I, α-dystroglycan staining is attenuated in all patients and is clearly lower in compound heterozygous versus homozygous patients [41]. While reduction of the amount of laminin-α2 is easily detectable immunohistochemically in the muscle of patients with profound hypoglycosylation, in most patients with the LGMD2I phenotype, the secondary reduction of laminin-α2 is detectable only by Western blot [35, 41].

After the deficiency of properly glycosylated α-dystroglycan has been confirmed, for WWS the best diagnostic strategy is to initially sequence POMT1, and POMT2, as they are the most frequent genes associated with WWS [13, 37]. Mutations in FKRP [19], fukutin [40], and LARGE [25] seem to be associated with WWS in rare cases. As noted before, in about half of WWS patients the causative gene is still elusive. POMGnT1 is most frequently associated with an MEB phenotype. However, it has to be noted again that it is likely that each of the phenotypes along this disease spectrum can be caused by mutations in a number of the genes identified as disease-causing along this pathway. In LGMD2I patients are frequently homozygous for the 826C > A mutation in the FKRP gene, while most of the remaining patients are compound heterozygous for this mutation with varying mutations on the other allele. With the exception of FKRP mutations in the LGMD2I phenotype, all the other phenotypes are associated with private mutations.

To confirm the pathogenicity of a mutation, especially when only one heterozygous mutation is identified, an enzymatic assay can be useful to measure the activity of the mutant protein in patient-derived cells. This assay is already available for POMGnT1 [42], and for POMT [43].

Most patients with WWS have mutations in the POMT1 and POMT2 genes, and several in POMGnT1 [37].

Therapeutic and preventative modalities

No specific treatments are available at this point. Orthopedic, respiratory, and nutritional management is similar to that for patients with primary laminin-α2 deficiency (see Laminin-α2 deficiency). Management of seizure follows general guidelines using medications appropriate for the focal mechanisms of onset.

Genetic counseling

The conditions in this category are inherited as autosomal recessive traits, so both parents can be assumed to be clinically asymptomatic carriers of one recessive mutation, thus a 25% recurrence risk will have to assumed for each future pregnancy.

Prenatal diagnosis can be obtained by direct sequencing of the gene if the mutation is known from the previously affected child. Other options that have been used in the absence of mutations on both alleles of a given gene include linkage analysis using DNA obtained from an ongoing pregnancy by chorionic villus sampling (CVS).

Future perspectives

There are currently no specific therapeutic alternatives available; however, Barresi *et al.* [44], demonstrated that overexpression of LARGE in Large/myd mice induced synthesis of glycan-enriched α-dystroglycan accompanied by increased affinity for extracellular ligands, thereby ameliorating the dystrophic pathology in these mice. Moreover, the authors demonstrated that overexpression of LARGE is able to bypass glycosylation defects in other forms of muscular dystrophies caused by abnormal glycosylation of dystroglycan. These data emphasize that manipulation of endogenous LARGE expression and activity represents a promising future therapeutic target for various muscular dystrophy syndromes caused by abnormal glycosylation of α-dystroglycan.

Genetic engineering of mice lacking POMGnT1 reproduces the phenotype observed in patients and will be of benefit in studying further aspects of molecular pathogenesis and the development of therapeutic strategies [45].

Integrin-α7 deficiency

Integrin-α7β1 [*600536] is a laminin-α2 receptor found on the surface of myocytes, participating in an important connection between the cell surface and the basal lamina. Integrin-α7β1 also functions to mediate the migration and proliferation of myoblasts [46]. More recently, the functional understanding of α7β1 has been extended to the development and maintenance of vascular smooth muscle [47]. Both α and β subunits are expressed in tissue-specific variants formed by differential splicing in a developmentally dependent manner [46]. The RNA coding for the cytoplasmic domain of integrin-α7 undergoes alternative splicing to generate two major forms, denoted α7A and α7B. The α7A and α7B variants are expressed to a large extent in skeletal muscle, specifically the myotendinous junctions, neuromuscular junctions, and the sarcolemma, although they are also found in cardiac and smooth muscle [48]. Integrin-α7B binds laminin within the plasma membrane forming an important support of structural and functional stability within the skeletal muscle [49, 50]. Recessive mutations in the gene for integrin α7 have been described on chromosome 12q13 in three Japanese patients [51] and probably one patient from Italy [52]. The discovery of the ITGA7 gene at locus 12q13 and the subsequent generation of a homozygous knockout mouse model were key steps in the determination of functional deficiencies created in the absence of integrin-α7 [53]. This condition appears to be very rare. The four patients described to date presented with significant developmental delay. One had mental retardation with impaired achievement of motor milestones, and a subtle increase in serum CK. Two other patients had similar motor delay without mental involvement, achieving ambulation after age 2 years, but were found to have torticollis, hip dislocation, and hypotonia during the first months of life. The fourth patient presented hypotonia with hip, wrist, and ankle contractures and died at 13 months of age from respiratory failure. Muscle biopsy changes ranged from myopathic to mildly dystrophic, with evidence for degeneration and regeneration.

The Italian patient was detected by systematic screening using antibodies against the intracellular domain of integrin-α7A and integrin-α7B in muscle biopsies from 210 patients with muscular dystrophy/myopathy of unknown etiology. Levels of integrin-α7A and integrin-α7B were found to be decreased in 35 of 210 patients (approximately 17%). Screening for the α7B mutation in 30 of 35 patients detected only one integrin-α7 missense mutation (the mutation on the second allele was not found) in a patient presenting with a CMD-like phenotype. Congenital myopathy and deficiency of integrin-α7-can be detected by immunocytochemical techniques, but from these data it seems that a secondary integrin-α7 deficiency is rather common in muscular dystrophy/myopathy of unknown etiology, emphasizing the multiple mechanisms that may modulate integrin function and stability.

Abnormalities of extracellular matrix proteins

Laminin-α2 deficiency

Definition of the entity or entities; basis for their classification

A specific form of CMD (MDC1A) [#607855] with absence of laminin-α2, the heavy chain isoform of laminin2 (also known as merosin) in skeletal muscle, was first described by Tomé *et al.* [54] in 13 patients with a classic non-Japanese form of congenital muscular dystrophy (the Japanese form being Fukuyama-type congenital muscular dystrophy, or FCMD). Muscle morphology showed a marked increase in endomysial connective tissue, and laminin-α2 was initially investigated as a candidate because it was known to be linked to the subsarcolemmal dystrophin-associated glycoproteins.

Salient diagnostic criteria

The classical form of CMD with primary laminin-α2 deficiency has a relatively homogeneous phenotype in patients with complete deficiency, characterized by severe muscle weakness, inability to achieve independent ambulation, markedly raised CK > 1000 U/l, and characteristic white matter hyperintensity on T_2-weighted images on cerebral MRI.

Molecular genetics and pathogenesis

Laminin is a heterotrimeric extracellular matrix protein consisting of three chains: α1 (LAMA1; 150320), β1 (LAMB1; 150240), and γ1, formerly called β2 (LAMC1; 150290). Several isoforms of each chain have been identified. Laminin-α2 is a heterotrimer composed of laminin subunits α2, β1, and γ1. It is the main laminin found in muscle fibers. The LAMA2 gene encodes the α2 chain of laminin-α2. The disease is inherited as an autosomal recessive trait caused by mutations in the *LAMA2* gene located at 6q22–q23 [55] [*156225]. Laminin-α2 is a protein specifically found in the basement membranes of striated muscle and Schwann cells. It is also found in the basement membrane of placental trophoblasts. The deduced amino acid sequence of the laminin-α2 polypeptide is similar to that of the C-terminal region of the laminin-α1 chain. The sequence identity between merosin and laminin is nearly 40% in this region. Like laminin, laminin-α2 is associated with the light chains laminin B1 and laminin B2, and the whole molecule has a cross-like structure similar to that of laminin. The spectrum of the phenotypes of CMD patients with partial laminin-α2 deficiency is wide and caused by homozygous missense mutations, homozygous in-frame deletions, or missense or in-frame deletions associated with a nonsense mutation [56].

Salient clinical phenotypical features

Clinical symptoms of muscle weakness are severe and are evident at birth or early infancy. In the more common classical form patients present with neonatal hypotonia with or without joint contractures, after which motor development is significantly delayed. Most affected children achieve the sitting position but are never able to walk. CK levels in blood are significantly raised >1000 U/l in most patients. On examination, weakness often affects upper limbs more severely than lower limbs, where antigravity movements are usually preserved. Contractures are nearly always present and flexion deformity at the hips, knees, elbows, and ankles, followed by rigidity and scoliosis of the spine, occur almost invariably, leading to increased limitations of functional abilities. Limitation of eye movements, in particular of upward gaze, are evident by the end of the first decade of life [10, 57].

In rare instances children may be able to stand or walk with some form of support. In most of the patients T_2-weighted MRI shows abnormalities of white matter affecting both hemispheres (Figure 12.3) but sparing the internal capsule, corpus callosum, basal ganglia, thalami, brain stem tracts, and cerebellum. White matter changes are limited to diffuse mild swelling of the cerebral white matter, and appear after the first 6 months of life and persist with time [58]. Patients with MDC1A also have diffusely abnormal, mildly swollen cerebral white matter in some cases giving rise to an MRI picture resembling megalencephalic leukoencephalopathy with subcortical cysts including evidence of myelin vacuolation [59]. However, a range of structural malformations such as occipital agyria, pontocerebellar hypoplasia or simply cerebellar hypoplasia can be seen in about 5% [60] of children with laminin-α2-deficient CMD. During follow-up most children show normal intelligence, but a subgroup of less than 10% may have moderate to severe mental retardation. Epilepsy is relatively frequent, affecting approximately 30% of cases [2], characterized mainly by complex partial seizures with atypical absences. Moreover, reduced motor nerve conduction velocity is a rather frequent finding in primary laminin-α2-deficient CMD [61]. It is currently not possible to establish confident percentages for the frequency of all individual symptoms because a number of studies published analyzing personal series and reviewing the literature run the risk of mixing primary and secondary laminin-α2 deficiency patients as there is no genetic confirmation of LAMA2 mutations in most studies [60]. Nevertheless, most published reports confirm that the typical white matter abnormalities on T_2-weighted MRI appear to be associated with the common classical phenotype of MDC1A [60]. However, about 12% of reported cases have later-onset LGMD-like presentations with slowly progressive weakness, in which cases the MRI can sometimes be normal. In addition, some clinical features are reported with relatively low frequency: mental retardation (∼6%), seizures (∼8%), subclinical cardiac involvement (3%–35%), and neuronal migration defects (4%). Between 10% and 20% of cases had maximum recorded CK levels of less than 1000 U/l.

More recently, mutations in the *LAMA2* gene in several patients with a LGMD phenotype and a partial laminin-α2 deficiency have been identified [62, 63], confirming that mutations in this gene can result in either a severe disease (MDC1A) or a mild LGMD-like disorder, depending on the type and location of the mutation within the gene.

a

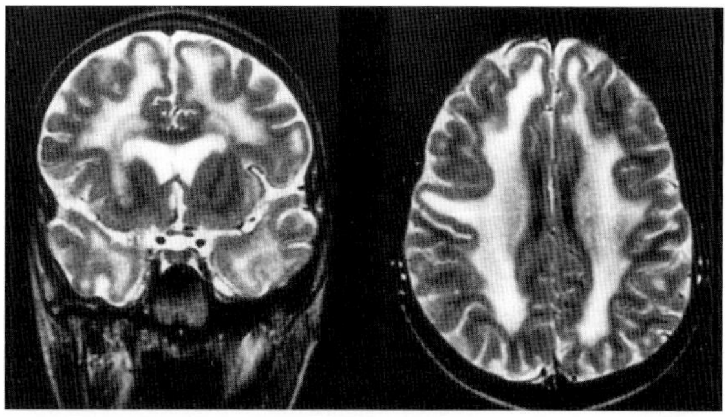

b

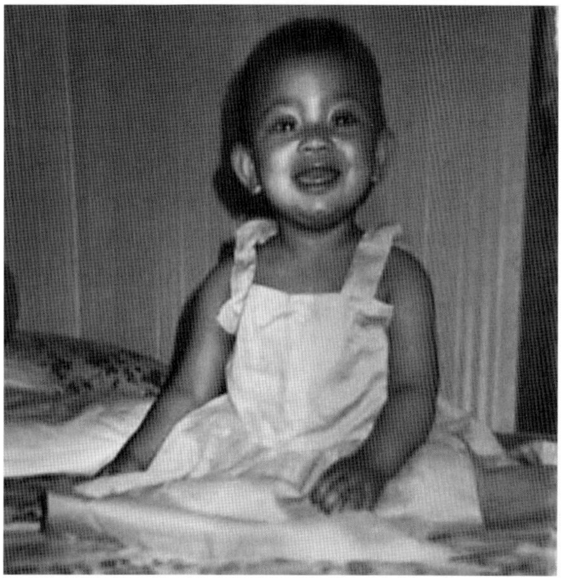

Figure 12.3a, b. MRI (a) and clinical aspect of a 1-year-old girl (b) affected by primary LAMA2 (merosin) deficiency. The child is able to sit alone and has normal cognitive development. The T_2-weighted MRI shows abnormal hyperintensity of the white matter sparing the U fibers and the internal capsule. There is a swollen appearance to the white matter.

Genotype–phenotype correlations

Analysis of the laminin-α2 chain cDNA or the *LAMA2* gene itself shows that nucleotide substitutions, small deletions, or insertions induce complete laminin-α2 deficiency. Most of the mutations are localized in the N-terminal domain (exons 1–31) and are predicted to result in the production of truncated protein. Changes of conserved cysteine residues of the short arm of the protein induce partial deficiency probably by inducing proteolysis or instability of the scaffold [56].

Most loss-of-function mutations have been reported in the severe variants, presenting with neonatal onset and absent immunostaining for laminin-α2 on the muscle biopsy. Patients with partial laminin-α2 deficiency, and yet presenting with a severe phenotype, may also have missense mutations in highly functional domains of the protein, such as the G (globular) domain, which is known to be important in binding to α-dystroglycan. Cases with a milder phenotype associated with partial laminin-α2 either show a homozygous in-frame deletion of the *LAMA2* chain gene on the basis of various splice site mutations or there is compound heterozygosity with a null allele and various splice site mutations again causing in-frame deletions [64, 65].

Diagnostic approaches (biochemistry, pathology, histochemistry, immunocytochemistry, fine structure, immunoblot, mutational analysis, imaging)

The diagnosis of laminin-α2-deficient CMD, especially in the cases with partial deficiency, should always be confirmed genetically by directed mutation analysis in the gene coding for the laminin-α2 chain (*LAMA2*). The general histological examination of the muscle biopsy shows dystrophic changes with a wide variation in fiber size and an increase in endomysial connective tissue and adipose tissue [54]. Inflammatory cellular infiltrates can be prominent, mimicking an inflammatory myopathy [66] (Figure 12.4a, b).

Laminin-α2 is found in skeletal muscle fibers, in basement membrane of Schwann cells, and in blood vessels within the brain. Immunostaining (Figure 12.4c, d) of the skeletal muscle for diagnostic purposes should be performed using antibodies that recognize both the 80-kDa fragment of laminin-α2 [MAB1922 (1:2000) Chemicon], in conjunction with a second antibody identifying a 300-kDa fragment such as the NCL-laminin-α2 antibody [(1(200) Novocastra] or Alexis (MAB4H8–2). The antibody detecting the 80-kDa fragment of laminin-α2 corresponds to the C-terminal part of the G globular domain of the human laminin-α2 and is the most commonly used antibody. The commercially available antibody from Alexis (MAB4H8–2) is reported to react predominantly with the 300-kDa N-terminal fragment while the Novocastra antibody (NCL-merosin) is raised against the whole laminin-α2 chain, however its precise epitope is unknown. Immunofluorescence in particular can readily demonstrate the reduction or absence of laminin-α2 chain immunoreactivity. In most cases, this laminin chain is totally absent or only present in traces. The detection of the laminin-α2 chain in cases with partial expression may depend on which, and how many, antibodies are used. The laminin-α2 chain is processed into two fragments on immunoblots, of 80 kDa and 300 kDa, and a reduction is often easier to observe with antibodies to the 300-kDa fragment or with the similarly behaving NCL-merosin antibody. This seems true also for immunofluorescence analysis using these two latter antibodies. The expression of laminin-α2 can also be demonstrated in the skin at the dermo-epidermal junction. The expression of this protein can therefore be studied in the skin when muscle is not available [67].

Generally absence of immunostaining for both antibodies correlates with the classical severe form of MDC1A while the milder cases show partial reduction of immunostaining when using one or both antibodies. Abnormalities on immunohistochemical analysis can also be confirmed by immunoblot.

Most of the mutations found in the *LAMA2* gene are private mutations, as there are no apparent mutational hot spots. Secondary reduction of laminin-α2 occurs in several

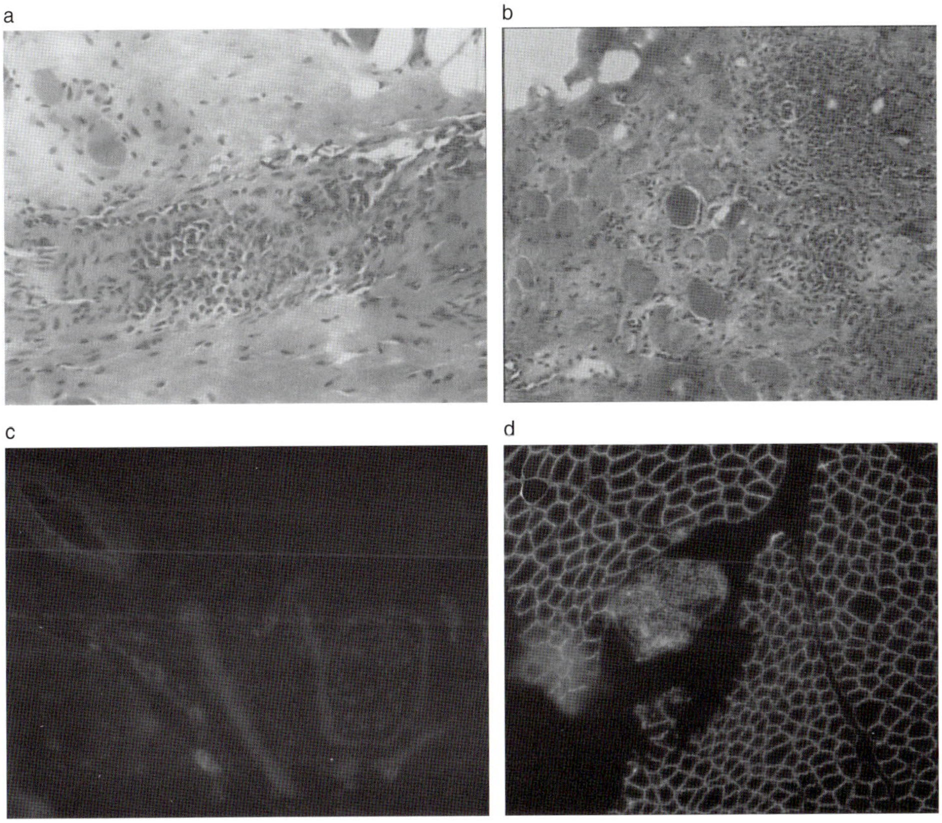

Figure 12.4a–d. Histological aspects of a muscle biopsy of a patient with primary LAMA2 (merosin) deficiency. H&E stain showing marked fibrosis (a) and inflammation (b). Immunohistochemistry using a monoclonal antibody recognizing the 80-kDa fragment of laminin-α2 (c) shows greatly reduced immunofluorescence of muscle fibers and a peripheral motor nerve in a patient compared to normal immunofluorescence in a control section (d).

CMD forms associated with reduced α-dystroglycan glycosylation [10] and also in other variants with atypical phenotypes not linked to the *LAMA2* locus [68]. As mentioned earlier it is therefore important to determine the primary defect in the *LAMA2* gene, particularly in families for which prenatal diagnosis is considered.

The best strategy for mutation analysis currently is to analyze genomic DNA extracted from blood by polymerase chain reaction (PCR) followed by direct sequencing of all 65 *LAMA2* exons. The fragments for direct sequencing can also be pre-selected by single-strand conformation polymorphism (SSCP) analysis as described [69].

Therapeutic and preventative modalities

Orthopedic management and follow-up is critical for children with MDC1A since most of them are not able to ambulate independently and are very prone to the development of kyphoscoliosis and joint contractures.

Respiratory function is often impaired such that respiratory insufficiency is frequently evident by the end of the first decade while night-time hypoventilation may be seen in early childhood. Clinical signs of nocturnal hypoventilation can be very subtle, so monitoring patients with overnight oxygen saturation studies is recommended in order to identify early symptoms and to institute night-time noninvasive positive pressure ventilation in a timely fashion.

Consideration of the nutritional status is important in any child with a primary muscle disorder. Children with MDC1A have difficulties at all stages of feeding that worsen with age. In long-term follow-up around 80% of patients have chewing and swallowing difficulties. Using video fluoroscopy studies some patients had an abnormal oral phase (breakdown and manipulation of food and transfer to the oropharynx) while others had an abnormal pharyngeal phase, with simply a delayed swallow reflex or aspiration. Some children showed recurrent chest infections and others gastroesophageal reflux [70]. Patients with critical swallowing dysfunction have a history of recurrent chest infections. Appropriate intervention, such as gastrostomy, for feeding reduces chest infections and improves weight gain.

Genetic counseling

MDC1A is inherited as an autosomal recessive trait, so both parents are generally asymptomatic carriers of recessive mutations.

Laminin-α2 chain is also expressed in fetal trophoblast, which provides a suitable tissue for prenatal diagnosis in families where the index case has total deficiency of the protein and if mutation analysis is not available. Depending on availability, protein and DNA analysis can be used either independently or in combination to provide accurate prenatal diagnosis of the MDC1A; however, identification of the disease-causing mutations should be attempted whenever possible [71].

Table 12.1. The congenital muscular dystrophies (CMD). CK, creatine kinase; CMD, congenital muscular dystrophy; IH, immunohistochemistry; LGMD, limb-girdle muscular dystrophy; MEB, muscle eye brain disease; UCMD, Ullrich congenital muscular dystrophy; WB, Western blot; WWS, Walker–Warburg syndrome.

Disease entity	Locus protein product Gene symbol	Helpful clinical features	CNS involvement	Laboratory testing
Primary merosin/laminin 2 deficiency				
CMD with primary laminin-2 (merosin) deficiency (MDC1A)	6q2 Laminin-α2 *LAMA2*	Sitting and standing with support as maximal motor ability if complete deficiency, neuropathy, epilepsy in about 30%, possible subclinical cardiomyopathy, generally normal mental development	Abnormal white matter signal (T_2 MRI), 5% occipital pachygyria or agyria, pontocerebellar atrophy (rare)	Mostly complete laminin-α2 deficiency on IH/WB, secondary reduction of integrin-α7 possible, mutation analysis*
α-Dystroglycanopathies – secondary merosin/laminin 2 deficiency				
CMD with partial merosin deficiency (MDC1B)	1q42 Not known	Rare, variety of severity, delayed onset possible, proximal girdle weakness, generalized muscle hypertrophy, early respiratory failure possible	Abnormal white matter and structural changes possible	Partial deficiency of laminin-α2 on IH/WB, α-DG significantly reduced on IH, linkage analysis
Fukutin related proteinopathy (MDC1C)	19q13 Fukutin related protein *FKRP*	Often reminiscent of MDC1A, but severity more variable, from severe CMD to LGMD as well as to WWS (see [14]), generally normal mental development, cases with structural brain involvement and mental retardation increasingly recognized, including MEB and WWS	Range from normal to significant structural abnormalities, ranging from cerebellar cysts to typical MEB and WWS	α-DG with diminished Mol. Wt. on WB, or reduction of IH using antibodies against glycosylated isotopes, secondary reductions in laminin-α2 on IH/WB, mutation analysis*
LARGE related CMD (MDC1D)	22q12 Acetylglucosaminyl transferase-like protein *LARGE*	So far only one patient described. Congenital muscular dystrophy with profound mental retardation may eventually blend with the MEB/WWS spectrum	White matter changes, hypoplastic brain stem, mild pachygyria (similar to MEB)	IH/WB comparable to MDC1C, mutation analysis*
Fukuyama CMD (FCMD)	9q31–q33 Fukutin *FCMD*	Frequent in Japanese population, never walk, mental retardation, epilepsy common – clinical overlap to MEB – see below	Lissencephaly type II/ pachygyria, hypoplastic brain stem, cerebellar abnormalities	IH/WB comparable to MDC1C, mutation analysis
Muscle eye brain disease (MEB)	1q33 Protein-*O*-linked mannose β1,2-*N*-acetylglucosaminyltranferase 1 POMGnT1 *FKRP*, Fukutin	Severe weakness and mental retardation, large head, prominent forehead, flat midface, walking rarely achieved, ocular involvement (e.g. severe myopia, retinal hypoplasia), deterioration because of spasticity	Lissencephaly type II/ pachygyria, eye malformations, brain stem and cerebellar abnormalities	IH/WB comparable to MDC1C, mutation analysis (genetic heterogeneity!)

Table 12.1. *(cont.)*

Disease entity	Locus protein product Gene symbol	Helpful clinical features	CNS involvement	Laboratory testing
Walker–Warburg syndrome (WWS)	9q34 Protein-*O*-mannosyltranferase 1 *POMT 1* *POMT2*, *FKRP*, Fukutin	Severe, lethal within first years of life because of severe CNS involvement	Lissencephaly type II, pachygyria, hydrocephalus, encephalocele, hypoplastic brain stem, cerebellar abnormalities, eye malformations	IH/WB comparable to MDC1C, mutation analysis (genetic heterogeneity!)
Other matrix disorders (merosin/laminin 2 positive)				
Ullrich CMD (UCMD)	21q22.3 and 2q37 α1/2 and α3 collagen VI *COL6A1*, *COL6A2*, *COL6A3*	Distal joint hyperextensibility, proximal contractures, motor abilities variable, precludes independent ambulation in severe cases, soft palmar skin	No	IH for collagen VI with severe to mild deficiency, mutation analysis*
Integrin α7	12q13 Integrin-α7 ITGA7	Very rare, delayed motor milestones, walking at 2–3 years	No	Absence of integrin-α7 on IH (secondary reduction possible), mutation analysis*
CMD with hyperlaxity (CMDH)	3p23–21 ITGA9	French-Canadian, presenting with weakness, proximal contractures, distal laxity, milder compared to UCMD with ambulation preserved into adulthood	No	Value of ITGA9 IH not clear yet
Other CMD				
Rigid spine muscular dystrophy (RSMD)	1p36–p35 Selenoprotein N *SEPN1*	Delayed walking, predominantly axial weakness with early development of rigidity of the spine, restrictive respiratory syndrome	No	Normal expression of laminin-α2, mutation analysis
Lamin-A/C-related CMD	1q21.2 *LMNA*	Absent motor development in severe cases, more typical: "dropped head" and axial weakness/rigidity, proximal upper and more distal lower extremity weakness, may show early phase of progression	No	Largely normal nuclear localization for lamin A/C on IH
CMD merosin-positive	4p16.3	Severe muscle weakness of trunk and shoulder girdle muscles, and mild to moderate involvement of facial, neck and proximal limb muscles. Normal intelligence	No	Normal expression of laminins, dystrophin, sarcoglycans and β-dystroglycan
CMD with microcephaly/calf hypertrophy	Not known	Joint contractures associated, severe psychomotor retardation, no walking, striking enlargement of the calf and quadriceps muscles, CK grossly elevated	Megacisterna magna, cerebellar hypoplasia, white matter changes	Mild to moderate partial deficiency of laminin α2 on IH

Table 12.1. *(cont.)*

Disease entity	Locus protein product Gene symbol	Helpful clinical features	CNS involvement	Laboratory testing
CMD with adducted thumbs	Not known	Rare, adducted thumbs, toe contractures, generalized weakness, delayed walking, ptosis, external ophthalmoplegia, mild mental retardation	Mild cerebellar hypoplasia	Normal expression of laminin-α2 and α-DG on IH
CMD with mental retardation and microcephaly	Not known, FKRP not yet excluded	Microcephaly, delayed psychomotor development, generalized muscular wasting and weakness with mild facial involvement, calf pseudohypertrophy, joint contractures, and severe mental retardation	Pontocerebellar hypoplasia, focal cortical dysplasia, white matter changes, cerebellar cysts	Normal expression of laminin-α2
CMD with cerebellar atrophy	Not known	Delayed motor milestones, mild intellectual impairment	Moderate to severe cerebellar hypoplasia, no white matter abnormalities	Normal expression of laminin-α2

Future perspectives

There currently is no direct therapy available for laminin-α2 deficiency. Therapeutic strategies are currently under preclinical development in animal models of the disease. A first mouse strain (dy/dy) with a mutation in the *lama2* gene was described by Michelson *et al.* [72]. Several other spontaneous and knockout mice models have become available later and are summarized in Shelton and Engvall [73].

Aiming to restore muscle function to a mouse model of LAMA2 deficiency, Moll *et al.* [74] designed a minigene of agrin, a protein known for its role in the formation of the neuromuscular junction. Moll *et al.* [74] demonstrated that this mini-agrin, which binds to laminin in the basement membrane and to α-dystroglycan (a member of the dystrophin–glycoprotein complex), amends muscle pathology by a mechanism that includes agrin-mediated stabilization of α-dystroglycan and the laminin-α5 chain, thus acting as a bridge between α-dystroglycan and an alternative laminin.

Suppression of apoptosis has been identified as another potential therapeutic strategy. Overexpression of the anti-apoptosis protein BCL2 in diseased muscles in the *Lama2*-null mice has been achieved by crossing these animals with transgenic mice that overexpressed human BCL2 under control of muscle-specific MyoD or MRF4 promoter. It was found that muscle-specific expression of BCL2 led to a several-fold increase in lifespan and an increased growth rate of the *Lama2*-null mice whereas no rescue was observed in the mdx mice [75]. This would open the door for potential anti-apoptotic pharmacological strategies as a treatment avenue in this disorder.

Collagen-VI-related myopathies

Definition of the entity or entities; basis for their classification

Ullrich disease (or Ullrich congenital muscular dystrophy – UCMD) is a severe disorder of congenital or infantile onset, with Bethlem myopathy (BM) as well as overlap phenotypes of intermediate severity representing an extension of the spectrum towards the milder end. Characteristic clinical features in the collagen-VI-related myopathies combine symptoms typical of disorders of muscle as well as those attributable to the connective tissue. Otto Ullrich described the condition now named after him in 1930 as "atonic-sclerotic muscular dystrophy" [76, 77], emphasizing the coexistence of striking laxity of the distal joints and more proximal contractures with the muscle weakness. As a disease classification it had mostly survived in the Japanese and European literature [2, 78, 79] before being brought back into focus with the discovery of collagen VI mutations in UCMD in 2001 [80]. BM was described in 1976 by van Bethlem and Wijngaarden [81] in the Netherlands as a dominant, relatively benign, myopathy with significant contractures. Collagen VI mutations were first identified in BM [82] and it is now clear that both UCMD and BM as well as phenotypes of intermediate severity are caused by mutations in the three known collagen VI genes *COL6A1*, *COL6A2*, and *COL6A3* [83]. Most patients with the classical phenotypes will have mutations in these genes; however, a small number of otherwise typical patients have no detectable mutations [84, 85] indicating that there will be a certain degree of genetic heterogeneity underlying an otherwise fairly typical phenotype. It is now emerging that the collagen-VI-related

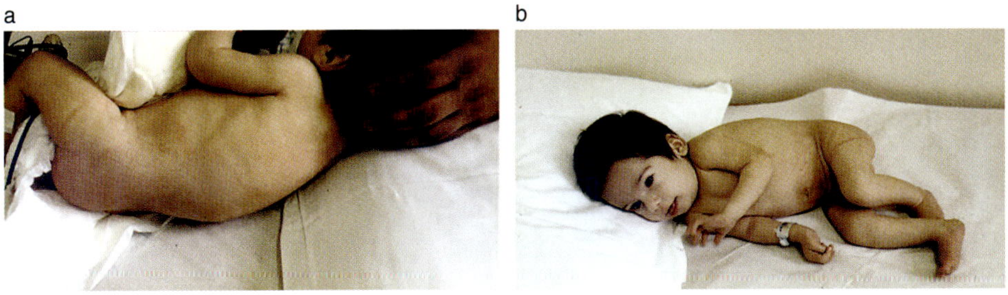

Figure 12.5a, b. Patient with Ullrich syndrome at birth. Note prominent kyphoscoliosis (a), elbow contractures, hip and knee contractures as well as lax hands, but no facial weakness (b).

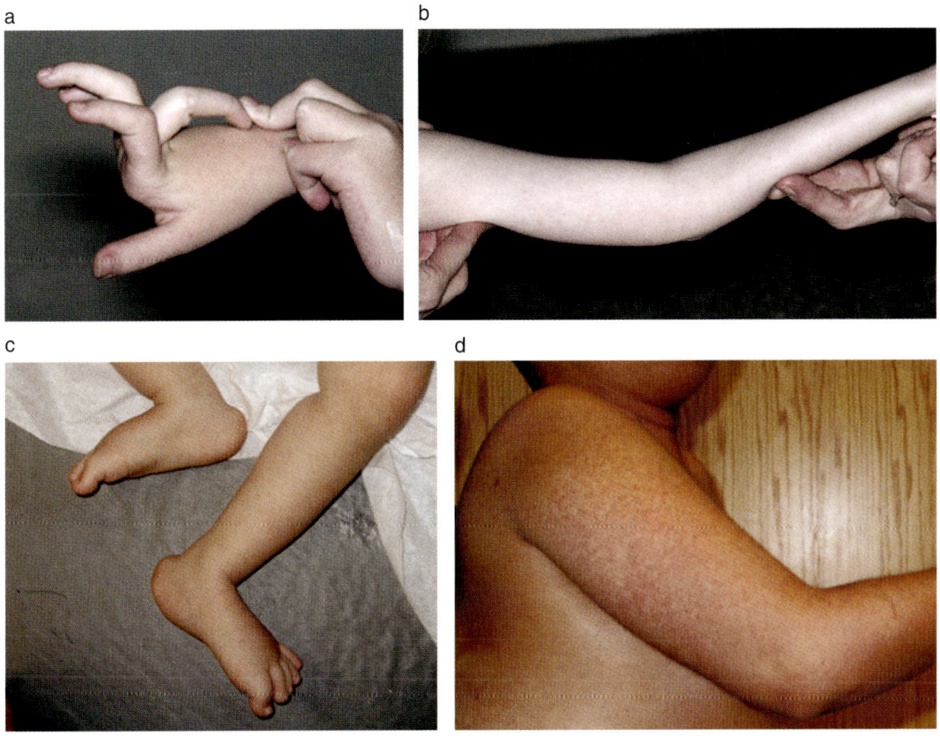

Figure 12.6a–d. Ullrich syndrome: prominent distal hypermobility (a), but coexisting elbow contractures in the same patient (b). There is a prominent calcaneus, associated with soft palmar skin (c). Keratosis pilaris on the proximal arm of a 21-year-old patient with Ullrich syndrome (d).

muscle disorders are among the most common entities subsumed under the category of CMD [86]. In this chapter we will be concentrating mostly on the congenital end of the spectrum (UCMD) while the later-onset condition (BM) will be described in greater detail in Chapter 14.

Salient diagnostic criteria

The typical diagnostic features of the congenital presentation in this group of disorders include congenital weakness and hypotonia, associated with striking joint laxity particularly of the distal joints, whereas more proximal joints such as hips and knees, elbows and spine may be affected by congenital contractures [87] (Figure 12.5). Early contractures may resolve but progressively reappear later. There are often dermatological findings such as soft and velvety skin on the palms of the hands and feet, keratosis pilaris on arms and legs, and abnormal scar formation [88] (Figure 12.6). Muscle biopsy findings range from the mildly myopathic, via findings suggestive of fiber type disproportion, to the more overtly dystrophic appearance. However, rarely is there much evidence for active degeneration and regeneration. Immunohistochemical analysis of the muscle biopsy may be helpful if collagen VI is found to be absent (as is the case in UCMD cases with null mutations on both alleles) [80, 89] or it may be mislocalized, i.e., no longer co-localizing with markers labeling the basement membrane (as is the case in dominantly acting mutations found in UCMD and Bethlem [90, 91] Figure 12.7). The diagnosis is finally confirmed by the demonstration of disease-causing mutation in the collagen VI genes.

Molecular genetics and pathogenesis

Collagen VI belongs to the nonfibrillar collagens that form a network of beaded microfibrils in the extracellular matrix [92, 93]. The major known collagen VI heterotrimer is composed of the α1 (VI), α2 (VI), and α3 (VI) chain, which are encoded by three genes: *COL6A1* and *COL6A2* on chromosome

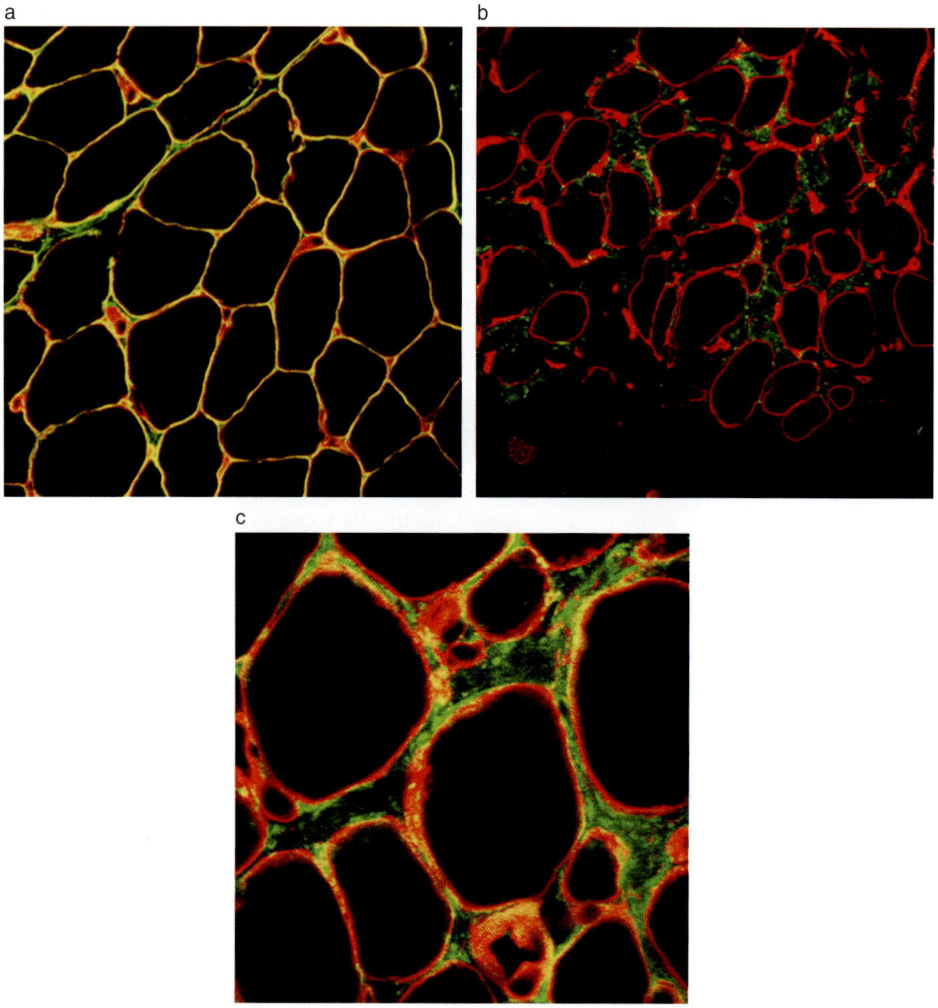

Figure 12.7a–c. Immunohistochemistry for collagen type VI (green label) with co-labeling of the basement membrane in red, using an anti-perlecan antibody. Note overlap of collagen VI and the basement membrane in normal muscle (yellow in a), but lack of overlap in the two patient biopsies. (b) A muscle biopsy from a patient with Ullrich syndrome; there is no co-localization between collagen VI and the basement membrane. (c) A patient with Bethlem myopathy, showing evidence of partial overlap between collagen VI and the basement membrane. Confocal microscopy.

21q22.3 and COL6A3 on chromosome 2q37 [94, 95]. All three chains have relatively short triple helical collagenous domains of 335–336 amino acids with single cysteine residues that are important for higher order assembly in the N-terminal part of the triple helical domains [96]. The α1 (VI) and α2 (VI) chains are related and likely arose by gene duplication on chromosome 21q22 where they are oriented head to tail [94]. Thus, they both have two C-terminal and one N-terminal globular von Willebrand factor A domains [97]. The α3 (VI) chain on chromosome 2q37 has a larger and extensively spliced N-terminal domain that is again rich in von Willebrand factor A domains [92]. The C-terminal domains of the α2 (VI) and the α3 (VI) undergo further splicing and post-translational processing. Recently three novel collagen VI chains, α4, α5, and α6, have been described [98].

Collagen VI undergoes a complex assembly inside and out of the cell [93, 99]. All three primary α chains have to combine to form a heterotrimeric monomer. Two monomers then associate in an anti-parallel arrangement mediated by a single cysteine residue located in the N-terminal part of the triple helical domain interacting with a cysteine residue in the C-globular domain [96, 100, 101]. Two dimers then associate in a parallel orientation [99], mediated by a similar triple helical cysteine to form a tetramer [96, 100, 102]. The tetramer is secreted into the extracellular space, where it associates end-to-end to form the beaded microfibrillar network of collagen VI that is characteristic of collagen VI in the extracellular space [97, 100, 103].

Collagen VI has a widespread distribution: it is found in most matrices and tissues, including muscle, vessels, skin, intervertebral disks, and other tissues. It shows a distinctly pericellular distribution in particular around tendon cells [104, 105] and has a particular affinity for basement membranes [106, 107] where it is found to overlap with markers of basement membranes [90]. Collagen VI appears to interact with a wide variety of molecules in the extracellular matrix [103]; however, the receptor or receptors for collagen VI in skeletal muscle are currently unknown. In a mouse model of collagen VI inactivation as well as in human cell culture models there is strong evidence for the occurrence of myofiber apoptosis mediated by mitochondria as a consequence of the lack of collagen VI [108, 109]. Blockers of the mitochondrial transition pore such as ciclosporin and its derivates are able to suppress this process, a therapeutic potential that remains to be further explored [108, 109]. Thus, an apoptotic mechanism rather than dystrophy due to an unstable plasma membrane appears to be a major contributor to myofiber degeneration in this condition. Pathways mediating between collagen VI in the matrix and the apoptosis control mechanisms are less clear and remain to be worked out in detail.

Salient clinical phenotypical features

Although the severe UCMD phenotype and the milder Bethlem phenotype are related and are linked by transitional phenotypes, in the context of this chapter we will focus on the congenital phenotype (UCMD), while the Bethlem phenotype is described in greater detail in Chapter 14.

UCMD [#254090] [76, 77]: there may be a history of perceived reduced prenatal movements, and symptoms are usually evident at birth [76, 77, 78, 79, 80, 83, 87]. Signs and symptoms at birth include hypotonia and weakness associated with extreme distal joint laxity while contractures can be seen at the same time in more proximal joints (Figure 12.6). There may be dislocated hips, torticollis, kyphoscoliosis as well as contractures of the hips, knees, and elbows. In contrast, hands, fingers, and feet are extremely hypermobile, allowing the finger to bend back onto the dorsum of the hands, and the feet are frequently found to bend back against the shin. A prominent calcaneus is often evident, although this is not a specific sign. Frequently the more prominent contractures found at birth will improve somewhat over the first several months of life; however, new and progressive contractures will often set in later (Figure 12.5). In the most severe cases walking is never achieved. A considerable number of affected children however will achieve the ability to walk, often with some delay [79]. However, walking is often lost again during childhood (starting as early as 4 years of age). Weakness is variable in its relative proximal versus distal distribution and is often quite diffuse. Antigravity strength in arms and legs seems initially preserved even in severely affected infants. It is often a combination of the progression of both weakness and contractures (in particular in the knees and hips) that will lead to the loss of the ability to ambulate. Even as the contractures progress to involve spine, pectoralis, elbows, hips, and knees, the hyperlaxity of the distal joints often persists to late stages of the disease. This hypermobility typically involves all interphalangeal joints, including the most distal ones; however, there will be increasing evidence of contractures of the long finger flexors. Scoliosis may become a serious and progressive problem, requiring surgical intervention in a number of patients. There are a number of notable dermatological findings [88] such as excessive scar formation including formation of keloids. Keratosis pilaris is seen on extensor surfaces of the limbs (Figure 12.6). Soft velvety skin is found on the palms of the hands and feet. Hyperhidrosis was commented upon by Ullrich [76, 77]. Respiratory involvement in the form of respiratory insufficiency progressively occurs in the majority of severely affected patients in the first decade of life and is based on a combination of restrictive lung disease and weakness so that noninvasive ventilation at least at night may become necessary. Frequently the respiratory situation after initiation of noninvasive ventilation is then quite stable over many years. Cardiac involvement does not seem to be prominent. Feeding difficulties and gastroesophageal reflux have been observed in more severely affected infants and have required G-tube feeding in a minority of the children.

Much of the natural history and of the late complications of severe collagen VI deficiency remain to be fully explored but will probably become clearer as patients now regularly survive given the institution of well-managed ventilatory support.

It has become apparent that there are patients with clinical presentations that are more severe compared to classic Bethlem but milder compared to classic Ullrich, thus representing transitional phenotypes on a spectrum bridging the two classic presentations. Patients in this transitional group between Ullrich and Bethlem present with significant weakness in childhood and will often show typical features of both presentations, including the Ullrich-like distal laxity of the distal interphalangeal joint as well as the Bethlem-like contractures of the long finger flexors. Ambulation is achieved but weakness can be considerable such that ambulation may be lost as the disease follows a slow progression. These patients are at higher risk for respiratory insufficiency compared to patients with classic Bethlem, in keeping with their more severe clinical involvement.

Genotype–phenotype correlations

Many mutations have been described in the three collagen VI genes in patients with both UCMD and BM so that a number of genotype–phenotype correlations are starting to emerge [83]. Mutations in BM have so far all been dominant and are described in Chapter 14.

The first mutations that were found to underlie UCMD were recessive null mutations, leading to absence of collagen VI in muscle biopsy sections [80, 89]. A larger variety of recessively acting mutations, mostly leading to premature termination codons, has subsequently been described, including some with milder manifestations because of their localization in alternatively spliced exons [86, 110, 111]. Splice site mutations may lead to out-of-frame exon skipping, thus acting as recessive null mutations [80, 112, 113]. Haploinsufficiency for one of the collagen VI chains in general does not lead to a clinical phenotype, so that carriers for these null mutations are not affected clinically. It has become evident more recently that de novo dominant mutations in all three collagen VI genes are responsible for a substantial proportion of patients presenting with sporadic UCMD [86, 91, 110, 113, 114]. These mutations are typically in-frame exon skipping mutations (splice site mutations or genomic deletions) of exons coding for the N-terminal part of the triple helical domain, sparing the cysteine residues responsible for higher order assembly of the basic heterotrimer into the dimer and tetramer states [91, 113, 115].

These deleted chains are thus effectively incorporated into the heterotrimeric monomer and into subsequent higher order structures up to the secretion of the tetramer into the extracellular matrix; therefore, these deleted chains act in a dominant negative way as 15/16 of tetramers will then include at least one mutant chain [91, 113, 115]. The dominant negative mutations in collagen VI are often associated with a phenotype close to the severity of recessive null mutations.

Diagnostic approaches (biochemistry, pathology, histochemistry, immunocytochemistry, fine structure, immunoblot, mutational analysis, imaging)

The first step to diagnosing a collagen-VI-related condition is recognition of the salient clinical features that raise the index of suspicion for the presence of UCMD or BM. The finding of a striking contractural phenotype is important in recognizing a collagen VI disorder in particular in the older patient with BM (see Chapter 14 for this phenotype and its differential diagnosis).

For the UCMD group usually the hyperlaxity of the distal joints is striking enough to raise suspicion of the presence of a collagen VI disorder. Core disorders such as multi-minicore disease or more severe neonatal central core disease can also lead to a high degree of joint laxity in some patients and may have to be considered in the differential diagnosis. Moreover multi-minicore disease caused by mutations in SEPN1 is likely in the presence of spinal rigidity associated with early respiratory failure. Similarly, the differential may also include the CMD presentation of LMNA mutations, in particular in cases with prominent axial involvement and rigidity (see below). The recently described CMD with joint hyperlaxity linked to chromosome 3 (see below) also figures in the differential. Skin findings as seen in the collagen-VI-related myopathies are not a feature in any of these conditions. Muscle imaging can be helpful as the collagen VI disorders present with a picture suggesting that the replacement of muscle with fatty and connective tissue starts around the fascia surrounding or traversing the muscle [116]. Thus, a peculiar "outside-in" picture of degeneration is seen on muscle imaging, which however may not be seen in all patients or may no longer be discernible in advanced cases [116]. A similar appearance can be seen on muscle ultrasound in collagen-VI-related myopathy, where the degeneration around the central fascia in the rectus femoris generates the appearance of a "central cloud" [117].

Muscle biopsy findings in the collagen-VI-related disorders can be quite variable and range from close to normal or mildly myopathic with some degree of fiber type disproportion, to more dramatically myopathic pictures with variability of fiber diameter including sometimes extremely atrophic fibers and build-up of extracellular connective and fat tissue. Evidence for myofiber degeneration also becomes more evident later in the disease although it is never a strikingly prominent aspect of the picture. Core-like abnormalities in the myofibers can also be seen on occasion and can be a source of confusion with the true core myopathies. Collagen VI immunohistochemistry on muscle biopsy sections can be done and may be very helpful, in particular in the recessive cases of UCMD in which the staining is absent or severely reduced. Changes tend to be more subtle in the case of dominant mutations in UCMD and BM, in which case careful double labeling of the basement membrane is important in order to assess collagen VI localization to the basement membrane (Figure 12.7). In the mutant case this overlap between collagen VI and the basement membrane will be lost. In the milder BM this lack of connection may only be partial and sometimes not apparent at all. Analysis of collagen VI production in dermal fibroblast cultures can also be very helpful in implicating collagen VI, ranging from completely absent or severely reduced in UCMD to more subtle abnormalities in BM [118]. Mutation analysis can now be achieved by genomic DNA sequencing of all exons for all three chains [110]. Not all sequence changes detected are immediately clear in their pathogenic significance as the collagen VI genes contain many polymorphic changes, many of which have not been completely catalogued yet. In doubtful cases it may be necessary to attempt to confirm the pathogenicity of a detected change in other ways, such as investigations in more family members or reverse transcriptase (RT) PCR analysis on RNA isolated from dermal fibroblasts to investigate potential abnormal splicing resulting from mutations located more deeply in the intron.

Therapeutic and preventative modalities

Therapeutic intervention in the collagen VI disorders at the time of writing consists mainly of careful clinical and preventive management of the various aspects of these conditions. Contractures are usually initially addressed by an aggressive stretching program and by dynamic splinting; however, rarely can their progression be stopped. Surgical release of the contractures can be helpful, in particular in the Achilles tendons to preserve normal walking in the intermediate phenotypes, although the contractures will have a tendency to recur. There is less experience with the surgical release of other joint contractures. Management of early and progressive scoliosis can be challenging. Bracing may have a temporizing effect but never actually stops the progression of the scoliosis. Careful respiratory monitoring and timely institution of respiratory support are of prime importance and will usually consist of noninvasive ventilatory support such as bi-level positive airway pressure (BiPAP). The respiratory insufficiency clearly is progressive, in particular during the first decade of life, but once ventilatory support is instituted there will be a long period of stability in the respiratory situation. Pharmacological agents that may counteract the propensity for the apoptosis that is part of the downstream effect of the collagen VI dysfunction will enter clinical trials in the near future. A recent study of five patients with collagen VI mutations treated with ciclosporin (acting as a blocker of the mitochondrial permeability transition pore) for 1 month showed decreased apoptosis and increased stability of the mitochondrial transition permeability pore, although strength improvement was not recorded [119]. Anti-apoptotic agents with less long-term toxicity are under clinical investigation.

Genetic counseling

Genetic counseling is greatly assisted by the positive identification of the disease-causing mutation as a more precise diagnosis in other family members will be possible to assess the degree of clinical variability in a given family. In the sporadic patient with UCMD both recessive mutations as well as a de novo dominant negative mutation can be expected with equal likelihood, with obviously greatly different recurrence risk estimations for the couple for future pregnancies. This would be 25% for the recessive scenario whereas for a de novo dominant mutation only the theoretical risk of germ-line mosaicism has to be assumed. Only the definitive identification of the causative mutations in the collagen VI genes will clarify this situation.

Future perspectives

Future perspectives for the collagen VI disorders center around rational treatment options in this group. Myofiber apoptosis has already been identified as a useful therapeutic target, but more analysis of the pathophysiological effect of the lack of collagen VI on muscle will need to be done to identify additional targets for treatment. A particular challenge lies in the predominance of dominant mutations in the combined collagen VI disorders (UCMD and BM). In this situation gene replacement approaches obviously will not work and other strategies such as inactivation of the dominant negative allele will have to be devised. Stem cell therapy will have to take account of the fact that the origin of collagen VI in muscle is predominantly the muscle interstitial fibroblast. As alluded to earlier, in a minority of UCMD patients mutations in the three collagen VI genes have been ruled out, such that there may be additional genes causing the phenotype that still await discovery. The role in health and disease of the newly discovered collagen VI chains will be another focus of future research.

Autosomal recessive congenital muscular dystrophy with joint hyperlaxity

More recently a form of autosomal recessive CMD with excessive joint laxity was recognized in the French-Canadian population and was mapped to chromosome 3p23–21 [85]. This form of CMD is characterized by neonatal hypotonia and contractures at birth. The achievement of independent ambulation was delayed to up to 3 years. Muscle weakness was slowly progressive, and some (3/14) patients lost the ability to ambulate with a range of 10–32 years of age. There was distal joint laxity (mostly in the fingers) and more proximal contractures. There was no spinal rigidity although scoliosis did develop in some, whereas other patients showed hypermobility of the cervical spine. There was reduced vital capacity in some patients but overt respiratory failure did not develop. CK was normal to mildly elevated; intelligence was largely normal. Muscle biopsies were notable for increased variability in fiber diameter, centrally placed nuclei, some rimmed vacuoles, and predominance of type I fibers. Collagen VI staining was normal on muscle sections. Thus, even though there are some clinical differences (in Figure 12.6 the degree of joint hyperlaxity looks somewhat less than what is typically seen in a UCMD patient), this disorder is an important differential diagnostic consideration for patients with an UCMD-like phenotype. It is expected that this disorder will eventually be seen outside of the French-Canadian population. Normal collagen VI immunohistochemical studies in a patient with a suitable phenotype will help when considering the diagnosis. There are three interesting candidate genes in the region: ITGA9 (integrin alpha 9), LAMR1 (laminin receptor 1) and ACVR2B (activin A IIB receptor, a receptor for the transforming growth factor-β growth factor family). All three of these candidates have a connection to the extracellular matrix.

Abnormalities of nuclear proteins

Lamin-A/C-associated congenital muscular dystrophy

Mutations in the lamin A/C gene [*150330] have been associated with a wide variety of different neuromuscular and non-neuromuscular conditions, ranging from autosomal dominant and recessive Emery Dreyfus muscular dystrophy (EDMD), LGMD1B, autosomal dominant cardiomyopathy with conduction system disease (DCM-CD), CMT2, familial partial lipodystrophy Dunnigan type (FPLD), mandibuloacral dysplasia, Hutchinson–Guilford progeria and related phenotypes, to restrictive dermopathy [120]. It now has become apparent that mutations in the gene coding for lamin A/C (LMNA) can also give rise to an early-onset muscle disease, best classified as a CMD.

Lamin A/C belongs to the A-type lamins that are part of the inner nuclear envelope and interact with emerin, the gene mutated in X-linked EDMD. How mutations in this system would cause muscle disease remains largely unclear but is the subject of intensive investigation.

The early-onset phenotype has been observed in single cases [121, 122, 123, 124] and has more recently been fully characterized in a larger group of patients [125]. The most extreme case of early-onset laminopathy is that of lethal fetal akinesia associated with homozygous stop mutations [126]. There are also cases that do not fall under the fetal akinesia group but still present with profound weakness at birth and virtually absent motor development [122]. In the more common and somewhat milder CMD presentation patients may achieve sitting, but have considerable axial weakness, often leading to an inability to hold the head upright ("dropped head" phenomenon). The weakness at that point tends to be more proximal in the upper extremity and more distal in the lower extremity, with relative sparing of the hip flexors and the quadriceps. Often there will be relatively rapid early progression of weakness, followed by a more stable phase. In particular respiratory insufficiency can be rapidly progressive leading to early necessity for mechanical ventilatory support. There typically will be significant spinal rigidity and scoliosis may also develop. Contractures develop mostly in the Achilles tendons and also in the knees, whereas the elbows are more variably affected by contractures and the fingers are usually free. Facial and extraocular muscles are spared. Cardiac involvement has been seen with more advanced disease, typically in the form of an arrhythmogenic cardiomyopathy. Depending on the clinical involvement of the muscle from which the biopsy was taken, muscle biopsy findings have ranged from just myopathic to more clearly dystrophic with evidence of degeneration and regeneration and prominent atrophic fibers. Immunohistochemistry for lamin A/C on the muscle biopsy has been normal as the mutations detected so far have been de novo dominant. Mutations have affected codons that are also mutated in the more typical EDMD, but with more severe and significant amino acid changes likely accounting for the more severe phenotype seen in this presentation.

Nesprin-associated congenital muscular dystrophy

Congenital muscular dystrophy with abducted thumbs is a rare syndrome described in two siblings from a single family originating from Sicily characterized by adducted thumbs, weakness, mental retardation, and ophthalmoplegia [127]. Both sibs, a boy and a girl, had congenital hypotonia and contractures of thumbs and toes in addition to the weakness. Moreover at birth the girl had to be briefly ventilated, whereas a poor suck was observed in the male. Subsequently there was delay of motor development, followed later by progressive decline in muscle strength. Muscle weakness in the limbs was more marked distally with near-complete wasting of the thenar, hypothenar, and interosseous muscles of the hands. Opposition of thumbs was impossible, and toes showed persistent lateral deviation. Electrophysiology showed normal motor and sensory nerve conduction. The muscle changes on histology showed an increased variation of fiber size with interspersed atrophic fibers, whirled and target fibers but no necrotic fibers. The number of internal nuclei was increased and there was a focal increase of endomysial fibrosis. Electron microscopy was not contributory.

Immunocytochemistry showed normal expression of muscle membrane proteins including laminin-α2, laminin-β2, and α-dystroglycan. Overall the findings were compatible with a chronic myopathic process and did not indicate a structural myopathy. Muscle MRI at midthigh level showed advanced fatty atrophy of all muscles with some preservation of the adductor longus, the semimembranosus, and semitendinosus muscles on both sides. In addition brain MRI showed mild global cerebellar hypoplasia.

By positional cloning the gene responsible for this condition was recently identified as that for nesprin-1 [*608441], a protein localized at the nuclear lamina and binding both emerin and lamins A/C [128]. Heterozygous missense mutations in the nesprin-1 and nesprin-2 genes have recently been related to Emery–Dreifuss muscular dystrophy phenotype [129].

Nesprin-1 and -2 (encoded by the genes SYNE1 and 2) are spectrin-repeat-containing proteins that are involved in nuclear anchorage and organelle migration [130]. They are widely distributed throughout cells, but have a particular role in linking the inner nuclear membrane where they bind to lamin A/C and emerin to the outer nuclear membrane and the cytoskeleton via the LINC complex [131]. Sequencing in patients with EDMD-like phenotypes has uncovered sequence changes that likely are mutations, although their pathogenicity is not completely clear at this point. The phenotype in the patients in three families was varied from almost asymptomatic to more severe dystrophic disease with dilated cardiomyopathy; however, congenital onset has not been described.

Abnormalities at the level of the endoplasmic reticulum: RSMD1 and selenocysteine

Salient diagnostic criteria

Rigid spine muscular dystrophy or RSMD1 [#602771] is a rare form of autosomal recessive CMD caused by mutations in the SEPN1 gene [132]. This condition was first described, at the 50th workshop of the European Consortium on CMD [133], as a subgroup of CMD distinguished by slowly progressive weakness, rigid spine, and early respiratory failure.

Molecular genetics and pathogenesis

The SEPN1 [*606210] gene encodes for selenoprotein N, which is a selenium-containing glycoprotein located within the endoplasmic reticulum [134]. Selenium is added to the peptide chain in the form of a single selenocysteine residue coded for by a distinctly recognized stop codon. Recognition of this codon and insertion of the selenocysteine residue is assisted by a unique sequence located in the 3′ UTR, referred to as the SECIS sequence (selenocysteine insertion sequence). Several other selenoproteins have been characterized, many of which are enzymes involved in oxidation–reduction reactions, and all of them have a selenocysteine at their active site. Full-length SEPN1 transcripts are expressed in a variety of tissues including skeletal muscle, brain, and lung. It is also found in the placenta and is more prevalent in fetal than adult tissue [135]. Little is known about the function of selenoproteins in skeletal muscle. Selenoprotein N with its localization in the endoplasmic reticulum may be involved in general metabolic pathways, such as protein post-translational modification. The reason why clinical manifestations are limited to muscle may have to do with muscle-specific pathways that are particularly dependent on SEPN1 function but are essentially unknown.

Inhibition of the sepn1 gene in the zebrafish during early development by injection of antisense morpholinos does not

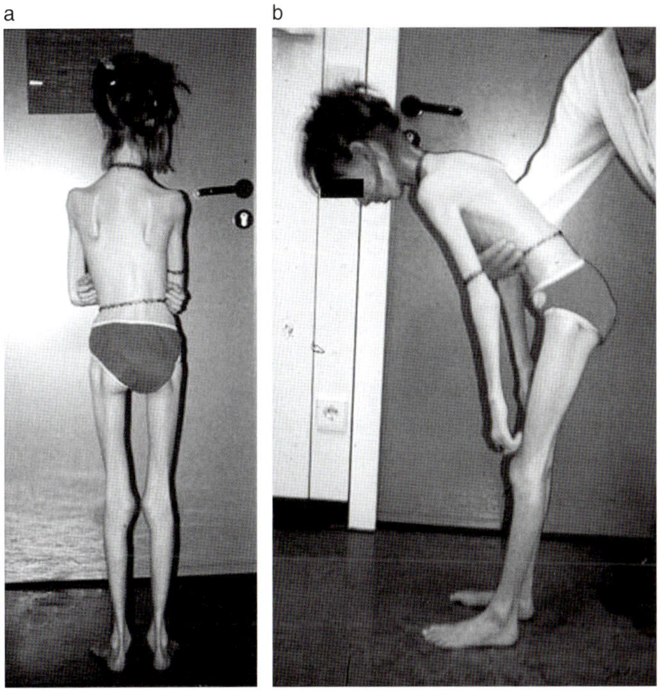

Figure 12.8a, b. Patient with a rigid spine syndrome due to SEPN1 mutations (RSMD1): generalized muscle wasting and extremely thin habitus is evident (a). There is considerable extensor rigidity of the entire spine when bending forward (b); note the contracture of the paraspinal cervical posterior neck muscles (b).

alter the fate of the muscular tissue, but causes muscle architecture disorganization and greatly reduced motility. Ultrastructural analysis of the myotomes reveals defects in muscle sarcomeric organization and in myofiber attachment, as well as altered myoseptum integrity. These studies demonstrate the important role of SEPN1 in muscle organization during early development [136].

Salient clinical phenotypical features

The distinctive clinical features are early rigidity of the spine and early onset of a restrictive respiratory syndrome (Figure 12.8). These children may have mild hypotonia and weakness in the first few months of life but generally achieve independent walking by 18 months of age. In some cases developmental milestones are normal but patients develop a rigid spine and Achilles tendon contractures in the first years.

On examination there is some weakness, mainly of the axial muscles and to a lesser extent the proximal muscles. Patients with RSMD1 generally do not become significantly weaker over time but often develop progressive and severe scoliosis as well as contractures which may require surgery. No muscle hypertrophy is noticed and serum CK is within the normal range.

Motor functional abilities may decrease because of the marked tendency to develop contractures, but patients rarely lose the ability to walk independently. Limitation of mouth opening and midface hypoplasia can also be observed. Due to palatal weakness, nasal speech is common.

Respiratory failure is an invariable and early feature, requiring nocturnal ventilatory support at the end of the first or in the second decade of life, when patients are still ambulant.

In a recent series of 11 juvenile patients from 8 families with SEPN1 mutations patients were followed for a mean period of 7.2 years, the age of first manifestations was variable within the first 2 years of life with muscle hypotonia, lack of head control, and delayed motor development. Further gross motor development was normal in 9/11 patients. All patients were ambulant at a mean age of 13.7 years. Eight patients exhibited a rigid spine diagnosed at a mean age of 10 years. All patients had respiratory impairment with a vital capacity ranging from 18% to 65%. Four patients were intermittently nocturnally ventilated at a mean age of 11 years. Body mass index was below 20 kg/m^2 in all patients. In this study there seemed to be no correlation between skeletal muscle weakness and respiratory failure [137]. Muscle MRI shows a typical pattern with adductors, sartorius, and biceps femoris more markedly involved and rectus femoris and gracilis relatively spared [138]. The atrophy of the adductor group in the thigh may also be apparent clinically, giving the impression of a "scooped out" inner thigh.

Genotype–phenotype correlations

Presently there are no firmly established genotype–phenotype correlations. Most mutations are private. *SEPN1* mutations in RSMD and MmD are predominantly truncating, with a few missense mutations typically affecting functionally important domains of the protein. Homozygous mutations are unexpectedly common even in families from nonconsanguineous backgrounds, due to the presence of few founder mutations in different European populations.

Diagnostic approaches (biochemistry, pathology, histochemistry, immunocytochemistry, fine structure, immunoblot, mutational analysis, imaging)

Skeletal muscle biopsies show nonspecific myopathic changes such as fiber diameter variability, prevalence of type 1 fibers, atrophy, and internalization of nuclei. Some specimens contain minicores typical of classical minicore myopathies [139] and others may show Mallory-body-like inclusions [140]. An early-onset, recessive form with Mallory-body-like inclusions (MB-DRMs) was first described in five related German patients [141] and had been classified among a heterogeneous group of muscle disorders denominated desmin-related myopathies (DRM) or myofibrillar myopathies. However, these patients were later shown to be homozygous for an SEPN1 mutation [140]. Recently a fourth morphological marker in muscle biopsy related to SEPN1 mutations in an RSMD1 patient was reported as congenital fiber-type disproportion. The patient also had insulin resistance [141, 142]. Even though there was morphological heterogeneity in the biopsies, clinically all the patients were quite consistent with the phenotype described above. Antibodies directed against the 70-kDa

SEPN1 can show absence of the protein in fibroblasts of patients with nonsense mutations. Screening for mutations in the *SEPN1* gene is required to establish the diagnosis of RSMD1.

Therapeutic and preventative modalities

Possible therapies have been elusive as the precise functions of SEPN1 in muscle are still elusive. Major complications such as early respiratory failure, impaired weight gain, and orthopedic problems need to be addressed following the principles outlined earlier for other conditions within CMD.

Genetic counseling

The gene is located on chromosome 1p36. This condition is inherited as an autosomal recessive trait, so both parents are generally asymptomatic carriers of the recessive mutations, resulting in a 25% recurrence risk for future pregnancies.

Future perspectives

Unlike other CMDs RSMD1 does not affect the basal lamina or laminin receptors. Novel pathogenic pathways will need to be explored as further work helps define the nature of this disease and its pathology. Gene replacement therapy appears to be an option when available, as the basis of the disease is loss of function of the protein.

Other rare forms

Congenital muscular dystrophy 1B (MDC1B): muscle hypertrophy and secondary laminin-α2 deficiency

This form, described in one United Arab Emirates family and one German family, is characterized by delayed motor milestones but acquisition of independent ambulation [143] [%604801]. There is predominantly axial and proximal muscle weakness with prominent head lag. Generalized muscle hypertrophy, combined with wasting of the neck muscle, was also observed. Serum CK was grossly elevated, and the muscle biopsy showed a partial deficiency of laminin-α2 and a deficiency of α-dystroglycan. Genetic studies have localized the locus responsible for this form of CMD to chromosome 1q42 in both families [68]. The responsible gene has not been identified yet.

Microcephaly-cortical-dysplasia peripheral neuropathy

Two separate families have been described with generalized muscle wasting and weakness, calf pseudohypertrophy and joint contractures, microcephaly, and severely delayed psychomotor development. These patients showed electrophysiological evidence of demyelinating peripheral neuropathy, with pontocerebellar hypoplasia in one family [144] and cerebellar hypoplasia in the other [145], bilateral opercular abnormalities and focal cortical dysplasia on brain MRI. Laminin-α2 expression in muscle was reportedly normal [144, 145]. Creatine kinase levels are elevated. Muscle biopsy showed dystrophic features with normal laminin-α2 staining. Ophthalmological and cardiac examinations were normal.

Congenital muscular dystrophy and cataracts

This form of CMD is characterized by mild mental retardation, bilateral cataracts, and normal cranial MRI [146]. It has been reported in two siblings originating from Brazil affected by a laminin-α2-positive CMD, cataracts, retinitis pigmentosa, diversion of the optic disk, but no cerebral anomalies, except for microcephaly and slight mental retardation. One child had epilepsy easily controlled by anticonvulsant therapy. Both children presented hypotonia from birth, delayed psychomotor development, generalized muscular weakness, and atrophy and joint contractures of knees and ankles. The course of the disease, apparently static during the first 10 years of life, became progressive during the second decade with loss of ambulation by the age of 13 years. Creatine kinase was increased in both children. Bilateral cataracts were diagnosed at 6 months of age. In spite of the occurrence of microcephaly, mental retardation was slight and the siblings acquired reading and writing skills after the age of 10. Marinesco–Sjögren syndrome is an important differential diagnostic consideration in this clinical scenario.

Congenital muscular dystrophy and cerebellar atrophy

This form of CMD is characterized by early-onset weakness, high CK, and marked cerebellar atrophy [#603323]. The muscle biopsy shows dystrophic changes, and immunohistochemical staining for laminin-α2, dystrophin, and dystrophin-related proteins is normal [147, 148]. Immunostaining for glycosylated α-dystroglycan appears to be normal in the patients in whom it was analyzed (Professor Carlo Trevisan, personal communication). The condition has been reported in familial cases with a likely autosomal recessive trait.

Congenital muscular dystrophy with short stature, mental retardation, and distal laxity

A form with distal laxity, early respiratory impairment, and a significant overlap with UCMD but associated with short stature and mental retardation has been described. Linkage to the collagen VI genes was negative [149].

References

1. F. E. Batten, The myopathies or muscular dystrophies. *Q. J. Med.* **3** (1909), 313.
2. T. Voit, Congenital muscular dystrophies: 1997 update. *Brain Dev.* **20**:2 (1998), 65–74.

3. K. Kobayashi, Y. Nakahori, M. Miyake, *et al.*, An ancient retrotransposal insertion causes Fukuyama-type congenital muscular dystrophy. *Nature* **394**:6691 (1998), 388–392.
4. A. Yoshida, K. Kobayashi, H. Manya, *et al.*, Muscular dystrophy and neuronal migration disorder caused by mutations in a glycosyltransferase, POMGnT1. *Dev. Cell.* **1**:5 (2001), 717–724.
5. M. Brockington, Y. Yuva, P. Prandini, *et al.*, Mutations in the fukutin-related protein gene (FKRP) identify limb girdle muscular dystrophy 2I as a milder allelic variant of congenital muscular dystrophy MDC1C. *Hum. Mol. Genet.* **10**:25 (2001), 2851–2859.
6. M. Brockington, D. J. Blake, P. Prandini, *et al.*, Mutations in the fukutin-related protein gene (FKRP) cause a form of congenital muscular dystrophy with secondary laminin alpha2 deficiency and abnormal glycosylation of alpha-dystroglycan. *Am. J. Hum. Genet.* **69**:6 (2001), 1198–1209.
7. D. Beltran-Valero De Bernabe, S. Currier, A. Steinbrecher, *et al.*, Mutations in the O-mannosyltransferase gene POMT1 give rise to the severe neuronal migration disorder Walker-Warburg syndrome. *Am. J. Hum. Genet.* **71**:5 (2002), 1033–1043.
8. C. Longman, M. Brockington, S. Torelli, *et al.*, Mutations in the human LARGE gene cause MDC1D, a novel form of congenital muscular dystrophy with severe mental retardation and abnormal glycosylation of alpha-dystroglycan. *Hum. Mol. Genet.* **12**:21 (2003), 2853–2861.
9. J. van Reeuwijk, M. Janssen, C. van den Elzen, *et al.*, POMT2 mutations cause alpha-dystroglycan hypoglycosylation and Walker Warburg syndrome. *J. Med. Genet.* **42**:12 (2005), 907–912.
10. F. Muntoni, T. Voit, The congenital muscular dystrophies in 2004: a century of exciting progress. *Neuromuscul. Disord.* **14**:10 (2004), 635–649.
11. D. E. Michele, R. Barresi, M. Kanagawa, *et al.*, Post-translational disruption of dystroglycan ligand interactions in congenital muscular dystrophies. *Nature* **418**:6896 (2002), 417–421.
12. E. Martin-Rendon, D. J. Blake, Protein glycosylation in disease: new insights into the congenital muscular dystrophies. *Trends. Pharmacol. Sci.* **24**:4 (2003), 178–183.
13. J. van Reeuwijk, S. Maugenre, C. van den Elzen, *et al.*, The expanding phenotype of POMT1 mutations: from Walker-Warburg syndrome to congenital muscular dystrophy, microcephaly, and mental retardation. *Hum. Mutat.* **27**:5 (2006), 453–459.
14. E. Mercuri, H. Topaloglu, M. Brockington, *et al.*, Spectrum of brain changes in patients with congenital muscular dystrophy and FKRP gene mutations. *Arch. Neurol.* **63**:2 (2006), 251–257.
15. A. D'Amico, A. Tessa, C. Bruno, *et al.*, Expanding the clinical spectrum of POMT1 phenotype. *Neurology* **66**:10 (2006), 1564–1567. discussion 461.
16. C. Godfrey, E. Clement, R. Mein, *et al.*, Refining genotype phenotype correlations in muscular dystrophies with defective glycosylation of dystroglycan. *Brain* **130**:Pt 10 (2007), 2725–2735.
17. L. Aravind, E. V. Koonin, The fukutin protein family – predicted enzymes modifying cell-surface molecules. *Curr. Biol.* **9**:22 (1999), R836–R837.
18. F. Muntoni, M. Brockington, D. J. Blake, S. Torelli, S. C. Brown, Defective glycosylation in muscular dystrophy. *Lancet* **360**:9343 (2002), 1419–1421.
19. D. Beltran-Valero de Bernabe, T. Voit, C. Longman, *et al.*, Mutations in the FKRP gene can cause muscle-eye-brain disease and Walker-Warburg syndrome. *J. Med. Genet.* **41**:5 (2004), e61.
20. H. Topaloglu, M. Brockington, Y. Yuva, *et al.*, FKRP gene mutations cause congenital muscular dystrophy, mental retardation, and cerebellar cysts. *Neurology* **60**:6 (2003), 988–992.
21. C. Diesen, A. Saarinen, H. Pihko, *et al.*, POMGnT1 mutation and phenotypic spectrum in muscle-eye-brain disease. *J. Med. Genet.* **41**:10 (2004), e115.
22. B. Balci, G. Uyanik, P. Dincer, *et al.*, An autosomal recessive limb girdle muscular dystrophy (LGMD2) with mild mental retardation is allelic to Walker-Warburg syndrome (WWS) caused by a mutation in the POMT1 gene. *Neuromuscul. Disord.* **15**:4 (2005), 271–275.
23. A. Yanagisawa, C. Bouchet, P. Y. Van den Bergh, *et al.*, New POMT2 mutations causing congenital muscular dystrophy: identification of a founder mutation. *Neurology* **69**:12 (2007), 1254–1260.
24. P. K. Grewal, P. J. Holzfeind, R. E. Bittner, J. E. Hewitt, Mutant glycosyltransferase and altered glycosylation of alpha-dystroglycan in the myodystrophy mouse. *Nat. Genet.* **28**:2 (2001), 151–154.
25. J. van Reeuwijk, P. K. Grewal, M. A. Salih, *et al.*, Intragenic deletion in the LARGE gene causes Walker-Warburg syndrome. *Hum. Genet.* **121**:6 (2007), 685–690.
26. R. Barresi, K. P. Campbell, Dystroglycan: from biosynthesis to pathogenesis of human disease. *J. Cell. Sci.* **119**:Pt 2 (2006), 199–207.
27. S. A. Moore, F. Saito, J. Chen, *et al.*, Deletion of brain dystroglycan recapitulates aspects of congenital muscular dystrophy. *Nature* **418**:6896 (2002), 422–425.
28. T. Toda, K. Kobayashi, E. Kondo-Iida, J. Sasaki, Y. Nakamura, The Fukuyama congenital muscular dystrophy story. *Neuromuscul. Disord.* **10**:3 (2000), 153–159.
29. T. Nakanishi, M. Sakauchi, Y. Kaneda, *et al.*, Cardiac involvement in Fukuyama-type congenital muscular dystrophy. *Pediatrics* **117**:6 (2006), e1187–e1192.
30. E. Kondo-Iida, K. Kobayashi, M. Watanabe, *et al.*, Novel mutations and genotype-phenotype relationships in 107 families with Fukuyama-type congenital muscular dystrophy (FCMD). *Hum. Mol. Genet.* **8**:12 (1999), 2303–2309.
31. C. Godfrey, D. Escolar, M. Brockington, *et al.*, Fukutin gene mutations in steroid-responsive limb girdle muscular dystrophy. *Ann. Neurol.* **60**:5 (2006), 603–610.
32. T. Murakami, Y. K. Hayashi, S. Noguchi, *et al.*, Fukutin gene mutations cause dilated cardiomyopathy with minimal muscle weakness. *Ann. Neurol.* **60**:5 (2006), 597–602.
33. B. Cormand, H. Pihko, M. Bayes, *et al.*, Clinical and genetic distinction between Walker-Warburg syndrome and muscle-eye-brain disease. *Neurology* **56**:8 (2001), 1059–1069.
34. W. B. Dobyns, R. A. Pagon, D. Armstrong, *et al.*, Diagnostic criteria for Walker-Warburg syndrome [see comments]. *Am. J. Med. Genet.* **32**:2 (1989), 195–210.

35. M. Poppe, J. Bourke, M. Eagle, *et al.*, Cardiac and respiratory failure in limb-girdle muscular dystrophy 2I. *Ann. Neurol.* **56**: 5 (2004), 738–741.

36. A. D'Amico, S. Petrini, F. Parisi, *et al.*, Heart transplantation in a child with LGMD2I presenting as isolated dilated cardiomyopathy. *Neuromuscul. Disord.* **18**:2 (2008), 153–155.

37. C. Bouchet, M. Gonzales, S. Vuillaumier-Barrot, *et al.*, Molecular heterogeneity in fetal forms of type II lissencephaly. *Hum. Mutat.* **28**:10 (2007), 1020–1027.

38. R. Biancheri, A. Falace, A. Tessa, *et al.*, POMT2 gene mutation in limb-girdle muscular dystrophy with inflammatory changes. *Biochem. Biophys. Res. Commun.* **363**:4 (2007), 1033–1037.

39. K. Taniguchi, K. Kobayashi, K. Saito, *et al.*, Worldwide distribution and broader clinical spectrum of muscle-eye-brain disease. *Hum. Mol. Genet.* **12**:5 (2003), 527–534.

40. F. Silan, M. Yoshioka, K. Kobayashi, *et al.*, A new mutation of the fukutin gene in a non-Japanese patient. *Ann. Neurol.* **53**:3 (2003), 392–396.

41. M. L. Sveen, M. Schwartz, J. Vissing, High prevalence and phenotype-genotype correlations of limb girdle muscular dystrophy type 2I in Denmark. *Ann. Neurol.* **59**:5 (2006), 808–815.

42. J. Vajsar, W. Zhang, W. B. Dobyns, *et al.*, Carriers and patients with muscle-eye-brain disease can be rapidly diagnosed by enzymatic analysis of fibroblasts and lymphoblasts. *Neuromuscul. Disord.* **16**:2 (2006), 132–136.

43. K. Akasaka-Manya, H. Manya, T. Endo, Mutations of the POMT1 gene found in patients with Walker-Warburg syndrome lead to a defect of protein O-mannosylation. *Biochem. Biophys. Res. Commun.* **325**:1 (2004), 75–79.

44. R. Barresi, D. E. Michele, M. Kanagawa, *et al.*, LARGE can functionally bypass alpha-dystroglycan glycosylation defects in distinct congenital muscular dystrophies. *Nat. Med.* **10**:7 (2004), 696–703.

45. J. Liu, S. L. Ball, Y. Yang, *et al.*, A genetic model for muscle-eye-brain disease in mice lacking protein O-mannose 1,2-N-acetylglucosaminyltransferase (POMGnT1). *Mech. Dev.* **123**:3 (2006), 228–240.

46. D. J. Burkin, S. J. Kaufman, The alpha7beta1 integrin in muscle development and disease. *Cell. Tissue. Res.* **296**:1 (1999), 183–190.

47. N. L. Flintoff-Dye, J. Welser, J. Rooney, *et al.*, Role for the alpha7beta1 integrin in vascular development and integrity. *Dev. Dyn.* **234**:1 (2005), 11–21.

48. P. T. Martin, S. J. Kaufman, R. H. Kramer, J. R. Sanes, Synaptic integrins in developing, adult, and mutant muscle: selective association of alpha1, alpha7A, and alpha7B integrins with the neuromuscular junction. *Dev. Biol.* **174**:1 (1996), 125–139.

49. R. D. Cohn, R. Herrmann, L. Sorokin, U. M. Wewer, T. Voit, Laminin alpha2 chain-deficient congenital muscular dystrophy: variable epitope expression in severe and mild cases. *Neurology* **51**:1 (1998), 94–100.

50. B. L. Patton, A. M. Connoll, P. T. Martin, *et al.*, Distribution of ten laminin chains in dystrophic and regenerating muscles. *Neuromuscul. Disord.* **9**:6–7 (1999), 423–433.

51. Y. K. Hayashi, F. -L. Chou, E. Engvall, *et al.*, Mutations in the integrin $\alpha7$ gene cause congenital myopathy. *Nat. Genet.* **19** (1998), 94–97.

52. E. Pegoraro, F. Cepollaro, P. Prandini, *et al.*, Integrin alpha 7 beta 1 in muscular dystrophy/myopathy of unknown etiology. *Am. J. Pathol.* **160**:6 (2002), 2135–2143.

53. U. Mayer, G. Saher, R. Fassler, *et al.*, Absence of integrin alpha 7 causes a novel form of muscular dystrophy. *Nat. Genet.* **17**:3 (1997), 318–323.

54. F. M. Tomé, T. Evangelista, A. Leclerc, *et al.*, Congenital muscular dystrophy with merosin deficiency. *C. R. Acad. Sci. Paris* **317**:4 (1994), 251–357.

55. D. Hillaire, A. Leclerc, S. Faure, *et al.*, Localization of merosin-negative congenital muscular dystrophy to chromosome 6q2 by homozygosity mapping. *Hum. Mol. Genet.* **3**:9 (1994), 1657–1661.

56. V. Allamand, P. Guicheney, Merosin-deficient congenital muscular dystrophy, autosomal recessive (MDC1A, MIM# 156225, LAMA2 gene coding for alpha2 chain of laminin). *Eur. J. Hum. Genet.* **10**:2 (2002), 91–94.

57. J. Philpot, F. Muntoni, Limitation of eye movement in merosin-deficient congenital muscular dystrophy [letter]. *Lancet* **353**:9149 (1999), 297–298.

58. J. Philpot, F. Cowan, J. Pennock, *et al.*, Merosin-deficient congenital muscular dystrophy: the spectrum of brain involvement on magnetic resonance imaging. *Neuromuscul. Disord.* **9**:2 (1999), 81–85.

59. I. Boor, M. Nagtegaal, W. Kamphorst, *et al.*, MLC1 is associated with the dystrophin-glycoprotein complex at astrocytic endfeet. *Acta Neuropathol.* **114**:4 (2007), 403–410.

60. K. J. Jones, G. Morgan, H. Johnston, *et al.*, The expanding phenotype of laminin alpha2 chain (merosin) abnormalities: case series and review. *J. Med. Genet.* **38**:10 (2001), 649–657.

61. Z. Shorer, J. Philpot, F. Muntoni, C. Sewry, V. Dubowitz, Demyelinating peripheral neuropathy in merosin-deficient congenital muscular dystrophy. *J. Child Neurol.* **10**:6 (1995), 472–475.

62. V. Allamand, Y. Sunada, M. A. Salih, *et al.*, Mild congenital muscular dystrophy in two patients with an internally deleted laminin alpha2-chain. *Hum. Mol. Genet.* **6**:5 (1997), 747–752.

63. I. Naom, M. D'Alessandro, C. A. Sewry, *et al.*, Mutations in the laminin alpha2-chain gene in two children with early-onset muscular dystrophy. *Brain* **123**:Pt 1 (2000), 31–41.

64. Z. Tezak, P. Prandini, M. Boscaro, *et al.*, Clinical and molecular study in congenital muscular dystrophy with partial laminin alpha 2 (LAMA2) deficiency. *Hum. Mutat.* **21**:2 (2003), 103–111.

65. C. Di Blasi, D. Piga, P. Brioschi, *et al.*, LAMA2 gene analysis in congenital muscular dystrophy: new mutations, prenatal diagnosis, and founder effect. *Arch. Neurol.* **62**:10 (2005), 1582–1586.

66. E. Pegoraro, P. Mancias, S. H. Swerdlow, *et al.*, Congenital muscular dystrophy with primary laminin alpha2 (merosin) deficiency presenting as inflammatory myopathy. *Ann. Neurol.* **40**:5 (1996), 782–791.

67. C. A. Sewry, J. Philpot, L. M. Sorokin, *et al.*, Diagnosis of merosin (laminin-2) deficient congenital muscular dystrophy by skin biopsy. *Lancet* **347**:9001 (1996), 582–584.

68. M. Brockington, C. A. Sewry, R. Herrmann, *et al.*, Assignment of a form of congenital muscular dystrophy with secondary

merosin deficiency to chromosome 1q42. *Am. J. Hum. Genet.* **66**:2 (2000), 428–435.

69. P. Guicheney, N. Vignier, X. Zhang, *et al.*, PCR based mutation screening in the laminin α2 chain gene (LAMA2): application to prenatal diagnosis and search for founder effects in congenital muscular dystrophy. *J. Med. Genet.* **35** (1998), 211–217.

70. J. Philpot, A. Bagnall, C. King, V. Dubowitz, F. Muntoni, Feeding problems in merosin deficient congenital muscular dystrophy. *Arch. Dis. Child.* **80**:6 (1999), 542–547.

71. M. Vainzof, P. Richard, R. Herrmann, *et al.*, Prenatal diagnosis in laminin alpha2 chain (merosin)-deficient congenital muscular dystrophy: a collective experience of five international centers. *Neuromuscul. Disord.* **15**:9–10 (2005), 588–594.

72. A. M. Michelson, E. S. Russell, P. J. Harman, Dystrophia muscularis: a hereditary primary myopathy in the house mouse. *Proc. Natl. Acad. Sci. U. S. A.* **41**:12 (1955), 1079–1084.

73. G. D. Shelton, E. Engvall, Canine and feline models of human inherited muscle diseases. *Neuromuscul. Disord.* **15**:2 (2005), 127–138.

74. J. Moll, P. Barzaghi, S. Lin, *et al.*, An agrin minigene rescues dystrophic symptoms in a mouse model for congenital muscular dystrophy. *Nature* **413**:6853 (2001), 302–307.

75. J. A. Dominov, A. J. Kravetz, M. Ardelt, C. A. Kostek, M. L. Beermann, J. B. Miller, Muscle-specific BCL2 expression ameliorates muscle disease in laminin {alpha}2-deficient, but not in dystrophin-deficient, mice. *Hum. Mol. Genet.* **14**:8 (2005), 1029–1040.

76. O. Ullrich, Kongenitale atonisch-sklerotische Muskeldystrophie, ein weiterer Typus der heredodegeneration Erkrankungen des neuromuskulären Systems. *Z. Ges. Neurol. Psychiat.* **126** (1930), 171–120.

77. O. Ullrich, Kongenitale atonisch-sklerotische Muskeldystrophie. *Monatsschr. Kinderheilkd.* **47** (1930), 502–510.

78. T. Furukawa, Y. Toyokura, Congenital, hypotonic sclerotic muscular dystrophy. *J. Med. Genet.* **14**:6 (1977), 426–429.

79. I. Nonaka, Y. Une, T. Ishihara, S. Miyoshino, T. Nakashima, H. Sugita, A clinical and histological study of Ullrich's disease (congenital atonic-sclerotic muscular dystrophy). *Neuropediatrics* **12**:3 (1981), 197–208.

80. O. Vanegas Camacho, E. Bertini, R. Z. Zhang, *et al.*, Ullrich scleroatonic muscular dystrophy is caused by recessive mutations in collagen type VI. *Proc. Natl. Acad. Sci. U. S. A.* **98**:13 (2001), 7516–7521.

81. J. Bethlem, G. K. Wijngaarden, Benign myopathy, wth autosomal dominant inheritance: a report on three pedigrees. *Brain* **99** (1976), 91–100.

82. G. J. Jöbsis, H. Keizers, J. P. Vreijling, *et al.*, Type VI collagen mutations in Bethlem myopathy, an autosomal dominant myopathy with contractures. *Nat. Genet.* **14** (1996), 113–115.

83. A. K. Lampe, K. M. Bushby, Collagen VI related muscle disorders. *J. Med. Genet.* **42**:9 (2005), 673–685.

84. S. Petrini, A. D'Amico, P. Sale, *et al.*, Ullrich myopathy phenotype with secondary ColVI defect identified by confocal imaging and electron microscopy analysis. *Neuromuscul. Disord.* **17**:8 (2007), 587–596.

85. M. Tetreault, A. Duquette, I. Thiffault, *et al.*, A new form of congenital muscular dystrophy with joint hyperlaxity maps to 3p23–21. *Brain* **129**:Pt 8 (2006), 2077–2084.

86. M. Okada, G. Kawahara, S. Noguchi, *et al.*, Primary collagen VI deficiency is the second most common congenital muscular dystrophy in Japan. *Neurology* **69**:10 (2007), 1035–1042.

87. E. Bertini, G. Pepe, Collagen type VI and related disorders: Bethlem myopathy and Ullrich scleroatonic muscular dystrophy. *Eur. J. Paediatr. Neurol.* **6**:4 (2002), 193–198.

88. J. Kirschner, I. Hausser, Y. Zou, *et al.*, Ullrich congenital muscular dystrophy: connective tissue abnormalities in the skin support overlap with Ehlers-Danlos syndromes. *Am. J. Med. Genet. A.* **132**:3 (2005), 296–301.

89. I. Higuchi, T. Shiraishi, T. Hashiguchi, *et al.*, Frameshift mutation in the collagen VI gene causes Ullrich's disease. *Ann. Neurol.* **50**:2 (2001), 261–265.

90. H. Ishikawa, K. Sugie, K. Murayama, *et al.*, Ullrich disease due to deficiency of collagen VI in the sarcolemma. *Neurology* **62**:4 (2004), 620–623.

91. T. C. Pan, R. Z. Zhang, D. G. Sudano, S. K. Marie, C. G. Bonnemann, M. L. Chu, New molecular mechanism for Ullrich congenital muscular dystrophy: a heterozygous in-frame deletion in the COL6A1 gene causes a severe phenotype. *Am. J. Hum. Genet.* **73**:2 (2003), 355–369.

92. M. L. Chu, T. C. Pan, D. Conway, *et al.*, The structure of type VI collagen. *Ann. N. Y. Acad. Sci.* **580** (1990), 55–63.

93. R. Timpl, M. L. Chu, Microfibrillar collagen type VI. In *Extracellular Matrix Assembly and Structure*, ed R. P. Mecham. (Orlando, FL: Academic Press, 1994), pp. 207–242.

94. M. Heiskanen, B. Saitta, A. Palotie, M. L. Chu, Head to tail organization of the human COL6A1 and COL6A2 genes by fiber-FISH. *Genomics* **29**:3 (1995), 801–803.

95. D. Weil, M. G. Mattei, E. Passage, *et al.*, Cloning and chromosomal localization of human genes encoding the three chains of type VI collagen. *Am. J. Hum. Genet.* **42**:3 (1988), 435–445.

96. M. L. Chu, D. Conway, T. C. Pan, *et al.*, Amino acid sequence of the triple-helical domain of human collagen type VI. *J. Biol. Chem.* **263**:35 (1988), 18601–18606.

97. M. L. Chu, R. Z. Zhang, T. C. Pan, *et al.*, Mosaic structure of globular domains in the human type VI collagen alpha 3 chain: similarity to von Willebrand factor, fibronectin, actin, salivary proteins and aprotinin type protease inhibitors. *EMBO J.* **9**:2 (1990), 385–393.

98. S. K. Gara, P. Grumati, A. Urciuolo, *et al.*, Three novel collagen VI chains with high homology to the alpha3 chain. *J. Biol. Chem.* **283**:16 (2008), 10658–10670.

99. E. Engvall, H. Hessle, G. Klier, Molecular assembly, secretion, and matrix deposition of type VI collagen. *J. Cell. Biol.* **102**:3 (1986), 703–710.

100. H. Furthmayr, H. Wiedemann, R. Timpl, E. Odermatt, J. Engel, Electron-microscopical approach to a structural model of intima collagen. *Biochem. J.* **211**:2 (1983), 303–311.

101. A. Colombatti, M T. Mucignat, P. Bonaldo, *et al.*, Secretion and matrix assembly of recombinant type VI collagen. *J. Biol. Chem.* **270**:22 (1995), 13105–13111.

102. P. Bonaldo, V. Russo, F. Bucciotti, R. Doliana, A. Colombatti, Structural and functional features of the alpha 3 chain indicate a bridging role for chicken collagen VI in connective tissues. *Biochemistry* **29**:5 (1990), 1245–1254.

103. C. Baldock, M. J. Sherratt, C. A. Shuttleworth, C. M. Kielty, The supramolecular organization of collagen VI microfibrils. *J. Mol. Biol.* **330**:2 (2003), 297–307.

104. K. Senga, M. Kobayashi, H. Hattori, *et al.*, Type VI collagen in mouse masseter tendon, from osseous attachment to myotendinous junction. *Anat. Rec.* **243**:3 (1995), 294–302.

105. T. M. Ritty, R. Roth, J. E. Heuser, Tendon cell array isolation reveals a previously unknown fibrillin-2-containing macromolecular assembly. *Structure* **11**:9 (2003), 1179–1188.

106. D. R. Keene, E. Engvall, R. W. Glanville, Ultrastructure of type VI collagen in human skin and cartilage suggests an anchoring function for this filamentous network. *J. Cell. Biol.* **107**:5 (1988), 1995–2006.

107. H. J. Kuo, C. L. Maslen, D. R. Keene, R. W. Glanville, Type VI collagen anchors endothelial basement membranes by interacting with type IV collagen. *J. Biol. Chem.* **272**:42 (1997), 26522–26529.

108. W. A. Irwin, N. Bergamin, P. Sabatelli, *et al.*, Mitochondrial dysfunction and apoptosis in myopathic mice with collagen VI deficiency. *Nat. Genet.* **35**:4 (2003), 367–371.

109. A. Angelin, T. Tiepolo, P. Sabatelli, *et al.*, Mitochondrial dysfunction in the pathogenesis of Ullrich congenital muscular dystrophy and prospective therapy with cyclosporins. *Proc. Natl. Acad. Sci. U. S. A.* **104**:3 (2007), 991–996.

110. A. K. Lampe, D. M. Dunn, A. C. von Niederhausern, *et al.*, Automated genomic sequence analysis of the three collagen VI genes: applications to Ullrich congenital muscular dystrophy and Bethlem myopathy. *J. Med. Genet.* **42**:2 (2005), 108–120.

111. E. Demir, P. Sabatelli, V. Allamand, *et al.*, Mutations in COL6A3 cause severe and mild phenotypes of Ullrich congenital muscular dystrophy. *Am. J. Hum. Genet.* **70**:6 (2002), 1446–1458.

112. L. Lucarini, B. Giusti, R. Z. Zhang, *et al.*, A homozygous COL6A2 intron mutation causes in-frame triple-helical deletion and nonsense-mediated mRNA decay in a patient with Ullrich congenital muscular dystrophy. *Hum. Genet.* **117**:5 (2005), 460–466.

113. A. K. Lampe, Y. Zou, D. Sudano, *et al.*, Exon skipping mutations in collagen VI are common and are predictive for severity and inheritance. *Hum. Mut.* **29**:6 (2008), 809–822.

114. N. L. Baker, M. Mörgelin, R. Peat, *et al.*, Dominant collagen VI mutations are a common cause of Ullrich congenital muscular dystrophy. *Hum. Mol. Genet.* **14**:2 (2005), 279–293.

115. N. L. Baker, M. Mörgelin, R A. Pace, *et al.*, Molecular consequences of dominant Bethlem myopathy collagen VI mutations. *Ann. Neurol.* **62** (2007), 390–405.

116. E. Mercuri, A. Lampe, J. Allsop, *et al.*, Muscle MRI in Ullrich congenital muscular dystrophy and Bethlem myopathy. *Neuromuscul. Disord.* **15**:4 (2005), 303–310.

117. C. G. Bonnemann, K. Brockmann, F. Hanefeld, Muscle ultrasound in Bethlem myopathy. *Neuropediatrics* **34**:6 (2003), 335–336.

118. C. Jimenez-Mallebrera, M. A. Maioli, J. Kim, *et al.*, A comparative analysis of collagen VI production in muscle, skin and fibroblasts from 14 Ullrich congenital muscular dystrophy patients with dominant and recessive COL6A mutations. *Neuromuscul. Disord.* **16**:9–10 (2006), 571–582.

119. L. Merlini, A. Angelin, T. Tiepolo, *et al.*, Cyclosporin A corrects mitochondrial dysfunction and muscle apoptosis in patients with collagen VI myopathies. *Proc. Natl. Acad. Sci. U. S. A.* **105**:13 (2008), 5225–5229.

120. J. Rankin, S. Ellard, The laminopathies: a clinical review. *Clin. Genet.* **70**:4 (2006), 261–274.

121. E. Mercuri, A. Y. Manzur, H. Jungbluth, *et al.*, Early and severe presentation of autosomal dominant Emery-Dreifuss muscular dystrophy (EMD2). *Neurology* **54**:8 (2000), 1704–1705.

122. E. Mercuri, M. Poppe, R. Quinlivan, *et al.*, Extreme variability of phenotype in patients with an identical missense mutation in the lamin A/C gene: from congenital onset with severe phenotype to milder classic Emery-Dreifuss variant. *Arch. Neurol.* **61**:5 (2004), 690–694.

123. E. Mercuri, S. C. Brown, P. Nihoyannopoulos, *et al.*, Extreme variability of skeletal and cardiac muscle involvement in patients with mutations in exon 11 of the lamin A/C gene. *Muscle Nerve* **31**:5 (2005), 602–609.

124. A. D'Amico, G. Haliloglu, P. Richard, *et al.*, Two patients with "Dropped head syndrome" due to mutations in LMNA or SEPN1 genes. *Neuromuscul. Disord.* **15**:8 (2005), 521–524.

125. B. Quijano-Roy, C. G. Mbielu, C. Bonnemann, *et al.*, Estournet: LMNA is responsible for a recognizable form of congenital muscular dystrophy associated with selective axial muscle weakness and progressive course (L-CMD). *Ann. Neurol.* **64** (2008), 177–186.

126. B. G. van Engelen, A. Muchir, C. J. Hutchison, A. J. van der Kooi, G. Bonne, M. Lammens, The lethal phenotype of a homozygous nonsense mutation in the lamin A/C gene. *Neurology* **64**:2 (2005), 374–376.

127. T. Voit, E. Parano, V. Straub, *et al.*, Congenital muscular dystrophy with adducted thumbs, ptosis, external ophthalmoplegia, mental retardation and cerebellar hypoplasia: a novel form of CMD. *Neuromuscul. Disord.* **12**:7–8 (2002), 623–630.

128. T. Voit, S. Cirak, S. Abraham, *et al.*, Congenital muscular dystrophy with adducted thumbs, mental retardation, cerebellar hypoplasia, and cataracts is caused by mutation of Enaptin (Nesprin-1): The third nuclear envelopathy with muscular dystrophy. [Abstract C O 4 presented at the 12th International Congress of the World Muscle Society Taormina, Italy.] *Neuromuscul. Disord.* **17** (2007), 1.

129. Q. Zhang, C. Bethmann, N. F. Worth, *et al.*, Nesprin-1 and -2 are involved in the pathogenesis of Emery Dreifuss muscular dystrophy and are critical for nuclear envelope integrity. *Hum. Mol. Genet.* **16**:23 (2007), 2816–2833.

130. D. T. Warren, Q. Zhang, P. L. Weissberg, C. M. Shanahan, Nesprins: intracellular scaffolds that maintain cell architecture and coordinate cell function? *Expert Rev Mol Med* **7**:11 (2005), 1–15.

131. G. Salpingidou, A. Smertenko, I. Hausmanowa-Petrucewicz, P. J. Hussey, C. J. Hutchison, A novel role for the nuclear membrane protein emerin in association of the centrosome to the outer nuclear membrane. *J. Cell. Biol.* **178**:6 (2007), 897–904.

132. B. Moghadaszadeh, N. Petit, C. Jaillard, *et al.*, Mutations in SEPN1 cause congenital muscular dystrophy with spinal rigidity and restrictive respiratory syndrome. *Nat. Genet.* **29**:1 (2001), 17–18.

133. V. Dubowitz, 50th ENMC International Workshop: congenital muscular dystrophy 28 February 1997 to 2 March 1997, Naarden, The Netherlands. *Neuromuscul. Disord.* 7:8 (1997), 539–547.

134. N. Petit, A. Lescure, M. Rederstorff, *et al.*, Selenoprotein N: an endoplasmic reticulum glycoprotein with an early developmental expression pattern. *Hum. Mol. Genet.* **12**:9 (2003), 1045–1053.

135. B. Moghadaszadeh, I. Desguerre, H. Topaloglu, *et al.*, Identification of a new locus for a peculiar form of congenital muscular dystrophy with early rigidity of the spine, on chromosome 1p35–36. *Am. J. Hum. Genet.* **62**:6 (1998), 1439–1445.

136. M. Deniziak, C. Thisse, M. Rederstorff, C. Hindelang, B. Thisse, A. Lescure, Loss of selenoprotein N function causes disruption of muscle architecture in the zebrafish embryo. *Exp. Cell. Res.* **313**:1 (2007), 156–167.

137. U. Schara, W. Kress, C. G. Bonnemann, *et al.*, The phenotype and long-term follow-up in 11 patients with juvenile selenoprotein N1-related myopathy. *Eur. J. Paediatr. Neurol.* **12**:3 (2008), 224–230.

138. E. Mercuri, B. Talim, B. Moghadaszadeh, *et al.*, Clinical and imaging findings in six cases of congenital muscular dystrophy with rigid spine syndrome linked to chromosome 1p (RSMD1). *Neuromuscul. Disord.* **12**:7–8 (2002), 631–638.

139. A. Ferreiro, S. Quijano-Roy, C. Pichereau, *et al.*, Mutations of the selenoprotein N gene, which is implicated in rigid spine muscular dystrophy, cause the classical phenotype of multiminicore disease: reassessing the nosology of early-onset myopathies. *Am. J. Hum. Genet.* **71**:4 (2002), 739–749.

140. A. Ferreiro, C. Ceuterick-de Groote, J. J. Marks, *et al.*, Desmin-related myopathy with mallory body-like inclusions is caused by mutations of the selenoprotein N gene. *Ann. Neurol.* **55**:5 (2004), 676–686.

141. A. Fidzianska, H. Drac, A. M. Kaminska, Familial inclusion body myopathy with desmin storage. *Acta. Neuropathol.* **97**:5 (1999), 509–514.

142. N. F. Clarke, W. Kidson, S. Quijano-Roy, *et al.*, SEPN1: associated with congenital fiber-type disproportion and insulin resistance. *Ann. Neurol.* **59**:3 (2006), 546–552.

143. F. Muntoni, J. Taylor, C. A. Sewry, I. Naom, V. Dubowitz, An early onset muscular dystrophy with diaphragmatic involvement, early respiratory failure and secondary alpha2 laminin deficiency unlinked to the LAMA2 locus on 6q22. *Eur. J. Paediatr. Neurol.* **2**:1 (1998), 19–26.

144. M. C. Belpaire-Dethiou, K. Saito, Y. Fukuyama, *et al.*, Congenital muscular dystrophy with central and peripheral nervous system involvement in a Belgian patient. *Neuromuscul. Disord.* **9**:4 (1999), 251–256.

145. V. Ruggieri, F. Lubieniecki, F. Meli, *et al.*, Merosin-positive congenital muscular dystrophy with mental retardation, microcephaly and central nervous system abnormalities unlinked to the Fukuyama muscular dystrophy and muscular-eye-brain loci: report of three siblings. *Neuromuscul. Disord.* **11**:6–7 (2001), 570–578.

146. U. C. Reed, A. M. Tsanaclis, M. Vainzof, *et al.*, Merosin-positive congenital muscular dystrophy in two siblings with cataract and slight mental retardation. *Brain Dev.* **21**:4 (1999), 274–278.

147. B. Echenne, F. Rivier, M. Tardieu, *et al.*, Congenital muscular dystrophy and cerebellar atrophy. *Neurology* **50**:5 (1998), 1477–1480.

148. C. P. Trevisan, E. Pastorello, S. Tonello, *et al.*, Ataxia and congenital muscular dystrophy: the follow-up of a new specific phenotype. *Brain Dev.* **23**:2 (2001), 108–114.

149. E. Mercuri, A. Lampe, V. Straub, *et al.*, Congenital muscular dystrophy with short stature, proximal contractures and distal laxity. *Neuropediatrics* **35**:4 (2004), 224–229.

Chapter 13

The congenital myopathies

Carina Wallgren-Pettersson and Nigel G. Laing

Introduction

In this chapter we first provide a general discussion of issues common to the congenital myopathies as a whole, and then address the specific entities individually.

Definition of the entities and basis for their classification

The congenital myopathies are a heterogeneous group of muscle diseases, usually present at birth or early infancy. They are characterized by muscle weakness and specific structural abnormalities in the muscle biopsy, often including abnormal placement/misplacement of organelles. The pathological hallmarks, after which the entities have been named, include central cores, multi-minicores, central nuclei, nemaline, and many other types of bodies. In some cases the histology simultaneously shows one or more of the specific abnormalities. The muscle fibers may be undifferentiated or predominantly type 1, with the type 1 fibers often being hypotrophic. Type 2 fibers, if any are present, are often hypertrophic, and thus, in many cases, a disproportion in size between the two fiber types is present, so-called fiber type or fiber size disproportion. Sometimes such aberrations in fiber type or size may be all that is seen. There may be myopathic features such as internal nuclei, splitting of fibers, and fibrosis, but necrosis and inflammatory components are usually not seen. The muscle pathology of the congenital myopathies has recently been excellently reviewed and illustrated [1].

The classification of congenital myopathies has traditionally been, and still is, based on the histological abnormalities in the muscle fibers. The discovery of many genes for congenital myopathies (Table 13.1) has clarified their genesis but is not yet and may never be the basis of their classification. The considerable genetic heterogeneity in the congenital myopathies, for example more than six genes for nemaline myopathy, makes a genetic categorization problematic.

Molecular genetics and pathogenesis

The last decade and a half, from the first identification of mutations in the ryanodine receptor gene (*RYR1*) in central core disease in 1993 until now, has been the age of gene discovery for the congenital myopathies, as for many other disease entities (Table 13.1). However, other genes are still to be identified, even for entities where multiple genes are already known. For example, there is at least one more gene for nemaline myopathy [33], another gene for core-rod disease on chromosome 15 [34] and at least a fourth gene for myotubular/centronuclear myopathy. In addition, no genes have yet been discovered for many other congenital myopathies (Table 13.2).

The molecular pathogenetic pathways of the congenital myopathies are still largely unknown, though investigation of animal (e.g., [40]), tissue culture (e.g., [41, 42, 43]) and in vitro models (e.g., [44, 45]), possible after the identification of the disease genes, are beginning to clarify the pathogenesis. Most is perhaps understood of the pathogenesis of central core disease caused by mutations in *RYR1*, since Ryr1 is an ion channel with better-known biology [46].

Salient clinical features

The congenital myopathies have similar clinical features, many patients presenting as floppy infants. Despite the term congenital myopathies, however, patients may present after the neonatal period, some even in adulthood.

Affected infants usually have myopathic facies, bulbar, neck flexor and proximal weakness, with a distal component present initially or at a later stage. Serum concentrations of creatine kinase (CK) are usually normal or only a few times higher than normal, while electromyography (EMG) shows normal, myogenic or, in severe neonatal cases or in distal muscles at later stages of the disease, "neurogenic" patterns (spontaneous activity, fibrillations, high-amplitude potentials).

Disorders of Voluntary Muscle, 8th edn., eds. George Karpati, David Hilton-Jones, Kate Bushby and Robert C. Griggs. Published by Cambridge University Press. © Cambridge University Press 2010.

Table 13.1. Congenital myopathies with identified causative genes

Congenital myopathy	Protein	Gene	Inheritance	Reference
Actin aggregate myopathy	α-actin, skeletal	*ACTA1*	AD	[2]
Cap myopathy	β-tropomyosin	*TPM2*	AD	[3, 4]
Central core disease	Ryanodine receptor 1	*RYR1*	AD	[5, 6]
	α-actin, skeletal	*ACTA1*	AD	[7]
Centronuclear myopathy	Amphiphysin 2	*BIN1*	AR	[8]
	Dynamin-2	*DNM2*	AD	[9]
	Ryanodine receptor 1	*RYR1*	AD	[10]
Congenital fiber-type disproportion	α-actin, skeletal	*ACTA1*	*De novo* dominant	[11]
	Selenoprotein N	*SEPN1*	AR	[12]
	α-tropomyosin, slow	*TPM3*	AD	[13]
Core-rod myopathy	Ryanodine receptor 1	*RYR1*	AD	[14, 15]
Intranuclear rod myopathy	α-actin, skeletal	*ACTA1*	AD *De novo* dominant	[2, 3, 4, 26, 27]
Mallory body myopathy	Selenoprotein N	*SEPN1*	AR	[16]
Multi-minicore disease	Ryanodine receptor 1	*RYR1*	AR	[17]
	Selenoprotein N	*SEPN1*	AR	[18]
Myosin storage myopathy (hyaline body myopathy)	β-myosin, slow cardiac	*MYH7*	AD	[19]
Myotubular (centronuclear) myopathy	Myotubularin	*MTM1*	X-linked	[20]
Nemaline myopathy	α-actin, skeletal	*ACTA1*	AD, AR, *de novo* dominant	[2]
	Cofilin	*CFL2*	AR	[21]
	Nebulin	*NEB*	AR	[22]
	α-tropomyosin, slow	*TPM3*	AD, AR	[23]
	β-tropomyosin	*TPM2*	AD	[24]
	Troponin T, slow	*TNNT1*	AR	[25]
Reducing body myopathy	Four and a half LIM domain protein 1	*FHL1*	X-linked	[28]
Sarcotubular myopathy	Tripartite motif-containing protein 32	*TRIM32*	AR	[29]
Spheroid body myopathy	Myotilin	*MYOT, TTID*	AD	[30]
Titin myopathy with cardiomyopathy	Titin	*TTN*	AR	[31]
X-linked autophagic vacuolar myopathy (Danon disease)	Lysosome-associated membrane protein-2	*LAMP2*	X-linked	[32]

Notes: AD, autosomal dominant; AR, autosomal recessive.

These neonates may have life-threatening respiratory and feeding problems requiring intensive support, and some do not survive beyond infancy (see Therapeutic and preventative modalities).

Polyhydramnios complicating pregnancy is rare, though more common in X-linked myotubular myopathy. Foot and chest deformities are often present. Distal arthrogryposis, characterized by contractures of distal joints and regarded by

Table 13.2. Congenital myopathies with no known genes

Broad A-band myopathy[q]	
Congenital myopathy with arrest of myogenesis prior to formation of myotubes	[35]
Congenital myopathy with diaphragmatic weakness not linked to SMARD1	[36]
Cylindrical spirals myopathy[a]	
Cytoplasmic body myopathy[a]	
Fingerprint body myopathy[a]	
Granulofilamentous body myopathy[a]	
Granulovacuolar lobular myopathy[q]	
Honeycomb myopathy[q]	
Minimal change myopathy[q]	
Mitochondria-jagged Z-line myopathy[q]	
Myopathy with hexagonally cross-linked tubular arrays	[37]
Nucleodegenerative myopathy[q]	
Reversed core myopathy[q]	
Rimmed vacuole myopathy[q]	
Samaritan myopathy	[38]
Sarcoplasmic body myopathy[a]	
Selective myosin degeneration myopathy[q]	
Syndromic nonspecific myopathies, e.g., King syndrome	
Trilaminar fiber myopathy[q]	
Tubular aggregate myopathy[a]	
Tubulomembranous inclusion myopathy[q]	
Z-band plaque myopathy[q]	

All entities reviewed in Goebel (1996) [39] unless otherwise noted.
Notes: [a]Accepted entity. [q]Questionable entity according to [39].

many as a separate group of disorders, may be a symptom of many congenital myopathies as well as of other neurological disorders, and causative mutations have been identified in some of the same gene families (tropomyosin, troponin, myosin) as are mutated in the congenital myopathies (see Distal arthrogryposis). While they may be present in very severe cases of the other congenital myopathies, multiple contractures of large joints at birth are common only in myotubular myopathy.

Cardiac involvement is rare [44, 47, 48], but should be sought, not only as part of the initial diagnosis but also during follow-up over the years. The spine is often hyperlordotic and there may be spinal rigidity. Scoliosis may develop, most commonly during the growth spurt preceding puberty, and may require surgical intervention to prevent lung collapse and to improve quality of life.

After infancy, the course of the diseases is usually static or only slowly progressive. Some patients, usually in the prepubertal period or later, will require the use of a wheelchair.

In childhood, respiratory infections are common and should be treated actively. Respiratory complications are the major cause of morbidity and mortality for many of these conditions and respiratory status requires life-long monitoring (see Therapeutic and preventative modalities) [49].

Genotype–phenotype correlations

Each of the congenital myopathies shows a phenotypic spectrum from severe disease, associated in some patients with almost complete paralysis at birth, through to adult-onset disease. The severity of the disease in each patient depends not so much on the gene mutated, but more on the exact mutation within the gene. This is clearly shown in nemaline myopathy, where different mutations in both skeletal muscle α-actin (*ACTA1*) and nebulin (*NEB*) can cause either severe or relatively benign disease (Figure 13.1), with similar nemaline bodies (Figure 13.2) [50, 51]. Further genetic heterogeneity (Table 13.1) is exemplified by mutations in *RYR1* and selenoprotein N (*SEPN1*) causing similar mini-cores, and mutations in *RYR1* and myotubularin (*MTM1*) resulting in similar central nuclei (Figure 13.3).

In another level of complication, different mutations in the same gene may be associated with different congenital myopathies (Table 13.3). For example, mutations in *SEPN1* are associated to date with congenital fiber-type disproportion [12], Mallory body myopathy [16] or multi-minicore disease [18].

Finally it is well known empirically that there are epigenetic and possibly also environmental modifiers of the congenital myopathies. The same mutation in different patients in one family may cause considerably different disease severity [27, 48, 54]. The epigenetic modifiers of disease severity in the congenital myopathies are largely unknown, however it was recently demonstrated that tissue-specific silencing of normal alleles for *RYR1* unmasks recessive mutations and causes core myopathies [55].

Diagnostic approaches

Because these muscle disorders are rare, the process of diagnosing congenital myopathies is best concentrated to specialist university centers. The diagnostic procedure is based on clinical features, determination of serum concentrations of CK, EMG patterns, and muscle biopsy findings. Examination of the muscle biopsy is by standard histochemical staining methods and, in some cases, immunohistochemical protein studies. Electron microscopy may be required for the confirmation of the presence of some of the specific abnormalities, such as accumulations of protein aggregates in actin myopathy or nemaline bodies if these are few and small.

A simplistic diagnostic algorithm for the congenital myopathies is provided in Figure 13.4. The first step is clinical evaluation, confirming the presence and pattern of muscle

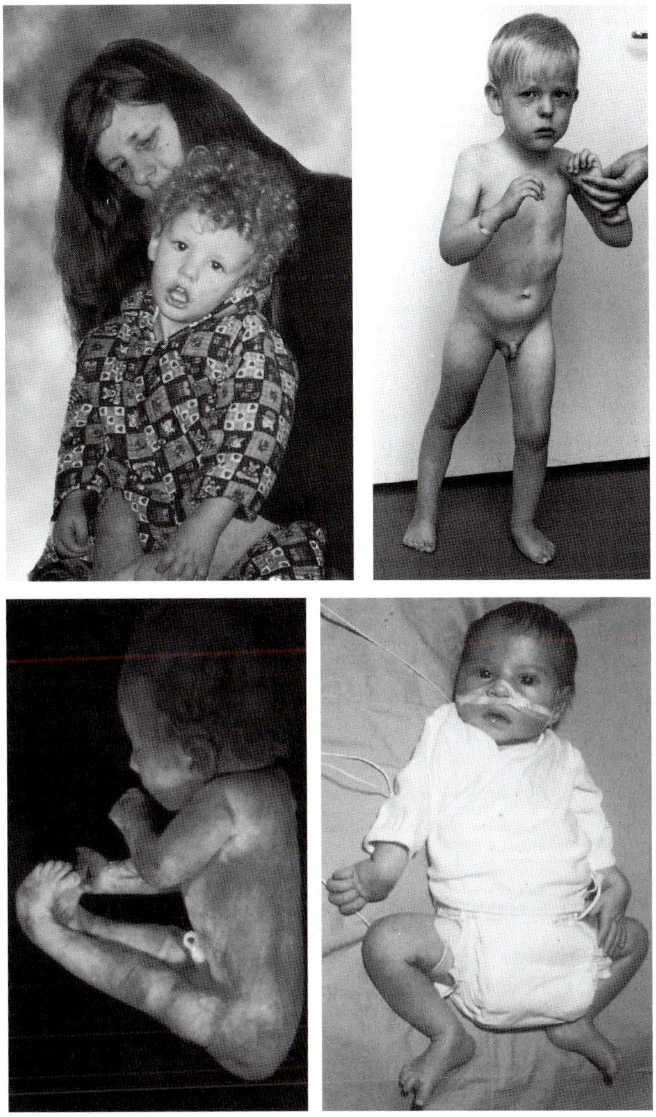

Figure 13.1. Similar grades of severity in patients with nemaline myopathy caused by mutations in *ACTA1* and *NEB*. Reproduced with permission.

weakness, normal or only moderately elevated CK, usually myogenic, but sometimes normal or even "neuropathic" EMG features. Muscle biopsy following the clinical diagnostic suspicion is the most crucial step, most often establishing the diagnosis. However, the histological aberrations seen in genetically proven cases of congenital myopathy may be highly variable, so that patients may have no specific findings on initial biopsy, or have one type of aberration, which subsequently evolves into another, characteristic, type of morphology at second biopsy [56]. Moreover, muscle biopsies from different sites in the one patient may show different pathologies. Thus, multiple biopsies, perhaps two at initial investigation, may be needed to make a definitive diagnosis.

If the biopsy shows histological hallmarks characteristic of one of the congenital myopathies, mutation detection, if genes are known for that congenital myopathy, is the next step. Mutation identification is becoming the gold standard for verifying the diagnosis in the congenital myopathies. Only genetic diagnosis provides certainty as to the cause of the disease in the patient, the mode of inheritance, and thus the recurrence risk in other family members. It also provides the possibility of carrier testing and prenatal diagnosis.

Molecular testing for the congenital myopathies is not however straightforward, because of the genetic heterogeneity and the size of some genes involved. For example, at 183 exons and a coding region of over 20 kb, *NEB* poses a significant problem for mutation screening [57].

There is increasing recognition of the diagnostic usefulness of magnetic resonance imaging/computer tomography (MRI/CT) in differentiating between the various congenital myopathies, especially in histologically equivocal cases. Imaging may mainly be used in patients who are old enough not to require anesthesia for the procedure. For congenital myopathies caused by *RYR1* [58], *ACTA1* or *NEB* mutations [59] and centronuclear myopathy caused by dynamin (*DNM2*) mutations [60], characteristic patterns of differential muscle involvement have been described. MRI was for example used to identify a patient diagnosed with centronuclear myopathy as having a mutation of *RYR1*: the MRI pattern of affected muscles being similar to that previously characterized in patients with *RYR1* mutations [10].

Diseases that may present as phenocopies of congenital myopathies – clinical differential diagnoses

Disorders of the central nervous system, chromosomal abnormalities, and metabolic disorders need to be excluded in the initial diagnostic work-up. Any severe case of congenital myopathy can be mistaken for spinal muscular atrophy because of "neurogenic" components on EMG [2, 48, 61]. In older children and adults, differential diagnoses include disorders of connective tissue causing slender build, muscle weakness, and long facies with high-arched palate (Table 13.4).

The myofibrillar myopathies, with disruption of myofibrils and accumulations of a variety of proteins including desmin, can sometimes present as a congenital myopathy. Differential diagnoses for the congenital myopathies are included in Table 13.4 and below under the headings for the specific disorders.

Therapeutic and preventative modalities

No primary prevention is currently feasible, therefore the treatment of patients with congenital myopathies is currently still symptomatic and should be managed by a specialized multidisciplinary team.

The most important issue in the care of patients with congenital myopathies is active respiratory monitoring and treatment. The favorable outcome documented for some

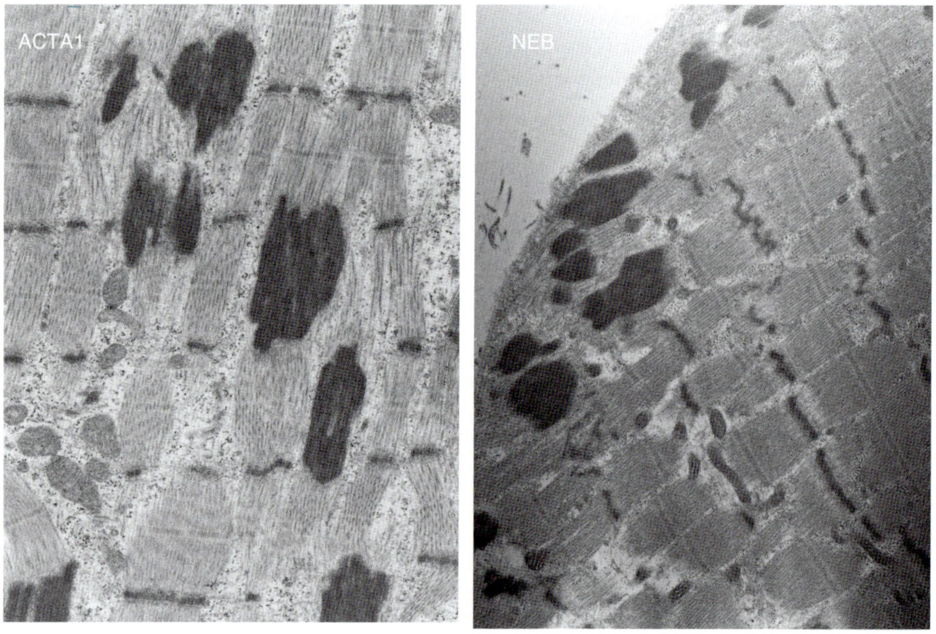

Figure 13.2. Nemaline bodies caused by mutation of either skeletal muscle α-actin (*ACTA1*) or nebulin (*NEB*) look very similar. Images courtesy of Professor Caroline Sewry.

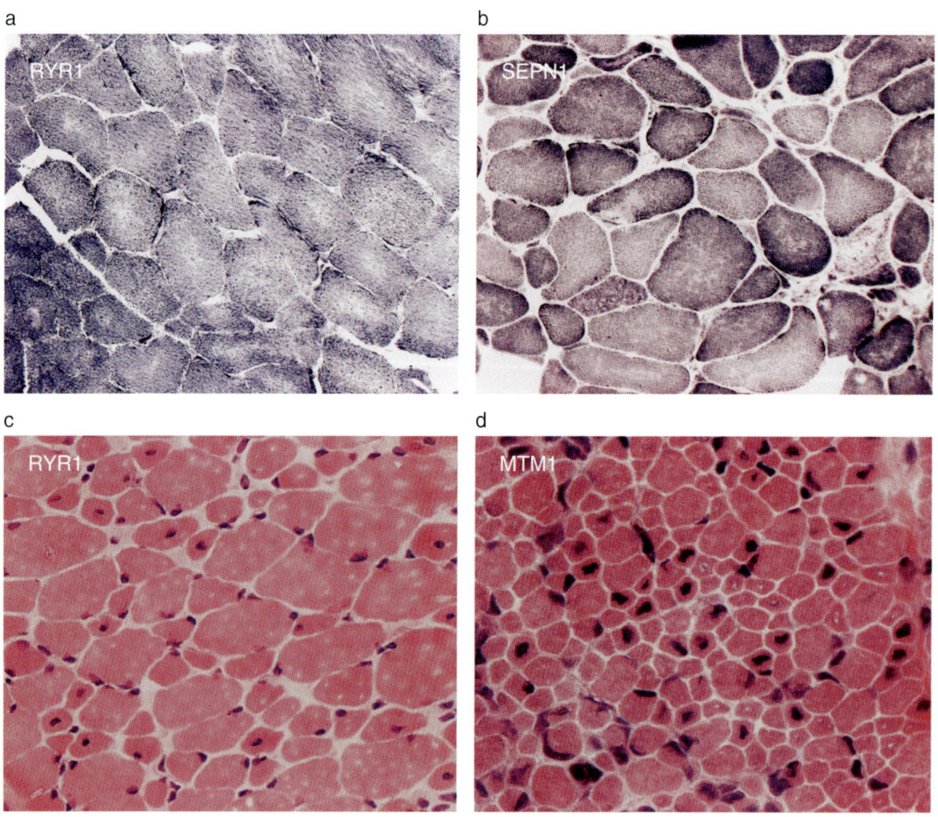

Figure 13.3a–d. Minicores caused by *RYR1* (a) or *SEPN1* (b) mutations, and central nuclei caused by *RYR1* (c) or *MTM1* (d) mutations can be very similar. Images courtesy of Professor Caroline Sewry.

patients with severe congenital forms suggests that active treatment is also warranted in this patient group, at least initially [49]; infants who fail to establish spontaneous respiration at birth may be able to breathe for themselves after a period of mechanical ventilation. Infections should be treated vigorously and immunization should be offered against influenza and pneumococcal infection.

Because of the possibility of respiratory insufficiency, respiratory capacity requires regular monitoring, with forced vital capacity (FVC) measured in both the erect and the supine

Table 13.3. Diseases caused by mutations in individual congenital myopathy disease genes, including diseases that are not classified as congenital myopathies

Gene	Symbol	Inheritance	Congenital myopathy	Other disease	Reference
α-actin, skeletal	ACTA1	*De novo* dominant	Actin aggregate myopathy		[2]
		AD, AR, *de novo* dominant	Nemaline myopathy		[2]
		AD, *de novo* dominant	Intranuclear rod myopathy		[2]
		AD	Core myopathy		[7]
		De novo dominant	Congenital fiber-type disproportion		[11]
Amphiphysin 2	BIN1	AR	Centronuclear myopathy		[8]
Cofilin	CFL2	AR	Nemaline myopathy		[21]
Dynamin-2	DNM2	AD	Centronuclear myopathy		[9]
Four and a half LIM domain protein 1	FHL1	X-linked	Reducing body myopathy		[28]
Lysosome-associated membrane protein-2	LAMP2	X-linked	Danon disease		[32]
Myosin, slow skeletal/beta cardiac	MYH7	AD, AR	Myosin storage myopathy		[19]
Myotilin	MYOT, TTID	AD	Spheroid body myopathy		[30]
Myotubularin	MTM1	X-linked	Myotubular myopathy		[20]
Nebulin	NEB	AR	Nemaline myopathy		[22]
		AR		Nebulin distal myopathy	[52]
Ryanodine receptor	RYR1	AD, AR, *de novo* dominant	Central core disease		[5, 6]
		AD	Core-rod myopathy		[14, 15]
		AD	Centronuclear myopathy		[10]
		AR	Multi-minicore disease		[17]
Selenoprotein N	SEPN1	AR	Multi-minicore disease		[18]
		AR	Congenital fiber-type disproportion		[12]
		AR	Mallory body myopathy		[16]
Titin	TTN	AR	Titin myopathy with cardiomyopathy		[31]
		AD		Tibial muscular dystrophy	OMIM 600334
		AD		Hereditary myopathy with early respiratory failure (HMERF)	OMIM 603689
		AR		Limb girdle muscular dystrophy 2J (LGMD2J)	OMIM 608807

Table 13.3. *(cont.)*

Gene	Symbol	Inheritance	Congenital myopathy	Other disease	Reference
Tripartite motif-containing protein 32	TRIM32	AR	Sarcotubular myopathy		[29]
		AR		Limb-girdle muscular dystrophy 2H	OMIM 254110
Tropomyosin-α slow	TPM3	AD, AR	Nemaline myopathy		[23]
Tropomyosin-β	TPM2	AD	Nemaline myopathy		[24]
		AD	Cap myopathy		[3, 4]
		AD	Congenital fiber-type disproportion		[13]
		AD		Distal arthrogryposis	[53]
Troponin T, slow	TNNT1	AR	Nemaline myopathy		[25]

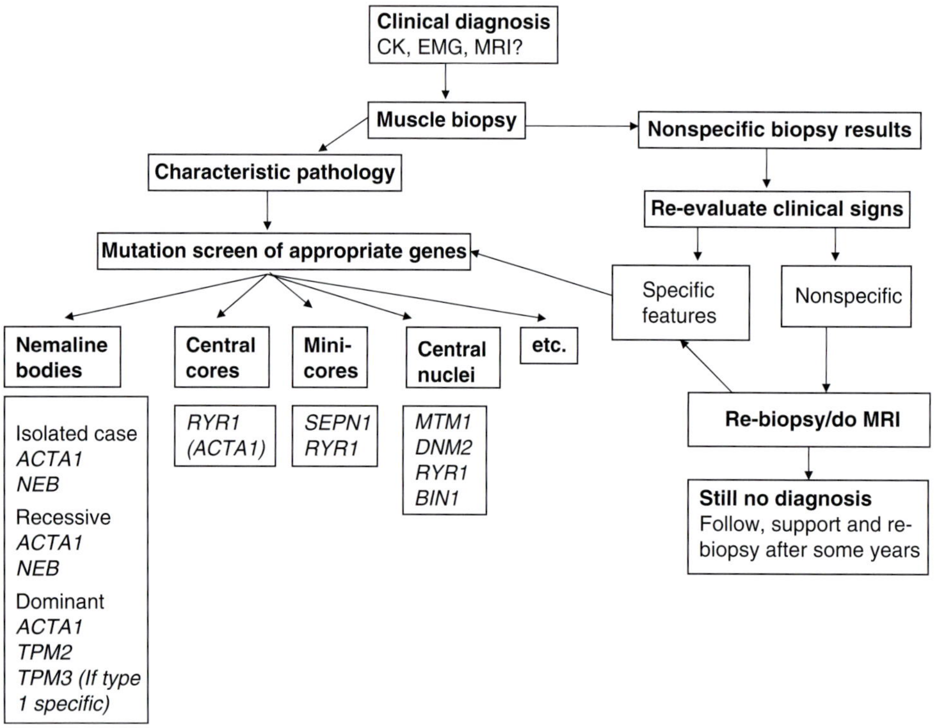

Figure 13.4. Simplistic diagnostic algorithm for the diagnosis of the congenital myopathies: clinical evaluation, muscle biopsy, genetic diagnosis. Where only one small gene or a small region of a large gene is known for a specific histopathology, e.g., *SEPN1* for Mallory body myopathy or *MYH7* mutations for myosin storage myopathy, the genetic testing algorithm is simple. Where multiple genes have been associated with the one histopathological hallmark, e.g., nemaline bodies, the pattern of inheritance, severity, etc. can guide which gene to test first. For example, if the pathology is restricted to type 1 fibers: screen *TPM3*.

position. Special attention should be paid to possible signs of insidious nocturnal hypoxia, such as morning headaches and nausea. The need for intermittent or permanent noninvasive mechanical ventilation should be continuously evaluated because of the risk of sudden respiratory failure on exertion or due to infection even in ambulant patients [49]. In other words, the weakness of the respiratory muscles may be way out of proportion to that of the muscles used for ambulation. Polysomnography should be performed annually when FVC is <60%, and more often when FVC is <40% [49].

Cardiac status requires monitoring, after an initial evaluation for uncommon structural abnormality. This is necessary both because of the risk of cor pulmonale [62] and the rare occurrence of early cardiomyopathy [31, 44, 47].

Early speech therapy is recommended to enhance the development of spontaneous speech, particularly for patients with dysarthria. Swallowing difficulties are common and may warrant training by a specialized speech therapist, tube feeding or even gastrostomy to prevent aspiration.

For scoliosis, early operation is preferable to bracing because of the tendency for bracing to restrict respiration still

Table 13.4. Diseases that may resemble congenital myopathies

Beals syndrome
Facioscapulohumeral muscular dystrophy
Marfan syndrome
Motor neuropathies
Myasthenic disorders
Myofibrillar myopathy
Myotonic dystrophy
Prader–Willi syndrome
Spinal muscular atrophy

further. Preoperative measures help to ensure safe surgery even for patients with severe respiratory compromise [63]. Other deformities and contractures should be treated conservatively, but actively, to avoid, as far as possible, surgical interventions requiring immobilization. Orthopedic treatment should be undertaken very selectively and only at centers with extensive experience with neuromuscular diseases, and the adverse effects of postoperative or post-traumatic immobilization ought to be rapidly counteracted by intensive physiotherapy.

Regular physiotherapy should aim for the preservation of muscle power and function, with emphasis on maintenance of cardiorespiratory capacity, thoracic mobility, coughing, and drainage. Further goals are the prevention of scoliosis, back pain, and contractures, and the maintenance of mobility, head control, and independence in the activities of daily living. In some patients calipers may be necessary to enhance the acquisition of walking ability. Assisted coughing should be provided and preferably supported by mechanical aids [49]. Recommendable exercises for improving cardiorespiratory function and endurance are swimming and horse riding.

Central core disease is associated with a greater than normal anesthetic risk of malignant hyperthermia (see below). A higher risk is not clearly associated with the other congenital myopathies, but the anesthesiologist should be aware of the patient's diagnosis and plan the anesthesia carefully, avoiding succinylcholine and volatile anesthetics [49], and have dantrolene readily to hand.

Occupations recommendable for patients in this disease group are those free from physical strain, a high risk of infection, and exposure to tobacco smoke and other inhaled irritants.

Patients with congenital myopathies have gone through pregnancy and delivery without significant problems, although intermittent deterioration has been reported in central core disease [64]. Pregnancies of affected women should be followed, with care coordinated cooperatively by the obstetrician and neurologist. Delivery must be carefully and individually planned, taking into account the patient's respiratory capacity, muscle weakness, and any contractures potentially complicating labor.

Genetic counseling

All families in which a congenital myopathy has been diagnosed should be offered genetic counseling. Precise information about mode of inheritance and risk of recurrence can only be given where the causative mutation(s) has been identified. Reliable carrier testing and prenatal diagnosis also require identification of the specific mutation(s) in the family. In counseling families regarding recurrence risks, it is to be noted that mosaicism has been documented for *ACTA1* nemaline myopathy [2], *MTM1* myotubular myopathy [65], and *RYR1* central core disease [66].

De novo mutations are frequent in the *ACTA1* gene [51] and relatively common in *RYR1*, but perhaps rarer in other genes for the congenital myopathies.

Nemaline myopathies and related disorders

Nemaline myopathy

Nemaline myopathy shows a spectrum of clinical phenotypes from fetal akinesia through to severe forms with patients lacking spontaneous respiration at birth to mild and even adult-onset disease (Figure 13.1) [48, 67]. In the International Consortium Database in Helsinki, the typical congenital form, characterized by congenital onset of muscle weakness, spontaneous respiration at birth, and motor milestones delayed but reached, appears to live up to its name by being the most common form. It is however paralleled in frequency by the neonatally severe form characterized at birth by inability to move or breathe, or by the presence of contractures or fractures at birth. The remaining four forms are rarer.

By definition [67] the muscle biopsy of every nemaline myopathy patient shows the presence of nemaline bodies, or rods, on Gomori trichrome staining. These are expansions and deposits of Z-disk and thin filament material (Figure 13.2). Toluidine-blue staining or even electron microscopy of plastic-embedded muscle biopsy sections may be necessary in some cases to detect very small numbers of nemaline bodies. The nemaline bodies are however not pathognomic, and the diagnosis of nemaline myopathy should only be made in the presence of muscle weakness and in the absence of other entities sometimes associated with similar rod formation [67].

Facial and bulbar weakness is common, in addition to neck flexor and proximal limb weakness, and many patients show a later distal component. Some patients have rigid spine. Cardiomyopathy is rare but has been reported [44].

To date, mutations in the genes for six thin filament proteins have been shown to cause nemaline myopathy. The genes, in the order in which they were identified, are slow α-tropomyosin (*TPM3*) [23], *NEB* [22], *ACTA1* [2] slow troponin T (*TNNT1*) [25], β-tropomyosin (*TPM2*) [24], and muscle-specific cofilin (*CFL2*) [21]. At least one more gene is yet to be found [33] and there will probably be more.

Mutations in *NEB* are thought to be the commonest cause of nemaline myopathy, followed by *ACTA1* [48]. Mutations in *TPM3*, although the first discovered, are rare causes of nemaline myopathy. It currently appears that mutations of *TPM3* are most often associated with a pathological diagnosis of congenital fiber-type disproportion without other, specific, aberrations (see below). Mutations in *TPM2* are also a rare cause of nemaline myopathy, while the only mutation identified to date in *TNNT1* is the null mutation that causes Amish recessive nemaline myopathy. Similarly, the only mutation identified in *CFL2* is in one family with recessive nemaline myopathy.

Thus, an isolated sporadic case of congenital nemaline myopathy most likely has recessive *NEB* mutations, with the next most likely cause being a de novo *ACTA1* mutation. It is practical to start mutation analysis from the *ACTA1* gene, because this is available as a service in multiple centers and the gene is small. In familial cases, autosomal recessive inheritance is most commonly associated with *NEB*, but sometimes with *ACTA1* or, uncommonly, *TPM3* (or *CFL2* or *TNNT1* as above). Autosomal dominant inheritance is most often associated with *ACTA1* but can be caused by *TPM2* or *TPM3*. Adult-onset cases may not be genetic in origin. The etiology awaits further clarification but pathological immune responses are involved in at least a proportion of cases [68].

NEB, with its 183 exons and with most families having two different private mutations anywhere along the length of the gene, is currently not suitable for routine diagnostic investigations [57, 69]. A notable exception is the deletion of exon 55 identified in a US Ashkenazi population [70] and found later to have worldwide occurrence [71] permitting screening for this mutation as a diagnostic service. Labeling of the biopsy from a patient with nebulin nemaline myopathy with antibodies against nebulin will not necessarily show any abnormality, because expression of the C-terminus of the protein is the rule despite truncating mutations.

Genotype–phenotype correlations have been published for nemaline myopathy caused by mutations in *ACTA1* and *NEB* [48, 51]. There are some general differences between patients with *ACTA1* mutations as a group and those with *NEB* mutations as a group, including different patterns of muscle involvement and that more severely affected patients have *ACTA1* mutations more often than *NEB* mutations [48, 59]. Only *ACTA1* mutation, not *NEB* mutation, has been associated with co-pathologies of intranuclear rods and actin aggregates and with cardiomyopathy [44].

Two nebulin knockout mouse models have been described, both surprisingly forming sarcomeres in the absence of nebulin, known to be a ruler for the length of the thin filament [72, 73]. The thin filaments were short, however, and maintenance of the sarcomere structure failed, the mice dying within 1–3 weeks after birth.

Recently a series of seven patients was described with recessive nemaline myopathy caused by homozygosity for *ACTA1* null mutations [74]. The clinical picture in these patients, who have no skeletal actin in their muscle, was not uniformly severe, with some having better muscle function than others. It was shown that all of the patients had retained expression of cardiac α-actin, which is the fetal isoform of actin in skeletal muscle. The level of cardiac actin correlated with the level of muscle function in the patients. Upregulation of cardiac actin had previously been documented in a patient with *ACTA1* recessive nemaline myopathy caused by compound heterozygosity for a missense mutation and a null mutation [75]. Thus, all patients with recessive *ACTA1* mutations may have no functional skeletal muscle α-actin.

Nemaline myopathy-related disorders

Actin aggregate myopathy

In actin aggregate myopathy the muscle pathology is characterized by accumulations of actin filaments, best seen on electron microscopy or with labeling of the filaments with antibodies against actin. Studies of this group of patients led to the identification of the first mutations in *ACTA1* [2]. Ten *ACTA1* mutations have now been associated with actin aggregate myopathy (N. G. Laing, unpublished observations). The clinical phenotype is most often severe, with death in the first few months, but two patients have been reported living at 7.5 and 10 years [51].

Cap disease

Cap myopathy is defined on the basis of the presence of cap-like structures at the periphery of muscle fibers, consisting of disarranged thin filaments with enlarged Z-disks (Figure 13.5a) [3, 4]. The diagnosis requires confirmation through immunolabeling and electron microscopy. Most patients follow a relatively stable course although there may be respiratory compromise disproportionate to the weakness of other muscles. The distribution of weakness may be similar to that of patients with *NEB* nemaline myopathy, and there may also be histological overlap [3, 4]. The first genetic cause of cap disease was independently identified by two groups as mutation of *TPM2* [3, 4]. A family with an affected sib pair showed no mutation in *TPM2*, indicating that there is at least one other gene for recessive cap myopathy [3].

Distal arthrogryposis

Mutations in β-tropomyosin (*TPM2*) and fast troponin I (*TNNI2*) [53] fast troponin T (*TNNT3*) [76] and embryonic myosin heavy chain (*MYH3*) [76] have all been shown to cause distal arthrogryposis. Aberrant TNNI2, TNNT3, and TPM2 proteins in such patients have been shown in *in vitro* experiments to increase contractility [78].

Distal nebulin myopathy

Homozygous missense mutations in *NEB* have recently been found to cause a novel distal myopathy [52]. Onset is

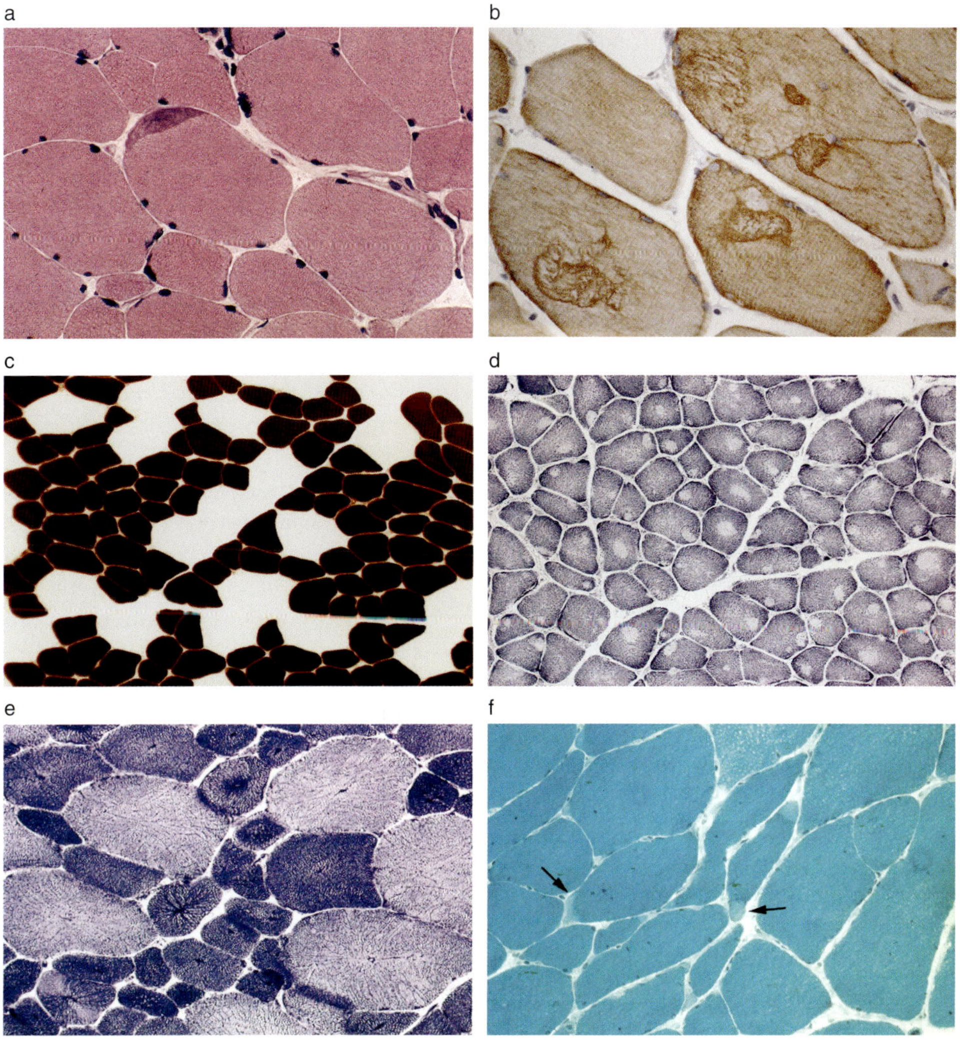

Figure 13.5a–f. (a) Cap disease caused by a mutation in *TPM2*. Courtesy of Professor Chantal Ceuterick-de Groote. (b) Chromosome 15 core-rod disease. Biopsy stained with anti-desmin. Courtesy of Dr. Vicki Fabian. (c) Congenital fiber-type disproportion caused by an *ACTA1* mutation demonstrated by ATPase pH 4.3. Courtesy of Professor Caroline Sewry. (d) Central core disease caused by an *RYR1* mutation – NADH-TR. Courtesy of Professor Caroline Sewry. (e) Radial strands in NADH-stained cross-section of muscle biopsy from the deltoid muscle of an adult patient with centronuclear myopathy caused by the recurrent mutation p.R465W in the middle domain of the *DNM2* gene. Courtesy of Dr. Marc Bitoun. (f) Myosin storage myopathy caused by a mutation in MYH7 – Gömöri trichrome. Courtesy of Professor Raf Sciot.

in childhood or adulthood of muscle weakness mainly affecting the ankle dorsiflexors, the finger extensors, and the neck flexors. The histological aberrations are unspecific and variable.

Intranuclear rod myopathy

In some nemaline myopathy patients both sarcoplasmic and intranuclear rods are seen, but in other patients rods are restricted to the nucleus. These latter patients may be designated as having intranuclear rod myopathy. The diagnosis is made using electron microscopy. To date, 12 different mutations in *ACTA1* have been associated with intranuclear rods. The prognosis for patients with this disorder is frequently, but not always, poor [27]. Recent experimental studies indicate that the vast majority of the mutant actin in intranuclear rod myopathy patients may be sequestered in the rod bodies in the nuclei [42, 43], perhaps allowing the sarcomeres to be composed largely of normal, nonmutant actin. Intranuclear rods may also be seen in other myopathies [79].

Mixed rod-core myopathies

One of the mixed congenital myopathies is rod-core disease or core-rod disease where both nemaline bodies and central cores are seen in the one biopsy. The first gene identified was *RYR1* [14, 15]. A patient with mild nemaline myopathy and a mutation in *ACTA1* showed core-like structures, too, in the muscle biopsy [80]. A third locus for rod-core disease has been linked to a region of chromosome 15 (Figure 13.5b) but the precise gene has not yet been identified [34].

Minicores along with nemaline bodies were seen in the patients with cofilin mutation [21].

Zebra body myopathy

Zebra bodies, which consist of alternating stripes of electron-dense and electron-lucent Z-disk and I-band material [1] were seen in three of seven patients with nemaline myopathy caused by absence of skeletal muscle actin [74]. It is possible therefore that patients diagnosed with zebra-body myopathy also lack actin, but this remains to be proved.

Congenital fiber-type disproportion

Congenital fiber-type disproportion (CFTD) is characterized by slow, type 1 muscle fibers being 12%, or, according to a more recent definition, 25% smaller than the fast type 2 fibers (Figure 13.5c) [81]. It is a phenomenon often encountered in patients with congenital myopathies, where they do have type 2 fibers at all, and in other neuromuscular disorders also. This being the case, many centers routinely do a later, second biopsy in young patients with CFTD as the only abnormal feature in the initial biopsy. Specific, additional findings in another biopsy may thus permit the diagnosis of a more well-defined muscle disorder. Some patients however still show no specific abnormality, and the diagnosis in these patients remains CFTD. The clinical features have recently been extensively reviewed [81]. The causative genes published to date have, not surprisingly, been genes previously known to cause congenital myopathies: *ACTA1* [11], *SEPN1* [12], and *TPM3* [13].

Central core disease and related disorders

Central core disease

Central core disease is one of the commonest congenital myopathies. The central cores consist of well-demarcated areas of low or absent oxidative activity running centrally along the longitudinal axis of the muscle fibers (Figure 13.5d) [1]. The disorder is frequently associated with congenital dislocation of the hips, and other orthopedic complications, and with the allelic condition malignant hyperthermia (see below). There is marked clinical variability even within the same family. Many patients present in infancy, rarely with very severe disease [82], but some only in adulthood, while others with similar histological findings remain asymptomatic but may still be susceptible to malignant hyperthermia caused by abnormal reaction to anesthetic agents.

Presentation of central core disease may be with muscle pain and weakness on exertion, and there are often contractures of the Achilles tendons and hypermobility of other joints. Facial and bulbar weakness may be less obvious than in the other congenital myopathies, while hip girdle involvement is prominent. Most affected persons remain ambulant throughout life. Temporary deterioration has been described during or after pregnancy [64].

Central core disease is due to mutations of *RYR1* in more than 90% of cases [83, 84]. Most of the mutations are heterozygous missense mutations [84]. Recessively inherited mutations in *RYR1* have been associated both with central core disease [46] and with multi-minicore disease [17]. Some of these patients have more severe disease, with ophthalmoplegia and depletion of the Ryr1 protein in muscle tissue, seen by Western blotting [46]. This more severe disease is modeled by the Ryr1 knockout mouse [85].

Although the 106-exon gene contains some hotspots, and diagnostic mutation analysis is best started by investigating these, mutation identification may in some cases require sequencing of the entire gene [83]. The pathogenetic mechanisms are thought to be related to changes in calcium homeostasis, possibly combined with altered excitability of muscle cells [84]. Genotype–phenotype correlations are complex [46], and in some cases epigenetic silencing plays an important pathogenetic role [86].

Multi-minicore disease

Multi-minicore disease [47, 87] is characterized by multiple, small (short in length and in cross-section), well-circumscribed areas of myofibrillar disruption with weak or absent oxidative enzyme staining due to absence of mitochondria (Figure 13.3). There is a clinical and histological overlap with central core disease, at least partly explained by the identification in some patients of mutations in the *RYR1* gene. Onset is usually perinatal but adult-onset cases have been described. An international consortium has classified multi-minicore disease into four categories [47].

In the classical form, most often caused by recessive mutations in *SEPN1* [18], patients have rigid spines, scoliosis, and early respiratory involvement, with "bracket-like" thighs due to wasting of the inner thigh muscles. Some patients who otherwise have similar clinical features to those in the first group may develop ophthalmoplegia over time. In the third category, the moderate form with hand involvement, which can be caused by recessive mutations in the *RYR1* gene [17], there is hip girdle weakness and hypotrophy of the hand muscles, with sparing of the respiratory and bulbar muscles and often normal spine. Again, ophthalmoplegia may be a later symptom. At least in this group of patients with multi-minicore disease, a potential risk for malignant hyperthermia has to be taken into account if the patient requires anesthesia. A rare severe form, the fourth group, is characterized by onset in utero, arthrogryposis, dysmorphic features, and respiratory insufficiency. A subset of patients with multi-minicore disease have cardiac involvement, either as a structural abnormality or as overt cardiomyopathy, which can be primary or secondary to respiratory compromise. It is to be noted however that no cases have been reported to date of cardiomyopathy in patients with mutations in *RYR1* or *SEPN1*.

Mutations in *SEPN1* are found all along the gene [18], although there are indications of founder mutations in some populations. The exact function of the protein is not known, but structural similarity with calcium-binding proteins may suggest a role for selenoprotein N in calcium homeostasis.

Malignant hyperthermia association

Malignant hyperthermia is allelic to central core disease, most cases being caused by mutations in *RYR1* [84]. This pathological reaction to succinylcholine and inhaled anesthetics may be aborted by early administration of the specific antagonist dantrolene sodium [88].

Congenital titin myopathy with cardiomyopathy

Homozygous mutations causing deletion of the C-terminus of titin may cause a congenital myopathy with minicores, central nuclei, and secondary calpain deficiency [31]. Later in life, at ages of 5–16 years, cardiomyopathy ensues. Biopsy findings become dystrophic with time. This novel congenital myopathy is the first truly recessive muscle disorder to be reported as being caused by mutations in the titin gene, previously known to cause cardiomyopathy, distal myopathy, and limb-girdle myopathy type 2J [OMIM 188840].

The myotubular/centronuclear myopathies

The myotubular/centronuclear myopathies (MTM/CNM) [61] are characterized histologically by central, often large, spaced nuclei surrounded by an area devoid of myofibrils but occupied by mitochondrial aggregates in small, rounded muscle fibers thus resembling fetal myotubes (Figure 13.3) [89]. These features are best seen on hematoxylin & eosin (HE) and nicotinamide adenine dinucleotide dehydrogenase (NADH) staining (where peripheral haloes are also shown), and using electron microscopy. The historical argument as to whether the X-linked form should have a separate name, myotubular versus centronuclear myopathy, reflects different hypotheses about whether the pathogenesis is one of defective maturation of the muscle fibers [61]. This argument, arisen long before any causative genes had been identified to permit objective analysis, may be resolved now that the genes are being identified and the pathogenetic mechanisms are thus becoming revealed.

Ophthalmoplegia, an unusual feature amongst patients with congenital myopathies, is often seen in MTM/CNM. In a floppy infant with ophthalmoplegia, the X-linked form is thus a diagnosis to consider. If the biopsy confirms the presence of central nuclei, differential diagnoses include the autosomal recessive forms of MTM/CNM and myotonic dystrophy (Table 13.4). It is to be noted that female carriers of the X-linked form may manifest overt muscle disease. Radial strands on NADH staining of the muscle biopsy may indicate the presence of a mutation in *DNM2* (Figure 13.5e).

The X-linked form

The X-linked form is caused by mutations in the myotubularin gene *MTM1* [20]. Pregnancy may be complicated by polyhydramnios, a feature otherwise seen only in rare, severe cases of the other congenital myopathies. Contractures of the hips and knees may be present. Affected boys are often long and light for gestational age, with large head circumferences, and their growth may be rapid. Genotype–phenotype studies in the X-linked form, in most cases neonatally very severe, showed that some missense mutations may be associated with a milder course [54]. A majority of mothers of affected boys are carriers, while others have shown mosaicism.

Autosomal forms

Recently, three of the genes for autosomal forms, *DNM2* [9], amphiphysin 2 (*BIN1)* [8], and *RYR1* [10] have been identified (Table 13.1) and their clinical pictures are currently being defined [9, 60, 90]. Interestingly, three of the genes for MTM/CNM, *MTM1*, *DNM2*, and *BIN1*, are implicated in the intracellular pathways of membrane and endosome trafficking and remodeling of T-tubules [8]. A direct functional link between the proteins encoded by the latter two has been identified [8]. The significance of the inactivating variants in the phosphoinositide phosphatase hJUMPY identified in two patients, one of whom also had a *DNM2* mutation, is unclear [91].

Magnetic resonance imaging findings can help direct mutational testing; selective involvement of the soleus, gastrocnemius, and tibialis anterior in the lower legs and the adductor longus, semimembranosus, biceps femoris, and vastus intermedius of the thighs has been noted in the *DNM2*-related form [60], while the patient with *RYR1* mutation showed almost a mirror image on MRI [10], similar to that of patients with central core disease and multi-minicore disease with ophthalmoplegia caused by mutations in *RYR1*.

Dominant form caused by mutations in dynamin 2: DNM2

Heterozygous missense mutations in *DNM2*, a gene previously associated with Charcot–Marie–Tooth disease type 2B [92], have been found to cause a dominantly inherited form of MTM/CNM [9]. The relationship between neurogenic and myogenic symptoms in patients with mutations in this gene is currently being explored [93]. Sufficient families have been described (e.g., [9, 60, 90, 93, 94]) to permit the delineation of a form with onset usually in adolescence or early adulthood. A few infants and children have been described also with mutations in *DNM2* [90, 94]. Weakness in some has been predominantly distal, with distal contractures, while in many it has been proximal. Pain on exercise, an unusual feature amongst the congenital myopathies, may be the first symptom. Most patients had ptosis, and some had involvement of extraocular muscles. To our knowledge, except in some of the children with neonatal onset [94], NADH-TR stains of muscle biopsies have consistently shown radial strands (Figure 13.5e) around the central nuclei, a feature so far not encountered in the forms caused by mutations in other genes.

Dominant form caused by mutation of the ryanodine receptor: RYR1

In a female patient with central nuclei in her first biopsy and additional central cores in the second, and an MRI pattern consistent with that of patients with *RYR1* mutations, a de novo heterozygous missense mutation was identified in *RYR1* [10]. Onset was in utero, with polyhydramnios, floppiness at birth, dysarthria, ophthalmoplegia, and delayed motor milestones.

Recessive form caused by mutations in amphiphysin 2: BIN1

Homozygosity for missense mutations in *BIN1* was recently found in five patients from three consanguineous families to cause recessive MTM/CNM [8]. Onset was congenital or in childhood. Weakness was predominantly proximal and severity was variable. In one family two out of three affected sibs died at ages of 18 hours and 1 year, respectively, whilst the third sib and the affected persons in the other two families had slowly progressive, predominantly proximal muscle weakness with retained respiratory independence. Two out of four had ptosis and one had ophthalmoplegia.

Other congenital myopathies for which genes have been identified

Danon disease

Danon disease is an X-linked disorder, characterized clinically by myopathy, cardiomyopathy, and mental retardation. The pathology shows a vacuolar myopathy with accumulation of autophagic material frequently, but not always, also including glycogen. Danon disease is caused by null mutations in the *LAMP2* (lysosomal-associated membrane protein 2) gene [32].

Mallory body myopathy

Mallory body myopathy is characterized by the presence on muscle biopsy of hyaline bodies similar to the Mallory bodies of alcoholic liver disease. The muscle Mallory bodies are immunoreactive for desmin and other proteins. The disease is autosomal recessive and is caused by mutations in the selenoprotein N gene (*SEPN1*) [16].

Myosin storage myopathy

Myosin storage myopathy is characterized by accumulations of myosin in type 1 fibers (Figure 13.5f), best seen by immunolabeling and electron microscopy. The clinical phenotype is highly variable, but weakness frequently shows a scapuloperoneal distribution. Myosin storage myopathy is caused by specific mutations in the "tail" of *MYH7* that may disrupt the assembly competence domain and interfere with myosin dimerization [19, 95].

Reducing body myopathy

The latest congenital myopathy for which a disease gene has been identified is reducing body myopathy, characterized by the presence of aggresome-like inclusion bodies that reduce nitro-blue-tetrazolium (NBT) and thus stain strongly with menadione-NBT [96]. Reducing body myopathy, similar to other congenital myopathies, may show a spectrum of phenotypes from severe neonatal to adult-onset forms [28, 95]. Schessl and co-workers [28] used for the first time proteomic techniques (laser capture microdissection to isolate the reducing bodies followed by tandem mass spectrometry) to identify a significant protein component of the reducing bodies as the X-chromosome protein four and half lim domain protein FHL1 and then demonstrated mutation of the *FHL1* gene in four separate families.

Sarcotubular myopathy

Sarcotubular myopathy, an autosomal recessive disease, manifests as multiple phenotypes including a limb-girdle phenotype with facial weakness. Onset may be in the first years of life or much later. The characteristic feature on biopsy is myriad small vacuoles in a segmental distribution. Electron microscopy and immuno-electron microscopy demonstrate that the vacuoles are expanded sarcoplasmic reticulum. Sarcotubular myopathy is caused by the same D487N mutation in *TRIM32* on the same haplotypic background as LGMD2H identified in the Hutterite population. Sarcotubular myopathy and LGMD2H are therefore manifestations of the same disease, with sarcotubular myopathy perhaps showing the more extreme vacuolar pathology [29].

Spheroid body myopathy

Spheroid body myopathy is an autosomal dominant disorder with onset from childhood to adulthood, where the biopsy shows characteristic spheroid bodies labeling with antibodies to myotilin. The causative mutation was identified as an S39F mutation in the serine-rich region of the myotilin gene which also shows mutations in LGMD1A and myofibrillar myopathy [30].

Congenital myopathies for which no genes have been identified

Congenital myopathies for which no genes have been identified are listed in Table 13.2. Some of these are questionable entities. Since many of these disorders are extremely rare, perhaps even seen in only one patient, but are the basis of the nosology, it is important to follow the patient(s) and report on the course of the disease and any new developments. Successful candidate gene analysis of classic cases has been achieved; for example, demonstrating that the original family described with myosin storage myopathy did have a mutation in *MYH7* [95]. Proteomic approaches such as that used by

Schessl and co-workers [28] might be particularly applicable in these disorders.

Conclusions and future directions

In the next few years further genes for the congenital myopathies should be discovered and their molecular pathology should be clarified. We can thus anticipate the rational development of effective therapies for the congenital myopathies. It may be possible for the congenital myopathies to piggy-back on successful investigation of possible therapies for Duchenne muscular dystrophy which is many years in advance [96].

Obtaining an accurate molecular genetic cause for the disorder in each patient is likely to become a prerequisite for specific gene- or mutation-based therapies. For example, successful therapies for actin-based nemaline myopathy are likely to be different from successful therapies for nebulin nemaline myopathy, and treatment modalities may be different for different mutations within the same gene. Anti-sense induced exon skipping, promising for Duchenne, may not be applicable to actin diseases, but may be applicable to nebulin diseases. Read-through of nonsense mutations may help patients with nonsense mutations, viral gene therapy may work for all the small genes, but inserting *RYR1*, *NEB* or especially *TTN* in a virus may not be possible. Muscle transplantation in the form of muscle stem cells may have the potential to help patients with all types of muscle disease as heart transplantation cures the parallel cardiomyopathies.

Studies of exercise in a mouse model of nemaline myopathy [98], initial reports of L-tyrosine use in nemaline myopathy [99], studies of upregulation of cardiac actin in a mouse model null for skeletal actin [100] and a pilot study of salbutamol for central core and multi-minicore disease [101] require confirmation of the potentially beneficial effects.

We can also anticipate further provision of the benefits to the community of discovering the genetic bases of the diseases. Useful applications will be available to more and more individual families as methodologies for screening even the large genes become more efficient and affordable. Benefits will involve further provision of accurate genetic diagnosis and counseling for individuals and families including those in high-incidence foci of recessive congenital myopathies.

The congenital myopathies, like many other muscle disease groups, are entering an interesting post gene-discovery era, with therapeutic clinical trials on the horizon.

Acknowledgments

N. G. L. is supported by the Australian National Health and Medical Research Council Fellowship 403904 and C. W. P. by grants from the Sigrid Jusélius Foundation, the Academy of Finland, the Finska Läkaresällskapet, the Association Francaise contre les Myopathies and the Liv och Hälsa Foundation. We thank Dr. Heinz Jungbluth and Professor Caroline Sewry for constructive comments on the manuscript.

References

1. V. Dubowitz, C. A. Sewry, *Muscle Biopsy A Practical Approach*. Third Edition. (Philadelphia, PA: Saunders Elsevier, 2007.)
2. K. J. Nowak, D. Wattanasirichaigoon, H. H. Goebel, *et al.*, Mutations in the skeletal muscle alpha-actin gene in patients with actin myopathy and nemaline myopathy. *Nat. Genet.* **23**:2 (1999), 208–212.
3. V. L. Lehtokari, C. Ceuterick-de Groote, P. de Jonghe, *et al.*, Cap disease caused by heterozygous deletion of the beta-tropomyosin gene TPM2. *Neuromuscul. Disord.* **17** (2007), 433–442.
4. H. Tajsharghi, M. Ohlsson, C. Lindberg, A. Oldfors, Congenital myopathy with nemaline rods and cap structures caused by a mutation in the beta-tropomyosin gene (TPM2). *Arch. Neurol.* **64**:9 (2007), 1334–1338.
5. K. A. Quane, J. M. S. Healy, K. E. Keating, *et al.*, Mutations in the ryanodine receptor gene in central core disease and malignant hyperthermia. *Nat. Genet.* **5** (1993), 51–55.
6. Y. Zhang, H. S. Chen, V. K. Khanna, *et al.*, A mutation in the human ryanodine receptor gene associated with central core disease. *Nat. Genet.* **5** (1993), 46–50.
7. A. M. Kaindl, F. Ruschendorf, S. Krause, *et al.*, Missense mutations of ACTA1 cause dominant congenital myopathy with cores. *J. Med. Genet.* **41**:11 (2004), 842–848.
8. A. S. Nicot, A. Toussaint, V. Tosch, *et al.*, Mutations in amphiphysin 2 (BIN1) disrupt interaction with dynamin 2 and cause autosomal recessive centronuclear myopathy. *Nat. Genet.* **39**:9 (2007), 1134–1139.
9. M. Bitoun, S. Maugenre, P. Y. Jeannet, *et al.*, Mutations in dynamin 2 cause dominant centronuclear myopathy. *Nat. Genet.* **37**:11 (2005), 1207–1209.
10. H. Jungbluth, H. Zhou, C. A. Sewry, *et al.*, Centronuclear myopathy due to a de novo dominant mutation in the skeletal muscle ryanodine receptor (RYR1) gene. *Neuromuscul. Disord.* **17**:4 (2007), 338–345.
11. N. G. Laing, N. F. Clarke, D. E. Dye, *et al.*, Actin mutations are one cause of congenital fibre type disproportion. *Ann. Neurol.* **56**:5 (2004), 689–694.
12. N. F. Clarke, W. Kidson, S. Quijano-Roy, *et al.*, SEPN1: associated with congenital fiber-type disproportion and insulin resistance. *Ann. Neurol.* **59**:3 (2006), 546–552.
13. N. F. Clarke, H. Kolski, D. E. Dye, *et al.*, Mutations in TPM3 are a common cause of congenital fiber type disproportion. *Ann. Neurol.* **63**:3 (2008), 329–339.
14. N. Monnier, N. B. Romero, J. Lerale, *et al.*, An autosomal dominant congenital myopathy with cores and rods is associated with a neomutation in the RYR1 gene encoding the skeletal muscle ryanodine receptor. *Hum. Mol. Genet.* **9**:18 (2000), 2599–2608.
15. P. C. Scacheri, E. P. Hoffman, J. D. Fratkin, *et al.*, A novel ryanodine receptor gene mutation causing both cores and rods in congenital myopathy. *Neurology* **55**:11 (2000), 1689–1696.
16. A. Ferreiro, C. Ceuterick-de Groote, J. J. Marks, *et al.*, Desmin-related myopathy with Mallory body-like inclusions is caused by mutations of the selenoprotein N gene. *Ann. Neurol.* **55**:5 (2004), 676–686.

17. A. Ferreiro, N. Monnier, N. B. Romero, *et al.*, A recessive form of central core disease, transiently presenting as multi-minicore disease, is associated with a homozygous mutation in the ryanodine receptor type 1 gene. *Ann. Neurol.* **51**:6 (2002), 750–759.

18. A. Ferreiro, S. Quijano-Roy, C. Pichereau, *et al.*, Mutations of the selenoprotein N gene, which is implicated in rigid spine muscular dystrophy, cause the classical phenotype of multiminicore disease: reassessing the nosology of early-onset myopathies. *Am. J. Hum. Genet.* **71**:4 (2002), 739–749.

19. H. Tajsharghi, L. E. Thornell, C. Lindberg, B. Lindvall, K. G. Henriksson, A. Oldfors. Myosin storage myopathy associated with a heterozygous missense mutation in MYH7. *Ann. Neurol.* **54** (2003), 494–500.

20. J. Laporte, L. J. Hu, C. Kretz, *et al.*, A gene mutated in X-linked myotubular myopathy defines a new putative tyrosine phosphatase family conserved in yeast. *Nat. Genet.* **13** (1996), 175–182.

21. P. B. Agrawal, R. S. Greenleaf, K. K. Tomczak, *et al.*, Nemaline myopathy with minicores caused by mutation of the CFL2 gene encoding the skeletal muscle actin-binding protein, cofilin-2. *Am. J. Hum. Genet.* **80**:1 (2007), 162–167.

22. K. Pelin, P. Hilpela, K. Donner, *et al.*, Mutations in the nebulin gene associated with autosomal recessive nemaline myopathy. *Proc. Natl. Acad. Sci. U. S. A.* **96**:5 (1999), 2305–2310.

23. N. G. Laing, S. D. Wilton, P. A. Akkari, *et al.*, A mutation in the α-tropomyosin gene TPM3 associated with autosomal dominant nemaline myopathy. *Nat. Genet.* **9** (1995), 75–79.

24. K. Donner, M. Ollikainen, M. Ridanpää, *et al.*, Mutations in the β-tropomyosin (TPM2) gene – a rare cause of nemaline myopathy. *Neuromuscul. Disord.* **12** (2002), 151–158.

25. J. J. Johnston, R. I. Kelley, T. O. Crawford, *et al.*, A novel nemaline myopathy in the Amish caused by a mutation in troponin T1. *Am. J. Hum. Genet.* **67**:4 (2000), 814–821.

26. D. A. Weeks, R. R. Nixon, V. Kaimaktchiev, G. W. Mierau, Intranuclear rod myopathy, a rare and morphologically striking variant of nemaline rod myopathy. *Ultrastruct. Pathol.* **27**:3 (2003), 151–154.

27. D. O. Hutchinson, A. Charlton, N. G. Laing, B. Ilkovski, K. N. North, Autosomal dominant nemaline myopathy with intranuclear rods due to mutation of the skeletal muscle ACTA1 gene: clinical and pathological variability within a kindred. *Neuromuscul. Disord.* **16**:2 (2006), 113–121.

28. J. Schessl, Y. Zou, M. J. McGrath, *et al.*, Proteomic identification of FHL1 as the protein mutated in human reducing body myopathy. *J Clin Invest.* **118**:3 (2008), 904–912.

29. B. G. Schoser, P. Frosk, A. G. Engel, U. Klutzny, H. Lochmuller, K. Wrogemann, Commonality of TRIM32 mutation in causing sarcotubular myopathy and LGMD2H. *Ann. Neurol.* **57**:4 (2005), 591–595.

30. T. Foroud, N. Pankratz, A. P. Batchman, *et al.*, A mutation in myotilin causes spheroid body myopathy. *Neurology* **65**:12 (2005), 1936–1940.

31. V. Carmignac, M. A. Salih, S. Quijano-Roy, *et al.*, C-terminal titin deletions cause a novel early-onset myopathy with fatal cardiomyopathy. *Ann. Neurol.* **61**:4 (2007), 340–351.

32. I. Nishino, J. Fu, K. Tanji, *et al.*, Primary LAMP-2 deficiency causes X-linked vacuolar cardiomyopathy and myopathy (Danon disease). *Nature* **406**:6798 (2000), 906–910.

33. P. Y. Jeannet, L. Mittaz, M. Dunand, J. A. Lobrinus, L. Bonafe, T. Kuntzer, Autosomal dominant nemaline myopathy: a new phenotype unlinked to previously known genetic loci. *Neuromuscul. Disord.* **17**:1 (2007), 6–12.

34. I. M. Gommans, M. Davis, K. Saar, *et al.*, A locus on chromosome 15q for a dominantly inherited nemaline myopathy with core-like lesions. *Brain* **126** (2003), 1545–1551.

35. U. P. Ketelsen, B. Brand-Saberi, B. Uhlenberg, M. Wagner, H. G. Laberke, H. Omran, Congenital myopathy with arrest of myogenesis prior to formation of myotubes. *Neuropediatrics* **36**:4 (2005), 246–251.

36. L. Hartley, M. Kinali, R. Knight, *et al.*, A congenital myopathy with diaphragmatic weakness not linked to the SMARD1 locus. *Neuromuscul Disord.* **17**:2 (2007), 174–179.

37. P. R. Bourque, B. Lach, S. Carpenter, P. Rippstein, Myopathy with hexagonally cross-linked tubular arrays: a new autosomal dominant or sporadic congenital myopathy. *Ann. Neurol.* **45**:4 (1999), 512–515.

38. D. Lev, M. Sadeh, N. Watemberg, *et al.*, A benign congenital myopathy in an inbred Samaritan family. *Eur. J. Paediatr. Neurol.* **10**:4 (2006), 182–185.

39. H. H. Goebel, Congenital myopathies. *Semin. Pediatr. Neurol.* **3**:2 (1996), 152–161.

40. M. A. Corbett, P. Anthony Akkari, A. Domazetovska, *et al.*, An alphatropomyosin mutation alters dimer preference in nemaline myopathy. *Ann. Neurol.* **57**:1 (2005), 42–49.

41. B. Ilkovski, K. J. Nowak, A. Domazetovska, *et al.*, Evidence for a dominant-negative effect in ACTA1 nemaline myopathy caused by abnormal folding, aggregation and altered polymerization of mutant actin isoforms. *Hum. Mol. Genet.* **13**:16 (2004), 1727–1743.

42. A. Domazetovska, B. Ilkovski, V. Kumar, *et al.*, Intranuclear rod myopathy: molecular pathogenesis and mechanisms of weakness. *Ann Neurol.* **62**:6 (2007), 597–608.

43. A. Domazetovska, B. Ilkovski, S. T. Cooper, *et al.*, Mechanisms underlying intranuclear rod formation. *Brain* **130**:Pt 12 (2007), 3275–3284.

44. A. D'Amico, C. Graziano, G. Pacileo, *et al.*, Fatal hypertrophic cardiomyopathy and nemaline myopathy associated with ACTA1 K336E mutation. *Neuromuscul. Disord.* **16**:9–10 (2006), 548–552.

45. N. F. Clarke, B. Ilkovski, S. Cooper, *et al.*, The pathogenesis of ACTA1-related congenital fiber type disproportion. *Ann. Neurol.* **61**:6 (2007), 552–561.

46. H. Zhou, H. Jungbluth, C. A. Sewry, *et al.*, Molecular mechanisms and phenotypic variation in RYR1-related congenital myopathies. *Brain* **130**:Pt 8 (2007), 2024–2036.

47. A. Ferreiro, B. Estournet, D. Chateau, *et al.*, Multi-minicore disease – searching for boundaries: phenotype analysis of 38 cases. *Ann. Neurol.* **48**:5 (2000), 745–757.

48. C. Wallgren-Pettersson, K. Pelin, K. J. Nowak, *et al.*, Genotype-phenotype correlations in nemaline myopathy caused by mutations in the genes for nebulin and skeletal muscle alpha-actin. *Neuromuscul. Disord.* **14**:8–9 (2004), 461–470.

49. C. Wallgren-Pettersson, K. Bushby, U. Mellies, A. Simonds, 117th ENMC workshop: ventilatory support in congenital neuromuscular disorders – congenital myopathies, congenital muscular dystrophies, congenital myotonic dystrophy and SMA (II) 4–6 April 2003, Naarden, The Netherlands. *Neuromuscul. Disord.* **14**:1 (2004), 56–69.

50. C. Wallgren-Pettersson, K. Donner, C. Sewry, *et al.*, Mutations in the nebulin gene can cause severe congenital nemaline myopathy. *Neuromuscul. Disord.* **12**:7–8 (2002), 674–679.

51. J. C. Sparrow, K. J. Nowak, H. J. Durling, *et al.*, Muscle disease caused by mutations in the skeletal muscle alpha-actin gene (ACTA1). *Neuromuscul. Disord.* **13** (2003), 519–531.

52. C. Wallgren-Pettersson, V. L. Lehtokari, H. Kalimo, *et al.*, Distal myopathy caused by homozygous missense mutations in the nebulin gene. *Brain* **130**:Pt 6 (2007), 1465–1476.

53. S. S. Sung, A. M. Brassington, K. Grannatt, *et al.*, Mutations in genes encoding fast-twitch contractile proteins cause distal arthrogryposis syndromes. *Am. J. Hum. Genet.* **72**:3 (2003), 681–690.

54. M. McEntagart, G. Parsons, A. Buj-Bello, *et al.*, Genotype-phenotype correlations in X-linked myotubular myopathy. *Neuromuscul. Disord.* **12**:10 (2002), 939–946.

55. H. Zhou, N. Yamaguchi, L. Xu, *et al.*, Characterization of recessive RYR1 mutations in core myopathies. *Hum. Mol. Genet.* **15**:18 (2006), 2791–2803.

56. C. A. Sewry, C. Muller, M. Davis, *et al.*, The spectrum of pathology in central core disease. *Neuromuscul. Disord.* **12**:10 (2002), 930–938.

57. K. Donner, M. Sandbacka, V. L. Lehtokari, C. Wallgren-Pettersson, K. Pelin, Complete genomic structure of the human nebulin gene and identification of alternatively spliced transcripts. *Eur. J. Hum. Genet.* **12**:9 (2004), 744–751.

58. H. Jungbluth, M. R. Davis, C. Muller, *et al.*, Magnetic resonance imaging of muscle in congenital myopathies associated with RYR1 mutations. *Neuromuscul. Disord.* **14**:12 (2004), 785–790.

59. H. Jungbluth, C. A. Sewry, S. Counsell, *et al.*, Magnetic resonance imaging of muscle in nemaline myopathy. *Neuromuscul. Disord.* **14**:12 (2004), 779–784.

60. J. Schessl, L. Medne, Y. Hu, *et al.*, MRI in DNM2-related centronuclear myopathy: evidence for highly selective muscle involvement. *Neuromuscul Disord.* **17**:1 (2007), 28–32.

61. C. Wallgren-Pettersson, A. Clarke, F. Samson, *et al.*, The myotubular myopathies: differential diagnosis of the X linked recessive, autosomal dominant, and autosomal recessive forms and present state of DNA studies. *J. Med. Genet.* **32**:9 (1995), 673–679.

62. C. Akiyama, I. Nonaka, A follow-up study of congenital non-progressive myopathies. *Brain Dev.* **18**:5 (1996), 404–408.

63. I. Gill, M. Eagle, J. S. Mehta, M. J. Gibson, K. Bushby, R. Bullock, Correction of neuromuscular scoliosis in patients with preexisting respiratory failure. *Spine* **31**:21 (2006), 2478–2483.

64. S. Rudnik-Schoneborn, B. Glauner, D. Rohrig, K. Zerres, Obstetric aspects in women with facioscapulohumeral muscular dystrophy, limb-girdle muscular dystrophy, and congenital myopathies. *Arch. Neurol.* **54**:7 (1997), 888–894.

65. J. Laporte, V. Biancalana, S. M. Tanner, *et al.*, MTM1 mutations in X-linked myotubular myopathy. *Hum. Mutat.* **15**:5 (2000), 393–409.

66. R. M. Quinlivan, C. R. Muller, M. Davis, *et al.*, Central core disease: clinical, pathological, and genetic features. *Arch. Dis. Child.* **88**:12 (2003), 1051–1055.

67. C. Wallgren-Pettersson, N. G. Laing, Report of the 70th ENMC International Workshop: Nemaline myopathy 11–13 June 1999, Naarden, The Netherlands, *Neuromuscul. Disord.* **10** (2000), 299–306.

68. N. Chahin, D. Selcen, A. G. Engel, Sporadic late onset nemaline myopathy. *Neurology* **65**:8 (2005), 1158–1164.

69. K. Pelin, K. Donner, M. Holmberg, H. Jungbluth, F. Muntoni, C. Wallgren-Pettersson, Nebulin mutations in autosomal recessive nemaline myopathy: an update. *Neuromuscul. Disord.* **12**:7–8 (2002), 680–686.

70. S. L. Anderson, J. Ekstein, M. C. Donnelly, *et al.*, Nemaline myopathy in the Ashkenazi Jewish population is caused by a deletion in the nebulin gene. *Hum. Genet.* **115**:3 (2004), 185–190.

71. V. L. Lehtokari, R. S. Greenleaf, E. T. DeChene, *et al.*, The exon 55 delection in the nebulin gene – one single founder mutation with worldwide occurrence. *Neuromusc. Disord.* **19**:3 (2009), 179–181.

72. M. L. Bang, X. Li, R. Littlefield, *et al.*, Nebulin-deficient mice exhibit shorter thin filament lengths and reduced contractile function in skeletal muscle. *J. Cell Biol.* **173**:6 (2006), 905–916.

73. C. C. Witt, C. Burkart, D. Labeit, *et al.*, Nebulin regulates thin filament length, contractility, and Z-disk structure in vivo. *EMBO J.* **25**:16 (2006), 3843–3855.

74. K. J. Nowak, C. A. Sewry, C. Navarro, *et al.*, Nemaline myopathy caused by absence of alpha-skeletal muscle actin. *Ann. Neurol.* **61**:2 (2007), 175–184.

75. P. B. Agrawal, C. D. Strickland, C. Midgett, *et al.*, Heterogeneity of nemaline myopathy cases with skeletal muscle alpha-actin gene mutations. *Ann. Neurol.* **56**:1 (2004), 86–96.

76. S. S. Sung, A. M. Brassington, P. A. Krakowiak, J. C. Carey, L. B. Jorde, M. Bamshad, Mutations in TNNT3 cause multiple congenital contractures: a second locus for distal arthrogryposis type 2B. *Am. J. Hum. Genet.* **73**:1 (2003), 212–214.

77. R. M. Toydemir, A. Rutherford, F. G. Whitby, L. B. Jorde, J. C. Carey, M. J. Bamshad, Mutations in embryonic myosin heavy chain (MYH3) cause Freeman-Sheldon syndrome and Sheldon-Hall syndrome. *Nat. Genet.* **38**:5 (2006), 561–565.

78. P. Robinson, S. Lipscomb, L. C. Preston, *et al.*, Mutations in fast skeletal troponin I, troponin T, and beta-tropomyosin that cause distal arthrogryposis all increase contractile function. *FASEB J.* **21**:3 (2007), 896–905.

79. B. L. Banwell, J. Russel, T. Fukudome, X. M. Shen, G. Stilling, A. G. Engel. Myopathy, myasthenic syndrome, and epidermolysis bullosa simplex due to plectin deficiency. *J. Neuropathol. Exp. Neurol.* **58**:8 (1999), 832–846.

80. H. Jungbluth, C. A. Sewry, S. C. Brown, *et al.*, Mild phenotype of nemaline myopathy with sleep hypoventilation due to mutation in the skeletal muscle a-actin (ACTA1) gene. *Neuromuscul. Disord.* **11** (2001), 35–40.

81. N. F. Clarke, K. N. North, Congenital fiber type disproportion – 30 years on. *J. Neuropathol. Exp. Neurol.* **62**:10 (2003), 977–989.

82. N. B. Romero, N. Monnier, L. Viollet, *et al.*, Dominant and recessive central core disease associated with RYR1 mutations and fetal akinesia. *Brain* **126**:Pt 11 (2003), 2341–2349.

83. S. Wu, M. C. Ibarra, M. C. Malicdan, *et al.*, Central core disease is due to RYR1 mutations in more than 90% of patients. *Brain* **129**:Pt 6 (2006), 1470–1480.

84. R. Robinson, D. Carpenter, M. A. Shaw, J. Halsall, P. Hopkins, Mutations in RYR1 in malignant hyperthermia and central core disease. *Hum. Mutat.* **27**:10 (2006), 977–989.

85. H. Takeshima, M. Iino, H. Takekura, *et al.*, Excitation-contraction uncoupling and muscular degeneration in mice lacking functional skeletal muscle ryanodine-receptor gene. *Nature* **369**:6481 (1994), 556–559.

86. H. Zhou, M. Brockington, H. Jungbluth, *et al.*, Epigenetic allele silencing unveils recessive RYR1 mutations in core myopathies. *Am. J. Hum. Genet.* **79**:5 (2006), 859–868.

87. A. Ferreiro, M. Fardeau, 80th ENMC International Workshop on Multi-Minicore Disease: 1st International MmD Workshop. 12–13th May, 2000, Soestduinen, The Netherlands. *Neuromuscul. Disord.* **12**:1 (2002), 60–68.

88. B. R. Fruen, J. R. Mickelson, C. F. Louis, Dantrolene inhibition of sarcoplasmic reticulum Ca^{2+} release by direct and specific action at skeletal muscle ryanodine receptors. *J. Biol. Chem.* **272**:43 (1997), 26965–26971.

89. C. Wallgren-Pettersson, N. S. Thomas, Report on the 20th ENMC sponsored international workshop: myotubular/centronuclear myopathy. *Neuromuscul. Disord.* **4**:1 (1994), 71–74.

90. P. Y. Jeannet, G. Bassez, B. Eymard, *et al.*, Clinical and histologic findings in autosomal centronuclear myopathy. *Neurology* **62**:9 (2004), 1484–1490.

91. V. Tosch, H. M. Rohde, H. Tronchere, *et al.*, A novel PtdIns3P and PtdIns(3,5)P2 phosphatase with an inactivating variant in centronuclear myopathy. *Hum. Mol. Genet.* **15**:21 (2006), 3098–3106.

92. S. Zuchner, M. Noureddine, M. Kennerson, *et al.*, Mutations in the pleckstrin homology domain of dynamin 2 cause dominant intermediate Charcot-Marie-Tooth disease. *Nat. Genet.* **37**:3 (2005), 289–294.

93. A. Echaniz-Laguna, A. S. Nicot, S. Carré, *et al.*, Subtle central and peripheral nervous system abnormalities in a family with centronuclear myopathy and a novel dynamin 2 gene mutation. *Neuromuscul. Disord.* **17**:11–12 (2007), 955–959.

94. M. Bitoun, J. A. Bevilacqua, B. Prudhon, *et al.*, Dynamin 2 mutations cause sporadic centronuclear myopathy with neonatal onset. *Ann. Neurol.* **62**:6 (2007), 666–670.

95. D. E. Dye, B. Azzarelli, H. H. Goebel, N. G. Laing, Novel slow-skeletal myosin (MYH7) mutation in the original myosin storage myopathy kindred. *Neuromuscul. Disord.* **16**:6 (2006), 357–360.

96. T. Liewluck, Y. K. Hayashi, M. Ohsawa, *et al.*, Unfolded protein response and aggresome formation in hereditary reducing-body myopathy. *Muscle Nerve* **35**:3 (2007), 322–326.

97. K. J. Nowak, K. E. Davies, Duchenne muscular dystrophy and dystrophin: pathogenesis and opportunities for treatment. *EMBO Rep.* **5**:9 (2004), 872–876.

98. J. E. Joya, A. J. Kee, V. Nair-Shalliker, *et al.*, Muscle weakness in a mouse model of nemaline myopathy can be reversed with exercise and reveals a novel myofiber repair mechanism. *Hum. Mol. Genet.* **13**:21 (2004), 2633–2645.

99. M. M. Ryan, C. Sy, S. Rudge, *et al.*, Dietary L-tyrosine supplementation in nemaline myopathy. *J. Child Neurol.* **23**:6 (2008), 609–613.

100. K. J. Nowak, G. Ravenscroft, C. Jackaman, *et al.*, Rescue of skeletal muscle a-actin null mice by cardiac (fetal) α-actin. *J. Cell Biol.* **183** (2009), 903–915.

101. S. Messina, L. Hartley, M. Main, *et al.*, Pilot trial of salbutamol in central core and multi-minicore diseases. *Neuropediatrics* **35**:5 (2004), 262–266.

Chapter

14 Muscle diseases with prominent muscle contractures

Gisèle Bonne and Anne K. Lampe

Introduction

Amongst the muscle diseases, muscle contractures are a rather common finding. However, whereas they may arise as secondary consequences of major muscular dystrophies, like in Duchenne muscular dystrophy (DMD) and congenital muscular dystrophies, contractures are prominent and occur in the early stages of the disease in two main groups of inherited disorders: (1) Emery–Dreifuss muscular dystrophies (EDMD) due to mutations in two genes encoding components of the nuclear envelope, emerin and the A-type lamins; and (2) Bethlem myopathy (BM) and Ullrich congenital muscular dystrophy (UCMD) due to mutations in the genes encoding the three peptide chains of collagen VI, a ubiquitous extracellular matrix protein which forms a microfibrillar network in close association with the basement membrane of most tissues. Thus defects of components of nuclear envelope (NE) and extracellular matrix (ECM) both lead to muscle diseases with prominent muscle contractures. Although the pathophysiological mechanisms of the respective primary defects (disruption of the NE versus ECM) are most probably different, the differential diagnosis between the various related clinical entities remains difficult.

Emery–Dreifuss muscular dystrophy (EDMD, Figure 14.1) is characterized by early-onset contractures, slowly progressive muscle weakness and cardiomyopathy with conduction defects and/or arrhythmias. The disease may have been described by Cestan and LeJonne in 1902 [1], and later on by Hauptmann and Thannhauser in 1941 [2]. In 1966, Emery reported a large Virginian family affected by an X-linked muscular dystrophy, which was previously reported by Dreifuss and Hogan as a form of DMD with unusual length of survival [3]. The disease observed in the family was quite distinct from DMD because of the unusual early contractures in elbows and Achilles tendons, cardiac abnormalities, and absence of muscle hypertrophy and intellectual impairment. The X-linked disorder was termed Emery–Dreifuss muscular dystrophy by Rowland *et al.* [4]. During the 1970s and the 1980s, several authors reported families where the EDMD phenotype appeared to be transmitted as an autosomal dominant trait (for review see [5]). The Hauptmann–Thannhauser eponym was sometimes suggested to be attached to autosomal dominant muscular dystrophy with early contractures and cardiomyopathy [2]. In the 1990s, the development of molecular genetics led to the identification of mutations in the *STA* gene (now called *EMD*) localized on chromosome Xq28 and encoding a new protein that was called emerin [6]. This protein was later found to be localized at the nuclear envelope [7, 8]. Soon after, mutations of the *LMNA* gene encoding the A-type lamins, other components of the nuclear envelope, were found to be responsible for the autosomal dominant as well as the very rare autosomal recessive forms of the disease, further confirming the implication of the nuclear envelope in the field of neuromuscular disorders [9, 10].

Ullrich congenital muscular dystrophy (UCMD, Figure 14.2f–k) was first described by Ullrich in 1930 who recognized a strikingly similar clinical phenotype consisting of severe muscle weakness of early onset with proximal joint contractures and striking hyperelasticity of distal small joints in two unrelated patients [11]. Highlighting the connective tissue involvement in his patients, he called the condition "congenital atonic-sclerotic muscular dystrophy" and also hypothesized that the parental consanguinity of his second case might play a causative role. Further case reports by colleagues [12, 13] and subsequent publications by other teams worldwide confirmed a likely autosomal recessive inheritance and a recognizable pattern of disease [14, 15, 16, 17]. Bethlem myopathy (BM, Figure 14.2a–e) was first described in 1976 by Bethlem and van Wijngaarden as a relatively mild dominantly inherited disorder characterized by the combination of slowly progressive proximal muscle weakness and long finger flexion contractures occurring in three Dutch pedigrees [18]. In 1978, the same group reported another family of Polish decent [19] and subsequently it has been reported worldwide (for review see [20]) with Mohire *et al.* proposing the name Bethlem myopathy when they described a French-Canadian family in 1988 [21]. In 1996 linkage studies in large BM families found significant linkage with loci on chromosome 21q22.3 [22] and 2q37 [23], identifying the collagen VI genes as candidate genes, and later

Disorders of Voluntary Muscle, 8th edn., eds. George Karpati, David Hilton-Jones, Kate Bushby and Robert C. Griggs. Published by Cambridge University Press.

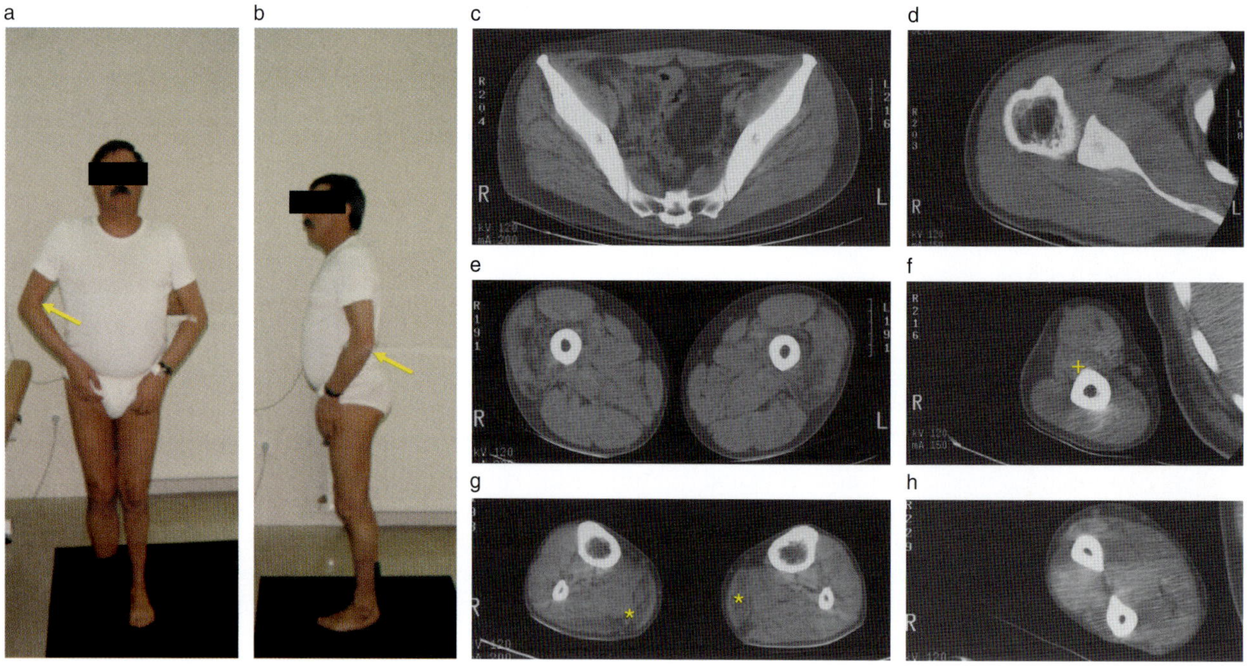

Figure 14.1a–h. Typical clinical features of EDMD (see text). (c–h). A lower and upper limbs muscle CT scan. Note the elbow contractures (a, b, arrows) and the predominantly affected medial head of the gastrocnemius and biceps brachialis muscles (*, +). Images kindly provided by Professors Bruno Eymard and Michel Fardeau (Reference center for neuromuscular disorders, Myology Institute, Paris, France).

in the same year mutations in these genes were found in three BM families [24]. However, it took until 2001 for the first autosomal recessively acting collagen VI gene mutations to be discovered in patients with the typical UCMD phenotype in whom collagen VI protein had been found to be almost completely absent on immunohistochemical analysis of their muscle biopsies [25, 26, 27]. Although originally believed to be entirely separate entities, it is now becoming clear that BM and UCMD probably represent two extremes of a clinical continuum in which individuals presenting with intermediate phenotypes could be considered to have either "mild UCMD" or "severe BM."

Emery–Dreifuss muscular dystrophy

Emery–Dreifuss muscular dystrophy is clinically characterized by the triad of: (1) early joint contractures involving elbows, Achilles tendons, and neck extensors resulting in limitation of neck flexion, followed by limitation of flexion of the entire spine, (2) slowly progressive wasting and weakness initially in a humeroperoneal distribution that later extends to the scapular and pelvic girdle muscles, and (3) by adult age, the development of a cardiac disease associated with conduction defects, arrhythmias, and dilated cardiomyopathy, which is the most serious and life-threatening clinical manifestation of the disease [28].

Emery–Dreifuss muscular dystrophy can be inherited in an X-linked recessive (XL-EDMD or EDMD1, MIM 310300), autosomal dominant (AD-EDMD or EDMD2, MIM 181350) or autosomal recessive (AR-EDMD or EDMD3, MIM 604929, the latter being extremely rare) way and is due to mutations in at least two genes, *EMD* encoding emerin (MIM 300384) for XL-EDMD [6], and *LMNA* encoding A-type lamins (MIM 150330) for the autosomal forms [9, 10].

Molecular genetics and pathogenesis

The *EMD* gene, localized to chromosome Xq28, is approximately 2 kb in size and is composed of six exons [6] (Figure 14.3). It encodes emerin, a 254-amino acid protein that is serine-rich and ubiquitously expressed, which belongs to the type II integral membrane protein family. Its hydrophobic tail anchors the protein to the inner nuclear membrane and the hydrophilic remainder of the molecule projects into the nucleoplasm, where it interacts with the nuclear lamina [7, 8] (Figure 14.4b). Emerin shares a homologous N-terminal domain with other nuclear envelope proteins, LAP2 family members and MAN1, which is termed LEM domain (for LAP2, Emerin, and MAN1) and confers the ability to bind to BAF, a DNA bridging protein involved in higher-order chromatin function and nuclear membrane assembly [29]. Emerin appears to have an inexhaustible list of binding partners, which currently include transcriptional repressors (GCL, Btf), RNA-splicing associated factors (YT521-B), the inner nuclear membrane isoforms of nesprins 1 and 2, nuclear actin, and lamins A, B, and C (Figure 14.4b). Characterization of the binding domain with these multiple partners strongly suggests that emerin may exist in several different multi-component protein complexes (for review see [29]).

The *LMNA* gene is localized to chromosome 1q21.2–q21.3 and composed of 12 exons that encode four A-type lamins

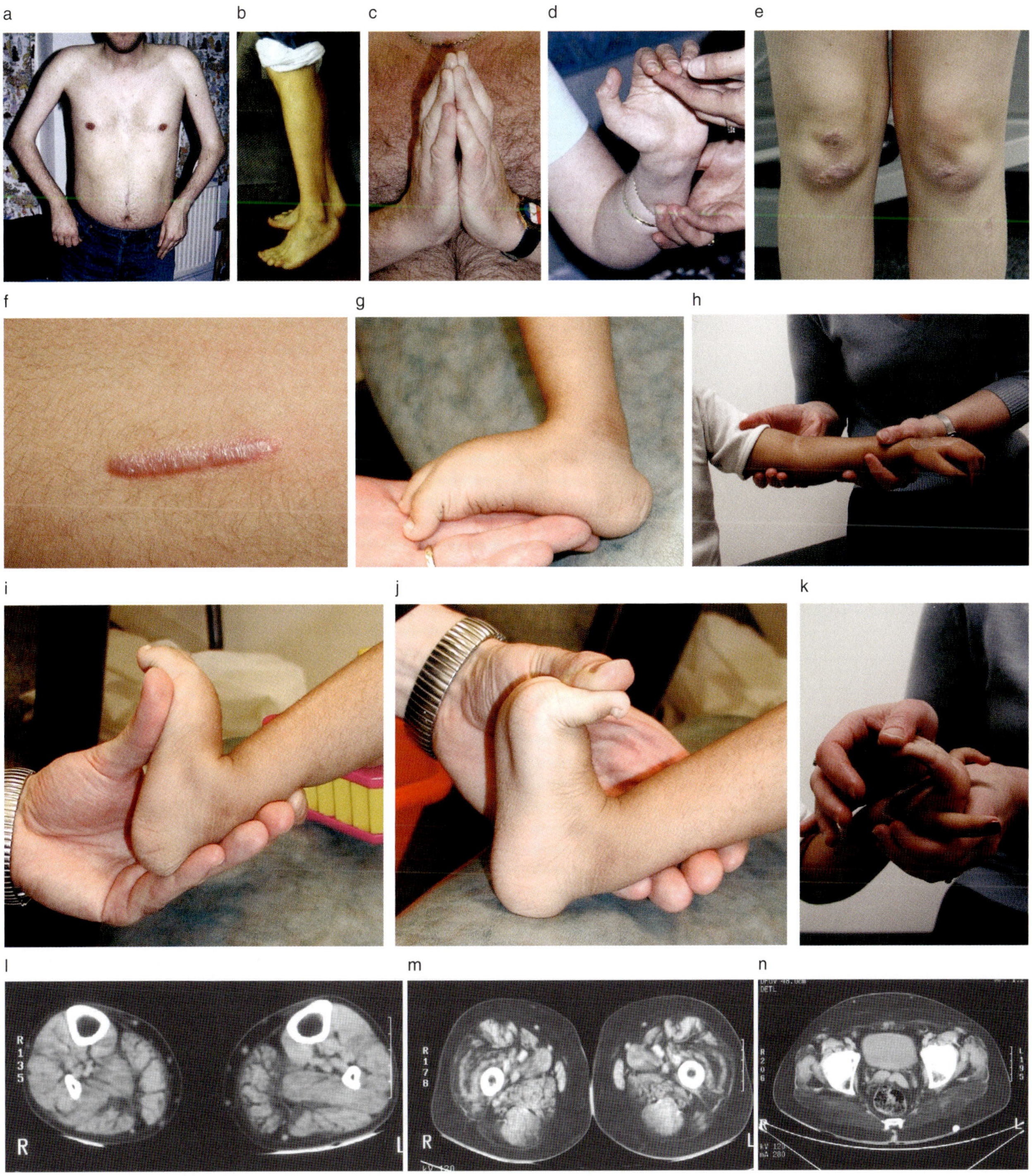

Figure 14.2a–n. Typical clinical features of Bethlem myopathy (a–e) and Ullrich congenital muscular dystrophy (f–k) (see text). CT scan of lower limbs of patient with Bethlem myopathy (l–n) shows a characteristic pattern of involvement of the peripheral region of the vasti muscles but relative sparing of their central parts and a central area of abnormal signal within the rectus femoris muscle (m). There is also relative sparing of sartorius, gracilis and adductor longus. Adapted from [20] *J. Med. Genet.* 2005; **42**(9): 673–85, reproduced with permission from the BMJ Publishing Group. CT scan images kindly provided by Dr. Tania Stojkovic (Reference center for neuromuscular disorders, Myology Institute, Paris, France).

(A, AΔ10, C, and C2) by alternative splicing. Lamin A and lamin C are the two main isoforms. They are identical for their 566 amino acids but are distinct at first their C-terminal domains (Figure 14.3). Lamin C has six unique C-terminal amino acids. Lamin A is synthesized as a precursor, prelamin A, which has 98 unique C-terminal amino acids. Prelamin A is farnesylated on the cysteine of a C-terminal CAAX box and then is endo-proteolytically processed by Zmpste24 protease to yield mature

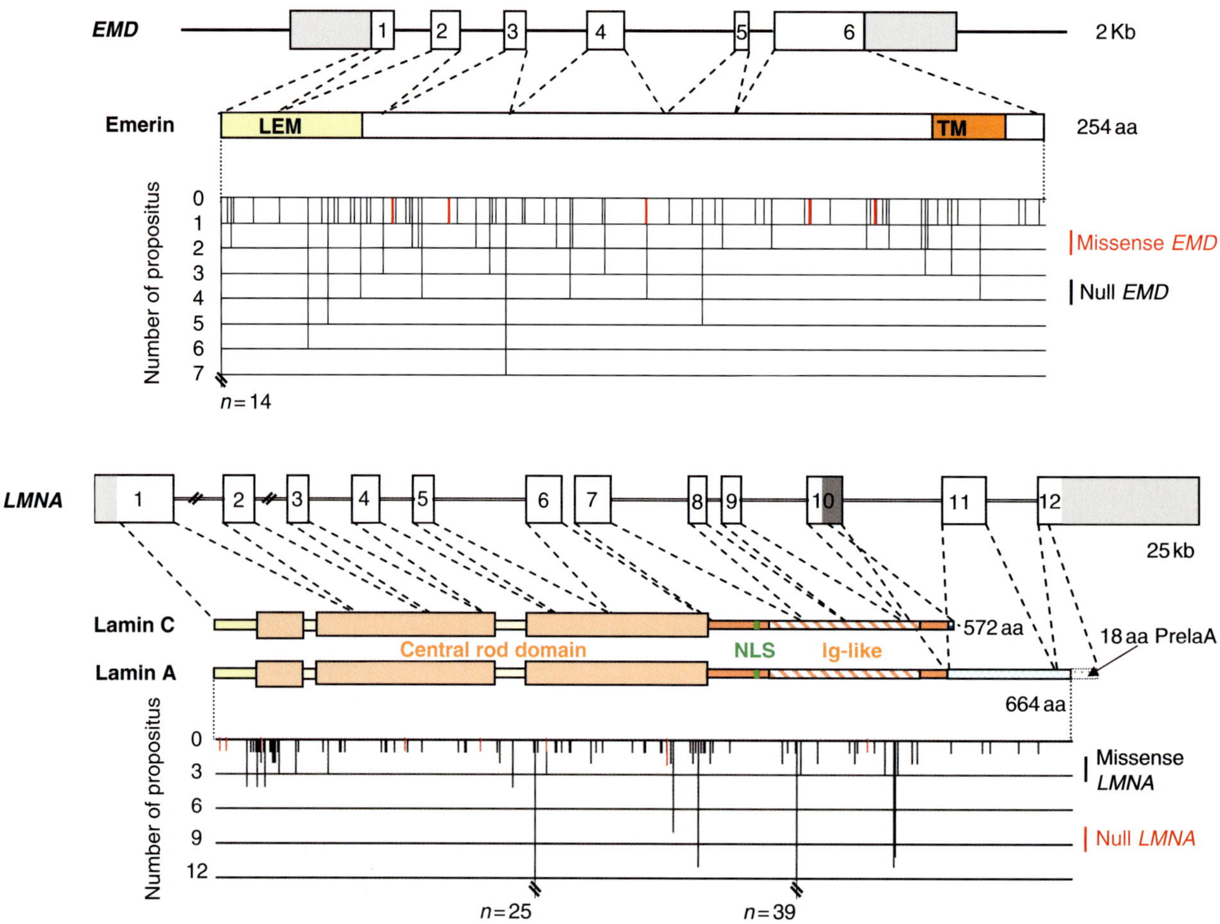

Figure 14.3. Schematic representation of emerin and lamins A/C gene structure and relative position of EDMD mutations. The six exons of *EMD* and the 12 exons of *LMNA* genes are represented by numbered boxes, with the gray boxes representing the untranslated regions of the genes. The main protein domains of emerin and lamins A and C are presented on each protein scheme: for emerin, the LEM domain and the transmembrane domain (TM), for lamins A/C, the central rod domain, the nuclear localization signal (NLS) and the Ig-like domain of the C-terminal tail [5]. The specific tails of lamin A and lamin C are represented by dash boxes and the 18 amino acids of prelamin A that are cleaved to produce mature lamin A are represented by a dot box. For each gene, mutations reported so far in familial or isolated EDMD patients are represented below the gene–protein schemes. Each bar represents a mutated position with the height of the bar corresponding to the number of propositus carrying the same mutation. For *EMD*, the less frequent type of mutation, i.e., missense mutations, is represented by a red bar and null mutations by a black bar (for details of the mutations see UMD-EMD mutation database at www.umd.be:2010). For *LMNA*, the less frequent null mutations are in red with the *LMNA* missense mutation being represented by black bars (for details of the mutations see UMD-*LMNA* mutation database at www.umd.be:2000).

lamin A, which lacks the last 18 amino acids [5]. Lamins A/C are widely expressed in most differentiated somatic cells but are absent in early embryos and some undifferentiated cells. A-type lamins together with B-type lamins (encoded by two other genes *LMNB1* and *LMNB2*) are type-V intermediate filaments that form the nuclear lamina, a fibrous network underlying the inner face of the internal nuclear membrane (Figure 14.4b). Lamins A/C interact also with multiple partners including emerin, MAN1, Rb, nesprins, histones (for review see [30, 31]). Although the precise functions of the lamins and the nuclear lamina remain to be established, they have been implicated in a wide range of processes, from providing structural support to the nucleus to regulating transcription and DNA replication. Data also suggest that lamins A/C are part of multi-component protein complexes involved in connections between the nucleus and cytoplasm, playing a crucial role in organizing the cytoskeleton [32].

Elucidation of the pathophysiology of EDMD still requires deciphering of the roles of lamins A/C, emerin, and their partners in the functional organization of the nuclear envelope. In most cases, *EMD* mutations are null (Figure 14.3) and lead to premature arrest of translation with no protein product. In the rare cases in which the protein is expressed, either the gene product is lacking the transmembrane domain (in-frame distal deletions) and is not able to target the nuclear membrane and thus is delocalized in the nucleoplasm or cytoplasm, or the mutated protein is present at the nuclear rim (missense mutations) but has weakened interactions with the lamina components [33]. Missense *LMNA* mutations (which form the majority of all *LMNA* mutations, Figure 14.3) lead to mutant protein of normal size carrying one modified amino acid. Western blot analysis of fibroblasts of affected individuals demonstrates a normal level of protein expression, strongly suggesting that mutant lamins A/C are expressed [34].

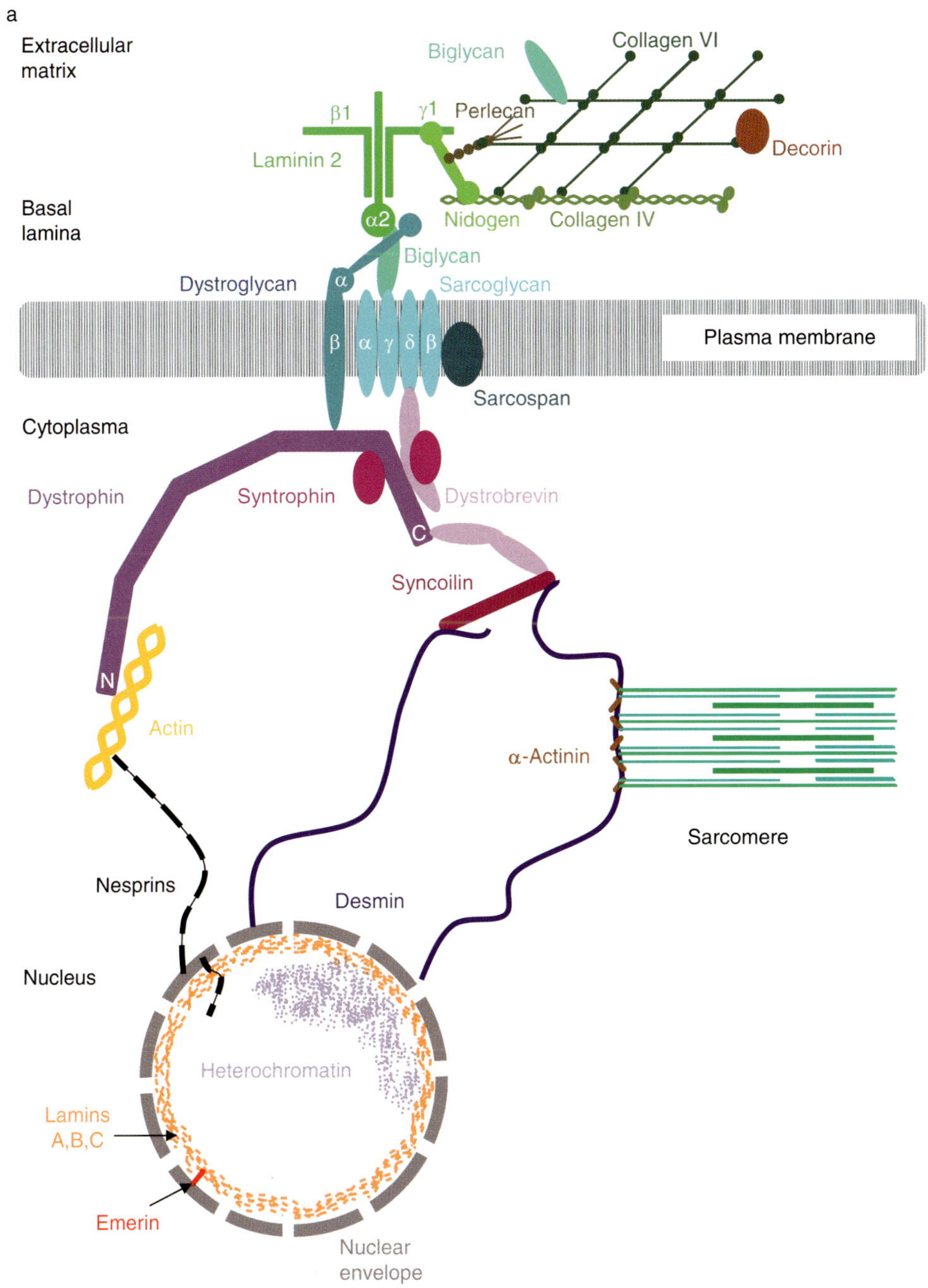

Figure 14.4a–c. (a) Possible link between the nuclear envelope and the extracellular matrix in striated muscle cells. (b) Schematic representation of the nuclear envelope, highlighting the multiple interactions of both emerin and lamins A and C (see text and [29, 30] for details on these interactions). (c) Schematic model of collagen VI assembly; see text, modified from [20] *J. Med. Genet.* 2005; **42**(9): 673–685; reproduced with permission from the BMJ Publishing Group.

Nonsense *LMNA* mutations also exist and lead to haploinsufficiency with expression of only the normal allele (50% of normal amount); the mutant allele is either not translated (because of degradation of abnormal mRNA) or is translated and degraded [35]. Analysis of cells or tissues from EDMD patients demonstrates abnormally shaped nuclei with increased fragility of their nuclear envelope [34, 36] as well as chromatin alterations [37].

Currently, experimental evidence supports two molecular mechanisms, not necessarily mutually exclusive, to explain the EDMD pathogenesis: (1) structural mechanisms caused by mechanical stress present in skeletal and cardiac striated muscles and (2) modification of gene expression secondary to abnormal chromatin organization associated with alteration of proliferation and/or differentiation of muscle cells [5, 35]. The abnormal shaped nuclei in both XL- and AD-EDMD

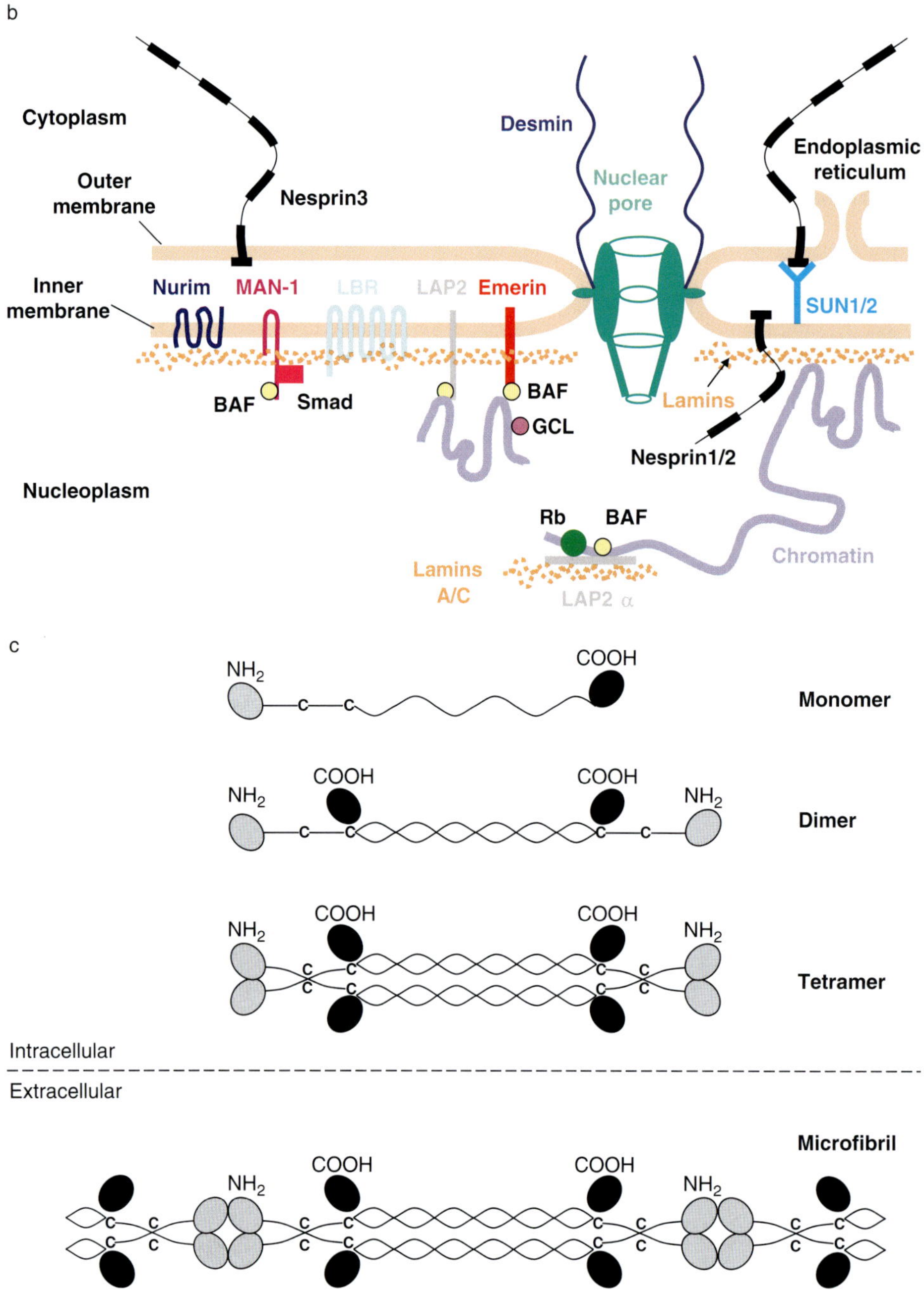

Figure 14.4a–c. *(cont.)*

patients suggests they are sensitive to mechanical stress [34, 36]. In the same line, embryonic fibroblasts from *Lmna*$^{-/-}$ and *Emd*$^{y/-}$ mice exhibit impaired nuclear mechanotransduction in response to strain [38, 39]. The gene expression hypothesis proposes that mutations lead to modified interactions within the emerin–lamin A/C multi-protein complexes, disrupting interactions at specific chromatin sites and/or with transcriptional regulators specific for the striated muscles, thus leading to downstream effects on chromatin organization and/or gene expression in muscles. Such changes in downstream gene expression have been reported in fibroblasts and myoblasts from both EDMD patients and mouse models of EDMD (for review see [33, 40]). Transcriptome analysis performed on regenerating muscle from *Emd*$^{y/-}$ mice and on muscle biopsies from EDMD patients revealed a perturbed cell cycle and delayed myogenic differentiation together with upregulation of retinoblastoma (Rb) and MyoD genes [41, 42]. These data highlight the role of nuclear structural proteins, i.e., emerin and lamins A/C, in the pathways involved in the cell cycle exit towards muscle differentiation. Another microarray analysis demonstrated the activation of mitogen-activated protein kinase signaling pathways in the hearts from both *Lmna*$^{H222P/H222P}$ and *Emd*$^{-/y}$ mice [43, 44]. This molecular pathway has been previously implicated in the development of heart failure and conduction defects and could, therefore, explain the cardiomyopathy in these animal models. Although these two main hypotheses, mechanical stress and gene expression alterations, form attractive models for how *EMD* and *LMNA* mutations may cause EDMD, more supporting data are necessary.

Salient clinical phenotypical features

AD-EDMD and XL-EDMD have similar, but not identical, neuromuscular and cardiac involvement (Figure 14.1). Joint contractures begin in early childhood in both XL- and AD-EDMD. However, in XL-EDMD, joint contractures are usually the first sign, whereas in AD-EDMD joint contractures may appear after the onset of muscle weakness. Joint contractures predominate in the elbows, ankles, and posterior cervical muscles followed by limitation in movement of the entire spine. The degree and the progression of contractures are variable and not always age related [45, 46]. Severe contractures may lead to loss of ambulation by limitation of joint movements, especially in spine and lower limbs. Slowly progressive muscle weakness and wasting are initially in a humeroperoneal distribution and always extend to the scapular and pelvic girdle muscles in the later stages. The progression of muscle wasting is usually slow in the first three decades of life, after which it becomes more rapid. Loss of ambulation can occur in AD-EDMD, but is rare in XL-EDMD [45].

Palpitations, presyncope and syncope, poor exercise tolerance or dyspnea may reveal cardiac involvement. A variable combination of supraventricular arrhythmias, disorders of atrioventricular conduction, ventricular arrhythmias, and dilated cardiomyopathy with a high risk of sudden death despite pacemaker implantation characterize EDMD-associated cardiac disease [47, 48]. Conduction defects include sinus bradycardia, and variable degrees of atrioventricular or bundle-branch blocks. Atrial arrhythmias (extrasystoles, atrial fibrillation or flutter, and atrial standstill) and ventricular arrhythmias (extrasystoles, ventricular tachycardia) are frequent [49]. In AD-EDMD, the risk of ventricular tachyarrhythmia and dilated cardiomyopathy appears to be higher than in XL-EDMD [50] and is associated with a higher risk of cerebral emboli and cardiac sudden death [48, 49]. Dilated cardiomyopathy often occurs in the later stages of the disease manifesting in symptoms of congestive heart failure [28].

Age of onset, severity, and progression of muscle and cardiac involvement demonstrate both inter- and intrafamilial variability [50, 51]. Clinical variability ranges from early and severe presentation in childhood to late onset and a slowly progressive course. In general, joint contractures appear during the first two decades, followed by muscle weakness and wasting. Cardiac involvement usually arises after the second decade of life with no obvious connection between neuromuscular impairment and cardiac involvement [49]. Respiratory function can be impaired in some individuals [28, 50]. Sudden cardiac death can be the first manifestation of the disorder especially in AD-EDMD [48].

Only one individual with genetically proven AR-EDMD (i.e., carrying a homozygous *LMNA* mutation) has been reported [10]. He had severe muscular dystrophy being wheelchair bound at 40 years of age. However, cardiac evaluation revealed no abnormalities [10].

Genotype–phenotype correlations

To date 86 different *EMD* mutations have been identified in 218 subjects from XL-EDMD families [male patients and female carriers reported in the literature and/or identified in the EDMD consortium (G. B., unpublished data), for details see UMD-*EMD* database at www.umd.be:2010, Figure 14.3]. The majority of mutations (95%) are null mutations: nonsense mutations, deletions/insertions, and splice site mutations that lead to exon skipping, frameshift, and premature arrest of translation, and, thus, to absence of emerin. However, intra- and interfamilial variability in the severity of the phenotype associated with null mutations can be observed [46]. A few missense mutations and in-frame deletions also exist, leading to decreased expression of emerin or to normal expression of a nonfunctional protein and resulting in a milder phenotype [33, 52]. No "hotspot" mutation is observed in the *EMD* gene; mutations are spread out along the gene virtually randomly.

More than 135 *LMNA* mutations have been identified to date in 335 EDMD patients [reported in the literature and/or identified in the EDMD consortium (G. B., unpublished data); for details see UMD-*LMNA* database at www.umd.be:2000; Figure 14.3]. The majority of mutations (81%) are missense mutations. Nonsense mutations, small deletions/insertions in-frame or with frameshift, and splice-site mutations also exist. Mutations are spread all along the gene. A few recurrent mutations exist [5] (Figure 14.3). It is important to note that besides its implication in EDMD, *LMNA* was also found mutated in more than ten other disorders, now called laminopathies [35]. Laminopathies can be broadly split into two groups: (1) neuromuscular disorders affecting specifically the striated muscles [EDMD, dilated cardiomyopathy with conduction system disease (DCM-CD), limb-girdle muscular dystrophy type 1B (LGMD1B)] or the peripheral nervous system (axonal type of Charcot–Marie–Tooth disease, CMT2) and (2) partial lipodystrophy syndrome with or without developmental abnormalities and premature aging (mandibuloacral dysplasia, Hutchison–Gilford progeria syndrome). *LMNA* mutations leading to EDMD represent around 46% of all identified *LMNA* mutations so far and EDMD patients represent up to 25% of all individuals carrying a *LMNA* mutation (UMD-*LMNA* database at www.umd.be:2000).

EDMD-related-*LMNA* mutations do not show a clear correlation between genotype and phenotype [5, 50]. Incomplete penetrance in families with AD-EDMD has been reported [53]. Marked intra- and interfamilial variability is observed for the same *LMNA* mutation [45, 51]. For example, within the same family the same *LMNA* mutation can lead to AD-EDMD,

LGMD1B, or isolated DCM-CD, i.e., various laminopathies involving striated muscle [5]. Rarely EDMD patients may present symptoms of lipodystrophy highlighting a possible overlap between the various types of laminopathies [54]. Severe EDMD has been reported in individuals with mutations in both *EMD* and *LMNA* [55]. A range of clinical presentations (i.e., CMT2, CMT2-EDMD, and isolated cardiopathy) were found in a large family in which mutations in both *EMD* and *LMNA* genes co-segregate [52] suggesting that digenism may partially explain the large clinical variability observed in some EDMD families. However, as for other genetic disease, modifier genes as well as environmental factors may also contribute to the complexity of EDMD.

Diagnostic approaches

The diagnosis of EDMD is not possible without molecular testing, as other findings are nonspecific. Creatine kinase levels are normal or moderately elevated (2–20 times the upper limit of normal); the highest values being usually observed at the beginning of the disease [45]. Electromyography usually shows myopathic features with normal nerve conduction studies, but neuropathic patterns have been described [56]. Muscle biopsy may show nonspecific myopathic or dystrophic changes, including variation in fiber size, increased internal nuclei, increased endomysial connective tissue, and necrotic fibers while electron microscopy may reveal specific alterations of the nuclear architecture [37]. Muscle imaging, rarely reported, shows a diffuse pattern of muscle involvement on CT scan affecting biceps, soleus, peroneal, external vasti, gluteus, and paravertebral muscles [57] (Figure 14.1). Characteristic findings in the calf muscles on MRI have been reported in AD-EDMD [58].

The diagnosis of XL-EDMD is based on immunodetection of emerin and molecular genetic testing of the *EMD* gene [59]. As emerin is ubiquitously expressed, it can be detected by immunofluorescence (IF) and/or by Western blot (WB) in various tissues: exfoliative buccal cells (IF), lymphocytes (WB), a lymphoblastoid cell line (WB), skin biopsy (IF, WB), or muscle biopsy (IF, WB) [59]. Emerin is absent in 95% (null allele) of the XL-EDMD patients and is absent in varying proportions of nuclei in XL-EDMD female carriers. WB is not reliable for carrier detection as it may show an either normal or reduced amount of emerin depending on the degree of X-inactivation [60]. The diagnosis of AD- and AR-EDMD is based on clinical findings, family history, and molecular genetic testing of *LMNA*. In individuals with AD-EDMD, emerin is normally expressed. The immunodetection of lamins A/C is not reliable for confirmation of the diagnosis of AD-EDMD as lamins A/C are always present, usually in normal amounts, in the nuclei of AD-EDMD individuals [34].

The differential diagnosis of EDMD includes several neuromuscular disorders that may result in a similar pattern of muscle involvement, joint contractures, or cardiac disease, but none is associated with the triad observed in EDMD [46]. Several myopathies with or without contractures and/or cardiac disease can resemble EDMD but have distinguishing features: congenital muscular dystrophies including those with partial merosin deficiency, rigid spine syndrome (especially SEPN1 and FKRP-related), some forms of LGMD2A with prominent contractures (calpain related), myotonic dystrophy type 1, dystrophinopathies, desmin-related myopathies, X-linked vacuolar myopathy with cardiomyopathy or Danon disease and myotonic dystrophy type 2 (PROMM) [46]. Although muscle MRI may help to differentiate between both conditions [58, 61] (Figures 14.1, 14.2) the collagen-VI-related disorders remain the closest and most difficult differential diagnosis, as clinical features in young or even adult EDMD patients still lacking cardiac involvement might be similar to those in UCMD/BM patients. It is thus important to perform an immunoanalysis for emerin and molecular analysis of the LMNA gene in any patient in whom a collagen-VI-related disorder is considered.

Therapeutic and preventative modalities

Evaluations following initial diagnosis of EDMD should include ECG, Holter-ECG monitoring, and echocardiography, especially in those patients showing overt cardiac involvement. An invasive electrophysiological cardiac study is often advisable; however, it is performed in selected individuals only on the basis of the clinical presentation and the results of noninvasive studies. Evaluation of respiratory function (vital capacity and other pulmonary volume measurements) and evaluation of metabolic functions (blood glucose, insulin, triglyceride, and cholesterol levels) are also recommended in order to detect any overlapping features [50]. The treatment of manifestations includes orthopedic surgery to release Achilles tendons and other contractures or scoliosis and the provision of mechanical aids (canes, walkers, orthoses, wheelchairs) to help ambulation. Specific treatments for cardiac manifestations (arrhythmias, AV conduction disorders, and congestive heart failure) includes antiarrhythmic drugs, cardiac pacemaker, implantable cardioverter defibrillator (ICD), and both pharmacological and nonpharmacological therapy for heart failure [49, 50, 62]. Heart transplantation may be necessary in the end stages of heart failure. Respiratory treatment interventions (respiratory muscle physiotherapy and mechanical ventilation) may also be required. Physiotherapy and stretching exercises can also promote mobility and help to prevent contractures. In AD-EDMD, it has been demonstrated that ICD implantation can reduce the risk of sudden death considerably [62]. Antithromboembolic drugs (vitamin K antagonists, warfarin, heparin) are probably required to prevent cerebral thromboembolism of cardiac origin in those individuals with either decreased left ventricular function or atrial arrhythmias [49].

Genetic counseling

For XL-EDMD, female carriers are usually asymptomatic, but they are at risk of developing cardiac disease, progressive muscular dystrophy, and/or a complete EDMD phenotype.

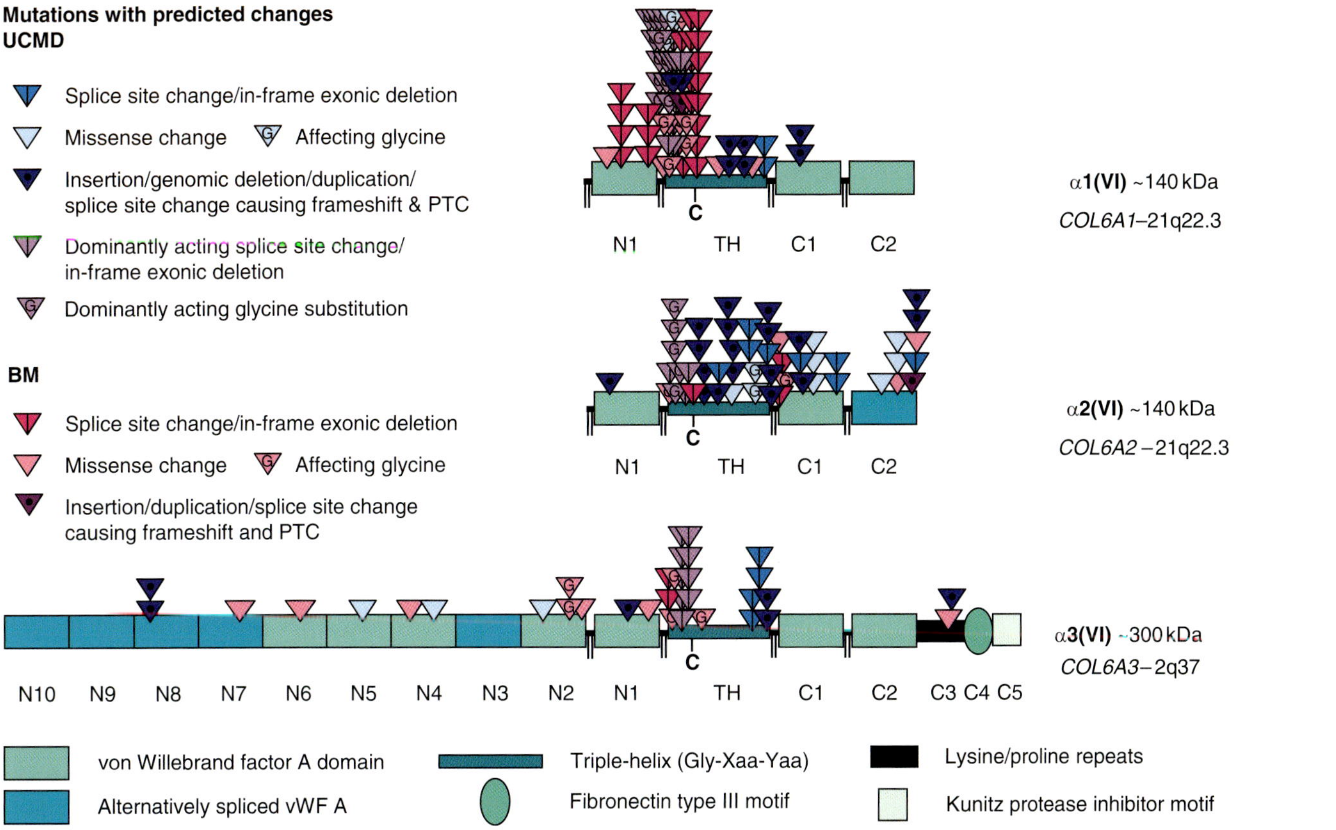

Figure 14.5. Genomic organization of collagen VI and localization of genomic changes reported for BM and UCMD to date (see text; modified from [20] *J. Med. Genet.* 2005; **42**(9): 673–85; reproduced with permission from the BMJ Publishing Group). The triple helical domains contain a single cysteine residue (depicted as "C") which is important for dimer assembly. The localization of the mutations reported for BM and UCMD to date is shown stratified by clinical phenotype and type of mutation with different shades of blue triangles depicting various types of recessively acting mutations described for UCMD patients; purple triangles indicating de novo dominantly acting mutations reported for UCMD patients; and different shades of pink triangles depicting dominantly acting mutations found in BM patients. For details of the mutations see [77].

Thus, cardiac evaluation is recommended in female carriers of XL-EDMD [50]. Similarly, in AD-EDMD families, a cardiac evaluation for first-degree relatives is highly recommended given that a high risk of cardiac complications, including sudden death, is observed in *LMNA* mutation carriers [49, 62].

Prenatal testing is possible if the causative *EMD* or *LMNA* mutation has been identified in an affected family member but the complexity of the genetics underlying EDMD has to be borne in mind, including de novo mutations (i.e., 76% of AD-EDMD probands have a de novo *LMNA* mutation [45]), germline mosaicism reported for both *EDM* [60] and *LMNA* [9], and possible digenism [52, 55].

Collagen-VI-related disorders

The collagen-VI-related muscle disorders include Bethlem myopathy (BM; MIM 158810) and Ullrich congenital muscular dystrophy (UCMD; MIM 254090).

Molecular genetics and pathogenesis

Mutations in *COL6A1*, *COL6A2* (both situated head to tail on chromosome 21q22.3), and *COL6A3* (located on chromosome 2q37) encoding the three peptide chains α1(VI), α2(VI) and α3(VI) have been demonstrated in both of these conditions [20]. All three chains contain a central short triple helical domain of 335–336 amino acids with repeating Gly-Xaa-Yaa sequences flanked by large N- and C-terminal globular domains made up of motifs of 200 amino acids each that are homologous to von Willebrand factor (vWF) type A domains (Figure 14.5). *COL6A2* and *COL6A3* undergo extensive alternative splicing.

The assembly of collagen VI is a complex multistep process. Intracellular equimolar association of α1(VI), α2(VI), and α3(VI) to form a triple helical monomer is followed by staggered assembly into disulfide-bonded antiparallel dimers, which then align to form tetramers, also stabilized by disulfide bonds (Figure 14.4c). Folding of the collagen VI triple helix from the C- to the N-terminus is nucleated by C-terminal Gly-Xaa-Yaa triplets, and single cysteine residues located in the triple-helical domain of each of the three chains are thought to be responsible for the formation and stability of dimers and tetramers [63, 64]. Outside the cell, the tetrameric secreted form of collagen VI associates end-to-end through overlapping N-terminal globular domains to form beaded microfibrils [65].

Collagen VI is a ubiquitous extracellular matrix protein which forms a highly branched interstitial and pericellular microfibrillar network in most tissues but is also found in close association with the basement membrane around muscle cells [66, 67]. By interacting with several other extracellular matrix constituents it is believed to anchor the basement membrane to the underlying connective tissue and to act as a scaffold for the formation of fibrillar collagen networks. Other roles attributed to collagen VI include cell cycle signaling and maintenance of tissue homeostasis, mediating interactions of cells with the extracellular matrix, and it is implicated in the development of the matrix supramolecular structure. In this way the collagen VI network may have an important role in repair processes such as wound healing as well as tissue development and architecture. As yet it remains unclear whether a reduction of the amount of collagen VI per se in the extracellular matrix can cause the clinical features of collagen-VI-related disorders or whether these might be attributable to the inability of structurally abnormal collagen VI microfibrils to form an extracellular network, to interact effectively with other extracellular matrix components, to form a connection with the sarcolemma or to interact with cells to prevent apoptosis.

Salient clinical phenotypical features

Bethlem myopathy is a relatively mild dominantly inherited disorder characterized by the combination of proximal muscle weakness and variable contractures, affecting most frequently the long finger flexors, elbows, and ankles [68]. BM patients typically become symptomatic within the first or second decade with moderate predominantly proximal muscle weakness and atrophy involving the extensors more than the flexors. Although BM is classically described as a mild disorder with its major impact in adult life it is often possible in retrospect to elicit a history of neonatal hypotonia or torticollis, delayed motor milestones or even decreased fetal movements [68]. Contractures may be of a strikingly dynamic nature during childhood, appearing and disappearing in various joints, but nearly all patients eventually develop flexion contractures of the fingers, wrists, elbows and ankles (Figure 14.2a–d) and these, in addition to weakness, contribute to disability. Strikingly, hypermobility of distal interphalangeal joints can be present together with long finger flexion contractures. The clinical course is usually slowly progressive and more than two-thirds of patients over 50 years of age will require aids to mobilize outdoors. Cardiac involvement is usually absent but respiratory muscle and especially diaphragmatic involvement necessitating nocturnal respiratory support is reported in association with severe weakness in later life [69].

Ullrich congenital muscular dystrophy is a clinically and genetically distinct entity within the congenital muscular dystrophies [20, 70, 71]. It was classically described as an exclusively autosomal recessive condition but recently cases with dominant mutations have been reported [72, 73]. The hallmarks of UCMD consist of severe muscle weakness of early onset with proximal joint contractures (Figure 14.2h) and striking hyperelasticity of distal small joints (Figure 14.2i–k). Posteriorly protruding calcanei are also common (Figure 14.2g) and at birth hip dislocations and a transient kyphosis can be present. Children typically either never achieve the ability to walk independently, or walk independently for only a short time. Spinal rigidity and scoliosis and variable proximal contractures usually develop with progression of the disease, as well as marked long finger flexion contractures and tight Achilles tendons [74]. Respiratory failure in the first or second decade frequently requires nocturnal respiratory support, but to date cardiac involvement has not been documented.

Distinctive skin features such as follicular hyperkeratosis and the tendency to keloid or cigarette paper scar formation may also be present in both UCMD as well as BM patients [75, 76] (Figure 14.2e, f).

Over the past decade it has become obvious that a clear clinical differentiation between UCMD and BM may be very difficult, especially in neonates and young children. BM can occur de novo and may present at birth. In addition, the patterns of joint hypermobility and contractures and the level of mobility found in some patients cannot be neatly categorized as either BM or UCMD. BM and UCMD are probably better regarded as representing opposite endpoints of a clinical continuum of collagen-VI-related disorders [20].

Genotype–phenotype correlations

The number of reported genetic changes for BM and UCMD is now well in excess of 100 [77] (Figure 14.5). Specific mutations mostly appear to be associated with either a clear BM or UCMD phenotype. However, the correlation of genotype and phenotype is complicated by the emergence of patients with an intermediate phenotype where some groups might describe a patient as "mild UCMD" who might be classified as suffering from "severe BM" by other groups.

With regards to BM, heterozygous single amino acid substitutions disrupting the Gly-Xaa-Yaa motif towards the N-terminus of the triple helix are a common mutation mechanism. Other missense mutations have been reported for a number of BM kindreds; however, additional confirmatory data are only available for very few of these [78]. Given the highly polymorphic nature of the collagen VI genes, pathogenicity of a novel missense change other than a glycine substitution within the triple helical domain has to be ascribed with care. Heterozygously occurring splice site mutations or large genomic deletions causing in-frame deletions have also been described for many kindreds and thus form another very frequent group of mutations in BM. It is currently not completely clear how much of the effect of this type of mutation is due to faulty higher order assembly and how much to haploinsufficiency.

Ullrich congenital muscular dystrophy was initially regarded as an exclusively autosomal recessive condition. The majority of the recessively acting mutations appear to result in premature termination codons. These patients are unable to assemble or secrete collagen VI tetramers, as all three chains are necessary to form functional monomers. Some recessively acting missense mutations have also been described but their effect on collagen biosynthesis and assembly has mostly not been studied in detail. In recent years heterozygously occurring in-frame deletions have been found to cause a dominant negative effect and result in a classical UCMD phenotype. These in-frame deletions are located within the N-terminal triple helical domain of any of the three collagen VI chains where they universally preserve a unique cysteine important for dimer or tetramer formation, allowing the mutant chains to be further incorporated into dimers and tetramers so that predominantly abnormal molecules are secreted which then exert a strong dominant negative effect on microfibrillar assembly and extracellular collagen VI matrix formation [72]. In addition, a number of recessively acting in-frame deletions within the C-terminal part of the triple helical domain have also been described for UCMD patients. These deletions appear to interfere with the initial C-terminal triple helical nucleation process that initiates formation of the basic hetero-trimeric monomer, thereby excluding the chains from the very first steps of assembly. Recessively acting missense mutations in the C-terminal triple helical domain in other UCMD patients presumably interfere with monomer formation in a similar way [63].

In this context it is interesting to note that virtually no BM mutations have been documented in the C-terminal part of the triple helix. Some of the UCMD patients with heterozygous N-terminal triple helical glycine substitutions are perhaps better characterized as affected by a "severe BM" clinical phenotype as their clinical descriptions do not allow for a convincing assignment as "classical" UCMD. Similarly, the clinical phenotype of some of the BM patients with heterozygous N-terminal triple helical glycine substitutions can be comparatively severe, suggesting that this type of mutation can often produce an intermediate phenotype.

It remains intriguing that the heterozygous parents of UCMD patients, in particular parents who carry a single copy of a nonsense mutation, are clinically unaffected. A study showed that although mRNA levels in fibroblasts with a single *COL6A2* nonsense mutation can be initially reduced, long-term collagen VI extracellular matrix deposition is virtually normal [79]. If haploinsufficiency does not lead to myopathic symptoms in parents of UCMD patients, it is difficult to understand how it could cause a BM phenotype [80]. It is tempting to speculate whether phenotypic variation may arise from alternative splicing, modifying polymorphisms or the influence of other genes but, as yet, this conundrum remains unresolved.

Diagnostic approaches

The diagnosis of BM and UCMD depends on the typical clinical features, with electromyography showing a nonspecific myopathic pattern and the serum creatine kinase concentration usually being normal or only mildly elevated (usually less than 5 times the upper limit of normal). Muscle histopathological features range from mild myopathic to more dystrophic changes, with conventional collagen VI immunolabeling of the endomysium and basal lamina generally normal in BM (with the exception of a few cases showing patchy minor abnormalities) and ranging from absent to moderately or markedly reduced in UCMD.

Studies using double immunostaining for collagen VI and collagen IV or perlecan have described collagen VI to be present in the interstitium but absent from the sarcolemma [72, 81, 82] in patients with collagen-VI-related disorders and dominantly acting mutations. A space between muscle fibers and connective tissue with folding of the plasma membrane and thickening of the basal lamina has been observed on electron microscopy of collagen-VI-negative UCMD muscle biopsies, indicating a loose connection between basal lamina and other ECM collagens [83]. For patients with a less severe (BM) phenotype collagen VI immunolabeling studies on dermal fibroblast cultures can be more sensitive than conventional muscle immunohistochemistry and are thus a useful adjunct.

Detection of mutations in the three collagen VI genes remains the gold standard for diagnosis. Mutation detection rates reach approximately 60% for BM and 78% for UCMD [78, 81, 84]. Due to the large size of the genes involved, diagnostic mutation analysis remains difficult. Since a large proportion of mutations cause triple helical deletions, these regions can be checked by RT-PCR prior to embarking on screening of all 107 coding exons. In the past linkage analysis has also been used for UCMD families, but the recent description of de novo dominant mutations causing UCMD means this can no longer be regarded as a reliable method to exclude collagen-VI-related disease.

Muscle magnetic resonance imaging (MRI) may also be a useful aid to diagnosis. In BM patients muscle MRI shows a characteristic pattern of involvement of the peripheral region of the vasti muscles but relative sparing of their central parts and a central area of abnormal signal within the rectus femoris muscle [61]. The involvement of the thigh muscles of UCMD patients appears more diffuse with relative sparing of sartorius, gracilis, and adductor longus but also the distinct pattern of involvement of the peripheral rim of the vastus lateralis [61].

The differential diagnosis for collagen-VI-related disorders includes forms of congenital muscular dystrophy and limb-girdle muscular dystrophy, EDMD, congenital myopathies, rigid spine syndromes, spinal muscular atrophy, forms of Ehlers–Danlos syndrome or Marfan syndrome. The characteristic hyperlaxity of distal interphalangeal joints together with normal intelligence and the absence of structural abnormalities or white matter changes on brain MRI can help to distinguish UCMD clinically from other forms of congenital muscular dystrophy which in addition are usually associated with higher creatine kinase levels. Spinal muscular atrophy can usually be diagnosed by demonstrating mutations in the *SMN* gene and the muscle biopsy shows features of denervation rather than myopathic or dystrophic changes. Muscle immunohistochemistry and/or molecular genetic testing can help to establish alternative diagnoses such as sarcoglycanopathy, calpainopathy, and dysferlinopathy as well as XL- and AD-EDMD and some CMD subtypes. Forms of Ehlers–Danlos syndrome or Marfan syndrome are usually not associated with significant muscle weakness or an abnormal muscle biopsy but may be confused with collagen-VI-related disorders because of joint laxity and skin features such as abnormal scar formation [75]. Ehlers–Danlos syndrome, kyphoscoliotic form (also known as type VIa or Nevo syndrome), can be diagnosed by demonstration of an increased ratio of deoxypyridinoline to pyridinoline crosslinks in urine measured by high-performance liquid chromatography.

As discussed before, XL- and AD-EDMD remain the closest and most difficult differential diagnosis for collagen-VI-related disorders, as clinical features in young or even adult EDMD patients still lacking cardiac involvement might be similar to those of UCMD/BM patients. It is thus important to perform an immunoanalysis for emerin and molecular analysis of the LMNA gene in any patient in whom a collagen-VI-related disorder is considered.

Therapeutic and preventative modalities

Treatment for patients with collagen-VI-related disorders is supportive, aiming to promote mobility and independence, and to treat complications such as scoliosis and respiratory failure. Regular stretching and splinting are used to keep contractures at bay and maintain mobility. Early mobilization of severely affected children with a UCMD phenotype in a standing frame is important to achieve upright posture and protect against the development of contractures. Their contractures tend to be aggressive and may require surgical release in order to maintain or achieve a certain level of mobility. In view of the dynamic nature of contractures in early childhood in milder BM patients [68] it appears advisable to delay surgical orthopedic management until established contractures emerge. Achilles tenotomy for established contractures occurring later on in childhood or adult life can perpetuate ambulation in these patients. However, because of the recurrence of contractures following surgery repeat procedures are often necessary in order to maintain a certain level of mobility. A progressive kyphoscoliosis often develops in severe UCMD patients in the first or second decade of life and may require active management including spinal surgery to prevent progression.

Respiratory failure in the first or second decade of life is a common complication in patients with UCMD [71] and intermediate phenotypes but occurs less frequently in BM where it appears to be related to more severe weakness in later life [74]. Follow-up with regular assessments of respiratory function, including spirometry and overnight pulse oximetry studies, is important for all patients with collagen-VI-related disorders to detect asymptomatic decline [85]. Respiratory support with nocturnal ventilation usually becomes necessary in the first or second decade for UCMD patients and can be effective in reducing symptoms and promoting quality of life [85]. In BM, respiratory failure with diaphragmatic involvement may supervene before loss of ambulation [69] and symptoms of nocturnal hypoventilation respond well to noninvasive respiratory support. Prophylaxis of chest infections with influenza and pneumococcal vaccination and physiotherapy, as well as early and aggressive use of antibiotics, may prevent further respiratory problems in both BM and UCMD [85].

Genetic counseling

In fully characterized multi-generation BM families genetic counseling is usually straightforward with BM being inherited in an autosomal dominant manner. However, dominantly acting mutations causing BM or intermediate phenotypes can also occur de novo and although UCMD was classically described as an autosomal recessive disorder, over recent years autosomal dominant de novo mutations have emerged as a common mechanism for UCMD [72, 77]. In a de novo dominant family constellation the recurrence risk for the parents thus ranges from the 25% applicable to an autosomal recessive disease to a theoretical germline mosaicism risk. Delineation of a specific mutation which has previously been consistently recognized as being associated with either BM or UCMD may help to resolve some of these counseling issues. Prenatal diagnosis for UCMD has been previously undertaken using haplotype analysis and immunohistochemical analysis of a chorionic villus biopsy in a consanguineous family [86]. For families where the muscle biopsy of the proband shows absence of collagen VI immunolabeling, examination of a chorionic villus biopsy can offer a potential route for prenatal diagnosis even if the causative mutation in the family is not known. However, linkage or haplotype analysis in small nuclear families is no longer a reliable method to exclude collagen-VI-related disease as this analysis is not valid for de novo mutations.

Future perspectives

There remain many unanswered questions concerning the etiology of EDMD and collagen-VI-related muscle disorders. Amongst them, in only 40% of patients clinically diagnosed with EDMD was a mutation found in either their emerin or lamin A/C genes, suggesting that other components of the various emerin–lamin A/C protein complexes are candidate genes [50]. Indeed, very recently missense mutations in the nesprin 1 and 2 genes were reported in patients with an EDMD-like phenotype [87], opening new avenues and new links between the nuclear envelope and the cytoplasm compartment. Numerous other candidates exist as at least 90 inner nuclear membrane proteins were detected through a proteomic approach of the nuclear envelope [88]. With regards to collagen-VI-related disorders, mitochondrial dysfunction and consequent apoptosis has been implicated in the pathogenesis of the myopathic phenotype in collagen-VI-deficient mice [89]. The muscle ultrastructural defects of the *Col6a1*$^{-/-}$ mouse model appeared to be at least partially reversible by treatment with ciclosporin [89], an inhibitor of the mitochondrial permeability transition pore in vitro, which itself is known to be involved in the mitochondrial switch to apoptosis. Further studies on muscle biopsies and myoblast cultures of patients [90] have since shown that apoptotic features and mitochondrial dysfunction could be normalized by treatment with ciclosporin or the addition of a ciclosporin derivative which does not affect calcineurin activity and could thus be expected to have fewer side-effects [90]. These findings clearly have potential implications with regard to pharmacological treatment options for collagen-VI-related disorders.

Further deciphering of the pathophysiological mechanisms of emerin, lamin A/C, and collagen VI defects are needed in order to better define the nosologic frontiers of EDMD and collagen-VI-related disorders and increase our knowledge of the various differential diagnoses for a better management and therapeutic care of the patients.

References

1. R. Cestan, N. J. Le Jonne, Une myopathie avec rétractions familiales. *Nouvelle Iconogr. Salpétrière* **15** (1902), 38–52.
2. A. Hauptmann, S. J. Thannhauser, Muscular shortening and dystrophy: a heredofamilial disease. *Arch. Neurol. Psychiatr.* **46** (1941), 654–664.
3. A. E. H. Emery, F. E. Dreifuss, Unusual type of benign X-linked muscular dystrophy. *J. Neurol. Neurosurg. Psychiatr.* **29** (1966), 338–342.
4. L. P. Rowland, M. Fetell, M. Olarte, A. Hays, N. Singh, F. E. Wanat, Emery-Dreifuss muscular dystrophy. *Ann. Neurol.* **5**:2 (1979), 111–117.
5. J. Broers, F. Ramaekers, G. Bonne, R. Ben Yaou, C. Hutchison, The nuclear lamins: laminopathies and their role in premature ageing. *Physiol. Rev.* **86**:3 (2006), 967–1008.
6. S. Bione, E. Maestrini, S. Rivella, *et al.*, Identification of a novel X-linked gene responsible for Emery-Dreifuss muscular dystrophy. *Nat. Genet.* **8** (1994), 323–327.
7. A. Nagano, R. Koga, M. Ogawa, *et al.*, Emerin deficiency at the nuclear membrane in patients with Emery-Dreifuss muscular dystrophy. *Nat. Genet.* **12** (1996), 254–259.
8. S. Manilal, T. M. Nguyen, C. A. Sewry, G. E. Morris, The Emery-Dreifuss muscular dystrophy protein, emerin, is a nuclear membrane protein. *Hum. Mol. Genet.* **5**:6 (1996), 801–808.
9. G. Bonne, M. R. di Barletta, S. Varnous, *et al.*, Mutations in the gene encoding lamin A/C cause autosomal dominant Emery-Dreifuss muscular dystrophy. *Nat. Genet.* **21**:3 (1999), 285–288.
10. M. R. di Barletta, E. Ricci, G. Galluzzi, *et al.*, Different mutations in the LMNA gene cause autosomal dominant and autosomal recessive Emery-Dreifuss muscular dystrophy. *Am. J. Hum. Genet.* **66**:4 (2000), 1407–1412.
11. O. Ullrich, Kongenitale, atonisch-sklerotische Muskeldystrophie, ein weiteres Typus der heredodegenerativen Erkrankungen des neuromuskulären Systems. *Z. Gesamte. Neurol. Psychiatr.* **126** (1930), 171–201.
12. E. Stoeber, Ueber atonisch-sklerotische Muskeldystrophie (Typ Ullrich). *Z. Kinderheilkd.* **60** (1939), 279–284.
13. H. Goett, E. Josten, Beitrag zur kongenitalen atonisch-sklerotischen Muskeldystrophie (Typ Ullrich). *Z. Kinderheilkd.* **75** (1954), 105–118.
14. G. Serratrice, J. Pellissier, A forgotten muscular dystrophy: Ullrich's disease. *Rev. Neurol. (Paris)* **139**:8–9 (1983), 523–525.
15. I. Nonaka, Y. Une, T. Ishihara, S. Miyoshino, T. Nakashima, H. Sugita, A clinical and histological study of Ullrich's disease (congenital atonic-sclerotic muscular dystrophy). *Neuropediatrics* **12**:3 (1981), 197–208.
16. L. De Paillette, J. Aicardi, F. Goutieres, Ullrich's congenital atonic sclerotic muscular dystrophy. A case report. *J. Neurol.* **236**:2 (1989), 108–110.
17. T. Furukawa, Y. Toyokura, Congenital, hypotonic-sclerotic muscular dystrophy. *J. Med. Genet.* **14**:6 (1977), 426–429.
18. J. Bethlem, G. Wijngaarden, Benign myopathy, with autosomal dominant inheritance. A report on three pedigrees. *Brain* **99**:1 (1976), 91–100.
19. W. Arts, J. Bethlem, W. Volkers, Further investigations on benign myopathy with autosomal dominant inheritance. *J. Neurol.* **217**:3 (1978), 201–206.
20. A. K. Lampe, K. M. Bushby, Collagen VI related muscle disorders. *J. Med. Genet.* **42**:9 (2005), 673–685.
21. M. Mohire, R. Tandan, T. Fries, B. Little, W. Pendlebury, W. Bradley, Early-onset benign autosomal dominant limb-girdle myopathy with contractures (Bethlem myopathy). *Neurology* **38**:4 (1988), 573–580.
22. G. Jöbsis, P. Bolhuis, J. Boers, *et al.*, Genetic localization of Bethlem myopathy. *Neurology* **46**:3 (1996), 779–782.
23. M. Speer, R. Tandan, P. Rao, *et al.*, Evidence for locus heterogeneity in the Bethlem myopathy and linkage to 2q37. *Hum. Mol. Genet.* **5**:7 (1996), 1043–1046.
24. G. Jöbsis, H. Keizers, J. Vreijling, *et al.*, Type VI collagen mutations in Bethlem myopathy, an autosomal dominant myopathy with contractures. *Nat. Genet.* **14**:1 (1996), 113–115.
25. I. Higuchi, T. Shiraishi, T. Hashiguchi, *et al.*, Frameshift mutation in the collagen VI gene causes Ullrich's disease. *Ann. Neurol.* **50**:2 (2001), 261–265.
26. I. Higuchi, M. Suehara, H. Iwaki, M. Nakagawa, K. Arimura, M. Osame, Collagen VI deficiency in Ullrich's disease. *Ann. Neurol.* **49**:4 (2001), 544.
27. O. Camacho Vanegas, E. Bertini, R. Z. Zhang, *et al.*, Ullrich scleroatonic muscular dystrophy is caused by recessive mutations in collagen type VI. *Proc. Natl. Acad. Sci. U. S. A.* **98**:13 (2001), 7516–7521.
28. A. E. H. Emery, Emery-Dreifuss muscular dystrophy – a 40 year retrospective. *Neuromusc. Disord.* **10** (2000), 228–232.

29. L. Bengtsson, K. L. Wilson, Multiple and surprising new functions for emerin, a nuclear membrane protein. *Curr. Opin. Cell Biol.* **16**:1 (2004), 73–79.

30. M. S. Zastrow, S. Vlcek, K. L. Wilson, Proteins that bind A-type lamins: integrating isolated clues. *J. Cell Sci.* **117**:Pt 7 (2004), 979–987.

31. S. Vlcek, R. Foisner, A-type lamin networks in light of laminopathic diseases. *Biochim. Biophys. Acta* **1773**:5 (2007), 661–674.

32. H. J. Worman, G. G. Gundersen, Here come the SUNs: a nucleocytoskeletal missing link. *Trends. Cell Biol.* **16**:2 (2006), 67–69.

33. J. A. Ellis, Emery-Dreifuss muscular dystrophy at the nuclear envelope: 10 years on. *Cell. Mol. Life Sci.* **63**:23 (2006), 2702–2709.

34. A. Muchir, J. Medioni, M. Laluc, *et al.*, Nuclear envelope alterations in fibroblasts from patients with muscular dystrophy, cardiomyopathy, and partial lipodystrophy carrying lamin A/C gene mutations. *Muscle Nerve* **30**:4 (2004), 444–450.

35. H. J. Worman, G. Bonne, "Laminopathies": a wide spectrum of human diseases. *Exp. Cell Res* **313**:10 (2007), 2121–2133.

36. E. A. Fairley, J. Kendrick-Jones, J. A. Ellis, The Emery-Dreifuss muscular dystrophy phenotype arises from aberrant targeting and binding of emerin at the inner nuclear membrane. *J. Cell Sci.* **112**:15 (1999), 2571–2582.

37. A. Fidzianska, Z. Glinka, Nuclear architecture remodelling in envelopathies. *Folia Neuropathol.* **45**:2 (2007), 47–55.

38. J. Lammerding, R. T. Lee, The nuclear membrane and mechanotransduction: impaired nuclear mechanics and mechanotransduction in lamin A/C deficient cells. *Novartis. Found. Symp.* **264** (2005), 264–273.

39. J. Lammerding, J. Hsiao, P. C. Schulze, S. Kozlov, C. L. Stewart, R. T. Lee, Abnormal nuclear shape and impaired mechanotransduction in emerin-deficient cells. *J. Cell Biol.* **170**:5 (2005), 781–791.

40. A. Muchir, H. J. Worman, Emery-Dreifuss muscular dystrophy. *Curr. Neurol. Neurosci. Rep.* **7**:1 (2007), 78–83.

41. M. Bakay, Z. Wang, G. Melcon, *et al.*, Nuclear envelope dystrophies show a transcriptional fingerprint suggesting disruption of Rb-MyoD pathways in muscle regeneration. *Brain* **129**:Pt 4 (2006), 996–1013.

42. G. Melcon, S. Kozlov, D. A. Cutler, *et al.*, Loss of emerin at the nuclear envelope disrupts the Rb1/E2F and MyoD pathways during muscle regeneration. *Hum. Mol. Genet.* **15**:4 (2006), 637–651.

43. A. Muchir, P. Pavlidis, G. Bonne, Y. Hayashi, H. Worman, Activation of MAPK in hearts of Emd null mice: similarities between mouse models of X-linked and autosomal dominant Emery-Dreifuss muscular dystrophy. *Hum. Mol. Genet.* **16**:15 (2007), 1884–1895.

44. A. Muchir, P. Pavlidis, V. Decostre, *et al.*, Activation of MAPK pathways links LMNA mutations to cardiomyopathy in Emery-Dreifuss muscular dystrophy. *J. Clin. Invest.* **117**:5 (2007), 1282–1293.

45. G. Bonne, E. Mercuri, A. Muchir, *et al.*, Clinical and molecular genetic spectrum of autosomal dominant Emery Dreifuss muscular dystrophy due to mutations of the lamin A/C gene. *Ann. Neurol.* **48**:2 (2000), 170–180.

46. G. Bonne, F. Leturcq, D. Recan-Budiartha, R. Ben Yaou, Emery- Dreifuss muscular dystrophy. In: *GeneReviews at GeneTests: Medical Genetics Information Resource* [database online] (updated April 2007). Copyright, University of Washington, Seattle 1997–2007. Available at http://www.Genetests.org.

47. T. Sanna, A. Dello Russo, D. Toniolo, *et al.*, Cardiac features of Emery-Dreifuss muscular dystrophy caused by lamin A/C gene mutations. *Eur. Heart. J.* **24**:24 (2003), 2227–2236.

48. J. H. Van Berlo, W. G. de Voogt, A. J. van der Kooi, *et al.*, Meta-analysis of clinical characteristics of 299 carriers of LMNA gene mutations: do lamin A/C mutations portend a high risk of sudden death? *J. Mol. Med.* **83**:1 (2005), 79–83.

49. G. Boriani, M. Gallina, L. Merlini, *et al.*, Clinical relevance of atrial fibrillation/flutter, stroke, pacemaker implant, and heart failure in Emery-Dreifuss muscular dystrophy: a long-term longitudinal study. *Stroke* **34**:4 (2003), 901–908.

50. G. Bonne, R. Ben Yaou, C. Beroud, *et al.*, 108th ENMC International Workshop, 3rd Workshop of the MYO-CLUSTER project: EUROMEN, 7th International Emery-Dreifuss Muscular Dystrophy (EDMD) Workshop, 13–15 September 2002, Naarden, The Netherlands. *Neuromusc. Disord.* **13** (2003), 508–515.

51. E. Mercuri, M. Poppe, R. Quinlivan, *et al.*, Extreme variability of phenotype in patients with an identical missense mutation in the lamin a/c gene: from congenital onset with severe phenotype to milder classic Emery-Dreifuss variant. *Arch. Neurol.* **61**:5 (2004), 690–694.

52. R. Ben Yaou, A. Toutain, T. Arimura, *et al.*, Multitissular involvement in a family with LMNA and EMD mutations: Role of digenic mechanism? *Neurology* **68**:22 (2007), 1883–1894.

53. M. Vytopil, E. Ricci, A. Dello Russo, *et al.*, Frequent low penetrance mutations in the Lamin A/C gene, causing Emery Dreifuss muscular dystrophy. *Neuromuscul. Disord.* **12**:10 (2002), 958–963.

54. A. J. van der Kooi, G. Bonne, B. Eymard, *et al.*, Lamin A/C mutations with lipodystrophy, cardiac abnormalities, and muscular dystrophy. *Neurology* **59**:4 (2002), 620–623.

55. F. Muntoni, G. Bonne, L. G. Goldfarb, *et al.*, Disease severity in dominant Emery Dreifuss is increased by mutations in both emerin and desmin proteins. *Brain* **129**:Pt 5 (2006), 1260–1268.

56. M. C. Walter, T. N. Witt, B. S. Weigel, *et al.*, Deletion of the LMNA initiator codon leading to a neurogenic variant of autosomal dominant Emery-Dreifuss muscular dystrophy. *Neuromuscul. Disord.* **15**:1 (2005), 40–44.

57. P. Graux, R. Carlioz, I. Krivosic, *et al.*, [Emery-Dreifuss muscular dystrophy with major conduction disorders and cardiac excitability.] *Ann. Cardiol. Angeiol. (Paris)* **42**:10 (1993), 554–560.

58. E. Mercuri, S. Counsell, J. Allsop, *et al.*, Selective muscle involvement on magnetic resonance imaging in autosomal dominant Emery-Dreifuss muscular dystrophy. *Neuropediatrics* **33**:1 (2002), 10–14.

59. S. Manilal, C. A. Sewry, N. T. Man, F. Muntoni, G. E. Morris, Diagnosis of X-linked Emery-Dreifuss muscular dystrophy by protein analysis of leucocytes and skin with monoclonal antibodies. *Neuromuscul. Disord.* **7**:1 (1997), 63–66.

60. S. Manilal, D. Recan, C. A. Sewry, *et al.*, Mutations in Emery-Dreifuss muscular dystrophy and their effects on emerin protein expression. *Hum. Mol. Genet.* **7**:5 (1998), 855–864.

61. E. Mercuri, A. Lampe, J. Allsop, *et al.*, Muscle MRI in Ullrich congenital muscular dystrophy and Bethlem myopathy. *Neuromuscul. Disord.* **15**:4 (2005), 303–310.

62. C. Meune, J. H. Van Berlo, F. Anselme, G. Bonne, Y. M. Pinto, D. Duboc, Primary prevention of sudden death in patients with lamin A/C gene mutations. *N. Engl. J. Med.* **354**:2 (2006), 209–210.

63. S. Lamandé, M. Mörgelin, C. Selan, G. Jöbsis, F. Baas, J. Bateman, Kinked collagen VI tetramers and reduced microfibril formation as a result of Bethlem myopathy and introduced triple helical glycine mutations. *J. Biol. Chem.* **277**:3 (2002), 1949–1956.

64. S. Lamandé, M. Mörgelin, N. Adams, C. Selan, J. Allen, The C5 domain of the collagen VI alpha3(VI) chain is critical for extracellular microfibril formation and is present in the extracellular matrix of cultured cells. *J. Biol. Chem.* **281**:24 (2006), 16607–16614.

65. C. Baldock, M. Sherratt, C. Shuttleworth, C. Kielty, The supramolecular organization of collagen VI microfibrils. *J. Mol. Biol.* **330**:2 (2003), 297–307.

66. H. von der Mark, M. Aumailley, G. Wick, R. Fleischmajer, R. Timpl, Immunochemistry, genuine size and tissue localization of collagen VI. *Eur. J. Biochem.* **142**:3 (1984), 493–502.

67. H. Kuo, C. Maslen, D. Keene, R. Glanville, Type VI collagen anchors endothelial basement membranes by interacting with type IV collagen. *J. Biol. Chem.* **272**:42 (1997), 26522–26529.

68. G. J. Jöbsis, J. M. Boers, P. G. Barth, M. de Visser, Bethlem myopathy: a slowly progressive congenital muscular dystrophy with contractures. *Brain* **122**:Pt 4 (1999), 649–655.

69. A. van der Kooi, W. de Voogt, E. Bertini, *et al.*, Cardiac and pulmonary investigations in Bethlem myopathy. *Arch. Neurol.* **63**:11 (2006), 1617–1621.

70. J. Schessl, Y. Zou, C. Bönnemann, Congenital muscular dystrophies and the extracellular matrix. *Semin. Pediatr. Neurol.* **13**:2 (2006), 80–89.

71. E. Mercuri, Y. Yuva, S. Brown, *et al.*, Collagen VI involvement in Ullrich syndrome: a clinical, genetic, and immunohistochemical study. *Neurology* **58**:9 (2002), 1354–1359.

72. T. Pan, R. Zhang, D. Sudano, S. Marie, C. Bönnemann, M. Chu, New molecular mechanism for Ullrich congenital muscular dystrophy: a heterozygous in-frame deletion in the COL6A1 gene causes a severe phenotype. *Am. J. Hum. Genet.* **73**:2 (2003), 355–369.

73. N. Baker, M. Mörgelin, R. Peat, *et al.*, Dominant collagen VI mutations are a common cause of Ullrich congenital muscular dystrophy. *Hum. Mol. Genet.* **14**:2 (2005), 279–293.

74. G. Pepe, E. Bertini, P. Bonaldo, *et al.*, Bethlem myopathy (BETHLEM) and Ullrich scleroatonic muscular dystrophy: 100th ENMC international workshop, 23–24 November 2001, Naarden, The Netherlands. *Neuromuscul. Disord.* **12**:10 (2002), 984–993.

75. J. Kirschner, I. Hausser, Y. Zou, *et al.*, Ullrich congenital muscular dystrophy: connective tissue abnormalities in the skin support overlap with Ehlers-Danlos syndromes. *Am. J. Med. Genet.* **132**:3 (2005), 296–301.

76. G. Pepe, M. de Visser, E. Bertini, *et al.*, Bethlem myopathy (BETHLEM) 86th ENMC international workshop, 10–11 November 2000, Naarden, The Netherlands. *Neuromuscul. Disord.* **12**:3 (2002), 296–305.

77. I. Fokkema, J. den Dunnen, P. Taschner, Leiden muscular dystrophy database COL6A1, 2 and 3 mutation data. http://www.dmd.nl/ LOVD: easy creation of a locus-specific sequence variation database using an "LSDB-in-a-box" approach. *Hum. Mutat.* **26**:2 (2005), 63–68.

78. N. Baker, M. Mörgelin, R. Pace, *et al.*, Molecular consequences of dominant Bethlem myopathy collagen VI mutations. *Ann. Neurol.* **62**:4 (2007), 390–405.

79. R. Zhang, P. Sabatelli, T. Pan, *et al.*, Effects on collagen VI mRNA stability and microfibrillar assembly of three COL6A2 mutations in two families with Ullrich congenital muscular dystrophy. *J. Biol. Chem.* **277**:46 (2002), 43557–43564.

80. S. Lamandé, J. Bateman, W. Hutchison, *et al.*, Reduced collagen VI causes Bethlem myopathy: a heterozygous COL6A1 nonsense mutation results in mRNA decay and functional haploinsufficiency. *Hum. Mol. Genet.* 7:6 (1998), 981–989.

81. M. Okada, G. Kawahara, S. Noguchi, *et al.*, Primary collagen VI deficiency is the second most common congenital muscular dystrophy in Japan. *Neurology* **69**:10 (2007), 1035–1042.

82. C. Jimenez-Mallebrera, M. Maioli, J. Kim, *et al.*, A comparative analysis of collagen VI production in muscle, skin and fibroblasts from 14 Ullrich congenital muscular dystrophy patients with dominant and recessive COL6A mutations. *Neuromuscul. Disord.* **16**:9–10 (2006), 571–582.

83. T. Niiyama, I. Higuchi, M. Suehara, *et al.*, Electron microscopic abnormalities of skeletal muscle in patients with collagen VI deficiency in Ullrich's disease. *Acta Neuropathol.* **104**:1 (2002), 67–71.

84. A. Lampe, D. Dunn, A. von Niederhausern, *et al.*, Automated genomic sequence analysis of the three collagen VI genes: applications to Ullrich congenital muscular dystrophy and Bethlem myopathy. *J. Med. Genet.* **42**:2 (2005), 108–120.

85. C. Wallgren-Pettersson, K. Bushby, U. Mellies, A. Simonds, 117th ENMC workshop: ventilatory support in congenital neuromuscular disorders – congenital myopathies, congenital muscular dystrophies, congenital myotonic dystrophy and SMA (II) 4–6 April 2003, Naarden, The Netherlands. *Neuromuscul. Disord.* **14**:1 (2004), 56–69.

86. M. Brockington, S. Brown, A. Lampe, *et al.*, Prenatal diagnosis of Ullrich congenital muscular dystrophy using haplotype analysis and collagen VI immunocytochemistry. *Prenat. Diagn.* **24**:6 (2004), 440–444.

87. Q. Zhang, C. Bethmann, N. F. Worth, *et al.*, Nesprin-1 and -2 are involved in the pathogenesis of Emery-Dreifuss Muscular Dystrophy and are critical for nuclear envelope integrity. *Hum. Mol. Genet.* **16**:23 (2007), 2816–2833.

88. E. C. Schirmer, L. Florens, T. Guan, J. R. Yates, L. Gerace 3rd, Nuclear membrane proteins with potential disease links found by subtractive proteomics. *Science* **301**:5638 (2003), 1380–1382.

89. W. Irwin, N. Bergamin, P. Sabatelli, *et al.*, Mitochondrial dysfunction and apoptosis in myopathic mice with collagen VI deficiency. *Nat. Genet.* **35**:4 (2003), 367–371.

90. A. Angelin, T. Tiepolo, P. Sabatelli, *et al.*, Mitochondrial dysfunction in the pathogenesis of Ullrich congenital muscular dystrophy and prospective therapy with cyclosporins. *Proc. Natl. Acad. Sci. U. S. A.* **104**:3 (2007), 991–996.

Chapter 15

Facioscapulohumeral dystrophy

Shannon L. Venance and Rabi Tawil

Introduction

Facioscapulohumeral muscular dystrophy (FSHD) is the third most common muscular dystrophy (after Duchenne and myotonic dystrophy) with an estimated prevalence of 1:20 000 [1]. The inheritance pattern is autosomal dominant, although 10%–30% of cases are sporadic or due to mosaicism [2]. Symptomatic onset may occur at any age, although typically is in adolescence [1]. Despite a wide range in severity and variability in progression, there is a distinctive descending evolution of weakness and wasting involving the facial, scapular, humeral, truncal, and finally anterolateral leg and pelvic girdle muscles in the majority of affected individuals [1, 3]. In general, life expectancy is not shortened, although 20% of individuals will require the use of a wheelchair for mobility. Identification of a contraction in a tandem repeat sequence known as D4Z4 [4] on the long arm of chromosome 4 [5] confirms FSHD in over 95% of affected individuals. The molecular pathogenesis, a topic of much research and discussion, remains unknown.

Clinical features

The phenotype of FSHD is broad, ranging from asymptomatic individuals with minimal signs on examination, to patients requiring a wheelchair and assistance for activities of daily living. While the age of onset is variable, penetrance is high, and more than 95% of affected individuals show signs by the end of the second decade. Classically, the distribution of weakness is asymmetrical, and the reason for this remains unclear but is not thought to be related to handedness [6].

In general, FSHD is characterized by a typical, asymmetrical, pattern of muscle weakness that begins with the face, before "descending" along the scapular, humeral, truncal, and lower-extremity muscle groups. Facial weakness alone rarely leads to medical consultation unless it is severe and infantile in onset. Adolescents or young adults present with difficulty elevating their arms overhead, with scapular winging due to weakness of the scapular fixators. There may be a history of difficulty in gym class with push-ups and sit-ups secondary to humeral and truncal weakness. On occasion, the initial complaint will be difficulty running or tripping secondary to footdrop and, less commonly, trouble climbing stairs due to pelvic girdle weakness.

Nevertheless, on direct questioning, many features of otherwise asymptomatic weakness of facial and scapulohumeral muscles can be elicited. Parents or bed partners may have appreciated the patient sleeping with their eyes not fully closed. There may be a history of soap irritating the eyes during a shower, an inability to whistle or difficulty using a straw. However, intrafamilial variability is well documented, and affected individuals in otherwise typical kindreds with FSHD may have facial sparing. Asking about athletic ability in school will often uncover otherwise asymptomatic weakness of the scapular stabilizers in students who did not like gym class and had difficulty keeping up with their peers on climbing rope and doing push-ups or "jumping jacks."

Inspection reveals a reduced facial expression (Figure 15.1). Careful examination often shows an asymmetrical inability to bury the eyelashes or imperfection in pursing the lips in mildly affected individuals (Figure 15.2). Observation of the upper trunk reveals rounding of the shoulders, straight clavicles and scapular winging, which is often asymmetrical. The scapulae move superiorly (sparing of the upper trapezius) and laterally (rhomboid weakness). The arms may be internally rotated, with the thumbs pointing (inward) towards the thighs, rather than forward. Pectoral atrophy leads to characteristic axillary creases, unilaterally or bilaterally. The biceps and triceps atrophy preferentially with relative preservation of the deltoid and forearm muscles, i.e., "Popeye" arms (Figure 15.3). Truncal weakness, often profound, may lead to a protuberant abdomen and an exaggerated lumbar lordosis (Figure 15.4). The anterolateral leg, as well as the quadriceps and hamstrings, may be atrophied with sparing of the posterior calf.

Examination confirms the facial weakness, with an inability to bury the eyelashes, a transverse smile, and weakness of lip pursing. There is no involvement of extraocular or bulbar muscles. Neck flexion is strong relative to neck extension. Flexion and abduction of the arms will demonstrate over-riding

Disorders of Voluntary Muscle, 8th edn., eds. George Karpati, David Hilton-Jones, Kate Bushby and Robert C. Griggs. Published by Cambridge University Press.

and winging of the scapula(e), if not readily apparent at rest (Figure 15.5). Shoulder abduction is strong, and activation of deltoid is easily demonstrated with the patient lying supine and gravity eliminated. Shoulder range of motion may be demonstrated by manually fixing the scapula to the chest wall, and then asking for arm elevation above the head (Figure 15.6). Elbow flexion and extension are impaired early. With progression, the distal wrist extensors may become involved. The inability to perform an unassisted sit-up reveals the abdominal muscle weakness. The lower abdominal muscles tend to be preferentially weaker, and the umbilicus moves cephalad with neck flexion in a supine position (Beevor sign; 95% sensitivity) [7, 8]. Classically, ankle dorsiflexor involvement occurs prior to pelvic girdle, although early and severe involvement of thigh and hip girdle muscles is well documented [6]. Unlike other dystrophies, contractures are not a feature of FSHD.

Other phenotypic considerations

Symptomatic extramuscular manifestations are uncommon in adolescent- or adult-onset FSHD [3]. In the majority of affected individuals, there is no cardiorespiratory involvement. Rarely, severely affected patients have pulmonary restriction and ineffective nocturnal ventilation [9, 10]. Potential predictors of chronic respiratory failure include wheelchair use and kyphoscoliosis. Subjective sleep quality was impaired in the absence of excessive daytime sleepiness in adults with FSHD, but polysomnography is needed to determine whether this is related to sleep-disordered breathing [11]. Infrequently 5%–10% of affected individuals have cardiac conduction defects, most commonly supraventricular tachyarrhythmias [12], that are not clearly correlated to disease severity or deletion size [13, 14]. High-frequency hearing loss (65%) and peripheral retinal vasculopathy (60%) have been described in adult-onset patients [15, 16], although rarely symptomatic. No difference was found in the prevalence of hearing impairment in adult-onset FSHD patients compared to the general population [17, 18]. However, while near tone hearing thresholds were largely normal in 24 adults with FSHD, evoked otoacoustic emissions were impaired consistent with cochlear dysfunction [19].

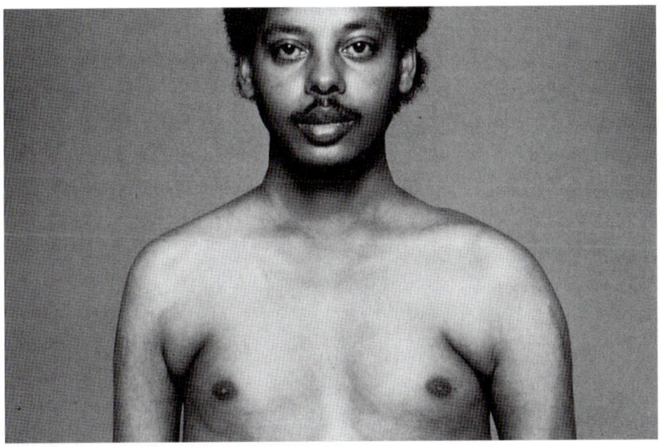

Figure 15.1. Patient with FSHD and typical myopathic facies, straight clavicles, and pectoral wasting with axillary creases.

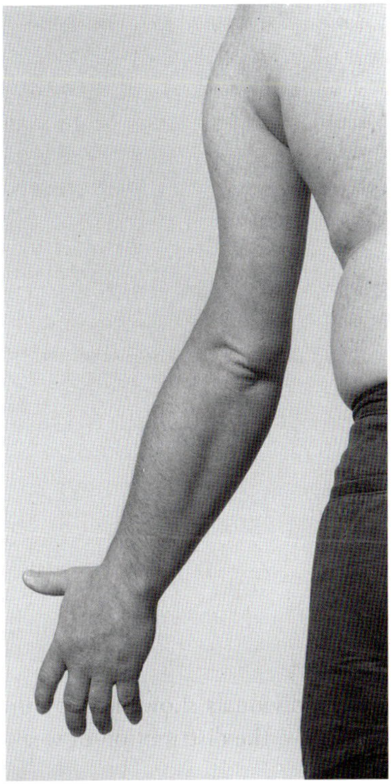

Figure 15.3. "Popeye" arms with selective atrophy of humeral muscles and preservation of forearm muscle bulk.

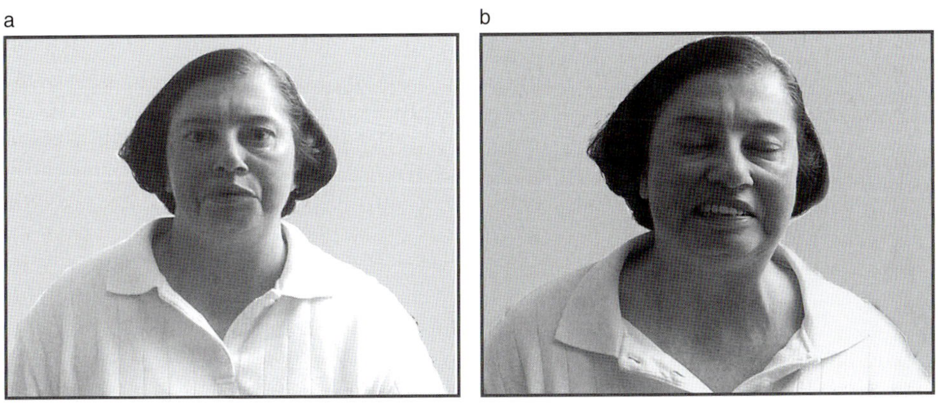

Figure 15.2a, b. Patient with FSHD and typical asymmetry of lip pursing (a) and eyelash burying (b).

Molecular genetics and pathogenesis

In 1991, through linkage analysis, FSHD was mapped to the sub-telomeric region of chromosome 4q35 [5, 20, 21]. Shortly thereafter, the causal genetic defect was identified as a deletion of an integral number of 3.3-kb polymorphic repeats known as D4Z4 [5, 22]. How loss of a critical number of these repetitive elements results in FSHD remains uncertain since it does not result in the disruption of a transcribed sequence. The prevailing hypotheses implicate complex epigenetic mechanisms resulting from the contraction of D4Z4 repeats that alter the expression of genes either contained within D4Z4 (*DUX4*) or upstream from the repeats (*FRG1*) (reviewed by van der Maarel *et al.* [23]).

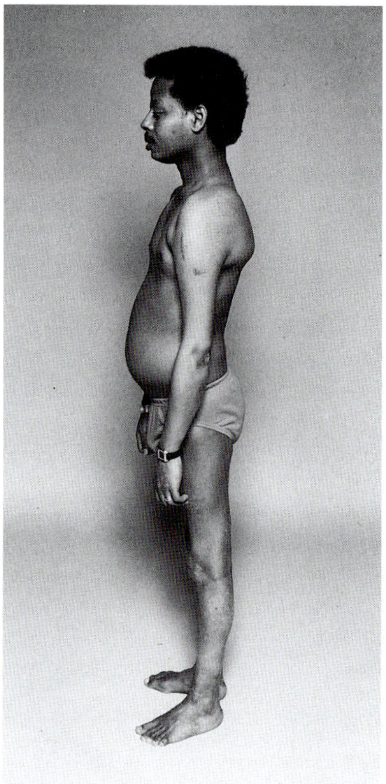

Figure 15.4. Patient with advanced FSHD demonstrating scapular winging at rest, forward sloping of the shoulders, weak abdominal muscles with resultant protuberant abdomen, and atrophy of the thigh muscles.

Applying the molecular genetics of FSHD in the clinic

Molecular diagnostic testing must be performed in the context of patient phenotype and a pretest probability [24]. Diagnostic testing involves separation of digested DNA fragments by Southern blot and hybridization or binding of a probe, p13E-11, to a fragment cut by the *Eco*RI restriction enzyme, which contains the D4Z4 repeat elements on chromosome 4q35 [5]. Both *Eco*RI fragments from each copy of 4q35 in control populations are >50–300+ kb in size whereas one *Eco*RI fragment in FSHD patients ranges from 10 to 38 kb due to the loss of a critical number of D4Z4 repeats.

The molecular diagnosis is complicated by the presence of a nonpathogenic repeat sequence on chromosome 10 that is highly homologous to D4Z4 on 4q35 [25, 26]. Additionally, 20% of the population have complex exchanges of these repeats between chromosomes 4 and 10 [27, 28, 29]. Fortunately, the *Eco*RI fragments on chromosomes 10 and 4 are differentially digested by the restriction enzymes *Bln*I and *Xap*I respectively [30]. This differential digestion allows the accurate assignment of a short *Eco*RI fragment as the disease-causing allele on chromosome 4 [30, 31]. To complicate matters

a b

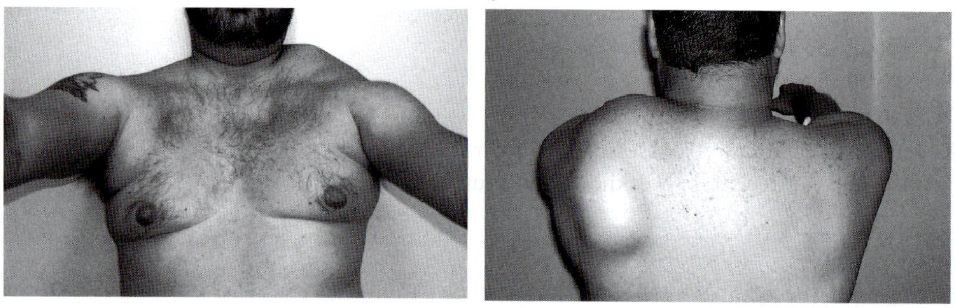

Figure 15.5a, b. Typical appearance of shoulder and upper chest with jutting up of the scapula on attempted shoulder forward flexion (a). Scapular winging showing the side-to-side asymmetry typical of FSHD (b). With permission, *Muscle and Nerve* 2006; **34**: 1–15.

a b

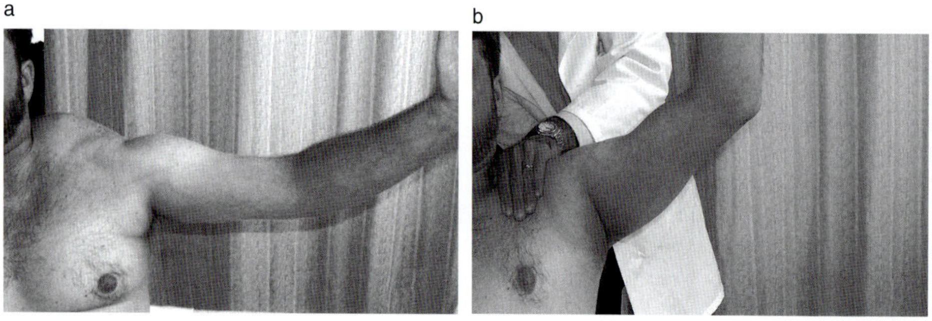

Figure 15.6a, b. Inability to abduct arm due to weakness of periscapular muscles (a). Bedside manual fixation of the scapula results in significant improvement of range of motion, mimicking the effect of surgical scapular fixation (b). With permission, *Muscle and Nerve* 2006; **34**: 1–15.

further, however, there is heterogeneity on chromosome 4q35 distal to the D4Z4 repeat sequence [32], and *only* when the contracted D4Z4 repeat resides on the A isoform of chromosome 4 (4qA) is there an association with FSHD [33, 34, 35]. While the 4qA and 4qB alleles occur with almost identical frequencies in the population [33], FSHD is solely associated with 4qA: the 4qB isoform is nonpathogenic.

In the majority of typical FSHD patients with an autosomal dominant family history, genetic testing is straightforward. However, a triple digest DNA analysis using pulsed-field gel electrophoresis (PFGE) rather than standard linear gel electrophoresis may be crucial in occasional cases of diagnostic uncertainty. In these instances, referral to an outside laboratory with additional testing capabilities may be indicated [23]. For example, false-negatives may be seen in cases of somatic mosaicism [36, 37] or when the deletion extends proximally to involve the p13E–11 hybridization site on the *Eco*RI fragment accounting for some of the apparent non-4q35 linked cases [27, 38, 39]. In an individual or kindred with typical FSHD and negative DNA analysis for D4Z4, testing with alternative probes to recognize the deletion may be required [40]. False-negatives may also be seen in at-risk, clinically unaffected individuals with germline mosaicism (for example, in a parent with clinically affected offspring) as the diagnostic testing is done on leukocyte DNA. Even less commonly, false-positives may be seen with complex 4q and 10q rearrangements or with short D4Z4 alleles carried on chromosome 4qB and segregating with unaffected family members [34]. Therefore, it remains critical to interpret the results of molecular diagnostic testing in the context of the clinical diagnosis.

Pathogenesis

Several pathogenic mechanisms have been proposed in FSHD. The D4Z4 repeats contain an open reading frame (*DUX4*) implying the presence of a putative gene but whether *DUX4* is actively transcribed is controversial [41, 42, 43]. Evidence of evolutionary conservation of the ORF supports a protein coding function [44]. Consequently *DUX4* remains a candidate gene for FSHD. The function of *DUX4* is uncertain but recent data indicate that it may play a role in cellular apoptotic mechanisms [43].

One epigenetic hypothesis concerning pathogenesis in FSHD suggests that contraction of the D4Z4 repeats affects transcription of adjacent genes. *FRG1* is the closest upstream gene to the D4Z4 repeats and is therefore a logical candidate gene. *FRG1* protein localizes to the nucleolus and appears to play a role in regulating transcription [45]. Data from Gabellini *et al.* suggest that loss of a repressor complex that normally binds D4Z4 results in transcriptional upregulation of nearby genes such as *FRG1* [46]. Moreover, a mouse overexpressing *FRG1* shows a myopathic phenotype [46, 47]. Although a tantalizing finding, further proof is needed to confirm that this mouse is an animal model of FSHD as upregulation of *FRG1* expression has not been reproduced by other investigators [48, 49, 50].

In an expression profiling study of FSHD skeletal muscle, selective upregulation of vascular and endothelial genes was observed [49]. This finding raises the possibility that skeletal muscle vascular pathology, similar to that seen in the retina, may be contributing to skeletal muscle pathology.

Another recent finding raises the possibility that FSHD may be a nuclear envelope disease. The telomere region of 4q (compared to none of the other chromosomes) is preferentially localized to the outer rim of the nuclear envelope at a region just proximal to D4Z4 [51, 52]. This preferential localization is lost in the absence of lamin A/C [51]. Recent microarray data reveal that mRNA transcriptomes for EDMD patients (both X-linked and autosomal dominant) were related to those obtained from FSHD patients [53] suggesting similar pathogenic mechanisms between EDMD and FSHD.

Diagnostic criteria

A clinical diagnosis of FSHD is based on the typical pattern of weakness and an autosomal dominant family history (in the absence of contractures, ocular, bulbar, and cardiorespiratory involvement). Confirmation is through genetic testing in over 95% of individuals by determining a D4Z4 allele size below 35 kb on chromosome 4qA in leukocyte-derived DNA using a triple digest [30]. In isolated or sporadic cases where the phenotype of affected individuals is indistinguishable from classic FSHD, DNA testing is also highly sensitive and specific [54]. Muscle biopsy in FSHD is no longer necessary in typical cases. There are no pathognomic features for FSHD. Pathology reveals a dystrophic picture with variability in fiber size with rounded atrophic and hypertrophic muscle fibers, internalized nuclei, rare necrotic fibers, and increased connective tissue deposition. Mild to moderate inflammation is well recognized. Electrodiagnostic studies may be normal or reveal small-amplitude, short-duration "myopathic" units. Other diagnostic considerations such as congenital myopathies, mitochondrial cytopathies, myofibrillar myopathy, inclusion body myositis or polymyositis are most often excluded by careful clinical assessment (in particular ruling out subtle asymmetrical facial weakness) and muscle biopsy [24].

Genotype–phenotype correlations

There is phenotypic heterogeneity with inter- and intrafamilial variability in FSHD ranging from asymptomatic carriers to early infantile onset. Cohort studies support anticipation (that is, earlier onset with increasing severity) in FSHD [2, 55, 56, 57]. Somatic mosaicism, which is not uncommon in FSHD [36, 37, 58], may partially explain some cases of apparent anticipation and why a parent may be minimally symptomatic with a clearly affected child. Germline mosaicism may account for asymptomatic parents of affected offspring [59, 60]. Women tend to be less severely affected than men [61], and, again, mosaicism may be partially responsible. It is important to detect mosaicism because of the implications for genetic counseling and the risk to future offspring [24]. De novo mutations are seen in up to 30% of affected individuals, and 1%–2% of affected individuals remain nonlinked to 4q35, suggesting locus heterogeneity.

There is a loose correlation for increasing severity of disease with larger deletions [55, 57], most evident in infantile-onset FSHD and large deletion size [1, 3]. Early-onset FSHD [62] have symptoms or signs of facial involvement developing before age 5 and shoulder girdle weakness before age 10. Infantile FSHD is associated with larger deletions, i.e., small D4Z4 allele sizes of 11–18 kb [63, 64]. Infantile-onset cases of FSHD may be sporadic or inherited from a parent with somatic mosaicism or with classic adult-onset FSHD [65]. Moderate to marked hearing impairment is common. In a large Japanese cohort, the early-onset patients with the largest deletions (10–11 kb allele size) had mental retardation (8/9), sensorineural hearing loss (6/9), and epilepsy (4/9), suggesting central nervous system involvement [64]. Coats syndrome, mental retardation, and deafness were the presenting features of two Norwegian children [66]. A cohort of seven infantile-onset FSHD patients followed in the UK showed a rapidly progressive course with a severe phenotype including sensorineural hearing loss, but without cardiac involvement, mental retardation or seizures [65]. FSHD is always a consideration in infants with severe facial diplegia: normal extraocular movements are helpful in excluding Mobius syndrome [64]. Rarely, dysphagia [67] and/or tongue atrophy [68] may be seen in early-onset FSHD.

Diagnostic approaches

When the clinical diagnosis of FSHD is suspected and there is a positive family history, the diagnostic work-up should proceed directly to confirmation by molecular DNA testing. In sporadic cases, a brief work-up to exclude other diagnoses is warranted before proceeding to DNA testing. Serum creatine kinase should be checked. It is typically mildly to modestly elevated (<1500 IU/l). A creatine kinase level > 2000 IU/l suggests an alternative diagnosis. Next electromyography (EMG) is performed. Nonspecific myopathic changes are typically seen on EMG while the presence of neurogenic changes or myotonia suggests an alternative diagnosis. If the work-up is still consistent with FSHD, DNA analysis in a clinical diagnostic laboratory for 4q35 D4Z4 allele size will confirm the diagnosis. Molecular testing is reported to be ~95% sensitive and ~95% specific [54, 69]. It should be kept in mind that this high specificity is based on data collected using strict research criteria. With more widespread testing in clinical practice using looser diagnostic criteria, the specificity drops; consequently clinicians need to keep in mind the possibility of a false-positive test as outlined in a previous section. Similarly, clinicians need to be aware of the small possibility of a false-negative test in an individual who may have a typical FSHD clinical profile. Additional testing by a specialized laboratory is indicated if either a false-positive or false-negative result is suspected. If the DNA test does not confirm the clinical suspicion of FSHD, a muscle biopsy is then in order to rule out other myopathic processes.

Therapeutic and preventative modalities

Currently there are no effective treatments to slow or halt progression of the muscle weakness and wasting in FSHD. Rational therapeutic trials are hindered by the lack of understanding of the specific underlying pathophysiology in FSHD.

Management centers on treatment of the individual patient's symptoms and careful monitoring for some of the known, if infrequent, extramuscular manifestations of the disease.

Pain is common in FSHD [70], is predominantly musculoskeletal in origin and should be managed accordingly. Shoulder pain arises due to changes in posture and overuse of a joint that is poorly supported by weak periscapular muscles. Recurrent shoulder dislocations can occur, as can brachial plexopathies. Lower back pain exacerbated by weak abdominal muscles and hyperlordosis is also common.

Several early uncontrolled studies demonstrated that exercise has no detrimental effects on muscle function in FSHD. This was confirmed recently in a controlled study of moderate-intensity strength training and albuterol [71] but this training had no effect on perceived pain or fatigue [72].

Assistive devices are indicated to maintain function and independence. Anterolateral compartment weakness resulting in foot drop and predisposing to ankle instability and falls may be managed with ankle–foot orthoses (AFO). With concomitant quadriceps weakness, the molded AFO hinders the ability to hyperextend and lock the knee. In such instances Floor Reaction AFOs may assist with knee extension. Any potential benefit of an orthotic device needs to be balanced against the additional weight of the device. Referral for physiatry assessment and then to an experienced custom orthotic specialist is helpful for developing an assistive device tailored to an individual's needs. Scapular fixation has been shown to improve arm range of motion in retrospective case series [73, 74, 75, 76, 77], although prospective, randomized data are lacking [78]. Patients with stable or slowly progressive disease, mild arm weakness and a significant increase in shoulder range of motion with bedside manual fixation are potential surgical candidates (Figure 15.6).

Respiratory compromise in FSHD is rare but clinicians should be alert to the early, subtle signs of chronic nocturnal hypoventilation. Forced vital capacity should be routinely monitored, both supine and sitting, in patients with significant truncal weakness, progressive kyphoscoliosis, and those who are wheelchair bound.

Hearing loss in FSHD is generally trivial and asymptomatic but can be severe in infantile FSHD. Undetected hearing loss in a child can result in cognitive developmental delays or may be misconstrued as mental retardation. Audiograms should be routinely done on patients with infantile-onset FSHD.

Retinal vasculopathy represents another rarely symptomatic problem in FSHD. Here again, patients with the infantile form may develop significant retinal vasculopathy with Coats disease that can result in retinal detachment, loss of vision and secondary painful glaucoma requiring enucleation of the eye [79]. Early detection and laser treatment can prevent such catastrophic complications. To this end, a careful dilated retinal exam, and if needed a fluoroscein angiogram, is essential in all patients with infantile FSHD.

Despite several clinical trials, no therapies have been shown to be beneficial in FSHD [80]. Challenges in clinical trial design include a need to identify suitable outcome measures for the relatively brief duration of a clinical trial for a disease that is only slowly progressive [81]. Prednisone, evaluated because of the inflammation seen on muscle biopsy, failed to show improvement in muscle strength or mass in a prospective, open label study [81]. The anabolic effects of the β-agonist, albuterol, were assessed in a randomized, placebo-controlled trial that failed to show a difference between treatment groups at 1 year [82]. An open-label pilot trial of diltiazem, a calcium channel blocker, in 20 patients with FSHD did not improve muscle strength or mass [83]. A 12-week open-label pilot trial of 5 mg/day folic acid and methionine 1 g/t.i.d., undertaken based on the hypomethylation of D4Z4 in FSHD [84], found no differences between nine subjects with FSHD and six healthy controls [84]. A phase II trial of MYO-029, a monoclonal antibody raised against human myostatin, in subjects with FSHD, Becker muscular dystrophy, and limb girdle muscular dystrophy was negative [89].

Genetic counseling

Because FSHD is an autosomal dominant condition, each child of an affected individual has a 50% chance of inheriting the contracted allele. Any individual with a genetic confirmation of FSHD should be offered genetic counseling. Prenatal diagnosis is readily available [86, 87] but pre-implantation diagnosis is not possible. In general, pregnancy outcomes are good in women affected with FSHD. Data from a mail-out questionnaire revealed an increased incidence of low-birth weight infants without a concomitant increase in premature births [88]. Pain and deterioration of muscle strength was reported in 25% of the 105 gestations. Despite the failure of these symptoms to resolve postpartum, the majority of the 38 women with FSHD indicated they would choose to conceive again [88].

Future perspectives

Understanding the underlying pathophysiology is critical for identifying potential therapeutic targets in FSHD. Several competing pathogenic hypotheses are being considered but need further study. Given the likelihood that FSHD is caused, at the molecular level, by an epigenetic mechanism, more than one cellular mechanism may account for the disease's pleomorphic manifestations. In the meantime, the development of therapeutic strategies to inhibit myostatin may offer ways to slow down disease progression until the time that targeted, FSHD-specific therapeutic interventions become a reality.

Acknowledgments

The authors acknowledge the generous support of The Fields Center for FSHD and Neuromuscular Research and the University of Rochester's Senator Paul D. Wellstone Muscular Dystrophy Cooperative Research Center.

References

1. G. W. Padberg, *Facioscapulohumeral Disease*. (Leiden, the Netherlands: The University of Leiden, 1982.)
2. M. Zatz, S. K. Marie, M. R. Passos-Bueno, *et al.*, High proportion of new mutations and possible anticipation in Brazilian facioscapulohumeral muscular dystrophy families. *Am. J. Hum. Genet.* **56** (1995), 99–105.
3. R. Tawil, D. A. Figlewicz, R. C. Griggs, B. Weiffenbach, Facioscapulohumeral dystrophy: a distinct regional myopathy with a novel molecular pathogenesis. FSH Consortium. *Ann. Neurol.* **43** (1998), 279–282.
4. J. E. Hewitt, R. Lyle, L. N. Clark, *et al.*, Analysis of the tandem repeat locus D4Z4 associated with facioscapulohumeral muscular dystrophy. *Hum. Mol. Genet.* **3** (1994), 1287–1295.
5. C. Wijmenga, J. E. Hewitt, L. A. Sandkuijl, *et al.*, Chromosome 4q DNA rearrangements associated with facioscapulohumeral muscular dystrophy. *Nat. Genet.* **2** (1992), 26–30.
6. R. Tawil, M. P. McDermott, J. R. Mendell, J. Kissel, R. C. Griggs, Facioscapulohumeral muscular dystrophy (FSHD): design of natural history study and results of baseline testing. FSH-DY Group. *Neurology* **44** (1994), 442–446.
7. G. I. Awerbuch, M. A. Nigro, R. Wishnow, Beevor's sign and facioscapulohumeral dystrophy. *Arch. Neurol.* **47** (1990), 1208–1209.
8. N. Shahrizaila, A. J. Wills, Significance of Beevor's sign in facioscapulohumeral dystrophy and other neuromuscular diseases. *J. Neurol. Neurosurg. Psychiatry* **76** (2005), 869–870.
9. G. T. Carter, T. D. Bird, Ventilatory support in facioscapulohumeral muscular dystrophy. *Neurology* **64** (2005), 401.
10. M. Wohlgemuth, E. L. van der Kooi, R. G van Kesteren, S. M. van der Maarel, G. W. Padberg, Ventilatory support in facioscapulohumeral muscular dystrophy. *Neurology* **63** (2004), 176–178.
11. G. Della Marca, R. Frusciante, C. Vollono, *et al.*, Sleep quality in facioscapulohumeral muscular dystrophy. *J. Neurol. Sci.* **263** (2007), 49–53.
12. W. G. Stevenson, J. K. Perloff, J. N. Weiss, T. L. Anderson, Facioscapulohumeral muscular dystrophy: evidence for selective, genetic electrophysiologic cardiac involvement. *J. Am. Coll. Cardiol.* **15** (1990), 292–299.
13. P. Laforet, C. de Toma, B. Eymard, *et al.*, Cardiac involvement in genetically confirmed facioscapulohumeral muscular dystrophy. *Neurology* **51** (1998), 1454–1456.
14. C. P. Trevisan, E. Pastorello, M. Armani, *et al.*, Facioscapulohumeral muscular dystrophy and occurrence of heart arrhythmia. *Eur. Neurol.* **56** (2006), 1–5.

15. R. B. Fitzsimons, E. B. Gurwin, A. C. Bird, Retinal vascular abnormalities in facioscapulohumeral muscular dystrophy. A general association with genetic and therapeutic implications. *Brain* **110**:Pt 3 (1987), 631–648.

16. G. W. Padberg, O. F. Brouwer, R. J. de Keizer, *et al.*, On the significance of retinal vascular disease and hearing loss in facioscapulohumeral muscular dystrophy. *Muscle Nerve* **2** (1995), S73–S80.

17. M. T. Rogers, F. Zhao, P. S. Harper, D. Stephens, Absence of hearing impairment in adult onset facioscapulohumeral muscular dystrophy. *Neuromuscul. Disord.* **12** (2002), 358–365.

18. C. P. Trevisan, E. Pastorello, M. Ermani, *et al.*, Facioscapulohumeral muscular dystrophy: a multicenter study on hearing function. *Audiol. Neurotol.* **13** (2008), 1–8.

19. D. G. Balatsouras, S. Korres, P. Manta, A. Panousopoulou, D. Vassilopoulos, Cochlear function in facioscapulohumeral muscular dystrophy. *Otol. Neurotol.* **28** (2007), 7–10.

20. B. Weiffenbach, R. Bagley, K. Falls, *et al.*, Linkage analyses of five chromosome 4 markers localizes the facioscapulohumeral muscular dystrophy (FSHD) gene to distal 4q35. *Am. J. Hum. Genet.* **51** (1992), 416–423.

21. C. Wijmenga, G. W. Padberg, P. Moerer, *et al.*, Mapping of facioscapulohumeral muscular dystrophy gene to chromosome 4q35-qter by multipoint linkage analysis and in situ hybridization. *Genomics* **9** (1991), 570–575.

22. J. C. van Deutekom, C. Wijmenga, E. A. van Tienhoven, *et al.*, FSHD associated DNA rearrangements are due to deletions of integral copies of a 3.2 kb tandemly repeated unit. *Hum. Mol. Genet.* **2** (1993), 2037–2042.

23. S. M. van der Maarel, R. R. Frants, G. W. Padberg, Facioscapulohumeral muscular dystrophy. *Biochim. Biophys. Acta* **1772** (2007), 186–194.

24. R. Tawil, S. M. van der Maarel, Facioscapulohumeral muscular dystrophy. *Muscle Nerve* **34** (2006), 1–15.

25. E. Bakker, C. Wijmenga, R. H. Vossen, *et al.*, The FSHD-linked locus D4F104S1 (p13E-11) on 4q35 has a homologue on 10qter. *Muscle Nerve* **2** (1995), S39–S44.

26. G. Deidda, S. Cacurri, P. Grisanti, E. Vigneti, N. Piazzo, L. Felicetti, Physical mapping evidence for a duplicated region on chromosome 10qter showing high homology with the facioscapulohumeral muscular dystrophy locus on chromosome 4qter. *Eur. J. Hum. Genet.* **3** (1995), 155–167.

27. R. J. Lemmers, S. M. van der Maarel, J. C. van Deutekom, *et al.*, Inter- and intrachromosomal sub-telomeric rearrangements on 4q35: implications for facioscapulohumeral muscular dystrophy (FSHD) aetiology and diagnosis. *Hum. Mol. Genet.* **7** (1998), 1207–1214.

28. J. C. van Deutekom, R. J. Lemmers, P. K. Grewal, *et al.*, Identification of the first gene (FRG1) from the FSHD region on human chromosome 4q35. *Hum. Mol. Genet.* **5** (1996), 581–590.

29. P. G. van Overveld, R. J. Lemmers, G. Deidda, *et al.*, Interchromosomal repeat array interactions between chromosomes 4 and 10: a model for subtelomeric plasticity. *Hum. Mol. Genet.* **9** (2000), 2879–2884.

30. R. J. L. Lemmers, P. de Kievit, M. van Geel, *et al.*, Complete allele information in the diagnosis of facioscapulohumeral muscular dystrophy by triple DNA analysis. *Ann. Neurol.* **50** (2001), 816–819.

31. Y. Zhang, J. Forner, S. Fournet, M. Jeanpierre, Improved characterization of FSHD mutations. *Ann. Genet.* **44** (2001), 105–110.

32. M. van Geel, M. C. Dickson, A. F. Beck, *et al.*, Genomic analysis of human chromosome 10q and 4q telomeres suggests a common origin. *Genomics* **79** (2002), 210–217.

33. R. J. Lemmers, P. de Kievit, L. Sandkuijl, *et al.*, Facioscapulohumeral muscular dystrophy is uniquely associated with one of the two variants of the 4q subtelomere. *Nat. Genet.* **32** (2002), 235–236.

34. R. J. Lemmers, M. Wohlgemuth, R. R. Frants, G. W. Padberg, E. Morava, S. M. van der Maarel, Contractions of D4Z4 on 4qB subtelomeres do not cause facioscapulohumeral muscular dystrophy. *Am. J. Hum. Genet.* **75** (2004), 1124–1130.

35. N. S. Thomas, K. Wiseman, G. Spurlock, M. MacDonald, D. Ustek, M. Upadhyaya, A large patient study confirming that facioscapulohumeral muscular dystrophy (FSHD) disease expression is almost exclusively associated with an FSHD locus located on a 4qA-defined 4qter subtelomere. *J. Med. Genet.* **44** (2007), 215–218.

36. R. J. Lemmers, M. J. van der Wielen, E. Bakker, G. W. Padberg, R. R. Frants, S. M. van der Maarel, Somatic mosaicism in FSHD often goes undetected. *Ann. Neurol.* **55** (2004), 845–850.

37. M. M. Tonini, R. J. Lemmers, R. C. Pavanello, *et al.*, Equal proportions of affected cells in muscle and blood of a mosaic carrier of facioscapulohumeral muscular dystrophy. *Hum. Genet.* **119** (2006), 23–28.

38. K. L. Deak, R. J. Lemmers, J. M. Stajich, *et al.*, Genotype-phenotype study in an FSHD family with a proximal deletion encompassing p13E-11 and D4Z4. *Neurology* **68** (2007), 578–582.

39. R. J. Lemmers, M. Osborn, T. Haaf, *et al.*, D4F104S1 deletion in facioscapulohumeral muscular dystrophy: phenotype, size, and detection. *Neurology* **61** (2003), 178–183.

40. M. Ehrlich, K. Jackson, K. Tsumagari, P. Camano, R. J. Lemmers, Hybridization analysis of D4Z4 repeat arrays linked to FSHD. *Chromosoma* **116** (2007), 107–116.

41. V. Alexiadis, M. E. Ballestas, C. Sanchez, *et al.*, RNAPol-ChIP analysis of transcription from FSHD-linked tandem repeats and satellite DNA. *Biochim. Biophys. Acta* **1769** (2007), 29–40.

42. M. Dixit, E. Ansseau, A. Tassin, *et al.*, DUX4, a candidate gene of facioscapulohumeral muscular dystrophy, encodes a transcriptional activator of PITX1. *Proc. Natl. Acad. Sci. U. S. A.* **104**:46 (2007), 18157–18162.

43. V. Kowaljow, A. Marcowycz, E. Ansseau, *et al.*, The DUX4 gene at the FSHD1A locus encodes a pro-apoptotic protein. *Neuromuscul. Disord.* **17** (2007), 611–623.

44. J. Clapp, L. M. Mitchell, D. J. Bolland, *et al.*, Evolutionary conservation of a coding function for D4Z4, the tandem DNA repeat mutated in facioscapulohumeral muscular dystrophy. *Am. J. Hum. Genet.* **81** (2007), 264–279.

45. S. van Koningsbruggen, K. R. Straasheijm, E. Sterrenburg, *et al.*, FRG1P-mediated aggregation of proteins involved in pre-mRNA processing. *Chromosoma* **116** (2007), 53–64.

46. D. Gabellini, M. R. Green, R. Tupler, Inappropriate gene activation in FSHD: a repressor complex binds a chromosomal repeat deleted in dystrophic muscle. *Cell* **110** (2002), 339–348.

47. D. Gabellini, G. D'Antona, M. Moggio, *et al.*, Facioscapulohumeral muscular dystrophy in mice overexpressing FRG1. *Nature* **439** (2006), 973–977.

48. G. Jiang, F. Yang, P. G. van Overveld, V. Vedanarayanan, S. van der Maarel, M. Ehrlich, Testing the position-effect variegation hypothesis for facioscapulohumeral muscular dystrophy by analysis of histone modification and gene expression in subtelomeric 4q. *Hum. Mol. Genet.* **12** (2003), 2909–2921.

49. R. J. Osborne, S. Welle, S. L. Venance, C. A. Thornton, R. Tawil, Expression profile of FSHD supports a link between retinal vasculopathy and muscular dystrophy. *Neurology* **68** (2007), 569–577.

50. S. T. Winokur, Y. W. Chen, P. S. Masny, *et al.*, Expression profiling of FSHD muscle supports a defect in specific stages of myogenic differentiation. *Hum. Mol. Genet.* **12** (2003), 2895–2907.

51. P. S. Masny, U. Bengtsson, S. A. Chung, *et al.*, Localization of 4q35.2 to the nuclear periphery: is FSHD a nuclear envelope disease? *Hum. Mol. Genet.* **13** (2004), 1857–1871.

52. R. Tam, K. P. Smith, J. B. Lawrence, The 4q subtelomere harboring the FSHD locus is specifically anchored with peripheral heterochromatin unlike most human telomeres. *J. Cell Biol.* **167** (2004), 269–279.

53. M. Bakay, Z. Wang, G. Melcon, *et al.*, Nuclear envelope dystrophies show a transcriptional fingerprint suggesting disruption of Rb-MyoD pathways in muscle regeneration. *Brain* **129** (2006), 996–1013.

54. R. W. Orrell, R. Tawil, J. Forrester, J. T. Kissel, J. R. Mendell, D. A. Figlewicz, Definitive molecular diagnosis of facioscapulohumeral dystrophy. *Neurology* **52** (1999), 1822–1826.

55. P. W. Lunt, P. E. Jardine, M. C. Koch, *et al.*, Correlation between fragment size at D4F104S1 and age at onset or at wheelchair use, with a possible generational effect, accounts for much phenotypic variation in 4q35-facioscapulohumeral muscular dystrophy (FSHD). *Hum. Mol. Genet.* **4** (1995), 951–958.

56. E. Ricci, G. Galluzzi, G. Deidda, *et al.*, Progress in the molecular diagnosis of facioscapulohumeral muscular dystrophy and correlation between the number of KpnI repeats at the 4q35 locus and clinical phenotype. *Ann. Neurol.* **45** (1999), 751–757.

57. R. Tawil, J. Forrester, R. C. Griggs, *et al.*, Evidence for anticipation and association of deletion size with severity in facioscapulohumeral muscular dystrophy. The FSH-DY Group. *Ann. Neurol.* **39** (1996), 744–748.

58. S. M. van der Maarel, G. Deidda, R. J. Lemmers, *et al.*, De novo facioscapulohumeral muscular dystrophy: frequent somatic mosaicism, sex-dependent phenotype, and the role of mitotic transchromosomal repeat interaction between chromosomes 4 and 10. *Am. J. Hum. Genet.* **66** (2000), 26–35.

59. J. Kohler, B. Rupilius, M. Otto, K. Bathke, M. C. Koch, Germline mosaicism in 4q35 facioscapulohumeral muscular dystrophy (FSHD1A) occurring predominantly in oogenesis. *Hum. Genet.* **98** (1996), 485–490.

60. M. Upadhyaya, J. Maynard, M. Osborn, P. Jardine, P. S. Harper, P. Lunt, Germinal mosaicism in facioscapulohumeral muscular dystrophy (FSHD). *Muscle Nerve* **2** (1995), S45–S49.

61. M. Zatz, S. K. Marie, A. Cerqueira, M. Vainzof, R. C. Pavanello, M. R. Passos-Bueno, The facioscapulohumeral muscular dystrophy (FSHD1) gene affects males more severely and more frequently than females. *Am. J. Med. Genet.* **77** (1998), 155–161.

62. O. F. Brouwer, G. W. Padberg, C. Wijmenga, R. R. Frants, Facioscapulohumeral muscular dystrophy in early childhood. *Arch. Neurol.* **51** (1994), 387–394.

63. O. F. Brouwer, G. W. Padberg, E. Bakker, C. Wijmenga, R. R. Frants, Early onset facioscapulohumeral muscular dystrophy. *Muscle Nerve* **2** (1995), S67–S72.

64. M. Funakoshi, K. Goto, K. Arahata, Epilepsy and mental retardation in a subset of early onset 4q35-facioscapulohumeral muscular dystrophy. *Neurology* **50** (1998), 1791–1794.

65. L. Klinge, M. Eagle, I. D. Haggerty, C. E. Roberts, V. Straub, K. M. Bushby, Severe phenotype in infantile facioscapulohumeral muscular dystrophy. *Neuromuscul. Disord.* **16** (2006), 553–558.

66. L. A. Bindoff, N. Mjellem, K. Sommerfelt, *et al.*, Severe facioscapulohumeral muscular dystrophy presenting with Coats' disease and mental retardation. *Neuromuscul. Disord.* **16** (2006), 559–563.

67. M. Wohlgemuth, B. J. de Swart, J. G. Kalf, F. B. Joosten, A. M. Van der Vliet, G. W. Padberg, Dysphagia in facioscapulohumeral muscular dystrophy. *Neurology* **66** (2006), 1926–1928.

68. G. Yamanaka, K. Goto, T. Matsumura, *et al.*, Tongue atrophy in facioscapulohumeral muscular dystrophy. *Neurology* **57** (2001), 733–735.

69. J. C. van Deutekom, E. Bakker, R. J. Lemmers, *et al.*, Evidence for subtelomeric exchange of 3.3 kb tandemly repeated units between chromosomes 4q35 and 10q26: implications for genetic counselling and etiology of FSHD1. *Hum. Mol. Genet.* **5** (1996), 1997–2003.

70. K. M. Bushby, C. Pollitt, M. A. Johnson, M. T. Rogers, P. F. Chinnery, Muscle pain as a prominent feature of facioscapulohumeral muscular dystrophy (FSHD): four illustrative case reports. *Neuromuscul. Disord.* **8** (1998), 574–579.

71. E. L. van der Kooi, O. J. Vogels, R. J. van Asseldonk, *et al.*, Strength training and albuterol in facioscapulohumeral muscular dystrophy. *Neurology* **63** (2004), 702–708.

72. E. L. van der Kooi, J. S. Kalkman, E. Lindeman, *et al.*, Effects of training and albuterol on pain and fatigue in facioscapulohumeral muscular dystrophy. *J. Neurol.* **254** (2007), 931–940.

73. C. T. Andrews, T. C. Taylor, V. H. Patterson, Scapulothoracic arthrodesis for patients with facioscapulohumeral muscular dystrophy. *Neuromuscul. Disord.* **8** (1998), 580–584.

74. W. H. Bunch, I. M. Siegel, Scapulothoracic arthrodesis in facioscapulohumeral muscular dystrophy. Review of seventeen procedures with three to twenty-one-year follow-up. *J. Bone Joint Surg. Am.* **75** (1993), 372–376.

75. S. Giannini, F. Ceccarelli, C. Faldini, S. Pagkrati, L. Merlini, Scapulopexy of winged scapula secondary to facioscapulohumeral muscular dystrophy. *Clin. Orthop. Relat. Res.* **449** (2006), 288–294.

76. S. G. Krishnan, R. J. Hawkins, J. D. Michelotti, R. Litchfield, R. B. Willis, Y. K. Kim, Scapulothoracic arthrodesis: indications, technique, and results. *Clin. Orthop. Relat. Res.* June **435** (2005), 126–133.

77. Y. G. Rhee, J. H. Ha, Long-term results of scapulothoracic arthrodesis of facioscapulohumeral muscular dystrophy. *J. Shoulder Elbow Surg.* **15** (2006), 445–450.

78. C. J. Mummery, S. A. Copeland, M. R. Rose, Scapular fixation in muscular dystrophy. *Cochrane Database Syst. Rev.* CD003278 (2003).

79. C. L. Shields, J. Zahler, N. Falk, *et al.*, Neovascular glaucoma from advanced Coats disease as the initial manifestation of facioscapulohumeral dystrophy in a 2-year-old child. *Arch. Ophthalmol.* **125** (2007), 840–842.

80. M. R. Rose, R. Tawil, Drug treatment for facioscapulohumeral muscular dystrophy. *Cochrane Database Syst. Rev.* CD002276 (2004).

81. R. Tawil, M. P. McDermott, S. Pandya, *et al.*, A pilot trial of prednisone in facioscapulohumeral muscular dystrophy. FSH-DY Group. *Neurology* **48** (1997), 46–49.

82. J. T. Kissel, M. P. McDermott, J. R. Mendell, *et al.*, Randomized, double-blind, placebo-controlled trial of albuterol in facioscapulohumeral dystrophy. *Neurology* **57** (2001), 1434–1440.

83. B. H. Elsheikh, E. Bollman, M. Peruggia, W. King, G. Galloway, J. T. Kissel, Pilot trial of diltiazem in facioscapulohumeral muscular dystrophy. *Neurology* **68** (2007), 1428–1429.

84. P. G. van Overveld, R. J. Lemmers, L. A. Sandkuijl, *et al.*, Hypomethylation of D4Z4 in 4q-linked and non-4q-linked facioscapulohumeral muscular dystrophy. *Nat. Genet.* **35** (2003), 315–317.

85. E. L. van der Kooi, J. C. de Greef, M. Wohlgemuth, *et al.*, No effect of folic acid and methionine supplementation on D4Z4 methylation in patients with facioscapulohumeral muscular dystrophy. *Neuromuscul. Disord.* **16** (2006), 766–769.

86. E. Bakker, M. J. Van der Wielen, E. Voorhoeve, *et al.*, Diagnostic, predictive, and prenatal testing for facioscapulohumeral muscular dystrophy: diagnostic approach for sporadic and familial cases. *J. Med. Genet.* **33** (1996), 29–35.

87. M. Upadhyaya, M. MacDonald, D. Ravine, Prenatal diagnosis for facioscapulohumeral muscular dystrophy (FSHD). *Prenat. Diagn.* **19** (1999), 959–965.

88. E. Ciafaloni, E. K. Pressman, A. M. Loi, *et al.*, Pregnancy and birth outcomes in women with facioscapulohumeral muscular dystrophy. *Neurology* **67** (2006), 1887–1889.

89. K. R. Wagner, V. L. Fleckenstein, A. A. Amato, *et al.*, A phase I/II trial of MYO-029 in adult subjects with muscular dystrophy. *Ann. Neurol.* **62** (2008), 561–571.

Chapter 16

Distal myopathies

Bjarne Udd

Definition and basis for classification

Distal myopathies are primary muscle disorders defined by onset of weakness in hands or feet usually followed by atrophy in muscles of the lower legs, forearm, feet or hands. Because all of the currently determined entities are progressive hereditary diseases with loss of muscle tissue replaced by fat and connective tissue, the distal myopathies are in fact muscular dystrophies. However, by tradition distal myopathy has remained the main collective term.

Distal myopathies are less frequent than proximal muscular dystrophies. However, as recent developments have shown, they have been underdiagnosed in the past. The previous edition of this corresponding chapter listed six entities in the group of distal myopathies. The number of defined entities has meanwhile increased almost threefold and the diversity of different entities for the clinician to consider has enlarged correspondingly. All of the entities detailed here have a molecular genetic definition and most of them are identified by gene and protein defect (Table 16.1). Older reports exist that are not further covered, even if some of these may represent separate entities [1, 2, 3, 4, 5, 6, 7, 8, 9, 10]. Myopathies that frequently show a distal phenotype but have been described by other terms are tabulated only (Table 16.2).

Why then do some dystrophic processes cause distal muscles to be preferentially involved? In some of the distal myopathies the high degree of distal selectivity may prevail throughout the lifetime. The reasons for the distal predilection are not clarified but there is a striking difference concerning the distribution of muscle proteins involved: while the more frequent proximal dystrophies often involve sarcolemmal proteins, the defective proteins causing distal myopathies are more often found in the sarcomere (Figure 16.1) [11].

Historically the first description of a distal myopathy patient is attributed to Gowers in 1902 [12]. However, there were reports even earlier and neither Gowers' patient nor the others can be proven to have had primary myopathies. The first published distal myopathy family later proven to be so is the large European-US family reported by Milhorat and Wolff in 1943 [13]. The disease was shown to be caused by a mutation in desmin 56 years later [14].

Previously the classification of distal myopathies relied on clinical and genetic findings of the different entities. These classifications have now been replaced by molecular genetic designations. However, grouping according to age of onset and inheritance pattern is still of some use because the further molecular genetic diagnostics can be directed based on these features (Table 16.1).

Welander distal myopathy (WDM)

Long before molecular genetics emerged Welander proved the existence of a true distal myopathy with her report on a large cohort of Swedish patients [15].

Salient diagnostic criteria

If no Scandinavian ancestry is present, the diagnosis remains possible if the clinical phenotype is present in dominant families, and probable where it is possible to show linkage to the established locus on chromosome 2p13. In Scandinavian patients molecular genetics is partly applicable in the diagnosis of Welander myopathy despite the lack of an exact gene defect. Because the large Scandinavian patient population shows one unique founder haplotype [16], genotyping of this haplotype can be used for diagnosis, particularly if family material is available.

Molecular genetics and pathogenesis

The autosomal dominant disease is linked to a locus on chromosome 2p13 [16]. Ever since linkage was established the search for the gene defect has continued. The region of interest is 1 Mb in size and lies just centromeric but outside the locus of the *dysferlin* gene. All genes in the linkage region have been sequenced without apparent mutations found (unpublished, Udd).

Salient clinical phenotypical features

The WDM phenotype is characteristic with very late onset between the ages of 40 and 60 years [15, 17]. In most cases

Disorders of Voluntary Muscle, 8th edn., eds. George Karpati, David Hilton-Jones, Kate Bushby and Robert C. Griggs. Published by Cambridge University Press.

Table 16.1. Molecularly defined distal myopathies

Description	Type	Reference/ OMIM #	Locus/Gene	Onset (age)	Early symptoms	CK	Pathology
Autosomal dominant distal myopathies	Welander myopathy	Welander [15]/604454	2p13	>40	Hands, finger extensors	1–3×	Dystrophic, rimmed vacuoles
	Tibial muscular dystrophy (Udd myopathy)	Udd *et al.* [20]/600334	2q31/titin	>35	Anterior lower leg	1–4×	Dystrophic, rimmed vacuoles in tibial anterior muscle
	Zaspopathy	Markesbery *et al.* [31]	10q22/ZASP	40–50	Clinically anterior but posterior lower leg on muscle imaging	1–4×	Myofibrillar myopathy, dystrophic, rimmed and nonrimmed vacuoles
	Myotilinopathy	Penisson-Besnier *et al.* [47]/609200	5q31/myotilin	50–60	Posterior more than anterior distal leg	13×	Myofibrillar myopathy, dystrophic, rimmed and nonrimmed vacuoles
	Desmin-related myopathy	Vicart [98]/608810	11q22/ B-crystallin	Variable	Distal leg and hands, cataracts, cardiomyopathy	1–3×	Myofibrillar myopathy, dystrophic, rimmed vacuoles
	Desminopathy	Milhorat and Wolf [13]/601419	2q35/Desmin	Variable	Distal lower leg weakness, respiratory, cardiomyopathy	1–4×	Myofibrillar myopathy, dystrophic, rimmed vacuoles
	Laing myopathy (MPD1)	Laing *et al.* [54]/ 160500	14q11.2/ beta-myosin MYH7	3–25	Anterior lower leg	1–3×	Mild to moderate dystrophic, fiber-type disproportion in proximal muscle
	Vocal cord and pharyngeal VCPDM (MPD2)	Feit *et al.* [89]/ 606070	5q31.2/Matrin 3	35–60	Anterior lower legs and hands, dysphonia	1–3x	Rimmed vacuoles
	Distal neuromyopathy	Servidei *et al.* [95]/601846	19p13	15–50	Anterior and posterior lower leg, dysphonia + dysphagia	2–6×	Rimmed vacuoles
	Adult distal myopathy (MPD3)	Mahjneh *et al.* [92]/610099	Both 8p–q and 12q linked	>30	Hands or lower legs	1–4×	Dystrophic, rimmed vacuoles + eosinophilic inclusions
	Distal myopathy with respiratory failure	Chinnery *et al.* [97]/607569	Linkage to all known loci excluded	32–75	Anterior lower leg in most, and proximal in some	1–2×	Dystrophic, rimmed vacuoles + eosinophilic inclusions, myofibrillar myopathy
	Early adult distal myopathy	Williams *et al.* [94]	Linkage to all known loci excluded	20–40	Hand grip, posterior and lateral compartment of lower legs	1–2×	Myopathic
Autosomal recessive distal myopathies	Nonaka myopathy	Nonaka *et al.* [62] 605820	9p12–p11/GNE	15–30	Anterior lower leg	3–4×	Dystrophic, prominent rimmed vacuoles
	Miyoshi myopathy	Liu [76]/254130	2p13/Dysferlin	15–30	Posterior lower leg, calf	20–150×	Dystrophic, dysferlin defect
	Distal nebulin myopathy	Wallgren-Pettersson *et al.* [88]	2q22/Nebulin	1–20	Anterior lower leg	1–3x	Myopathic, group atrophy, no rods on light microscopy

the first symptom is weakness of the index finger extension, followed by weakness of the other fingers (Figure 16.2). Later moderate to severe muscle atrophy of thenar and hand muscles appears together with weakness of finger flexors [15]. In about one-third of patients the disease may start in the lower legs with ankle dorsiflexion weakness, not infrequently asymmetrical. Proximal muscles are usually not involved to a degree that would cause clinical disability regarding ambulation [15]. The most disabling weakness late in the course is that of the hands with corresponding problems for activities of daily living

Table 16.2. Other myopathies frequently presenting with distal phenotype

1. VCP mutated (scapulo-)peroneal syndromes
2. FSHD
3. Dynamin2-mutated centronuclear myopathy
4. Myotonic dystrophy type 1
5. Telethoninopathy
6. Branching and de-branching glycogenoses
7. Caveolinopathy
8. Oculopharyngodistal myopathy
9. Nemaline myopathy
10. Sporadic inclusion body myositis (s-IBM)

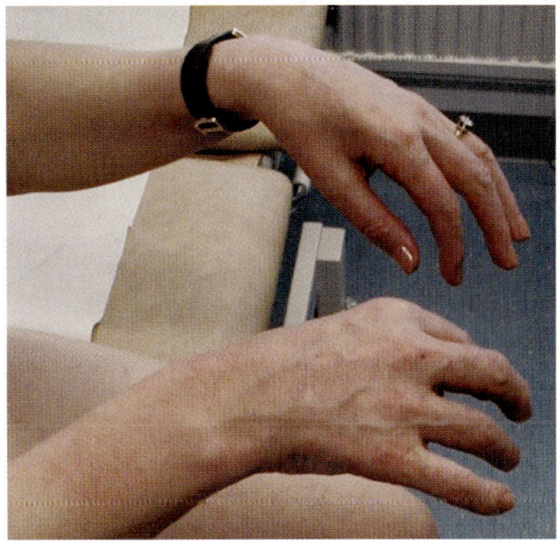

Figure 16.2. Hands of a 55-year-old woman with Welander distal myopathy showing weakness of finger extension most prominent in index fingers and atrophy of interossei, thenar, and hypothenar muscles.

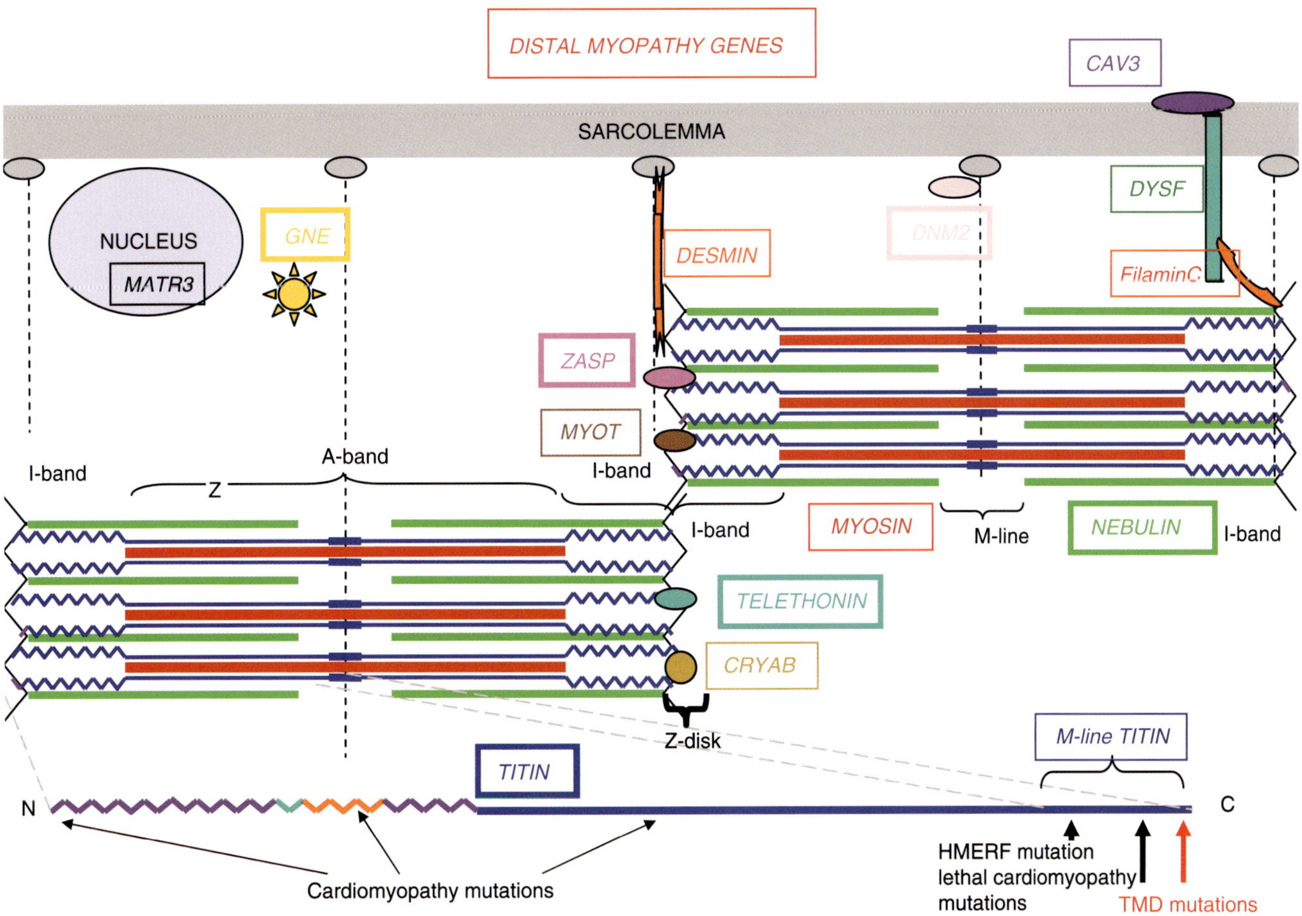

Figure 16.1. Schematic drawing of the muscle cell sarcomeres indicating the location of proteins known to cause distal myopathy when defective.

(ADL). Facial weakness, respiratory or dysphagia problems have not been reported. Tendon reflexes are preserved except for ankle reflexes, which may be lost later in the disease. Sensory system clinical examination is usually normal. The progression of disease is typically slow, and most patients continue full activities and have a normal life span. Cardiomyopathy does not occur. Rare homozygous patients have more severe disease with early age at onset, proximal muscle weakness, and wheelchair dependency [18].

Diagnostic approaches

Serum creatine kinase (CK) level is normal or twofold to threefold elevated. Needle electromyography (EMG) reveals small, brief motor unit potentials with early recruitment. Fibrillations and complex repetitive discharges may occur [17]. Although routine nerve conduction studies are normal, mild abnormalities in sural nerve biopsies and deficits in vibration and temperature examination by quantitative sensory testing suggest underlying asymptomatic, length-dependent, predominantly sensory small-fiber neuropathy [17].

Imaging

Muscle imaging of lower leg muscles always shows fatty degenerative involvement of the posterior and inconsistently of the anterior compartment muscles, frequently with considerable asymmetry (Figure 16.3) [19]. Proximal muscles in the thigh and pelvic region are usually not involved. Imaging of forearm muscles shows atrophy without as much replacement change.

Pathology

Muscle biopsy shows dystrophic features with fiber size variability, increase in connective and fat tissue, central nuclei, and split fibers. Rimmed vacuoles and 15- to 18-nm cytoplasmic and nuclear filaments are seen in patients with moderate to severe weakness [17]. Absence of inflammation helps distinguish Welander myopathy from inclusion body myositis.

Mutational analysis

As indicated above no gene has yet been identified and no general molecular diagnosis is available, except for patients of Scandinavian origin in whom screening for the founder haplotype can be done.

Therapeutic and preventative modalities

Patients usually manage with their disease when provided with practical measures to overcome finger and hand weakness with the help of the occupational and physical therapists. Orthoses for severe footdrop may also be needed.

Genetic counseling

When linkage is established with the known Scandinavian founder haplotype, family members can be offered genetic counseling on the basis of molecular testing. Presymptomatic and prenatal testing procedures are not indicated.

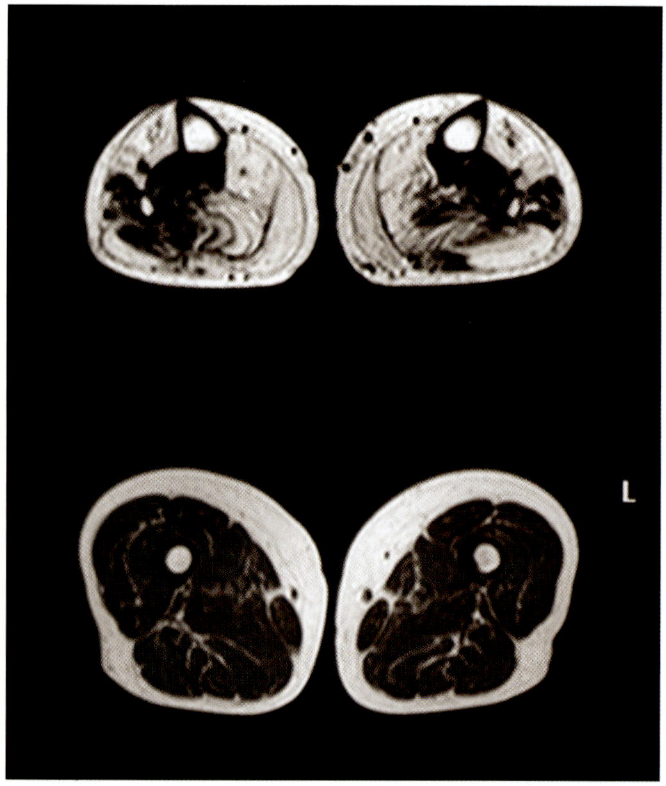

Figure 16.3. MRI scans of lower leg and thigh muscles in an advanced form of Welander distal myopathy in a 74-year-old woman showing severe fatty degeneration of posterior calf muscles, soleus and lateral gastrocnemius, as well as of anterior compartment muscles. In contrast the proximal thigh muscles show no abnormality for the age.

Future perspectives

The next step is identify the responsible gene.

Tibial muscular dystrophy (TMD, OMIM #600334 Udd myopathy)

Tibial muscular dystrophy (TMD) was first described in Finnish patients [20], and has since been identified in various European populations and in North America, both in descendants of Finnish immigrants as well in families with other separate mutations [21, 22, 23]. The prevalence of TMD is very high, over 10/100 000, in Finland where it is the most common muscle disease [24].

Salient diagnostic criteria

The final key for diagnosis relies on molecular genetic verification of the disease-causing mutation in C-terminal titin. In new, unrelated TMD patients, searching for mutations by sequencing the last titin exons may be productive.

Molecular genetics and pathogenesis

Tibial muscular dystrophy is caused by mutations in C-terminal titin physically located in the M-line of the sarcomere.

All Finnish patients carry one common founder mutation (FINmaj), a complex 11-bp deletion–insertion mutation changing four amino acids without frameshift [25]. A point mutation changing a lysine to proline was found in French families in the same last exon 363 (Mex6) of titin [25]. A third point mutation in the same exon 363 has been described in a Belgian TMD family [22], and more recently three other mutations in the last exon 363 and second last exon 362 (Mex5) have been identified in Spanish and other French families [23]. Mutant titin is transcribed, translated, and incorporated into the sarcomere. However, the mutations alter the protein over a larger C-terminal portion than the specific domains harboring the mutations. Since C-terminal antibodies for the last three domains do not recognize their epitopes at all the C-terminus may be completely cleaved off [11].

Titin is the third most abundant protein after myosin and actin in the muscle and makes the third filament system of the sarcomere. Titin binds, among other proteins, calpain-3 in the N2A-line of I-band titin and in its C-terminus. The role of calpain-3 in TMD is unsettled, but homozygously inherited C-terminal titin mutations cause a completely different severe limb-girdle muscular dystrophy (LGMD) phenotype with marked secondary calpain-3 deficiency [26]. Since this phenotype segregates in a recessive fashion, it has been designated LGMD2J [27]. In primary calpain-3 defect, LGMD2A, perturbations of IκBα/NF-κB pathway and apoptotic myonuclei have been observed [28]. In TMD/LGMD2J similar changes with clusters of apoptotic myonuclei were also found, suggesting similar molecular pathology [26]. The titin C-terminus contains motifs for signaling, and a catalytic kinase domain with interacting signaling molecules is physically very close to the ultimate c-terminus with mutations causing TMD [29].

Salient clinical phenotypical features

Symptoms in TMD present after age 35 with weakness in ankle dorsiflexion and later visible atrophy of anterior compartment lower leg muscles (Figure 16.4) [20]. At onset symptoms and signs may be asymmetrical. Progression is slow; 10–15 years after onset long toe extensors also become weak and there is a moderate footdrop. After age 70 one-third of patients have proximal weakness in lower extremities, but only rarely become wheelchair-bound even late in life [20]. Sparing of short toe extensors (extensor digitorum brevis) is a significant clinical finding and hand muscles are rarely affected.

Genotype–phenotype correlations

The common TMD phenotype is fairly stereotyped but a recent study of 207 mutation-confirmed patients with the one identical FINmaj mutation showed considerable phenotype variations in 9% of the patients [27]. This variation has no further explanation but other genetic or exogenic modifying factors need to be involved to account for the different outcome. The completely different LGMD2J phenotype without cardiomyopathy seen in homozygotes is unusual and not clarified at the molecular level, but an additional loss-of-function mechanism starting earlier than the dominant gain-of-function caused by heterozygosity is implied. The secondary loss of calpain-3 explicitly in these homozygous patients is one possible mechanism to account for the early-onset loss-of-function mechanism. The recently evaluated frameshift mutation in the second last exon 362 (Mex5) is of interest as it is associated with a clearly more severe TMD phenotype [23]. The muscles preferentially involved are the same but onset is earlier, after age 20, and progression to proximal muscles is earlier and more severe. This indicates that the complete loss of the last domain of the protein causes a more severe phenotype than amino acid changes or truncations within the last domain. Of interest are the recently reported truncating mutations further upstream in titin exons 360 and 358. Children homozygous for this develop lethal cardiomyopathy with severe generalized skeletal myopathy, but the heterozygote parents are unaffected carriers [30].

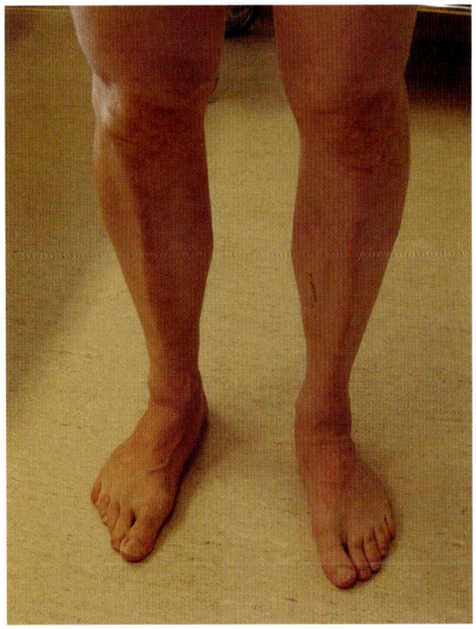

Figure 16.4. Lower legs of a 50-year-old man with tibial muscular dystrophy (Udd distal myopathy) and symptoms of ankle dorsiflexion weakness for 10 years and moderate footdrop on both legs.

Diagnostic approaches

Serum CK is normal or mildly elevated. In affected muscles EMG shows low-amplitude, short-duration motor unit potentials on moderate activity, frequent fibrillation potentials, and occasional high-frequency and complex repetitive discharges. In unaffected upper limbs polyphasic potentials may be recorded [20].

Imaging

Computer tomography (CT) and magnetic resonance (MRI) imaging show fatty degeneration at the time of clinical weakness in the anterior tibial muscles. Later lesions appear in the long toe extensor muscles, and in hamstring muscles. Clinically

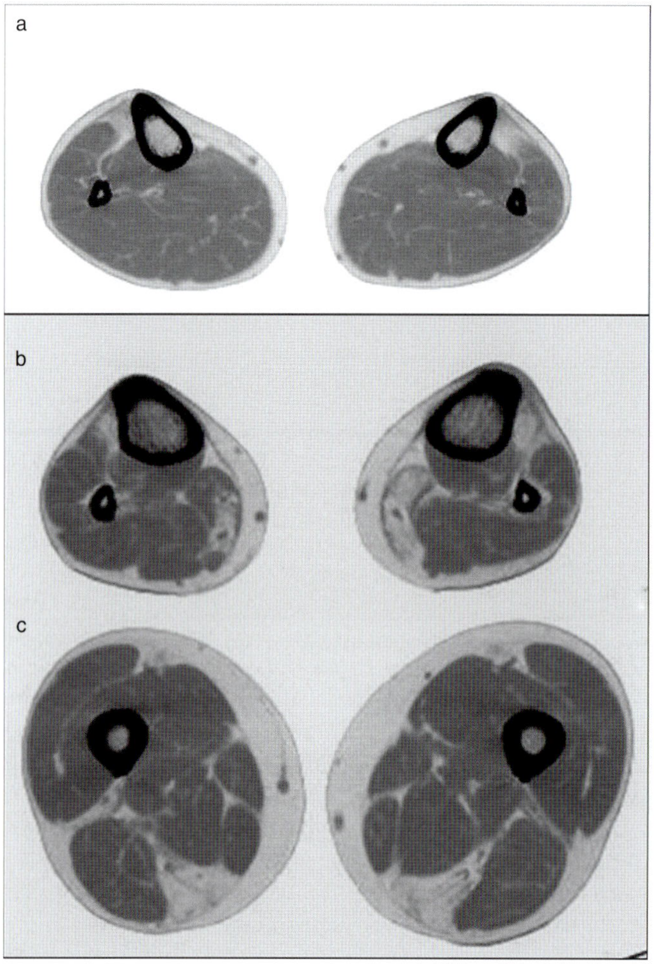

Figure 16.5a–c. CT scans (inverted) of lower legs in (a) a 45-year-old TMD male patient showing selective fatty degeneration of tibialis anterior muscle on both sides, and in a 57-year-old TMD male patient (b) with slightly more severe disease showing involvement of medial gastrocnemius muscles as well as tibialis anterior lesions. In the same patient scans of thigh muscles (c) reveal involvement of hamstring muscles usually appearing at later age points.

inapparent focal lesions may occur in soleus and medial gastrocnemius (Figure 16.5). The pattern of involvement is different in the aberrant phenotypes [27].

Pathology

Muscle pathology includes variation of fiber size, thin atrophic fibers, central nuclei, structural changes within the fibers, endomysial fibrosis, usually rimmed vacuoles in the tibial anterior, and fatty replacement in the end-stage muscle. Necrotic fibers, some showing phagocytosis, are rare in TMD. Both major fiber types are equally involved in the pathological process [20]. There were no neurogenic findings. Many rimmed vacuoles were acid phosphatase positive, while others were ubiquitin positive and, with rare exceptions, they were not lined by sarcolemmal membrane proteins. Congo red stains and immunohistochemistry for beta-amyloid and amyloid precursor protein remained negative in contrast to hereditary inclusion body myopathy (HIBM). Ultrastructural studies in TMD revealed overall well-preserved sarcomere structure, even in the homozygote LGMD2J mutants [27]. Autophagy and occasional tubulofilamentous inclusions were encountered in the vacuolated fibers.

Mutational analysis

The current diagnostic procedure in patients of Finnish descent is direct DNA testing of the founder mutation (FINmaj). In patients without Scandinavian background the direct sequencing of the two to three last exons of titin is necessary.

Therapeutic and preventative modalities

The life expectancy of TMD patients is not diminished and patients usually manage with their disease when provided with practical measures to overcome ankle dorsiflexion weakness and later footdrop, first with the help of orthoses. If footdrop is severe a surgical procedure of transposition of the posterior tibial tendon to the anterior insertion on the foot has been applied successfully.

Genetic counseling

After diagnosis is clarified by DNA methods genetic counseling is recommended. However, because of the mild phenotype, no presymptomatic or prenatal testing procedures are indicated.

Future perspectives

Clarification of the molecular pathogenesis in TMD is of scientific and practical interest. In populations with a high frequency of heterozygotes children with new severe LGMD2J will be born for whom currently no curative therapy is available. Since C-terminal titin is important for signaling functions and there is a lack of information essential to our understanding of muscle protein turnover regulation and rapid adaptation to large variations in physical demand, the investigation of C-terminal titin mutations is of great general interest.

ZASPopathy

The classic textbook example of distal myopathy, besides WDM, is a large family described in the USA in the 1970s [31]. This family was long thought to be associated with titinopathy because of early indications of linkage to the titin locus [32]. However, the pathology was more myofibrillar myopathy and titin was not the causative gene. Instead, mutations in ZASP have recently been identified as being responsible for the disease in this classic distal myopathy family and in many other families of European descent [33]. The other genes known to cause myofibrillar myopathy can, besides distal myopathy [34], also cause other phenotypes, but so far the only clinical presentation of ZASP mutations is the distal phenotype (see Chapter 25).

Salient diagnostic criteria

The combination of late-onset dominant distal myopathy and muscle pathology indicative of myofibrillar myopathy should lead directly to molecular genetic DNA testing for mutations in ZASP and myotilin. However, because of the very late onset in some patients the familial dominant inheritance may be missed and patients seem to be sporadic.

Molecular genetics and pathogenesis

Two mutations in exon 6 of the ZASP gene (Z-disk alternatively spliced PDZ-domain containing protein, also termed *LDB3* gene) associated with this type of distal myopathy are frequently recurring [33, 35]. The causative A165V mutation in the Markesbery–Griggs family was shown to be an ancient European founder mutation based on a relatively short common haplotype around the mutation in six unrelated families tested [33]. The other recurring ZASP mutation, A147T, causes an identical phenotype.

ZASP is an integrated protein of the Z-disk with direct binding to α-actinin, ALP, and FATZ protein [36, 37]. Interactions were also shown with nebulette and protein kinase C [38]. All members of the PDZ/LIM family of proteins are also involved in actin dynamics [38]. What exactly goes wrong due to the mutations in exon 6 is not known, but this region of the protein is important for skeletal-muscle-specific isoforms and it contains the conserved ZM-domain needed for α-actinin binding [36]. Interestingly, our evaluation of myofibrillar protein aggregations revealed that all the other proteins in this group, i.e., myotilin, αB-crystallin, and desmin, show more aggregation than ZASP itself [33]. This indicates a ruler-organizing function of ZASP that, when defective, leads to more abnormal aggregations of these other myofibrillar proteins. This is supported by the fact that ZASP knockout mice have a severe phenotype whereas myotilin knockout mice have a mild phenotype [39].

Salient clinical phenotypical features

This late-onset, dominantly inherited distal myopathy has been identified in families of English, French, and German descent. Symptoms usually begin after age 40 years with ankle weakness causing tripping [33]. As the disease progresses lower legs become atrophic with mild footdrop as the leading sign even if posterior calf muscles are more severely involved. Finger and wrist extensors will follow and, later in life, moderate proximal weakness usually occurs. Occasionally the disease may progress rapidly after onset. The ability to walk can be lost after 15 or 20 years of disease, progressing to complete incapacity some 30 years after onset [33]. One patient in the index family had cardiomyopathy with heart block requiring a pacemaker [31]. Facial, bulbar, and respiratory muscles are not affected.

Genotype–phenotype correlations

So far only two recurrent mutations are known, A165V and A147T, which are located in the same functional domain encoded by exon 6, and also cause identical phenotypes. There is a third mutation reported in exon 9 but until this has been verified in familial material no further conclusions can be made. Mutations in other parts of ZASP are known to cause cardiomyopathy without reported skeletal myopathy [40].

Diagnostic approaches

Serum CK levels can be normal or threefold to fourfold elevated. EMG reveals small, brief-duration motor-unit potentials with early recruitment in affected muscles [31].

Imaging

At onset of the disease muscle imaging shows early changes in the posterior compartment of the lower legs with preference for soleus and medial gastrocnemius (Figure 16.6). Later changes include severe involvement of all lower leg muscles and moderate involvement in proximal leg muscles [33].

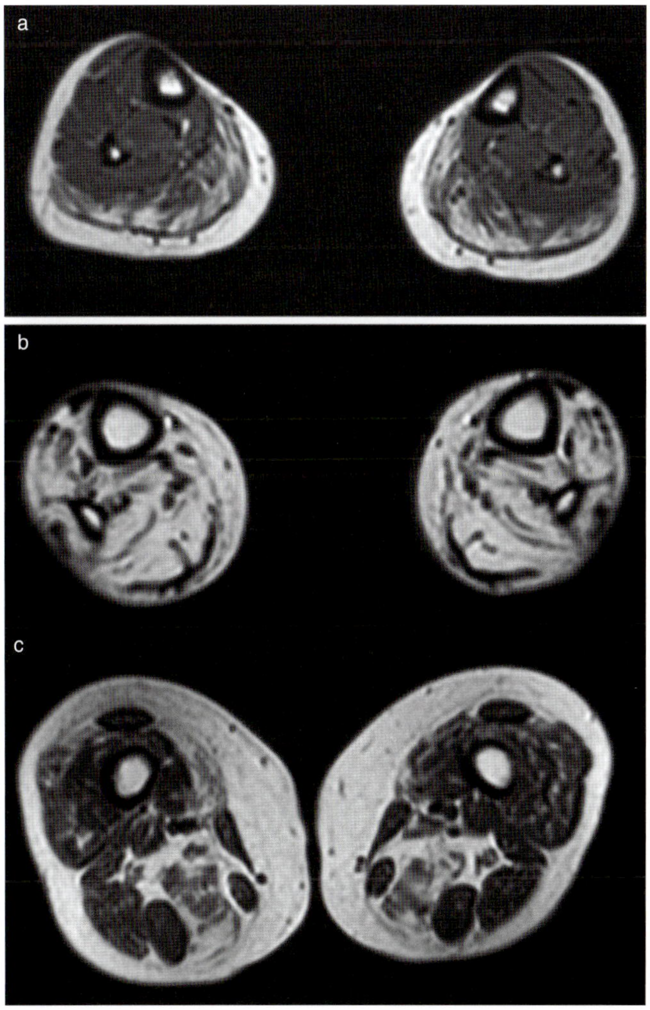

Figure 16.6a–c. MRI scans of lower legs in a 52-year-old ZASPopathy woman at onset of the disease with minimal symptoms of ankle instability and no findings of muscle weakness (a) showing early fatty degeneration of posterior soleus muscle, and scans of a 74-year-old woman with ZASPopathy at an advanced stage showing involvement of all lower leg muscles (b) and less severe lesions proximally in quadriceps and hamstrings (c).

a

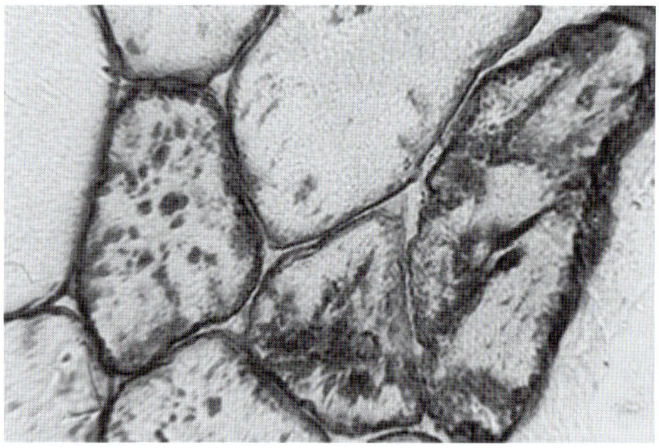

b

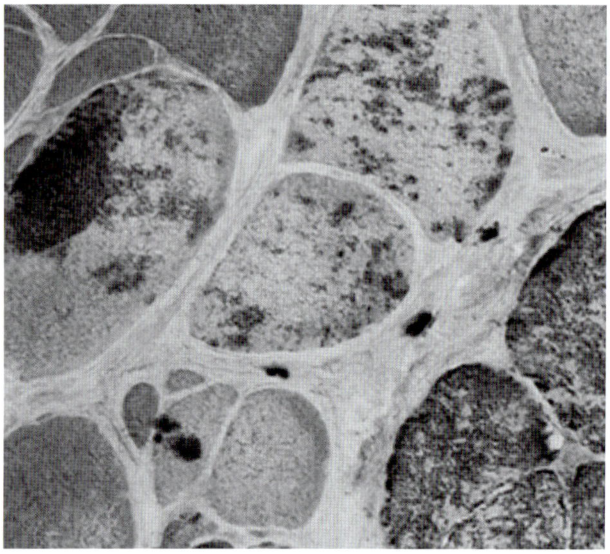

Figure 16.7a, b. Dystrophin and myotilin immunohistochemistry in a ZASP-opathy frozen muscle section showing ectopic cytoplasmic expression of dystrophin (a) and variable accumulations as larger areas or irregular distributions of myotilin (b) in the abnormal muscle fibers.

Pathology

Muscle biopsy shows prominent myofibrillar myopathy changes with dark material on Gömöri trichrome (GTC) staining in addition to hyaline parts and large vacuolations, both rimmed and non-rimmed. Immunohistochemical stains for desmin, myotilin, and αB-crystallin reveal abnormal cytoplasmic aggregations corresponding to the dark GTC regions and these also reveal ectopic dystrophin expression (Figure 16.7) [33]. Ultrastructural studies were extensive in the index family in the 1970s showing a wide range of myofibrillar disorganization, accumulating granulomatous material, and vast degradative features [41]. Immunoblots for the ZASP and the other myofibrillar proteins show no changes specific for the ZASPopathy [33].

Mutational analysis

As indicated above the clinical and pathology phenotype together should be indicative of either ZASPopathy or myotilinopathy. Currently, no specific finding can clearly make a distinction between these two. On the other hand first-line molecular genetics can be restricted to two exons in both genes, and if nothing is found in the first gene the lab should know to proceed to the second gene.

Therapeutic and preventative modalities

Patients usually manage with their disease when provided with practical measures to overcome ankle, finger, and hand weakness with the help of the occupational and physical therapists. Orthoses for severe footdrop may also be needed.

Genetic counseling

After diagnosis is clarified by DNA methods genetic counseling is recommended. No presymptomatic or prenatal testing procedures are warranted.

Future perspectives

The ruling-organizing role of ZASP in the Z-disk needs further clarification in order to elucidate how mutated ZASP can cause myotilin, CRYAB, and desmin to aggregate. Knowing the mechanism may open avenues for therapeutic intervention.

Distal myotilinopathy

Mutations in myotilin were first identified in families with a proximal phenotype, autosomal dominant LGMD1A [42]. Work on the genetic background of the morphological category of myofibrillar myopathy revealed that 10% of patients with this pathology in fact had mutations in myotilin (see Chapter 25) [43]. More recently the dominant myopathy called spheroid body myopathy [44] also proved to be caused by mutations in the myotilin gene [45]. The later experience has shown that the most common phenotype with myotilinopathy is the late-onset distal myopathy [46]. The first family with late-onset distal myopathy later shown to be a myotilinopathy was described in France [47].

Salient diagnostic criteria

Recognition requires molecular genetic diagnosis. The clinical phenotype of distal myotilinopathy may be indistinguishable from that of ZASPopathy. The combination of late-onset dominant distal myopathy and muscle pathology findings indicating myofibrillar myopathy should direct the clinician towards molecular genetic investigations to clarify MYOT and ZASP in the first place. However, because of the very late onset in some patients the familial dominant inheritance may be missed and patients seem to be sporadic.

Molecular genetics and pathogenesis

Almost all reported mutations in myotilin (myofibrillar protein with titin-like Ig domains) are dominant missense mutations located in the serine-rich second domain (residues 28–124), no matter what the clinical phenotype. Mutations most often involve serine and threonine residues. In our own cohort of late-onset distal myopathy patients we have observed recurrence of the mutations S60F and S60C. Myotilin is a 57-kDa Z-disk component that interacts with α-actinin [48], filamin-C, FATZ [49], and actin [50]. It also controls sarcomere assembly [51]. The α-actinin binding site resides between myotilin residues 79 and 150, and the filamin-C binding site is located in the second Ig-like domain. Myotilin dimerizes via its C-terminal half, which may be necessary for the actin-bundling activity. Myotilin is strongly expressed in skeletal muscle and weakly in cardiac muscle [50]. Intramuscular nerve fibers show myotilin expression [51].

Salient clinical phenotypical features

Onset can be very late, even after age 60. Atrophy of calf muscles can be the first sign even before subjective symptoms of weakness, but in many patients the fatty replacement masks the atrophy [47]. Despite more posterior than anterior involvement of lower legs, in some families the first symptom was loss of ankle dorsiflexion followed by plantar flexion weakness, but in others weakness and atrophy of calf muscles was the prominent finding after a period of pain and cramps [47, 52]. Involvement of upper limbs or proximal leg muscles was moderate or severe at later stages. Progression of muscle weakness can be fairly severe with considerable disability 10 years after onset. Dysphonia or respiratory defect is usually not part of the distal phenotype. Ankle reflexes are usually lost because of the calf involvement. Mild late cardiomyopathy may occur [43].

Genotype–phenotype correlations

Numerous families with late-onset distal myopathy have mutations in different serine or threonine residues in exon 2 [43, 46, 52]. The S55F mutation found in one of the two published LGMD1A families with early onset is also known to cause late-onset distal myopathy. The reason for the phenotype variation is not known. The previously described spheroid body myopathy family had a slightly more N-terminal mutation, S39F [45], than usually seen in most distal families. Mechanistic explanation for the slightly different pathology is lacking but patients with spheroid body myopathy also had distal weakness.

Diagnostic approaches

Serum CK levels range from normal to less than twofold elevated. EMG shows myopathic changes with fibrillations and complex repetitive discharges. Neurogenic components and mild neuropathy have also been observed [43].

Imaging

Muscle imaging paralleled clinical findings with extensive fatty degenerative changes in calf muscles and milder proximal leg muscle involvement [52]. In fact, the pattern of involvement is very similar to that of ZASPopathy showing soleus and medial gastrocnemius to be the most severely affected muscles on the lower legs, followed by anterior and lateral compartments and deep flexors. In thigh muscles semimembranosus, biceps femoris, and adductor magnus are the first targets of involvement [52].

Pathology

Myofibrillar myopathy changes were apparent: large non-rimmed vacuoles, and focal cytoplasmic HE-basophilic and trichrome-dark material in both fiber types [43, 46, 47]. There are occasional rimmed vacuoles and some fiber splitting but rare fiber necrosis. Electron microscopy showed autophagic vacuoles and large zones of myofibrillar disorganization with peculiar semi-dark longitudinal structures replacing filaments of the sarcomere. Inclusion-body-myositis-type 15- to 18-nm tubular filaments were occasionally observed [43]. Early changes included widening of dark material and loss of electron density in the Z-disk. Of the different proteins associated with myofibrillar myopathy myotilin showed the highest degree of abnormal aggregation.

Mutational analysis

Sequencing the relevant exons of myotilin is the gold standard to achieve molecular determination of the diagnosis.

Therapeutic and preventative modalities

Patients usually manage with their disease in the early stages when provided with practical measures for ambulation to overcome ankle weakness with the help of the occupational and physical therapists. Later the disability may become severe but respiratory problems or dysphagia are not apparent.

Genetic counseling

After diagnosis is clarified by DNA analysis genetic counseling is recommended. No presymptomatic or prenatal testing procedures are needed.

Future perspectives

Myotilin is involved in many dynamic aspects of sarcomeric integrity and thus is of high interest in myology. This said, it is of interest to note that the knockout mouse is not severely affected, indicating that lack of myotilin is less harmful than abnormal myotilin.

Desminopathy

Desminopathies and desmin-related disorders have long been known to frequently display a distal skeletal muscle phenotype with onset in the anterior muscles of the lower legs. In fact, the first ever reported distal myopathy family, and later confirmed to be so, was a large Jewish family living on both sides of the Atlantic ocean [13]. However, the distal phenotype is rarely the main problem in desminopathy because cardiomyopathy and respiratory failure usually dominate the clinical setting.

Since myofibrillar myopathy as a morphological concept is covered extensively in a separate chapter, only diagnostic aspects are briefly covered here (see Chapter 25 for comprehensive description of desminopathy).

Diagnostic criteria and pitfalls

Juvenile or early adult onset of distal leg weakness with signs of cardiomyopathy and/or respiratory failure, and fairly rapid progression of symptoms suggest a mutation in the desmin gene. Identification of desmin gene mutation is currently mandatory for a diagnosis of desminopathy. Most desminopathies show increased cytoplasmic desmin aggregations together with general myofibrillar myopathy findings. However, recently the classic scapuloperoneal syndrome of Stark–Kaeser, reported as a neurogenic syndrome, was identified as desmin-mutated disease [53]. In this family the myofibrillar pathology, including rimmed vacuolar changes, was very mild, and aberrant cytoplasmic protein aggregations were minimal. The message from this family is that the pathology is not always typical in desminopathy. On the other hand, minor focal accumulation of desmin can be a nonspecific finding. It can be observed in many neuromuscular diseases, including neurogenic target fibers, spinal muscular atrophy, congenital myotonic dystrophy, myotubular myopathy, and nemaline myopathy. Another type of increased diffuse cytoplasmic desmin expression is observed in regenerating muscle fibers of any etiology.

Laing distal myopathy (MPD1)

The first distal myopathy to be identified and determined by molecular genetic methods was the early-onset distal myopathy genetically linked to a locus on chromosome 14q in 1995 [54].

Salient diagnostic criteria

The final diagnosis of Laing distal myopathy relies on gene mutation identification in slow beta-myosin gene MYH7.

Molecular genetics and pathogenesis

The disease was linked to chromosome 14q11 in 1995 and 10 years later the responsible gene, MYH7, was published [55]. MYH7 encodes slow beta-myosin heavy chain protein which is the main myosin isoform in type 1 slow muscle fibers and in cardiac muscle fibers. All nine mutations currently known to cause early-onset distal myopathy are located in the C-terminal near-tail region of the slow beta-myosin heavy chain molecule. Almost all mutations involve lysine residues. The pathogenic effect of mutations, such as proline substitution for lysine which introduces knicking of the alpha-helix, is easy to imagine in terms of improper dimerization. The mechanism through which certain selected muscles become atrophic due to continuous loss of muscle fibers is far from understood. All tails of the myosin subunit are piled up in the M-line of the sarcomere, physically close to the C-terminus of titin, where mutations cause late-onset dystrophic damage in the same set of muscles in the leg (see "Tibial muscular dystrophy") [11]. The same myosin heavy chain tail region has been proposed to have direct interaction with C-terminal titin but the interaction has never been confirmed. Mutations in middle and N-terminal parts of the protein may cause cardiomyopathy with or without skeletal myopathy, and mutations in the ultimate C-terminus are known to cause hyaline body myopathy [56].

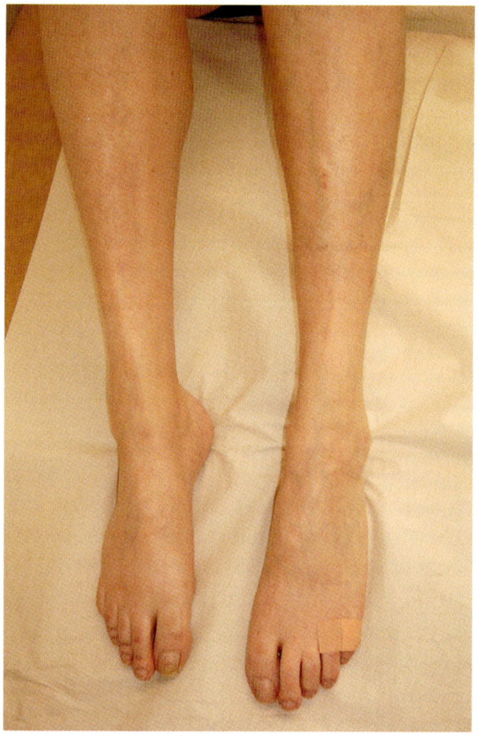

Figure 16.8. Lower legs of a 32-year-old woman with distal myosinopathy (Laing myopathy) starting with reduced ankle dorsiflexion and hanging big toe in her teens.

Salient clinical phenotypical features

The main symptom of mild footdrop and hanging big toe usually begins between the ages of 2 and 25 years (Figure 16.8). Inheritance is autosomal dominant. Since the first report of a family with English–Welsh ancestry in 1995 [54], many more families have been identified [57, 58, 59, 60]. Weakness is prominent in ankle dorsiflexors, toe extensors, and neck flexors. Finger extensors and shoulder muscles are affected later in the disease. The course is protracted, and most patients remain ambulatory. In milder forms patients remain without disability into late adulthood, whereas the severe forms include scoliosis, ankle contractures, abnormal head posture, and major disabilities. Recently an Austrian family was reported with a similar distribution of muscles involved but with late onset of the disease [61].

Genotype–phenotype correlations

Mutations causing cardiomyopathy occur throughout the beta-myosin subunit, although clearly the majority are located towards the neck and head region of the heavy chain monomer. Equally the pathological features of hyaline bodies [56], restricted to type 1 fibers and containing slow myosin, are caused by mutations in the far end of the C-terminus, indicating that these mutations make it difficult for the monomer to be correctly incorporated into the thick filament structure. However, many of the clinical features in patients with hyaline body myopathy resemble those of Laing distal myopathy. The mutations underlying Laing distal myopathy are all in the C-terminal tail just upstream of the mutations causing hyaline body (HB) myopathy. Interestingly almost all are associated with deletions, insertions or exchanges of lysine residues. Many of the mutations are de novo mutations such as the common re-occurring K1617del mutation.

Diagnostic approaches

Even if the disease is autosomal dominant a family history is frequently lacking because many mutations are de novo. Serum CK level is normal or mildly elevated (up to threefold). EMG shows short, brief myopathic potentials.

Imaging

Muscle imaging of lower legs always shows highly selective atrophy and degeneration of anterior tibialis muscles. If the atrophy occurred early in life the space for this muscle may have become minimal and the lesion can be overlooked. In late adulthood the atrophy and degeneration (with less fatty replacement compared to the previously discussed distal myopathies) spread to the other anterior compartment muscles and the medial gastrocnemius is also frequently involved. Proximal muscles show only minor abnormality.

Pathology

Muscle biopsy shows variable findings [60]. Most frequently a biopsy from a less affected proximal muscle shows features of fiber-type disproportion [54]. Rimmed vacuoles are usually not observed but may occasionally be found. On immunohistochemistry using myosin heavy chain (MyHC) antibodies the fiber types may be abnormally distributed in the target muscle, tibialis anterior. Instead of predominance of type 1 fibers this muscle may show expression of fast myosin in all fibers including the many groups of highly atrophic type 1 slow myosin fibers that are hybrids expressing fast MyHC as well [60].

Mutational analysis

Sequencing and identification of the mutation in the C-terminal part of the MYH7 gene is the method of choice for the molecular diagnosis.

Therapeutic and preventative modalities

Many patients with mild disease manage when provided with practical measures to overcome footdrop, finger, and hand weakness with the help of occupational and physical therapists. However, some young patients with a severe condition need surgery for ankle contractures and thoraco-scoliosis, which also may impair respiratory function. Because of abnormal back posture and neck flexor weakness the head can be abnormally retropositioned with subsequent problems for ADL functions.

Genetic counseling

After molecular diagnosis is clarified genetic counseling is recommended. No presymptomatic or prenatal testing procedures are needed.

Future perspectives

Myosin is one of the major molecules in striated muscle fibers and clarification of all functions of myosin is of vital interest for the neuromuscular field.

Distal myopathy with rimmed vacuoles (DRMV, Nonaka myopathy)

In addition to Miyoshi distal myopathy, another recessive distal myopathy was identified in Japanese patients in the 1970s [62]. The gene associated with quadriceps-sparing myopathy–hereditary inclusion body myopathy (HIBM), *GNE*, was identified [63], and soon after it became clear that Nonaka myopathy is caused by the same gene [64, 65, 66]. Thus, HIBM and Nonaka myopathy are the same disease (see Chapter 17). These patients differ from those with sporadic inclusion body myopathy by their earlier age at onset, initial symptom of footdrop, autosomal recessive inheritance, and absence of inflammation on muscle biopsy.

Salient diagnostic criteria

Molecular genetic diagnosis is necessary for a definitive diagnosis of DRMV.

Molecular genetics and pathogenesis

Nonaka myopathy and HIBM are linked to chromosome 9p12–p11. The (UDP-*N*-acetyl)-2-epimerase/*N*-acetylmannosamine kinase (GNE) gene defect was first clarified in patients with HIBM, and later shown to also cause Nonaka distal myopathy [64, 65, 66]. In Japanese patients one mutation is more frequent, the founder mutation V572L [64]. Families of other ethnic origins (Asian Indian, North American, and Caribbean) are usually heterozygous for distinct missense mutations in the kinase and epimerase domains of the GNE. As indicated by the name, GNE is a bifunctional enzyme that catalyzes the first two steps in the biosynthesis of *N*-acetylneuraminic acid or sialic acid. GNE is exclusively shared by vertebrates and bacteria. There is no GNE ortholog in *Drosophila melanogaster*, *Caenorhabditis elegans*, or yeast. The two enzymatic activities of GNE are carried out by separate proteins in bacteria. GNE has been shown to be the rate-limiting enzyme in the sialic acid biosynthetic pathway. Sialic acid modification of glycoproteins and glycolipids expressed at the cell surface is crucial for their function in many biological processes, including cell adhesion and signal transduction. Hyposialylation of proteins in affected muscles has been proposed in Nonaka myopathy [67], but was not confirmed by others [68]. Recently a GNE-deficient mouse model was reported to replicate features of the disease including hyposialylation [69]. Immunohistochemistry results indicate that GNE protein localization and expression is not altered in patient muscle [70].

Salient clinical phenotypical features

Onset of symptoms is in the second or third decade, with an average age of 26 years in the Japanese population [62]. Later onset has been reported. Weakness is first observed in ankle dorsiflexors and toe extensors, causing footdrop and steppage gait. Within 5–10 years patients may develop proximal weakness, and most patients lose ambulation 10–15 years after disease onset [62]. However, the quadriceps muscles remain relatively spared. Neck flexors are affected while other cranial muscles are not involved. Cardiac arrhythmia is not a regular feature of the disease.

Genotype–phenotype correlations

Besides mutations reported in DMRV or HIBM disease new mutations were reported to cause a proximal phenotype, in contrast to the conventional distal weakness and atrophy known to occur with GNE mutations [71]. Mutations in the C-terminal part of the enzyme cause sialuria disease with completely different phenotype. Sialuria does not occur in DMRV/HIBM patients.

Diagnostic approaches

Serum CK level is elevated threefold to fourfold. EMG shows small, brief motor-unit potentials and fibrillation potentials [62]. Recently, a new Western-blotting-based method was reported to complement other diagnostic methods. Hyposialylation of neural cell adhesion molecule (NCAM) occurs in the tissue of GNE-mutated patients and can be assayed by Western blots, showing a band with considerably lower molecular weight compared to the fully sialylated NCAM [72].

Imaging

Muscle imaging shows the initial, extensive fatty degenerative changes in lower leg anterior compartment muscles later followed by proximal leg muscle involvement largely sparing the quadriceps muscles. The pattern of involvement is clearly indicative of a GNE-mediated disease in recessive/sporadic patients.

Pathology

Muscle biopsy is characterized by prominent rimmed vacuoles and dystrophic changes [73, 74]. The vacuoles exhibit acid phosphatase activity and in some focal ubiquitin expression as well [73, 74]. Electron microscopy reveals 15- to 18-nm filamentous inclusions in the nucleus and cytoplasm [75].

Mutational analysis

Sequencing the GNE gene is the gold standard for molecular diagnosis.

Therapeutic and preventative modalities

Patients have considerable disabilities in the later course of the disease, and need a large arsenal of rehabilitative support. Major respiratory failure or dysphagia has not been reported to directly follow the severely progressive limb muscle weakness and atrophy.

Genetic counseling

After diagnosis is clarified by DNA analysis genetic counseling is recommended.

Future perspectives

Current attempts to clarify the role of hyposialylation of secondary proteins caused by the primary GNE defect could, if proven, lead to direct therapeutic interventions to overcome the sialylation defect.

Distal dysferlinopathy – Miyoshi myopathy

The first ever gene discovered to be associated with distal myopathy was *dysferlin* in patients with Miyoshi myopathy [76]. Early reports of Miyoshi myopathy came from Japan [77]. Subsequently, the disease has been reported in many ethnic groups all over the world. The prevalence is not fully established but the overall frequency of dysferlinopathy is in the magnitude of 1/106 (see Chapter 2).

Salient diagnostic criteria

Confirmed mutations on both chromosomes in the patient are the final criteria for a definite molecular genetic diagnosis. However, loss of dysferlin protein on Western blotting is also considered sufficient for diagnosis, whereas loss of protein on immunofluorescence sections should be interpreted with great care.

Molecular genetics and pathogenesis

Different mutations throughout the large gene all lead to loss of protein in patient muscle. Dysferlin is expressed in many tissues, including heart, skeletal muscle, kidney, stomach, liver, spleen, lung, uterus and, to a lesser extent, brain and spinal cord [78]. Dysferlin is expressed in the embryonic tissues from the earliest time point examined [78], and it is mainly localized to the plasma membrane. However, dysferlin does not interact with dystrophin or the sarcoglycans or dystroglycans.

The presence of C2 domains in dysferlin suggests that it may play an important role in signaling pathways. C2 domains bind calcium, triggering signal transduction and membrane trafficking events. Immunoprecipitation studies revealed that dysferlin interacts with caveolin-3 [79]. Dysferlin staining was reduced in two *LGMD1 C* muscles reported. Thus, caveolin-3 defects may cause secondary dysferlin deficiency [79]. Possible caveolin-3-binding domains have been identified in dysferlin. Dysferlin also interacts with filamin-C, recently shown to be mutated in one form of myofibrillar myopathy. Further studies on dysferlin indicated essential functions in membrane repair mechanisms [80].

The spontaneous dysferlin deficiency mouse model (SJL-Dysf) [81] carries mutations in the fourth C2 domain. These mice develop muscle weakness, atrophy, and histopathology reminiscent of the human condition.

Salient clinical phenotypical features

Clinical features shared by the different phenotypes are early age at onset, recessive inheritance, and a marked rise in serum CK levels [77]. The patterns of muscle involvement in Miyoshi myopathy are quite distinct at onset. Symptoms usually begin between 15 and 25 years of age [77]. Inheritance is autosomal recessive. Initial symptoms are in the calf muscles (gastrocnemius). Patients complain that they cannot walk on their toes or climb stairs. Aching or discomfort in the calves is common to the extent of swelling and pains. Subsequently gastrocnemius and soleus muscles become atrophic, and ankle reflexes are lost [77]. The anterior compartment muscles are spared initially but later become involved. The early involvement of the posterior compartment in Miyoshi myopathy distinguishes it from other distal myopathies. As the disease progresses, proximal muscles in legs and arms are affected, and the two phenotypes in dysferlinopathy, Miyoshi myopathy and LGMD2B, merge into one. Progression of the disease appears to correlate better with disease duration than with age at onset. About one-third of patients are confined to a wheelchair within 10–15 years after onset.

Genotype–phenotype correlations

Identical mutations in the *dysferlin* gene on chromosome 2p13 may cause different phenotypes: distal Miyoshi myopathy, proximal LGMD2B, or distal myopathy with clinical onset in anterior tibial muscles [82]. The reason for such diverse phenotypes caused by similar gene defects is not known, although in dysferlinopathy these clinical differences are present in the early stages only. Recently, observations of preserved protein levels even with pathogenic mutations have been discussed but this issue is not settled.

Not all patients with Miyoshi-like phenotype have dysferlinopathy. Both in families with typical phenotype and in families with adult and later onset of symptoms, linkage to the locus 2p has been excluded [83, 84].

Diagnostic approaches

Serum CK levels are markedly increased in Miyoshi myopathy compared to other distal myopathies. Serum CK levels range from 20 to 150 times the upper normal limit [77]. Elevated CK levels may also be detected prior to symptoms or signs in these patients. EMG shows small, brief myopathic motor-unit potentials and early recruitment. Very weak and atrophic gastrocnemius muscles may show long-duration polyphasic motor-unit potentials with reduced recruitment [77].

Imaging

Muscle imaging paralleled clinical findings, with extensive fatty degenerative changes in calf muscles and milder proximal leg muscle involvement. The pattern of involvement can be similar to that of ZASPopathy showing soleus and medial gastrocnemius to be the most severely affected muscles on the lower legs, followed by anterior and lateral compartments and deep flexors. In thigh muscles semimembranosus, biceps femoris, and adductor magnus are the first targets of involvement.

Pathology

In severely affected gastrocnemius muscle the findings may be severe "end-stage" pathology with widespread fibrosis, fatty replacement, and loss of most muscle fibers [77]. At earlier stages biopsies in calf muscles may show inflammatory infiltrates frequently leading to a diagnosis of "polymyositis" [85]. Suggested targets for diagnostic biopsy are the hamstrings. Rimmed vacuoles are not common in these patients. With dysferlin antibodies, the diagnosis of Miyoshi myopathy can now be established by showing loss of protein. Dysferlin normally localizes to the plasma membrane of muscle fibers. In patients with Miyoshi myopathy and LGMD2B, dysferlin is absent in the plasma membrane, whereas scattered granular staining in the cytoplasm or nuclear membrane may be observed. Western blotting of the protein is a more reliable method for diagnostic purposes. On electron microscopy, structural abnormalities of the sarcolemma, including subsarcolemmal vacuoles and papillary projections, have been reported in patients with Miyoshi myopathy [86].

Mutational analysis

Loss of dysferlin in muscle biopsy together with a phenotype is considered sufficient for diagnosis but should be followed by sequencing of the gene to characterize the specific mutation. Gene sequencing by cDNA is the preferred method in those rare instances without total loss of protein or if genomic sequencing was inconclusive.

Therapeutic and preventative modalities

Patients usually manage with their disease in the early stages when provided with practical measures for ambulation to overcome ankle weakness with the help of occupational and physical therapists. Later the disability may become severe but respiratory problems or dysphagia are not apparent.

Genetic counseling

After diagnosis is clarified at least by Western blotting and better by DNA analysis, genetic counseling is recommended.

Future perspectives

Dysferlin appears to be involved in many dynamic aspects of sarcolemmal integrity and signaling and is thus of high interest in myology. How interventions can restore the loss of function is unknown.

Distal nebulin myopathy

Mutations in nebulin are known to cause autosomal recessive nemaline myopathy (see Chapter 4) [87]. It was therefore surprising to find pathogenic mutations in nebulin as the cause of a much milder distal myopathy phenotype. The clue is that different types of mutations are responsible for the phenotype variation.

Salient diagnostic criteria

Confirmed mutations on both chromosomes in the patient are required for a definite molecular genetic diagnosis.

Molecular genetics and pathogenesis

The molecular etiology of the distal phenotype is missense mutation on both chromosomes in nebulin [88]. Why mutations other than missense mutations cause abundant nemaline rods in the muscle fibers while the missense mutations do not is not further clarified at the molecular level. Apparently, disruptive and truncating mutations form protein aggregations that are more difficult to dissolve compared with those formed by missense mutations.

Salient clinical phenotypical features

The leading symptom or sign is onset of footdrop starting in early childhood or not later than in adolescence [88]. The progression is slow and weakness may remain restricted to lower legs even in later adulthood. However, in most cases the evolution of the disease includes weakness and atrophy of hands and forearm muscles and mild neck flexor weakness [88]. Major disability has not been observed. The oldest living patient was still ambulant at the age of 74 years, without respiratory problems or dysphagia [88].

Genotype–phenotype correlations

Different mutations along the large nebulin gene are known to cause congenital nemaline myopathy [87]. The mutations involved have been of all kinds but, in retrospect, after always finding two missense mutations as the cause of mild distal nebulin myopathy, it turns out that in all known cases of congenital nemaline myopathy either both or at least one of the mutant alleles carries a severely disruptive mutation that is not missense.

Diagnostic approaches

Serum CK levels are normal or mildly increased. EMG shows small, brief myopathic motor-unit potentials and early recruitment in most of the affected muscles [88]. Findings were not always easy to interpret and loss of motor units was also stated as neurogenic in the past.

Imaging

Imaging of lower limb muscles can reveal patterns very similar to those in TMD titinopathy (see above) with selective involvement of the anterior tibialis muscle and later involvement of long toe extensors and medial gastrocnemius [88]. In cases with very early onset the compartment of anterior tibialis has almost disappeared and the loss of muscle can be overlooked.

Pathology

Muscle biopsy has shown variable nonspecific myopathy with atrophic fibers and without rimmed vacuolar changes. In none of the cases studied were nemaline rods ever observed on light microscopy. In more severely affected extensor muscles group atrophies suggestive of neurogenic atrophy were also encountered. After knowing the gene defect a retrospective analysis of semi-thin sections and ultrastructure disclosed a few rare rods in four out of six, not enough to suggest the diagnosis of nemaline myopathy [88]. One of the patients had four different biopsies over the years and in none of them could nemaline rods be detected. Findings on electron microscopy were those of myofibrillar disintegration, some Z-disk streaming, and semidense longitudinal structures replacing the organized filaments of the sarcomere.

Mutational analysis

Sequencing the nebulin gene in the search of unknown missense mutations is not a valid option as yet. In cases with compatible phenotype without a dominant family history the current option is to assay for known missense mutations in the gene. In a family situation where there are two or more members affected, linkage analysis can be applied and, if positive, it is possible to continue with gene sequencing.

Therapeutic and preventative modalities

Patients usually manage with their disease when provided with practical measures for ambulation to overcome ankle weakness with the help of occupational and physical therapists.

Genetic counseling

After diagnosis by DNA-genetic analysis, genetic counseling is recommended.

Future perspectives

The big nebulin protein is central to thin filament structure and function, as well as for Z-disk properties. Clarification of the mechanisms behind cell loss due to malfunctions in nebulin may help in finding strategies to avoid damage, because replacement of the defective protein is not yet feasible.

Other molecularly defined distal myopathies

Vocal cord and pharyngeal distal myopathy (VCPDM, MPD2)

In 1998 Feit *et al.* described an autosomal dominant myopathy characterized by distal upper- and lower-extremity weakness and prominent symptoms of vocal cord and pharyngeal weakness [89]. Onset of symptoms varied from 35 to 60 years starting with weakness in ankle dorsiflexors and toe extensors in most patients and with finger extensors first in other patients. At onset weakness may be very asymmetrical [89].

Laboratory findings

Serum CK levels ranged from normal to eightfold increased levels. Electrophysiology showed mild slowing of velocities and myopathic potentials were recorded on EMG [89]. Morphological findings on muscle biopsy included rimmed vacuolated fibers.

Molecular genetics

The disorder has been linked to a region on chromosome 5q overlapping the locus for *LGMD1A* [89]. However, mutations in myotilin were carefully excluded and recently a mutation in the nuclear matrix gene MATR3 was proposed [90, 91].

Adult-onset dominant distal myopathy (MPD3)

A new type of dominant distal myopathy in a Finnish family was described by Mahjneh *et al.* [92]. Symptoms started around age 30 either with weakness of the intrinsic hand muscles and thenar atrophy or with asymmetrical weakness in the anterior compartment muscles of the lower legs. Muscle biopsy showed that abundant rimmed vacuoles were frequent and some of these contained prominent eosinophilic inclusions. Known distal myopathies were excluded by genome-wide screen (GWS) linkage, which resulted in a complex finding as chromosomes segregated completely identically in two different loci, 8p22–q11 and 12q13–q22, with a significant LOD score >3 for both loci [93].

Early adult dominant distal myopathy

A large Australian family with a clearly separate dominant distal myopathy was reported by Williams *et al.* [94]. In this disease early signs may be loss of forced strength of the hand grip in adolescence later followed by involvement of posterior-lateral calf muscles. Anterior lower leg muscles are spared as shown also by muscle imaging. CK was only mildly elevated and dysferlin staining was normal. Molecular genetic studies excluded all known distal myopathy loci [94].

Dominant distal neuromyopathy

In an Italian family with ten affected members in three generations, a distal myopathy with additional neurogenic features including areflexia and pes cavus was reported by Servidei *et al.* [95]. Weakness in the lower legs started between the second and sixth decades of life and progressed to upper limbs and proximal muscles. Dysphagia and dysphonia were early signs. The disease in this family was linked to 19p13 with a LOD score of 3.03 [95]. Rimmed vacuoles were frequent on muscle biopsy together with dystrophic changes, and features of both lysosomal and nonlysosomal degradation have been reported [96].

Distal myopathy with respiratory failure

A large UK family spanning three generations in which patients presented with weakness in ankle dorsiflexion starting in mid-adult life was reported by Chinnery *et al.* [97]. Suggestive anticipation was observed as the second generation of patients had an earlier age at onset and more rapid progression than the first generation. In many patients respiratory failure early in the disease course was a prominent symptom [97]. All known candidate gene loci for distal myopathies at the time were excluded in this family. Muscle pathology showed eosinophilic inclusions and minor rimmed vacuolation. Muscle imaging showed unusual, relative sparing of soleus and medial gastrocnemius, while at the thigh level semitendinosus and rectus femoris were selectively affected [97].

Distal phenotypes in myopathies defined by other terms

Several muscular dystrophies and myopathies may present with a marked distal phenotype either regularly as with myotonic dystrophy type 1 and dynaminopathy, or occasionally as with facioscapulohumeral muscular dystrophy, caveolinopathy, telethoninopathy or VCP mutated syndrome. These disorders are listed in Table 16.2.

References

1. C. M. Campbell, A case of muscular dystrophy affecting hands and feet. *Rev. Neurol. Psychiatry* **4** (1906), 192.
2. W. G. Spiller, Myopathy of the distal type and its relation to the neural form of muscular atrophy (Charcot-Marie-Tooth type). *J. Nerv. Ment. Dis.* **34** (1907), 14.
3. F. E. Batten, Distal type of myopathy in several members of a family. *Proc. R. Soc. Med.* **3** (1910), 93.
4. L. Rimbaud, G. Giraud, Myopathie familiale du type peronier ou distal. *Rev. Neurol.* **37** (1921), 1004.
5. F. Naville, E. Christin, E. Frommel, Les myopathies distales tardives. *Encephale* **18** (1923), 182.
6. K. H. Krabbe, Late forms of familial progressive myopathy. *J. Neurol. Psychopathol.* **10** (1930), 289.
7. J. Ley, J. Titeca, Deux cas familiaux de myopathie distale tardive. *Scalpel* **86** (1933), 595.
8. K. R. Magee, R. N. Dejong, Hereditary distal myopathy with onset in infancy. *Arch. Neurol.* **13** (1965), 387.
9. A. E. M. Van der Does de Willebois, J. Bethlem, A. E. F. H. Meyer, A. J. R. Simons, Distal myopathy with onset in early infancy. *Neurology* **18** (1968), 383.

10. H. Heyck, C. J. Luders, M. Wolter, Über eine kongenitale distale Muskeldystrophie mit benigner Progredienz. *Nervenarzt.* **39** (1968), 549.

11. B. Udd, Molecular biology of distal muscular dystrophies – sarcomeric proteins on top. *Biochim. Biophys. Acta* **1772** (2007), 145–158.

12. W. R. Gowers, A lecture on myopathy and a distal form. *Br. Med. J.* **2** (1902), 89–92.

13. A. T. Milhorat, H. G. Wolff, Studies in diseases of muscle. XIII. Progressive muscular dystrophy of atrophic distal type. Report on a family. Report of autopsy. *Arch. Neurol. Psychiatry* **49** (1943), 655.

14. G. Sjöberg, C. Saavedra-Matiz, D. Rosen, *et al.*, A missense mutation in the desmin rod domain is associated with autosomal dominant distal myopathy, and exerts a dominant negative effect on filament formation. *Hum. Mol. Genet.* **8** (1999), 2191–2198.

15. L. Welander, Myopathia distalis tarda hereditaria. *Acta Med. Scand.* **141**: Suppl. 265 (1951), l.

16. G. Ahlberg, D. Tell, K. Borg, *et al.*, Genetic linkage of Welander distal myopathy to chromosome 2p13. *Ann. Neurol.* **46** (1999), 399–404.

17. K. Borg, G. Ahlberg, J. Borg, L. Edström, Welander's distal myopathy. Clinical, neurophysiological and muscle biopsy observations in young and middle aged adults with early symptoms. *J. Neurol. Neurosurg. Psychiatry* **54** (1991), 494.

18. L. Welander, Homozygous appearance of distal myopathy. *Acta Genet.* 7 (1957), 321.

19. I. Mahjneh, A. Lamminen, B. Udd, *et al.*, Magnetic resonance imaging shows distinct patterns of involvement in Welander distal myopathy and Tibial muscular dystrophy. *Acta Neurol. Scand.* **110** (2004), 87–93.

20. B. Udd, J. Partanen, P, Halonen, *et al.*, Tibial muscular dystrophy. Late adult-onset distal myopathy in 66 Finnish patients. *Arch. Neurol.* **50** (1993), 604–608.

21. J. de Seze, B. Udd, H. Haravuori, *et al.*, The first European tibial muscular dystrophy family outside the Finnish population. *Neurology* **51** (1998), 1746–1748.

22. P. Van den Bergh, O. Bouquiaux, C. Verellen, *et al.*, Tibial muscular dystrophy in a Belgian family. *Ann. Neurol.* **54** (2003), 248–251.

23. P. Hackman, S. Marchand, J. Sarparanta, *et al.*, Truncating mutations in Cterminal titin may cause more severe tibial muscular dystrophy (TMD). *Neuromusc. Disord.* **18**:12 (2008), 922–928.

24. B. Udd, Distal myopathies. In *Clinical Handbook of Neurology*. Third Edition. Volume: Myopathies and Muscle diseases, eds. D. Hilton-Jones, F. Mastaglia. (Amsterdam: Elsevier, 2007), pp. 215–242.

25. P. Hackman, A. Vihola, H. Haravuori, *et al.*, Tibial muscular dystrophy is a titinopathy caused by mutations in TTN, the gene encoding the giant skeletal-muscle protein titin. *Am. J. Hum. Genet.* **71** (2002), 492–500.

26. H. Haravuori, A. Vihola, V. Straub, *et al.*, Secondary calpain3 deficiency in 2q linked muscular dystrophy – titin is the candidate gene. *Neurology* **56** (2001), 869–877.

27. B. Udd, A. Vihola, J. Sarparanta, *et al.*, Titinopathies and extension of the M-line mutation phenotype beyond distal myopathy and LGMD2J. *Neurology* **64** (2005), 636–642.

28. I. Richard, O. Broux, V. Allamand, *et al.*, Mutations in the proteolytic enzyme calpain3 cause limb-girdle muscular dystrophy type 2A. *Cell* **81** (1995), 27–40.

29. P. Hackman, A. Vihola, B. Udd, The role of titin in muscular disorders. *Ann. Med.* **35** (2003), 434–441.

30. V. Carmignac, M. Salih, S. Quijano-Roy, *et al.*, C-terminal titin deletions cause a novel early-onset myopathy with fatal cardiomyopathy. *Ann. Neurol.* **61** (2007), 340–351.

31. W. R. Markesbery, R. C. Griggs, R. P. Leach, *et al.*, Late onset hereditary distal myopathy. *Neurology* **23** (1974), 127.

32. H. Haravuori, P. Mäkelä-Bengs, D. Figlewicz, *et al.*, Tibial muscular dystrophy and late-onset distal myopathy are linked to the same locus on chromosome 2. *Neurology* **50**: Suppl 4 (1998), A186 [abstract].

33. R. Griggs, A. Vihola, P. Hackman, *et al.*, ZASPopathy in a large classic late onset distal myopathy family. *Brain* **130** (2007), 1477–1484.

34. D. Selcen, K. Ohno, A. G. Engel, Myofibrillar myopathy clinical, morphological and genetic studies in 63 patients. *Brain* **127** (2004), 439–451.

35. D. Selcen, A. G. Engel, Mutations in ZASP define a novel form of muscular dystrophy in humans. *Ann. Neurol.* **57** (2005), 269–276.

36. T. Klaavuniemi, J. Ylanne, Zasp/Cypher internal ZM-motif containing fragments are sufficient to co-localize with alpha-actinin. Analysis of patient mutations. *Exp. Cell. Res.* **312** (2006), 1299–1311.

37. C. Huang, Q. Zhou, P. Liang, *et al.*, Characterization and in vivo functional analysis of splice variants of cypher. *J. Biol. Chem.* **278** (2003), 7360–7365.

38. A. J. Te Velthuis, C. P. Bagowski, PDZ and LIM domain-encoding genes molecular interactions and their role in development. *Sci. World J.* 7 (2007), 1470–1492.

39. Q. Zhou, P. -H. Chu, C. Huang, *et al.*, Ablation of Cypher, a PDZ-LIM domain Z-line protein, causes a severe form of congenital myopathy. *J. Cell. Biol.* **155** (2001), 605–612.

40. M. Vatta, B. Mohapatra, S. Jimenez, *et al.*, Mutations in Cypher/ZASP in patients with dilated cardiomyopathy and left ventricular non-compaction. *J. Am. Coll. Cardiol.* **42** (2003), 2014–2027.

41. W. R. Markesbery, R. C. Griggs, B. Herr, Distal myopathy. Electron microscopic and histochemical studies. *Neurology* **27** (1977), 727–729.

42. M. A. Hauser, S. K. Horrigan, P. Salmikangas, *et al.*, Myotilin is mutated in limb girdle muscular dystrophy 1A. *Hum. Mol. Genet.* **9** (2000), 2141–2147.

43. D. Selcen, A. G. Engel, Mutations in myotilin cause myofibrillar myopathy. *Neurology* **62** (2004), 1363–1371.

44. H. H. Goebel, A. N. D'Agostino, J. Wilson, *et al.*, Spheroid body myopathy revisited. *Muscle Nerve* **20** (1997), 1127–1136.

45. T. Foroud, N. Pankratz, A. P. Batchman, *et al.*, A mutation in myotilin causes spheroid body myopathy. *Neurology* **65** (2005), 1936–1940.

46. M. Olive, L. G. Goldfarb, A. Shatunov, *et al.*, Myotilinopathy refining the clinical and myopathological phenotype. *Brain* **128** (2005), 2315–2326.

47. I. PenissonBesnier, C. Dumez, D. Chateau, *et al.*, Autosomal dominant late adult onset distal leg myopathy. *Neuromuscul. Disord.* **8** (1998), 459–466.

48. P. Salmikangas, O. M. Mykkänen, M. Grönholm, *et al.*, Myotilin, a novel sarcomeric protein with two Ig-like domains, is encoded by a candidate gene for limb girdle muscular dystrophy. *Hum. Mol. Genet.* **8** (1999), 1329–1336.

49. Y. Gontier, A. Taivanen, L. Fontao, *et al.*, The Z-disc proteins myotilin and FATZ interact with each other and are potentially connected to the sarcolemmal membrane via muscle-specific filamins. *J. Cell. Sci.* **118** (2005), 3769–3780.

50. P. von Nandelstadh, M. Grönholm, M. Moza, *et al.*, Actin-organising properties of the muscular dystrophy protein myotilin. *Exp. Cell. Res.* **310**:1 (2005), 131–139.

51. P. Salmikangas, P. F. van der Ven, M. Lalowski, *et al.*, Myotilin, the limb-girdle muscular dystrophy 1A (LGMD1A) protein, cross-links actin filaments and controls sarcomere assembly. *Hum. Mol. Genet.* **12** (2003), 189–203.

52. I. Penisson-Besnier, K. Talvinen, C. Dumez, *et al.*, Myotilinopathy in a family with late onset myopathy. *Neuromuscul. Disord.* **16** (2006), 427–431.

53. M. C. Walter, P. Reilich, A. Huebner, *et al.*, Scapuloperoneal syndrome type Kaeser and a wide phenotypic spectrum of adult-onset, dominant myopathies are associated with the desmin mutation R350P. *Brain* **130** (2007), 1485–1496.

54. N. Laing, B. Laing, C. Meredith, *et al.*, Autosomal dominant distal myopathy. Linkage to chromosome 14. *Am. J. Hum. Genet.* **56** (1995), 422–427.

55. C. Meredith, R. Herrmann, C. Parry, *et al.*, Mutations in the slow skeletal muscle fiber myosin heavy chain gene (MYH7) cause Laing early-onset distal myopathy (MPD1). *Am. J. Hum. Genet.* **75** (2004), 703–708.

56. H. Tajsharghi, L. E. Thornell, C. Lindberg, *et al.*, Myosin storage myopathy associated with a heterozygous missense mutation in MYH7. *Ann. Neurol.* **54** (2003), 494–500.

57. T. Voit, P. Kutz, B. Leube, *et al.*, Autosomal dominant distal myopathy. Further evidence of a chromosome 14 locus. *Neuromuscul. Disord.* **11** (2001), 11–19.

58. F. Zimprich, A. Djamshidian, J. Hainfellner, *et al.*, An autosomal dominant early adult onset distal muscular dystrophy. *Muscle Nerve* **23** (2000), 1876–1879.

59. P. Hedera, E. Petty, M. Bui, *et al.*, The second kindred with autosomal dominant distal myopathy linked to chromosome 14q genetic and clinical analysis. *Arch. Neurol.* **60** (2003), 1321–1325.

60. P. Lamont, B. Udd, F. Mastaglia, *et al.*, Laing early-onset distal myopathy – slow myosin defect with variable abnormalities on muscle biopsy. *J. Neurol. Neurosurg. Psychiatry* **77** (2006), 208–215.

61. M. Auer Grumbach, E. John, W. Wallefeld, *et al.*, A novel slow-skeletal myosin (MYH7) mutation in a large Austrian family presenting as late onset distal myopathy. *Neuromuscul. Disord.* **17** (2007), 883.

62. I. Nonaka, N. Sunohara, E. Satoyoshi, *et al.*, Autosomal recessive distal muscular dystrophy. A comparative study with distal myopathy with rimmed vacuole formation. *Ann. Neurol.* **17** (1985), 51–59.

63. I. Eisenberg, N. Avidan, T. Potikha, *et al.*, The UDP-N-acetylglucosamine 2-epimerase/N-acetylmannosamine kinase gene is mutated in recessive hereditary inclusion body myopathy. *Nat. Genet.* **29** (2001), 83–87.

64. H. Tomimitsu, K. Ishikawa, J. Shimizu, *et al.*, Distal myopathy with rimmed vacuoles novel mutations in the GNE gene. *Neurology* **59** (2002), 451–454.

65. T. Kayashima, H. Matsuo, A. Satoh, *et al.*, Nonaka myopathy is caused by mutations in the UDP-N-acetylglucosamine-2-epimerase/N-acetylmannosamine kinase gene (GNE). *J. Hum. Genet.* **47** (2002), 77–79.

66. I. Nishino, S. Noguchi, K. Murayama, *et al.*, Distal myopathy with rimmed vacuoles is allelic to hereditary inclusion body myopathy. *Neurology* **59** (2002), 1689–1693.

67. I. Nishino, M. C. Malicdan, K. Murayama, *et al.*, Molecular pathomechanism of distal myopathy with rimmed vacuoles. *Acta Myol.* **24** (2005), 80–83.

68. I. Salama, S. Hinderlich, Z. Shlomai, *et al.*, No overall hyposialylation in hereditary inclusion body myopathy myoblasts carrying the homozygous M712T GNE mutation. *Biochem. Biophys. Res. Commun.* **328** (2005), 221–226.

69. D. Gagiannis, A. Orthmann, I. Danssmann, *et al.*, Reduced sialylation status in UDP-N-acetylglucosamine-2-epimerase/N-acetylmannosamine kinase (GNE)-deficient mice. *Glycoconj. J.* **24**:2–3 (2007), 125–130.

70. S. Krause, A. Aleo, S. Hinderlich, *et al.*, GNE protein expression and subcellular distribution are unaltered in HIBM. *Neurology* **69** (2007), 655–659.

71. Y. Motozaki, K. Komai, M. Hirohata, *et al.*, Hereditary inclusion body myopathy with a novel mutation in the GNE gene associated with proximal leg weakness and necrotizing myopathy. *Eur. J. Neurol.* **14** (2007), 14–15.

72. E. Ricci, A. Broccolini, T. Gidaro, *et al.*, NCAM is hyposialylated in hereditary inclusion body myopathy due to GNE mutations. *Neurology* **66** (2006), 755–758.

73. I. Nonaka, N. Sunohara, E. Satoyoshi, *et al.*, Autosomal recessive distal muscular dystrophy. A comparative study with distal myopathy with rimmed vacuole formation. *Ann. Neurol.* **17** (1985), 51–56.

74. N. Murakami, Y. Ihara, I. Nonaka, Muscle fiber degeneration in distal myopathy with rimmed vacuoles. *Acta Neuropathol.* **89** (1995), 29–34.

75. H. Mizusawa, H. Kurisaki, M. Takatsu, *et al.*, Rimmed vacuolar distal myopathy. An ultrastructural study. *J. Neurol.* **234** (1987), 137–147.

76. J. Liu, M. Aoki, I. Illa, *et al.*, Dysferlin, a novel skeletal muscle gene, is mutated in Miyoshi myopathy and limb girdle muscular dystrophy. *Nat. Genet.* **20** (1998), 31–36.

77. K. Miyoshi, M. Iwasa, H. Kawai, *et al.*, Autosomal recessive distal muscular dystrophy. A new variety of distal muscular dystrophy predominantly seen in Japan. *Nippon Rinsho. Tokyo* **35** (1977), 3922–3926.

78. L. Anderson, K. Davison, J. Moss, *et al.*, Dysferlin is a plasma membrane protein and is expressed early in human development. *Hum. Mol. Genet.* **8** (1999), 855–861.

79. C. Matsuda, Y. Hayashi, M. Ogawa, *et al.*, The sarcolemmal proteins dysferlin and caveolin-3 interact in skeletal muscle. *Hum. Mol. Genet.* **10** (2001), 1761–1766.

80. D. Bansal, K. P. Campbell, Dysferlin and the plasma membrane repair in muscular dystrophy. *Trends. Cell. Biol.* **14** (2004), 206–213.

81. R. Bittner, L. Anderson, E. Burkhardt, *et al.*, Dysferlin deletion in SJL mice (SJL-Dysf) defines a natural model for limb girdle muscular dystrophy 2B. *Nat. Genet.* **23** (1999), 141–142.

82. I. Illa, C. Serrano-Munuera, E. Gallardo, *et al.*, Distal anterior compartment myopathy. A dysferlin mutation causing a new muscular dystrophy phenotype. *Ann. Neurol.* **49** (2001), 130–134.

83. W. Linssen, M. de Visser, N. Notermans, *et al.*, Genetic heterogeneity in Miyoshi type distal muscular dystrophy. *Neuromuscul. Disord.* **8** (1998), 317–320.

84. J. K. Jaiswal, G. Marlow, G. Summerill, *et al.*, Patients with a non-dysferlin Miyoshi myopathy have a novel membrane repair defect. *Traffic* **8** (2007), 77–88.

85. E. Gallardo, R. Rojas-Garcia, N. de Luna, *et al.*, Inflammation in dysferlin myopathy immunohistochemical characterization of 13 patients. *Neurology* **57** (2002), 2136–2138.

86. D. Selcen, G. Stilling, A. Engel, The earliest pathologic alterations in dysferlinopathy. *Neurology* **56** (2001), 1472–1481.

87. C. Wallgren-Pettersson, K. Pelin, K. J. Nowak, *et al.*, Genotype-phenotype correlations in nemaline myopathy caused by mutations in the genes for nebulin and skeletal muscle alpha-actin. *Neuromuscul. Disord.* **14** (2004), 461–470.

88. C. Wallgren-Pettersson, V. -L. Lehtokari, H. Kalimo, *et al.*, Distal myopathy caused by homozygous missense mutations in the nebulin gene. *Brain* **130** (2007), 1465–1476.

89. H. Feit, A. Silbergleit, L. Schneider, *et al.*, Vocal cord and pharyngeal weakness with autosomal dominant distal myopathy. Clinical description and gene localization to 5q31. *Am. J. Hum. Genet.* **63** (1998), 1732–1742.

90. S. M. Garvey, J. Senderek, J. S. Beckmann, *et al.*, Myotilin is not the causative gene for vocal cord and pharyngeal weakness with distal myopathy (VCPDM). *Ann. Hum. Genet.* **70** (2006), 414–416.

91. J. Senderek, S. M. Garvey, M. Krieger, *et al.*, Autosomal-dominant distal myopathy associated with a recurrent missense mutation in the gene encoding the nuclear matrix protein, matrin 3. *Am. J. Hum. Genet.* **84** (2009), 511–518.

92. I. Mahjneh, H. Haravuori, A. Paetau, *et al.*, A distinct phenotype of distal myopathy in a large Finnish family. *Neurology* **61** (2003), 87–92.

93. H. Haravuori, A. Siitonen, I. Mahjneh, *et al.*, Linkage to two separate loci in a family with a novel distal myopathy phenotype (MPD3). *Neuromuscul. Disord.* **14** (2004), 183–187.

94. D. R. Williams, K. Reardon, L. Roberts, *et al.*, A new dominant distal myopathy affecting posterior leg and anterior upper limb muscles. *Neurology* **64** (2005), 1245–1254.

95. S. Servidei, F. Capon, M. Spinazzola, *et al.*, A distinctive autosomal dominant vacuolar neuromyopathy linked to 19p13. *Neurology* **53** (1999), 830–837.

96. C. Di Blasi, B. Moghadaszadeh, C. Ciano, *et al.*, Abnormal lysosomal and ubiquitin-proteasome pathways in 19p13.3 distal myopathy. *Ann. Neurol.* **56** (2004), 133–138.

97. P. Chinnery, M. Johnson, T. Walls, *et al.*, A novel autosomal dominant distal myopathy with early respiratory failure. Clinicopathologic characteristics and exclusion of linkage to candidate genetic loci. *Ann. Neurol.* **49** (2001), 443–452.

Chapter

17

Oculopharyngeal muscular dystrophy

Bernard Brais

Definition

The common autosomal dominant form of oculopharyngeal muscular dystrophy (OPMD) is a late-onset **genetic muscle disease** that usually presents in the fifth and sixth decade with eyelid ptosis and dysphagia [1, 2]. With time a variable degree of limb-girdle proximal weakness appears. A rarer recessive form has a similar presentation that can be milder [3, 4] or more severe [5] than dominant OPMD. Both forms are allelic, being caused by variable size expansions of (GCN) triplets coding for alanine in the first exon of the polyadenylation binding protein nuclear 1 (PABPN1, previously referred to as PABP2) (Figure 17.1) [6, 7]. Dominant and recessive OPMD are caused by mitotically and meiotically stable short triplet repeat expansions of a $(GCN)_{10}$, and more rarely point mutations, leading to a lengthening of a polyalanine stretch in the protein [6, 8].

Autosomal dominant OPMD was first clearly reported in a Bostonian family of French-Canadian descent [9]. OPMD became a distinct muscular dystrophy in 1962 [10]. André Barbeau established the existence of a large French-Canadian cluster due to a founder effect [11]. In 1980, Tomé and Fardeau identified by electron microscopy unique filamentous intranuclear inclusions (INI) in deltoid muscles biopsies from three unrelated OPMD patients (Figure 17.2) [12]. Since then, these INI have been considered the specific histological marker of OPMD [13]. Dominant OPMD has a worldwide distribution with cases described in more than 35 countries [2]. Only in three populations has the prevalence of OPMD been estimated: 1:200 000 in France [14], 1:1000 in the French-Canadian population of the Canadian province of Quebec [15], and 1:600 in Bukhara Jews living in Israel [16]. In the United States, though many cases are of French-Canadian extraction, there is a very large concentration of cases in the south-western states [17, 18]. The predicted prevalence of the recessive form is in the order of 1:10 000 in France, Quebec, and Japan based on the allele frequency of the $(GCN)_{11}$ recessive mutation in these populations [6].

Salient diagnostic criteria

When the following three clinical criteria are met, it establishes that a patient is affected by OPMD: a positive family history with involvement of two or more generations; the presence of ptosis (defined as either vertical separation of at least one palpebral fissure that measures less than 8 mm at rest) or previous corrective surgery for ptosis; and the presence of dysphagia, defined as swallowing time greater than seven seconds when drinking 80 ml of ice-cold water [15]. The decade-specific penetrances of these criteria for carriers of a dominant $(GCN)_{13}$ mutation are: 1% (<40), 6% (40–49), 31% (50–59), 63% (60–69), 99% (>69) [19]. The age of onset of autosomal dominant OPMD is variable and often difficult to pinpoint. A study of 72 French-Canadian symptomatic carriers of a $(GCN)_{13}$ mutation established a mean age of onset for ptosis of 48.1 (26–65) years and for dysphagia of 50.7 (40–63) years [20]. Other signs observed as the disease progresses are: proximal upper-extremity weakness (38%), facial muscle weakness (43%), limitation of upper gaze (61%), dysphonia (67%), proximal lower-extremity weakness (71%), and tongue atrophy and weakness (82%) [20]. The relative percentage of cases with the different associated findings varies between cohorts [21]. Mutation analysis has also defined three subgroups of patients with more severe phenotypes [6]. The most severe of all forms is observed in homozygotes for two dominant mutations [22]. In these children of two carrier parents, symptoms start in the twenties and progress to include leg weakness in their thirties. Patients that are compound heterozygotes for a dominant $(GCN)_{12-17}$ and a $(GCN)_{11}$ recessive mutation also have a more severe phenotype with symptoms starting in the late thirties or early forties and symptomatic leg weakness before the age of 55 [6]. Lastly, 18% of patients will have a similar phenotype to compound heterozygotes but are only carriers of a dominant mutation. These cases usually cluster in families suggesting that other genetic factors can influence the severity of OPMD. These three forms of severe OPMD will lead to earlier surgical treatment and often to wheelchair use.

Disorders of Voluntary Muscle, 8th edn., eds. George Karpati, David Hilton-Jones, Kate Bushby and Robert C. Griggs. Published by Cambridge University Press.

Molecular genetics and pathogenesis

How mutations in the *PABPN1* gene lead to a late-onset muscular dystrophy that is more significant in certain muscles is still unknown. Various nuclear-inclusion-dependent and -independent mechanisms have been proposed [1, 2]. Though most hypotheses suggest that the expansion of the polyalanine stretch leads to a gain of function of the protein, there is growing evidence that the INIs may not be the culprit but more a byproduct of the cell's reaction to the abnormal protein [23]. PABPN1 is a ubiquitous polyadenylation factor essential for the formation of poly(A) tails of eukaryotic mRNA [24]. The protein shuttles between the nucleus and the cytoplasm [25, 26, 27, 28]. PABPN1 is a multidomain protein. The role of the polyalanine tract and its expansion on PABPN1 structure and function is still unknown. PABPN1 was shown to be an integral part of the INIs in OPMD skeletal muscle [12]. These INIs are also composed of molecular chaperones, components of the ubiquitin–proteasome pathway, poly(A)-RNA [28, 29, 30] and transcription co-factors [31].

The increasing aggregative biophysical property of polyalanine stretches as they grow in size has served to support the most prevalent hypothesis that the OPMD expansion mutations lead to aggregation of PABPN1 and some of its partners [32, 33, 34, 35]. However, it has been reported that overexpressing PABPN1 with a normal 10-alanine size domain, or even without an alanine domain, can lead to PABPN1 nuclear aggregation [31]. Furthermore, in normal physiological circumstances PABPN1 can form intranuclear accumulations [36] and cause cellular toxicity even if there is no apparent aggregate formation in cell lines [23] and in an OPMD fly model [37]. It has been suggested that it may be more the INI-independent micro-aggregation of free PABPN1 that plays a role in the pathology rather than the presence of INI, which may in fact be protective [23]. Different authors have proposed INI-independent mechanisms, including: interference with myogenic factors [38, 39], accumulation of defective mRNA leading to cell cycle impairment [40], and overall disturbance of mRNA maturation machinery [2, 25].

It has now been well established that the overexpression of PABPN1 in cellular, mice, and drosophila models induces the formation of INIs and leads to cell death [29, 30, 31, 37, 38, 41, 42, 43, 44]. The PABPN1-containing INIs are usually filamentous and share features of OPMD muscle INIs though they are less well structured [2]. In different cellular and animal models of OPMD, investigators have shown that some molecules reduced cellular toxicity. In a cellular model it was shown that inducing heat shock protein expression using $ZnSO_4$, 8-hydroxyquinoline, ibuprofen, and indomethacin [45], or exposing cells to anti-PABPN1 antibodies that interfere with oligomerization [46] could prevent cell deaths. In a mouse transgenic model of OPMD, investigators have reduced inclusion formation and cell death with agents that interfere with protein aggregation such as Congo red, doxycycline [41], and trehalose [47].

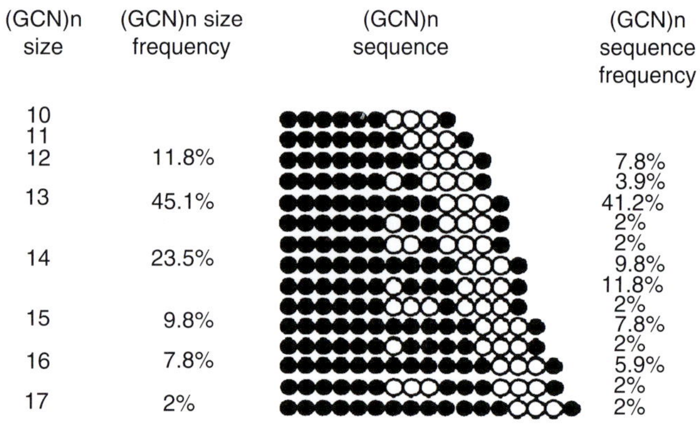

Figure 17.1. Graphic representation of *PABPN1* OPMD mutations. Description and frequency of the 13 different dominant *PABPN1* $(GCN)_{12-17}$ mutations observed in an international cohort of 51 families from various populations. A single case was included from the following three populations with known founder effects: French-Canadian, Uruguayan, and Bukhara Jews. No case of point mutation is depicted. GCG: black dots; GCA: white dots.

Genotype–phenotype correlations

Though some studies have suggested that the larger $(GCN)_n$ mutations cause earlier onset and more severe phenotypes [48, 49], there is no published statistical evidence to support this conclusion. This probably reflects the fact that there is only a one or two triplet difference between the three most common mutations worldwide [i.e., $(GCN)_{13-15}$] limiting the investigator's power to demonstrate significant differences. The most

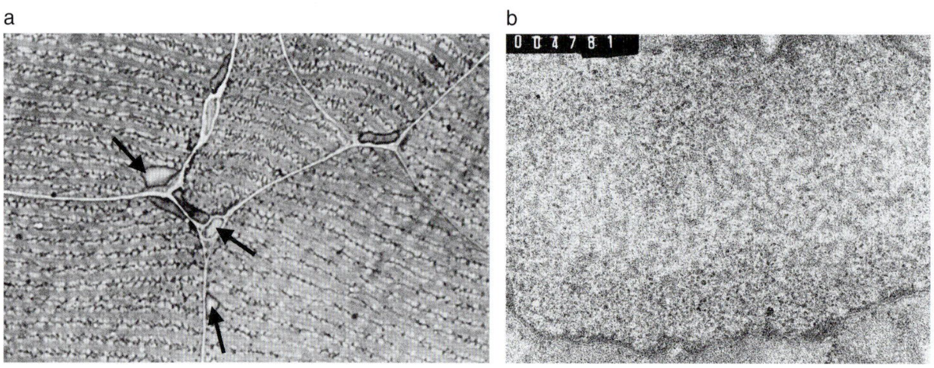

Figure 17.2a, b. Intranuclear inclusions (INI) in oculopharyngeal muscular dystrophy. (a) Clear zones occupied by INI can be seen in two nuclei on a semi-thin section (×1600). (b) By electron microscopy, the INI can be seen to comprise palisading tubular filaments, which often form tangles (× 63 000). (Photographs kindly provided by F. M. S. Tomé.)

severe OPMD presentation was reported for individuals homozygous for two autosomal dominant OPMD mutations with, on average, an onset 18 years earlier than that experienced by the $(GCN)_{13}$ heterozygote siblings [6, 22]. Some of the individuals with clearly more severe autosomal dominant OPMD phenotypes were shown to be compound heterozygotes for a $(GCN)_{12-17}$ mutation and a recessive $(GCN)_{11}$ *PABPN1* mutation [3, 48, 49]. This polymorphism has a prevalence of 1%–2% in North America, Europe, and Japan [3]. There are conflicting reports as to whether recessive $(GCN)_{11}$ OPMD cases have a more severe or a later onset and milder presentation than dominant cases [3, 5]. In one study, only the carrier of the smaller and rarer $(GCN)_{12}$ mutation seemed to have a later onset at the age of 70 [48].

Diagnostic approaches

Until the identification of the OPMD *PABPN1* mutations, a definitive diagnosis relied on the electron microscopy observation of OPMD INI [50]. This approach as now been supplanted by DNA testing [6]. As autosomal dominant and recessive OPMD are allelic, the molecular diagnosis of both conditions is quite straightforward. A single polymerase chain reaction (PCR) is required to establish if the $(GCN)_{10}$ region is expanded [6]. The test has a 99% sensitivity and specificity. In a negative case with a very suggestive presentation, the first exon of PABPN1 should be sequenced to exclude the possibility that a point mutation has converted the (GGG)/glycine in position 12 into a (GGC)/alanine coding for an uninterrupted stretch of 12 alanine residues (Figure 17.1). This mutation was observed in one dominant family [8]. The test is offered by many commercial and university laboratories worldwide. The major indications for DNA testing of a symptomatic individual are: (1) confirmation of the diagnosis in a family never tested; (2) the clinical picture presents a diagnostic dilemma; (3) the patient has a more severe form than the affected parents raising the possibility that he or she is a compound heterozygote for a dominant and recessive mutation or there is a secondary expansion of the polyalanine stretch; and (4) the patient may suffer from recessive OPMD. On the other hand, much care should be taken before requesting the predictive testing of an at-risk asymptomatic individual. It is unclear whether these individuals will benefit from the test, considering there is no medical therapy or prevention for this disease. Presymptomatic testing should be performed in a context in which genetic counseling and psychological support are offered. Electromyography (EMG) shows myopathic changes, but may also demonstrate mild neurogenic changes, in particular in older patients. Creatine kinase (CK) is often elevated to 2–5 times the upper normal value.

Histopathology

Rimmed vacuoles (RV) and intranuclear inclusions (INI) are the two main morphological changes observed in OPMD (Figure 17.2) [13]. RV are readily detected by light microscopy. They were first described in OPMD but have been observed since in other myopathies, in particular in inclusion body myositis (IBM) [51, 52]. The RV are non-membrane bound and are believed to be autophagic. They are found in 90% of biopsies in both normal and atrophied fibers but are not specific for OPMD [13]. On semi-thin sections INI can be observed as clear zones in 2%–5% (mean 4.9%) of heterozygote deltoid muscle nuclei (Figure 17.2a) and 9.4% of homozygote muscle [22]. The percentage of nuclei observed with INI is believed to correlate with the limited volume occupied by the filaments [13]. The OPMD intranuclear inclusions consist of tubular filaments often arranged in palisades or tangles (Figure 17.2b) [12]. The filaments are up to 0.25 µm in length, and have an external diameter of 8.5 nm and internal diameter of 3 nm. They are exclusively nuclear and have not been found in the nuclei of other tissues. They are different from the 15- to 18-nm-diameter IBM nuclear and cytoplasmic filaments. However, cytoplasmic and more rarely nuclear IBM filaments are also seen in OPMD [13]. Since the discovery of the mutated gene, the nuclear inclusions have been shown to contain PABPN1 [28, 53, 54], components of the ubiquitin-proteasome pathway [29, 55], poly(T)RNA [28], transcription factors such as SNW1 (SKIP) important in myogenesis [38] and other mRNA binding proteins such as CUGP1, SFRS3, and FKP1A [31]. Other nonspecific pathological changes observed in OPMD include: atrophied small angulated muscle fibers with type 1 predominance, and very rarely necrotic fibers [13].

Molecular biology

The dominant OPMD locus was mapped to chromosome 14q11.2 using three large French-Canadian families [15]. Linkage to the same markers was confirmed by four other groups [56, 57, 58, 59]. Linkage studies further support that dominant OPMD is a genetically homogeneous condition. A positional cloning strategy relying on the French-Canadian founder effect led to the identification of short $(GCN)_{12-17}$ expansions in the *PABPN1* gene in all dominant OPMD cases [6]. These expanded repeats are mitotically and meiotically stable. Based on the study of a large group of French-Canadian families the estimated rate of a second expansion of an existing OPMD mutation is in the order of 1:500 meioses [6]. The *PABPN1* mutations were first described as pure (GCG) expansions of a $(GCG)_6$ stretch coding for six alanine residues in the first exon of the gene [6]. However, it has become clear that approximately 25% of these mutations consist of (GCN) insertions or cryptic synonymous expansions [7] that do not modify the impact on the PABPN1 protein because all four (GCN) triplets code for alanine (Figure 17.1). Dominant mutations consist of lengthening the (GCN)/polyalanine stretch from 10 to 12–17 alanine residues. The study of 51 OPMD families originating from 17 different ethno-cultural populations documented the existence of 13 different dominant mutations (Figure 17.1).

Therapeutic and preventive modalities

There is no medical treatment yet available for OPMD. A high protein diet is recommended. This is particularly important as the dysphagia becomes severe and patients shy away from sources of animal proteins such as meats. Special attention should be made to prevent the frequent social withdrawal of patients as their dysphagia progresses. They should be advised to eat prior to or after social gatherings. They should be reassured about the risk of fatal choking, which is exceedingly small. Aspiration pneumonia being a frequent cause of death, patients should be advised to consult early on if they have a productive cough accompanied by fever. Exercises that maintain a good cardiovascular condition should be encouraged but strenuous exercises should not be promoted. A wheelchair will be needed by the more severe cases. An even larger percentage of patients will use, late in the course of the disease, either a cane or a walker. Prevention of traumatic fractures due to falls is paramount.

The surgical treatments presently available are used to correct the eyelid ptosis and improve swallowing in moderately to severely affected individuals. Two types of operation are used to correct the ptosis with overall good results: resection of the levator palpebral aponeurosis and frontal suspension of the eyelids. Resection of aponeurosis is easily done but usually needs to be repeated once or twice [60, 61, 62, 63]. Frontal suspension of the eyelids consists of using a thread of skeletal muscle fascia or a synthetic fiber as a sling that is inserted in the tarsal plate of the upper eyelid and attached at its ends in the frontalis muscle, which is relatively preserved in OPMD [60, 61, 62, 63]. Its major advantage is that it is permanent. When fascia is taken from a limb muscle it requires general anesthesia. Surgery is recommended when the ptosis interferes with vision or cervical pain appears secondary to the constant dorsiflexion of the neck. Contraindications to blepharoplasty are marked ophthalmoplegia, a dry-eye syndrome or a poor orbicularis function. Surgical evaluation of symptomatic dysphagia should be prompted by severe dysphagia, marked weight loss, near-fatal choking or recurrent pneumonia. Cricopharyngeal myotomy will alleviate symptoms in most cases [62, 64, 65]. Unfortunately, dysphagia will slowly reappear. Severe dysphonia and lower esophageal sphincter incompetence are contraindications to surgery [64, 66]. Repetitive dilatations of the upper esophageal sphincter using endoscopy or a bougie usually only provides temporary benefits [67]. Botulinum injections of the upper esophageal sphincter cricopharyngeal muscle has been used by some, but no study has been published on its efficacy or its complications [68].

Genetic counseling

The absence of preventive therapy has largely limited genetic testing to the laboratory confirmation of the OPMD diagnosis. Therefore, testing of presymptomatic individuals at risk has not been performed in most cases. In the author's experience, the test has never been used for prenatal diagnosis. Clearly if the test is used for presymptomatic and prenatal diagnosis the results should be shared with the individual in a clinical environment where genetic counselors and psychologists are available.

Future perspectives

The major clinical challenge in OPMD is to uncover medical treatments that will delay its onset and slow its progression. Despite the fact that OPMD is one of the few muscular dystrophies for which excellent surgical treatments are available to alleviate some of the major symptoms, there is still no treatment for the limb-girdle muscular dystrophy that further limits the quality of life in later years. The study of cellular and animal models has already identified available molecules that could be studied in the setting of clinical trials. The further study of these models to screen new molecules should accelerate the uncovering of potential drugs. To ensure the success of these trials in humans there is a need for a validated OPMD clinical scale. A better understanding of OPMD's molecular pathophysiology will undoubtedly help in the uncovering of new therapeutic molecules. Through an understanding of the key biological processes that are disrupted in OPMD, more targeted treatments will undoubtedly be designed.

References

1. A. Abu-Baker, G. A. Rouleau, Oculopharyngeal muscular dystrophy: recent advances in the understanding of the molecular pathogenic mechanisms and treatment strategies. *Biochim. Biophys. Acta* **1772**:2 (2007), 173–185.
2. B. Brais, Oculopharyngeal muscular dystrophy: a late-onset polyalanine disease. *Cytogenet. Genome Res.* **100**:1–4 (2003), 252–260.
3. B. Brais, *et al.*, Short GCG expansions in the PABP2 gene cause oculopharyngeal muscular dystrophy. *Nat. Genet.* **18**:2 (1998), 164–167.
4. S. Hebbar, *et al.*, Siblings with recessive oculopharyngeal muscular dystrophy. *Neuromuscul. Disord.* **17**:3 (2007), 254–257.
5. A. Semmler, *et al.*, Variability of the recessive oculopharyngeal muscular dystrophy phenotype. *Muscle Nerve* **35**:5 (2007), 681–684.
6. B. Brais, *et al.*, Short GCG expansions in the PABP2 gene cause oculopharyngeal muscular dystrophy. *Nat. Genet.* **18** (1998), 164–167.
7. M. Nakamoto, *et al.*, Unequal crossing-over in unique PABP2 mutations in Japanese patients: a possible cause of oculopharyngeal muscular dystrophy. *Arch. Neurol.* **59**:3 (2002), 474–477.
8. D. O. Robinson, *et al.*, Oculopharyngeal muscular dystrophy: a point mutation which mimics the effect of the PABPN1 gene triplet repeat expansion mutation. *J. Med. Genet.* **43**:5 (2006), e23.
9. E. W. Taylor, Progressive vagus-glossopharyngeal paralysis with ptosis: a contribution to the group of family diseases. *J. Nerv. Mental Dis.* **42**:42 (1915), 129–139.
10. M. Victor, R. Hayes, R. D. Adams, Oculopharyngeal muscular dystrophy: a familial disease of late life characterized by dysphagia and progressive ptosis of the eyelids. *New Engl. J. Med.* **267** (1962), 1267–1272.

11. J. P. Bouchard, Andre Barbeau and the oculopharyngeal muscular dystrophy in French Canada and North America. *Neuromuscul. Disord.* 7: Suppl 1 (1997), S5–S11.

12. F. M. S. Tomé, M. Fardeau, Nuclear inclusions in oculopharyngeal muscular dystrophy. *Acta Neuropathol.* **49** (1980), 85–87.

13. F. M. Tomé, *et al.*, Morphological changes in muscle fibers in oculopharyngeal muscular dystrophy. *Neuromuscul. Disord.* **7**: Suppl 1 (1997), S63–S69.

14. G. Brunet, *et al.*, Dytrophie musculaire oculo-pharyngée. Recensement des familles françaises et étude généalogique. *Rev. Neurol.* **146** (1990), 425–429.

15. B. Brais, *et al.*, The oculopharyngeal muscular dystrophy locus maps to the region of the cardiac alpha and beta myosin heavy chain genes on chromosome 14q11.2-q13. *Hum. Mol. Genet.* **4**:3 (1995), 429–434.

16. S. C. Blumen, *et al.*, Epidemiology and inheritance of oculopharyngeal muscular dystrophy in Israel. *Neuromuscul. Disord.* 7 (1997), S38–S40.

17. M. W. Becher, *et al.*, Oculopharyngeal muscular dystrophy in Hispanic New Mexicans. *J. Am. Med. Assoc.* **286**:19 (2001), 2437–2440.

18. R. P. Grewal, *et al.*, Mutation analysis of oculopharyngeal muscular dystrophy in Hispanic American families. *Arch. Neurol.* **56** (1999), 1378–1381.

19. B. Brais, *et al.*, Using the full power of linkage analysis in 11 French Canadian families to fine map the oculopharyngeal muscular dystrophy gene. *Neuromuscul. Disord.* **7** (1997), S70–S75.

20. J. P. Bouchard, *et al.*, Recent studies on oculopharyngeal muscular dystrophy in Quebec. *Neuromuscul. Disord.* **7**: Suppl 1 (1997), S22–S29.

21. S. Ruegg, *et al.*, Oculopharyngeal muscular dystrophy – an under-diagnosed disorder? *Swiss Med. Wkly.* **135**:39–40 (2005), 574–586.

22. S. C. Blumen, *et al.*, Homozygotes for oculopharyngeal muscular dystrophy have a severe form of the disease. *Ann. Neurol.* **46**:1 (1999), 115–118.

23. C. Messaed, *et al.*, Soluble expanded PABPN1 promotes cell death in oculopharyngeal muscular dystrophy. *Neurobiol. Dis.* **26**:3 (2007), 546–557.

24. U. Kuhn, E. Wahle, Structure and function of poly(A) binding proteins. *Biochim. Biophys. Acta* **1678**:2–3 (2004), 67–84.

25. D. G. Bear, *et al.*, Nuclear poly(A)-binding protein PABPN1 is associated with RNA polymerase II during transcription and accompanies the released transcript to the nuclear pore. *Exp. Cell Res.* **286**:2 (2003), 332–344.

26. A. Calado, M. Carmo-Fonseca, Localization of poly(A)-binding protein 2 (PABP2) in nuclear speckles is independent of import into the nucleus and requires binding to poly(A) RNA. *J. Cell Sci.* **113**:Pt 12 (2000), 2309–2318.

27. A. Calado, *et al.*, Deciphering the cellular pathway for transport of poly(A)-binding protein II. *RNA* **6**:2 (2000), 245–256.

28. A. Calado, *et al.*, Nuclear inclusions in oculopharyngeal muscular dystrophy consist of poly(A) binding protein 2 aggregates which sequester poly(A) RNA. *Hum. Mol. Genet.* **9**:15 (2000), 2321–2328.

29. A. Abu-Baker, *et al.*, Involvement of the ubiquitin-proteasome pathway and molecular chaperones in oculopharyngeal muscular dystrophy. *Hum. Mol. Genet.* **12**:20 (2003), 2609–2623.

30. Y. P. Bao, *et al.*, Congo red, doxycycline, and HSP70 overexpression reduce aggregate formation and cell death in cell models of oculopharyngeal muscular dystrophy. *J. Med. Genet.* **41**:1 (2004), 47–51.

31. L. P. Corbeil-Girard, *et al.*, PABPN1 overexpression leads to upregulation of genes encoding nuclear proteins that are sequestered in oculopharyngeal muscular dystrophy nuclear inclusions. *Neurobiol. Dis.* **18**:3 (2005), 551–567.

32. S. E. Blondelle, *et al.*, Polyalanine-based peptides as models for self-associated B-pleated-sheet complexes. *Biochemistry* **36** (1997), 8393–8400.

33. K. Giri, N. P. Bhattacharyya, S. Basak, pH-dependent self-assembly of polyalanine peptides. *Biophys. J.* **92**:1 (2007), 293–302.

34. T. Scheuermann, *et al.*, Trinucleotide expansions leading to an extended poly-L-alanine segment in the poly (A) binding protein PABPN1 cause fibril formation. *Protein Sci.* **12**:12 (2003), 2685–2692.

35. L. M. Shinchuk, *et al.*, Poly-(L-alanine) expansions form core beta-sheets that nucleate amyloid assembly. *Proteins* **61**:3 (2005), 579–589.

36. M. T. Berciano, *et al.*, Oculopharyngeal muscular dystrophy-like nuclear inclusions are present in normal magnocellular neurosecretory neurons of the hypothalamus. *Hum. Mol. Genet.* **13**:8 (2004), 829–838.

37. A. Chartier, B. Benoit, M. Simonelig, A Drosophila model of oculopharyngeal muscular dystrophy reveals intrinsic toxicity of PABPN1. *Embo J.* **25**:10 (2006), 2253–2262.

38. Y. J. Kim, *et al.*, The product of an oculopharyngeal muscular dystrophy gene, poly(A)-binding protein 2, interacts with SKIP and stimulates muscle-specific gene expression. *Hum. Mol. Genet.* **10**:11 (2001), 1129–1139.

39. Q. Wang, J. Bag, Ectopic expression of a polyalanine expansion mutant of poly(A)-binding protein N1 in muscle cells in culture inhibits myogenesis. *Biochem. Biophys. Res. Commun.* **340**:3 (2006), 815–822.

40. J. D. Wirtschafter, D. A. Ferrington, L. K. McLoon, Continuous remodeling of adult extraocular muscles as an explanation for selective craniofacial vulnerability in oculopharyngeal muscular dystrophy. *J. Neuroophthalmol.* **24**:1 (2004), 62–67.

41. J. Davies, *et al.*, Doxycycline attenuates and delays toxicity of the oculopharyngeal muscular dystrophy mutation in transgenic mice. *Nat. Med.* **6** (2005), 672–677.

42. H. Hino, *et al.*, Myopathy phenotype in transgenic mice expressing mutated PABPN1 as a model of oculopharyngeal muscular dystrophy. *Hum. Mol. Genet.* **13**:2 (2004), 181–190.

43. B. Ravikumar, R. Duden, D. C. Rubinsztein, Aggregate-prone proteins with polyglutamine and polyalanine expansions are degraded by autophagy. *Hum. Mol. Genet.* **11**:9 (2002), 1107–1117.

44. V. Shanmugam, *et al.*, PABP2 polyalanine tract expansion causes intranuclear inclusions in oculopharyngeal muscular dystrophy. *Ann. Neurol.* **48**:5 (2000), 798–802.

45. Q. Wang, D. D. Mosser, J. Bag, Induction of HSP70 expression and recruitment of HSC70 and HSP70 in the nucleus reduce aggregation of a polyalanine expansion mutant of PABPN1 in HeLa cells. *Hum. Mol. Genet.* **14**:23 (2005), 3673–3684.

46. P. Verheesen, *et al.*, Prevention of oculopharyngeal muscular dystrophy-associated aggregation of nuclear polyA-binding protein with a single-domain intracellular antibody. *Hum. Mol. Genet.* **15**:1 (2006), 105–111.

47. J. E. Davies, S. Sarkar, D. C. Rubinsztein, Trehalose reduces aggregate formation and delays pathology in a transgenic mouse model of oculopharyngeal muscular dystrophy. *Hum. Mol. Genet.* **15**:1 (2006), 23–31.

48. T. Muller, *et al.*, Genetic heterogeneity in 30 German patients with oculopharyngeal muscular dystrophy. *J. Neurol.* **253**:7 (2006), 892–895.

49. D. O. Robinson, *et al.*, Oculopharyngeal muscular dystrophy (OPMD): analysis of the PABPN1 gene expansion sequence in 86 patients reveals 13 different expansion types and further evidence for unequal recombination as the mutational mechanism. *Hum. Genet.* **116**:4 (2005), 267–271.

50. F. M. S. Tomé, M. Fardeau, Oculopharyngeal muscular dystrophy. In *Myology*, eds. A. G. Engel, C. Franzini-Armstrong. (New York: McGraw-Hill, 1994), pp. 1233–1245.

51. V. Askanas, W. K. Engel, New advances in the understanding of sporadic inclusion-body myositis and hereditary inclusion-body myositis. *Curr. Opin. Rheumatol.* 7 (1995), 486–496.

52. V. Dubowitz, M. H. Brooke, *Muscle Biopsy. A Modern Approach.* (Philadelphia: Saunders, 1973), pp. 231–241.

53. M. W. Becher, *et al.*, Intranuclear inclusions in oculopharyngeal muscular dystrophy contain poly(A) binding protein 2. *Ann. Neurol.* **48**:5 (2000), 812–815.

54. E. Uyama, *et al.*, Nuclear accumulation of expanded PABP2 gene product in oculopharyngeal muscular dystrophy. *Muscle Nerve* **23**:10 (2000), 1549–1554.

55. Y. P. Bao, *et al.*, Mammalian, yeast, bacterial, and chemical chaperones reduce aggregate formation and death in a cell model of oculopharyngeal muscular dystrophy. *J. Biol. Chem.* **277**:14 (2002), 12263–12269.

56. R. P. Grewal, *et al.*, Genetic mapping and haplotype analysis of oculopharyngeal muscular dystrophy. *Neuroreport* **9**:6 (1998), 961–965.

57. H. Porschke, *et al.*, Oculopharyngeal muscular dystrophy and carnitine deficiency in a Nothern German family. *Neuromuscul. Disord.* 7 (1997), S57–S62.

58. J. M. Stajich, *et al.*, Confirmation of linkage of oculopharyngeal muscular dystrophy to chromosome 14q11.2-q13 in American families suggests the existence of a second causal mutation. *Neuromuscul. Disord.* 7: Suppl 1 (1997), S75–S81.

59. B. T. Teh, *et al.*, Oculopharyngeal muscular dystrophy (OPMD) – report and genetic studies of an Australian kindred. *Clin. Genet.* **51**:1 (1997), 52–55.

60. F. Codère, Oculopharyngeal muscular dystrophy. *Can. J. Ophthalmol.* **28**:1 (1993), 1–2.

61. F. Codère, *et al.*, Oculopharyngeal muscular dystrophy: what's new? *Orbit* **20**:4 (2001), 259–266.

62. H. G. Pellerin, *et al.*, Postoperative complications in patients with oculopharyngeal muscular dystrophy: a retrospective study. *Can. J. Anaesth.* **54**:5 (2007), 361–365.

63. D. Rodrigue, Y. M. Molgat, Surgical correction of blepharoptosis in oculopharyngeal muscular dystrophy. *Neuromuscul. Disord.* 7 (1997), S82–S84.

64. C. Brigand, *et al.*, Risk factors in patients undergoing cricopharyngeal myotomy. *Br. J. Surg.* **94**:8 (2007), 978–983.

65. L. Coiffier, *et al.*, Long-term results of cricopharyngeal myotomy in oculopharyngeal muscular dystrophy. *Otolaryngol. Head Neck Surg.* **135**:2 (2006), 218–222.

66. A. Duranceau, Cricopharyngeal myotomy in the management of neurogenic and muscular dysphagia. *Neuromuscul. Disord.* 7 (1997), S85–S89.

67. J. Mathieu, *et al.*, A pilot study on upper esophageal sphincter dilatation for the treatment of dysphagia in patients with oculopharyngeal muscular dystrophy. *Neuromuscul. Disord.* 7: Suppl 1 (1997), S100–S104.

68. D. A. Restivo, *et al.*, Successful botulinum toxin treatment of dysphagia in oculopharyngeal muscular dystrophy. *Gastroenterology* 119:**5** (2000), 1416.

Chapter 18

Myotonic dystrophy

John Day and Charles Thornton

The clinical, genetic, and pathophysiological complexities of myotonic dystrophy have been defined over the 100 years since it was identified, but a coherent understanding of the disease has only recently begun to take shape. Steinert [1], and Batten and Gibb [2] independently described what is now known as myotonic dystrophy (or dystrophia myotonica, DM) in 1909, focusing on the skeletal muscle weakness and atrophy that differentiated it from Thomsen's previously identified familial myotonia [3]. Multisystemic features have been gradually identified in DM, clearly differentiating it from other forms of muscular dystrophy [4] as well as from the nondystrophic myotonias. A near-certain diagnosis can be made clinically, before genetic testing, if highly characteristic features are present in multiple generations of a family: myotonia, a particular pattern of weakness, a specific type of cataract, cardiac conduction defects, and stereotyped involvement of gut, skin, brain, and the endocrine system.

Genetic heterogeneity in myotonic dystrophy was unsuspected until 1992 when an untranslated CTG expansion in the DMPK gene on chromosome 19 [5, 6] was determined to cause most cases of DM. Subsequently, multisystemic myotonic disorders in families that did not carry the chromosome 19 mutation were variously referred to as having proximal myotonic myopathy (PROMM) [7, 8, 9], proximal myotonic dystrophy (PDM) [10], or myotonic dystrophy type 2 (DM2) [11, 12] to emphasize differences or similarities with the chromosome 19 form of DM. These novel disorders were subsequently shown to all result from an untranslated CCTG [13] expansion in the *ZNF9* gene on chromosome 3, which led to the revised nomenclature [14] in which myotonic dystrophy type 1 (dystrophia myotonica type 1, or DM1) refers to the chromosome 19 form of the disease, and DM2 refers to the multisystemic disease caused by the chromosome 3 mutation. To date, only two genetic causes of myotonic dystrophy have been identified, though features of myotonic dystrophy have been described in families and individuals without either DM1 or DM2 mutations, suggesting that a third dominantly inherited form of the disease may exist, or even that sporadic patients may manifest features of DM due to other genetic causes. Although a family with a complex multisystemic disorder has been reported to have DM3, subsequent investigation showed that affected individuals have hereditary inclusion body myopathy with Paget disease of bone and frontotemporal dementia caused by mutation in the *VCP* gene [15].

Diagnostic criteria

To different degrees of certainty myotonic dystrophy can be diagnosed clinically, histologically or by directly testing for the DM1 or DM2 mutations. Although the gold standard for the diagnosis is identification of either the DM1 or DM2 expansion in genomic DNA, a combination of clinical assessment with genetic testing of affected family members provides sufficient accuracy for many clinical circumstances.

Even without genetic identification in a family member, hallmark elements of the DM phenotype are strongly suggestive of the diagnosis; electrophysiological verification of myotonia in a patient with weakness progressing in a pattern characteristic of DM strongly suggests the diagnosis, which can be immediately substantiated by the presence of degenerative changes in the ocular lens on direct ophthalmoscopy (further refined by slit lamp examination), cardiac conduction defects on ECG, and serological validation of specific multisystemic involvement, as discussed below. In a single patient without affected family members these abnormalities do not, of course, verify the existence of an underlying unifying cause, but this constellation of unusual features is sufficiently uncommon that it strongly indicates myotonic dystrophy even in those without a known family history. Furthermore, in individuals who prove not to carry DM1 or DM2 expansions this same constellation of features may lead to the identification of additional causes of DM.

In addition to initial clinical assessment, routinely processed muscle biopsies can be highly suggestive of myotonic dystrophy, though as opposed to many limb-girdle forms of muscular dystrophy routine methods do not have sufficient sensitivity or specificity to definitively diagnose DM. Nonetheless, even without additional clinical information, DM cases

Disorders of Voluntary Muscle, 8th edn., eds. George Karpati, David Hilton-Jones, Kate Bushby and Robert C. Griggs. Published by Cambridge University Press.

Table 18.1. Myotonic dystrophy genetic diagnosis

Disease	Gene and location	Repeat motif	Normal	Borderline	Expanded
DM1	DMPK, 3′ UTR, Chm 19.21	CTG/CAG	5–37	38–60	60–3000
DM2	ZNF9, Intron 1, Chm 3.21	CCTG/CAGG	10–26	26–75	75–11 000
			104–176bp	176–350 bp	>350 bp (mean ~20 kb)

can be appropriately ascertained if the light microscopic features are recognized as characteristic and subsequent RNA fluorescence *in situ* hybridization (RNA-FISH) reveals the CUG and CCUG transcripts that cause DM1 and DM2, respectively. In the appropriate clinical setting, these transcripts can be detected in muscle tissue or fibroblasts [16, 17]. Theoretically a diagnosis could be histologically substantiated by RNA-FISH studies of various cells or tissue, although the utility of FISH as a primary diagnostic tool is unclear. In theory RNA-FISH could be an important assay for identifying some novel genetic forms of DM.

The definitive diagnosis of DM is genetic, but testing can be difficult due to the instability and somatic mosaicism of the DM repeats. For both genetic forms of DM, routine polymerase chain reaction (PCR) amplification across the repeat is useful for excluding the diagnosis of DM. Because repeat sizes vary in the normal population, most unaffected individuals carry alleles of different size; routine PCR demonstration of two different but normally sized alleles eliminates the chance an individual harbors a DM expansion. Because routine PCR is ineffective across a large expansion no observable band is produced from mutated alleles, and affected individuals have only a single PCR product reflecting the normal allele – the expanded repeat preventing amplification of the pathogenic allele. Unfortunately, a proportion of normal individuals also have a single PCR band because they carry two alleles of equal size, making their PCR results indistinguishable from those of affected individuals. Consequently, individuals with a single PCR product require Southern analysis of genomic DNA, with which an expansion can be visualized, to distinguish affected individuals from normal individuals with identically sized alleles. Combined, routine PCR and Southern analysis are sufficiently sensitive and specific to diagnose DM1, but a third method is often required to accurately diagnose DM2 because dramatic somatic mosaicism can obscure results of the Southern analysis; a genetic diagnosis of DM2 can also be confirmed by a PCR amplification into the repeat, rather than across it, to verify existence of a CCTG expansion though not its overall size [18]. The results of genetic testing are often reported in terms of size of the Southern analysis band, but these results must be recognized as estimates because expanded alleles inevitably result in marked somatic mosaicism (Table 18.1); DM1 results are typically reported as numbers of CTG repeats, but DM2 repeat length is typically measured in nucleotides (kilobases, or kb) rather than estimating a number of CCTG repeats because a nonpathogenic but highly variable sequence adjacent to the CCTG expansion interferes with sizing by routine methods. Both DM1 and DM2 are variably severe but highly penetrant disorders in adults with full mutations, though individuals with DM2 expansions and those with smaller DM1 expansions may not have clinical signs of the disease during childhood and adolescence.

Dynamic instability of the expanded CTG repeat in DM1

The human genome contains around 1.1 million loci of di-, tri-, or tetra-nucleotide repeats [19]. The frequency of these simple sequence repeats (SSRs) in the genome is enormously higher than expected by chance alone, yet the evolutionary origin and function of these repetitive elements is not well understood. For the purpose of this chapter, the key feature of SSRs is that they are inherently prone to mutation. For many of these elements, the rate of mutation is more than a thousand-fold higher than the genome-wide average. The mechanism for increased mutability of SSRs is thought to involve slippage of DNA replication machinery [20]. Whereas most replication slippage errors are quickly repaired by mismatch repair proteins, those errors that are not repaired lead to changes in length of the repeat tract, usually by addition or subtraction of a single repeat unit. When DNA mismatch repair pathways are dysfunctional, as occurs in individuals who carry mutations in *MSH2* or *MSH3* mismatch repair genes, there is a genome-wide increase in the frequency of SSRs mutations.

As compared to SSR elements, the genetic instability of expanded CTG repeats at the DM1 locus is further increased. For example, a parent with classical DM1 is almost certain to transmit a mutant allele that differs in size from the one that they inherited, and intergenerational changes of 200 or more repeats are routinely observed [21]. Furthermore, the direction of instability is strongly biased, with expansions far outnumbering contractions. This hyper-mutability is an intrinsic property of the expanded CTG repeat, which does not depend on an underlying general defect of DNA replication or repair, and which is not associated with increased instability of SSRs elsewhere in the genome. Indeed, when mismatch repair proteins MSH2 or MSH3 are eliminated in mice, this has the unexpected effect of stabilizing an expanded CTG repeat [22, 23]. Thus, instead of protecting against mutations, as is the case for most SSRs, it appears that these proteins may actually promote the instability of expanded CTG repeats in DM1.

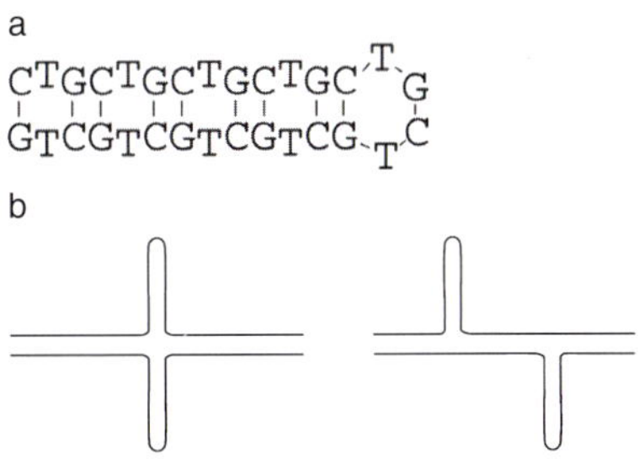

Figure 18.1a, b. (a) Diagram showing stem-loop (hairpin) structure formed within a single strand of DNA that contains CTG repeats. The duplex in the stem of the hairpin is stabilized by C•G and G•C base pairs. (b) Separation of DNA strands within an expanded CTG•CAG repeat, as occurs during DNA replication, repair, or transcription, may lead to formation of "looped out" or slipped strand structure. Each looped out segment is a hairpin of CTG or CAG repeats.

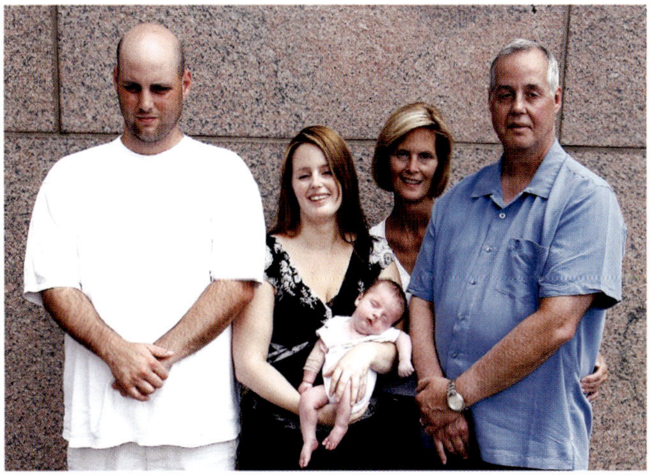

Figure 18.2. Anticipation and clinical variability are demonstrated in this DM1 family diagnosed after the proband was born with profound hypotonia and weakness. The infant required 1 week of gavage feeding and had weak ventilation but never needed ventilatory support, before gradually improving after the first week of life (photo shows him at age 1 month, with, from left to right, his affected uncle, mother, affected grandmother, and affected great uncle). Features of the individuals were: proband – diffuse hypotonia and weakness including face, ptosis, ventilation, trunk, and limb muscles; uncle – gastroparesis, balding at 16 years, attention deficit disorder, grip myotonia, weakness and ptosis already more severe than his uncle's, and a sleep abnormality diagnosed as "narcolepsy"; mother – ptosis, distal weakness, early cataracts, percussion and grip myotonia, weakness similar to that of her uncle, gastroparesis, hypersomnia; grandmother – cataracts extracted at 50 years, mild ptosis and neck flexor weakness, percussion myotonia though no grip myotonia by history or examination; great uncle – weakness including neck, finger flexors and ankle dorsiflexors, ptosis, cataracts, hypersomnia, and gastrointestinal symptoms – the lack of normal finger flexion tone is suggested in the photograph.

Out of around 100 000 trinucleotide repeats in the human genome [19], only 15 have been associated with repeat expansion diseases. Of these, 14 are caused by expansions of CTG:CAG or CGG:CCG repeats, raising the question of why these particular DNA motifs are more likely to have a disease association. The answer relates partly to the biophysical properties of triplet repeat DNA. In a single strand of DNA, CNG repeats (where N = A, C, T, or G) have the propensity to form hairpin structures (Figure 18.1a), in which there is intrastrand G•C and G•C base pairing in the stem. When DNA strands are separated during replication or transcription, this property may lead to formation of "looped out" or slipped strand structures that are relatively stable (Figure 18.1b) [24]. Though mechanisms are not fully defined, evidence suggests that the action of DNA repair proteins on these slipped strand structures may lead to changes in repeat length, with the potential for adding many repeat units in a single event [25].

Families with DM1 show a systematic tendency for symptom onset to occur at an earlier age in successive generations (Figure 18.2). This genetic phenomenon, know as anticipation, was first recognized in DM1. While anticipation is a general feature of dynamic mutations caused by unstable repeat expansions, it is more pronounced in DM1 than in any other genetic disease. For example, a study of 61 parent–child pairs showed that the mean age at symptom onset occurred 29 years earlier in offspring than in parents [26]. Despite the flagrant nature of anticipation in DM1, it is noteworthy that this unusual genetic behavior was generally dismissed by geneticists as an artifact of ascertainment bias, probably because it did not fit with prevailing concepts of DNA replication and heritability. When the DM1 mutation was identified in 1992, however, it displayed three properties that could account for anticipation: the CTG repeat was unstable, it showed a bias for expansion over contraction, and disease onset and severity was partly a function of repeat length. Thus, the existence of anticipation only became generally accepted when its biological basis was uncovered.

When viewed across several generations, DM1 tends to follow stereotypical patterns of clinical involvement within families. Relatively small expansions of 50–80 repeats are often transmitted with minor changes, and these alleles cause late-onset symptoms of mild weakness, cataracts, and possibly changes in cognition and sleep regulation. Unless others in the family have classical DM1, these symptoms are usually attributed to aging and the diagnosis of DM1 is rarely considered. These small CTG expansions may constitute a reservoir of unrecognized DM1 alleles in a population. Because small expansions show greater instability during spermatogenesis than oogenesis, the transition from this minimal phenotype to classical DM1 usually occurs when the disease is transmitted through the male germline [27]. Once the expansion exceeds 100 repeats, instability is very pronounced with either maternal or paternal transmission. For example, the average increase in expansion size in 66 parent–child pairs was 459 repeats [21], with no difference between male and female transmission when congenital cases were excluded. However, there is a bias against very large expansions during spermatogenesis, whereas no such restriction applies during oogenesis [28]. Since congenital DM1 is usually associated with repeat expansions greater than 1000 repeats, this may explain why congenital DM1 is nearly always transmitted through the female germline. Owing to these parent-of-origin effects, a common scenario in DM1 families is a mildly affected grandfather, a mother with classical disease, and a severely affected infant, with the infant's illness being the triggering event that leads to simultaneous recognition of DM1 in three generations.

Followed to its biological conclusion, anticipation culminates in severely affected individuals whose reproductive fitness is low. Through this mechanism, DM1 will reach a point of nontransmissibility, and therefore expanded alleles are continuously lost from the gene pool. This process of attrition-by-anticipation raises the questions of what maintains the disease in the population, and whether the prevalence of DM1 is stable over time. Although the instability of the expanded repeat is not strictly unidirectional, in that contractions are observed in 4% of transmissions [21], these events are probably too infrequent to counter the attrition of DM1 alleles. The existence of founder populations in which DM1 has stably propagated for greater than 12 generations argues for a reservoir of pre-manifest DM1 alleles [29]. The nature of this reservoir, however, has not been determined. It may consist of "borderline" alleles (38–60 repeats) that are transmitted with relatively stability, or a pool of "large normal" alleles (18–37 repeats) that occasionally will transition into the borderline or disease-causing range (>60 repeats) [30].

The pattern of DM1 inheritance in a family is determined by the dynamics of repeat instability in cells of the germline. A related phenomenon is the instability of expanded CTG repeats in somatic cells, which may have important implications for disease progression and organ involvement in an individual. Classical DM1 is usually transmitted by gametes that carry 100–700 CTG repeats in *DMPK* [31, 32]. By contrast, the repeat expansions found at autopsy in skeletal muscle, heart, and cerebral cortex are much larger, typically around 3000–4000 CTG repeats [33]. This implies that the size of the expanded repeat has increased dramatically between conception and death, but exactly when and how this occurs has not been clearly defined. Based on examination of fetuses or infants with congenital DM1, it appears that the extent of somatic instability during prenatal development, a period of intense DNA replication, is fairly limited (reviewed by Wong and Ashizawa [34]), suggesting that much of the somatic expansion occurs during postnatal life. Age-dependent growth of the expanded repeat is probably a general feature in somatic cells, but the rate and extent may vary widely among tissues. A surprising finding was that CTG repeat expansions in skeletal muscle, a tissue with low rates of cell division, were 3- to 13-fold larger than in blood leukocytes, a cell population that depends on active cell proliferation [33, 35]. Paradoxically, whereas serial sampling of peripheral blood from an individual reveals growth of the expanded repeat over time [36], the three instances in which the same muscle was sampled at intervals 7–15 years apart showed no change in expansion size [33, 37]. These results, together with studies of CAG:CTG expansions in Huntington disease and transgenic mouse models, suggest that somatic instability can occur in either dividing or nondividing cells [25]. In nondividing cells the process driving instability is probably DNA repair, whereas in proliferating cells the instability may occur through either DNA replication or repair. The somatic growth of the expanded repeat in skeletal muscle may occur primarily in the presymptomatic phase of the disease, perhaps during childhood and adolescent development, eventually reaching a plateau of around 3000–4000 repeats [37]. It is unknown, however, whether this plateau reflects a stabilization of highly expanded repeats, or a process of elimination in which alleles exceeding a size threshold can trigger demise of myonuclei. Also, it is unclear how the expansion size may correlate with muscle impairment at different ages. It seems likely that age-dependent growth of the CTG expansion in somatic cells is an important determinant of onset and progression of DM1, but this aspect of the disease has not been carefully studied.

Dynamic instability of the expanded CCTG repeat in DM2

As compared to DM1, the instability of expanded repeats in DM2 is more extreme. For example, CCTG expansions can range up to 11 000 repeats, and blood samples from an individual often display multiple discrete expanded alleles of different size [18]. While serial changes in CCTG length in individuals with DM2 have not been examined in detail, cross-sectional studies indicate that the length of the repeat does correlate with age [18], consistent with a model in which expansions in peripheral blood cells increase by 2000–4000 repeats per decade. This age-dependency of expansion length complicates efforts to monitor intergenerational changes or establish the relationship between repeat number and disease severity. For example, in contrast to DM1, longer CCTG repeats correlated with later symptom onset in DM2 [18]. However, multivariate analysis showed that this correlation was driven entirely by the age at which the blood sample was drawn. Similarly, analysis of parent–child pairs showed a bias toward CCTG contraction rather than expansion in offspring [18], but this again may be explained by sampling of parents at a later age. Clinical anticipation has been reported in DM2 [38], although it is less pronounced than in DM1, does not correlate with intergenerational differences in CCTG repeat length [18], and is not associated with congenital disease. Presently there is little information about how the DM2 expansion length in peripheral blood may correlate with expansions in affected tissue, such as skeletal muscle.

RNA-mediated disease in DM1

The expanded CTG repeat is the only mutation in *DMPK* that gives rise to DM1. The location of the mutation outside of the protein-coding sequence, in the 3′ untranslated region, is quite unusual for a dominantly inherited disease. Analysis of the mutant mRNA in DM1 cells has confirmed that it encodes normal DMPK protein [39], and that it contains an expanded CUG repeat [40]. Thus, the circumstance that prevails in DM1 is that cells express two kinds of *DMPK* transcripts, one having an expanded CUG repeat, the other having 5–37 CUG repeats, and both encoding normal protein. This situation is contrary to conventional ideas about the mechanism for genetic dominance, which usually involve loss- or gain-of-function by mutant protein. Moreover, DM1 phenotypes were not accurately reproduced in mice either by eliminating or overexpressing DMPK protein [41, 42]. Taken together, these results indicate that DM1 does not primarily result from too much, too little, or abnormal DMPK protein. The finding that mutant DMPK mRNA was retained in the nucleus in RNA nuclear (ribonuclear) inclusions [16] raised the possibility of an unconventional mechanism in which mutant RNA has a deleterious effect. Transgenic mouse models devised to test this possibility were able to reproduce key aspects of DM1 [43, 44]. The discovery of the DM2 mutation added further support for an RNA gain-of-function mechanism [13]. Thus, a considerable body of evidence now supports the idea that DM1 and DM2 are RNA-dominant disorders in which pathogenic effects are mediated by RNAs containing an expanded repeat [45].

As discussed above, the genetic instability of DM1 may derive from looped out hairpins of CTG repeat DNA. Toxicity of the mutant RNA may relate to formation of similar hairpin structures in CUG^{exp} RNA. Biophysical studies indicated, and X-ray crystallography subsequently confirmed, that purified CUG^{exp} transcripts form extended hairpins in vitro [46, 47, 48]. Like the triplet repeat DNA, the stem of the RNA hairpin is a duplex stabilized by C•G and G•C base pairs, which accommodates the periodic U•U mismatch with very little distortion of the RNA double helix. Yet, as discussed below, some perturbation of the duplex must exist, because RNA binding proteins in the Muscleblind (MBNL) family recognize this imperfect duplex in preference to double-strand RNAs that are perfectly complementary [49, 50]. The stability of the CUG^{exp} hairpin is very high, and the CUG^{exp}-MBNL complexes can be directly observed in DM1 tissue [51], indicating that these RNA hairpins structures do occur in vivo.

Elucidation of disease mechanisms in DM1 has relied heavily on transgenic mouse and fly models. While none of the current models provides an ideal rendering of the DM1 phenotype, one consistent finding that has emerged is that many of the biochemical and physiological features of DM1 are reproduced by expression of CUG repeat RNA in skeletal or cardiac muscle, even if the repeat tract is expressed in a transcript that has no other similarity to DMPK [43, 44, 52]. These findings indicate that the critical element leading to RNA-dominant disease is the CUG repeat itself. However, the toxicity of mutant mRNA is modulated by several factors, including the length of the CUG repeat, the amount and distribution of mutant RNA in cells, and other sequences that are present in the repeat-containing RNA [53, 54].

Alternative splicing is a process whereby one gene may give rise to multiple transcripts and proteins, depending on which exons are included in the mRNA and where particular exon boundaries are drawn. Alternative splicing constitutes an important tier of gene expression regulation, and is subject to tight developmental controls [55]. This process is regulated by proteins that bind to the primary transcript, influencing how it is handled by the spliceosome. Tissue-specific patterns of alternative splicing are established through differences in the amount and activity of different splicing regulatory factors.

Abnormal regulation of alternative splicing, or spliceopathy, is a primary biochemical abnormality in DM1. This derangement was first observed in cardiac muscle for cardiac troponin T [56], and has subsequently been confirmed in transcripts from more than 15 other genes expressed in DM1 muscle, heart, and brain [57]. More examples of genes that are subject to splicing misregulation are being identified through high throughput technologies, suggesting that more than a hundred different transcripts are affected. In most cases the effect of the spliceopathy is to alter the ratio of two alternative splice isoforms. In every case investigated so far, the effect of the spliceopathy is the reemergence in adult tissue of splice products that are characteristic of fetal or neonatal development [58]. This finding implies that the spliceopathy is not a general defect of RNA processing, but a specific derangement of developmentally regulated alternative splicing.

Effects of DM1 on RNA processing involve alternative splicing events that are highly conserved between distantly related species, suggesting that they are functionally important. For some genes the effects on protein function of including or skipping a particular exon may be subtle, and the clinical impact of the spliceopathy difficult to discern. In other cases alternative splice isoforms may have functions that are radically different, and for these events the possibility exists that a particular splicing change can be linked to a specific aspect of the DM1 phenotype. For example, the muscle-specific chloride channel, ClC-1, acts to stabilize the transmembrane potential during muscle activity. Its absence results in generalized recessive myotonia congenita. The splice isoform of ClC-1 expressed in DM1 muscle includes an additional exon, designated exon 7a, which results in a truncated channel protein that has no chloride ion conductance activity [59, 60]. In mouse models of DM1, reversal of this splicing defect, by using antisense oligonucleotides to block the inclusion of exon 7a, restores the sarcolemmal chloride conductance to its normal level and eliminates the myotonia [61]. This finding suggests that the myotonia in DM1 results primarily from abnormal alternative splicing of the muscle-specific chloride channel.

While the biological utility of synthesizing a ClC-1 transcript that encodes a nonfunctional protein is puzzling, studies show that this splice variant is not an anomaly, it is a naturally occurring isoform that is normally expressed during late fetal development. Notably, the role of ClC-1 in maintaining the electrical stability of the muscle fiber is closely linked to functions of the transverse tubule system (TSS). In prenatal muscle the TSS is a rudimentary structure. During this window of development the requirement for ClC-1 channels is low and the transcript is spliced in a manner that relegates the mRNA to a discard pathway. During postnatal maturation, splicing of ClC-1 switches from isoforms that include exon 7a to those in which this exon is skipped, resulting in production of a full-length, functional channel protein [62]. This switch in splicing coincides with the development of the TSS, and fulfills the increased requirement for ClC-1 channels to maintain electrical stability of muscle fibers. For ClC-1, therefore, the functional consequences of expressing fetal splice products in adult muscle are particularly dramatic and deleterious.

A second example of spliceopathy giving rise to a clinical feature of DM1 involves the insulin receptor (IR). The isoform of IR that normally predominates in mature skeletal muscle has greater insulin signaling capacity than the fetal (nonmuscle) isoform, owing to increased inclusion of exon 11. In DM1 the proportion of exon 11-skipped transcripts is increased, which may contribute to insulin resistance in skeletal muscle [63].

The recognition of a toxic gain-of-function by mutant RNA initiated a search for proteins that interact with CUG repeats. The first such protein to be identified was CUG binding protein 1 (CUGBP1), named for its ability to interact with short CUG repeats in vitro [64]. This protein is implicated in DM1 pathogenesis but the exact manner of its involvement is complex. CUGBP1 is a multifunctional RNA binding protein that regulates gene expression at several levels. In the nucleus it binds to pre-mRNA to regulate alternative splicing, whereas in the cytoplasm it regulates translation and decay of mRNA. Although initially envisioned as a protein that binds to mutant DMPK transcripts, it is unclear whether such an interaction occurs in vivo. The RNA binding domains in CUGBP1 are of the type that recognize single-strand RNA, rather than duplex structures that are suspected to predominate for CUG^{exp} RNA [65]. CUGBP1 does not localize to ribonuclear foci of CUG^{exp} RNA in DM1 cells [66], but it remains possible that it interacts with a fraction of mutant DMPK transcripts that are not retained in nuclear inclusions, or with short CUG repeats that are degradation products of the mutant mRNA. Unexpectedly, the concentration and activity of CUGBP1 was found to be increased in DM1 cells [63, 67]. Through an unknown mechanism, the expression of mutant DMPK mRNA results in activation of a signaling pathway that leads to phosphorylation of CUGBP1 [68]. This post-translation modification stabilizes the protein, causing it to accumulate to higher levels in the nucleus. This alteration may contribute to splicing misregulation or perturb other aspects of nuclear function.

Muscleblind-like (MBNL) proteins constitute a second group of CUG-interacting proteins [49]. Biochemical characterization of this family has focused on MBNL1, the predominant MBNL protein expressed in skeletal muscle. This protein regulates alternative splicing for a group of genes expressed in muscle, heart, and brain [69]. It performs this function by binding to a primary transcript at a point close to an alternative exon, thereby promoting or repressing the inclusion of the exon. In regulating its physiological targets, the structural feature of RNA that is recognized by MBNL1 is a short double-stranded RNA that contains a mismatched pyrimidine [50, 70]. Notably, this structural feature is mimicked by CUG^{exp} RNA. Not only does MBNL1 bind to CUG^{exp} RNA with high affinity, but the binding site is highly reiterated, allowing each mutant DMPK transcript to interact with a huge molar excess of MBNL1 proteins. This interaction can be directly visualized in DM1 tissue, where MBNL1 is recruited into the nuclear foci of CUG^{exp} RNA so extensively that its levels elsewhere in the nucleus are markedly reduced [71, 72]. Evidence suggests that this process of MBNL1 sequestration is a critical step in the pathogenesis of DM1. For example, elimination of MBNL1 protein in mice, by deleting part of the MBNL1 gene, causes changes in alternative splicing regulation that are strikingly similar to those that occur in DM1 [58, 73]. Also, increasing the expression of MBNL1 protein, to levels that exceed the protein binding capacity of CUG^{exp} RNA, can improve the DM1-like phenotype in transgenic mouse and fly models of DM1 [52, 74]. In contrast, decreasing the expression of MBNL1 protein in DM1 cells inhibits the formation of CUG^{exp} nuclear foci [75]. This observation suggests that an interaction of MBNL1 protein with CUG^{exp} RNA is the primary event that triggers the formation of ribonuclear inclusions.

Evidence linking MBNL1 protein to DM1 pathogenesis is strong, but it is unlikely that sequestration of a single protein can provide a unitary explanation for the complex phenotype. MBNL1 knockout mice display multisystemic features of DM1, including myotonic myopathy, cataracts, and cardiac defects, but they do not develop progressive muscle wasting, suggesting that other effects of the mutant RNA underlie this aspect of the disease [73]. For example, muscle wasting may require additive effects of CUGBP1 overexpression [44]. Alternatively, two other members of the MBNL family, MBNL2 and MBNL3, are structurally similar to MBNL1, and also bind avidly to CUG^{exp} RNA [76]. Their sequestration may also have a role in the disease process.

While abnormal regulation of alternative splicing is the major biochemical abnormality that is currently recognized in DM1 muscle, it is likely that effects of CUG^{exp} RNA extend beyond RNA processing. For example, upregulation of CUGBP1 may influence the translation and turnover of specific transcripts in the cytoplasm [77]. Expression of CUG^{exp} RNA may also cause abnormal regulation of transcription [78]. DM1 has been associated with upregulation of NKX2–5, a cardiac-specific transcription factor that normally is not expressed in skeletal muscle [79]. Also, expansion of the repeat alters chromatin structure at the DM1 locus, decreasing the expression of *SIX5*, a neighboring gene that encodes a transcription factor [80]. Alternatively, it is possible that expanded CUG repeats are cleaved to small fragments that act as short interfering RNAs (siRNAs) [81]. These siRNAs would be expected to induce degradation of the numerous cellular mRNAs that contain CAG repeats.

RNA-mediated disease in DM2

The discovery of the expanded CCTG repeat in the first intron of *ZNF9*, together with observations that expanded CCUG repeats (CCUG^{exp}) form ribonuclear inclusions in DM2 myonuclei [13], gave strong impetus to the theory of RNA-dominant pathogenesis in DM. Indeed, while the nucleic acid binding protein encoded by *ZNF9* is essential for neural development [82], there is no compelling evidence that the DM2 mutation has a significant impact on expression of ZNF9 protein [83, 84]. Despite the remarkable length of CCTG expansions, the repeat does not block transcription of the *ZNF9* gene. Moreover, the first intron of *ZNF9*, including the expanded repeat, is properly excised from the primary transcript, allowing for expression of a normal mRNA from the mutant *ZNF9* allele. These findings make it difficult to construe DM2 as a disease of ZNF9 deficiency, and suggest that the phenotypic similarities of DM1 and DM2 stem from a shared RNA-dominant mechanism. Additional support for a common mechanism comes from observations that MBNL1 also interacts with CCUG^{exp} RNA [50], and becomes sequestered in nuclear foci in DM2 cells, and that alternative splicing changes in DM2 skeletal muscle appear very similar to those observed in DM1 [58]. However, if both disorders share a common pathogenetic mechanism, it has not been determined why there are important phenotypic differences between DM1 and DM2. In particular, as ZNF9 is expressed early in development, it is unclear why DM2 is not associated with developmental defects similar to those observed in congenital DM1.

Clinical features

The DM clinical presentation is complicated by variable multisystemic features and a large range in age of onset and rate of progression. As previously noted, a primary difference between the two genetic forms of DM is that DM2 does not affect individuals in the first years of life, during which DM1 can cause severe abnormalities (Figure 18.2). Although the molecular and cellular mechanisms of the variably severe congenital DM1 features remain controversial, their time course (as typified by mental retardation) is indicative of abnormal development in that deficits present at birth are subsequently static. Distinct from these congenital or developmental abnormalities, both forms of DM cause variably severe disabilities in adulthood that follow a degenerative course, which are the only clinical features of DM2 and true adult-onset DM1 (Table 18.2). These complexities of disease time course and pathogenesis, coupled with profound differences in patient, family, and physician awareness and recognition of DM, inevitably undercut attempts to categorize individuals based on "age of onset," but nonetheless DM1 subjects are typically considered to have congenital, juvenile or adult forms of disease, though DM2 only causes an adult-onset disorder [18].

Time course of myotonic dystrophy

Neonatal onset

The pregnancies of congenitally affected DM1 infants, as described by Harper [85], are complicated by polyhydramnios, and the children are born with potentially severe neurological, neuromuscular, and musculoskeletal abnormalities. They have craniofacial abnormalities, including tapered chin, high-arched palate and prominent brow, and may be born with talipes, diffuse arthrogryposis or other orthopedic abnormalities [4], and commonly mental retardation and global cerebral atrophy. The development of congenitally affected offspring in minimally affected mothers was the most salient clinical feature that led to recognition of genetic anticipation, now recognized as secondary to marked repeat expansion during maternal transmission.

Juvenile onset

Cases of DM1 that come to medical attention during childhood typically manifest developmental abnormalities that are similar to, but less severe than those seen in congenital onset cases [86]. Many of these patients have cognitive deficits and learning abnormalities [87], as well as craniofacial and skeletal abnormalities that are milder than in congenitally affected individuals, but which nonetheless distinguish them from the true adult-onset DM1 and DM2 individuals.

Adult onset

DM1 patients come to medical attention during adulthood either because they have affected family members (all too often congenitally affected children) or because they develop symptoms of their degenerative disease (e.g., weakness, myotonia, cataracts, cardiac arrhythmia or gonadal failure). On examination, some adult-onset patients have no recognizable developmental defects, but others manifest abnormalities, including the craniofacial changes, a highly arched palate or congenital talipes that indicate developmental effects of their disease. The degenerative features of the disease occur in all adult-onset cases over time, but can progress at different rates, with some middle-aged individuals succumbing to the disease over several years and others having a relatively static course for decades [88, 89]. DM2, given the absence of developmental effects, typically comes to medical attention in adulthood, though myotonia, myalgias, and cataracts can occur within the first two decades of life, and like adult-onset DM1 can develop a relatively rapidly progressive disability with death occurring in mid-life, or can follow a much more protracted course with gradually evolving weakness. Though developmental features clearly distinguish DM1 from DM2, degenerative features of the two disorders may also differ, though previous studies may have obscured disease-specific differences by comparing DM2 to DM1 patients affected by both developmental and degenerative disabilities. Only comparison

Table 18.2. Myotonic dystrophy clinical features

		DM2	DM1
Skeletal muscle features			
Myotonia	On EMG	+++	+++
	Grip and percussion myotonia	+	+++
Weakness	Facial weakness	+	++
	Neck flexors	+++	+++
	Thumb or deep finger flexors	+++	+++
	Hip flexors	++	+
	Deep knee bend	+++	+
Bulk	Diffuse or focal atrophy	+	+++
	Diffuse or focal hypertrophy	++	–
Multisystemic features			
Cardiac	Conduction defect on ECG	+	++
Cataracts	By slit lamp	+++	+++
Serology	Elevated CK	++	++
	Elevated AST/ALT	++	++
	Elevated GGT	+	+
	Low IgG/IgM	++	++
	Male low testosterone/high FSH	++	++
	Insulin insensitivity	++	++
CNS	Mental retardation	–	+
	Executive function loss	++	++
	MRI white matter abnormalities	++	++
Grading system for features			

Keys: – Not clearly associated with the disease. + In some individuals at some point in disease. ++ In many individuals sometime in the disease. +++ Expected in all individuals sometime in the disease.
Notes: ALT, alanine aminotransferase; AST, aspartate aminotransferase; CK, creatine kinase; ECG, electrocardiography; EMG, electromyography; FSH, follicle-stimulating hormone; GGT, gamma glutamyltranspeptidase.

of DM2 and true adult-onset DM1 will allow identification of differences in progressive and degenerative aspects of these two similar disorders.

Skeletal muscle involvement in myotonic dystrophy

Clinical features

The skeletal muscle features in both genetic forms of myotonic dystrophy include progressive weakness, stereotyped changes on biopsy [4, 18, 90, 91], and myotonia. Muscle pain can be a significant feature of both disorders [4, 18], though has been more commonly noted in DM2. The pattern of muscle weakness in DM1 and DM2 is detailed in Table 18.2: at onset both forms of DM affect neck flexors, flexor pollicis longus, and flexor digitorum profundus to the index finger [18, 92]. DM1 is accurately listed as a "distal myopathy" because it affects forearm muscles prior to shoulder girdle muscles, but weakness does not simply follow a distal to proximal gradient, as evidenced by both the early involvement of neck flexors and the fact that intrinsic hand muscles commonly weaken later than volar forearm musculature. As the disease progresses, involvement of the triceps typically, though not invariably, precedes involvement of shoulder abductors in both DM1 and DM2. In the lower extremities DM1 is more likely to affect ankle dorsiflexors than pelvic girdle muscle, as distinct from many DM2 patients who come to medical attention because of early pelvic girdle involvement, which led to the name proximal myotonic myopathy (PROMM) [93]. In later stages of both diseases, diffuse profound weakness can develop, though DM1 involves bulbar, ventilatory, and pelvic floor more notably than does DM2 [4, 18].

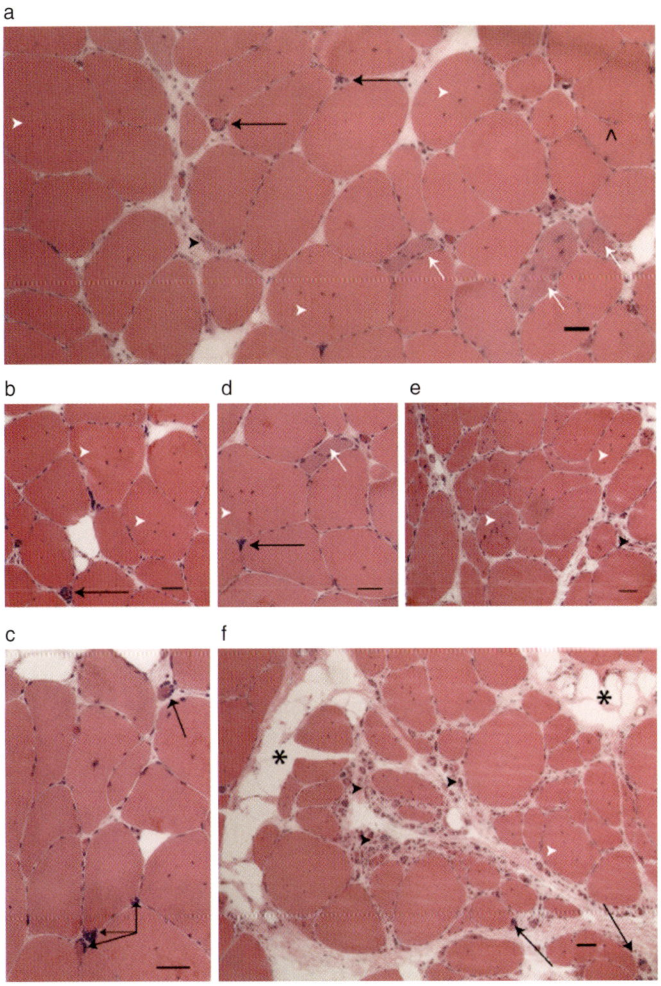

Figure 18.3a–f. Characteristic hematoxylin and eosin histology in DM2 (a–d) and DM1 (e, f). White arrows, atrophic regenerating fibers; black arrows, severely atrophic nuclear clump or bag fibers; white arrowheads, proliferation of central nuclei; black arrowheads, endomysial fibrosis with grouped atrophic fibers; open arrowhead, central nuclei in a splitting fibers; asterisk, adipose deposition.

A notable difference between DM1 and DM2 relates to muscle bulk, in that DM1 commonly results in markedly thin musculature, initially involving the temporalis, sternocleidomastoid and volar forearm musculature, and later becoming more diffuse. The extent to which reduced bulk reflects either atrophy or hypotrophy is variable between patients. In DM1 of early onset, muscles probably never attain their normal size. In contrast, DM2 can result in muscle hypertrophy that is similar to that in nondystrophic myotonias, which occurs rarely in DM1. Although muscle wasting is not obvious early in the course of DM2, the sternocleidomastoid and volar forearm muscles are often thinner and weaker than other muscles, indicating a similar pattern of involvement in DM1 and DM2, though the two diseases differ in severity.

Difference in severity of myotonia also distinguish DM1 and DM2. Although almost all patients with both diseases have electrical myotonia, grip and percussion myotonia are more common in DM1. DM2 subjects commonly note stiffness of hip and thigh musculature, which may relate to myotonia, but clinically significant grip, jaw, and tongue myotonia are much less common in DM2 than DM1. EMG studies confirmed the proximal localization of myotonia in DM2 compared to the more common distal myotonia in DM1 [94]. Myotonia is less severe and less frequently requires treatment in DM than in myotonia congenita.

Muscle histology

Although not pathognomonic, routine histological features of affected muscle are sufficiently stereotyped to suggest DM but may not distinguish between DM1 and DM2 (Figure 18.3). In addition to degenerating, regenerating and necrotic fibers, and fibrosis that is less severe than in limb-girdle muscular dystrophies, additional features characterize DM: (1) presence of severely atrophic fibers that are clumps of pyknotic nuclei with scant myofibril preservation; (2) presence of hypertrophic fibers, sometimes exceeding 200 μm in diameter with secondary fiber splitting; (3) marked increase of internally located nuclei, sometimes exceeding 10 nuclei per cross-section and occurring in chains when viewed longitudinally. Even without clinical information these histological features can lead to an appropriate diagnosis that can be verified genetically, or further investigated with chloride channel immunofluorescence or FISH studies [59, 95]. Fiber type differences can help differentiate muscle from DM1 and DM2 patients, in that type 1 fibers are atrophic in DM1, and severely atrophic fibers in DM2 are more likely type 2 as evidenced by myosin staining [90].

Other organ system involvement in myotonic dystrophy

Central nervous system

Although DM was identified because of its effects on skeletal muscle, and its alteration of cardiac and ventilatory function can be fatal, the CNS abnormalities in DM have increasingly been recognized as an important source of morbidity [96, 97]. Mental retardation is a recognized feature of congenital and juvenile-onset DM1 [4] but has not been causally associated with DM2. In addition to these developmental CNS abnormalities in DM1, both DM1 and DM2 may affect behavior and in both disorders CNS white matter abnormalities have been associated with abnormal executive function [98, 99] (Figure 18.4). Central hypersomnia is a common feature of DM1 [100] that has not yet been specifically investigated in DM2, though daytime sleepiness has been reported [12].

Cardiac

The most common cardiac effects of DM are atrioventricular and intraventricular conduction abnormalities, and arrhythmias [18, 101, 102, 103, 104] all of which occur in both DM1

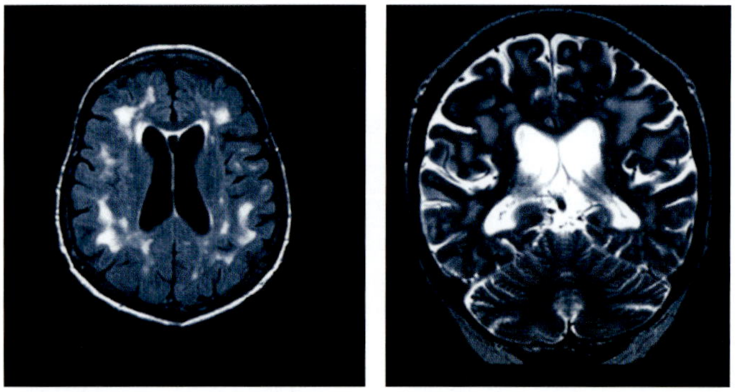

Figure 18.4a, b. Characteristic DM white matter abnormalities on brain MRI. The axial (a, FLARE) and coronal (b, T_2-weighted) images of this 59-year-old woman with DM1 show patchy high signal intensity in large subcortical and periventricular regions of the cerebrum.

and DM2. These abnormalities can persist without consequence for years, or can be associated with sudden death at any age [105, 106]. The development of cardiomyopathy in DM is less clear since it may be secondary to arrhythmias and ventilatory dysfunction rather than a primary feature of the disease, and may occur more commonly in DM2 than in DM1 [107, 108].

Ocular

The cataracts in both forms of DM are stereotypic and indistinguishable, resulting in posterior subcapsular opacities that are iridescent on slit lamp examination [4, 18]. Cataracts are commonly identifiable by careful examination in the second or third decade of life, and can be symptomatic during the second decade of life or later; congenital cataracts are not a recognized part of DM. Vision improves with cataract extraction, but postoperative calcifications are common and can recur [109, 110]. Ptosis and slow saccades are a feature of DM1, but frank ophthalmoplegia is not causally related to either form of DM [111, 112].

Gastrointestinal

Gastrointestinal features are frequent in both forms of DM, though are much more severe and thoroughly characterized in DM1. Dysphagia may reflect pharyngeal or esophageal dysfunction [113], and may respond to sodium channel blockers. Gastroparesis can be frequent and severe [114], causing postprandial pain and bloating that can lead to inadequate nutritional intake if not treated successfully with prokinetic agents; misdiagnosis of gastroparesis as mechanical bowel obstruction can lead to inappropriate and contraindicated surgery that further impairs bowel function and exposes the patient to the myriad risks of anesthesia and postoperative care. Serum transaminase elevation is common in both DM1 and DM2 and often misattributed to liver abnormalities rather than being more likely myogenic, but gamma-glutamyl transferase is also often increased in both forms of DM, and possible hepatocellular involvement has not been excluded [115].

Other

Various other features are common to DM1 and DM2, including primary testicular failure with both hypotestosteronism and oligospermia, hypogammaglobulinemia (serum levels of both IgG and IgM are reduced), and insulin resistance [18, 115]. Hypothyroidism is not clearly caused by DM, but can exacerbate DM1 and DM2 if it develops secondarily [116]. Various neoplastic disorders have been identified in DM patients, but a causal association has not been strongly indicated other than for pilomatrixoma, a typically benign skin tumor [117], though associations have been postulated for basal cell carcinoma, atypical adenoma, thymoma, and hyperparathyroidism with parathyroid adenoma [118, 119, 120, 121, 122, 123]. The risks of anesthesia and postoperative complications in DM cannot be overstated and have been long noted [124]; persistent and often needless morbidity and mortality relate to inadequate appreciation of excessive sensitivity of DM patients to sedative and analgesic medication, and inadequate postoperative monitoring of airway and ventilatory function.

Treatment of type 1 and type 2 myotonic dystrophy

No treatment has been shown to stop or slow the progression of DM. Accordingly, treatment of individuals with DM is focused on genetic counseling, managing symptoms, maximizing independence and function, and preventing cardiac and surgical complications.

One of the most important therapeutic goals in DM1 is to recognize the risk of impending heart block and insert a pacemaker before severe bradycardia or cardiac arrest can occur [125]. While there is agreement that periodic electrocardiograms (ECG) or prolonged ECG monitoring are useful to monitor changes in the conduction system, there are no generally accepted criteria to determine when a patient should be referred for invasive electrophysiology studies or insertion of a pacemaker. Syncopal symptoms, progressive widening of the PR interval and QRS duration, and second-degree heart block likely merit cardiologic evaluation, but whether lesser degrees of heart block require any specific intervention, other than educating patients to recognize and act promptly on symptoms of arrhythmia, has not been determined. Furthermore, because DM1 is also associated with atrial and ventricular tachyarrhythmias, placement of a pacemaker does not fully protect against cardiac events [104]. It is likely that some individuals may benefit from an implantable defibrillator, but it is unclear how to predict which patients are at risk for ventricular tachyarrhythmia.

There is less information about risks and prevention of cardiac complications in DM2. The frequency of major conduction disease is lower than in DM1 [18], but periodic ECG monitoring is nevertheless justified. Sudden death and cardiomyopathy have been reported in a few individuals with DM2, even at an early stage of the disease [105]. These complications are uncommon, and further studies are needed to identify patients at high risk for these events.

Hypersomnolence can be a prominent and disabling feature in DM1. Small trials have suggested benefit from psychostimulant agents [126].

Loss of manual dexterity is an important functional limitation in DM1. The relative contribution of weakness and myotonia in causing this impairment varies considerably among patients and in the same individual over time. When a person with DM1 performs tasks that require repetitive or forceful movement of the fingers, an observer would often conclude that myotonia is causing significant impairment. However, it is noteworthy that many patients do not regard myotonia as an important limitation. Small studies or uncontrolled case series suggest that mexiletene or phenytoin may provide partial relief of myotonia [127], but definitive studies have not been carried out to determine how effective this can be for improving pain, function, or quality of life. It is possible that a subgroup of individuals may derive sufficient benefit to justify anti-myotonia treatment, at least in some stages of the illness, but the long-term safety and consequences of treatment with these agents have not been determined.

Without a clear understanding of mechanisms for muscle wasting in DM1, efforts to improve muscle weakness, or slow its progression, have focused mainly on nonspecific measures to promote muscle growth or regeneration. While some success has been achieved in increasing muscle mass, using testosterone, growth hormone, or insulin-like growth factor 1, to date there are no compelling indications that these agents have improved muscle strength or function [128, 129].

The role of exercise in maintaining function in DM is not clearly defined. In contrast to dystrophies associated with defects in the dystrophin glycoprotein complex, where fragility and necrosis of muscle fibers may predispose to use-dependent muscle damage, there is little reason to postulate that exercise would be harmful to muscle in DM. While limited studies have suggested that progressive resistive exercise can increase muscle strength in DM1 [130], there is no evidence that such interventions improve mobility, function, or quality of life [131]. However, there is also no evidence that exercise causes harm. A small study suggested benefit from resistive training of respiratory muscles [132].

The diaphragm is among the muscles selectively affected by DM1, which may lead to supine respiratory impairment and nocturnal hypoventilation. When coupled with pharyngeal weakness and abnormal CNS control of sleep and respiration, DM1 is associated with complex patterns of sleep-related breathing disorder that may reflect central or obstructive sleep apnea in addition to weakness of inspiratory muscles [133, 134]. Nocturnal hypoventilation can be treated with noninvasive ventilatory support, and should be considered in patients with symptoms of supine dyspnea, daytime hypersomnolence or morning headaches, or with signs of paradoxical diaphragm movement or reduced supine vital capacity. Overnight home oximetry is often useful in evaluation, but in some individuals formal sleep studies are necessary [133].

Genetic counseling

As understanding of DM genetics has expanded, the importance of genetic counseling for DM family care has become increasingly clear. Because it is a dominantly inherited disorder, each child of an affected individual has an approximately 50% chance of inheriting the mutation; for both forms of DM, genetic penetrance is nearly complete, so individuals who inherit the mutation can be expected to develop features of the disease. Furthermore, given the marked anticipation commonly evident in DM1, undiagnosed adults frequently have severely affected children, which demonstrates both the importance of improved diagnosis of minimally affected individuals entering their reproductive years, and the need for effective communication of their diagnosis by a trained genetic counselor. Preimplantation genetic testing can successfully differentiate embryos with DM1 or DM2 expansions after in vitro fertilization, allowing patients to procreate safely [135, 136, 137]. Currently, genetic testing of asymptomatic children at risk for DM is typically discouraged, though development of meaningful treatment, or improved management of the multisystemic features of DM1 and DM2 may make genetic testing appropriate at all ages in the near future [138, 139, 140].

Future perspectives

In the interval since the last edition of this volume, remarkable progress has been made in understanding how an expanded repeat in a non-protein-coding region can give rise to progressive neuromuscular disease. Indeed, research on DM1 and DM2 has opened a new chapter in human genetics by revealing an RNA-mediated mechanism for genetic dominance. This stands as an unusual example in which human genetics provided insight into a fundamental genetic mechanism that was not previously suspected in any other species.

While a provisional understanding of some aspects of DM has been achieved, the disease process appears quite complex, as befits a disorder with one of the most complex and variable phenotypes in all of human genetics. While current understanding of molecular pathogenesis is far from complete, insight into RNA-dominant disease mechanisms has reached a point where therapeutic strategies to target the underlying biochemical defects and alter the course of the disease can be formulated. These strategies include methods to reduce the cellular burden of mutant RNA using antisense or siRNA [141, 142], to inhibit the interaction of CUG^{exp} RNA with MBNL1 protein, or to modify signaling pathways to block the phosphorylation of CUGBP1 [68]. If the example of myotonia is a guide, it appears possible that symptoms of DM could prove to be unusually reversible [61].

Because genetic testing for CTG or CCTG expansions can be performed in high throughput and at relatively low cost, complete ascertainment of DM1 and DM2 is technically feasible, either through newborn screening or population-based screening at a later age. The development of any successful therapeutic strategy, such as methods to target the mutant RNA for destruction or neutralize its deleterious effects, will inevitably raise the question of when, during the course of the illness, treatment should be initiated, including the possibility of treating individuals prior to symptom onset. An important barrier for implementation is that relatively little is known about the presymptomatic phase of the disease, in terms of molecular pathology or attitudes and desires of individuals with pre-manifest DM.

References

1. H. Steinert, Myopathologische Beitrage 1. Uber das klinischeund anatomische Bild des Muskelschwunds der Myotoniker. *Dtsch. Z. Nervenheilkd.* **37** (1909), 58–104.
2. F. Batten, H. Gibb, Myotonia atrophica. *Brain* **32** (1909), 187–205.
3. J. Thomsen, Tonische krampfe in sillkurlich beweglichen Muskeln infole von erebter paychischer disposition (ataxia muscularis). *Arch. Psychiatr. Nervenkr.* **6** (1876), 702–718.
4. P. S. Harper, *Myotonic Dystrophy*. (London: WB Saunders, 2001.)
5. J. D. Brook, M. E. McCurrah, H. G. Harley, *et al.*, Molecular basis of myotonic dystrophy: expansion of a trinucleotide (CTG) repeat at the 3′ end of a transcript encoding a protein kinase family member. *Cell* **68** (1992), 799–808.
6. Y. H. Fu, A. Pizzuti, R. G. Fenwick, Jr., *et al.*, An unstable triplet repeat in a gene related to myotonic muscular dystrophy. *Science* **255** (1992), 1256–1258.
7. K. Ricker, M. C. Koch, F. Lehmann-Horn, *et al.*, Proximal myotonic myopathy: a new dominant disorder with myotonia, muscle weakness, and cataracts. *Neurology* **44** (1994), 1448–1452.
8. C. A. Thornton, R. C. Griggs, R. T. Moxley, Myotonic dystrophy with no trinucleotide repeat expansion. *Ann. Neurol.* **35** (1994), 269–272.
9. R. Moxley, Proximal myotonic myopathy: mini-review of a recently delineated clinical disorder. *Neuromuscul. Disord.* **6** (1996), 87–93.
10. B. Udd, R. Krahe, C. Wallgren-Petterson, B. Falck, H. Kalimo, Proximal myotonic dystrophy – a family with autosomal dominant muscular dystrophy, cataracts, hearing loss and hypogonadism: heterogeneity of proximal myotonic syndromes? *Neuromuscul. Disord.* **7** (1997), 217–228.
11. L. Ranum, P. Rasmussen, K. Benzow, M. Koob, J. Day, Genetic mapping of a second myotonic dystrophy locus. *Nat. Genet.* **19** (1998), 196–198.
12. J. W. Day, R. Roelofs, B. Leroy, I. Pech, K. Benzow, L. P. Ranum, Clinical and genetic characteristics of a five-generation family with a novel form of myotonic dystrophy (DM2). *Neuromuscul. Disord.* **9** (1999), 19–27.
13. C. Liquori, K. Ricker, M. L. Moseley, *et al.*, Myotonic dystrophy type 2 caused by a CCTG expansion in intron 1 of ZNF9. *Science* **293** (2001), 864–867.
14. IMD Consortium, New nomenclature and DNA testing guidelines for myotonic dystrophy type 1 (DM1). The International Myotonic Dystrophy Consortium (IDMC). *Neurology* **54** (2000), 1218–1221.
15. L. Guyant-Marechal, A. Laquerriere, C. Duyckaerts, *et al.*, Valosin-containing protein gene mutations: clinical and neuropathologic features. *Neurology* **67** (2006), 644–651.
16. K. L. Taneja, M. McCurrach, M. Schalling, D. Housman, R. H. Singer, Foci of trinucleotide repeat transcripts in nuclei of myotonic dystrophy cells and tissues. *J. Cell Biol.* **128** (1995), 995–1002.
17. C. L. Liquori, K. Ricker, M. L. Moseley, *et al.*, Myotonic dystrophy type 2 caused by a CCTG expansion in intron 1 of ZNF9. *Science* **293** (2001), 864–867.
18. J. W. Day, K. Ricker, J. F. Jacobsen, *et al.*, Myotonic dystrophy type 2: molecular, diagnostic and clinical spectrum. *Neurology* **60** (2003), 657–664.
19. Y. D. Kelkar, S. Tyekucheva, F. Chiaromonte, K. D. Makova, The genome-wide determinants of human and chimpanzee microsatellite evolution. *Genome Res.* **18** (2008), 30–38.
20. H. Ellegren, Microsatellites: simple sequences with complex evolution. *Nat. Rev. Genet.* **5** (2004), 435–445.
21. J. B. Redman, R. G. Fenwick, Jr., Y. H. Fu, A. Pizzuti, C. T. Caskey, Relationship between parental trinucleotide GCT repeat length and severity of myotonic dystrophy in offspring. *J. Am. Med. Assoc.* **269** (1993), 1960–1965.
22. C. Savouret, C. Garcia-Cordier, J. Megret, R. H. te Riele, C. Junien, G. Gourdon, MSH2-dependent germinal C T G repeat expansions are produced continuously in spermatogonia from DM1 transgenic mice. *Mol. Cell. Biol.* **24** (2004), 629–637.
23. L. Foiry, L. Dong, C. Savouret, *et al.*, Msh3 is a limiting factor in the formation of intergenerational CTG expansions in DM1 transgenic mice. *Hum. Genet.* **119** (2006), 520–526.
24. C. E. Pearson, R. R. Sinden, Alternative structures in duplex DNA formed within the trinucleotide repeats of the myotonic dystrophy and fragile X loci. *Biochemistry* **35** (1996), 5041–5053.
25. C. E. Pearson, E. K. Nichol, J. D. Cleary, Repeat instability: mechanisms of dynamic mutations. *Nat. Rev. Genet.* **6** (2005), 729–742.
26. C. J. Howeler, H. F. Bisch, J. P. Geraedts, M. F. Niermeijer, A. Staal, Anticipation in myotonic dystrophy: fact or fiction? *Brain* **112** (1989), 779–797.
27. H. G. Brunner, H. T. Bruggenwirth, W. Nillesen, *et al.*, Influence of sex of the transmitting parent as well as of parental allele size on the CTG expansion in myotonic dystrophy (DM). *Am. J. Hum. Genet.* **53** (1993), 1016–1023.
28. G. Jansen, P. Willems, M. Coerwinkel, *et al.*, Gonosomal mosaicism in myotonic dystrophy patients: involvement of mitotic events in (CTG)n repeat variation and selection against extreme expansion in sperm. *Am. J. Hum. Genet.* **54** (1994), 575–585.
29. V. Yotova, D. Labuda, E. Zietkiewicz, *et al.*, Anatomy of a founder effect: myotonic dystrophy in Northeastern Quebec. *Hum. Genet.* **117** (2005), 177–187.

30. S. A. Tishkoff, A. Goldman, F. Calafell, *et al.*, A global haplotype analysis of the myotonic dystrophy locus: implications for the evolution of modern humans and for the origin of myotonic dystrophy mutations. *Am. J. Hum. Genet.* **62** (1998), 1389–1402.

31. L. Martorell, J. Gamez, M. L. Cayuela, *et al.*, Germline mutational dynamics in myotonic dystrophy type 1 males: allele length and age effects. *Neurology* **62** (2004), 269–274.

32. N. De Temmerman, K. Sermon, S. Seneca, *et al.*, Intergenerational instability of the expanded CTG repeat in the DMPK gene: studies in human gametes and preimplantation embryos. *Am. J. Hum. Genet.* **75** (2004), 325–329.

33. C A. Thornton, K. Johnson, R T. Moxley 3rd., Myotonic dystrophy patients have larger CTG expansions in skeletal muscle than in leukocytes. *Ann. Neurol.* **35** (1994), 104–7.

34. L. J. Wong, T. Ashizawa, Instability of the (CTG)n repeat in congenital myotonic dystrophy. *Am. J. Hum. Genet.* **61** (1997), 1445–1448.

35. T. Ashizawa, J. R. Dubel, Y. Harati, Somatic instability of CTG repeat in myotonic dystrophy. *Neurology* **43** (1993), 2674–2678.

36. L. Martorell, D. G. Monckton, J. Gamez, *et al.*, Progression of somatic CTG repeat length heterogeneity in the blood cells of myotonic dystrophy patients. *Hum. Mol. Genet.* **7** (1998), 307–312.

37. M. Zatz, M. R. Passos-Bueno, A. Cerqueira, *et al.*, Analysis of the CTG repeat in skeletal muscle of young and adult myotonic dystrophy patients: when does the expansion occur? *Hum. Mol. Genet.* **4** (1995), 401–406.

38. C. Schneider, A. Ziegler, K. Ricker, *et al.*, Proximal myotonic myopathy: evidence for anticipation in families with linkage to chromosome 3q. *Neurology* **55** (2000), 383–388.

39. R. Krahe, T. Ashizawa, C. Abbruzzese, *et al.*, Effect of myotonic dystrophy trinucleotide repeat expansion on DMPK transcription and processing. *Genomics* **28** (1995), 1–14.

40. B. M. Davis, M. E. McCurrach, K. L. Taneja, R. H. Singer, D. E. Housman, Expansion of a CUG trinucleotide repeat in the 3′ untranslated region of myotonic dystrophy protein kinase transcripts results in nuclear retention of transcripts. *Proc. Natl. Acad. Sci. U. S. A.* **94** (1997), 7388–7393.

41. G. Jansen, P. J. T. A. Groenen, D. Bachner, *et al.*, Abnormal myotonic dystrophy protein kinase levels produce only mild myopathy in mice. *Nat. Genet.* **13** (1996), 316–324.

42. S. Reddy, D. B. J. Smith, M. M. Rich, *et al.*, Mice lacking the myotonic dystrophy protein kinase develop a late onset progressive myopathy. *Nat. Genet.* **13** (1996), 325–334.

43. A. Mankodi, E. Logigian, L. Callahan, *et al.*, Myotonic dystrophy in transgenic mice expressing an expanded CUG repeat. *Science* **289** (2000), 1769–1773.

44. J. P. Orengo, P. Chambon, D. Metzger, D. R. Mosier, G. J. Snipes, T. A. Cooper, Expanded CTG repeats within the DMPK 3′ UTR causes severe skeletal muscle wasting in an inducible mouse model for myotonic dystrophy. *Proc. Natl. Acad. Sci. U. S. A.* **105** (2008), 2646–2651.

45. R. J. Osborne, C. A. Thornton, RNA-dominant diseases. *Hum. Mol. Genet.* **15**: Spec No 2 (2006), R162–R169.

46. M. Napierala, W. J. Krzyzosiak, CUG repeats present in myotonin kinase RNA form metastable slippery hairpins. *J. Biol. Chem.* **272** (1997), 31079–31085.

47. B. Tian, R. J. White, T. Xia, *et al.*, Expanded CUG repeat RNAs form hairpins that activate the double-stranded RNA-dependent protein kinase PKR. *RNA* **6** (2000), 79–87.

48. B. H. Mooers, J. S. Logue, J. A. Berglund, The structural basis of myotonic dystrophy from the crystal structure of CUG repeats. *Proc. Natl. Acad. Sci. U. S. A.* **102** (2005), 16626–16631.

49. J. W. Miller, C. R. Urbinati, P. Teng-Umnuay, *et al.*, Recruitment of human muscleblind proteins to (CUG)(n) expansions associated with myotonic dystrophy. *EMBO J.* **19** (2000), 4439–4448.

50. Y. Yuan, S. A. Compton, K. Sobczak, *et al.*, Muscleblind-like 1 interacts with RNA hairpins in splicing target and pathogenic RNAs. *Nucleic Acids Res.* **35** (2007), 5474–5486.

51. A. Mankodi, P. Teng-Umnuay, M. Krym, D. Henderson, M. Swanson, C. A. Thornton, Ribonuclear inclusions in skeletal muscle in myotonic dystrophy types 1 and 2. *Ann. Neurol.* **54** (2003), 760–768.

52. M. de Haro, I. Al-Ramahi, B. De Gouyon, *et al.*, MBNL1 and CUGBP1 modify expanded CUG-induced toxicity in a Drosophila model of myotonic dystrophy type 1. *Hum. Mol. Genet.* **15** (2006), 2138–2145.

53. J. D. Amack, M. S. Mahadevan, The myotonic dystrophy expanded CUG repeat tract is necessary but not sufficient to disrupt C2C12 myoblast differentiation. *Hum. Mol. Genet.* **10** (2001), 1879–1887.

54. M. S. Mahadevan, R. S. Yadava, Q. Yu, *et al.*, Reversible model of RNA toxicity and cardiac conduction defects in myotonic dystrophy. *Nat. Genet.* **38** (2006), 1066–1070.

55. D. L. Black, Mechanisms of alternative pre-messenger RNA splicing. *Annu. Rev. Biochem.* **72** (2003), 291–336.

56. A. V. Philips, L. T. Timchenko, T. A. Cooper, Disruption of splicing regulated by a CUG-binding protein in myotonic dystrophy. *Science* **280** (1998), 737–741.

57. L. P. Ranum, T. A. Cooper, RNA-mediated neuromuscular disorders. *Annu. Rev. Neurosci.* **29** (2006), 259–277.

58. X. Lin, J. W. Miller, A. Mankodi, *et al.*, Failure of MBNL1-dependent postnatal splicing transitions in myotonic dystrophy. *Hum. Mol. Genet.* **15**:13 (2006), 2087–2097.

59. A. Mankodi, M. P. Takahashi, H. Jiang, *et al.*, Expanded CUG repeats trigger aberrant splicing of ClC-1 chloride channel pre-mRNA and hyperexcitability of skeletal muscle in myotonic dystrophy. *Mol. Cell.* **10** (2002), 35–44.

60. N. Charlet, R. S. Savkur, G. Singh, A. V. Philips, E. A. Grice, T. A. Cooper, Loss of the muscle-specific chloride channel in type 1 myotonic dystrophy due to misregulated alternative splicing. *Mol. Cell* **10** (2002), 45–53.

61. T. M. Wheeler, J. D. Lueck, M. S. Swanson, R. T. Dirksen, C. A. Thornton, Correction of ClC-1 splicing eliminates chloride channelopathy and myotonia in mouse models of myotonic dystrophy. *J. Clin. Invest.* **117** (2007), 3952–3957.

62. J. D. Lueck, C. Lungu, A. Mankodi, *et al.*, Chloride channelopathy in myotonic dystrophy resulting from loss of post-transcriptional regulation for CLCN1. *Am. J. Physiol. Cell. Physiol.* **292**:4 (2007), C1291–C1297.

63. R. S. Savkur, A. V. Philips, T. A. Cooper, Aberrant regulation of insulin receptor alternative splicing is associated with insulin resistance in myotonic dystrophy. *Nat. Genet.* **29** (2001), 40–47.

64. L. T. Timchenko, J. W. Miller, N. A. Timchenko, *et al.*, Identification of a (CUG)n triplet repeat RNA-binding protein and its expression in myotonic dystrophy. *Nucleic Acids Res.* **24** (1996), 4407–4414.

65. S. Michalowski, J. W. Miller, C. R. Urbinati, M. Paliouras, M. S. Swanson, J. Griffith, Visualization of double-stranded RNAs from the myotonic dystrophy protein kinase gene and interactions with CUG-binding protein. *Nucleic Acids Res.* **27** (1999), 3534–3542.

66. M. Fardaei, K. Larkin, J. D. Brook, M. G. Hamshere, In vivo co-localisation of MBNL protein with DMPK expanded-repeat transcripts. *Nucleic Acids Res.* **29** (2001), 2766–2771.

67. N. A. Timchenko, Z. J. Cai, A. L. Welm, S. Reddy, T. Ashizawa, L. T. Timchenko, RNA CUG repeats sequester CUGBP1 and alter protein levels and activity of CUGBP1. *J. Biol. Chem.* **276** (2001), 7820–7826.

68. N. M. Kuyumcu-Martinez, G. S. Wang, T. A. Cooper, Increased steady-state levels of CUGBP1 in myotonic dystrophy 1 are due to PKC-mediated hyperphosphorylation. *Mol. Cell* **28** (2007), 68–78.

69. T. H. Ho, B. N. Charlet, M. G. Poulos, G. Singh, M. S. Swanson, T. A. Cooper, Muscleblind proteins regulate alternative splicing. *EMBO J.* **23** (2004), 3103–3112.

70. M. B. Warf, J. A. Berglund, MBNL binds similar RNA structures in the CUG repeats of myotonic dystrophy and its pre-mRNA substrate cardiac troponin T. *RNA* **13**:12 (2007), 2238–2251.

71. X. Lin, J. W. Miller, A. Mankodi, *et al.*, Failure of MBNL1-dependent post-natal splicing transitions in myotonic dystrophy. *Hum. Mol. Genet.* **15** (2006), 2087–2097.

72. H. Jiang, A. Mankodi, M. S. Swanson, R. T. Moxley, C. A. Thornton, Myotonic dystrophy type 1 is associated with nuclear foci of mutant RNA, sequestration of muscleblind proteins and deregulated alternative splicing in neurons. *Hum. Mol. Genet.* **13** (2004), 3079–3088.

73. R. N. Kanadia, K. A. Johnstone, A. Mankodi, *et al.*, A muscleblind knockout model for myotonic dystrophy. *Science* **302** (2003), 1978–1980.

74. R. N. Kanadia, J. Shin, Y. Yuan, *et al.*, Reversal of RNA missplicing and myotonia after muscleblind overexpression in a mouse poly(CUG) model for myotonic dystrophy. *Proc. Natl. Acad. Sci. U. S. A.* **103** (2006), 11748–11753.

75. W. Dansithong, S. Paul, L. Comai, S. Reddy, MBNL1 is the primary determinant of focus formation and aberrant insulin receptor splicing in DM1. *J. Biol. Chem.* **280** (2005), 5773–5780.

76. M. Fardaei, M. T. Rogers, H. M. Thorpe, *et al.*, Three proteins, MBNL, MBLL and MBXL, co-localize in vivo with nuclear foci of expanded-repeat transcripts in DM1 and DM2 cells. *Hum. Mol. Genet.* **11** (2002), 805–814.

77. N. A. Timchenko, P. Iakova, Z. J. Cai, J. R. Smith, L. T. Timchenko, Molecular basis for impaired muscle differentiation in myotonic dystrophy. *Mol. Cell. Biol.* **21** (2001), 6927–6938.

78. A. Ebralidze, Y. Wang, V. Petkova, K. Ebralidse, R. P. Junghans, RNA leaching of transcription factors disrupts transcription in myotonic dystrophy. *Science* **303** (2004), 383–387.

79. R. S. Yadava, C. D. Frenzel-McCardell, Q. Yu, *et al.*, RNA toxicity in myotonic muscular dystrophy induces NKX2–5 expression. *Nat. Genet.* **40** (2008), 61–68.

80. T. R. Klesert, A. D. Otten, T. D. Bird, S. J. Tapscott, Trinucleotide repeat expansion at the myotonic dystrophy locus reduces expression of DMAHP. *Nat. Genet.* **16** (1997), 402–406.

81. J. Krol, A. Fiszer, A. Mykowska, K. Sobczak, M. de Metzer, W. J. Kyzyzosiak, Ribonuclease dicer cleaves triplet repeat hairpins into shorter repeats that silence specific targets. *Mol. Cell 25*:4 (2007), 575–586.

82. W. Chen, Y. Liang, W. Deng, *et al.*, The zinc-finger protein CNBP is required for forebrain formation in the mouse. *Development* **130** (2003), 1367–1379.

83. J. M. Margolis, B. G. Schoser, M. L. Moseley, J. W. Day, L. P. Ranum, DM2 intronic expansions: evidence for CCUG accumulation without flanking sequence or effects on ZNF9 mRNA processing or protein expression. *Hum. Mol. Genet.* **15** (2006), 1808–1815.

84. A. Botta, S. Caldarola, L. Vallo, *et al.*, Effect of the [CCTG] n repeat expansion on ZNF9 expression in myotonic dystrophy type II (DM2). *Biochim. Biophys. Acta* **1762** (2006), 329–334.

85. P. S. Harper, Congenital myotonic dystrophy in Britain. Clinical aspects. I. *Arch. Dis. Child.* **50** (1975), 505–513.

86. T. A. O'Brien, P. S. Harper, Course, prognosis and complications of childhood-onset myotonic dystrophy. *Dev. Med. Child. Neurol.* **26** (1984), 62–67.

87. J. Steyaert, C. de Die-Smulders, J. P. Fryns, E. Goossens, D. Willekens, Behavioral phenotype in childhood type of dystrophia myotonica. *Am. J. Med. Genet.* **96** (2000), 888–889.

88. C. E. de Die-Smulders, C. J. Howeler, C. Thijs, *et al.*, Age and causes of death in adult-onset myotonic dystrophy. *Brain* **121**: Pt 8 (1998), 1557–1563.

89. J. Mathieu, P. Allard, L. Potvin, C. Prevost, P. Begin, A 10-year study of mortality in a cohort of patients with myotonic dystrophy. *Neurology* **52** (1999), 1658–1662.

90. A. Vihola, G. Bassez, G. Meola, *et al.*, Histopathological differences of myotonic dystrophy type 1 (DM1) and PROMM/DM2. *Neurology* **60** (2003), 1854–1857.

91. B. G. Schoser, C. Schneider-Gold, W. Kress, *et al.*, Muscle pathology in 57 patients with myotonic dystrophy type 2. *Muscle Nerve* **29** (2004), 275–281.

92. J. Mathieu, H. Boivin, D. Meunier, M. Gaudreault, P. Begin, Assessment of a disease-specific muscular impairment rating scale in myotonic dystrophy. *Neurology* **56** (2001), 336–340.

93. K. Ricker, M. Koch, F. Lehmann-Horn, *et al.*, Proximal myotonic myopathy: clinical features of a multisystem disorder similar to myotonic dystrophy. *Arch. Neurol.* **52** (1995), 25–31.

94. E. L. Logigian, E. Ciafaloni, L. C. Quinn, *et al.*, Severity, type, and distribution of myotonic discharges are different in type 1 and type 2 myotonic dystrophy. *Muscle Nerve* **35** (2007), 479–485.

95. A. Mankodi, C. R. Urbinati, Q. P. Yuan, *et al.*, Muscleblind localizes to nuclear foci of aberrant RNA in myotonic dystrophy types 1 and 2. *Hum. Mol. Genet.* **10** (2001), 2165–2170.

96. C. Gagnon, Social factors in DM1 in Quebec. In: NIH Burden of Muscle Disease Workshop, 2005.

97. T. Ashizawa, Myotonic dystrophy as a brain disorder. *Arch. Neurol.* **55** (1998), 291–293.

98. E. Hund, O. Jansen, M. C. Koch, *et al.*, Proximal myotonic myopathy with MRI white matter abnormalities of the brain. *Neurology* **48** (1997), 33–37.

99. G. Meola, V. Sansone, D. Perani, *et al.*, Executive dysfunction and avoidant personality trait in myotonic dystrophy type 1 (DM-1) and in proximal myotonic myopathy (PROMM/DM-2). *Neuromuscul. Disord.* **13** (2003), 813–821.

100. E. Ciafaloni, E. Mignot, V. Sansone, *et al.*, The hypocretin neurotransmission system in myotonic dystrophy type 1. *Neurology* **70** (2008), 226–230.

101. M. F. Phillips, P. S. Harper, Cardiac disease in myotonic dystrophy. *Cardiovasc. Res.* **33** (1997), 13–22.

102. J. A. Colleran, R. J. Hawley, E. E. Pinnow, P. F. Kokkinos, R. D. Fletcher, Value of the electrocardiogram in determining cardiac events and mortality in myotonic dystrophy. *Am. J. Cardiol.* **80** (1997), 1494–1497.

103. G. Bassez, A. Lazarus, I. Desguerre, *et al.*, Severe cardiac arrhythmias in young patients with myotonic dystrophy type 1. *Neurology* **63** (2004), 1939–1941.

104. W. J. Groh, M. R. Groh, C. Saha, *et al.*, Electrocardiographic abnormalities and sudden death in myotonic dystrophy type 1. *N. Engl. J. Med.* **358** (2008), 2688–2697.

105. B. G. Schoser, K. Ricker, C. Schneider-Gold, *et al.*, Sudden cardiac death in myotonic dystrophy type 2. *Neurology* **63** (2004), 2402–2404.

106. A. Lazarus, J. Varin, D. Babuty, F. Anselme, J. Coste, D. Duboc, Long-term follow-up of arrhythmias in patients with myotonic dystrophy treated by pacing: a multicenter diagnostic pacemaker study. *J. Am. Coll. Cardiol.* **40** (2002), 1645–1652.

107. K. Wahbi, C. Meune, G. Bassez, *et al.*, Left ventricular non-compaction in a patient with myotonic dystrophy type 2. *Neuromuscul. Disord.* **18** (2008), 331–333.

108. O. Vignaux, A. Lazarus, J. Varin, *et al.*, Right ventricular MR abnormalities in myotonic dystrophy and relationship with intracardiac electrophysiologic test findings: initial results. *Radiology* **224** (2002), 231–235.

109. K. M. Baig, M. Discepola, Recurrent capsular opacification after Nd:YAG laser treatment in myotonic dystrophy. *Can. J. Ophthalmol.* **42** (2007), 489–490.

110. D. K. Newman, Severe capsulorhexis contracture after cataract surgery in myotonic dystrophy. *J. Cataract. Refract. Surg.* **24** (1998), 1410–1412.

111. R. Osanai, M. Kinoshita, K. Hirose, Eye movement disorders in myotonic dystrophy type 1. *Acta Otolaryngol. Suppl.* (2007), 78–84.

112. S. Shaunak, R. Orrell, L. Henderson, C. Kennard, Saccades and smooth pursuit in myotonic dystrophy. *J. Neurol.* **246** (1999), 600–606.

113. I. Modolell, F. Mearin, J. S. Baudet, J. Gamez, C. Cervera, Malagelada, Jr., Pharyngo-esophageal motility disturbances in patients with myotonic dystrophy. *Scand. J. Gastroenterol.* **34** (1999), 878–882.

114. M. Bellini, P. Alduini, F. Costa, *et al.*, Gastric emptying in myotonic dystrophic patients. *Dig. Liver Dis.* **34** (2002), 484–488.

115. C. R. Heatwole, J. Miller, B. Martens, R. T. Moxley, 3rd, Laboratory abnormalities in ambulatory patients with myotonic dystrophy type 1. *Arch. Neurol.* **63** (2006), 1149–1153.

116. V. Sansone, R. C. Griggs, R. T. Moxley, 3rd, Hypothyroidism unmasking proximal myotonic myopathy. *Neuromuscul. Disord.* **10** (2000), 165–172.

117. J. L. Geh, A. L. Moss, Multiple pilomatrixomata and myotonic dystrophy: a familial association. *Br. J. Plast. Surg.* **52** (1999), 143–145.

118. M. R. Draper, J. M. Pickles, Pleomorphic adenoma and myotonic dystrophy: an association? *J. Laryngol. Otol.* **114** (2000), 985–987.

119. A. E. Saponaro, M. A. Marini, G. C. Rossi, J. G. Casas, Multiple basal cell carcinomas in a patient with myotonic dystrophy type 1. *Int. J. Dermatol.* **45** (2006), 87–88.

120. R. M. Azurdia, J. L. Verbov, Myotonic dystrophy and basal cell carcinoma-a true association? *Br. J. Dermatol.* **141** (1999), 941–942.

121. T. Sugio, K. Jinnai, T. Ohara, *et al.*, Myotonic dystrophy associated with insulinoma. *Intern. Med.* **38** (1999), 504–506.

122. E. Bell, A. R. Lorimer, J. Hinnie, Association between myotonic dystrophy and primary hyperparathyroidism. *J. Int. Med. Res.* **22** (1994), 296–298.

123. L. Carlin, J. Biller, Myotonic dystrophy and thymoma. *J. Neurol. Neurosurg. Psychiatry* **44** (1981), 852–853.

124. B. J. Mudge, P. B. Taylor, A. F. Vanderspek, Perioperative hazards in myotonic dystrophy. *Anaesthesia* **35** (1980), 492–495.

125. G. Gregoratos, J. Abrams, A. E. Epstein, *et al.*, ACC/AHA/NASPE 2002 guideline update for implantation of cardiac pacemakers and antiarrhythmia devices: summary article: a report of the American College of Cardiology/American Heart Association Task Force on Practice Guidelines (ACC/AHA/NASPE Committee to Update the 1998 Pacemaker Guidelines). *Circulation* **106** (2002), 2145–2161.

126. D. Annane, D. H. Moore, P. R. Barnes, R. G. Miller, Psychostimulants for hypersomnia (excessive daytime sleepiness) in myotonic dystrophy. *Cochrane Database Syst. Rev.* **3** (2006), CD003218.

127. H. Kwiecinski, B. Ryniewicz, A. Ostrzycki, Treatment of myotonia with antiarrhythmic drugs. *Acta Neurol. Scand.* **86** (1992), 371–375.

128. R. C. Griggs, S. Pandya, J. M. Florence, *et al.*, Randomized controlled trial of testosterone in myotonic dystrophy. *Neurology* **39** (1989), 219–222.

129. E. Vlachopapadopoulou, J. J. Zachwieja, J. M. Gertner, *et al.*, Metabolic and clinical response to recombinant human insulin-like growth factor I in myotonic dystrophy–a clinical research center study. *J. Clin. Endocrinol. Metab.* **80** (1995), 3715–3723.

130. A. Tollback, S. Eriksson, A. Wredenberg, *et al.*, Effects of high resistance training in patients with myotonic dystrophy. *Scand. J. Rehabil. Med.* **31** (1999), 9–16.

131. E. Lindeman, P. Leffers, F. Spaans, *et al.*, Strength training in patients with myotonic dystrophy and hereditary motor and sensory neuropathy: a randomized clinical trial. *Arch. Phys. Med. Rehabil.* **76** (1995), 612–620.

132. V. Ugalde, E. H. Breslin, S. A. Walsh, H. W. Bonekat, R. T. Abresch, G. T. Carter, Pursed lips breathing improves ventilation in myotonic muscular dystrophy. *Arch. Phys. Med. Rehabil.* **81** (2000), 472–478.

133. S. P. Kumar, D. Sword, R. K. Petty, S. W. Banham, K. R. Patel, Assessment of sleep studies in myotonic dystrophy. *Chron. Respir. Dis.* **4** (2007), 15–18.

134. P. Begin, J. Mathieu, J. Almirall, A. Grassino, Relationship between chronic hypercapnia and inspiratory-muscle weakness in myotonic dystrophy. *Am. J. Respir. Crit. Care. Med.* **156** (1997), 133–139.

135. W. Verpoest, M. De Rademaeker, K. Sermon, *et al.*, Real and expected delivery rates of patients with myotonic dystrophy undergoing intracytoplasmic sperm injection and preimplantation genetic diagnosis. *Hum. Reprod.* **23** (2008), 1654–1660.

136. N. L. Dean, S. L. Tan, A. Ao, Instability in the transmission of the myotonic dystrophy CTG repeat in human oocytes and preimplantation embryos. *Fertil. Steril.* **86** (2006), 98–105.

137. N. L. Dean, S. L. Tan, A. Ao, The development of preimplantation genetic diagnosis for myotonic dystrophy using multiplex fluorescent polymerase chain reaction and its clinical application. *Mol. Hum. Reprod.* **7** (2001), 895–901.

138. S. Fokstuen, J. Myring, C. Evans, P. S. Harper, Presymptomatic testing in myotonic dystrophy: genetic counselling approaches. *J. Med. Genet.* **38** (2001), 846–850.

139. A. C. Magee, A. E. Hughes, A. Kidd, *et al.*, Reproductive counselling for women with myotonic dystrophy. *J. Med. Genet.* **39** (2002), E15.

140. L. Martorell, A. M. Cobo, M. Baiget, M. Naudo, J. J. Poza, J. Parra, Prenatal diagnosis in myotonic dystrophy type 1. Thirteen years of experience: implications for reproductive counselling in DM1 families. *Prenat. Diagn.* **27** (2007), 68–72.

141. M. A. Langlois, C. Boniface, G. Wang, *et al.*, Cytoplasmic and nuclear retained DMPK mRNAs are targets for RNA interference in myotonic dystrophy cells. *J. Biol. Chem.* **280** (2005), 16949–16954.

142. D. Furling, G. Doucet, M. A. Langlois, *et al.*, Viral vector producing antisense RNA restores myotonic dystrophy myoblast functions. *Gene. Ther.* **10** (2003), 795–802.

Chapter

19 Mitochondrial myopathies

Patrick F. Chinnery and Eric A. Shoubridge

Introduction

Mitochondria are intimately involved in various aspects of cellular homeostasis, and have a fundamental role in cellular energy metabolism, including fatty acid β oxidation and the urea cycle. However, the term "mitochondrial disorder" refers to pathological defects of the final common pathway of energy production - oxidative phosphorylation (OXPHOS). Although some patients present with clinical phenotype restricted to skeletal muscle (i.e., isolated mitochondrial myopathy), multisystem involvement is the hallmark of mitochondrial disease. Cardiomyopathy is common, central and peripheral neurological disease is a frequent finding, and many patients have ocular manifestations, hearing loss, and endocrine dysfunction (particularly diabetes mellitus). As a result, patients with a mitochondrial disorder can present to many different hospital specialists, and the underlying myopathy is often missed, being overshadowed by the presenting feature in a different organ system. The extramuscular features can be extremely disabling, and some respond well to treatment. It is therefore probably better to refer to patients as having "mitochondrial disease," alerting nonspecialist clinicians to the possibility of other systems involvement.

The first human mitochondrial disease was described in a patient with nonthyroidal hypermetabolism (Luft disease) nearly 50 years ago [1]. Only a few patients have been described with this elusive condition, but this clinical description and biochemical studies paved the way for three decades of clinical and pathological research on cases of suspected mitochondrial disease. Initially patients were classified into groups based upon the pattern of clinical involvement, histological and ultrastructural abnormalities of mitochondria, or biochemical assays of mitochondrial function. Specific clinical syndromes were recognized such as the Kearns–Sayre syndrome (KSS) or chronic progressive external ophthalmoplegia (CPEO), but it soon became clear that many patients did not fit neatly into a specific syndromic diagnosis. The inheritance pattern also varied. Some patients appeared to be sporadic cases, whereas others were clearly familial, showing either autosomal or maternal inheritance. Different groups attempted to subdivide suspected mitochondrial disease into discrete categories (the "splitters" [2]) and those who thought of all mitochondrial disease as a single, if wide, spectrum of disorders (the "lumpers" [3]). At this early stage it was apparent that mitochondrial disorders were a heterogeneous group: clinically, histologically, biochemically, and probably genetically.

The human mtDNA sequence was published in 1981 [4], and in 1988 the first pathogenic mtDNA mutations were identified [5, 6]. This work laid the foundations for the description of over 150 different pathogenic point mutations and a larger number of different rearrangements of mtDNA in patients with OXPHOS disease [7]. Shortly after the first description of primary mtDNA disorders, it became clear that some patients inherited the propensity to develop secondary mtDNA abnormalities in a autosomal dominant manner [8, 9], and some biochemical defects were transmitted as a recessive trait. These studies led to the clinical, biochemical, and genetic classification of a growing group of nuclear genetic mitochondrial disorders. Many of these diseases are rare and have only been described in single families and affect structural subunits of the respiratory chain or their assembly [10]. However, disorders of the replication and repair of mtDNA have emerged as a major group, and the gene coding for the mtDNA polymerase γ (*POLG*) is a common cause of mitochondrial disease presenting at any age [11, 12]. Other recent new categories include nuclear genetic disorders of intra-mitochondrial protein synthesis, defects of the lipid mitochondrial membrane (including Barth syndrome, and disorders of protein import as in the Mohr–Tranjeberg syndrome), and disorders of mitochondrial fusion and fission (such as dominant optic atrophy, and Charcot–Marie–Tooth disease type 2A) [13]. Thus, the emphasis on disease classification has moved towards the molecular level, identifying discrete categories of genetic disease, with overlapping pathological mechanisms and clinical phenotypes. In many ways, the "lumpers" and "splitters" were both right and wrong.

Mitochondria are involved in the pathophysiology of many other inherited disorders, including X-linked sideroblastic

Disorders of Voluntary Muscle, 8th edn., eds. George Karpati, David Hilton-Jones, Kate Bushby and Robert C. Griggs. Published by Cambridge University Press.

anemia [14], Friedreich ataxia (*FRDA*) [15], hereditary spastic paraplegia (*SPG7*) [16] and Wilson disease (*ATP7B*) [17]. In addition, structural, biochemical and genetic mitochondrial defects have also been described in common neurodegenerative diseases [18, 19], and in healthy aged individuals [20]. It is currently not clear whether these abnormalities are primarily involved in the pathophysiology of these disorders, or whether mitochondrial dysfunction contributes to the aging process [21]. This debate is beyond the scope of this chapter, but the clinician must be aware of the possibility of these "secondary" mitochondrial abnormalities when investigating patients with suspected mitochondrial disease. There are many examples where patients with unexplained neuromuscular phenotypes were given a diagnosis of mitochondrial disease after the detection of subtle secondary mitochondrial abnormalities, which were subsequently found to be secondary to another disease process or were age-related. Making a confident diagnosis of mitochondrial disease remains a major challenge in some patients, made all the more difficult by the expanding clinical phenotype.

Abbreviations used in this chapter are summarized in Table 19.1.

Table 19.1. Abbreviations

adPEO	Autosomal dominant PEO
AHS	Alpers–Huttenlocher syndrome
arPEO	Autosomal recessive PEO
ATP	Adenosine triphosphate
bp	Base pairs
COX	Cytochrome *c* oxidase
CPEO	Chronic progressive external ophthalmoplegia
ICC	Immunocytochemistry
KSS	Kearns–Sayre syndrome
LHON	Leber hereditary optic neuropathy
LS	Leigh syndrome
MELAS	Mitochondrial encephalomyopathy with lactic acidosis and stroke-like episodes
MERRF	Myoclonic epilepsy with ragged-red fibers
MIRAS	Mitochondrial recessive ataxia syndrome
MNGIE	Mitochondrial neurogastrointestinal encephalomyopathy
mtDNA	Mitochondrial DNA
nDNA	Nuclear DNA
OXPHOS	Oxidative phosphorylation
PCR	Polymerase chain reaction
PEO	Progressive external ophthalmoplegia
POLG	Polymerase gamma
PS	Pearson syndrome
RFLP	Restriction fragment length polymorphism
SANDO	Sensory ataxic neuropathy with dysarthria and ophthalmoparesis
SNP	Single nucleotide polymorphism

Epidemiology of mitochondrial diseases

Until relatively recently, mitochondrial disorders were thought of as being extremely rare, perhaps only affecting one or two per million of the population. However, recent population-based surveys have established mitochondrial disorders as being amongst the most common inherited diseases. Current data indicate that mitochondrial disorders affect at least ~1 in 5000 of the population [22, 23, 24, 25]. These studies show that, in general, patients with mitochondrial disease presenting in adult life have an underlying mtDNA defect responsible for their disease, whereas the majority of children have a proven or presumed nuclear genetic defect responsible for their mitochondrial disease. The most common pathogenic mtDNA mutations cause Leber hereditary optic neuropathy (LHON, due to the following point mutations m.11778A > G, m.14484T > C or m.3460A > G), accounting for half of all adults. The remainder are equally distributed into three groups: single mtDNA deletions, disease due to the m.3243A > G tRNA Leu^{UUR} gene point mutation of mtDNA, and other mtDNA point mutations. However, these figures underestimate the prevalence, as the published studies do not include the large number of patients with nuclear gene defects in *POLG* that are currently being defined [11]. By contrast, mtDNA defects have only been detected in ~15% of children presenting with mitochondrial disease [26]. A range of nuclear gene defects account for the remainder, including mutations in *POLG*.

Mitochondrial biology and biogenesis

Mitochondrial structure and morphology

Mitochondria are cytoplasmic organelles about 0.5–1.0 μm in diameter, similar in size to the α-proteobacteria from which they derived by endosymbiosis more than a billion years ago. The mitochondrial matrix is enclosed by a double membrane system: an outer membrane that is permeable to most small molecules less than 10 kDa, and an impermeable inner membrane across which an electrochemical gradient is formed to drive ATP synthesis. The outer membrane contains a number of proteins including porin, monoamine oxidase, enzymes of phospholipid biosynthesis, and part of the protein import system, and its lipid composition is similar to that of other microsomal membranes. The inner membrane is a highly specialized structure containing the protein complexes of the electron transport system and numerous carriers involved in moving metabolites into and out of the matrix compartment. It is rich in cardiolipin and highly convoluted into foldings called cristae, which greatly increase its surface area. The shape and pattern of the cristae are cell-type specific; muscle fibers typically have a large number of flattened cristae necessary to support the high metabolic demands of muscle. The matrix space enclosed by the inner membrane contains the pyruvate dehydrogenase complex and enzymes for the tricarboxylic acid cycle, β-oxidation of fatty acids, heme biosynthesis, the urea cycle, ketone and amino acid metabolism. It also contains mtDNA and the machinery necessary for its replication and expression.

Mitochondria take on a variety of shapes ranging from simple spheres to large interconnected reticular networks, and undergo active fission and fusion (reviewed in [27]). Many of the proteins involved in this process have been identified and two involved in fusion are associated with human disease: OPA1 with dominantly inherited optic atrophy [28] and mitofusin2 with CMT Type 2A [29] and CMT Type 6 [30].

Mitochondria in skeletal muscle are conventionally classified as either subsarcolemmal or inter-myofibrillar, indicating the locations in the myofiber where they are found. Mitochondrial volume fraction varies from about 2% to 5% in human skeletal muscle, a difference that is associated with different fiber types and energy requirements. In human muscle the volume fraction of mitochondria usually varies by a factor of 2–3 between fiber types. Subsarcolemmal mitochondria consist of what appear to be independent organelles clustered between the myofibrils and the plasma membrane. Intermyofibrillar mitochondria are interspersed between myofibers, and on cross-section appear as pairs in the half I-bands adjacent to the Z-line. In three dimensions there are in fact bracelets that encircle the myofiber.

Mitochondrial biogenesis

Proteomic and bioinformatic studies suggest that between 1000 and 1500 proteins are necessary for mitochondria to perform their diverse biochemical activities. As only a handful are encoded by mtDNA, the vast majority, which are synthesized on cytosolic ribosomes, must be transported to the mitochondrion and inserted into the correct location in the mitochondrion. In the case of the respiratory chain enzymes, this must be coordinated with the expression of the mtDNA-encoded polypeptides. Four different transport systems have been characterized that are responsible for targeting proteins to the matrix, inner and outer mitochondrial membranes, and the intermembrane space (reviewed in [31]). The mitochondrial content of muscle, which can be up- or down-regulated by a variety of stimuli such as endurance training or disuse, is coordinated through the master regulatory protein PGC1α [32].

The process by which new mitochondrial membranes are elaborated is much less well understood than the protein import pathways. Cardiolipin, a phospholipid unique to mitochondria, is synthesized in mitochondria. The other major phospholipids in mitochondrial membranes (phosphatidylserine, -ethanolamine, -choline, and -inositol) are transferred from their site of synthesis in the endoplasmic reticulum via regions of membrane continuity.

Electron transport and oxidative phosphorylation

The electron transport–oxidative phosphorylation system is located in the inner mitochondrial membrane. Functionally the system is composed of five enzyme complexes: NADH CoQ reductase (I), succinate CoQ reductase (II), ubiquinol cytochrome *c* reductase (III), cytochrome *c* oxidase (COX) (IV), and ATP synthase (V). These complexes are large oligomers composed of 89 polypeptides in total. Complexes I–IV make up the respiratory chain; coenzyme Q (CoQ) and cytochrome *c* act as shuttle molecules to move electrons between the complexes. Electrons derived from the oxidation of glucose or fatty acids enter the chain as NADH or $FADH_2$ at complex I or II, and are passed to carriers of progressively greater electron affinity and ultimately accepted by molecular oxygen to form water. Complex I transfers electrons through a series of redox groups which include flavin mononucleotide (FMN) and six iron-sulfur clusters. It is composed of about 43 subunits, 7 of which are encoded in mtDNA. Complex II performs a key reaction in the tricarboxylic acid cycle in which succinate is dehydrogenated to fumarate and the electrons are donated to CoQ. It is located on the matrix side of the membrane, and its four subunits are encoded by nuclear genes. Complex III transfers electrons between the two shuttle molecules, CoQ and cytochrome *c*. It is composed of 11 subunits, only one of which (cytb) is encoded in mtDNA. Complex IV accepts electrons from cytochrome *c* and donates them to molecular oxygen. Three of its 13 subunits are encoded in mtDNA. At three stages along this chain (complexes I, III, and IV) energy is conserved by pumping protons across the inner mitochondrial membrane from the matrix space, which establishes an electrochemical gradient for protons across this membrane. The energy conserved in this gradient is then used to synthesize ATP in the ATP synthase (V) reaction, functionally coupling electron transport along the respiratory chain to oxidative phosphorylation. Complex V is composed of two parts, an F_1 segment that catalyzes the synthesis of ATP, and an F_o component that translocates protons into the mitochondrial matrix. It consists of 12–13 subunits, 2 of which are mitochondrially encoded. Some of the individual respiratory chain complexes are organized into supercomplexes, the so-called respirasome, the major one being composed of I:III:IV in a 1:2:1 ratio in mammals [33]. This is thought to increase the efficiency of energy transduction.

Mitochondrial genetics

Structure, genetic code and organization of mtDNA

mtDNA is a double-stranded circular DNA molecule of ~16.5 kb in all mammals in which it has been sequenced. The two stands are referred to as heavy (H) and light (L) reflecting their behavior in density gradients. Mammalian mtDNA codes for 13 polypeptides, all of which are subunits of the enzyme complexes of the oxidative phosphorylation system, and 22 tRNAs and 2 rRNAs, which constitute part of the dedicated mitochondrial translation machinery. The genetic code of mammalian mtDNA is different than the "universal" genetic code: UGA, the universal STOP, is Trp, AUA is Met, AGA and AGG (universal Arg) are STOP codons. Thus genes encoded in mtDNA cannot be translated on cytosolic ribosomes. The genome is exceedingly compact; there are no introns, and there is only one noncoding (control) region of ~1 kb that contains the replication origin for leading strand synthesis (O_H), and the promoters for transcription of the H- and L-strands. The mtDNA copy number in somatic cells is generally in the range of 10^3–10^4 copies per cell, packaged in a DNA–protein structure called the nucleoid at approximately 2–10 copies per nucleoid [34]. Gametes are a notable exception: mature oocytes contain approximately 2×10^5 mtDNAs [35, 36, 37] and sperm about 102 [38]. The mitochondrial nucleoid in higher eukaryotes is reported to contain more than 30 core nucleoid proteins including many of those involved in transcription and replication [39]. The transcription factor mtTFA is a basic protein of the HMG box family that is also thought to package mtDNA Kaufmann [40]. Decreasing mtTFA levels results in loss of mtDNA; likewise cells devoid of mtDNA contain no detectable mtTFA, leading to the suggestion that mtDNA levels are controlled by mtTFA [41].

Heteroplasmy and threshold expression

Most mammals have a single mtDNA sequence variant in all of their cells, a condition referred to as mtDNA homoplasmy. New mutations lead to the occurrence of more than one sequence variant in an individual, a condition known as mtDNA heteroplasmy. The vast majority of patients with mtDNA mutations are heteroplasmic, and the proportion of mutant mtDNAs varies both in space and time in ways that are specific to particular mutations, but not well understood. As mtDNA is a multi-copy genome, the proportion of genomes carrying a particular pathogenic mutation is important for the expression of a biochemical and clinical phenotype. Studies in cultured cells have determined that such thresholds for common point mutations are generally high (>80% mutant mtDNAs) [42], suggesting that intra-mitochondrial genetic complementation is a common feature. However, in vivo studies of the $tRNA^{leu}$ mutation associated with MELAS suggest that in tissues the thresholds for expression of a biochemical defect may be very low or even nonexistent [43, 44].

Replication

The mechanism of mtDNA replication has been the subject of recent controversy. The conventional, strand-displacement model developed over the past two decades by Clayton and colleagues [45] was suggested to be an artifact of biased incorporation of ribonucleotides into the L-strand [46], and a coupled, strand-synchronous mechanism was proposed in its stead [47, 48]. In the strand-displacement model, leading strand synthesis of the H-strand starts from O_H in the control region and proceeds about two-thirds the way around the molecule until a second origin (O_L) is exposed allowing synthesis of the L-strand to proceed. The alternative model proposes that replication is strand-coupled, originating from a broad zone around O_H [47]. A recent study in which atomic force microscopy was used to examine mtDNA replicative intermediates in mouse liver was entirely consistent with the strand-displacement model, and did not show any evidence of the theta structures that would be predicted from the strand-coupled model [49]. The same study also provided evidence for alternative L-strand origins, and it was suggested that their presence, in addition to the propensity for branch migration in replicating DNA, might account for the patterns observed by 2D gel electrophoresis that were interpreted as evidence for strand-coupled replication [49].

Replication is catalyzed by a distinct nuclear-encoded polymerase, the γ-DNA polymerase, which is a heterotrimeric molecule consisting of one subunit of the catalytic subunit (encoded by *POLG*, also called *POLG1*), and two accessory subunits encoded by *POLG2*. Leading strand synthesis at O_H is primed by a short piece of RNA generated by transcription from the L-strand promoter. It is not known how replication is primed on the L-strand. Phylogenetic analysis of eukaryotic homologs of the Twinkle helicase suggests that the domains associated with primase function are not well conserved in mammals [50], and recent biochemical studies failed to demonstrate primase activity associated with Twinkle [51]. A minimal mtDNA replisome can be reconstituted with γ-DNA polymerase, mitochondrial single-stranded binding protein, and the Twinkle helicase [52].

mtDNA copy number varies widely from cell to cell, and is tightly regulated in a cell-specific fashion; however, replication of mtDNA is not tightly coupled to the cell cycle [53]. Thus, during mitosis some templates may replicate more than once, others not at all. This behavior, coupled with the random distribution of mtDNAs to daughter cells at cytokinesis, provides a mechanism for the segregation of mtDNA sequence variants. Replicative segregation of mtDNA also occurs in post-mitotic cells, as mtDNA replication and turnover is an ongoing process throughout their lifetime [54].

Transcription

mtDNA is transcribed as three polycistronic units: the entire H- and L-strands and the two rRNAs, by a single subunit, phage-like RNA polymerase [55]. The rRNAs are transcribed 10–60 times more frequently than the entire H-strand, a process controlled by a specific termination factor that binds to both the transcription initiation site, and a termination site located 3′ to the 16S rRNA in the gene coding for $tRNA^{leu(UUR)}$ [56]. Mitochondrial transcription has been reconstituted in vitro and requires only the presence of two transcription factors, mtTFA and mtTFB (either B1 or B2), and the single subunit RNA polymerase [57, 58]. Maturation of the mitochondrial transcripts requires an RNAase P activity, and it is thought that the tRNA genes, which are interspersed between many of the protein coding genes, act as signal sequences in this process [59].

Translation

The mitochondrial translation system has evolved as a specialized system to translate the handful of hydrophobic inner mitochondrial membrane proteins coded in mtDNA. Translation of these polypeptides requires recruitment of the mRNAs, ribosomes and the rest of the translational machinery to the inner mitochondrial membrane where the nascent polypeptides are most probably co-translationally inserted into the inner membrane with the aid of molecular chaperones. Many of the features of mitochondrial translation are similar to those found in prokaryotes; however, there are striking differences in the composition and structure of mitoribosomes, and in the structure of the mRNAs. Defects in mitochondrial translation are the most common cause of all oxidative phosphorylation diseases; however, most that have so far been reported are due to mtDNA mutations in tRNA and rRNA genes.

The antibiotic sensitivity of mitoribosomes is generally similar to that of prokaryotic ribosomes, however they contain a much higher protein/RNA ratio than bacterial ribosomes [60]. The protein constituents of both mammalian ribosomal subunits have been identified in their entirety. The translation process requires a number of initiation, elongation, and termination (or release) factors and all have been cloned and sequenced in several mammalian species, including humans.

Transmission of mtDNA

mtDNA is maternally inherited in mammals [61], so new sequence variants are transmitted along maternal lineages without the benefit of recombination with male mtDNA. A single case of paternal transmission of a pathogenic mtDNA mutation has been reported in an individual with a severe muscle myopathy [62], but this is likely to be an extremely rare event in human biology. The relative rarity of mtDNA heteroplasmy and the high degree of population polymorphism suggest that new germline mtDNA sequence variants are rapidly segregated in maternal lineages. This observation seemed paradoxical given the high mtDNA copy number ($\sim 2 \times 10^5$) in mature oocytes, and the relatively small number of cell divisions in the development of the female germline, and suggested the existence of a genetic bottleneck for the transmission of mitochondria and mtDNA, a concept first proposed by Hauswirth and Laipis [63] to explain the rapid segregation of a mtDNA D-loop sequence variant in several maternal lineages of Holstein cows.

The mechanism that produces the bottleneck has been investigated in mouse models of heteroplasmy using single-cell PCR techniques [35, 36, 64]. Replication of mtDNA does not appear to restart until after implantation [65, 66], resulting in an almost 1000-fold reduction in mtDNA copy number to about 200 mtDNAs in the earliest primordial germ cells (PGCs) [36]. Little intercellular variation in the degree of mtDNA heteroplasmy was found amongst individual PGCs in one study, and all of the genotypic variance in the subsequent generation was already generated by the time primary oocytes were formed in early postnatal life [64]. These studies are consistent with the idea that replicative segregation during the mitotic expansion of the PGC population can account for the variation in heteroplasmy levels in the next generation; however, it is not possible to eliminate the hypothesis that the mechanism involves replication of a subpopulation of mtDNAs at some point during oocyte development.

The mean level of heteroplasmy in a large sample of offspring from single mothers was not significantly different than the level of heteroplasmy in the mother, suggesting that mtDNA segregation between generations, at least for polymorphic sequence variants, is stochastic [64]. Random genetic drift also appears, for the most part, to account for the pattern of transmission of six of the most common pathogenic mtDNA point mutations in human pedigrees [67]. However, two studies have investigated oocytes or early embryos from mothers carrying the T8993C NARP (neuropathy, ataxia, and retinitis pigmentosa) mutation in the ATP6 gene, and shown almost complete segregation of this mutation, suggesting that genetic drift alone may not explain the transmission of all pathogenic mutations [68]. Consistent with extreme skewing of heteroplasmy in the germline in these cases, a disproportionate number of reports of apparently de novo mutations in the ATP6 gene have appeared [69].

It has not been possible to construct animal models segregating specific pathogenic mtDNAs at will, as a method to transform mammalian mitochondria has remained elusive. This problem has been circumvented in one instance by transferring naturally occurring large-scale mtDNA deletions to one-cell embryos using enucleated cytoplasts as the transfer vehicle [70]. These large deletions are usually associated with progressive external ophthalmoplegia (PEO) or Kearns–Sayre syndrome (KSS), both of which are nearly always sporadic diseases [71]. The mice were able to transmit the deleted species of mtDNA at high levels (greater than 80% mutant mtDNAs in some animals) through three generations, clearly showing that there is no barrier to the transmission of large-scale mtDNA deletions in this model. By contrast, the risk of transmitting a large-scale mtDNA deletion in humans is only about 4% [72]. It is not known why the human and mouse differ in their ability to transmit these particular mtDNA mutations, but it likely reflects the fact that humans with high proportions of large-scale mtDNA deletions have a severe clinical phenotype and rarely reproduce.

The spectrum of human mtDNA mutations that are associated with diseases is not a random sampling of the mitochondrial genome, and this observation prompted Wallace and co-workers to compare the transmission of severe versus mild mtDNA mutations, which they were able to isolate from murine cell lines and introduce into the female germline [73]. Strikingly, they found evidence for strong selection against a severe mtDNA mutation, suggesting that a mechanism exists to filter these out at some point during oocyte development. Stewart *et al.* reached a similar conclusion using a completely different strategy [74]. They mated female mice carrying a *POLG1* transgene with defective proofreading activity with wild-type males and tracked the evolution of mtDNA mutations in successive backcross generations. They observed a significant bias against non-synonymous mutations in protein-coding genes in successive generations, supporting the concept of purifying selection in the female germline. It thus appears that the spectrum of human mtDNA mutations that have been associated with disease may include only those that are able to escape this filter in germline development.

Segregation of mtDNA in somatic cells

Although there is abundant opportunity for mitotic segregation of mutant mtDNAs during fetal development, studies of fetal tissues in individuals carrying pathogenic mtDNA mutations show little tissue-to-tissue variation in the proportion of mutant and wild-type mtDNAs [75]. Similar observations have been made in heteroplasmic mice in which there is little variation in heteroplasmy among tissues at birth, but strong, tissue-specific selection for alternate mtDNA genotypes as the animal ages [76].

In contrast to the situation during development, mitotic segregation of pathogenic mtDNA sequence variants occurs throughout postnatal life. The load of mtDNA mutations inherited at birth undoubtedly plays an important role in the clinical phenotype of patients with pathogenic mtDNA mutations, but tissue-specific segregation can modify the proportions of mutant and wild-type mtDNAs significantly, and this is often associated with a worsening clinical course. There is good evidence for increases in the proportions of some pathogenic mtDNA mutations [77, 78] with age in the skeletal muscle of patients with mitochondrial encephalomyopathies in whom mutant mtDNAs are often undetectable in actively dividing cells in the same individuals. This had led to the suggestion that there may be feedback mechanisms that promote the replication of mutant mtDNAs in post-mitotic cells, reflecting a futile attempt to restore oxidative phosphorylation function, and selection against cells with a growth disadvantage due to the presence of the mutants in actively mitotic cells. It is interesting to note that the most dramatic segregation patterns are observed in sporadic cases, where mutant mtDNAs are often only detectable in skeletal muscle [5, 79, 80].

Clinical presentation of mitochondrial disorders

Neuromuscular features often dominate the clinical picture in mitochondrial disease. The signs may fall into a well-recognized clinical syndrome (Table 19.2), but often this is not the case, with only one organ system being involved, or there may be a complex multisystem disorder that is not instantly recognizable as a mitochondrial disease. In general, a mitochondrial disorder should be considered in patients presenting with an unexplained combination of neuromuscular and/or non-neuromuscular symptoms which often involve hearing, visual failure, cardiomyopathy, and diabetes mellitus. Liver failure and renal tubular defects are also well-recognized features of mitochondrial disease, particularly in childhood.

Myopathy in mitochondrial disease

Although myopathy can be the presenting or only feature, skeletal muscle weakness is often overshadowed by other neurological signs as part of a classical mitochondrial syndrome (see below) or as part of a multisystem syndrome that does not neatly fit into one of these specific categories. Slowly progressive proximal limb-girdle muscle weakness is the most common finding, usually causing fatigue and weakness, with exercise intolerance. The pattern usually follows that typical for a metabolic disorder, but focal symmetrical muscle weakness and atrophy have been described mimicking limb-girdle muscular dystrophy [81], and although uncommon, the loss of muscle fibers with fatty replacement has been reported on numerous occasions [82]. Muscle pain and rhabdomyolysis are common in patients with mutations in the *MTCYB* gene [83]. Distal myopathic presentations have been described in adult life [84], but are uncommon. Neonatal and infantile generalized hypotonia are well-recognized presenting features, and arthrogryposis has also been described [85].

Classic clinical syndromes

Chronic progressive external ophthalmoplegia (CPEO)

Chronic progressive external ophthalmoplegia (CPEO) is an ocular myopathy leading to ophthalmoplegia and ptosis [3, 86] which often begins in adult life and is slowly progressive, often remaining asymmetrical and causing transient diplopia [87]. Some patients develop proximal muscle weakness in later life [86]. Dysphagia is common, but not as prominent as in oculopharyngeal muscular dystrophy [88]. The presence of additional neurological features has led some to use the term "PEO-plus," particularly if there is a peripheral sensorimotor neuropathy. These disorders probably form a spectrum of severity which includes KSS (see below). In general, PEO of early onset is associated with a more progressive clinical course and the development of additional neurological features [86].

Progressive external ophthalmoplegia usually affects sporadic cases, but it can be maternally transmitted [72], or recessive or dominantly inherited [12, 89, 90]. In autosomal dominant (AD) and recessive (AR) PEO there may be additional features including severe sensory ataxia, cerebellar ataxia, intractable seizures, parkinsonism, and premature ovarian failure (see *POLG* disease described below).

Kearns–Sayre syndrome (KSS)

Kearns–Sayre syndrome is characterized by early-onset PEO, cerebellar ataxia, bilateral sensorineural deafness, and pigmentary retinopathy before the age of 20 years. Other features include cerebellar ataxia, proximal myopathy, complete heart block, cardiomyopathy, endocrinopathies, short stature, deafness, dysphagia [88], and an elevated CSF protein. KSS is usually a sporadic disease.

Table 19.2. Clinical syndromes associated with mitochondrial disease

Syndrome	Primary features	Additional features
Alpers-Huttenlocher syndrome	Encephalopathy with seizures, liver failure	Developmental delay and hypotonia
Chronic progressive external ophthalmoplegia	External ophthalmoplegia and bilateral ptosis	Mild proximal myopathy
Kearns–Sayre syndrome	Progressive external ophthalmoplegia onset before age 20 with pigmentary retinopathy	Bilateral deafness
	Plus one of the following: cerebrospinal fluid protein greater than 1 g/l, cerebellar ataxia, or heart block	Myopathy
		Dysphagia
		Diabetes mellitus
		Hypoparathyroidism
		Dementia
Pearson syndrome	Sideroblastic anemia of childhood	Renal tubular defects
	Pancytopenia	
	Exocrine pancreatic failure	
Mitochondrial encephalomyopathy with lactic acidosis and stroke-like episodes (MELAS)	Stroke-like episodes before age 40 years	Diabetes mellitus
	Seizures and/or dementia	Cardiomyopathy
	Ragged-red fibers and/or lactic acidosis	Bilateral deafness
	Pigmentary retinopathy	
	Cerebellar ataxia	
Mitochondrial neurogastrointestinal encephalomyopathy (MNGIE)	Gastrointestinal pseudo obstruction	
	Myopathy	
	Leukoencephalopathy	
	Peripheral neuropathy	
Myoclonic epilepsy with ragged-red fibers (MERRF)	Myoclonus	Dementia
	Seizures	Optic atrophy
	Cerebellar ataxia	Bilateral deafness
	Myopathy	Peripheral neuropathy
		Spasticity
		Multiple lipomas
Leber hereditary optic neuropathy	Subacute bilateral visual failure; males: females approximately 4:1	Dystonia
	Median age of onset 24 years	Cardiac pre-excitation syndromes
Leigh syndrome	Subacute relapsing encephalopathy with cerebellar and brain stem signs	Basal ganglia lucencies
Infantile myopathy and lactic acidosis	Hypotonia	Cardiomyopathy $\pm$ Toni–Fanconi–Debre syndrome

Pearson (bone marrow pancreas) syndrome (PS)

Pearson syndrome is a rare multisystem disorder characterized by sideroblastic anemia with pancytopenia, vacuolization of marrow precursors, and exocrine pancreatic dysfunction. It is a disease that presents in infancy and frequently results in early death. Survival through childhood leads to an improvement in anemia but patients then develop the characteristic features of KSS. PS is usually sporadic.

Mitochondrial encephalopathy lactic acidosis and stroke-like episodes (MELAS)

The syndrome MELAS is characterized by recurrent occipito-parietal stroke-like episodes, often following a migrainous prodrome, and associated with encephalopathy and seizures [91]. Deafness, diabetes mellitus, myopathy, cardiomyopathy, gastrointestinal dysmotility, and basal ganglia calcification are also common features in either the index case or oligosymptomatic family members [92]. The term "stroke-like episode" is somewhat misleading because the focal deficits are rarely acute in onset, and brain imaging reveals evolving and resolving high signal in regions crossing vascular territories [93], which are probably due to focal encephalopathy. Cases can be sporadic, or there may be a relevant maternal family history.

Myoclonic epilepsy with ragged red fibers (MERRF)

The syndrome MERRF is a progressive encephalomyopathy with associated epilepsy, myoclonus, and ataxia [94, 95]. Visual failure and optic atrophy are common, and the ataxia usually evolves from a pure cerebellar form to a mixed ataxia due to an emerging sensorimotor neuropathy, often with associated pyramidal tract signs, and eventually a dementia. Some families also demonstrate multiple lipomatas (Ekbom syndrome) [96, 97]. Cardiomyopathy is also well described. The disorder can appear as a sporadic case, or there may be a maternal family history.

Leigh syndrome (LS)

In the strict sense, Leigh syndrome is an autopsy diagnosis based on the presence of symmetrical necrotic lesions in the brain stem and basal ganglia, which were first described on post-mortem tissue. The basal ganglia lesions are often visible on brain MRI, and LS is often diagnosed in children with an unexplained encephalopathy and characteristic MR appearances. The phenotype can be highly variable, from a relapsing-remitting brain stem encephalopathy with ataxia, to a more generalized encephalopathy with muscle hypotonia. Dystonia is often a feature and can dominate the picture, particularly in late-onset cases in adult life. The clinical course can follow a stepwise deterioration with moderate recovery of developmental skills between episodes of regression, or a slowly progressive decline. Cases can be sporadic, recessive, X-linked or maternally inherited [98, 99, 100].

Neuropathy, ataxia, and retinitis pigmentosa (NARP)

Originally described in patients with developmental delay, retinitis pigmentosa, dementia, seizures, ataxia, proximal neurogenic muscle weakness, and sensory neuropathy in four members of a single family [101], the phenotype has now been expanded to include cardiomyopathy and Leigh syndrome [102].

Leber hereditary optic neuropathy (LHON)

Leber hereditary optic neuropathy (LHON, also called Leber optic atrophy) typically presents in young adult life with sequential bilateral visual failure with a predilection for males [103, 104]. Approximately one-third of cases present with no family history, with the remainder having affected maternal relatives [105]. Visual failure is the sole symptom in the vast majority of cases, but dystonia, peripheral neuropathy, and cardiac conduction defects have been described in some patients [106, 107].

Mitochondrial neurogastrointestinal encephalopathy syndrome (MNGIE)

The syndrome MNGIE is a rare recessive disorder characterized by PEO, gastrointestinal pseudo-obstruction, diffuse leukoencephalopathy, peripheral neuropathy, and proximal myopathy. Histological and biochemical studies of MNGIE patients have confirmed the involvement of mitochondria in this disorder. The inheritance is autosomal recessive and it is due to mutations in the thymidine phosphorylase (*TP*) gene [108].

Alpers–Huttenlocher syndrome (AHS)

Alpers–Huttenlocher is an autosomal recessive hepatocerebral syndrome characterized clinically by severe mutations in *POLG*/psychomotor regression, intractable seizures, and liver failure, which is usually fatal in childhood [109, 110]. Sodium valproate should be avoided in all patients with AHS and suspected AHS because it can precipitate fulminant hepatic necrosis [111]. Myoclonic epilepsy is common, can be refractory to treatment, and leads to a progressive neurological deterioration with associated cortical blindness [112]. Adult-onset cases have been described, with Leigh-like lesions on brain MRI [113].

POLG disease

Since 2004 it has become clear that mutations in *POLG* are a major cause of mitochondrial disease which can present at any stage of life. *POLG* codes for polymerase γ (pol γ), which is the only DNA polymerase present within mitochondria [114]. *POLG* mutations cause secondary defects of mtDNA (mtDNA depletion, multiple mtDNA deletions or multiple point mutations) in clinically affected tissues leading to disorders which resemble primary mtDNA diseases. Given the emerging high prevalence of these disorders, the clinical presentation merits specific consideration. A number of different specific phenotypes have been described in patients with *POLG* mutations

Table 19.3. Defined clinical syndromes described in patients with *POLG* mutations

Alpers–Huttenlocher syndrome (AHS)
Chronic progressive external ophthalmoplegia (CPEO)
Infantile hypotonia/spinal muscular atrophy (SMA)
Mitochondrial encephalomyopathy with ragged-red fibers (MERRF)
Mitochondrial encephalomyopathy with lactic acidosis and stroke-like episodes (MELAS)
Mitochondrial neurogastrointestinal encephalomyopathy (MNGIE)
Mitochondrial recessive ataxia syndrome (MIRAS)
Sensory ataxic neuropathy with dysarthria and ophthalmoparesis (SANDO)

(Table 19.3). In general, acute encephalopathy and hepatic involvement is more common in childhood, ataxia and epilepsy present in the late-teens or early adult life, and PEO presents in middle-age or later [84]. However, there is considerable overlap creating a spectrum of *POLG* disease from neonatal life to old age [11].

Autosomal dominant progressive external ophthalmoplegia

The first pathogenic mutations in *POLG* were identified in families with autosomal dominant chronic progressive external ophthalmoplegia (adPEO) [12]. A high incidence of psychiatric disease, a parkinsonian syndrome, and primary gonadal failure have also been documented in some families transmitting dominant *POLG* mutations [115, 116].

Autosomal recessive progressive external ophthalmoplegia

Compound heterozygous and homozygous recessive *POLG* mutations have also been identified in patients with sporadic and recessive PEO [12]. These cases often present in late adult life with mild PEO and ptosis [84].

Autosomal recessive epilepsy and ataxia

Many recessive cases have cerebellar ataxia and a profound peripheral neuropathy, which is axonal in the vast majority of cases. This is similar to the previously described SANDO syndrome (sensory ataxic neuropathy with dysarthria and ophthalmoparesis) [117]. Recessive *POLG* mutations also present with adult-onset ataxia without ophthalmoplegia (also called mitochondrial recessive ataxia syndrome, MIRAS) [118, 119], which, in Scandinavia, is more common than Friedreich ataxia [118]. Epilepsy or complicated migraine with occipital aura are very common features, often pre-dating the development of ataxia by many years [118, 120]. The epilepsy is often focal, typically affecting the right limb and presenting as epilepsia partialis continua. Status epilepticus has a very poor prognosis, being the terminal event in many patients. Characteristic neuroimaging findings are currently being defined which can resemble the MELAS syndrome [121].

Alpers–Huttenlocher syndrome (AHS, see above)

The vast majority of cases of AHS, if not all, are due to compound heterozygous or homozygous recessive mutations in *POLG* [111, 122, 123, 124, 125, 126, 127]. In ~50% of cases, sodium valproate had been used before the onset of the liver failure, indicating the importance of avoiding this drug in children with unexplained encephalopathy.

Other phenotypes

There is a growing list of unusual phenotypes that have been described in families with *POLG* disease including neonatal hypotonia, a spinal-muscular atrophy-like disorder, distal isolated muscle weakness, and axonal Charcot–Marie–Tooth disease, broadening the phenotypic spectrum.

Clinical investigation of suspected mitochondrial disorders

Despite major advances in understanding the pathophysiology and molecular basis of mitochondrial disease, mitochondrial medicine is a strongly clinical specialty. The clinical assessment will initiate and guide subsequent investigations, which are often complex and expensive. A detailed clinical history and examination are therefore critically important, supplemented by careful questioning about relevant features in other family members. Relatives may only have one or two features of mitochondrial disease, such as diabetes mellitus or cardiac failure. Although common in the general population, knowledge of these features, and particularly the age at presentation, provides key evidence leading to the clinical diagnosis.

In some patients, the initial presentation alone may point to a specific mitochondrial disorder that can be confirmed with blood DNA testing. However, many patients do not have an instantly recognizable clinical syndrome, prompting a series of clinical and laboratory tests aimed at defining the phenotype, demonstrating a biochemical defect, and ultimately leading to a molecular diagnosis. Identifying the causative gene defect is of major importance. Mitochondrial disorders can be autosomal dominant, autosomal recessive, X-linked recessive, and maternally inherited, having profound implications for the index case and family members (Tables 19.4, 19.5). Although there have been major advances in molecular diagnostics over the last decade, it is still not possible to make a molecular diagnosis in a substantial group of patients. This is because many recently defined nuclear disease genes are only tested in the research setting, or because the underlying disease gene has yet to be identified.

General clinical investigations

Routine blood tests play only a minor role in the diagnosis of the mtDNA disorders but may provide supporting evidence

Table 19.4. Primary mitochondrial DNA defects causing human disease

	Inheritance pattern
Rearrangements (large-scale partial deletions and duplications)	
Chronic progressive external ophthalmoplegia (CPEO)	S or M
Kearns–Sayre syndrome	S or M
Diabetes and deafness	S
Pearson marrow–pancreas syndrome	S or M
Sporadic tubulopathy	S
Point mutations	
Protein-encoding genes	
LHON (11778G > A, 14484T > C, 3460G > A)	M
NARP/Leigh syndrome (8993T > G/C)	M
tRNA genes	
MELAS (3243A > G, 3271T > C, 3251A > G)	M
MERRF (8344A > G, 8356T > C)	M
CPEO (3243A > G, 4274T > C)	M
Myopathy (14709T > C, 12320A > G)	M
Cardiomyopathy (3243A > G, 4269A > G, 4300A > G)	M
Diabetes and deafness (3243A > G, 12258C > A)	M
Encephalomyopathy (1606G > A, 10010T > C)	M
rRNA genes	
Nonsyndromic sensorineural deafness (7445A > G)	M
Aminoglycoside induced nonsyndromic deafness (1555A > G)	M
Point mutations	
Protein-encoding genes	
LHON (11778G > A, 14484T > C, 3460G > A)	M
NARP/Leigh syndrome (8993T > G/C)	M
tRNA genes	
MELAS (3243A > G, 3271T > C, 3251A > G)	M

Notes: M, maternal; S, sporadic. mtDNA nucleotide positions refer to the L-chain, and are taken from the Cambridge reference sequence. CPEO, chronic progressive external ophthalmoplegia; KSS, Kearns–Sayre syndrome; LHON, Leber hereditary optic neuropathy; MELAS, mitochondrial encephalomyopathy with lactic acidosis and stroke-like episodes; MERRF, myoclonic epilepsy with ragged-red fibers; NARP, neurogenetic weakness with ataxia and retinitis pigmentosa.

Table 19.5. Nuclear genes causing mitochondrial disease

Nuclear genetic disorders of the mitochondrial respiratory chain, mutations in structural subunits:
Leigh syndrome (complex I deficiency – mutations in *NDUFS1, NDUFS4, NDUFS7, NDUFS8, NDUFV1*. Complex II deficiency, *SDHA*)
Cardiomyopathy and encephalopathy (complex I deficiency, mutations in *NDUFS2*)
Optic atrophy and ataxia (complex II deficiency – mutations in *SDHA*)
Hypokalemia and lactic acidosis (complex III, mutations in *UQCRB*)
Nuclear genetic disorders of the mitochondrial respiratory chain, mutations in assembly factors:
Leigh syndrome (mutations in *SURF* I and the mRNA binding protein *LRPPRC*)
Hepatopathy and ketoacidosis (mutations in *SCO1*)
Cardiomyopathy and encephalopathy (mutations in *SCO2*)
Leukodystrophy and renal tubulopathy (mutations in *COX10*)
Hypertrophic cardiomyopathy (mutations in *COX15*)
Encephalopathy, liver failure, renal tubulopathy (with complex III deficiency, mutations in *BCS1L*)
Encephalopathy (with complex V deficiency, mutations in *ATP12*)
Nuclear genetic disorders of intra-mitochondrial protein synthesis:
Leigh syndrome, liver failure and lactic acidosis (mutations in *EFG1*)
Lactic acidosis, developmental failure and dysmorphism (mutations in *MRPS16*)
Myopathy and sideroblastic anemia (mutations in *PUS1*)
Leukodystrophy and polymicrogyria (mutations in *EFTu*)
Edema, hypotonia, cardiomyopathy, and tubulopathy (mutations in *MRPS22*)
Hypotonia, renal tubulopathy, lactic acidosis (mutations in *RRM2B*)
Nuclear genetic disorders of mitochondrial DNA maintenance (causing multiple mtDNA deletions or mtDNA depletion):
Autosomal progressive external ophthalmoplegia (mutations in *POLG, POLG2, PEO1*, and *SLC25A4*)
Mitochondrial neurogastrointestinal encephalomyopathy (thymidine phosphorylase deficiency – mutations in *ECGF1*)
Alpers–Huttenlocher syndrome (mutations in *POLG* and *MPV*)
Infantile myopathy/spinal muscular atrophy (mutations in *TK2*)
Encephalomyopathy and liver failure (mutations in *DGUOK*)
Hypotonia, movement disorder, and/or Leigh syndrome with methylmalonic aciduria (mutations in *SUCLA2*)

Optic atrophy, ophthalmoplegia, ataxia, peripheral neuropathy (mutations in *OPA1*)

Others

Coenzyme Q10 deficiency (mutations in *COQ2*)

Barth syndrome (mutations in *TAZ*)

Cardiomyopathy and lactic acidosis (mitochondrial phosphate carrier deficiency, mutations in *SLC25A3*)

for the clinical diagnosis and help define the extent of the phenotype. Initial investigations should include serum creatine kinase, resting blood lactate, plasma electrolytes, full blood count, thyroid and liver function, bone chemistry, fasting blood glucose, and glycosylated hemoglobin (HbA1c). Creatine kinase levels can vary greatly, but are typically normal or only modestly elevated (below 500 U/l). Levels exceeding 1000 U/l are rare but can occur, particularly in the presence of renal disease or seizures.

Cardiac complications are frequent in mitochondrial disease, so all patients should have an electrocardiogram and an echocardiogram to detect asymptomatic cardiac conduction defects or cardiomyopathy. Peripheral neurophysiological studies can be helpful, but may be normal. Electromyography may reveal myogenic or neurogenic features, and nerve conduction studies may reveal a neuropathy which is usually of the mixed axonal type, although demyelinating neuropathies and a spinal muscular atrophy phenotype are well recognized. Central nervous system neurophysiology can be helpful in defining the phenotype. The electroencephalogram is usually normal, but can reveal generalized slow waves, indicative of a subacute or subclinical encephalopathy. Brain imaging can be helpful, and both computed tomography (CT) and MRI are indicated to determine whether there is basal ganglia calcification, focal or generalized atrophy, or high signal especially in the basal ganglia or brain stem [128]. Detailed brain imaging is essential to make the clinical diagnosis of Leigh syndrome (Figure 19.1).

A strong clinical suspicion based on the history and examination findings is sufficient to prompt further investigation. Immediate molecular genetic testing in blood or urinary epithelial cells is indicated in patients with a specific phenotype (Table 19.4), but if the phenotype is less clear-cut, then further investigations are required in skeletal muscle, cultured skin fibroblasts, or clinically affected tissue such as liver.

Specific biochemical investigations in blood, urine or cerebrospinal fluid

Lactate may be increased in blood, urine or cerebrospinal fluid, particularly in children during a period of acute illness, leading to a systemic acidosis [129]. Lactate measurements are usually normal in adults or in children in between periods of acute illness [130]. The results must be interpreted with caution because abnormal lactate levels are common in patients with a number of acute medical illnesses such as stroke, sepsis or following generalized seizures.

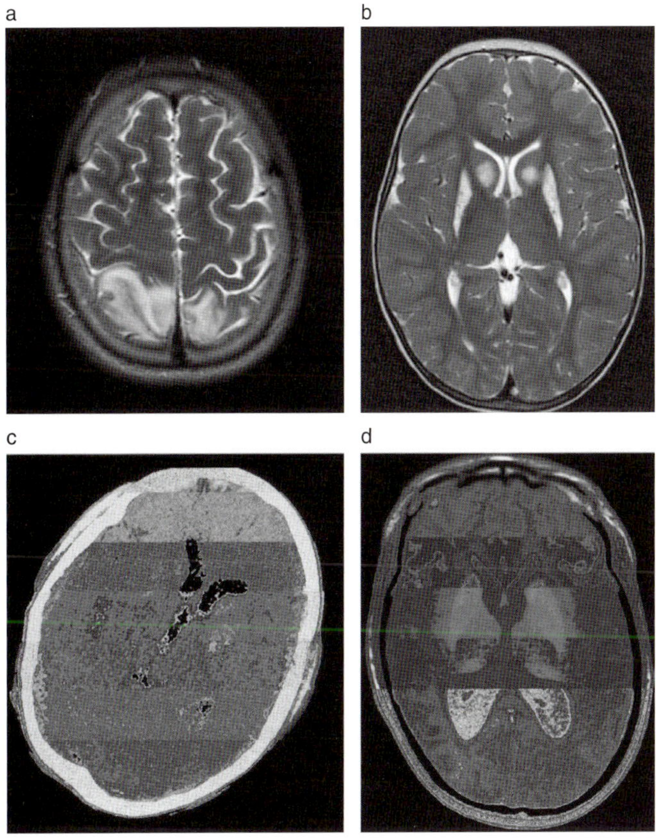

Figure 19.1a–d. Brain imaging in mitochondrial disorders. (a) MRI showing occipital high signal during a stroke-like episode in MELAS (with thanks to Dr. Andrew Schaefer, University of Newcastle upon Tyne). (b) Axial T_2 and coronal FLAIR MR imaging from a child with Leigh syndrome showing hyperintensity of caudate and putamen (with thanks to Dr. Robert McFarland, University of Newcastle upon Tyne). (c) Brain CT showing basal ganglia calcification in a patient harboring the 3243A > G MELAS mutation. (d) Brain MRI from the same subject showing generalized atrophy and increased signal in the basal ganglia.

Muscle pathology

Adults with mitochondrial disease often have an abnormal muscle biopsy, and skeletal muscle histopathology is the mainstay of investigation of adult mitochondrial disease. However, a normal muscle biopsy does not exclude mitochondrial disease, particularly in children and adults with localized phenotypes or tissue-specific mitochondrial disorder. The muscle biopsy should be taken with care, carefully oriented and frozen for a series of histochemical stains.

Hematoxylin and eosin may reveal nonspecific myopathic features including focal muscle fiber atrophy and an increase in the range of muscle fiber sizes. Acutely necrotic fibers are rare. In severe mitochondrial myopathy there may be muscle fiber loss and replacement with fibrous connective tissue and fat resembling a muscular dystrophy [131]. Punctate lipid within myofibers is a frequent finding in patients with PEO

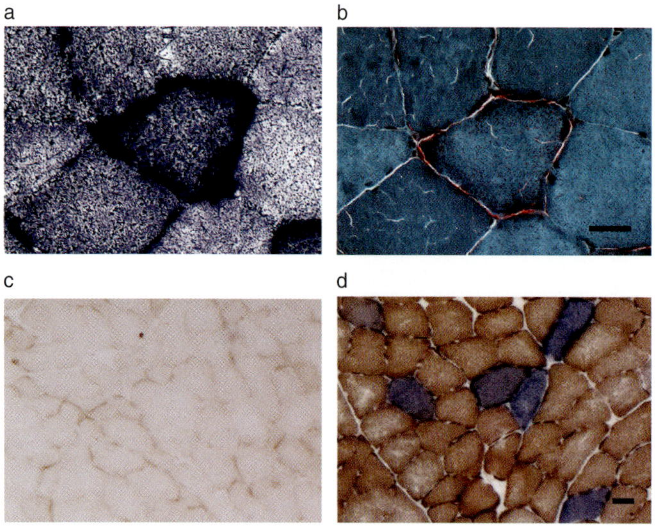

Figure 19.2a–d. Muscle pathology in mitochondrial disorders. Cryostat sections (20 μm) of quadriceps skeletal muscle showing (a) succinate dehydrogenase (SDH) histochemistry in a patient with a heteroplasmic mtDNA defect, showing sub-sarcolemmal proliferation of mitochondria corresponding to a ragged-red fiber. (b) Ragged-red fiber shown by Gömöri trichrome staining. (c) Global reduction in cytochrome *c* oxidase (COX) activity in a patient with a nuclear gene defect. (d) Mosaic COX defect demonstrated by sequential COX-SDH histochemistry in a patient with a heteroplasmic pathogenic mtDNA mutation. (a, b) Scale bar = 50 m as shown in (b, c, d) Scale bar = 25 μm as shown in (d) (With thanks to Professor Robert Taylor).

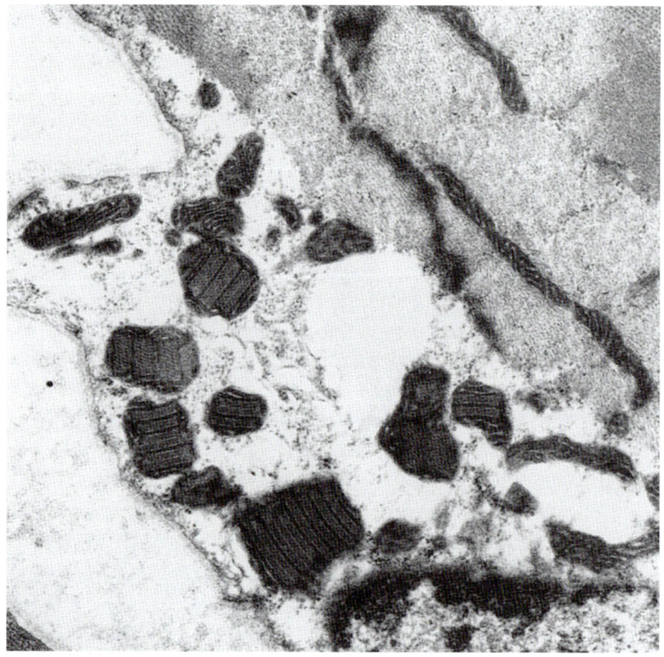

Figure 19.3. Electron microscopy of mitochondrial paracrystalline inclusions which contain the mitochondrial isoform of creatine kinase between the inner and outer mitochondrial membranes in skeletal muscle.

and KSS but not in MELAS or MERRF. Myofibrillar ATPase staining may reveal neurogenetic features.

Histochemical stains often provide the first definitive clue of a mitochondrial disorder. The subsarcolemmal collection of abnormal mitochondria leads to a red appearance with the Gömöri trichrome stain (so called ragged-red fibers, Figure 19.2b). Although performed routinely in some laboratories, the same feature is readily seen on muscle histochemistry, particularly by the succinate dehydrogenase (SDH) reaction (Figure 19.2a). SDH is a component of respiratory chain complex II, which only contains nuclear-encoded subunits.

Cytochrome *c* oxidase (COX) histochemistry is extremely valuable, especially in adults with mitochondrial disease. COX, or complex IV of the respiratory chain, contains mitochondrial DNA-encoded subunits. Patients with a mtDNA defect often show a mosaic COX defect which may co-segregate with ragged-red fibers (Figure 19.2d). However, some patients with MELAS or point mutations in non-COX structural subunits such as the complex I genes [132] or cytochrome *b* genes [83] may have normal COX activity. In normal individuals, the level of COX activity varies between muscle fiber types, and it can be difficult to distinguish COX-deficient type II (glycolytic) fibers from normal. The sequential COX-SDH approach was developed to circumvent this difficulty [133], allowing the easy identification of sometimes infrequent COX-deficient muscle fibers. A global decrease in the activity of COX is usually suggestive of a nuclear mutation in one of the ancillary proteins required for COX assembly and function such as *SURF1* [134, 135] although a similar pattern is observed in some patients presenting with pathogenic, homoplasmic mitochondrial tRNA gene mutations [136] (Figure 19.2c).

Great care should be taken when interpreting mild histochemical defects or infrequent COX-deficient fibers which could be secondary to another disease (such as myotonic dystrophy or inclusion body myositis). A low frequency of COX-deficient fibers is also seen in muscle taken from healthy aged control subjects. These fibers arise through the clonal expansion of somatic mtDNA mutations, and the abnormal fibers themselves cannot be distinguished from those found in patients with mitochondrial disease [137]. The age of the patient must therefore be taken into account when interpreting the biopsy, and the presence of $<5\%$ COX-deficient fibers in subjects >50 years of age should be interpreted with great caution. On the other hand, patients with well-recognized phenotypes such as MELAS or CPEO [138] can have normal muscle histochemistry, as can patients with an established *POLG* mutation [139].

Patients with mitochondrial disease often have abnormalities on electron microscopy, including abnormal mitochondrial morphology or distribution, and paracrystalline inclusions. However, these findings are nonspecific, and can also be found in other disorders (Figure 19.3).

Respiratory chain biochemistry

The biochemical assessment of respiratory chain function is technically demanding. Subtle differences in the methodology between laboratories can have a major impact on the absolute values measured for each complex, and there are well-recognized cases where the diagnosis made in one laboratory cannot be confirmed in another. It is strongly advised that diagnostic mitochondrial biochemistry should only be carried out in a specialized laboratory.

Respiratory chain studies should be carried out on a clinically affected tissue because some mitochondrial disorders are strikingly tissue-specific. In children this may not be possible, and the first step usually involves cultured skin fibroblasts.

The preparation of intact muscle mitochondria is the preferred approach by many laboratories. Rates of flux, substrate oxidation, and ATP production are measured by polarography or using ^{14}C-labeled substrates.

Children with mitochondrial disease usually have a biochemical abnormality in a clinically affected tissue or organ, but the biochemical defect is usually more subtle in adults, possibly falling within the normal reference range. Multiple enzyme defects involving complexes I, III, and IV are sometimes seen in patients harboring single, large-scale mtDNA deletions, mtDNA tRNA mutations or nuclear factors involved in mitochondrial translation.

Molecular diagnosis of mitochondrial disorders

Mitochondrial DNA studies and specific nuclear genetic studies are widely available, but the results must be interpreted with caution. This is all the more important when the result is negative because some well-recognized mtDNA defects are tissue-specific and cannot be reliably detected in a blood DNA sample. In addition, the genetic analysis is far from comprehensive in many laboratories – a problem that is compounded by the growing list of pathogenic nuclear genes (Table 19.5), most of which are only tested in the research setting. Interpreting novel sequence changes also presents a particular challenge for the highly polymorphic mitochondrial genome, and for novel nuclear disease genes where the range of polymorphic variability has yet to be established.

The vast majority of adults with mitochondrial disease have a primary or secondary abnormality mtDNA (Tables 19.4, 19.5). The standard approach in adults is therefore to start molecular investigations on mtDNA unless there is a specific phenotype and inheritance pattern pointing to a specific nuclear gene such as *POLG*. mtDNA abnormalities are much less common in children. Under these circumstances, biochemical studies guide the molecular genetic approach.

Mitochondrial DNA defects

Specific mtDNA mutations are associated with specific clinical syndromes (Tables 19.4, 19.5). Under these circumstances it is appropriate to test for specific mtDNA point mutations. This can be carried out in a standard blood DNA sample (no specific mitochondrial DNA extraction is required), remembering that the percentage level of the mtDNA mutation may be low or even undetectable in blood. Urinary epithelium provides an reliable alternative [140].

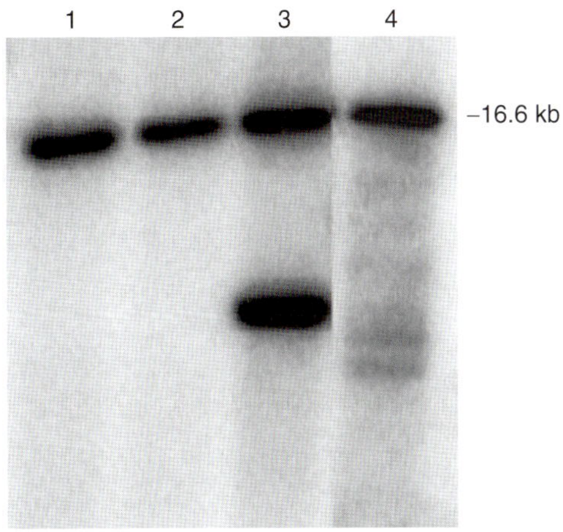

Figure 19.4. Southern blot of mitochondrial DNA. Southern blot of skeletal muscle DNA probed with a mtDNA-specific probe. Lanes 1 and 2 = healthy controls, lane 3 = known single heteroplasmic mtDNA deletion, lane 4 = multiple mtDNA deletions. Adapted from [141].

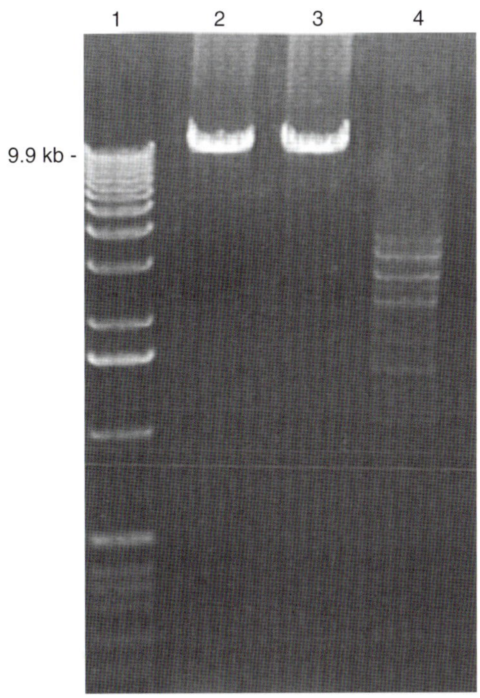

Figure 19.5. Long-range PCR of skeletal muscle DNA amplifying a 9.9-kb fragment across the major mtDNA arc (nucleotide positions 6249–16215). Lane 1 = DNA size marker; lanes 2 and 3 = control muscle; lane 4 = muscle from II-1 showing multiple mtDNA deletions. Adapted from [143].

The first step is to look for rearrangements of mtDNA in a clinically affected tissue (usually muscle). Traditionally this has been carried out using Southern blot analysis (Figure 19.4; [141]) looking for single deletions or duplications, multiple mtDNA deletions or the loss of mtDNA (depletion). Many laboratories now use a more rapid approach, screening for deletions using long-range PCR [142], or real-time PCR, and measuring mtDNA quantity by real-time PCR (Figure 19.5; [143]). The results of these analyses must be interpreted with caution because low levels of mtDNA deletions are detected in healthy aged muscle, and long-range PCR preferentially amplifies deleted mtDNA giving the impression that it is the dominant species. Long-range PCR techniques using shorter extension times may be more valuable in differentiating the deletions seen in aging from those observed in patients with multiple mtDNA deletions syndrome [144]. Finally, in some cases where the clinical and histochemical findings are suggestive of a multiple mtDNA deletion disorder, the relative amount of deleted mtDNA can be determined in individual COX-deficient and COX-positive muscle fibers by real-time PCR [145]. The identification of clear-cut multiple mtDNA deletions (Figures 19.4, 19.5) or mtDNA depletion prompts nuclear genetic testing of genes involved in mitochondrial DNA maintenance (Table 19.5).

Standard molecular techniques are used to detect specific mtDNA point mutations in the diagnostic setting. Different laboratories test for a range of different point mutations, usually because these mutations have been previously detected in the local population (Table 19.4). Again the results must be interpreted with caution because the causative mutation may be present at low or undetectable levels in the tissue being studied. If no common mtDNA mutations are detected in patients with phenotypes typical of mitochondrial disease, then the standard approach is to sequence the entire mitochondrial genome. This often reveals a previously described pathogenic mtDNA mutation, however many sporadic cases have unique or private mtDNA point mutations. Proving that these substitutions are pathogenic can be a challenge, particularly if they are homoplasmic. The entire mtDNA sequence should be interpreted in the context of known genetic variation in the local population and world mtDNA phylogeny (for example [146]). Showing that the mutation affects a highly conserved nucleotide residue, alters the amino acid sequence, and segregates with the clinical or biochemical phenotype is essential [147]. In patients with a mosaic histochemical defect it is possible to micro-dissect normal and biochemically deficient fibers and show that higher percentage levels of mutated mtDNA or a loss of wild-type mtDNA segregates with the biochemical phenotype (single-fiber PCR). Functional studies in cell lines, or the identification of the same mutation in an otherwise genetically distinct family provides final confirmatory evidence, but this is not routinely carried out in diagnostic practice.

Nuclear gene defects

Defects in nuclear-encoded genes associated with the structure or assembly of the respiratory chain have historically been more difficult to identify than defects in mtDNA because of the large number of potential genes involved and the genetic heterogeneity underlying similar biochemical defects. Linkage analysis has been useful in identifying some of these gene defects, especially in consanguineous families where homozygosity mapping can be informative. However, many patients are isolated cases, and in such instances complementation cloning strategies, such as microcell-mediated chromosome transfer, are the only alternatives for mapping the defective gene.

The majority of defects that have been reported (Table 19.5) result in compromised assembly of one or more of the respiratory chain complexes, and analysis of mitochondria from an affected tissue or cell type by Blue-Native gel electrophoresis, which permits evaluation of the assembly of all of the complexes, is probably the best frontline screen to identify the biochemical defect. Defining the nature of the biochemical defect is essential for further molecular analysis. There is a bewildering array of clinical phenotypes that result from mutations in genes even in the same part of an assembly pathway for the same enzyme complex. Uncovering the molecular basis for this diversity remains a major scientific challenge.

Gene defects in structural components of the respiratory chain

Most mutations in the structural components of the respiratory chain have been found in patients with isolated complex I deficiency, the most common biochemical deficiency reported in the respiratory chain. Disease-causing mutations have been found in all of the seven highly conserved nuclear-encoded core subunits of complex I (NDUFS1, NDUFS2, NDUFS3, NDUFS7, NDUFS8, NDUFV1, and NDUFV2) and in four of the supernumerary subunits (NDUFS4, NDUFS6, NDUFA1, NDUFA11) (reviewed in [148]). The majority of these mutations are associated with Leigh syndrome, Leigh-like disease, or cardioencephalomyopathy. Mutations in these genes account for 20%–30% of patients presenting with a complex I deficiency and another 20% have a defect in a mitochondrially encoded gene. Therefore, the molecular basis of complex I deficiency remains unknown in about half of cases, implying that factors involved in the assembly and regulation of complex I are important in human disease. In every case in which the assembly status of complex I in patients with known structural subunit mutations has been examined by Blue-Native polyacrylamide gel electrophoresis (PAGE), a defect in the assembly of the complex has been found. While it has been argued that catalytic mutants of complex I exist, [149] no mutation has been found in a nuclear gene that definitively causes a change in the catalytic ability of the enzyme without affecting its assembly.

Complex II is the only respiratory chain complex whose subunits are entirely encoded by nuclear genes and it is relatively rarely reported as an isolated enzyme deficiency. Nevertheless mutations have been reported in all four subunits. Only those in *SDHA*, which encodes the flavoprotein, have so far been associated with neurological disease (Leigh syndrome [150]). Mutations in the other subunits are associated with rare forms of cancer such as hereditary paragangliomas and pheochromocytomas.

Mutations in two complex III structural subunits have been reported: UQCRB, the ubiquinol cytochrome *c* reductase binding protein, subunit VI in a patient with hypoglycemia and lactic acidosis [151]; and in the *UQCRQ* gene (subunit VII), in a large consanguineous kindred with severe psychomotor retardation and extrapyramidal signs [152].

Searches for mutations in the nuclear-encoded subunits of complex IV in several large groups of patients failed to reveal any mutations, suggesting that they were either very rare or incompatible with live birth. Very recently the first such mutation was identified in subunit COX6B1 associated with a severe infantile encephalomyopathy [153].

Assembly factor defects

Mutations in assembly factors appear to be the most common cause of isolated COX (complex IV) deficiency, and to date six such factors have been associated with human disease. The first such gene, identified by functional complementation cloning, was *SURF1*, the most common cause of classical Leigh syndrome in patients with COX deficiency [134, 154]. All of the patients with SURF1 mutations appear to be null for the protein, with residual COX activities in the range of 15%–20%. Although the exact function of the protein in COX assembly is not known, studies of the homolog in the bacterium *Rhodobacter sphaeroides* suggest that it may play a role in heme *a* addition to the COI subunit [155]. Integrative genomic studies on the French Canadian form of Leigh syndrome identified mutations in LRPPRC [156]. This form of Leigh syndrome is associated with severe COX deficiency in brain and liver, and modest deficiencies in heart, skeletal muscle, and kidney [157]. LRPPRC is a homolog of Pet 309, a specific translational activator of the COX1 subunit in *Saccharomyces cerevisiae*, and is part of a family of proteins that are involved in RNA–protein interactions in mitochondria. Consistent with this, LRPPRC has been shown to bind both nuclear and mitochondrial RNA in vivo. Fibroblasts carrying the common missense mutation found in these patients display reduced amounts of LRPPRC protein, translational defects in COX I, and the presence of an abnormal translation product that has not yet been identified [158]. Interestingly, LRPPRC has also been found in a complex with PGC-1α [159] that was shown to regulate expression of genes in gluconeogenesis and several mitochondrial genes.

Mutations in both genes coding for the enzymes involved in the synthesis of heme *a* (*COX10*, *COX15*) have been found in COX-deficient patients [160, 161]. These patients present with a variety of different clinical phenotypes, including Leigh syndrome, leukodystrophy, hypertrophic cardiomyopathy, and anemia. Two paralogous genes, *SCO1* and *SCO2*, coding for metallochaperones that are necessary for the delivery of copper to the Cu_A site on the CO II subunit, have also been associated with isolated COX deficiency. Both *SCO1* and *SCO2* are essential in humans, with mutations in either gene causing a severe, isolated COX deficiency that results in early-onset disease with a fatal clinical outcome. *SCO2* mutations are associated primarily with neonatal encephalocardiomyopathy [162, 163], while *SCO1* mutations cause neonatal hepatic failure and ketoacidotic coma [164]. These distinct clinical phenotypes are not a result of tissue-specific expression of the two genes, as *SCO1* and *SCO2* are ubiquitously expressed and exhibit a similar expression pattern in different human tissues. Molecular, genetic, and biochemical analyses of *SCO1* and *SCO2* patient cell lines have demonstrated that the SCO proteins have independent but cooperative functions in the biogenesis of the Cu_A site [165]. Both SCO1 and SCO2 appear to have additional regulatory roles in the maintenance of cellular copper homeostasis [166]. Tissue-specific cellular copper deficiencies are seen in the context of mutants in both proteins, and this serves to exacerbate the COX deficiency that results from the crippled metallochaperone function of both proteins.

Mutations in the complex III assembly factor were initially reported in patients with renal tubulopathy, encephalopathy, and liver failure [167], and were subsequently found in patients with GRACILE syndrome (intrauterine growth retardation, aminoaciduria, cholestasis, iron overload, lactic acidosis) [168] and in patients with Bjornstad syndrome (sensorineural hearing loss, pili torti) [169]. While all known mutations in *BCS1L* disrupt complex III assembly, the different clinical manifestations have been suggested to result from different rates of production of reactive oxygen species [169].

In yeast five factors have been identified that are important in the assembly of the complex V. Two of these, ATP11 and ATP12, have mammalian orthologs, and function in mediating the assembly of the F_1 subcomplex [170]. A number of patients have been identified with isolated complex V deficiencies of nuclear origin [171], all of which have reduced levels of the complex, but the genetic defect in these patients remains unknown in all but a single pedigree with a mutation in *ATP12* [172]. The clinical phenotype of these patients is strikingly different from those with *ATP6* mutations; cardiomyopathy is a prominent feature, but Leigh syndrome has not been reported.

The identification of complex I assembly factors has lagged behind the discovery of factors for the other respiratory complexes, in large part due to the lack of complex I in the model organism *S. cerevisiae*. The question of whether a single common gene is responsible for most of these cases has been addressed using complementation analysis: in a study of ten unrelated patients, two had mitochondrial DNA mutations, and the remaining eight fell into seven complementation groups ruling out the effect of an unidentified common gene in complex I deficiency [173].

Two assembly factors, CIA30 and CIA84, were found in the aerobic yeast *Neurospora crassa* that associate with the membrane arm of the protein [174]. CIA30 has a human homolog, NDUFAF1. Low levels of NDUFAF1 protein were discovered in a complex-I-deficient patient with cardiomyopathy, developmental delay, and lactic acidosis, and two novel heterozygous mutations in the *NDUFAF1* gene were identified [175]. A protein that co-purifies with NDUFAF1, Ecsit, was also shown to be necessary for complex I assembly [176], but no mutations have so far been reported in this gene in complex-I-deficient patients. A comparative genomics analysis of different yeast species led to the identification of *NDUFA12L* (B17.2L), a paralog of a small structural subunit of complex I,

NDUFA12 (B17.2), that is found in the matrix arm of the enzyme [177]. Investigation of NDUFA12L in cases of complex I deficiency identified a patient with a severe childhood-onset progressive encephalopathy, who lacked detectable NDUFA12L protein and assembled very little mature complex I [177]. The B17.2L protein was shown to associate specifically with a subassembly of complex I of about 830 kDa in several patients with complex I assembly defects, suggesting that it stabilizes this intermediate late in the assembly process. The clinical presentation of this patient is an unusual one for a mitochondrial disease, sharing most of the diagnostic criteria for vanishing white matter disease.

Another complex I assembly factor, C6ORF66, was identified by homozygosity mapping in patients with infantile mitochondrial encephalomyopathy, but its function remains unknown [178]. An enzyme of the size and complexity of complex I is likely to have many more assembly factors. Candidates for some of these factors were suggested by a recent analysis of the evolution of complex I [179], which identified several paralogs of complex I structural genes including NDUFA12L.

Multiple enzyme defects of oxidative phosphorylation

Deficiencies in the activity of multiple complexes of the oxidative phosphorylation system are nearly as common as isolated deficiencies, and in theory could derive from a number of different problems including: a failure to maintain an adequate mtDNA copy number, defects in expression of mtDNA (transcription or translation), the accumulation of mutations in mtDNA, or a defect in an accessory factor involved in the biosynthesis of a common prosthetic group, such as an Fe–S cluster or heme. Pulse labeling of the mitochondrial translation products with [^{35}S]methionine in cells with multiple defects is a simple screen to characterize whether the defect is due to a translation factor.

Mitochondrial translation defects

Mutations in the mitochondrial elongation factor EFG1 have been found in two pedigrees in patients who presented with combined defects in the activities of respiratory chain enzymes associated with a hepatoencephalopathy [180]. The effects of the mutation on mitochondrial translation were polypeptide-specific, but the molecular explanation for this remains unknown. Analysis of the respiratory chain complexes by Blue-Native PAGE in a patient who was a compound heterozygote for a missense and a nonsense mutation in EFG1 showed striking differences in the nature and severity of the biochemical defect amongst tissues. Whereas heart muscle showed only a mild deficiency in complex IV assembly, both complexes IV and V were severely reduced in skeletal muscle and there was a small decrease in complex I. Complexes I and IV were severely reduced in fibroblasts and liver, and there was a more modest reduction in complex V [181]. Consistent with these results, immunoblot analysis demonstrated that EFG1 was reduced in heart tissue, but was undetectable in skeletal muscle and liver. These results suggest a different organization and control of mitochondrial translation in different tissues. However, the identification of *EFG1* mutations in a patient with Leigh syndrome but no liver disease [182], and of the identical mutation in EFTs in two patients with completely different clinical phenotypes (encephalomyopathy, hypertrophic cardiomyopathy) [183] strongly suggests the existence of genetic modifiers. Further complicating this picture, a mutation in the elongation factor EFTu has been identified in a patient with infantile macrocystic leukodystrophy and micropolygyria [182].

Mutations have so far been identified in two mitochondrial ribosomal proteins in humans, (MRPS16) [184] and MRPS22 [185]. The MRPS16 patient, from a consanguineous family, presented with intractable lactic acidosis, agenesis of the corpus callosum, dysmorphism, and marked decreases in the activities of complexes I and IV. Mitochondrial translation in patient fibroblasts was impaired, and there was a marked reduction in the steady-state level of the 12S rRNA. DNA sequence analysis of the genes coding for small ribosomal subunit proteins that are conserved between *Escherichia coli* and mammals revealed a homozygous premature stop codon in MRPS16. This is one of the most highly conserved proteins between mammals and yeast and it is 40% identical to the bacterial homologue. S16 has been shown to play a role in assembly of the small ribosomal subunit in *Thermus thermophilus* [186], but its role in the mitoribosome is unknown. The MRPS22 patients presented at birth with muscle hypotonia, lactic acidemia, and hyperammonemia, and subsequently developed tubulopathy and hypertrophic cardiomyopathy. MRPS22 does not have a bacterial homolog and its function in the mitoribosome is unknown.

The unexpected involvement of an AAA-protease in mitochondrial ribosome assembly has been reported by Langer and colleagues [187]. Mitochondria contain two AAA-protease activities, directed to opposite surfaces of the inner membrane, that are important in quality control of inner mitochondrial membrane proteins [188]. The matrix-directed protease is composed of two subunits, which in humans are called AFG3l2 and paraplegin [189]. Loss-of-function mutations in paraplegin are associated with a dominant form of hereditary spastic paraplegia [16], a neurodegenerative disease caused by axonal degeneration of motor neurons of the corticospinal tracts. The ribosomal protein MrpL32 was shown to be a substrate for the matrix-directed AAA-protease in yeast and in the mouse [187], and it was demonstrated that proteolytic processing of this protein was essential for the recruitment of preassembled ribosomal particles and completion of ribosomal assembly. When the protease is defective, maturation of MrpL32 is prevented and a translation deficiency results [187].

A missense mutation in the *PUS1* gene, coding for pseudouridine synthase 1, has been reported in families with mitochondrial myopathy and sideroblastic anemia [14]. Cell lines from these patients lack Pus1 activity and both cytoplasmic and mitochondrial tRNAs lack pseudouridine at sites known to be modified by Pus1 [190]. Pus1 is found in the nucleus, cytoplasm and in mitochondria, so the phenotype caused by mutations in this gene could be much broader than just an oxidative phosphorylation deficiency; however, the fact that patient muscles show combined respiratory chain defects [191] demonstrates that mitochondrial dysfunction is a major part of the disease.

mtDNA depletion syndromes

mtDNA depletion syndromes result from an inability to maintain adequate steady-state copy number for mtDNA (review in [192]). These syndromes, which are inherited as autosomal recessive traits, are invariably early onset and severe, with a fatal outcome. At least eight different genes have so far been implicated in these syndromes and they either affect the supply or balance of the deoxynucleotide pool – the building blocks for mtDNA – or are part of the mtDNA replisome. Like most other mitochondrial diseases, there is a great deal of tissue specificity in the deficiency, most of which is not well understood. There are three major clinical presentations of mtDNA depletion syndrome: myopathic, hepatocerebral, and encephalomyopathic.

Mutations in the thymidine kinase-2 gene (*TK2*) are associated with myopathic mtDNA depletion syndrome [193], although these account for only 20% of reported cases. TK2 is a mitochondrial deoxyribonucleoside kinase that is responsible for phosphorylation of thymidine, deoxycytidine, and deoxyuridine. Most of the reported TK2 mutations are missense and they result in a greater than 70% reduction in the activity of the enzyme. Mutations in mitochondrial deoxyguanosine kinase (*DGUOK*) were the first described genetic defects in patients with hepatocerebral mtDNA depletion syndrome [194]. Many of the mutations in these patients are nonsense mutations. Although the basis for the different tissue susceptibilities in patients with *TK2* versus *DGUOK* is not known with certainty, it has been suggested that the cytosolic enzyme dCK, whose activity is low in brain and liver, might compensate for the loss of mitochondrial enzyme activity in muscle [195]. On the other hand, as all TK2 patients express at least one missense allele, residual activities might be high enough in brain and liver to support adequate DNA replication.

A new genetic cause of mtDNA depletion in muscle was recently uncovered by homozygosity mapping in a large inbred family with severe muscle mtDNA depletion (1%–2% residual levels) [196]. Sequencing of candidate genes in the single autozygous region on chromosome 8q identified a homozygous nonsense mutation, encoding a subunit of a p53-inducible ribonucleotide reductase (*RRM2B*), and the enzyme responsible for the conversion of ribonucleoside 5′-diphosphates to deoxyribonucleoside 5′-diphosphates. Additional mutations (splice site, missense) were identified in three other small families. The clinical phenotype involved severe neurological disorder with or without renal involvement. Analysis of the knockout mouse showed marked reductions in mtDNA in kidney muscle and liver, but no overt respiratory chain deficiency.

As described elsewhere in this chapter, mutations in *POLG* produce a very wide spectrum of clinical phenotypes, with both dominant and recessive inheritance, that depend, at least in part, on where the mutations are located in the POLG protein. Alpers-Huttenlocher syndrome is a form of hepatocerebral mtDNA depletion that appears to be almost entirely due to specific combinations of POLG alleles, at least one of which is in the region that links the proofreading domain with the polymerase domain [84]. Recessive mutations in another component of the mtDNA replisome, Twinkle helicase (*PEO1*), have also been reported in one family with hepatocerebral mtDNA depletion syndrome [197].

In a search for additional genetic causes of the hepatocerebral form of mtDNA depletion, a new locus was mapped to chromosome 2p21–23 [198]. Using an integrative genomics mitochondrial prediction program (Maestro) [199], *MPV17* was identified as a candidate gene in which missense mutations segregated with the disease phenotype. Additional missense and nonsense mutations have recently been reported in three ethnically diverse pedigrees [200]. Interestingly the *MPV17* gene product was previously annotated as a peroxisomal protein based on investigation of a retroviral insertion at the *MPV17* locus in a mouse model, despite the clear inner mitochondrial membrane location for the yeast ortholog (sym1). The MPV17 protein is predicted to have four transmembrane helices and studies of the human protein showed that it is targeted to mitochondria and behaves biochemically like an integral membrane protein. A re-evaluation of the mouse model showed tissue-specific depletions of mtDNA, the liver being the most severely affected. At present it is unclear what the exact function of this protein is in humans; however, as there was no detectable immunoreactive protein in two patients analyzed with an R50Q mutation, it appears that MPV17 protein is not absolutely essential to mtDNA maintenance. One possibility is that it plays a role in tethering the mitochondrial nucleoid to the inner mitochondrial membrane, and that its complete loss can be only partially compensated by other proteins with which it interacts. Alternatively, it could exert some influence on transport of the mtDNA deoxyribonucleotides into the matrix.

A mutation in *MPV17* has also been shown to underlie the neurohepatopathy in the Navajo population [201]. This phenotype, which has an estimated birth incidence of 1:1600 in the western Navaho Reservation, is characterized by liver disease and sensory and motor neuropathy. Interestingly all individuals examined had the same R50Q mutation seen in some juvenile Italian patients, suggesting a founder effect mutation; however, subsequent haplotype analysis showed that the mutation arose independently in the two populations [202]. Clinical investigations had described three distinct forms of the disease: so-called infantile, juvenile, and classic (adult-onset) forms of the disease. As all of these are due to the same pathogenic mutation, there must be genetic, epigenetic or environmental factors that influence expression of the clinical phenotype.

The genetic cause of an encephalomyopathic form of mtDNA depletion syndrome in an Arab family was identified in the *SUCLA2* gene, which encodes a β-subunit of the mitochondrial matrix enzyme succinyl CoA ligase [203]. A much more severe clinical phenotype of fatal infantile lactic acidosis caused by mtDNA depletion is associated with mutations in the *SUCLA1* gene that encodes the α-subunit of the same enzyme [204]. The SUCL enzyme is an αβ heterodimer that catalyzes the substrate-level phosphorylation of either ATP or GTP, in which the β-subunit determines specificity for the ADP/ATP or GDP/GTP couple. It is not obvious from such an activity how this would result in mtDNA depletion. However, the enzyme complex has been shown to immunoprecipitate with nucleoside diphosphate kinase, an enzyme that is essential for creating the nucleoside triphosphates for mtDNA synthesis.

Multiple mtDNA deletion syndromes

Multiple mtDNA deletion syndromes are inherited as autosomal dominant or recessive traits and share many of the same features as single-deletion syndromes. Several gene defects are now known including: the muscle heart-specific isoform of the adenine nucleotide translocase (*ANT1*), Twinkle helicase (*PEO1*), the catalytic subunit of the gamma-polymerase (*POLG1*), the accessory subunit of the gamma-polymerase (*POLG2*), and the thymidine phosphorylase gene (*ECGF1*) (reviewed in [205]). *ANT1* was the first gene to be discovered in multiple mtDNA deletion syndrome in patients with autosomal dominant PEO [89], but the mechanism by which it causes these mutations remains a bit of a mystery. The transporter exchanges ATP for ADP and is thus required for import of ADP into the matrix for oxidative phosphorylation and export of ATP to the cytosol, and how this might influence intramitochondrial deoxynucleotide pools remains uncertain. An autosomal recessive form of *ANT1* disease has also been reported [206]. Skeletal muscle pathology in *ANT1* patients typically shows ragged-red fibers, in which clonal expansions of usually single mtDNA deletions can be detected. Twinkle is a helicase that forms an essential part of the mtDNA replisome. Patients with autosomal dominant disease usually have uncomplicated PEO [90]. A recessive Twinkle mutation is the cause of a Finnish disease known as IOSCA (infantile-onset spinocerebellar ataxia) [207].

As discussed elsewhere in this chapter, mutations in *POLG1* are a major cause of mitochondrial disease. They produce a wide range of autosomally dominant or recessive phenotypes depending, at least in part, on where the mutation is located. Mutations in this gene are reported to cause about 50% of autosomal dominant PEO and most of the recessive cases [205].

Mutations in the thymidine phosphorylase gene produce an autosomal recessive disease known as MNGIE (mitochondrial neurogastrointestinal encephalomyopathy) [108]. These patients have a serious clinical phenotype that is characterized by PEO, neuropathy, leukodystrophy, and intestinal dysmotility. Interestingly, the enzyme is hardly expressed in muscle, and this led to the idea that the pathology results from the accumulation of toxic metabolites, two of which were identified in blood: thymidine and deoxyuridine [208]. Large-scale deletions and the point mutations accumulate in the skeletal muscle of MNGIE patients [209], the latter due to next-nucleotide effects and dislocation mutagenesis, presumably the result of increased concentrations of the metabolites. Allogeneic bone marrow transplantation has been suggested as a treatment for this devastating disorder, as a means of restoring thymidine phosphorylase activity to leukocytes [210].

CoQ deficiency

The CoQ biosynthetic pathway comprises a series of nine enzymes that are required to synthesize CoQ. In addition to its role in transferring electrons from complex I to complex III in the respiratory chain, it also accepts electrons from complex II, and from ETF-DH in the beta-oxidation pathway. CoQ deficiency is associated with a very heterogeneous clinical presentation. It is important to identify patients with CoQ deficiency as most respond to supplementation. Mutations in four enzymes in the pathway (*COQ2*, *PDSS1*, *PDSS2*, *CABC1*) have been reported in children with primary CoQ deficiency (reviewed in [211]). Mutations in apraxin [212] and in ETF-DH deficiency [213] have also been identified as secondary causes of CoQ deficiency.

Cardiolipin abnormalities

The formation of mitochondrial supercomplexes is sensitive to the lipid environment of the mitochondrial inner membrane. As previously discussed, cardiolipin is a unique component of this membrane. Barth syndrome, an X-linked disorder that presents with myopathy, cardiomyopathy, neutropenia, and growth retardation, is caused by mutations in the Tafazzin gene, which codes for a phospholipid acyltransferase that is important for cardiolipin biosynthesis [214]. Mitochondrial supercomplexes are destabilized in cells from Barth syndrome patients [215].

Clinical management of mitochondrial disease

There is currently no treatment known to influence the natural history of mitochondrial disease. However, the importance of an accurate diagnosis cannot be underestimated, and ideally this should be at the genetic level to allow confident genetic counseling and subsequent surveillance for mutation-specific complications, which can minimize disability.

Genetic counseling and prenatal diagnosis

mtDNA is only inherited down the maternal line, so men with a primary mtDNA disorder can be reassured that their offspring will not be affected by mtDNA disease.

mtDNA defects can be sporadic or maternally inherited. The recurrence risk for mtDNA deletions is low (~4%), and may be related to the presence of mtDNA duplications [72]. Some muscle-specific mtDNA mutations also do not appear to be transmitted (for example, [78]); however, most mtDNA are transmitted down the maternal line. Women with homoplasmic mtDNA mutations only pass mutant mtDNA to their offspring. The most common homoplasmic mtDNA mutations cause Leber hereditary optic neuropathy, which has well-established gender-specific recurrence risks determined empirically from large clinical studies [216, 217]. Women with heteroplasmic mtDNA mutations pass a variable proportion of mutant mtDNA to their offspring. Retrospective studies have shown a relationship between the proportion of mutant mtDNA in the mother and the risk of clinical recurrence [69, 218], but prospective comprehensive studies have not been carried out, limiting the clinical applicability of these data. Empirical recurrence risks are currently being developed through multi-national consortia.

The identification of autosomal dominant, autosomal recessive, and X-linked recessive nuclear genetic defects allows appropriate genetic counseling (Table 19.5). Although this is usually straightforward, the penetrance of recently identified dominant mutations may not be known, and putative genetic modifiers may complicate the situation in certain circumstances (for example [11]).

There is limited worldwide experience in prenatal diagnosis [219, 220, 221]. Established nuclear gene defects can be tested in a chorionic villus biopsy or in cultured amniocytes [222]. Prenatal biochemical tests may be possible in families without a molecular diagnosis where it was possible to identify a clear-cut biochemical defect. However, a negative result must be interpreted with caution because some biochemical defects are not expressed in all tissues, even if they are caused by a nuclear gene defect [222]. The prenatal diagnosis of mtDNA defects presents a particular challenge because, in theory, the proportion of mutant mtDNA in a cellular sample may not reflect the level found in clinically relevant tissues. Work carried out on preimplantation mouse embryos [220] and recent studies carried out human embryos [223] suggests that the level of heteroplasmy is evenly distributed before implantation. This provides some hope for preimplantation genetic diagnosis, which has been carried out in some centers. Limited pathological studies of post-mortem human embryos have also shown an even distribution of pathogenic mtDNA mutations throughout the embryo, including the placenta [75]. This work has prompted a number of European centers to offer prenatal diagnosis, but there has been insufficient time to allow long-term follow-up studies. Even if the level of heteroplasmy in the biopsy sample does reflect the rest of the developing embryo, it is difficult to interpret the result. There is general agreement that very high (>80%) and very low (<20%) levels of m.3243A > G and m.8993T > G/C probably correspond to a very high, and low risk of recurrence, respectively [224], but there are limited clinical data to support this. Unfortunately, many patients have intermediate heteroplasmy values (between 20% and 80%) of uncertain significance. Prenatal diagnosis of mtDNA disease is therefore not considered to be part of routine clinical service at present.

Surveillance and management of complications

Specific mtDNA mutations are associated with a spectrum of complications, some of which can be detected before they present clinically with appropriate diagnostic tests, leading to preventative management [225]. Patients should have regular fasting blood glucose or HbA1c measurements. An annual ECG is advisable in all patients (apart from those with Leber hereditary optic neuropathy), and echocardiography every 2 years is recommended in patients with disorders associated with cardiomyopathy. The detection of asymptomatic cardiac hypertrophy should prompt standard therapy with angiotensin converting enzyme inhibitors. Patients should be asked about hearing loss, and audiometry should be carried out if there is any concern. High-frequency hearing loss often remains undetected until advanced, but responds well to amplification and cochlear implantation in selected cases [226]. Patients should be asked about symptoms suggestive of nocturnal hypoventilation, prompting overnight oximetry or a full sleep study, and leading to a trial of nocturnal ventilation if appropriate. Ptosis and persistent diplopia due to ophthalmoplegia can be treated surgically [227].

Exercise therapy

There is emerging evidence that exercise therapy is beneficial in mitochondrial myopathy. Aerobic exercise increases strength and stamina, decreases symptoms of fatigue, and improves quality of life in some patients [228, 229]. The improvement probably occurs by reversing the effects of deconditioning that usually accompany mitochondrial myopathy [230]. A program of exercise therapy has been shown to increase the muscle capillary bed, thus enhancing oxygen delivery [229]. Recent studies of endurance training failed to confirm previous reports of improved respiratory chain activity, a decrease in the frequency of COX-negative fibers, or alterations in mtDNA [228, 229].

Strength training has achieved much attention because of the potential benefits of reversing the biochemical defect through the activation of muscle satellite cells, which contain low percentage levels of mutant mtDNA. Single case studies have demonstrated the potential benefits of this approach [231, 232], but one study showed an increase in the proportion of mutated mtDNA in some cases following treatment [233], raising concerns about the longer-term consequences of this approach.

Dietary supplements and pharmacological management

Many different vitamins, co-factors, and dietary supplements have been used in patients with mitochondrial disease. With the exception of primary coenzyme Q10 deficiency, there is no clear evidence that any of these agents have an objective clinical benefit. Patients with recessive molecular defects affecting enzymes in the coenzyme Q10 biosynthetic pathway report clinical improvement with sustained oral coenzyme Q10 therapy [213, 234]. A recent Cochrane systematic review of over 650 case reports and clinical trials only identified six placebo-controlled clinical trials [235]. Two trials studied the effects of coenzyme Q10 (ubiquinone), one reporting a subjective improvement and a significant increase in a global scale of muscle strength [236], but the other trial did not show any benefit [237]. Two trials used creatine, with one reporting improved measures of muscle strength and post-exercise lactate [238], but the other reported no benefit [239]. One trial of dichloroacetate showed an improvement in secondary outcome measures of mitochondrial metabolism [240], and one trial using dimethylglycine showed no significant effect [241]. Since the Cochrane review, a randomized controlled clinical trial using dichloracetate in MELAS patients had to be terminated because of drug toxicity, particularly affecting the peripheral nerves [242]. Part of the difficulty in developing new treatments for mitochondrial disease relates to the heterogeneous nature of the disease, and a lack of natural history data. The establishment of multi-center collaborations in Europe and North America will hopefully address some of these issues and lead to treatment trials in the near future.

Acknowledgments

P.F.C. is a Wellcome Trust Senior Fellow in Clinical Science who also receives funding from the Medical Research Council (UK), United Mitochondrial Diseases Foundation, an unconditional research grant from the United States Army, The Parkinson's Disease Society (UK), and the European Union FP6 program EUmitocombat and MITOCIRCLE.

References

1. R. Luft, D. Ikkos, G. Palmieri, L. Ernster, B. Afzelius, A case of severe hypermetabolism of nonthyroid origin with a defect in the maintenance of mitochondrial respiratory control: a correlated clinical, biochemical and morphological study. *J. Clin. Invest.* **41** (1962), 1776–1804.
2. L. P. Rowland, A. P. Hays, S. Di Mauro, *et al.*, Diverse clinical disorders associated with abnormalities of mitochondria. In *Mitochondrial Pathology in Muscle Diseases*, eds. G. Scarlato, C. Cerri. (Padova: Piccin, 1983), pp. 141–158.
3. R. K. Petty, A. E. Harding, J. A. Morgan-Hughes, The clinical features of mitochondrial myopathy. *Brain* **109**:Pt 5 (1986), 915–938.
4. S. Anderson, A. T. Bankier, B. G. Barrell, *et al.*, Sequence and organization of the human mitochondrial genome. *Nature* **290** (1981), 457–465.
5. I. Holt, A. E. Harding, J. A. Morgan-Hughes, Deletion of muscle mitochondrial DNA in patients with mitochondrial myopathies. *Nature* **331** (1988), 717–719.
6. D. C. Wallace, G. Singh, M. T. Lott, *et al.*, Mitochondrial DNA mutation associated with Leber's hereditary optic neuropathy. *Science* **242** (1988), 1427–1430.
7. S. Servidei, Mitochondrial encephalomyopathies: gene mutation. *Neuromuscul. Disord.* **14** (2004), 107–116.
8. M. Zeviani, Nucleus-driven mutations of human mitochondrial DNA. *J. Inher. Metab. Dis.* **15** (1992), 456–471.
9. M. Zeviani, N. Bresolin, C. Gellera, *et al.*, Nucleus-driven multiple large-scale deletions of the human mitochondrial genome: a new autosomal dominant disease. *Am. J. Hum. Genet.* **47** (1990), 904–914.
10. E. A. Shoubridge, Nuclear genetic defects of oxidative phosphorylation. *Hum. Mol. Genet.* **10** (2001), 2277–2284.
11. P. F. Chinnery, M. Zeviani, 155th ENMC workshop: polymerase gamma and disorders of mitochondrial DNA synthesis, 21–23 September 2007, Naarden, The Netherlands. *Neuromuscul. Disord.* **18**:3 (2008), 259–267.
12. G. Van Goethem, B. Dermaut, A. Lofgren, J. J. Martin, C. Van Broeckhoven, Mutation of POLG is associated with progressive external ophthalmoplegia characterized by mtDNA deletions. *Nat. Genet.* **28** (2001), 211–212.
13. M. Zeviani, S. Di Donato, Mitochondrial disorders. *Brain* **127** (2004), 2153–2172.
14. Y. Bykhovskaya, K. Casas, E. Mengesha, A. Inbal, N. Fischel-Ghodsian, Missense mutation in pseudouridine synthase 1 (PUS1) causes mitochondrial myopathy and sideroblastic anemia (MLASA). *Am. J. Hum. Genet.* **74** (2004), 1303–1308.
15. A. Rotig, P. de Lonlay, D. Chretien, *et al.*, Aconitase and mitochondrial iron-sulphur protein deficiency in Friedreich ataxia. *Nat. Genet.* **17** (1997), 215–217.
16. G. Casari, M. De Fusco, S. Ciarmatori, *et al.*, Spastic paraplegia and OXPHOS impairment caused by mutations in paraplegin, a nuclear-encoded mitochondrial metalloprotease. *Cell* **93** (1998), 973–983.
17. S. Lutsenko, M. J. Cooper, Localization of the Wilson's disease protein product to mitochondria. *Proc. Natl. Acad. Sci. U.S.A.* **95** (1998), 6004–6009.
18. A. Bender, K. J. Krishnan, C. M. Morris, *et al.*, High levels of mitochondrial DNA deletions in substantia nigra neurons in aging and Parkinson disease. *Nat. Genet.* **38**:5 (2006), 515–517.
19. Y. Kraytsberg, E. Kudryavtseva, A. C. McKee, C. Geula, N. W. Kowall, K. Khrapko, Mitochondrial DNA deletions are abundant and cause functional impairment in aged human substantia nigra neurons. *Nat. Genet.* **38** (2006), 518–520.
20. E. Nekhaeva, N. D. Bodyak, Y. Kraytsberg, *et al.*, Clonally expanded mtDNA point mutations are abundant in individual cells of human tissues. *Proc. Natl. Acad. Sci. U.S.A.* **99** (2002), 5521–5526.
21. K. Khrapko, J. Vijg, Mitochondrial DNA mutations and aging: a case closed? *Nat. Genet.* **39** (2007), 445–446.
22. P. F. Chinnery, M. A. Johnson, T. M. Wardell, *et al.*, Epidemiology of pathogenic mitochondrial DNA mutations. *Ann. Neurol.* **48** (2000), 188–193.
23. N. Darin, A. Oldfors, A. R. Moslemi, E. Holme, M. Tulinius, The incidence of mitochondrial encephalomyopathies in childhood: clinical features and morphological, biochemical, and DNA abnormalities. *Ann. Neurol.* **49** (2001), 377–383.

24. A. M. Schaefer, R. McFarland, E. L. Blakely, *et al.*, Prevalence of mitochondrial DNA disease in adults. *Ann. Neurol.* **63** (2008), 35–39.

25. D. Skladal, F. P. Bernier, J. L. Halliday, D. R. Thorburn, Birth prevalence of mitochondrial respiratory chain defects in children. *J. Inher. Metab. Dis.* **23** (2000), 138.

26. D. Skladal, J. Halliday, D. R. Thorburn, Minimum birth prevalence of mitochondrial respiratory chain disorders in children. *Brain* **126** (2003), 1905–1912.

27. S. A. Detmer, D. C. Chan, Functions and dysfunctions of mitochondrial dynamics. *Nat. Rev. Mol. Cell. Biol.* **8** (2007), 870–879.

28. C. Alexander, M. Votruba, U. E. Pesch, *et al.*, OPA1, encoding a dynamin-related GTPase, is mutated in autosomal dominant optic atrophy linked to chromosome 3q28. *Nat. Genet.* **26** (2000), 211–215.

29. S. Zuchner, P. De Jonghe, A. Jordanova, *et al.*, Axonal neuropathy with optic atrophy is caused by mutations in mitofusin 2. *Ann. Neurol.* **59** (2006), 276–281.

30. S. Zuchner, J. M. Vance, Mechanisms of disease: a molecular genetic update on hereditary axonal neuropathies. *Nat. Clin. Pract. Neurol.* **2** (2006), 45–53.

31. W. Neupert, J. M. Herrmann, Translocation of proteins into mitochondria. *Annu. Rev. Biochem.* **76** (2007), 723–749.

32. C. Handschin, B. M. Spiegelman, Peroxisome proliferator-activated receptor gamma coactivator 1 coactivators, energy homeostasis, and metabolism. *Endocr. Rev.* **27** (2006), 728–735.

33. H. Schagger, R. de Coo, M. F. Bauer, S. Hofmann, C. Godinot, U. Brandt, Significance of respirasomes for the assembly/stability of human respiratory chain complex I. *J. Biol. Chem.* **279** (2004), 36349–36353.

34. M. Satoh, T. Kuroiwa, Organisation of multiple nucleoids and DNA molecules in mitochondria of a human cell. *Exp. Cell Res.* **196** (1991), 137–140.

35. L. Cao, H. Shitara, T. Horii, *et al.*, The mitochondrial bottleneck occurs without reduction of mtDNA content in female mouse germ cells. *Nat. Genet.* **39** (2007), 386–390.

36. L. M. Cree, D. C. Samuels, S. Chuva de Sousa Lopes, *et al.*, A reduction in the number of mitochondrial DNA molecules during embryogenesis explains the rapid segregation of genotypes. *Nat. Genet.* **40** (2008), 249–254.

37. L. Piko, L. Matsumoto, Number of mitochondria and some properties of mitochondrial DNA in the mouse egg. *Dev. Biol.* **49** (1976), 1–10.

38. N. B. Hecht, H. Liem, K. C. Kleene, R. J. Distel, S. M. Ho, Maternal inheritance of the mouse mitochondrial genome is not mediated by a loss or gross alteration of the paternal mitochondrial DNA or by methylation of the oocyte mitochondrial DNA. *Dev. Biol.* **102** (1984), 452–461.

39. D. F. Bogenhagen, D. Rousseau, S. Burke, The layered structure of human mitochondrial DNA nucleoids. *J. Biol. Chem.* **283** (2008), 3665–3675.

40. T. I. Alam, T. Kanki, T. Muta, *et al.*, Human mitochondrial DNA is packaged with TFAM. *Nucleic Acids Res.* **31** (2003), 1640–1645.

41. M. I. Ekstrand, M. Falkenberg, A. Rantanen, *et al.*, Mitochondrial transcription factor A regulates mtDNA copy number in mammals. *Hum. Mol. Genet.* **13** (2004), 935–944.

42. L. Boulet, G. Karpati, E. A. Shoubridge, Distribution and threshold expression of the tRNA(Lys) mutation in skeletal muscle of patients with myoclonic epilepsy and ragged-red fibers (MERRF). *Am. J. Hum. Genet.* **51** (1992), 1187–1200.

43. P. F. Chinnery, D. J. Taylor, D. T. Brown, D. Manners, P. J. Styles, R. Lodi, Very low levels of the mtDNA A3243G mutation associated with mitochondrial dysfunction in vivo. *Ann. Neurol.* **47** (2000), 381–384.

44. F. Dubeau, N. De Stefano, B. G. Zifkin, D. L. Arnold, E. A. Shoubridge, Oxidative phosphorylation defect in the brains of carriers of the tRNAleu(UUR) A3243G mutation in a MELAS pedigree. *Ann. Neurol.* **47** (2000), 179–185.

45. D. A. Clayton, Replication of animal mitochondrial DNA. *Cell* **28** (1982), 693–705.

46. M. Y. Yang, M. Bowmaker, A. Reyes, *et al.*, Biased incorporation of ribonucleotides on the mitochondrial L-strand accounts for apparent strand-asymmetric DNA replication. *Cell* **111** (2002), 495–505.

47. M. Bowmaker, M. Y. Yang, T. Yasukawa, *et al.*, Mammalian mitochondrial DNA replicates bidirectionally from an initiation zone. *J. Biol. Chem.* **278** (2003), 50961–50969.

48. I. J. Holt, H. E. Lorimer, H. T. Jacobs, Coupled leading- and lagging-strand synthesis of mammalian mitochondrial DNA. *Cell* **100** (2000), 515–524.

49. T. A. Brown, D. A. Clayton, Genesis and wanderings: origins and migrations in asymmetrically replicating mitochondrial DNA. *Cell Cycle* **5** (2006), 917–921.

50. T. E. Shutt, M. W. Gray, Twinkle, the mitochondrial replicative DNA helicase, is widespread in the eukaryotic radiation and may also be the mitochondrial DNA primase in most eukaryotes. *J. Mol. Evol.* **62** (2006), 588–599.

51. G. Farge, T. Holmlund, J. Khvorostova, R. Rofougaran, A. Hofer, M. Falkenberg, The N-terminal domain of TWINKLE contributes to single-stranded DNA binding and DNA helicase activities. *Nucleic Acids Res.* **36** (2008), 393–403.

52. M. Falkenberg, N. G. Larsson, C. M. Gustafsson, DNA replication and transcription in mammalian mitochondria. *Annu. Rev. Biochem.* **76** (2007), 679–699.

53. D. A. Clayton, Replication and transcription of vertebrate mitochondrial DNA. *Ann. Rev. Cell. Biol.* **7** (1992), 453–478.

54. N. J. Gross, G. S. Getz, M. Rabinowitz, Apparent turnover of mitochondrial deoxyribonucleic acid and mitochondrial phospholipids in the tissues of the rat. *J. Biol. Chem.* **244** (1969), 1552–1562.

55. G. S. Schadel, D. A. Clayton, Mitochondrial DNA maintenance in vertebrates. *Annu. Rev. Biochem.* **66** (1997), 409–435.

56. P. Fernandez-Silva, R. Acin-Perez, E. Fernandez-Vizarra, A. Perez-Martos, J. A. Enriquez, In vivo and in organello analyses of mitochondrial translation. *Methods Cell Biol.* **80** (2007), 571–588.

57. M. Falkenberg, M. Gaspari, A. Rantanen, A. Trifunovic, N. G. Larsson, C. M. Gustafsson, Mitochondrial transcription factors B1 and B2 activate transcription of human mtDNA. *Nat. Genet.* **31** (2002), 289–294.

58. M. Gaspari, M. Falkenberg, N. G. Larsson, C. M. Gustafsson, The mitochondrial RNA polymerase contributes critically to promoter specificity in mammalian cells. *EMBO J.* **23** (2004), 4606–4614.

59. D. Ojala, J. Montoya, G. Attardi, tRNA punctuation model of RNA processing in human mitochondria. *Nature* **290** (1981), 470–474.

60. T. W. O'Brien, Evolution of a protein-rich mitochondrial ribosome: implications for human genetic disease. *Gene* **286** (2002), 73–79.

61. R. E. Giles, H. Blanc, H. M. Cann, D. C. Wallace, Maternal inheritance of human mitochondrial DNA. *Proc. Natl. Acad. Sci. U.S.A.* **77** (1980), 6715–6719.

62. M. Schwartz, J. Vissing, Paternal inheritance of mitochondrial DNA. *N. Engl. J. Med.* **347** (2002), 576–580.

63. W. M. Hauswirth, P. J. Laipis, Mitochondrial DNA polymorphism in a maternal lineage of Holstien cows. *Proc. Natl. Acad. Sci. U.S.A.* **79** (1982), 4686–4690.

64. J. Jenuth, A. C. Peterson, K. Fu, E. A. Shoubridge, Random genetic drift in the female germ line explains the rapid segregation of mammalian mitochondrial DNA. *Nat. Genet.* **14** (1996), 146–151.

65. L. Piko, K. D. Taylor, Amounts of mitochondrial DNA and abundance of some mitochondrial gene transcripts in early mouse embryos. *Dev. Biol.* **123** (1987), 364–374.

66. J. Thundathil, F. Filion, L. C. Smith, Molecular control of mitochondrial function in preimplantation mouse embryos. *Mol. Reprod. Dev.* **71** (2005), 405–413.

67. P. F. Chinnery, D. R. Thorburn, D. C. Samuels, *et al.*, The inheritance of mitochondrial DNA heteroplasmy: random drift, selection or both? *Trends Genet.* **16** (2000), 500–505.

68. R. B. Blok, D. A. Gook, D. R. Thorburn, H. H. Dahl, Skewed segregation of the mtDNA nt 8993 (T to G) mutation in human oocytes. *Am. J. Hum. Genet.* **60** (1997), 1495–1501.

69. S. L. White, V. A. Collins, R. Woolfe, *et al.*, Genetic counseling and prenatal diagnosis for the mitochondrial DNA mutations at nucleotide 8993. *Am. J. Hum. Genet.* **65** (1999), 474–482.

70. K. Inoue, K. Nakada, A. Ogura, *et al.*, Generation of mice with mitochondrial dysfunction by introducing mouse mtDNA carrying a deletion into zygotes [In Process Citation]. *Nat. Genet.* **26** (2000), 176–181.

71. S. DiMauro, E. A. Schon, Mitochondrial respiratory-chain diseases. *N. Engl. J. Med.* **348** (2003), 2656–2668.

72. P. F. Chinnery, S. DiMauro, S. Shanske, *et al.*, Risk of developing a mitochondrial DNA deletion disorder. *Lancet* **364** (2004), 592–596.

73. W. Fan, K. G. Waymire, N. Narula, *et al.*, A mouse model of mitochondrial disease reveals germline selection against severe mtDNA mutations. *Science* **319** (2008), 958–962.

74. J. B. Stewart, C. Freyer, J. L. Elson, *et al.*, Strong purifying selection in transmission of mammalian mitochondrial DNA. *PLoS Biol.* **6** (2008), e10.

75. P. M. Matthews, J. Hopkin, R. M. Brown, J. B. Stephenson, D. Hilton-Jones, G. K. Brown, Comparison of the relative levels of the 3243 (A— > G) mtDNA mutation in heteroplasmic adult and fetal tissues. *J. Med. Genet.* **31** (1994), 41–44.

76. J. P. Jenuth, A. C. Peterson, E. A. Shoubridge, Tissue-specific selection for different mtDNA genotypes in heteroplasmic mice. *Nat. Genet.* **16** (1997), 93–95.

77. N. G. Larsson, E. Holme, B. Kristiansson, A. Oldfors, M. Tulinius, Progressive increase of the mutated mitochondrial DNA fraction in Kearns-Sayre syndrome. *Pediatr. Res.* **28** (1990), 131–136.

78. K. Weber, J. N. Wilson, L. Taylor, *et al.*, A new mtDNA mutation showing accumulation with time and restriction to skeletal muscle. *Am. J. Hum. Genet.* **60** (1997), 373–380.

79. K. Fu, R. Hartlen, T. Johns, A. Genge, G. Karpati, E. A. Shoubridge, A novel heteroplasmic tRNAleu(CUN) mtDNA point mutation in a sporadic patient with mitochondrial encephalomyopathy segregates rapidly in skeletal muscle and suggests an approach to therapy. *Hum. Mol. Genet.* **5** (1996), 1835–1840.

80. C. T. Moraes, F. Ciacci, E. Bonilla, *et al.*, Two novel pathogenic mitochondrial DNA mutations affecting organelle number and protein synthesis. Is the tRNA(Leu(UUR)) gene an etiologic hot spot? *J. Clin. Invest.* **92** (1993), 2906–2915.

81. R. McFarland, A. M. Schaefer, J. L. Gardner, *et al.*, Familial myopathy: new insights into the T14709C mitochondrial tRNA mutation. *Ann. Neurol.* **55** (2004), 478–484.

82. D. B. Olsen, A. Langkilde, J. Vissing, Muscle fat infiltration is a common finding in patients with a mitochondrial myopathy. *J. Neurol. Sci.* **187** (2001), S1113.

83. A. L. Andreu, M. G. Hanna, H. Reichmann, *et al.*, Exercise intolerance due to mutations in the cytochrome b gene of mitochondrial DNA. *N. Engl. J. Med.* **341** (1999), 1037–1044.

84. R. Horvath, G. Hudson, G. Ferrari, *et al.*, Phenotypic spectrum associated with mutations of the mitochondrial polymerase gamma gene. *Brain* **129** (2006), 1674–1684.

85. E. McPherson, C. Zabel, Mitochondrial mutation in a child with distal arthrogryposis. *Am. J. Med. Genet. A.* **140** (2006), 184–185.

86. K. Aure, H. Ogier de Baulny, P. Laforet, C. Jardel, B. Eymard, A. Lombes, Chronic progressive ophthalmoplegia with large-scale mtDNA rearrangement: can we predict progression? *Brain* **130** (2007), 1516–1524.

87. C. Y. Yu Wai Man, T. Smith, P. F. Chinnery, D. M. Turnbull, P. G. Griffiths, Assessment of visual function in chronic progressive external ophthalmoplegia. *Eye* **20**:5 (2006), 564–568.

88. C. Kornblum, R. Broicher, E. Walther, *et al.*, Cricopharyngeal achalasia is a common cause of dysphagia in patients with mtDNA deletions. *Neurology* **56** (2001), 1409–1412.

89. J. Kaukonen, J. K. Juselius, V. Tiranti, *et al.*, Role of adenine nucleotide translocator 1 in mtDNA maintenance. *Science* **289** (2000), 782–785.

90. J. N. Spelbrink, F. Y. Li, V. Tiranti, *et al.*, Human mitochondrial DNA deletions associated with mutations in the gene encoding Twinkle, a phage T7 gene 4-like protein localised in mitochondria. *Nat. Genet.* **28** (2001), 223–231.

91. M. Hirano, E. Ricci, M. R. Koenigsberger, *et al.*, Melas: an original case and clinical criteria for diagnosis. *Neuromuscul. Disord.* **2** (1992), 125–135.

92. E. Ciafaloni, E. Ricci, S. Shanske, *et al.*, MELAS: clinical features, biochemistry, and molecular genetics. *Ann. Neurol.* **31** (1992), 391–398.

93. T. Iizuka, F. Sakai, S. Kan, N. Suzuki, Slowly progressive spread of the stroke-like lesions in MELAS. *Neurology* **61** (2003), 1238–1244.

94. J. M. Shoffner, M. T. Lott, A. M. Lezza, P. Seibel, S. W. Ballinger, D. C. Wallace, Myoclonic epilepsy and ragged-red fiber disease (MERRF) is associated with a mitochondrial DNA tRNA(Lys) mutation. *Cell* **61** (1990), 931–937.

95. G. Silvestri, C. T. Moraes, S. Shanske, S. J. Oh, S. DiMauro, A new mtDNA mutation in the tRNA(Lys) gene associated with myoclonic epilepsy and ragged-red fibers (MERRF). *Am. J. Hum. Genet.* **51** (1992), 1213–1217.

96. N. G. Larsson, M. H. Tulinius, E. Holme, A. Oldfors, Pathogenetic aspects of the A8344G mutation of mitochondrial DNA associated with MERRF syndrome and multiple symmetric lipomas. *Muscle Nerve* **3** (1995), S102–S106.

97. J. Traff, E. Holme, K. Ekbom, B. Y. Nilsson, Ekbom's syndrome of photomyoclonus, cerebellar ataxia and cervical lipoma is associated with the tRNA(Lys) A8344G mutation in mitochondrial DNA. *Acta Neurol. Scand.* **92** (1995), 394–397.

98. S. DiMauro, D. C. DeVivo, Genetic heterogeneity in Leigh syndrome. *Ann. Neurol.* **40** (1996), 5–7.

99. A. A. M. Morris, J. V. Leonard, G. K. Brown, *et al.*, Deficiency of respiratory chain complex I is a common cause of Leigh disease. *Ann. Neurol.* **40** (1996), 25–30.

100. S. Rahman, R. B. Blok, H. H. Dahl, *et al.*, Leigh syndrome: clinical features and biochemical and DNA abnormalities. *Ann. Neurol.* **39** (1996), 343–351.

101. I. J. Holt, A. E. Harding, R. K. Petty, J. A. Morgan-Hughes, A new mitochondrial disease associated with mitochondrial DNA heteroplasmy. *Am. J. Hum. Genet.* **46** (1990), 428–433.

102. G. Uziel, I. Moroni, E. Lamantea, *et al.*, Mitochondrial disease associated with the T8993G mutation of the mitochondrial ATPase 6 gene: a clinical, biochemical, and molecular study in six families. *J. Neurol. Neurosurg. Psychiatry* **63** (1997), 16–22.

103. N. Howell, Leber hereditary optic neuropathy: how do mitochondrial DNA mutations cause degeneration of the optic nerve? *J. Bioenerget. Biomembr.* **29** (1997), 165–173.

104. E. K. Nikoskelainen, K. Huoponen, V. Juvonen, T. Lamminen, K. Nummelin, M. L. Savontaus, Ophthalmologic findings in Leber hereditary optic neuropathy, with special reference to mtDNA mutations. *Ophthalmology* **103** (1996), 504–514.

105. P. Y. Man, P. G. Griffiths, D. T. Brown, N. Howell, D. M. Turnbull, P. F. Chinnery, The epidemiology of Leber hereditary optic neuropathy in the north East of England. *Am. J. Hum. Genet.* **72** (2003), 333–339.

106. R. McFarland, P. F. Chinnery, E. L. Blakely, *et al.*, Homoplasmy, heteroplasmy, and mitochondrial dystonia. *Neurology* **69** (2007), 911–916.

107. E. K. Nikoskelainen, K. Huoponen, V. Juvonen, T. Lamminen, K. Nummelin, M. -L. Savontaus, Ophthalmologic findings in Leber hereditary optic neuropathy, with special reference to mtDNA mutations. *Ophthalmology* **103** (1996), 540–514.

108. I. Nishino, A. Spinazzola, M. Hirano, Thymidine phosphorylase gene mutations in MNGIE, a human mitochondrial disorder. *Science* **283** (1999), 689–692.

109. B. J. Alpers, Diffuse progressive degeneration of the gray matter of the cerebrum. *Arch. Neurol. Psychiatry* **25** (1931), 469–505.

110. P. R. Huttenlocher, G. B. Solitare, G. Adams, Infantile diffuse cerebral degeneration with hepatic cirrhosis. *Arch. Neurol.* **33** (1976), 186–192.

111. K. V. Nguyen, E. Ostergaard, S. H. Ravn, *et al.*, POLG mutations in Alpers syndrome. *Neurology* **65** (2005), 1493–1495.

112. A. E. Harding, I. J. Holt, J. M. Cooper, *et al.*, Mitochondrial myopathies: genetic defects. *Biochem. Soc. Trans.* **18** (1990), 519–522.

113. B. N. Harding, N. Alsanjari, S. J. Smith, *et al.*, Progressive neuronal degeneration of childhood with liver disease (Alpers' disease) presenting in young adults. *J. Neurol. Neurosurg. Psychiatry* **58** (1995), 320–325.

114. L. S. Kaguni, DNA polymerase gamma, the mitochondrial replicase. *Annu. Rev. Biochem.* **73** (2004), 293–320.

115. P. Luoma, A. Melberg, J. O. Rinne, *et al.*, Parkinsonism, premature menopause, and mitochondrial DNA polymerase gamma mutations: clinical and molecular genetic study. *Lancet* **364** (2004), 875–882.

116. A. T. Pagnamenta, J. W. Taanman, C. J. Wilson, *et al.*, Dominant inheritance of premature ovarian failure associated with mutant mitochondrial DNA polymerase gamma. *Hum. Reprod.* **21**:10 (2006), 2467–2473.

117. G. Van Goethem, J. J. Martin, B. Dermaut, *et al.*, Recessive POLG mutations presenting with sensory and ataxic neuropathy in compound heterozygote patients with progressive external ophthalmoplegia. *Neuromuscul. Disord.* **13** (2003), 133–142.

118. A. H. Hakonen, S. Heiskanen, V. Juvonen, *et al.*, Mitochondrial DNA polymerase W748S mutation: a common cause of autosomal recessive ataxia with ancient European origin. *Am. J. Hum. Genet.* **77** (2005), 430–441.

119. S. Winterthun, G. Ferrari, L. He, *et al.*, Autosomal recessive mitochondrial ataxic syndrome due to mitochondrial polymerase gamma mutations. *Neurology* **64** (2005), 1204–1208.

120. C. Tzoulis, B. A. Engelsen, W. Telstad, *et al.*, The spectrum of clinical disease caused by the A467T and W748S POLG mutations: a study of 26 cases. *Brain* **129** (2006), 1685–1692.

121. M. Deschauer, S. Tennant, A. Rokicka, *et al.*, MELAS associated with mutations in the POLG1 gene. *Neurology* **68** (2007), 1741–1742.

122. G. Davidzon, P. Greene, M. Mancuso, *et al.*, Early-onset familial parkinsonism due to POLG mutations. *Ann. Neurol.* **59** (2006), 859–862.

123. G. Davidzon, M. Mancuso, S. Ferraris, *et al.*, POLG mutations and Alpers syndrome. *Ann. Neurol.* **57** (2005), 921–923.

124. G. Ferrari, E. Lamantea, A. Donati, *et al.*, Infantile hepatocerebral syndromes associated with mutations in the mitochondrial DNA polymerase-gammaA. *Brain* **128** (2005), 723–731.

125. G. Kollberg, A. R. Moslemi, N. Darin, *et al.*, POLG1 mutations associated with progressive encephalopathy in childhood. *J. Neuropathol. Exp. Neurol.* **65** (2006), 758–768.

126. R. K. Naviaux, K. V. Nguyen, POLG mutations associated with Alpers' syndrome and mitochondrial DNA depletion. *Ann. Neurol.* **55** (2004), 706–712.

127. K. V. Nguyen, F. S. Sharief, S. S. Chan, W. C. Copeland, R. K. Naviaux, Molecular diagnosis of Alpers syndrome. *J. Hepatol.* **45**:1 (2006), 108–116.

128. M. C. Bianchi, G. Sgandurra, M. Tosetti, R. Battini, G. Cioni, Brain magnetic resonance in the diagnostic evaluation of mitochondrial encephalopathies. *Biosci. Rep.* **27** (2007), 69–85.

129. A. Munnich, A. Rotig, D. Chretien, *et al.*, Clinical presentation of mitochondrial disorders in childhood. *J. Inher. Metab. Dis.* **19** (1996), 521–527.

130. M. J. Jackson, J. A. Schaefer, M. A. Johnson, A. A. M. Morris, D. M. Turnbull, L. A. Bindoff, Presentation and clinical investigation of mitochondrial respiratory chain disease. *Brain* **118** (1995), 339–357.

131. D. B. Olsen, A. R. Langkilde, M. C. Orngreen, E. Rostrup, M. Schwartz, J. Vissing, Muscle structural changes in mitochondrial myopathy relate to genotype. *J. Neurol.* **250** (2003), 1328–1334.

132. A. L. Andreu, K. Tanji, C. Bruno, *et al.*, Exercise intolerance due to a nonsense mutation in the mtDNA ND4 gene. *Ann. Neurol.* **45** (1999), 820–823.

133. M. Sciacco, E. Bonilla, E. A. Schon, S. DiMauro, C. T. Moraes, Distribution of wild-type and common deletion forms of mtDNA in normal and respiration-deficient muscle fibers from patients with mitochondrial myopathy [published erratum appears in *Hum Mol Genet* 1994 Apr;3(4):687]. *Hum. Mol. Genet.* **3** (1994), 13–19.

134. V. Tiranti, K. Hoertnagel, R. Carrozzo, *et al.*, Mutations of SURF-1 in Leigh disease associated with cytochrome c oxidase deficiency. *Am. J. Hum. Genet.* **63** (1998), 1609–1621.

135. Z. Zhu, J. Yao, T. Johns, *et al.*, SURF1, encoding a factor involved in the biogenesis of cytochrome c oxidase, is mutated in Leigh syndrome. *Nat. Genet.* **20** (1998), 337–343.

136. R. McFarland, K. M. Clark, A. A. Morris, *et al.*, Multiple neonatal deaths due to a homoplasmic mitochondrial DNA mutation. *Nat. Genet.* **30** (2002), 145–146.

137. E. J. Brierley, M. A. Johnson, R. N. Lightowlers, O. F. James, D. M. Turnbull, Role of mitochondrial DNA mutations in human aging: implications for the central nervous system and muscle. *Ann. Neurol.* **43** (1998), 217–223.

138. A. M. Schaefer, R. W. Taylor, D. M. Turnbull, P. F. Chinnery, The epidemiology of mitochondrial disorders – past, present and future. *Biochim. Biophys. Acta* **1659** (2004), 115–120.

139. G. Van Goethem, P. Luoma, M. Rantamaki, *et al.*, POLG mutations in neurodegenerative disorders with ataxia but no muscle involvement. *Neurology* **63** (2004), 1251–1257.

140. M. T. McDonnell, A. M. Schaefer, E. L. Blakely, *et al.*, Noninvasive diagnosis of the 3243A > G mitochondrial DNA mutation using urinary epithelial cells. *Eur. J. Hum. Genet.* **12** (2004), 778–781.

141. G. Hudson, A. M. Schaefer, R. W. Taylor, *et al.*, Mutation of the linker region of the polymerase gamma-1 (POLG1) gene associated with progressive external ophthalmoplegia and Parkinsonism. *Arch. Neurol.* **64** (2007), 553–557.

142. B. Fromenty, G. Manfredi, J. Sadlock, L. Zhang, M. P. King, E. A. Schon, Efficient and specific amplification of identified partial duplications of human mitochondrial DNA by long PCR. *Biochim. Biophys. Acta* **1308** (1996), 222–230.

143. T. Harrower, J. D. Stewart, G. Hudson, *et al.*, POLG1 mutations manifesting as autosomal recessive axonal Charcot-Marie-Tooth disease. *Arch. Neurol.* **65** (2008), 133–136.

144. P. T. Luoma, N. Luo, W. N. Loscher, *et al.*, Functional defects due to spacer-region mutations of human mitochondrial DNA polymerase in a family with an ataxia-myopathy syndrome. *Hum. Mol. Genet.* **14** (2005), 1907–1920.

145. L. He, P. F. Chinnery, S. E. Durham, *et al.*, Detection and quantification of mitochondrial DNA deletions in individual cells by real-time PCR. *Nucleic Acids Res.* **30** (2002), e68.

146. C. Herrnstadt, J. L. Elson, E. Fahy, *et al.*, Reduced median network analysis of complete mtDNA coding region sequences for the major African, Asian, and European haplogroups. *Am. J. Hum. Genet.* **70** (2002), 1152–1171.

147. S. DiMauro, E. A. Schon, Mitochondrial DNA mutations in human disease. *Am. J. Med. Genet.* **106** (2001), 18–26.

148. M. Lazarou, D. R. Thorburn, M. T. Ryan, M. McKenzie, Assembly of mitochondrial complex I and defects in disease. *Biochim. Biophys. Acta* **1793** (2009), 78–88.

149. C. Ugalde, R. Hinttala, S. Timal, *et al.*, Mutated ND2 impairs mitochondrial complex I assembly and leads to Leigh syndrome. *Mol. Genet. Metab.* **90** (2007), 10–14.

150. T. Bougeron, P. Rustin, M. Birch-Machin, *et al.*, A mutation of nuclear succinate dehydrogenase gene results in mitochondrial respiratory chain deficiency. *Nat. Genet.* **11** (1995), 144–149.

151. S. Haut, M. Brivet, G. Touati, *et al.*, A deletion in the human QP-C gene causes a complex III deficiency resulting in hypoglycaemia and lactic acidosis. *Hum. Genet.* **113** (2003), 118–122.

152. O. Barel, Z. Shorer, H. Flusser, *et al.*, Mitochondrial complex III deficiency associated with a homozygous mutation in UQCRQ. *Am. J. Hum. Genet.* **82** (2008), 1211–1216.

153. V. Massa, E. Fernandez-Vizarra, S. Alshahwan, *et al.*, Severe infantile encephalomyopathy caused by a mutation in COX6B1, a nucleus-encoded subunit of cytochrome c oxidase. *Am. J. Hum. Genet.* **82** (2008), 1281–1289.

154. Z. Zhu, J. Yao, T. Johns, *et al.*, SURF1, encoding a factor involved in the biogenesis of cytochrome c oxidase, is mutated in Leigh syndrome. *Nat. Genet.* **20** (1998), 337–343.

155. D. Smith, J. Gray, L. Mitchell, W. E. Antholine, J. P. Hosler, Assembly of cytochrome-c oxidase in the absence of assembly protein Surf1p leads to loss of the active site heme. *J. Biol. Chem.* **280** (2005), 17652–17656.

156. V. K. Mootha, P. Lepage, K. Miller, *et al.*, Identification of a gene causing human cytochrome c oxidase deficiency by integrative genomics. *Proc. Natl. Acad. Sci. U.S.A.* **100** (2003), 605–610.

157. F. Merante, R. Petrova-Benedict, N. MacKay, *et al.*, A biochemically distinct form of cytochrome oxidase (COX) deficiency in the Saguenay-Lac-Saint-Jean region of Quebec. *Am. J. Hum. Genet.* **53** (1993), 481–487.

158. F. Xu, C. Morin, G. Mitchell, C. Ackerley, B. H. Robinson, The role of the LRPPRC (leucine-rich pentatricopeptide repeat cassette) gene in cytochrome oxidase assembly: mutation causes lowered levels of COX (cytochrome c oxidase) I and COX III mRNA. *Biochem. J.* **382** (2004), 331–336.

159. M. P. Cooper, L. Qu, L. M. Rohas, *et al.*, Defects in energy homeostasis in Leigh syndrome French Canadian variant through PGC-1alpha/LRP130 complex. *Genes Dev.* **20** (2006), 2996–3009.

160. H. Antonicka, A. Mattman, C. G. Carlson, *et al.*, Mutations in COX15 produce a defect in the mitochondrial heme biosynthetic

pathway, causing early-onset fatal hypertrophic cardiomyopathy. *Am. J. Hum. Genet.* **72** (2003), 101–114.

161. I. Valnot, J. C. von Kleist-Retzow, A. Barrientos, A mutation in the human heme A:farnesyltransferrase gene (COX 10) causes cytochrome c oxidase deficiency. *Hum. Mol. Genet.* **9** (2000), 1245–1249.
162. M. Jaksch, I. Ogilvie, J. Yao, *et al.*, Mutations in SCO2 are associated with a distinct form of hypertrophic cardiomyopathy and cytochrome c oxidase deficiency. *Hum. Mol. Genet.* **9** (2000), 795–801.
163. L. C. Papadopoulou, C. M. Sue, M. M. Davidson, *et al.*, Fatal infantile cardioencephalomyopathy with COX deficiency and mutations in SCO2, a COX assembly gene. *Nat. Genet.* **23** (1999), 333–337.
164. I. Valnot, S. Ormond, N. Gigarel, Mutations of the SCO 1 gene in mitochondrial cytochrome c oxidase (COX) deficiency with neonatal-onset hepatic failure and encephalopathy. *Am. J. Hum. Genet.* **67** (2000), 1104–1109.
165. S. C. Leary, B. A. Kaufman, G. Pellecchia, *et al.*, Human SCO1 and SCO2 have independent, cooperative functions in copper delivery to cytochrome c oxidase. *Hum. Mol. Genet.* **13** (2004), 1839–1848.
166. S. C. Leary, P. A. Cobine, B. A. Kaufman, *et al.*, The human cytochrome c oxidase assembly factors SCO1 and SCO2 have regulatory roles in the maintenance of cellular copper homeostasis. *Cell. Metab.* **5** (2007), 9–20.
167. P. de Lonlay, I. Valnot, A. Barrientos, *et al.*, A mutant mitochondrial respiratory chain assembly protein causes complex III deficiency in patients with tubulopathy, encephalopathy and liver failure. *Nat. Genet.* **29** (2001), 57–60.
168. I. Visapaa, V. Fellman, J. Vesa, *et al.*, GRACILE syndrome, a lethal metabolic disorder with iron overload, is caused by a point mutation in BCS1L. *Am. J. Hum. Genet.* **71** (2002), 863–876.
169. J. T. Hinson, V. R. Fantin, J. Schonberger, *et al.*, Missense mutations in the BCS1L gene as a cause of the Bjornstad syndrome. *N. Engl. J. Med.* **356** (2007), 809–819.
170. S. H. Ackerman, Atp11p and Atp12p are chaperones for F(1)-ATPase biogenesis in mitochondria. *Biochim. Biophys. Acta* **1555** (2002), 101–105.
171. W. Sperl, P. Jesina, J. Zeman, *et al.*, Deficiency of mitochondrial ATP synthase of nuclear genetic origin. *Neuromuscul. Disord.* **16** (2006), 821–829.
172. L. De Meirleir, S. Seneca, W. Lissens, *et al.*, Respiratory chain complex V deficiency due to a mutation in the assembly gene ATP12. *J. Med. Genet.* **41** (2004), 120–124.
173. D. M. Kirby, R. Salemi, C. Sugiana, *et al.*, NDUFS6 mutations are a novel cause of lethal neonatal mitochondrial complex I deficiency. *J. Clin. Invest.* **114** (2004), 837–845.
174. R. Kuffner, A. Rohr, A. Schmiede, C. Krull, U. Schulte, Involvement of two novel chaperones in the assembly of mitochondrial NADH:ubiquinone oxidoreductase (complex I). *J. Mol. Biol.* **283** (1998), 409–417.
175. C. J. Dunning, M. McKenzie, C. Sugiana, *et al.*, Human CIA30 is involved in the early assembly of mitochondrial complex I and mutations in its gene cause disease. *EMBO J.* **26** (2007), 3227–3237.
176. R. O. Vogel, R. J. Janssen, M. A. van den Brand, *et al.*, Cytosolic signaling protein Ecsit also localizes to mitochondria where it interacts with chaperone NDUFAF1 and functions in complex I assembly. *Genes Dev.* **21** (2007), 615–624.
177. I. Ogilvie, N. G. Kennaway, E. A. Shoubridge, A molecular chaperone for mitochondrial complex I assembly is mutated in a progressive encephalopathy. *J. Clin. Invest.* **115** (2005), 2784– 2792.
178. A. Saada, S. Edvardson, M. Rapoport, *et al.*, C6ORF66 is an assembly factor of mitochondrial complex I. *Am. J. Hum. Genet.* **82** (2008), 32–38.
179. T. Gabaldon, D. Rainey, M. A. Huynen, Tracing the evolution of a large protein complex in the eukaryotes, NADH:ubiquinone oxidoreductase (Complex I). *J. Mol. Biol.* **348** (2005), 857–870.
180. M. J. Coenen, H. Antonicka, C. Ugalde, *et al.*, Mutant mitochondrial elongation factor G1 and combined oxidative phosphorylation deficiency. *N. Engl. J. Med.* **351** (2004), 2080–2086.
181. H. Antonicka, F. Sasarman, N. G. Kennaway, E. A. Shoubridge, The molecular basis for tissue specificity of the oxidative phosphorylation deficiencies in patients with mutations in the mitochondrial translation factor EFG1. *Hum. Mol. Genet.* **15** (2006), 1835–1846.
182. L. Valente, V. Tiranti, R. M. Marsano, *et al.*, Infantile encephalopathy and defective mitochondrial DNA translation in patients with mutations of mitochondrial elongation factors EFG1 and EFTu. *Am. J. Hum. Genet.* **80** (2007), 44–58.
183. J. A. Smeitink, O. Elpeleg, H. Antonicka, *et al.*, Distinct clinical phenotypes associated with a mutation in the mitochondrial translation elongation factor EFTs. *Am. J. Hum. Genet.* **79** (2006), 869–877.
184. C. Miller, A. Saada, N. Shaul, *et al.*, Defective mitochondrial translation caused by a ribosomal protein (MRPS16) mutation. *Ann. Neurol.* **56** (2004), 734–738.
185. A. Saada, A. Shaag, S. Arnon, *et al.*, Antenatal mitochondrial disease caused by mitochondrial ribosomal protein (MRPS22) mutation. *J. Med. Genet.* **44**:12 (2007), 784–786.
186. P. Allard, A. V. Rak, B. T. Wimberly, *et al.*, Another piece of the ribosome: solution structure of S16 and its location in the 30S subunit. *Structure* **8** (2000), 875–882.
187. M. Nolden, S. Ehses, M. Koppen, A. Bernacchia, E. I. Rugarli, T. Langer, The m-AAA protease defective in hereditary spastic paraplegia controls ribosome assembly in mitochondria. *Cell* **123** (2005), 277–289.
188. K. Leonhard, J. M. Herrmann, R. A. Stuart, G. Mannhaupt, W. Neupert, T. Langer, AAA proteases with catalytic sites on opposite membrane surfaces comprise a proteolytic system for the ATP-dependent degradation of inner membrane proteins in mitochondria. *EMBO J.* **15** (1996), 4218–4229.
189. L. Atorino, L. Silvestri, M. Koppen, *et al.*, Loss of m-AAA protease in mitochondria causes complex I deficiency and increased sensitivity to oxidative stress in hereditary spastic paraplegia. *J. Cell. Biol.* **163** (2003), 777–787.
190. J. R. Patton, Y. Bykhovskaya, E. Mengesha, C. Bertolotto, N. Fischel-Ghodsian, Mitochondrial myopathy and sideroblastic anemia (MLASA): missense mutation in the pseudouridine synthase 1 (PUS1) gene is associated with the loss of tRNA pseudouridylation. *J. Biol. Chem.* **280** (2005), 19823–19828.
191. A. Zeharia, N. Fischel-Ghodsian, K. Casas, *et al.*, Mitochondrial myopathy, sideroblastic anemia, and lactic acidosis: an

autosomal recessive syndrome in Persian Jews caused by a mutation in the PUS1 gene. *J. Child Neurol.* **20** (2005), 449–452.

192. S. Alberio, R. Mineri, V. Tiranti, M. Zeviani, Depletion of mtDNA: syndromes and genes. *Mitochondrion* **7** (2007), 6–12.

193. A. Saada, E. Ben-Shalom, R. Zyslin, C. Miller, H. Mandel, O. Elpeleg, Mitochondrial deoxyribonucleoside triphosphate pools in thymidine kinase 2 deficiency. *Biochem. Biophys. Res. Commun.* **310** (2003), 963–966.

194. H. Mandel, R. Szargel, V. Labay, *et al.*, The deoxyguanosine kinase gene is mutated in individuals with depleted hepatocerebral mitochondrial DNA. *Nat. Genet.* **29** (2001), 337–341.

195. A. Saada, Deoxyribonucleotides and disorders of mitochondrial DNA integrity. *DNA Cell Biol.* **23** (2004), 797–806.

196. A. Bourdon, L. Minai, V. Serre, *et al.*, Mutation of RRM2B, encoding p53-controlled ribonucleotide reductase (p53R2), causes severe mitochondrial DNA depletion. *Nat. Genet.* **39** (2007), 776–780.

197. E. Sarzi, S. Goffart, V. Serre, *et al.*, Twinkle helicase (PEO1) gene mutation causes mitochondrial DNA depletion. *Ann. Neurol.* **62**:6 (2007), 579–587.

198. A. Spinazzola, C. Viscomi, E. Fernandez-Vizarra, *et al.*, MPV17 encodes an inner mitochondrial membrane protein and is mutated in infantile hepatic mitochondrial DNA depletion. *Nat. Genet.* **38** (2006), 570–575.

199. S. Calvo, M. Jain, X. Xie, *et al.*, Systematic identification of human mitochondrial disease genes through integrative genomics. *Nat. Genet.* **38** (2006), 576–582.

200. L. J. Wong, N. Brunetti-Pierri, Q. Zhang, *et al.*, Mutations in the MPV17 gene are responsible for rapidly progressive liver failure in infancy. *Hepatology* **46** (2007), 1218–1227.

201. C. L. Karadimas, T. H. Vu, S. A. Holve, *et al.*, Navajo neurohepatopathy is caused by a mutation in the MPV17 gene. *Am. J. Hum. Genet.* **79** (2006), 544–548.

202. A. Spinazzola, V. Massa, M. Hirano, M. Zeviani, Lack of founder effect for an identical mtDNA depletion syndrome (MDS)-associated MPV17 mutation shared by Navajos and Italians. *Neuromuscul. Disord.* **18** (2008), 315–318.

203. O. Elpeleg, C. Miller, E. Hershkovitz, *et al.*, Deficiency of the ADP-forming succinyl-CoA synthase activity is associated with encephalomyopathy and mitochondrial DNA depletion. *Am. J. Hum. Genet.* **76** (2005), 1081–1086.

204. E. Ostergaard, E. Christensen, E. Kristensen, *et al.*, Deficiency of the alpha subunit of succinate-coenzyme A ligase causes fatal infantile lactic acidosis with mitochondrial DNA depletion. *Am. J. Hum. Genet.* **81** (2007), 383–387.

205. A. Spinazzola, M. Zeviani, Disorders of nuclear-mitochondrial intergenomic communication. *Biosci. Rep.* **27** (2007), 39–51.

206. L. Palmieri, S. Alberio, I. Pisano, *et al.*, Complete loss-of-function of the heart/muscle-specific adenine nucleotide translocator is associated with mitochondrial myopathy and cardiomyopathy. *Hum. Mol. Genet.* **14** (2005), 3079–3088.

207. K. Nikali, A. Suomalainen, J. Saharinen, *et al.*, Infantile onset spinocerebellar ataxia is caused by recessive mutations in mitochondrial proteins Twinkle and Twinky. *Hum. Mol. Genet.* **14** (2005), 2981–2990.

208. M. Hirano, Y. Nishigaki, R. Marti, Mitochondrial neurogastrointestinal encephalomyopathy (MNGIE): a disease of two genomes. *Neurologist* **10** (2004), 8–17.

209. Y. Nishigaki, R. Marti, W. C. Copeland, M. Hirano, Site-specific somatic mitochondrial DNA point mutations in patients with thymidine phosphorylase deficiency. *J. Clin. Invest.* **111** (2003), 1913–1921.

210. M. Hirano, R. Marti, C. Casali, *et al.*, Allogenic stem cell transplantation corrects biochemical derangements in MNGIE. *Neurology* **67**:8 (2006), 1458–1460.

211. C. M. Quinzii, S. DiMauro, M. Hirano, Human coenzyme Q10 deficiency. *Neurochem Res* **32** (2007), 723–727.

212. I. Le Ber, O. Dubourg, J. F. Benoist, *et al.*, Muscle coenzyme Q10 deficiencies in ataxia with oculomotor apraxia 1. *Neurology* **68** (2007), 295–297.

213. K. Gempel, H. Topaloglu, B. Talim, *et al.*, The myopathic form of coenzyme Q10 deficiency is caused by mutations in the electron-transferring-flavoprotein dehydrogenase (ETFDH) gene. *Brain* **130** (2007), 2037–2044.

214. M. Schlame, M. Ren, Barth syndrome, a human disorder of cardiolipin metabolism. *FEBS Lett.* **580** (2006), 5450–5455.

215. M. McKenzie, M. Lazarou, D. R. Thorburn, M. T. Ryan, Mitochondrial respiratory chain supercomplexes are destabilized in Barth syndrome patients. *J. Mol. Biol.* **361** (2006), 462–469.

216. A. E. Harding, M. G. Sweeney, G. G. Govan, P. Riordan-Eva, Pedigree analysis in Leber hereditary optic neuropathy families with a pathogenic mtDNA mutation. *Am. J. Hum. Genet.* **57** (1995), 77–86.

217. C. Macmillan, T. Kirkham, K. Fu, *et al.*, Pedigree analysis of Leber's hereditary optic neuropathy families with the T14484C mtDNA mutation. *Neurology* **49** (1997), A245.

218. P. F. Chinnery, N. Howell, R. N. Lightowlers, D. M. Turnbull, MELAS and MERRF: the relationship between maternal mutation load and the frequency of clinically affected offspring. *Brain* **121** (1998), 1889–1894.

219. D. T. Brown, M. Herbert, V. K. Lamb, *et al.*, Transmission of mitochondrial DNA disorders: possibilities for the future. *Lancet* **368** (2006), 87–89.

220. N. L. Dean, B. J. Battersby, A. Ao, *et al.*, Prospect of preimplantation genetic diagnosis for heritable mitochondrial DNA diseases. *Mol. Hum. Reprod.* **9** (2003), 631–638.

221. E. A. Shoubridge, T. Wai, Mitochondrial DNA and the mammalian oocyte. *Curr. Top. Dev. Biol.* **77** (2007), 87–111.

222. D. R. Thorburn, H. H. M. Dahl, Mitochondrial disorders: genetics, counseling, prenatal diagnosis and reproductive options. *Am. J. Med. Genet.* **106** (2001), 102–114.

223. J. Steffann, N. Gigarel, J. Corcos, *et al.*, Stability of the m8993T- > G mtDNA mutation load during human embryofetal development has implications for the feasibility of prenatal diagnosis in NARP syndrome. *J. Med. Genet.* **44** (2007), 664–669.

224. J. Poulton, D. M. Turnbull, 74th ENMC International workshop: mitochondrial diseases. *Neuromuscul. Disord.* **10** (2000), 460–462.

225. P. F. Chinnery, L. A. Bindoff, 116th ENMC international workshop: the treatment of mitochondrial disorders, 14th–16th

March 2003, Naarden, The Netherlands. *Neuromuscul. Disord.* **13** (2003), 757–764.

226. A. R. Sinnathuray, V. Raut, A. Awa, A. Magee, J. G. Toner, A review of cochlear implantation in mitochondrial sensorineural hearing loss. *Otol. Neurotol.* **24** (2003), 418–426.

227. V. Biousse, N. J. Newman, Neuro-ophthalmology of mitochondrial diseases. *Curr. Opin. Neurol.* **16** (2003), 35–43.

228. T. D. Jeppesen, M. Schwartz, D. B. Olsen, *et al.*, Aerobic training is safe and improves exercise capacity in patients with mitochondrial myopathy. *Brain* **129** (2006), 3402–3412.

229. T. Taivassalo, J. L. Gardner, R. W. Taylor, *et al.*, Endurance training and detraining in mitochondrial myopathies due to single large-scale mtDNA deletions. *Brain* **129** (2006), 3391–3401.

230. T. Taivassalo, T. D. Jensen, N. Kennaway, S. DiMauro, J. Vissing, R. G. Haller, The spectrum of exercise tolerance in mitochondrial myopathies: a study of 40 patients. *Brain* **126** (2003), 413–423.

231. K. Clark, L. A. Bindoff, R. N. Lightowlers, *et al.*, Correction of a mitochondrial DNA defect in human skeletal muscle. *Nat. Genet.* **16** (1997), 222–224.

232. K. Fu, R. Hartien, T. Johns, A. Genge, G. Karpati, E. A. Shoubridge, A novel heteroplasmic tRNAleu(UUR) mtDNA point mutation in a sporadic patient with mitochondrial encephalomyopathy segregates rapidly in muscle and suggests an approach to therapy. *Hum. Mol. Genet.* **5** (1996), 1835–1840.

233. T. Taivassalo, E. A. Shoubridge, J. Chen, *et al.*, Aerobic conditioning in patients with mitochondrial myopathies: physiological, biochemical, and genetic effects. *Ann. Neurol.* **50** (2001), 133–141.

234. C. Quinzii, A. Naini, L. Salviati, *et al.*, A mutation in para-hydroxybenzoate-polyprenyl transferase (COQ2) causes primary coenzyme Q10 deficiency. *Am. J. Hum. Genet.* **78** (2006), 345–349.

235. P. F. Chinnery, K. Majamaa, D. M. Turnbull, D. R. Thorburn, Treatment for mitochondrial disorders. *Cochrane Database Syst. Rev.* **1** (2006), CD004426.

236. R. S. Chen, C. C. Huang, N. S. Chu, Coenzyme Q10 treatment in mitochondrial encephalomyopathies. Short-term double-blind, crossover study. *Eur. Neurol.* **37** (1997), 212–218.

237. W. Muller, C. D. Reimers, T. Berninger, *et al.*, Coenzyme Q10 in ophthalmoplegia plus – a double blind, cross over therapeutic trial. *J. Neurol. Sci. Suppl.* **98** (1990), 442.

238. M. A. Tarnopolsky, B. D. Roy, J. R. MacDonald, A randomized, controlled trial of creatine monohydrate in patients with mitochondrial cytopathies. *Muscle Nerve* **20** (1997), 1502–1509.

239. T. Klopstock, V. Querner, F. Schmidt, *et al.*, A placebo-controlled crossover trial of creatine in mitochondrial diseases. *Neurology* **55** (2000), 1748–1751.

240. N. DeStefano, P. M. Matthews, B. Ford, A. Genge, G. Karpati, D. L. Arnold, Short-term dichloracetate treatment improves indices of cerebral metabolism in patients with mitochondrial disorders. *Neurology* **45** (1995), 1193–1198.

241. J. M. Liet, V. Pelletier, B. H. Robinson, *et al.*, The effect of short-term dimethylglycine treatment on oxygen consumption in cytochrome oxidase deficiency: a double-blind randomized crossover clinical trial. *J. Pediatr.* **142** (2003), 62–66.

242. P. Kaufmann, K. Engelstad, Y. Wei, *et al.*, Dichloroacetate causes toxic neuropathy in MELAS: a randomized, controlled clinical trial. *Neurology* **66** (2006), 324–330.

Chapter 20

Metabolic myopathies

Defects of carbohydrate and lipid metabolism

John Vissing, Stefano Di Donato and Franco Taroni

Introduction

The metabolic myopathies are a group of muscle disorders caused by inherited defects in the biochemical pathways that produce adenosine triphosphate (ATP), the "energy currency" of the cell. Although all cells require energy, cardiac and skeletal muscle are particularly vulnerable to ATP depletion due to their high energy requirements [1]. The hydrolysis of ATP to adenosine diphosphate (ADP) and inorganic phosphor (P_i) supplies energy for muscle contraction and relaxation. ATP can be regenerated from ADP and the high-energy compound phosphocreatine, but during long-term exercise, re-phosphorylation of ADP to ATP requires the oxidative combustion of carbohydrates (glucose and glycogen), lipids (fatty acids, FA), and ketones. Although anaerobic glycogenolysis in the cytosol can generate ATP up to 100 times faster than aerobic oxidation of glucose, it yields only 2 mol of ATP per mole of glucose as compared to 38 mol of ATP per mole of glucose yielded by mitochondrial oxidative phosphorylation (OXPHOS). Furthermore, it rapidly leads to the accumulation of toxic fatigue-promoting metabolic end products. Therefore, OXPHOS is the primary energy source for the regeneration of ATP during muscle work.

Although both carbohydrate and FA catabolic pathways converge into acetyl-coenzyme A (acetyl-CoA) for final intramitochondrial oxidation through the tricarboxylic acid cycle (TCA, also known as the citric acid cycle or Krebs cycle) and the respiratory chain (OXPHOS), the pattern of muscle fuel utilization is determined primarily by the intensity and duration of exercise. At rest, most muscle energy is provided by mitochondrial oxidation of long-chain (C_{14}–C_{20}) FA (LCFA) [2]. The heart is also largely dependent on LCFA oxidation for its functional activity. During the early phase of exercise, energy is derived mainly from catabolism of muscle glycogen stores and blood glucose. After approximately 90 min of exercise at an intensity of approximately 70% of maximum oxygen uptake (VO_{2max}), muscle and hepatic glycogen stores are depleted and there is a gradual shift from glucose to FA utilization. After a few hours, more than 70% of the skeletal muscle energy requirement is met by the oxidation of FA. Although the mobilization and rate of energy production from FA are slow, compared with those of glycogen, complete oxidation of a FA molecule is highly exergonic. For example, the oxidation of one molecule of palmitate ($C_{16:0}$) has a net yield of 129 ATPs [2].

Because of the many biochemical reactions required to produce cellular energy, numerous causes of metabolic myopathies exist, resulting from failed energy production related to defects in substrate utilization (disorders of glycogen and lipid metabolism) or mitochondrial OXPHOS (mitochondrial myopathies, see Chapter 19). Inherited defects of glycogen and FA metabolism in muscle cause two main clinical presentations (Figure 20.1): (1) acute, recurrent, reversible muscle dysfunction, manifesting as exercise intolerance, with myalgia and cramps often culminating in muscle breakdown (rhabdomyolysis) and myoglobinuria; and (2) static, often progressive weakness, sometimes simulating dystrophic, inflammatory, and even neurogenic processes. These muscle manifestations typically occur in older children and adults, whereas newborns and infants exhibit severe multisystem disorders characterized by episodes of hypoglycemia, encephalopathy, and sudden death.

Early recognition and treatment of these conditions is important to prevent morbidity and mortality. The field of metabolic myopathies has changed rapidly in recent years, and many diagnostic tools are now available to the clinician for the identification of the metabolic defect (Table 20.1). Biochemical investigations such as the detection of metabolites in urine and plasma both at rest and during acute episodes, and the measurement of muscle release of lactate and ammonia following forearm exercise may point to the likely metabolic block. In vitro enzyme analyses in muscle tissue, leukocytes, or cultured fibroblasts usually allows a specific diagnosis to be established. Finally, genetic analysis with the identification of the disease-causing mutation is now possible for almost all of the disorders of glycogen and FA metabolism, thus allowing direct molecular diagnosis, genetic counseling, genotyping of at-risk individuals, and prenatal testing.

Disorders of Voluntary Muscle, 8th edn., eds. George Karpati, David Hilton-Jones, Kate Bushby and Robert C. Griggs. Published by Cambridge University Press.

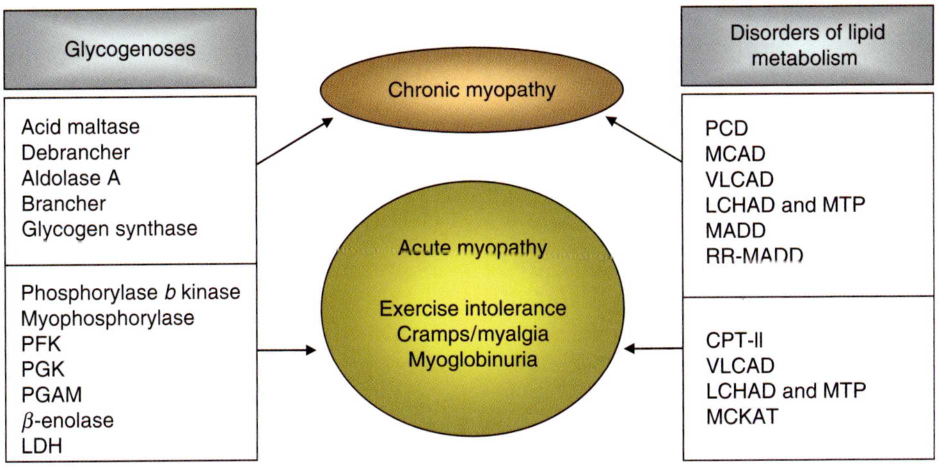

Figure 20.1. The two major myopathic phenotypes associated with defects of muscle substrate utilization. PFK, phosphofructokinase; PGK, phosphoglycerate kinase; PGAM, phosphoglycerate mutase; LDH, lactate dehydrogenase; PCD, primary carnitine deficiency (carnitine transporter deficiency); MCAD, medium-chain acyl-CoA dehydrogenase; VLCAD, very-long-chain acyl-CoA dehydrogenase; LCHAD, long-chain L-3-hydroxyacyl-CoA dehydrogenase; MTP, mitochondrial trifunctional protein; MADD, multiple acyl CoA dehydrogenase deficiency; RR-MADD, riboflavin-responsive multiple acyl-CoA dehydrogenase deficiency; CPT-II, carnitine palmitoyl-transferase II; MCKAT, medium-chain 3-ketoacyl-CoA thiolase.

Table 20.1. Laboratory investigations in patients with suspected metabolic myopathy

General investigations
Blood
Creatine kinase
At rest
During metabolic decompensation
CBC
Electrolytes, glucose
Calcium, potassium, phosphate
BUN, creatinine
Lactate, pyruvate (with lactate/pyruvate ratio)
Lactate dehydrogenase
Liver amino transferases (ALT, AST)
Carnitine: free, total, free/total ratio
Ketones
Myoglobin[a]
Uric acid
Urine
Myoglobin[a]
Ketones
Specific investigations
Cardiac evaluation
Electrocardiogram
Echocardiogram
Lipid metabolism defects
Blood glucose, ammonia
Plasma carnitine – free, total, free/total ratio
Plasma acylcarnitines
Plasma free fatty acids
Plasma and urine ketones
Plasma free fatty acid/ketone ratio
Urine organic acids (dicarboxylic acids)
Urine acylglycines
Skin fibroblast culture for enzyme assay
Muscle biopsy (histologic examination, enzyme assay)
EMG/NCS
Biochemical/molecular studies
Glycolytic/glycogenolytic defects
CBC, reticulocyte count, bilirubin
Ischemic forearm exercise test
EMG/NCS
Muscle/skin biopsy (histological examination, enzyme assay)
Biochemical/molecular studies

Notes: [a]If pigmenturia occurs.
ALT, alanine transaminase; AST, aspartate transaminase; BUN, blood urea nitrogen; CBC, complete blood count; EMG, electromyogram; NCS, nerve conduction studies.

Disorders of carbohydrate metabolism

Most known disorders of muscle carbohydrate metabolism were discovered in the three decades following Dr. McArdle's description in 1951 of the first metabolic myopathy, myophosphorylase deficiency [3]. Only three new defects of carbohydrate metabolism, aldolase A deficiency [4], β-enolase deficiency [5], and muscle glycogen storage disease type 0 [6], have been described in the last 27 years. The total number of known inborn errors of muscle glycogen and glucose metabolism is 12. Many more enzymatic steps than these 12 are involved in the metabolism of glycogen and glucose, and it is therefore likely that more conditions will be discovered. All disorders are quite rare, even the commonest, McArdle disease, which has a prevalence of about 1:100 000. While the conditions may be rare, the dynamic symptoms of exercise intolerance, exercise-induced pain and cramps, which are typical of most glycogenoses, are very common in the general population. It is therefore important to know the symptoms and diagnostic strategies used to identify patients with disorders of carbohydrate metabolism, not only to be able to help this patient group specifically, but also to avoid expensive and invasive diagnostic procedures in the large group of patients presenting with "glycogenoses-like" symptoms.

The disorders are inherited as autosomal recessive traits, with the exception of phosphoglycerate kinase and phophorylase *b* kinase deficiencies, which are X-linked recessive. In the following, the description of individual defects will be grouped into those with static (muscle wasting and weakness) and dynamic (exercise-related) symptoms. Although this division of glycogenoses based on clinical presentation is helpful from a diagnostic and descriptive point of view, it should be acknowledged that patients with dynamic symptoms may also present with some muscle wasting (McArdle disease and phosphofructokinase deficiency), and patients with static symptoms may also have exercise-related symptoms of fatigue and pain.

Glycogenoses with exercise-induced symptoms

In accordance with the normal pattern of fuel utilization during exercise described in the introduction, patients with glycogenoses and exercise-related symptoms all develop symptoms early in exercise. Rhabdomyolysis, myoglobinuria, and renal failure may occur in almost all conditions. However, the exercise intensity at which symptoms are elicited varies according to the residual activity of the affected enzyme. Patients with McArdle disease and phosphofructokinase deficiency typically have no functional enzyme left, and, accordingly, have the worst exercise intolerance of all the glycogenoses.

The methods used to diagnose these conditions are similar, and are therefore described in a separate paragraph at the end of the description of specific diseases.

Myophosphorylase deficiency (McArdle disease)

In 1951, Dr. Brian McArdle elegantly showed in a patient the lack of lactate production from an arm that had performed ischemic exercise, and at the same time demonstrated that norepinephrine-induced mobilization of glucose from the liver was intact [3]. He correctly concluded that the patient had a disorder of muscle glycogen breakdown. Myophosphorylase deficiency was subsequently identified in 1959.

Clinical phenotype

Patients have a low maximal work capacity of approximately a third or half of normal [7], and suffer from muscle cramps and fatigue early in exercise. Muscle cramps periodically lead to myoglobinuria in about two-thirds of cases, and a fraction of these have experienced renal failure requiring hospitalization. A third of patients develop fixed weakness, predominantly of the proximal upper extremities, after age 40. It is still enigmatic why only a third develop this weakness, and why it is localized predominantly to the shoulder girdle. A characteristic feature of the condition is the second wind phenomenon, which is pathognomonic for the disease [7]. About three-quarters of patients spontaneously report experiencing this phenomenon, but all patients show it on testing [7]. During a second wind, patients feel that previously fatiguing exercise suddenly feels easy. The phenomenon is attributable to improved delivery of extra-muscular glucose and FA to the working muscle. After the second wind, most patients can almost double their work effort [8]. Patients have an increased incidence of gout.

Genetics

The myophosphorylase gene (*PYGM*) on chromosome 11 was discovered in 1984. Since then, more than 80 different disease-causing mutations have been reported [9]. The most common mutation is the Arg50stop mutation, which is very common in Northern Europe (about 75% of mutant alleles), less common in the USA and Germany (60%), and Italy and Spain (30%) [9]. The R50X nonsense mutation does not occur in Japanese patients, who instead carry a common single-codon deletion in exon 17 in 73% of all cases. A number of other mutations also occur with increased rate. Nearly all mutations result in a totally dysfunctional enzyme, and, therefore, muscle glycogen breakdown is completely blocked in this disease. Maybe for that reason, a genotype–phenotype relationship has not been established for the disease [10]. In rare instances, however, mutations may occur that permit some functional myophosphorylase, and in these variant cases, although still prone to muscle cramps and myoglobinuria, patients have a much higher work capacity than "classical" McArdle patients [8]. There is evidence indicating that carriers of single *PYGM* mutation do not get symptoms of McArdle disease [11], although this has been suggested several times, but the evidence has been anecdotal.

Treatment

A number of treatments for McArdle disease have proved ineffective, including gene transfer, supplementation with branched-chain amino acids, creatine, B6 vitamin, or a high protein diet [9, 12]. The most important thing is to make the patient aware of the condition, so that they can avoid muscle injury by slowly warming up muscles in order to achieve a second wind. If more vigorous exercise is anticipated, as for instance sexual intercourse, an oral supplement of glucose shortly before exercise dramatically improves exercise performance, but the treatment is short-lived and cannot be repeated too often due to the high caloric load [13]. Exercise performance can be improved by a diet high in carbohydrate, and by supervised aerobic conditioning [9].

Phosphorylase *b* kinase (PHK) deficiency

Phosphorylase *b* kinase catalyzes the conversion of myophosphorylase from the inactive (*b*) to the active (*a*) form, and thus facilitates muscle glycogenolysis. The enzyme consists of four subunits, each encoded by separate genes. There has been some confusion in the past about the many different phenotypes associated with PHK deficiency, but in recent years it has become clear that the myopathic form is caused by mutations in the gene on the X-chromosome for the α-subunit of PHK (*PHKA1*). Another peculiarity in patients with the myopathic form of PHK deficiency has been the finding of normal lactate and ammonia responses on forearm exercise testing, which has questioned whether PHK deficiency really is a metabolic myopathy. Alternative activation of myophosphorylase during maximal exercise may, however, be responsible for this surprising finding. Thus, muscle PHK deficiency due to pathogenic alterations in *PHKA1* is, without question, a true muscle glycogenosis.

The pure muscle form of this condition has been described in fewer than 20 men, and only 5 patients with confirmed mutations in *PHKA1* have been reported to date [14]. Generally the symptoms resemble those found in other partial defects of muscle glycolysis, i.e., mild exercise intolerance with near-normal maximal oxygen uptake, myoglobinuria (not common), and muscle pain and cramps on exercise. This muscle mild glycogenosis with exercise-related symptoms may turn out to be much more common than it appears at the moment, now that phenotype–genotype correlations and the reason for a normal forearm exercise test have been recognized.

Muscle phosphofructokinase (PFK) deficiency (Tarui disease)

Phosphofructokinase deficiency was first described in Japanese patients [15]. Fewer than 150 cases have been reported worldwide. Symptoms are almost indistinguishable from those of McArdle disease, although exercise intolerance in most cases is more severe, and patients do not experience a second wind during exercise [16]. The frequency of muscle weakness is unknown, but likely is higher than in McArdle disease.

Phosphofructokinase is a tetrameric enzyme, found in three isoforms. Only the muscle isoform of the enzyme is expressed in skeletal muscle. PFK is the rate-limiting enzyme of glycolysis. For other enzymes of glycolysis and glycogenolysis, only a small amount of functional enzyme is necessary to maintain normal glycolytic flux. It is therefore not surprising that the existence of symptomatic carriers of single gene mutations in genes controlling muscle glycogenolysis has never been proven [11]. For PFK deficiency, however, one can speculate that the situation might be rather different, since the enzyme is rate-limiting for glycolysis, but once again symptomatic carriers have not been reported. PFK deficiency is caused by mutations in the gene on chromosome 1 that codes for the muscle isoform of PFK. More than 20 different mutations have been described in the gene, and there do not seem to be any mutational hotspots.

The muscle isoform of PFK is also expressed in high concentrations in erythrocytes, brain and heart, and in the typical presentation of the disease, this red cell involvement gives rise to a hemolytic anemia with increased bilirubin and reticulocyte count. Heart and brain on the other hand are not clinically involved, except in the rare infantile form of the disease. The biochemical and genetic basis of the severe infantile form of PFK deficiency is still unknown.

Experimentally, a lipid infusion improves and a glucose infusion impairs work capacity [17]. However, no dietary intervention, which the patients can use themselves, has been found to be helpful.

Muscle phosphoglycerate kinase (PGK) deficiency

The muscle form of PGK deficiency was identified in 1981 [18]. Like PHK deficiency, PGK deficiency has an X-linked inheritance, and mutation analyses indicate genetic heterogeneity. The most common presentation has onset in infancy with severe hemolytic anemia, seizures, and mental retardation. Approximately ten patients with a myopathic form, with or without slight hemolytic anemia, have been reported [19]. Symptoms in these rare patients are indistinguishable from those of other partial glycolytic defects, and include intolerance to brief intense exercise, and exertional myoglobinuria and cramps.

Unlike most other glycolytic enzymes, PGK only exists in one isoform (except in spermatogenic cells). It is, therefore, surprising that phenotypes may vary considerably in this condition. In infantile cases, the multisystem affection, most notably the central nervous system (CNS) symptoms, may mask any myopathic component, but it is still enigmatic why multisystem affection is absent in myopathic cases. The different phenotypes cannot be explained by differences in residual enzyme activity or location of the mutation in the PGK gene.

Muscle phosphoglycerate mutase (PGAM) deficiency

The condition was described in 1981 [20]. PGAM is a dimeric enzyme, which is present in muscle (M) and brain (B) isoforms. The isoforms are mixed in most tissues, but the M-isoform predominates in sperm cells, and skeletal and cardiac muscles. Symptoms, however, only develop in skeletal muscle, and are uniform, consisting of intolerance to sudden vigorous exercise, cramps, and episodic myoglobinuria [21]. Approximately 14 patients have been reported so far [21]. African-Americans predominate, but the condition has also been described in Italian and Pakistani patients [21]. Molecular studies indicate genetic heterogeneity [21]. Patients have about 5% residual PGAM activity in muscle, attributable to the presence of the B-isoform. As in other partial defects of glycolysis, exercise capacity is only mildly affected [21].

Dantrolene alleviates exercise-induced cramps, but treatment is generally not warranted. When diagnosed, patients learn to shun sudden vigorous exercise.

Muscle lactate dehydrogenase (LDH) deficiency

Lactate dehydrogenase deficiency was discovered in 1980, prompted by the dissociation between exercise-induced myoglobinuria/high plasma creatine kinase (CK) levels, and low plasma LDH levels in a patient [22]. LDH exists in five isoforms, and muscle LDH deficiency is caused by mutations in the gene for the muscle-specific subunit of LDH (LDH-A) on chromosome 11. Fewer than ten patients with LDH deficiency have been reported so far, most of Japanese descent. Symptoms mimic those in PGAM deficiency, but in addition to the muscle symptoms, patients typically also have an erythematous skin rash. Genetic heterogeneity also prevails in this condition.

Muscle β-enolase deficiency

Muscle β-enolase deficiency has only been described in one patient, a 47-year-old Italian man with onset in adulthood of exercise-induced myalgia without overt cramps [23]. Muscle strength and bulk were normal, but CK was consistently elevated, without episodes of myoglobinuria. The condition was caused by mutations in the gene for the β-subunit of enolase (*ENO3*), which predominates in muscle. Lactate production was blocked on forearm exercise testing.

Diagnosis of glycogenoses with exercise-related symptoms

As indicated below, there are several possible diagnostic approaches. Some are nonspecific with respect to the glycogenosis; thus glycogen accumulation may be seen in several types, and biochemical studies such as forearm exercise and magnetic resonance spectroscopy may show similar abnormalities in different disorders. DNA-based diagnosis is specific, but not practical for everyday diagnosis given the lack of common mutations. Bicycle exercise studies are specific for McArdle disease, but few centers have experience in its use. Immunohistochemistry for McArdle and PFK disease is specific, cheap, and easy to perform. Given that McArdle disease is by far the commonest of these rare disorders, it is reasonable to consider muscle biopsy with immunohistochemistry as the first investigation in a patient with a typical history and raised serum CK, reserving other investigations for the rarer glycogenoses and research purposes.

Muscle morphology

The muscle, particularly in McArdle disease and PFK deficiency, may exhibit myopathic features with an increased number of central nuclei and variability in fiber size, increased glycogen content on periodic acid Schiff (PAS) staining, and during attacks, cell necrosis, and macrophage invasion. Between attacks, the muscle biopsy may be normal in patients with partial defects of glycolysis. Presence of myophosphorylase and PFK can be examined histochemically on frozen muscle sections. The myophosphorylase stain fades within 24 h, and needs immediate assessment. Tubular aggregates, visible on trichrome stain and electron microscopy (EM), are present in about a third of PGAM deficiency cases [21], and have never been observed in other glycogenoses.

Forearm exercise test

Although originally carried out under ischemic conditions to maximize muscle glycogenolysis, this test is better carried out without ischemia, because the diagnostic value is just as good, and muscle injury can be avoided [24]. A catheter must be placed in the median cubital vein of the arm to be exercised. Placement elsewhere will likely result in lactate and ammonia responses that are too low. In 1 min, the patient has to perform 30 maximal handgrips lasting 1 s, with 1-s intervals. Blood samples for lactate and ammonia assessments should be drawn before, immediately after and in the first and third minute after exercise.

An exaggerated amount of ammonia is produced by contracting muscle when glycolysis is impaired, because of increased deamination of ADP via the myokinase reaction. It is therefore important to measure ammonia as well as lactate in venous effluent blood, to be able to distinguish low lactate responses caused by a glycogenoses (high ammonia) from sluggish lactate responses due to low work effort (low ammonia). In McArdle disease and PFK deficiency, the forearm test shows a flat lactate response, and marked hyperammonemia. In partial glycolytic defects, lactate responses are blunted, but not abolished, while the ammonia response is severely exaggerated. PHK deficiency may be missed by a forearm exercise test. Often lactate and ammonia responses are normal with a forearm test in this condition. This is so since myophosphorylase may be activated by other mechanisms besides PHK, especially during maximal contractions where AMP and Ca^{2+} are potent stimulators of phosphorylase [14].

Cycle ergometry

Incremental exercise to exhaustion on a cycle ergometer will show severely impaired maximal oxidative capacity in McArdle disease and PFK deficiency, but close to normal capacities in the other glycolytic defects. At a constant submaximal workload (25–45 watts), a second wind (spontaneous drop in heart rate) will invariably appear after 6–8 min of exercise in McArdle disease (Figure 20.2) [7]. In PFK deficiency, there is no second wind, but a flat lactate response. Cycle ergometry is uninformative in the other glycolytic defects, except in PHK deficiency, where impaired lactate production may be identified, which can be missed on the forearm exercise test [14].

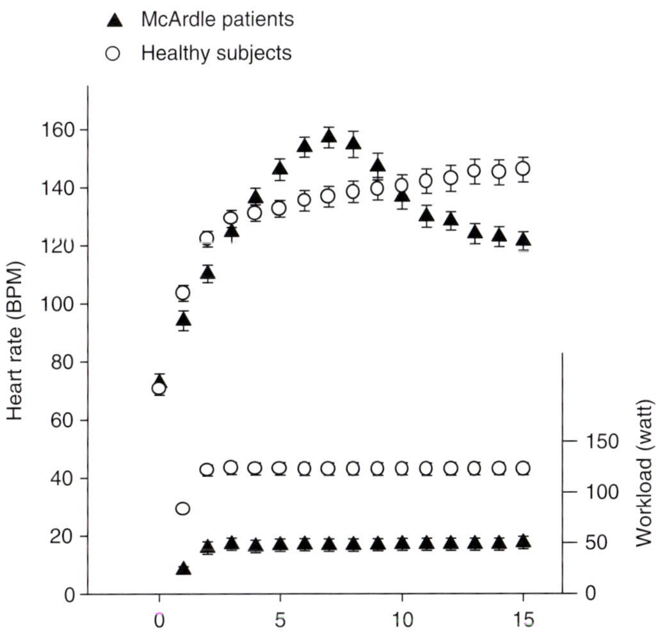

Figure 20.2. Heart rate response to a constant workload on a cycle ergometer in 12 patients with McArdle disease and in 12 healthy subjects. Workloads for the two groups are shown in the two lower graphs. Healthy subjects show the typical, slowly progressive rise in heart rate with continued exercise, whereas McArdle patients all showed an initial peak heart rate in the seventh minute of exercise, followed by a 38 beats per minute drop in heart rate with continued exercise. This second wind phenomenon is pathognomonic for McArdle disease.

Phosphorus magnetic resonance spectroscopy

This test can elegantly show lack of muscle acidification during exercise in McArdle disease and PFK deficiency, and characteristic accumulations of phospho-monoesters in muscle of PFK deficiency, and more distal defects of glycolysis [25]. However, MR spectroscopy is technically complicated and very expensive, and should not be considered a routine diagnostic tool in the diagnosis of metabolic myopathies.

Plasma creatine kinase (CK)

It is an exception to find normal CK levels in patients with McArdle disease and PFK deficiency, even between attacks. CK levels are typically 5 times upper reference level or higher, but may increase much more during attacks. In glycogenoses with partial enzyme defects, CK levels are normal or marginally elevated between attacks, but are periodically very high during attacks.

Biochemical and molecular genetic investigations

All muscle glycogenoses can be tested biochemically for the enzyme activity in question, and all corresponding genes can be sequenced for mutation detection. Final diagnosis always rests on biochemical verification of the enzyme deficiency and/or genetic analysis.

Glycogenoses associated with weakness

Pompe disease (acid maltase deficiency)

The defective enzyme in Pompe disease, α-glucosidase, is a lysosomal enzyme. The *GAA* gene, on chromosome 17, codes for the enzyme. A common mutation, c.-32–13T > G, is present on 75% of mutant alleles in adult cases, but more than 250 different mutations have been described [26]. A phenotype-genotype correlation exists. The exact function of α-glucosidase is unknown. Pathogenesis may be related to: (1) large accumulation of glycogen in muscle, displacing cellular organelles, (2) abnormal lysosomal activity which promotes autophagy, or (3) effects on intermediary metabolism.

Clinical presentation

The disease has three clinical presentations: (1) an early infantile form, with progressive weakness, enlargement of the tongue, heart and liver, and respiratory insufficiency with death before the age of two, if untreated; (2) a childhood or juvenile form associated primarily with skeletal muscle involvement affecting respiratory and proximal muscles; and (3) an adult form, which phenotypically resembles the juvenile form. A presenting symptom of respiratory distress occurs in about a third of all adult cases [27].

Diagnosis

Muscle biopsy shows a vacuolar myopathy with massive glycogen accumulation in infantile cases. This accumulation is less prominent in late-onset cases and occasionally the biopsy may be normal or show only increased acid phosphatase activity without obvious glycogen accumulation. CK levels are consistently elevated. Determination of α-glucosidase activity on muscle and cultured fibroblasts has increasingly been replaced by screening of blood spots with a fluorometric enzymatic assay [28].

Therapy

Treatment of Pompe disease in infantile, and to a lesser extent juvenile, cases with recombinant human α-glucosidase has dramatically improved prognosis [29]. The treatment has a clear effect, not only on skeletal muscle function, but also on the severe cardiomyopathy in infantile patients. Prognosis is also related to how early treatment starts. The outcome of treatment in adult-onset Pompe disease is much less certain, and cost-effectiveness may be an issue. Anecdotal reports suggest it may stabilize respiratory function and muscle strength, but publication of peer-reviewed trial data is still awaited.

Debrancher deficiency

Debrancher enzyme is needed to release glucose units from glycogen, and catalyzes two enzymatic reactions, an amylo-1,6-glucosidase and an oligo-1,4 →1,4-glucantransferase. The gene encoding debrancher enzyme (*AGL*) is localized on chromosome 1p21, and has been sequenced [30]. Numerous mutations have been identified in the gene.

The condition is usually benign in nature, and is associated with four biochemical variants. In the most common variant (85% of cases), which is also the one with muscle manifestations, both amylo-1,6-glucosidase and oligo-1,4 → 1,4-glucantransferase activities are deficient in liver and muscle (type IIIa). In a less frequent type (IIIb), both enzymes are also deficient, but only in liver. The molecular basis for the different tissue involvement is unknown. Likewise, the pathogenesis of the disorder is unclear. Structural changes due to vacuoles are unlikely to explain why weakness develops. It is unknown to what extent patients have true exercise intolerance related to impaired glycogenolysis.

Type IIIa most often results in a phenotype with childhood growth retardation, hepatomegaly, and fasting hypoglycemia. These symptoms usually resolve when the child is in the teens. In the third or fourth decade, about two-thirds of the patients develop a mild, primarily distal muscle weakness and wasting. Almost as frequent as the childhood onset is an adult onset with muscle weakness. Patients with weakness can also develop cardiomyopathy and have elevated CK levels, and muscle biopsy shows a vacuolar myopathy with glycogen deposits. Neurophysiologic evidence suggests that the weakness may be partially neurogenic in nature.

Treatment of debrancher deficiency is symptomatic, with emphasis on avoiding fasting in infants to prevent hypoglycemia.

Brancher deficiency

Branching deficiency is also called glycogenosis type IV, 1,4-α-D-glucan 6-α-D-[1,4-D-glucano] transferase deficiency, Andersen disease, amylopectinosis, and adult polyglucosan body disease. As suggested by the many synonyms, the disease is associated with many phenotypes [31]. As with PGK deficiency, this is surprising considering that branching enzyme only exists in one isoform, coded for by *GBE1*, which spans 16 exons and is localized on chromosome 3p14. Fewer than 100 cases have been reported.

The classical, and most common, form has onset in infancy with progressive hepatic fibrosis leading to hepatomegaly, and the children rarely live past age 4. A more rare neuromuscular debut presents with floppiness, severe muscle, and neuronal involvement, leading to death in the neonatal period. With onset in childhood, cardiomyopathy is usually the primary presenting feature. Childhood cases have only been documented in Ashkenazi Jews. In adult cases (adult polyglucosan body disease), which have been observed in multiple ethnic groups, the dominating features are progressive upper and lower motor neuron involvement and sensory loss, and a high incidence of dementia.

Raised liver enzymes and CK in blood and deposits of basophilic, intensely PAS-positive material on muscle biopsy suggest the diagnosis. Final diagnosis rests on biochemical demonstration of reduced branching enzyme activity in liver, cultured fibroblasts or leukocytes, and detection of pathogenic mutations in *GBE1*.

Treatment is symptomatic. Liver transplantation was considered beneficial in ten children [32], and heart transplantation has been performed in a few patients.

Aldolase A deficiency

Aldolase A deficiency has been described in four patients, but with muscle symptoms in just two [4, 33]. Aldolase A is one of three isoforms of aldolase, which converts fructose-1, 6-bisphosphate to glyceraldehyde-3-phosphate and dihydroxyacetone phosphate in the glycolytic pathway. The aldolase A isoform predominates in muscle and erythrocytes, and accordingly both patients also had anemia. The debut was in early infancy in both. Both had permanent proximal muscle weakness and atrophy and with episodes of exacerbated weakness and exercise intolerance triggered by febrile episodes.

Glycogen storage disease 0

This disease has been known since 1963, giving rise to fasting-sensitive hypoglycemia in children, caused by defects in the gene for the liver-specific isoform of glycogen synthetase (*GYS2*). This isoform is expressed exclusively in the liver. The other isoform, muscle glycogen synthase (encoded by the glycogen synthase 1 gene *GYS1*), is more ubiquitously expressed, but has recently been described to give rise to exercise intolerance, muscle weakness and wasting, and hypertrophy of heart and disturbed pump function during exercise in a consanguineous family from Syria [6]. The debut was in childhood. The condition is not a true glycogenosis, since glycogen is depleted. Preliminary reports have indicated myopathic forms of glycogen storage disease 0 in Algerian and Italian patients as well.

Disorders of mitochondrial fatty-acid oxidation

Since the first description in 1973 [34], 15 defects of mitochondrial FA oxidation have been identified, involving almost all enzyme steps in the pathway (Tables 20.2 and 20.3). With the exception of medium-chain acyl-CoA dehydrogenase (MCAD) deficiency, which has a relatively high frequency (1:13 000–1:30 000) among Northern European Caucasians [35], these disorders are uncommon and the prevalence rate is unknown for most of them.

Pathophysiology

Mitochondrial FA oxidation is a complex process that requires a concerted series of enzymatic reactions [2, 36]. The pathway is discussed in detail in Chapter 3 and outlined in Figure 20.3. The vulnerability of muscle to the metabolic block may depend on the activity [2]. When patients exercise for a prolonged period or fast (and in particular if they do both), glycogen stores may be exhausted and acute rhabdomyolysis may occur. Rhabdomyolysis and myoglobinuria are ultimately caused by reduced availability of ATP, necessary for sarcolemmal integrity, and increased Ca^{2+} permeability of sarcoplasmic reticulum due to the detergent effect of accumulated long-chain intermediates (acylcarnitines or esterified FAs). Nonoxidized

Table 20.2. Main clinical features of fatty-acid β-oxidation disorders

Disorder		Myopathic symptoms			Hepatic symptoms			Other features	MIM No.[c]
		Acute[a]	Chronic	Cardiomyopathy	Hypoketotic Hypoglycemia	Metabolic Encephalopathy[b]	Abnormal Organic acids		
Long-chain fatty-acid oxidation	Fatty-acid transport								
	CT	–	++	+++	+	+	–	Endocardial fibroelastosis	212140
	CPT-I	–	–	–	+++	+++	–	Renal tubular acidosis	255120
	CACT	?	++	+++[d]	+++	+++	+/–		212138
	CPT-II, type 1 (muscular)	+++	–	–	–	–	–		255110
									600650
	CPT-II, type 2 (hepatocardiomuscular)	+/–	++	++	++	++	+/–	Recurrent pancreatitis	600649
									600650
	CPT-II, type 3 (lethal neonatal)	–	++	+++	+++	+++	+/–	Brain and kidney dysplasia	600649
	β-Oxidation spiral								
	VLCAD[e]	+	++	++	++	–+	+++		201475
	ACAD9 [f]	+/–	+/–	+	++	++	++[g]	Brain atrophy, cerebellar infarct, chronic thrombocytopenia	611126
	MTP, type 1 (LCHAD)	++	++	++	+++	+++	+++	Retinitis pigmentosa, AFLP, HELLP, lactic acidemia	600890
	MTP, type 2 (LCEH/LCHAD/LCKT)	++	++	++	+++	+++	+++	Retinitis pigmentosa, peripheral neuropathy, hypoparathyroidism	143450
Medium- and short-chain fatty-acid oxidation	MCAD	+/–	+/–	–	+++	+++	+++		201450

Table 20.2. *(cont.)*

Disorder		Myopathic symptoms			Hepatic symptoms			Other features	MIM No.[c]
		Acute[a]	Chronic	Cardiomyopathy	Hypoketotic Hypoglycemia	Metabolic Encephalopathy[b]	Abnormal Organic acids		
	SCAD	–	?[h]	–	+/–	+/–	++	Hypotonia, hypertonia, mental retardation	201470
	SCHAD	–	–	–	++[i]	+/–	+++		601609
	MCKAT	++	–	–	++[i]	+/–	+++	Vomiting, hyperammonemia	602199
Unsaturated fatty-acid oxidation	2,4-Dienoyl-CoA reductase	–	?[j]	–	–	–	–[k]	Microcephaly, dysmorphism	222745
	Multiple acyl-CoA dehydrogenation defects								
	ETF or ETF:QO, severe	–	–	–	+++	+++	+++[l]	Congenital anomalies, renal dysplasia, dysmorphism	231680
									130410
									231675
	ETF or ETF:QO, mild	–	+	+/–	+++	+++	+++[l,m]		231680
									130410
									231675
	Riboflavin-responsive MADD[n]	–	+++	–	+++	+	+++	Leukodystrophy, coenzyme Q10 deficiency	

Notes: CT, carnitine transporter; CPT, carnitine palmitoyl-transferase; CACT, carnitine:acylcarnitine translocase; VLCAD, very-long-chain acyl-CoA dehydrogenase; ACAD9, acyl-CoA dehydrogenase 9; MTP, mitochondrial trifunctional protein; LCHAD, long-chain 3-hydroxyacyl-CoA dehydrogenase; LCEH, long-chain 2-enoyl-CoA hydratase; LCKT, long-chain 3-ketoacyl-CoA thiolase; MCAD and SCAD, medium- and short-chain acyl-CoA dehydrogenase, respectively; SCHAD, short-chain 3-hydroxyacyl-CoA dehydrogenase; MCKAT, medium-chain 3-ketoacyl-CoA thiolase; ETF, electron transferring flavoprotein; ETF:QO, ETF: coenzyme Q oxidoreductase; MADD, multiple acyl-CoA dehydrogenation deficiency; AFLP, acute fatty liver of pregnancy; HELLP, hypertension or hemolysis, elevated liver enzymes, and low platelets.
[a]Myoglobinuria; [b]Reye-like episodes; [c]*Mendelian Inheritance in Man* (MIM; McKusick, V. A. *Mendelian Inheritance in Man: A Catalog of Human Genes and Genetic Disorders*, 12th edn. Baltimore, MD: Johns Hopkins University Press; 1998.). Online MIM database (OMIM™): www.ncbi.nlm.nih.gov/sites/omim; [d]Ventricular arrhythmias in most cases; [e]Includes cases previously reported as defects of the long-chain acyl-CoA dehydrogenase; [f]Mostly active against unsaturated long-chain acyl-CoA substrates; [g]Abnormal unsaturated long-chain acylcarnitines ($C_{18:1}$ and $C_{18:2}$) in postmortem liver extract; [h]Hypotonia; [i]Ketotic hypoglycemia; [j]The only patient reported had persistent hypotonia in the neonatal period; [k]Urinary excretion of the unusual carnitine ester decadienoylcarnitine; [l]Glutaric aciduria type II (GAII); [m]Ethylmalonic-adipic aciduria; [n]Some patients have mutations in the *ETFDH* (ETF:QO) gene (see text for details); other patients have been reported to have coenzyme Q deficiency and mutations in the *ETFDH* gene (see text for details).

Table 20.3. Molecular genetics of fatty-acid β-oxidation disorders

Deficiency		MIM No.[a]	Gene name	Chromosomal localization	Gene structure	cDNA, coding region	Mutations identified	Prevalent mutation
Long-chain fatty-acid oxidation	Fatty-acid transport							
	CT	212140	*SLC22A5*	5q31.1	10 exons	1674 bp	++	None
	CPT-I, liver	255120	*CPT1A*	11q13.1–q13.5	20 exons	2322 bp	+	None
	CACT	212138	*SLC25A20*	3p21.31	9 exons	903 bp	+	None
	CPT-II	255110	*CPT2*	1p32	5 exons	1974 bp	++	c.439C > T
		600650						p.Ser113Leu
		600649						
	β-Oxidation spiral							
	VLCAD	201475	*ACADVL*	17p13	20 exons	1968 bp	+++	None
	ACAD9	611126	*ACAD9*	3c26	22 exons	1866 bp	+	None
	MTP, type 1 (LCHAD)	600890	*HADHA*	2p23	20 exons	2289 bp	+	c.1528G > C
								p.Glu474Gln
	MTP, type 2 (LCEH/LCHAD/LCKT)	143450	*HADHB*	2p23	16 exons	1422 bp	+	None
Medium- and short-chain fatty-acid oxidation	MCAD	201450	*ACADM*	1p31	12 exons	1263 bp	+++	c.985A > G
								p.Lys304Glu
	SCAD	201470	*ACADS*	12q22	10 exons	1239 bp	+	c.625G > A
								p.Gly185Ser
								c.511C > T
								p.Arg147Trp
	SCHAD	231530	*HADH*	4q22–q26	8 exons	945 bp	–	nd
	MCKAT	602199	–	nd	nd	nd	–	nd
Unsaturated fatty-acid oxidation	2,4-Dienoyl-CoA reductase	222745	*DECR1*	8q21.3	10 exons	1008 bp	–	nd

Table 20.3. *(cont.)*

Deficiency		MIM No.[a]	Gene name	Chromosomal localization	Gene structure	cDNA, coding region	Mutations identified	Prevalent mutation
Multiple acyl-CoA dehydrogenation defects	ETF							
	α-subunit	231680	*ETFA*	15q23–q25	12 exons	1002 bp	+	c.797C > T p.Thr266Met
	β-subunit	130410	*ETFB*	19q13.3	6 exons	768 bp	+	none
	ETF:QO	231675	*ETFDH*	4q32–q35	13 exons	1854 bp	+	none
	Riboflavin-responsive MADD[b]	–	–	nd	nd	nd	–	nd

Notes: nd, not determined; CT, carnitine transporter; CPT, carnitine palmitoyl-transferase; CACT, carnitine/acylcarnitine translocase; VLCAD, very-long-chain acyl-CoA dehydrogenase; ACAD9, acyl-CoA dehydrogenase 9; MTP, mitochondrial trifunctional protein; LCHAD, long-chain 3-hydroxyacyl-CoA dehydrogenase; LCEH, long-chain 2-enoyl-CoA hydratase; LCKT, long-chain 3-ketoacyl-CoA thiolase; MCAD and SCAD, medium- and short-chain acyl-CoA dehydrogenase, respectively; SCHAD, short-chain 3-hydroxyacyl-CoA dehydrogenase; MCKAT, medium-chain 3-ketoacyl-CoA thiolase; ETF, electron transferring flavoprotein; ETF:QO, ETF:coenzyme Q oxidoreductase; MADD, multiple acyl-CoA dehydrogenation disorders.

[a]*Mendelian Inheritance in Man* [MIM; McKusick, V. A. *Mendelian Inheritance in Man: A Catalog of Human Genes and Genetic Disorders*, 12th edn. Baltimore, MD: Johns Hopkins University Press; 1998]. Online MIM database (OMIM™): www.ncbi.nlm.nih.gov/sites/omim; [b]some patients have mutations in the *ETFDH* gene (see text for details); other patients have been reported to have coenzyme Q deficiency and mutations in the *ETFDH* gene (see text for details).

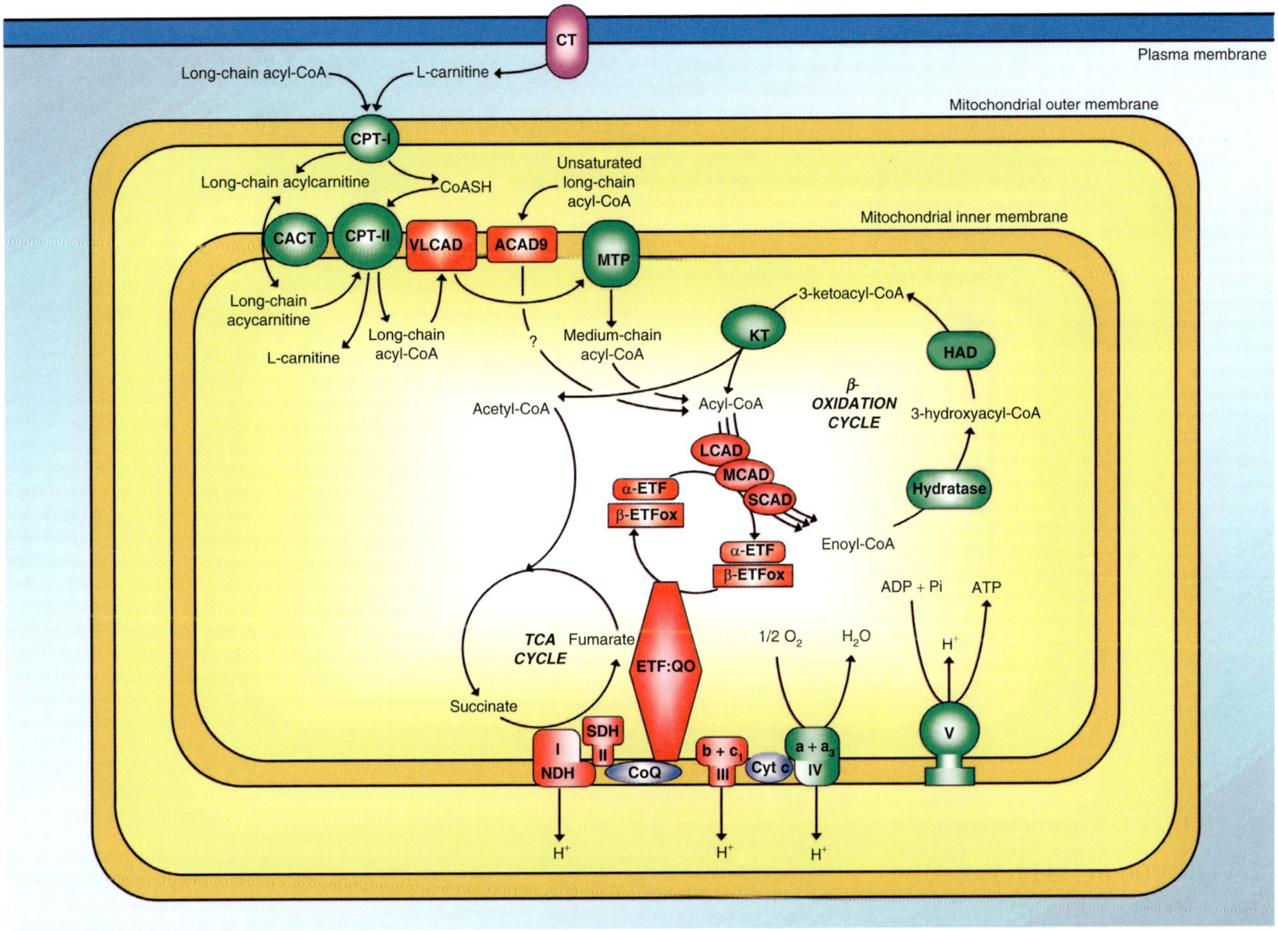

Figure 20.3. Schematic representation of the functional and physical organization of fatty-acid β-oxidation enzymes in mitochondria. CT, plasma membrane high-affinity sodium-dependent carnitine transporter (OCTN2); CPT-I, carnitine palmitoyl-transferase I; CACT, carnitine/acylcarnitine translocase; CPT-II, carnitine palmitoyl-transferase II; VLCAD, LCAD, MCAD, SCAD, very-long-, long-, medium-, and short-chain acyl-CoA dehydrogenase, respectively; ACAD9, acyl-CoA dehydrogenase 9; MTP, mitochondrial trifunctional protein; hydratase, 2-enoyl-CoA hydratase; HAD, L-3-hydroxyacyl-CoA dehydrogenase; KT, 3-ketoacyl-CoA thiolase; ETF, electron transferring flavoprotein (ox, oxidized; red, reduced); ETF:QO, ETF:coenzyme Q oxidoreductase; I, respiratory chain complex I (NDH, NADH:coenzyme Q reductase); II, respiratory chain complex II (SDH, succinate dehydrogenase); CoQ, coenzyme Q; III, respiratory chain complex III (b, cytochrome *b*; c_1, cytochrome c_1); Cyt c, cytochrome *c*; IV, respiratory chain complex IV (cytochrome *c* oxidase) (a, cytochrome a; a_3, cytochrome a_3); V, respiratory chain complex V (ATP synthase). Enzymes which use FAD as a coenzyme are indicated in red.

fatty acyl-CoAs are diverted to triacylglycerol synthesis causing the formation of lipid vacuoles (Figure 20.4a, b, e).

Cardiac involvement in patients with LCFA oxidation defects is characterized by myocardial damage caused by inadequate energy supply and arrhythmogenesis due to the toxic effects, via direct Ca^{2+} channel concentration of long-chain acylcarnitines [37].

Clinical features

Defects of mitochondrial FA β-oxidation are autosomal recessive disorders. Their classification and main clinical features are illustrated in Tables 20.2 and 20.3. Clinical manifestations range from a predominantly myopathic disease, either acute or chronic, to life-threatening systemic metabolic dysfunction (Table 20.4).

Two main clinical phenotypes can be observed in muscle (Figure 20.1): (1) a chronic myopathy usually characterized by abnormal accumulation of lipid in muscle fibers (lipid storage myopathy; approximately 35% of cases; e.g., PCD and CACT deficiency); or (2) acute, recurrent, reversible muscle dysfunction with exercise intolerance and rhabdomyolysis with myoglobinuria (approximately 65% of cases; e.g., deficiencies of CPT-II, VLCAD, or MTP) [2]. Because of the importance of LCFA oxidation in heart and skeletal muscle, cardiomyopathy (typically hypertrophic, but sometimes dilated) and skeletal muscle myopathy are commonly observed in LCFA oxidation defects while they are extremely rare in disorders of medium- and short-chain FA oxidation. Short- and medium-chain FA oxidation disorders most commonly cause episodic nonketotic hypoglycemia and liver-associated encephalopathy, which, if not treated promptly, may lead to coma and death. Since FA oxidation defects have similar effects on metabolism, the clinical features of different enzyme defects may overlap (Table 20.2).

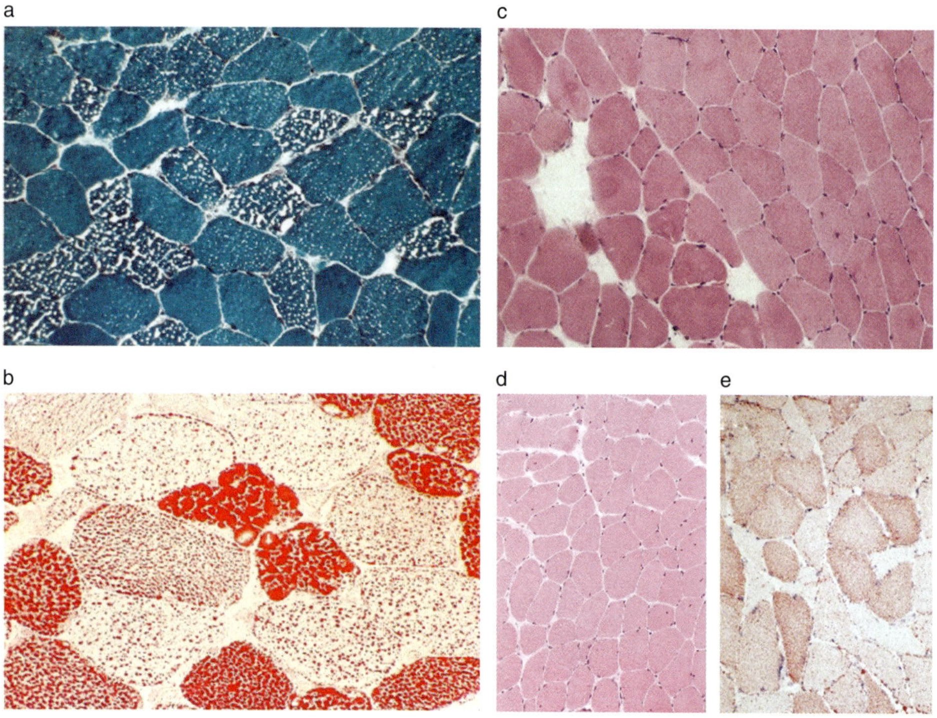

Figure 20.4a–e. Muscle biopsies from patients with fatty-acid oxidation defects. a, b. Lipid storage myopathy in a patient with primary carnitine deficiency (PCD) caused by a defect of the high-affinity plasma carnitine transporter (CT). (a) Modified Gömöri's trichrome staining showing numerous vacuoles mostly in type-1 fibers; ×160. (b) Oil red O stain showing numerous large lipid droplets within fibers; ×250. (c) Recurrent paroxysmal myoglobinuria in a young adult with CPT-II deficiency, harboring the common p.Ser113Leu mutation in the *CPT2* gene. Muscle biopsy performed 10 days after an acute episode shows mild nonspecific morphological alterations. There is evidence of fiber loss and modest variability of fiber diameter. Some fibers show central nuclei; hematoxylin & eosin, ×160. (d, e) Recurrent paroxysmal myoglobinuria and interictal chronic proximal myopathy in a young woman with VLCAD deficiency. (d) Hematoxylin & eosin stain shows mild nonspecific morphological alterations. There is fine vacuolization in some fibers and fiber diameter variability; ×160. (e) Oil red O stain shows signs of mild lipid accumulation with numerous fine droplets within most fibers. Lipid droplets exhibit a subsarcolemmal distribution; ×250.

Carnitine transporter deficiency (primary carnitine deficiency, PCD)

L-Carnitine (β-hydroxy-γ-*N*-trimethylamino-butyrate) is required for the active transport of LCFA into mitochondria. Primary carnitine deficiency (PCD) is caused by deficiency of the high-affinity plasma membrane carnitine transporter OCTN2, and is characterized by increased urinary carnitine loss and severely decreased carnitine concentration in plasma, heart, and skeletal muscle. The disease has a frequency of 1:37 000–1:100 000 newborns [37].

Clinical features

Two major clinical presentations are associated with PCD [37]. The most common phenotype is characterized by slowly progressive hypertrophic or dilated cardiomyopathy with lipid storage myopathy (Figure 20.4a, b), occurring between 1 and 7 years of age. A second phenotype, more frequent before 2 years of age, is characterized by acute recurrent episodes of non-ketotic hypoglycemic encephalopathy. These two phenotypes are not mutually exclusive, as both metabolic and cardiomuscular presentations have been described in some families [2].

Laboratory findings

Primary carnitine deficiency has to be distinguished from secondary carnitine deficiency that can be associated with a number of acquired or inherited diseases, including other FA oxidation defects [2]. In PCD, carnitine content is very low (<5% of normal) both in tissues (muscle, heart, liver) and in plasma, and analysis of plasma and urine does not show an abnormal acylcarnitine profile or dicarboxylic aciduria, which are usually seen in patients with other FA oxidation defects [2]. Once suspected, the transporter defect should be ultimately confirmed by carnitine uptake assay in cultured skin fibroblasts or by molecular analysis [38].

Molecular genetics

Primary carnitine deficiency is caused by mutations in the *SLC22A5* gene encoding the carnitine transporter OCTN2. Most of the mutations are nonsense mutations associated with no residual carnitine transport activity [37], but "leaky" missense mutations associated with residual transporter activity have also been identified, indicating a lack of genotype–phenotype correlation [38].

Therapy

If therapy is started before irreversible organ damage occurs, PCD patients respond very well to high-dose oral L-carnitine supplementation (usually 100–600 mg/kg per day) [37], which may prevent the need for cardiac transplantation. Hypoglycemic episodes also tend to disappear [37].

Carnitine palmitoyltransferase (CPT) deficiency

The CPT system is composed of two distinct acyltransferases, CPT-I on the outer mitochondrial membrane, and CPT-II on the inner mitochondrial membrane [39, 40]. CPT-I deficiency manifests in infants with encephalopathy and hypoketotic

Table 20.4. Clinical features associated with mitochondrial fatty acid β-oxidation disorders

Hepatic signs	Hypoglycemia associated with low ketones (hypoketotic hypoglycemia)
	Reye-like syndrome
	Steatosis
	Acute hepatic failure
	Sudden infant death syndrome (SIDS)
Muscle signs	Hypotonia
	Weakness and wasting
	Proximal myopathy with lipid storage
	Exercise intolerance and muscle pain with increased levels of creatine kinase
	Episodic rhabdomyolysis (with occasional paroxysmal myoglobinuria)
Cardiac signs	Hypertrophic and dilated cardiomyopathy
	Progressive heart failure
	Arrhythmias
	Cardiac arrest
	Sudden infant death syndrome (SIDS)
Nervous system signs	Permanent brain damage due to hypoglycemia, arrhythmias, or cardiac arrest
	Microgyria, cortical atrophy, and neuronal heterotopia
	Pigmentary retinopathy
	Peripheral sensorimotor neuropathy
Malformations	Renal dysplasia and nephromegaly[a]
	Polycystic kidney
	Facial dysmorphism
	Brain malformations

Note: [a]Proximal and distal tubulopathy is observed in CPT-I deficiency.

hypoglycemia with no cardiomuscular involvement [39, 41] (Table 20.2).

CPT-II deficiency

Clinical features

Three different clinical phenotypes are associated with CPT-II deficiency (Table 20.1): (1) a benign myopathic form with juvenile-adult onset, (2) a life-threatening infantile form with hepatocardiomuscular involvement, and (3) a lethal neonatal form with developmental abnormalities [2, 39, 40].

The "muscular" form of CPT-II deficiency is one of the most common inherited disorders of mitochondrial FA oxidation [41], and a major cause of hereditary recurrent myoglobinuria in both children and young adults [39, 40]. The clinical hallmark of the disease is paroxysmal myoglobinuria associated with pain and stiffness without cramps. Persistent weakness is very uncommon [2]. Attacks are most often precipitated by prolonged exercise. Unlike patients with glycolytic defects, patients with CPT-II deficiency do not show reduced tolerance to brief strenuous exercise and do not experience a second wind phenomenon (switch to utilization of fatty acids). Prolonged fasting, infections, and/or fever are the primary precipitating factors in the younger patients [39, 40]. In approximately 20% of cases, attacks may occur without any apparent cause.

The classic "muscular" form of CPT-II deficiency is usually a benign disease with a favorable evolution, provided that acute renal insufficiency, a complication that may develop in patients excreting more than 1000 ng/ml of myoglobin, is adequately managed [42]. There are usually no clinical signs of liver dysfunction. Fasting hypoglycemia is never observed and cardiac involvement is very unusual [2].

Laboratory findings

Outside episodes of myoglobinuria and at rest, serum CK levels are normal. During acute episodes of rhabdomyolysis, there are massively elevated urinary excretion of myoglobin ($\geq$200 ng/ml) and greatly increased levels of serum CK (20- to 400-fold) of muscle origin (CK-MM). Prolonged fasting or mild exercise may also provoke an increase in serum CK (2- to 20-fold above normal). Glycemia, ketonemia, ketonuria, urinary organic acid profile, and serum and muscle carnitine levels are usually normal. Following attacks, serum CK levels usually return to normal within 8–10 weeks. In most cases, muscle biopsies in interictal periods are normal or may show mild signs of muscle involvement with regenerating fibers (Figure 20.4c). Diagnosis is ultimately made by demonstrating the enzyme defect in muscle or, more conveniently, in peripheral blood leukocytes [2].

Molecular genetics

Approximately 60 mutations in the *CPT2* gene have been identified [39, 40, 43]. Most of the mutations are "private." However, a "common" mutation (p.Ser113Leu) accounts for $\geq$50% of mutant alleles in patients of different ethnic origins, and can be identified in approximately 90% of patients with muscular CPT-II deficiency [2, 44]. There is some genotype–phenotype correlation. The muscular form of the disease is always associated with residual CPT-II activity, whereas mutations which abolish enzyme activity are invariably found in patients with the lethal early-onset form [39, 40].

Therapy

Effective prevention of attacks may be accomplished by instituting a high-carbohydrate diet with low amount of long-chain fats, and with frequent and regularly scheduled meals, by avoiding the known precipitating factors (fasting, cold, prolonged exercise), and by increasing slow-release carbohydrate intake during intercurrent illness or sustained exercise [40, 41, 45].

Very-long-chain acyl-CoA dehydrogenase (VLCAD) deficiency

Clinical features

Very-long-chain acyl-CoA dehydrogenase deficiency has been described in more than 100 cases [35]. The defect is clinically heterogeneous. Overall, acute metabolic decompensation with recurrent episodes of hypoketotic hypoglycemia is the most frequent presentation and most VLCAD-deficient patients suffer from a severe cardiomyopathic form with early onset and poor outcome [35]. The disease may manifest with a myopathic phenotype characterized by exercise-induced rhabdomyolysis and myoglobinuria. Myalgia is more severe and episodes more numerous than in CPT-II deficiency.

Laboratory findings

In the muscle form, serum CK markedly increases during attacks (20- to more than 200-fold). However, patients do not exhibit hypoketotic hypoglycemia or dicarboxylic aciduria, and an increase of plasma long-chain acylcarnitines is rarely observed [2]. Plasma LCFA profile by gas chromatograhy-mass spectrometry (GC-MS) can be helpful for diagnosis because it may reveal an increase of tetradecenoic ($C_{14:1}$) acid, which persists even after the patient has fully recovered [46]. As in CPT-II deficiency, muscle biopsy may not provide any clue to the diagnosis. It may show mild nonspecific morphological alterations with no evidence of lipid accumulation (Figure 20.4d) or may demonstrate a diffuse increase of fat droplets mostly in type-1 fibers [46] (Figure 20.4e).

Molecular genetics

More than 60 disease-causing mutations have been identified in the *ACADVL* gene, none of which seems to predominate [35]. There is some genotype–phenotype correlation, and mutations that result in some residual enzyme activity are usually found in patients with the milder phenotypes [35].

Therapy

Patients with VLCAD deficiency should be treated with a dietary regimen consisting of avoidance of fasting plus a high-carbohydrate, low-LCFA diet. The beneficial effect of medium-chain triglycerides (MCT) is controversial and available evidences indicate that MCT ingestion does not ameliorate exercise performance in VLCAD-deficient myopathic patients [47].

Mitochondrial trifunctional protein (MTP) deficiency

Mitochondrial trifunctional protein is a complex enzyme composed of four α-subunits, harboring long-chain 2-enoyl-CoA hydratase (LCEH) and long-chain L-3-hydroxyacyl-CoA dehydrogenase (LCHAD) activities, and four β-subunits harboring long-chain 3-ketoacyl-CoA thiolase (LCKT) activity. MTP deficiency is relatively frequent, with more than 60 patients reported.

Clinical features

The clinical manifestations of the disease are characteristically associated with urinary excretion of C_6–C_{14} 3-hydroxydicarboxylic acids. Patients can be classified into two groups [48].

LCHAD deficiency

The vast majority (≥85%) of MTP-deficient patients have an isolated deficiency of LCHAD activity [48]. LCHAD deficiency appears to be a relatively common β-oxidation defect (1 in 50 000 births in Northern Europe) [48]. The disease is clinically heterogeneous. In infancy and early childhood, hypoglycemic encephalopathy with or without severe hepatic involvement and cardiomyopathy is the most common presentation. Mortality is high (~50%). However, cardiomyopathy in patients who survive acute episodes tends to resolve with dietary therapeutic measures [48]. Later in childhood, the predominant manifestation is paroxysmal rhabdomyolysis and myoglobinuria. Among the distinctive features of LCHAD deficiency are progressive pigmentary retinopathy and peripheral neuropathy, which are not observed in patients with any other β-oxidation defect [2, 48]. Also characteristic of this disorder is the occurrence of acute fatty liver disease in pregnant women with an affected fetus [48].

MTP deficiency (combined enzyme deficiency)

In a smaller group of patients, all the three activities harbored by MTP are deficient. Clinical manifestations are similar to those observed in patients with isolated LCHAD deficiency, although, in general, the clinical presentation is more severe with a higher mortality rate [48].

Molecular genetics

A prevalent missense mutation (1528G > C) in the LCHAD domain of the α-subunit gene (*HADHA*) can be detected in approx. 90% of LCHAD-deficient alleles [48], thus making molecular screening for the disease quite feasible. However, the relative frequency of this mutation appears to be lower in some geographical areas [e.g., Southern Europe (S. DiDonato and F. Taroni, unpublished observation)]. No apparent genotype–phenotype correlation has been observed, as patients homozygous for this mutation show widely different phenotypes [48].

Unlike LCHAD deficiency, the molecular basis of MTP deficiency is heterogeneous and different mutations have been identified in both *HADHA* and *HADHB* genes with poor genotype–phenotype correlation [48].

Therapy

The mainstay of therapy is avoidance of fasting plus a high-carbohydrate, low-LCFA diet associated with MCT oil supplementation [49]. Deficiency of docosahexaenoic acid (DHA), an essential *n*-3 polyunsaturated FA necessary for nerve myelination, has been documented in MTP-deficient patients, and an encouraging response to cod liver oil extract, high in DHA content, has been observed [50, 51].

Riboflavin-responsive multiple acyl-CoA dehydrogenase deficiency

Riboflavin (vitamin B_2) is the precursor of the coenzyme flavin adenine dinucleotide (FAD), which is the redox prosthetic group of several flavoproteins including the acyl-CoA dehydrogenases of the β-oxidation system (SCAD, MCAD, LCAD, VLCAD, and ACAD9) and the electron transferring flavoproteins ETF and ETF:QO [52] (Figure 20.3).

Clinical features

Riboflavin-responsive multiple acyl-CoA dehydrogenase deficiency (RR-MADD) is characterized by impaired oxidation of fatty acids due to multiple deficiencies of SCAD, MCAD, LCAD, and VLCAD. There are two major clinical phenotypes: (1) an "infantile form" with nonketotic hypoglycemia, hypotonia, failure to thrive, and acute metabolic episodes reminiscent of Reye syndrome; and (2) a "juvenile form" characterized by progressive proximal lipid storage myopathy [52].

Laboratory findings

There is usually a complex abnormal pattern of urinary excretion of organic acids [glutaric aciduria type II (GAII) or ethylmalonic-adipic aciduria] which indicates a multiple acyl-CoA dehydrogenation defect [2]. Activities and protein levels of SCAD, MCAD, and VLCAD are reduced in isolated muscle mitochondria [52].

Molecular genetics

Little information is available on the molecular bases of this disorder. Recessive mutations in the *ETFDH* gene encoding ETF:QO have been identified in some RR-MADD patients presenting with encephalopathy or muscle weakness, or a combination of the two [53]. Whether *ETFDH* mutations represent a common cause of RR-MADD remains to be elucidated. *ETFDH* mutations have also been reported in some patients with coenzyme Q (CoQ) deficiency presenting with lipid storage myopathy and late-onset GAII [54]. In these cases, however, response to therapy was not uniform, with some patients improving following riboflavin or CoQ_{10} (150–500 mg/day) monotherapy, and others requiring the combined therapy. Furthermore, *ETFDH* mutations are also observed in GAII patients who do not respond to riboflavin [2] (see below and Table 20.2).

Therapy

The clinical, morphological, and biochemical responses to oral riboflavin supplementation (100–400 mg/day) are usually dramatic [2, 52], with rapid improvement of muscle weakness and wasting and disappearance of signs of lipid accumulation at muscle biopsy. A prompt response to riboflavin treatment is also observed in encephalopathic patients [53].

Other disorders of fatty-acid β-oxidation

In a number of other defects of mitochondrial FA oxidation, skeletal and cardiac muscle involvement is either absent or a minor feature of clinical phenotypes dominated by systemic metabolic disturbances (Tables 20.2, 20.3). Thus, myopathy and cardiomyopathy are not observed in ***carnitine palmitoyltransferase I (CPT-I) deficiency*** [39, 41] (see above) or ***short-chain L-3-hydroxyacyl-CoA dehydrogenase (SCHAD) deficiency*** [2, 55], and mild acute or chronic skeletal myopathy, but not cardiomyopathy, has been only occasionally described in ***medium-chain acyl-CoA dehydrogenase (MCAD) deficiency*** [2, 41]. Signs of cardiomuscular involvement can be variably observed in ***carnitine:acylcarnitine translocase (CACT) deficiency*** (muscle weakness and high serum CK) [37], ***short-chain acyl-CoA dehydrogenase (SCAD)*** and ***2,4-dienoyl-CoA reductase deficiencies*** (persistent hypotonia), ***medium-chain 3-ketoacyl-CoA thiolase (MCKAT) deficiency*** (terminal rhabdomyolysis and myoglobinuria), and ***acyl-CoA dehydrogenase 9 (ACAD9) deficiency*** (cardiomyopathy and recurrent rhabdomyolysis) [56]. Progressive lipid storage myopathy can be observed in the milder form of ***multiple acyl-CoA dehydrogenase deficiency*** (glutaric aciduria type II, GAII) caused by mutations in ETF or ETF:QO [2].

Evaluation of patients with suspected FA oxidation disorders

Biochemical evaluation

Most reliable results are obtained if blood and urine specimens for metabolic investigations are collected during episodes of acute catabolic crises before glucose administration, during periods of fasting, or following exercise [57]. The initial laboratory studies usually include plasma CK, blood glucose, ammonia, bicarbonate, serum ketones, liver aminotransferases, electrolytes, creatinine, myoglobin, and urinary levels of ketones and myoglobin (Table 20.1). Besides these routine tests, which, though not specific, may be helpful in the differential diagnosis, quantitative profiling of carnitine, acylcarnitines, and FAs in plasma, and organic acids and acylglycines in urine are the methods of choice to pursue a biochemical diagnosis for most FA oxidation disorders [55, 56]. Plasma acylcarnitine analysis by tandem-mass spectrometry (MS/MS) is particularly useful, as acylcarnitine concentration in the blood reflects the concentration of those fatty acyl-CoA species which accumulate in mitochondria, hence not only indicating whether impairment of FA oxidation exists, but also providing information about the level of the enzyme defect. Diagnosis is ultimately made by demonstrating the enzyme defect in the patients' tissue(s) [57, 58], confirmed, when available, by molecular analysis.

Muscle biopsy

When a metabolic myopathy involving FA catabolism is suspected, muscle biopsy should not be performed before obtaining preliminary metabolic tests (plasma free fatty acid, urinary organic acid, and plasma and urinary acylcarnitine profiles). Chronic progressive myopathy associated with FA oxidation defects is usually characterized by lipid (mostly triglycerides) accumulation within muscle fibers (lipid storage myopathy), which represents a prominent pathological alteration (Figure 20.4a, b, e). In patients, lipid accumulation usually correlates with the oxidative capacity of muscle fibers, being most marked in type 1 fibers, less marked in type 2A fibers, and least conspicuous in type 2B fibers [2].

The histological evaluation of muscle following an episode of metabolic myoglobinuria is often not contributive. There may be some unspecific myopathic changes and isolated necrotic fibers (Figure 20.4c, d). By contrast, muscle specimens obtained several weeks or months after an acute episode are usually normal. The muscle glycogen content is normal and lipid accumulation, if any, is significantly less than in classical lipid storage myopathy (e.g., carnitine transporter deficiency; compare Figure 20.4b and e).

Molecular diagnosis

Almost all of the genes encoding the enzymes involved in mitochondrial FA catabolism have been identified and characterized. In most of the related disorders, the molecular defect has also been delineated, making molecular diagnosis feasible (Table 20.3). Molecular testing is particularly useful in CPT-II, LCHAD, MCAD, and SCAD deficiencies, as a single disease-causing mutation can be found in 50%–90% of the alleles [35, 59].

Genetic counseling and prenatal diagnosis

All known FA oxidation disorders are inherited as autosomal recessive traits, with a recurrence risk of 25% in the offspring of heterozygous parents. As with the glycogenoses, carriers are asymptomatic as 50% residual enzyme activity is adequate for normal function. Prenatal diagnosis is feasible for most disorders, provided that an index case has been appropriately characterized. Although biochemical and enzymatic methods can be used [60], direct molecular analysis is the most reliable approach to prenatal testing.

Management of patients with FA oxidation defects

Treatment options for FA oxidation disorders are, in general, satisfactory and are mainly based on diet, lifestyle recommendations (avoidance of fasting and strenuous exercise), and, in selected cases, administration of L-carnitine or riboflavin [42, 61].

Prevention and management of acute metabolic decompensation

Avoidance of precipitating factors (prolonged aerobic exercise >30 min, fasting, infection, and exposure to cold) is the most important therapeutic measure. At all times, but especially during an intercurrent illness, it is of outmost importance to guarantee suppression of lipolysis by ensuring sufficient carbohydrate supplementation. During acute metabolic attacks, intravenous glucose should be administered at a rate of ~7–10 mg/kg per minute. A high rate of glucose intake rapidly suppresses lipolysis, thus preventing the production of toxic metabolites such as long-chain acylcarnitines and dicarboxylic acids. The suggested intervention for the treatment of acute myoglobinuria and the prevention of acute renal failure is an intravenous infusion of hypotonic sodium chloride (110 mmol/l) and sodium bicarbonate (40 mmol/l) in 5% glucose–1% mannitol solution. In a young adult of 75 kg weight, the solution should be infused at the rate of 12 l/day in order to obtain a diuresis of 8 l/day and maintain pH above 6.5 [42].

Dietary treatment

A high-carbohydrate, low-fat diet – 70%–75% complex carbohydrates and 10%–15% fat – with frequent and regularly scheduled meals is recommended [45, 61]. The fat content should be restricted to the American Dietetic Association minimal nutritional requirements for age. For long-term increase of glycemia, slow-release carbohydrate-derived calories can be easily obtained from orally administered uncooked cornstarch snacks (1.5–2.0 g/kg per dose). Except for the studies in patients with LCHAD deficiency [62], current belief that supplementation of MCT (from 0.5 g/kg per day to 1–1.5 g/kg per day) can be beneficial in defects of LCFA oxidation is based on anecdotal evidence and descriptive case reports without controls [42, 61]. In any case, MCT should never be given to patients with medium- or short-chain fatty-acid oxidation disorder. Docosahexaenoic acid supplementation in patients with LCHAD deficiency and retinopathy or severe neuropathy has no adverse effect and has been associated with clinical and electrophysiological improvement [50, 51]. Replacing medium-even-chain triglycerides by medium-odd-chain triglycerides, such as precursors of acetyl-CoA and anaplerotic propionyl-CoA, has been shown to improve cardiac and skeletal muscle function in patients with VLCAD deficiency [63]. Emerging potential therapies include the use of fibrates to increase the expression of LCFA oxidation enzymes [64].

L-carnitine and riboflavin supplementation

Carnitine transporter deficiency represents the only condition in which L-carnitine supplementation (100–600 mg/kg per day) is mandatory. Although low plasma or muscle levels of free carnitine (25% to 50% of normal) can be observed also in other FA oxidation disorders, in these cases the beneficial effects of carnitine supplementation have not been systematically documented and its use has been questioned because of the potential increase of the toxic long-chain acylcarnitines [65]. Riboflavin (vitamin B_2) should always be given to patients with MADD. As discussed earlier, a subset of MADD patients promptly respond to riboflavin treatment. However, its efficacy in the treatment of other acyl-CoA dehydrogenase deficiencies has not been demonstrated.

References

1. M. Hirano, S. DiMauro, Metabolic myopathies. *Adv. Neurol.* **88** (2002), 217–234.
2. S. DiDonato, F. Taroni, Disorders of lipid metabolism. In *Myology*, Third Edition, eds. A. G. Engel, C. Franzini-Armstrong. (New York: McGraw-Hill, 2004), pp. 1587–1621.
3. B. McArdle, Myopathy due to a defect in muscle glycogen breakdown. *Clin. Sci. Lond.* **10** (1951), 13–32.
4. J. Kreuder, A. Borkhardt, R. Repp, *et al.*, Inherited metabolic myopathy and hemolysis due to a mutation in aldolase a. *N. Engl. J. Med.* **334** (1996), 1100–1104.
5. G. P. Comi, F. Fortunato, S. Lucchiari, *et al.*, β-enolase deficiency, a new metabolic myopathy of distal glycolysis. *Ann. Neurol.* **50** (2001), 202–207.
6. G. Kollberg, M. Tulinius, T. Gilljam, *et al.*, Cardiomyopathy and exercise intolerance in muscle glycogen storage disease 0. *N. Engl. J. Med.* **357** (2007), 1507–1514.
7. J. Vissing, R. G. Haller, A diagnostic cycle test for McArdle's disease. *Ann. Neurol.* **54** (2003), 539–542.
8. R. G. Haller, J. Vissing, Spontaneous "second wind" and glucose-induced second "second wind" in McArdle disease – oxidative mechanisms. *Arch. Neurol.* **59** (2002), 1395–1402.
9. R. Quinlivan, J. Vissing, 144th ENMC International Workshop: Outcome Measures in McArdle Disease, 29 September to 1 November 2006, Naarden, the Netherlands. *Neuromusc. Disord.* **17** (2007), 94–98.
10. R. Aquaron, J. L. Bergé-Lefranc, J. F. Pellissier, *et al.*, Molecular characterization of myophosphorylase deficiency (McArdle disease) in 34 patients from Southern France: identification of 10 new mutations. Absence of genotype-phenotype correlation. *Neuromuscul. Disord.* **17** (2007), 235–241.
11. S. T. Andersen, M. Dunø, M. Schwartz, J. Vissing, Do carriers of PYGM mutations have symptoms of McArdle disease? *Neurology* **67** (2006), 716–718.
12. R. M. Quinlivan, R. J. Beynon, Pharmacological and nutritional treatment of McArdle's disease (glycogen storage disease V). *Cochrane Database Syst. Rev.* **3** (2004), CD003458.
13. J. Vissing, R. G. Haller, The effect of oral sucrose on exercise tolerance in patients with McArdle's disease. *N. Engl. J. Med.* **349** (2003), 2503–2509.
14. M. C. Ørngreen, H. J. Schelhaas, T. D. Jeppesen, *et al.*, Is muscle glycogenolysis impaired in X-linked phosphorylase b kinase deficiency? *Neurology* **70** (2008), 1876–1882.
15. S. Tarui, G. Okuno, Y. Ikura, *et al.*, Phosphofructokinase deficiency in skeletal muscle: a new type of glycogenosis. *Biochem. Biophys. Res. Commun.* **34** (1965), 77–83.
16. R. G. Haller, J. Vissing, No spontaneous second wind in muscle phosphofructokinase deficiency. *Neurology* **62** (2004), 82–86.
17. R. G. Haller, S. F. Lewis, Glucose-induced exertional fatigue in muscle phosphofructokinase deficiency. *N. Engl. J. Med.* **324** (1991), 364–369.
18. S. DiMauro, M. Dalakas, A. F. Miranda, Phosphoglycerate kinase deficiency: a new cause of recurrent myoglobinuria. *Trans. Am. Neurol. Assoc.* **106** (1981), 202–205.
19. S. DiMauro, A. P. Hays, S. Tsujino, Nonlysosomal glycogenoses. In *Myology*, Third Edition, eds. A. G. Engel, C. Franzini-Armstrong. (New York: McGraw-Hill, 2004), pp. 1535–1558.
20. S. DiMauro, A. F. Miranda, S. Khan, K. Gitlin, R. Friedman, Human muscle phosphoglycerate mutase deficiency: newly discovered metabolic myopathy. *Science* **212** (1981), 1277–1279.
21. A. Naini, A. Toscano, O. Musumeci, J. Vissing, H. O. Akman, S. DiMauro, Muscle phosphoglycerate mutase (PGAM) deficiency revisited. *Arch. Neurol.* **66** (2009), 394–398.
22. T. Kanno, K. Sudo, I. Takeuchi, *et al.*, Hereditary deficiency of lactate dehydrogenase M-subunit. *Clin. Chim. Acta.* **108** (1980), 267–276.
23. G. P. Comi, F. Fortunato, S. Lucchiari, *et al.*, β-enolase deficiency, a new metabolic myopathy of distal glycolysis. *Ann. Neurol.* **50** (2001), 202–207.
24. P. Kazemi-Esfarjani, E. Skomorowska, T. D. Jensen, R. G. Haller, J. Vissing, A nonischemic forearm exercise test for McArdle disease. *Ann. Neurol.* **52** (2002), 153–159.
25. R. G. Haller, J. Vissing, Functional evaluation of metabolic myopathies. In *Myology*, Third Edition, eds. A. G. Engel, C. Franzini-Armstrong. (New York: McGraw-Hill, 2004), pp. 665–679.
26. M. Kroos, R. J. Pomponio, L. van Vliet, *et al.*, Update of the Pompe disease mutation database with 107 sequence variants and a format for severity rating. *Hum. Mutat.* **29** (2008), E13–E26.
27. M. L. Hagemans, L. P. Winkel, P. A. Van Doorn, *et al.*, Clinical manifestation and natural course of late-onset Pompe's disease in 54 Dutch patients. *Brain* **128** (2005), 671–677.
28. Pompe Disease Diagnostic Working Group, Methods for a prompt and reliable laboratory diagnosis of Pompe disease: report from an international consensus meeting. *Mol. Genet. Metab.* **93** (2008), 275–281.
29. J. M. Van den Hout, J. H. Kamphoven, L. P. Winkel, *et al.*, Long-term intravenous treatment of Pompe disease with recombinant human alpha-glucosidase from milk. *Pediatrics* **113** (2004), e448–457.
30. J. Shen, Y. Bao, H. M. Liu, P. Lee, J. V. Leonard, Y. T. Chen, Mutations in exon 3 of the glycogen debranching enzyme gene are associated with glycogen storage disease type III that is differentially expressed in liver and muscle. *J. Clin. invest.* **98** (1996), 352–357.
31. S. W. Moses, R. Parvari, The variable presentations of glycogen storage disease type IV: a review of clinical, enzymatic and molecular studies. *Curr. Mol. Med.* **2** (2002), 177–188.
32. R. Selby, T. E. Starzl, E. Yunis, *et al.*, Liver transplantation for type IV glycogen storage disease. *N. Engl. J. Med.* **324** (1991), 39–42.
33. D. C. Yao, D. R. Tolan, M. F. Murray, *et al.*, Hemolytic anemia and severe rhabdomyolysis caused by compound heterozygous mutations of the gene for erythrocyte/muscle isozyme of aldolase, ALDOA(Arg303X/Cys338Tyr). *Blood* **103** (2004), 2401–2403.
34. S. DiMauro, P. Melis-DiMauro, Muscle carnitine palmitoyltransferase deficiency and myoglobinuria. *Science* **182** (1973), 929–931.

35. N. Gregersen, B. S. Andresen, M. J. Corydon, *et al.*, Mutation analysis in mitochondrial fatty acid oxidation defects: Exemplified by acyl-CoA dehydrogenase deficiencies, with special focus on genotype-phenotype relationship. *Hum. Mutat.* **18** (2001), 169–189.

36. K. Bartlett, S. Eaton, Mitochondrial beta-oxidation. *Eur. J. Biochem.* **271** (2004), 462–469.

37. N. Longo, C. Amat di San Filippo, M. Pasquali, Disorders of carnitine transport and the carnitine cycle. *Am. J. Med. Genet. C. Semin. Med. Genet.* **142** (2006), 77–85.

38. Y. Wang, F. Taroni, B. Garavaglia, N. Longo, Functional analysis of mutations in the OCTN2 transporter causing primary carnitine deficiency: lack of genotype-phenotype correlation. *Hum. Mutat.* **16** (2000), 401–407.

39. J. P. Bonnefont, F. Djouadi, C. Prip-Buus, S. Gobin, A. Munnich, J. Bastin, Carnitine palmitoyltransferases 1 and 2: biochemical, molecular and medical aspects. *Mol. Aspects Med.* **25** (2004), 495–520.

40. M. Deschauer, F. Taroni, Carnitine palmitoytransferase II deficiency. In *MedLink Neurology*, ed. S. Gilman. (San Diego, CA: MedLink Corporation, 2006), available at www.Medlink.com

41. J. M. Saudubray, D. Martin, P. de Lonlay, *et al.*, Recognition and management of fatty acid oxidation defects: a series of 107 patients. *J. Inherit. Metab. Dis.* **22** (1999), 488–502.

42. C. Angelini, A. Federico, H. Reichmann, A. Lombes, P. Chinnery, D. Turnbull, Task force guidelines handbook: EFNS guidelines on diagnosis and management of fatty acid mitochondrial disorders. *Eur. J. Neurol.* **13** (2006), 923–929.

43. P. J. Isackson, M. J. Bennett, G. D. Vladutiu, Identification of 16 new disease-causing mutations in the CPT2 gene resulting in carnitine palmitoyltransferase II deficiency. *Mol. Genet. Metab.* **89** (2006), 323–331.

44. F. Taroni, E. Verderio, F. Dworzak, P. J. Willems, P. Cavadini, S. DiDonato, Identification of a common mutation in the carnitine palmitoyltransferase II gene in familial recurrent myoglobinuria patients. *Nat. Genet.* **4** (1993), 314–320.

45. M. C. Orngreen, R. Ejstrup, J. Vissing, Effect of diet on exercise tolerance in carnitine palmitoyltransferase II deficiency. *Neurology* **61** (2003), 559–561.

46. R. Pons, P. Cavadini, S. Baratta, *et al.*, Clinical and molecular heterogeneity in very-long-chain acyl-CoA dehydrogenase deficiency. *Pediatr. Neurol.* **22** (2000), 98–105.

47. M. C. Orngreen, M. G. Norgaard, B. G. van Engelen, B. Vistisen, J. Vissing, Effects of IV glucose and oral medium-chain triglyceride in patients with VLCAD deficiency. *Neurology* **69** (2007), 313–315.

48. S. E. Olpin, S. Clark, B. S. Andresen, *et al.*, Biochemical, clinical and molecular findings in LCHAD and general mitochondrial trifunctional protein deficiency. *J. Inherit. Metab. Dis.* **28** (2005), 533–544.

49. M. B. Gillingham, W. E. Connor, D. Matern, *et al.*, Optimal dietary therapy of long-chain 3-hydroxyacyl-CoA dehydrogenase deficiency. *Mol. Genet. Metab.* **79** (2003), 114–123.

50. C. O. Harding, M. B. Gillingham, S. C. van Calcar, J. A. Wolff, J. N. Verhoeve, M. D. Mills, Docosahexaenoic acid and retinal function in children with long-chain 3-hydroxyacyl-CoA dehydrogenase deficiency. *J. Inherit. Metab. Dis.* **22** (1999), 276–280.

51. I. Tein, J. Vajsar, L. MacMillan, W. G. Sherwood, Long-chain L-3-hydroxyacyl-coenzyme A dehydrogenase deficiency neuropathy: response to cod liver oil. *Neurology* **52** (1999), 640–643.

52. C. Antozzi, B. Garavaglia, M. Mora, *et al.*, Late-onset riboflavin-responsive myopathy with combined multiple acyl coenzyme A dehydrogenase and respiratory chain deficiency. *Neurology* **44** (1994), 2153–2158.

53. R. K. Olsen, S. E. Olpin, B. S. Andresen, *et al.*, ETFDH mutations as a major cause of riboflavin-responsive multiple acyl-CoA dehydrogenation deficiency. *Brain* **130** (2007), 2045–2054.

54. K. Gempel, H. Topaloglu, B. Talim, *et al.*, The myopathic form of coenzyme Q10 deficiency is caused by mutations in the electron-transferring-flavoprotein dehydrogenase (ETFDH) gene. *Brain* **130** (2007), 2037–2044.

55. P. Rinaldo, D. Matern, M. J. Bennett, Fatty acid oxidation disorders. *Annu. Rev. Physiol.* **64** (2002), 477–502.

56. M. He, S. L. Rutledge, D. R. Kelly, *et al.*, A new genetic disorder in mitochondrial fatty acid beta-oxidation: ACAD9 deficiency. *Am. J. Hum. Genet.* **81** (2007), 87–103.

57. K. G. Sim, J. Hammond, B. Wilcken, Strategies for the diagnosis of mitochondrial fatty acid beta-oxidation disorders. *Clin. Chim. Acta.* **323** (2002), 37–58.

58. M. J. Bennett, Assays of fatty acid beta-oxidation activity. *Methods Cell. Biol.* **80** (2007), 179–197.

59. N. Gregersen, B. S. Andresen, P. Bross, Prevalent mutations in fatty acid oxidation disorders: diagnostic considerations. *Eur. J. Pediatr.* **159** (2000), S213–S218.

60. P. Rinaldo, A. L. Studinski, D. Matern, Prenatal diagnosis of disorders of fatty acid transport and mitochondrial oxidation. *Prenat. Diagn.* **21** (2001), 52–54.

61. R. Pons, D. C. De Vivo, Mitochondrial disease. *Curr. Treat. Options Neurol.* **3** (2001), 271–288.

62. M. B. Gillingham, B. Scott, D. Elliott, C. O. Harding, Metabolic control during exercise with and without medium-chain triglycerides (MCT) in children with long-chain 3-hydroxy acyl-CoA dehydrogenase (LCHAD) or trifunctional protein (TFP) deficiency. *Mol. Genet. Metab.* **89** (2006), 58–63.

63. C. R. Raoe, L. Sweetman, D. S. Roe, F. David, H. Brunengraber, Treatment of cardiomyopathy and rhabdomyolysis in long-chain fat oxidation disorders using an anaplerotic odd-chain triglyceride. *J. Clin. Invest.* **110** (2002), 259–269.

64. S. Gobin-Limballe, F. Djouadi, F. Aubey, *et al.*, Genetic basis for correction of very-long-chain acyl-coenzyme A dehydrogenase deficiency by bezafibrate in patient fibroblasts: toward a genotype-based therapy. *Am. J. Hum. Genet.* **81** (2007), 1133–1143.

65. S. Primassin, F. Ter Veld, E. Mayatepek, U. Spiekerkoetter, Carnitine supplementation induces acylcarnitine production in tissues of very long-chain acyl-CoA dehydrogenase-deficient mice, without replenishing low free carnitine. *Pediatr. Res.* **63** (2008), 632–637.

Chapter 21

Muscle ion channelopathies and related disorders

Bertrand Fontaine and Michael G. Hanna

Nondystrophic myotonias

Nondystrophic myotonias refer to all myotonic syndromes of muscle origin excluding dystrophia myotonica (DM1, DM2) [1]. This distinction is important in clinical practice for two reasons: (1) nondystrophic myotonias are less frequent than dystrophia myotonica (prevalence estimated at 1/50 000), and (2) nondystrophic myotonias do not affect the heart, in contrast to dystrophia myotonica. Therefore, a physician should think first of dystrophia myotonica and perform a molecular diagnosis (DM1 and DM2) if necessary [2].

The diagnosis of subtypes of nondystrophic myotonias is complex but has been greatly simplified by the progress of functional electromyography (EMG) combined with molecular diagnosis (Figure 21.1) as we will detail in the following paragraphs [3, 4, 5].

Myotonia is a muscular symptom caused by impaired muscle relaxation. Patients complain of stiffness, often painless, occurring immediately after contraction. Myotonia is caused by a functional defect of the muscle membrane: instead of silencing after muscle contraction, the muscle membrane displays repetitive firings which result in prolonged muscle contraction. This phenomenon can be induced by a voluntary movement or a mechanical stimulation of the muscle (hammer percussion for example). The origin of the muscle membrane defect is now known: a proper functioning of the muscle membrane requires a coordinated depolarization and repolarization. The depolarization is induced by release of acetylcholine at the neuromuscular junction and subsequent propagation of action potentials by opening and closure of sodium and potassium channels all along the muscle membrane. Mutations in chloride or sodium channels disrupt this cycle of membrane excitability by slowing the repolarization of the membrane after depolarization enabling the sodium channels to re-open and produce nonevoked action potentials causing myotonia [6, 7]. The term channelopathies has been proposed as a reference to the pathophysiology of these disorders [8, 9].

Different types of nondystrophic myotonias have been described; some with a clinical definition, others with a molecular definition. Due to the progress of functional EMG and molecular diagnosis, we have today the opportunity to simplify the classification of nondystrophic myotonias and retain only three major categories: myotonia congenita, paramyotonia congenita, and sodium-channel myotonia, with a definition which includes clinical features, EMG and gene defects (Figure 21.1).

Myotonia congenita

Myotonia congenita was first defined clinically in the second part of the nineteenth century [10]. Myotonia is more pronounced after rest and *improves with exercise*, the so-called warm-up phenomenon. Myotonia can be evidenced by asking the patient to repeat the opening and closure of his or her eyes. Slow to start with, the movement will become normal after a few trials. When asked to look quickly downward, the eyelids will not follow the movement of the eyes and it will be possible to see the sclera (lid-lag sign). This sign is not specific to myotonic syndromes and may be observed in other muscle conditions such as both hyper- and hypokalemic periodic paralysis or even in normal persons. Even if this sign is too sensitive and not specific, it is useful in clinical practice because it suggests the existence of myotonia of any type when the myotonia is mild and difficult to evidence clinically in other body parts. In this occurrence, clinical suspicion will be confirmed by EMG which will definitively establish the diagnosis of myotonia by showing myotonic discharges. Myotonia can also be elicited by percussion. Striking the belly of a muscle with a reflex hammer provokes a contraction with delayed relaxation. Percussion of the tongue is classical, but may be unpleasant for the patient.

The main cause of myotonia congenita is the presence of mutations in the chloride channel gene *CLCN1*. Two modes of inheritance are known: autosomal dominant and recessive. Autosomal dominant myotonia congenita was described by the Danish physician Thomsen in his own family [10]. Symptoms usually appear within the first few years of life and are often noted by the parents when the eyes of the infant remain closed when crying, or when muscle stiffness is present for the first steps. Autosomal recessive myotonia congenita was

Disorders of Voluntary Muscle, 8th edn., eds. George Karpati, David Hilton-Jones, Kate Bushby and Robert C. Griggs. Published by Cambridge University Press.

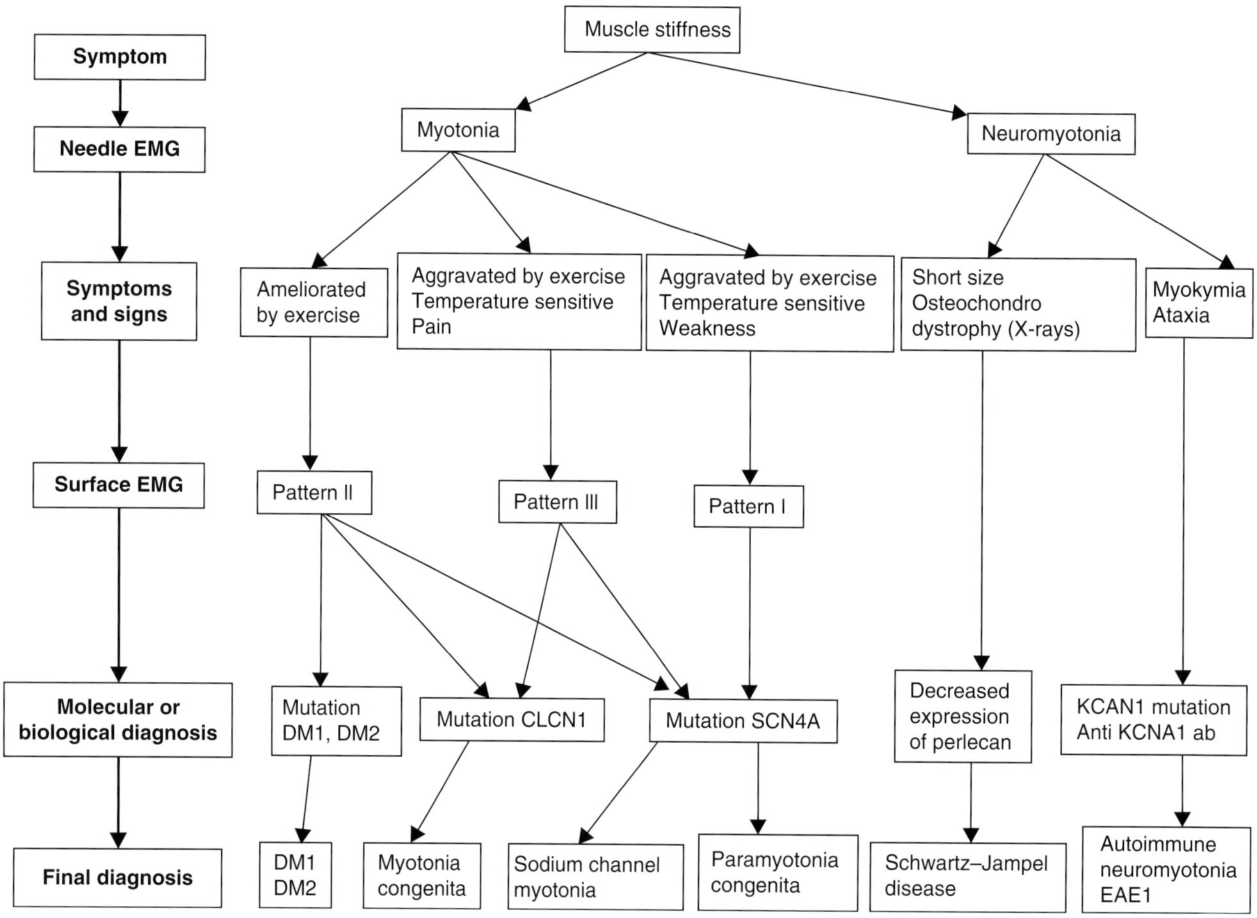

Figure 21.1. Diagnostic algorithm for myotonias.

described by the German physician Becker almost a century later [11]. It is usually considered as more severe than the dominant form. However, minor forms of autosomal recessive myotonia congenita (myotonia levior), or even asymptomatic (incidental discovery by EMG), have been described [12]. Muscle hypertrophy may be observed and is related to the trophic effect of muscle activity on muscle fibers. A dystrophic variant has been anecdotally described [13]. A transient muscle weakness is usually associated with the most severe forms of myotonia congenita. It occurs after rest or after the initiation of the first contraction, only lasts a few seconds, and rapidly improves with repetition of muscle contraction. It can be evidenced by asking the patient to raise and sit several times from the chair without using his or her arms. When clinically measured in an exercising muscle, the muscle force is usually normal. As noted above, most of the patients with a clinical profile of myotonia congenita carry one (dominant) or two chloride channel mutations (recessive). Nonsense mutations are always pathogenic. Missense mutations are more difficult to distinguish from benign polymorphisms, and *in vitro* expression in oocytes might be helpful in difficult cases. With availability of molecular diagnosis, the discovery that a yet undetermined proportion of patients actually carried a sodium channel mutation came as a surprise (Figure 21.1). In myotonia congenita, myotonia is usually painless but a yet undetermined fraction of patients also have muscle pain. This seems to be more frequent with sodium channel mutations but the exact figures are not known [14].

Needle EMG recordings of patients with myotonia congenita show "myotonic discharges," i.e., repetitive firing after nerve impulses have ceased that wax and wane. Functional EMGs, i.e., surface EMG recordings of compound muscle action potentials (CMAP) after short exercise or cooling, have shown distinct patterns that are highly linked to gene mutations [3, 4]. Patients with myotonia congenita display a pattern II, which is characterized by a transient decrease of muscle action potential after short exercise and no effect of the long exercise test [3, 5]. In autosomal dominant myotonia congenita, muscle cooling potentiates the transient decrease of muscle action potentials [4]. Surface EMG might also help elucidate the pathophysiology of myotonia congenita but its usage in practical diagnosis remains to be further evaluated [15].

The understanding of the pathophysiology of myotonia congenita has benefited from the study of animal models. Electrophysiological studies performed in vitro on muscle fibers from animal models of myotonia (myotonic goats, mouse strain *adr*) showed increased resistance of the muscle membrane due to a specific reduction in the membrane conductance for chloride ions. Lowering the chloride conductance with specific pharmacological agents induced membrane hyperexcitability and myotonic discharges [16, 17]. The skeletal muscle chloride channel gene thus appeared to be a good candidate gene for myotonia congenita. In 1991, the characterization of the rat skeletal muscle chloride channel gene permitted the testing of this hypothesis [18]. A transposon was discovered to functionally inactivate the skeletal chloride channel gene in the *adr* mouse strain [19]. Genetic linkage studies established that both autosomal dominant and recessive forms of myotonia congenita in humans mapped to chromosome 7q35, where the skeletal muscle chloride channel gene (*CLCN1*) was also localized [20, 21]. Subsequently, mutations were found in the skeletal muscle chloride channel gene *CLCN1* establishing it as the gene responsible for both forms of the disease [21, 22]. A large number of missense, splice-site and nonsense mutations have now been identified in the muscle chloride channel gene [23, 24, 25, 26, 27, 28, 29, 30, 31].

In vitro co-expression in *Xenopus* oocytes of mutant and wild-type chloride channels suggests that the muscle chloride channel functions as a homo-multimer [32, 33, 34]. Accordingly, nonsense mutations or mutations affecting a splice site result in nonfunctional gene products, suggesting that a loss-of-function underlies the recessive form of myotonia congenita [35, 36, 37, 38]. Missense (or dominant) mutations dramatically alter the functioning of the chloride channel by exerting a dominant negative effect on an oligomer composed of wild-type and mutant subunits [33, 39]. The notion of dominance and recessivity has been challenged by myotonia congenita since chloride channel mutations may display either a dominant or a recessive mode of inheritance as well as incomplete penetrance [40, 41]. The fact that an identical mutation causes both dominant and recessive myotonia congenita suggests that the composition of the oligomer forming the functional chloride channel may vary in individual muscle fibers. According to this hypothesis, if the oligomer comprises a high proportion of mutant subunits, the expression of the disease will be dominant, whereas if the oligomer is composed mostly of wild-type subunits, the expression of the disease would be recessive because of the compensatory effect of the wild-type subunits [42]. Alternative hypotheses are also possible since not all players involved in the complete cycle of muscle membrane excitability are fully known: compensatory mechanisms with other gene products (other channels or ionic pumps, for example) might also intervene. The fact that chloride channel mutations are not predictive of the mode of inheritance raises a specific difficulty in genetic counseling when only one chloride channel mutation is found and the mode of inheritance cannot be deduced from the analysis of the genealogy of the family. This is particular true for isolated cases. In this occurrence, it is impossible to predict whether the disease will be transmitted with a recessive or a dominant mode of inheritance. As mentioned above, functional EMG has shown a distinctive pattern in autosomal dominant myotonia congenita [4]. Functional EMG may therefore help with the genetic counseling. However, the sensitivity of this observation is not yet known and it is too early to use this observation to establish the mode of transmission of myotonia congenita on an individual basis.

It is well established that chloride channels play a role in the repolarization of the muscle membrane and thus participate in the maintenance of resting potential. Their inactivation by mutations modifies the cycle of excitability of the muscle membrane, shifting it towards hyperexcitability by slowing the return of the membrane potential to the resting level after depolarization. Myotonia is directly correlated to the repetitive firing of sodium channels caused by this state of hyperexcitability. It is therefore readily understandable that sodium channel blockers are drugs that are efficient in myotonia. Of course complete blockers of the sodium channel are lethal and the ones that can be used in therapy are those which block particular states of the sodium channel, such as blockers of the open state. The most efficient drug used in clinical practice is mexiletene, followed by carbamazepine and diphenylhydantoin [43, 44, 45]. Future approaches may implicate new strategies such as ribozymes to repair RNA defects but practical therapeutic applications remain under investigation [46].

Paramyotonia congenita

Paramyotonia congenita (PC) was clinically described by Von Eulenburg in the German literature at the end of the nineteenth century [47]. Myotonia is present at birth or is noted by the parents in the first years of life. *The distinction from myotonia congenita relates to the effect of exercise, which aggravates myotonia* (so-called *paradoxical myotonia* or *paramyotonia*). Muscle stiffness is exacerbated not only by exercise, but also by *cold*. It is usually predominant in the face and the upper extremities. A careful examination of the face is important in the diagnosis of myotonia in PC since myotonic features are almost constantly present in the face even if they are mild in the limbs. A lid-lag sign can be evidenced as in other myotonic syndromes. More specifically, when patients are asked to close and open their eyes, they cannot open them after a series of repeated lid closures (paradoxical myotonia). When exposed to cold, they have difficulties with opening their eyes ("Chinese eyes"). Myotonia can be evidenced by percussion of muscles but this sign may be absent since some patients may only have clinically obvious abnormalities when exposed to cold. Pharyngeal muscles can also be affected and the patient may have difficulties with eating ice or swallowing cold beverages. In addition to myotonia, patients with PC also present *attacks of muscle weakness which typically follow attacks of stiffness after prolonged exercise in a cold environment*. A cold-induced attack of weakness can be severe and last for several hours even if the muscles are re-warmed. It usually ends with a sensation of stiffness which may sometimes be painful. Variations in clinical features are observed among patients, some of them being more disturbed by weakness and others by stiffness. Sometimes, symptoms only manifest in the cold and with exercise. Some patients are constantly affected. There are variations not only between patients but also during a patient's life. A case of PC was reported with abnormal cardiac repolarization but the responsibility of the sodium channel mutation for the cardiac abnormalities is still under question [48].

Needle EMG displays myotonic discharges which confirm the clinical diagnosis in myotonia. Functional EMG shows the existence of post-exercise myotonic potentials. Exercise induced a prolonged decrease of compound muscle action potentials (pattern I), which is exacerbated by cooling [3, 4]. Muscle conduction is slowed and abnormal sodium shifts may be evidenced by MRI but the place of these findings in the practical management of PC remains to be established [49, 50].

Soon after genetic linkage between hyperkalemic periodic paralysis and the muscle sodium channel at a locus on chromosome 17 was demonstrated [8], linkage was established between PC and the same locus [51, 52, 53]. PC has been associated with several missense mutations in the gene encoding the voltage-gated sodium channel SCN4A [54, 55, 56]. Mutations affecting codons 1313 and 1448 are the most frequent [57, 58, 59, 60, 61, 62, 63, 64].

In vitro expression of sodium channels with mutations causing PC changes the biophysical properties of the mutated channel: slowed inactivation and incomplete closure of the channel compared to the control are observed [65, 66, 67, 68, 69, 70, 71, 72, 73, 74, 75, 76]. These new biophysical properties confer on the sodium channel the property of rendering the muscle membrane more excitable (gain of function) since leaking channels shift the membrane towards depolarization. The increased number of action potentials due to the increased numbers of sodium channel openings correlates with myotonia. It is therefore of no surprise that the drugs active in myotonia congenita are also active against the muscle stiffness caused by PC, through their blocking of the sodium channels in their open state [77, 78, 79, 80, 81, 82, 83]. They thus decrease the availability of sodium channels for depolarization. Acetazolamide was used with success to prevent the attacks of weakness by analogy to periodic paralysis. It is hypothesized that acetazolamide acts by acidification of the cell content, which results in a general slowing of all ion channels' kinetics. Acetazolamide may also improve myotonia in addition to weakness in some cases.

Sodium channel myotonias

Sodium channel myotonias are by definition myotonias caused by sodium channel mutations [62, 84]. In contrast with the definition of myotonia congenita and PC, which is only clinical, the term of sodium channel myotonia implies a molecular diagnosis. In this category were grouped different myotonic syndromes for which a sodium channel mutation was identified. The mode of inheritance is autosomal dominant. Some of the phenotypes did not attract enough attention to be specifically termed whereas others bear specific names [85, 86, 87, 88, 89, 90, 91, 92, 93].

A small number of patients with clinical and EMG (pattern II) features undistinguishable from those of myotonia congenita were shown to have a sodium channel mutation (Figure 21.1). These patients shifted from the diagnosis of myotonia congenita which was suspected on clinical and EMG grounds to the one of sodium channel myotonia (Figure 21.1). In other words, sodium channel mutation may in rare cases lead to myotonia with a warm-up phenomenon [94].

However, most of the patients with sodium channel myotonia find that exercise either does not affect them or it aggravates them. They do not present weakness and are not always cold-sensitive. Some of them may also complain of muscle pain or cramps. The functional EMG pattern is different from the two distinctive ones described above: no variation of compound muscle action potentials induced by cold or short-term exercise (pattern III) [4]. The most frequent sodium channel mutations in these cases affect codons 445, 1293 or 1306.

Some of the phenotypes that now belong to the group of sodium channel myotonias have been specifically termed [62, 84]. *Myotonia fluctuans* begins in adolescence. Myotonia is induced by exercise but usually occurs with a delayed onset, during immediate rest after exercise. Stiffness severity tends to fluctuate from day to day. While ingestion of potassium markedly aggravates myotonic symptoms (*potassium-aggravated myotonia*), cold has generally no effect. Mutations in the voltage-gated sodium channel SCN4A associated with myotonia fluctuans are S804F and G1306A. In *myotonia permanens*, myotonia is permanent and severe. Myotonia is so severe that patients may be suspected to have Schwartz–Jampel disease. Ventilation impairment may arise from severe stiffness of respiratory muscles or of the diaphragm. This phenotype has been associated with a de novo mutation of the voltage-gated sodium channel SCN4A (G1306E) [62]. *Acetazolamide-responsive myotonia* begins in childhood. Patients complain of intermittent painful muscle stiffness which lasts several hours. Fasting, potassium ingestion and, to a lesser degree exertion and cold, induce myotonia. Symptoms worsen with age. Acetazolamide markedly alleviates symptoms. The I1160V mutation of the voltage-gated sodium channel is associated with this phenotype [65].

Nondystrophia myotonica and anesthesia

Some precautions should be advised to patients with a channelopathy when they undergo general anesthesia. A careful check of the blood electrolytes should be recommended as well as temperature monitoring for those who are temperature-sensitive.

Anesthetic incidents occur more frequently in patients with a sodium channelopathy compared with a control population. Depolarizing agents can provoke severe stiffness of the

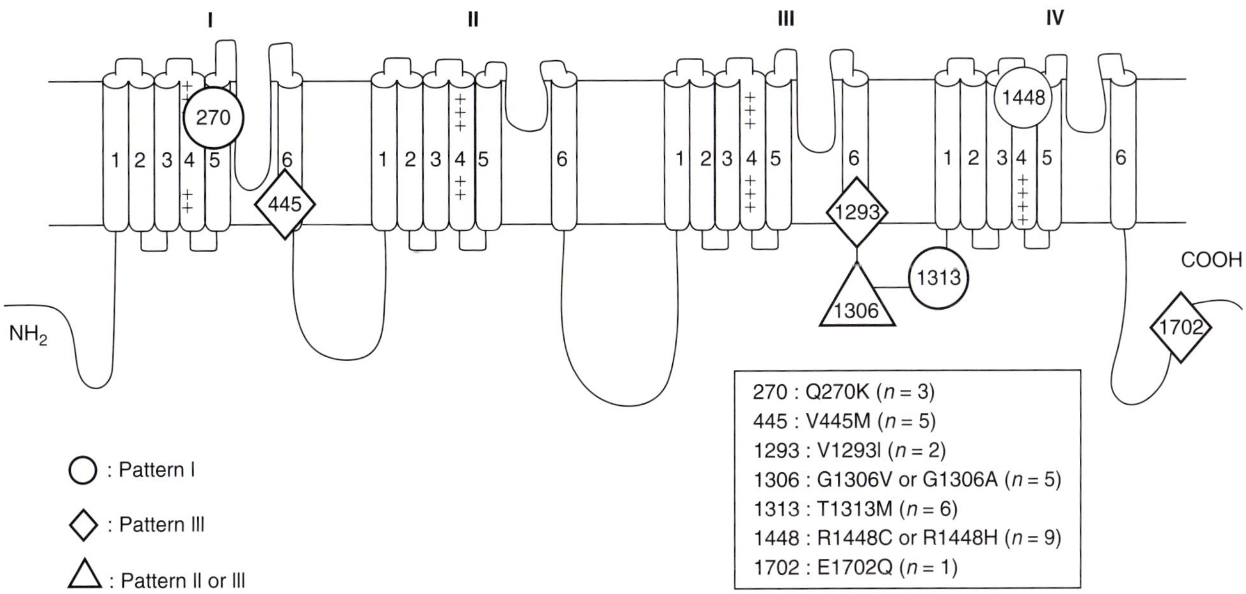

Figure 21.2. Structure of the muscle sodium channel with the most frequent mutations causing myotonia and the corresponding EMG patterns (with thanks to Damien Sternberg, Marianne Arzel-Hézode and Emmanuel Fournier).

respiratory muscles and may cause blood oxygen desaturation because of myotonia of the diaphragm. This muscle contracture might also affect the masseter and may render intubation difficult; in this case the trismus does not indicate malignant hyperthermia [95].

Nondystrophia myotonica and pregnancy and labor

Nonstriated muscles are spared and delivery is usually normal because of the normal uterine contractions. Patients with a sodium channelopathy should be advised not to recruit voluntary muscle to aid the delivery because the paradoxical myotonia may lead to permanent contracture of the striated muscles that may be severe enough to have negative consequences for the baby's oxygenation. Some patients complain of aggravation of myotonia during pregnancy.

Diagnosing nondystrophia myotonica

Progress made in both functional EMG and molecular diagnosis has changed the approach to diagnosing myotonia (Figures 21.1 and 21.2). Clinical challenging of the patient by cooling or potassium ingestion, which used to be done, have been efficiently replaced by functional EMG. The molecular diagnosis can be guided by functional EMG as proposed in Figures 21.1 and 21.2.

At the end of this diagnostic reasoning, we propose that only three categories should be retained: myotonia congenita, paramyotonia congenita, and sodium channel myotonia (Figure 21.1). The justification of this distinction into three categories is based on treatment outcome or follow-up data. Patients with paramyotonia congenita and sodium channel myotonia may be ameliorated by acetazolamide, which is not the case for patients with myotonia congenita. Depending on the severity of myotonia or weakness, mexiletene and acetazolamide should be discussed as drugs of first choice. Patients with paramyotonia congenita and sodium channel myotonia have increased sensitivity to variations in electrolyte levels, anesthetic depolarizing agents, and the cold. They should be informed and followed more closely during intubation or anesthesia.

Schwartz–Jampel disease

Schwartz–Jampel disease (SJD) was described by two ophthalmologists in 1962 and clinical features were further refined by Aberfeld and Beighton [96, 97, 98]. SJD is rare: approximately 100 cases have been reported in the medical literature. It is a genetic condition of autosomal recessive inheritance (Figure 21.3). *SJD is characterized by the association of a severe muscle stiffness, caused at least partly by myotonia, and chondrodysplasia.* The signs become obvious during the *first years of life.* The disease course is slowly progressive until mid-adolescence and then remains stable. The most recognizable feature is a "mask-like face" with a blepharospasm, pursed lips, and reduced mobility of the facial muscles. Osteoarticular deformities with pectus carinatum, kyphoscoliosis, lumbar lordosis, bowing of the long bones, and light dwarfism distinguish SJD from other myotonic disorders. However, some cases without obvious bone changes also exist [99]. Patients are usually smaller than their normal sibs. Radiographic features consist of decreased bone age, platyspondyly with frequent coronal cleft vertebrae, epimetaphyseal dysplasia, bilateral coxa vara and iliac base shortening with acetabular dysplasia, as well as anterior bowing of the diaphyses, metaphyseal widening,

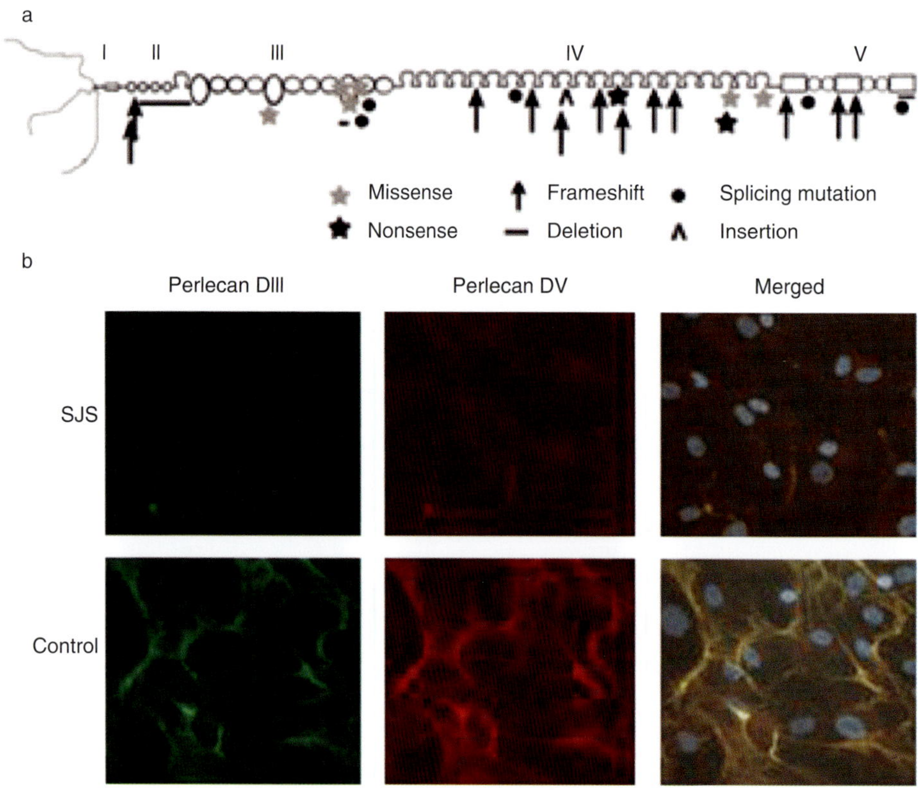

Figure 21.3a, b. Patients with Schwartz–Jampel disease mutations in the gene encoding perlecan and decreased expression of perlecan in cultured fibroblast cells (with thanks to Sophie Nicole).

and flattening of the epiphyses of the long bones. EMG reveals a permanent muscle activity which is thought to be of neurogenic origin (neuromyotonia) [100].

Schwartz–Jampel disease is caused by hypomorphic mutations in the gene HSPG2 (1p35-p36.1) encoding perlecan, the major heparan sulfate proteoglycan of basement membranes [101, 102]. Thirty mutations, including splicing, nonsense and missense mutations, and large genomic deletions, have been described [102, 103, 104]. They are located along the entire gene (Figure 21.3).

Perlecan is a secreted proteoglycan that is ubiquitously expressed. SJD mutations are hypomorphic and allow residual secretion of normal perlecan. In the neuromuscular system, perlecan is present in the muscle and nerve basement membrane. It is accumulated at the neuromuscular junction where it is crucial to the anchorage of acetylcholinesterase through its interaction with the ColQ collagenous subunit of this enzyme and γ-dystroglycan. Indeed, acetylcholinesterase is lacking at the neuromuscular junction in SJD in humans and in mouse models [105]. Abnormal neuromuscular junctions with absence of the normal pretzel-like shape and prominent denervation are also seen. How this remodeling of the neuromuscular junction leads to the abnormal neuromuscular activity in SJD remains to be determined.

To establish the diagnosis of SJD, neuromyotonia has to be confirmed by EMG. Chondrodysplasia confirmed by X-ray analysis is a strong argument in favor of the diagnosis and allows the exclusion of severe forms of nondystrophic myotonia [100]. The wide spectrum of mutations in the *HSPG2* gene and the large size of the gene renders mutation screening extremely laborious. An attractive approach to molecular diagnosis is the demonstration of decreased expression of perlecan in a primary cell culture of fibroblasts established from a patient skin biopsy [104].

Sodium channel blockers may improve the condition of patients. Carbamazepine, phenytoin, and procainamide have been tried with some success, carbamazepine being apparently the most efficient. For unknown reasons, these medications have to be taken for several weeks or months before observing a beneficial effect [106].

Periodic paralysis

The primary periodic paralyses are genetic skeletal muscle disorders in which patients experience attacks of muscle weakness lasting from a few minutes to several days. The weakness can be generalized or focal. Initially muscle strength returns to normal after an attack, but as the diseases progresses significant fixed muscle weakness often develops. Delay in accurate diagnosis and treatment is common because of variability in symptoms [107].

In all forms of periodic paralysis (PP), electrophysiological examination during an attack reveals the skeletal muscle fiber membrane to be in a partially depolarized and inexcitable state. The genetic forms of PP are caused by dysfunction of membrane-bound voltage-gated ion channels which play a key

Table 21.1. Features of periodic paralysis and ATS

	Hypokalemic periodic paralysis	Hyperkalemic periodic paralysis	Andersen–Tawil syndrome
Gene	CACNA1S SCN4A	SCN4A	KCJN2
Serum potassium at onset	Low	Normal or high	Normal, low or high
Age of onset	First or second decade	Usually first decade	First or second decade
Duration of episodes	Hours to days	Minutes to hours	Variable usually hours
Triggers	Exercise and then rest	Exercise and then rest	Exercise and then rest
	Carbohydrate load may cause weakness	Prolonged fast may cause weakness	Carbohydrates may trigger
Myotonia	No	Sometimes	No
Special physical characteristics	N/A	N/A	Yes but may be subtle
ECG	N/A	N/A	"U" waves, apparent prolonged QT
Muscle biopsy	May be normal, or vacuolar change or tubular aggregates	May be normal, or vacuolar change or tubular aggregates	May be normal, or vacuolar change or tubular aggregates
Response to acetazolamide	Yes but some patients with sodium channel mutations experience adverse response	Yes	Yes

role in determining membrane potential, muscle excitability, and excitation–contraction coupling.

Traditionally PP has been classified according to serum potassium levels at the onset into hypo- and hyperkalemic PP (hypoPP and hyperPP, respectively). This serum potassium-based classification is clinically useful but has now been supplemented by the molecular genetic classification described here.

Familial hypokalemic periodic paralysis (HypoPP)

Hypokalemic PP is the most common form of familial PP with a prevalence of 0.4 to 1 in 100 000 in Europe [108, 109, 110]. It is inherited in an autosomal dominant fashion with reduced penetrance in women giving a male:female ratio of ~3:1 [111].

Three genes have been implicated in familial hypoPP including *CACNA1S*, *SCN4A*, and *KCNJ2*. Mutations in the voltage-gated calcium channel gene *CACNA1S* cause most cases (~70%) [112, 113]. Approximately 10% of cases have mutations in the voltage-gated sodium channel gene *SCN4A* [113, 114, 115, 116]. Point mutations in *KCNJ2* encoding an inward rectifying potassium channel can cause Andersen–Tawil syndrome which is described in detail below [117].

Hypokalemic PP usually presents between the ages of 5 and 20 years, typically in the teenage years [112, 113] (see Table 21.1). Onset over the age of 20 has been reported [113]. Attacks tend to last from several hours up to 2–3 days. HypoPP attacks are longer and more severe than in hyperPP, although this is our experience and a recent retrospective study did not confirm this, but treatment effect could have been a confounding variable [113].

Typically in hypoPP the patient wakes in the night or in the early morning with generalized weakness. Intake of a carbohydrate-rich meal or strenuous exercise the preceding day or night can often be a triggering factor. Focal episodes of weakness, for example involving only one limb, are more common in hyperPP. In all forms of PP tendon reflexes are diminished or absent in an attack. Cranial muscles are consistently spared. Impairment of speech, visual symptoms or alterations in consciousness are not expected and suggest other diagnostic possibilities. Respiratory muscles are mostly spared although a reduction in vital capacity and consequent respiratory failure have been reported [118, 119, 120]. Strength gradually improves over the course of the next day or two although some patients indicate it takes up to a week to recover. Attacks become less frequent and severe in later life and in common with hyperPP a permanent myopathy may develop [121]. Interestingly, fixed weakness has been described in patients without a strong history of frequent paralytic attacks [116]. It remains unproven whether active treatment to reduce the frequency of attacks prevents the development of fixed weakness.

A useful feature to distinguish between hypoPP and hyperPP clinically is the absence of (true) myotonia in hypoPP.

A number of factors may induce or exacerbate attacks. These include exercise followed by rest, ingestion of carbohydrates, administration of insulin, and epinephrine injections [118, 119, 122]. Stress and excitement and exposure to cold are also triggers [113]. Menstruation and pregnancy have also been reported to trigger attacks [123, 124]. Although serum potassium levels are often reduced, especially at the beginning of an attack, they may not be below the normal range. Serum creatine kinase (CK) may be normal or slightly elevated in between attacks. During paralytic attacks there can be a moderate rise in CK [125].

Changes on ECG have been observed with very low potassium, including prominent U waves, flattening of T waves, and ST depression. Interictal ECG is usually normal. The presence of prominent U waves, frequent ventricular ectopic beats or arrhythmias should alert the clinician to the possibility of Andersen–Tawil syndrome (ATS) (see below). Familial HypoPP is not associated with cardiomyopathy [126].

Familial hyperkalemic periodic paralysis (HyperPP)

Familial hyperPP is due to mutations in *SCN4A* encoding the α-subunit of the skeletal muscle voltage-gated sodium channel $Na_v1.4$. HyperPP patients have attacks of limb weakness lasting for minutes to hours. In contrast to hypoPP the attacks frequently happen during the daytime but nocturnal attacks may occur [127, 128]. As a general guide frequent short daytime attacks favor a diagnosis of hyperPP and nocturnal prolonged attacks may slightly favor hypoPP. The onset of symptoms is most often during the first decade and attacks become milder and less frequent with age. A persistent mild myopathy may develop later in the course of the disease [129, 130, 131].

The rise in potassium during attacks may be subtle and transient and may not exceed the normal range [61]. Normokalemic PP was considered to be a distinct disorder based on descriptions of a few families [132, 133, 134]. We analyzed the original 1961 North East of England family and showed that they harbored the common M1592V hyperPP *SCN4A* mutation [135]. We consider normokalemic PP to be a variant of hyperPP.

Hyperkalemic PP, potassium-aggravated myotonia (PAM), and paramyotonia congenita are allelic sodium channel disorders and their phenotypes overlap to varying degrees [128, 136]. In hyperPP and paramyotonia congenita women may be less severely affected [128].

Patients who have both PP and myotonia often find it difficult to distinguish between stiffness and weakness, and attacks are often initially dominated by stiffness leading to paralysis later. EMG myotonia can be demonstrated in at least 50% of patients with the two most common *SCN4A* mutations T704M and M1592V [3, 61, 113] but myotonia on clinical examination is detected in a smaller percentage [61]. Interestingly myotonic symptoms are frequently experienced and easily elicited in the cranial musculature (myotonic lid-lag, eye closure myotonia), which is not usually involved in the paralytic attack. Consciousness is preserved and respiratory and cranial musculature is usually spared. Identified triggers include rest following exercise, fasting, cold, stress, intercurrent infection, and anesthesia. Hormonal changes may also play a role as menstruation, oral contraception, and pregnancy have been associated with an increase in symptoms [65, 128, 137].

a

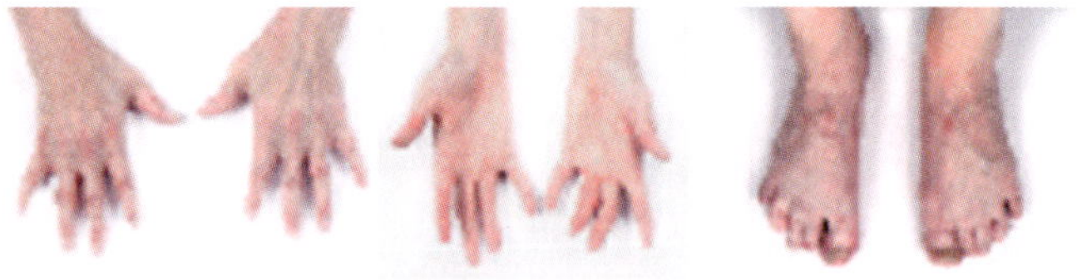

b

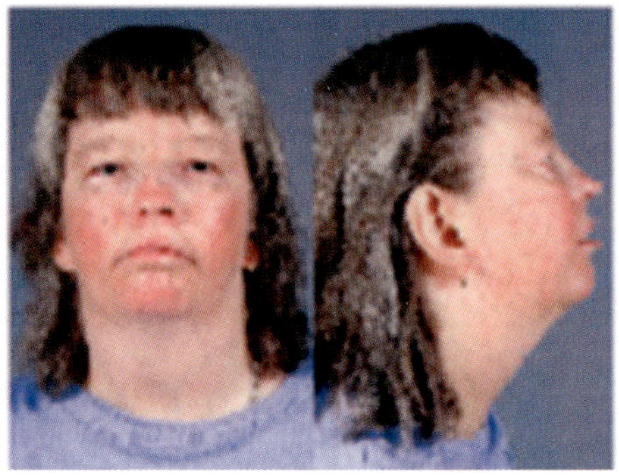

Figure 21.4a, b. (a) Hands and feet in Andersen–Tawil syndrome (ATS): small hands and feet, hand clinodactyly, foot syndactyly. (b) Facial features in ATS: Low-set ears, hypertelorism, broad forehead, and mandibular hypoplasia.

Andersen–Tawil syndrome (ATS)

First described by Andersen *et al.* [138] ATS is characterized by a triad of PP, ventricular arrhythmia, and distinctive physical features (see Figure 21.4 and Table 21.1). Many patients do not have all of these features and there can be marked intrafamilial variation [117]. It is the least common form of PP. Mutations in *KCNJ2* encoding the inward rectifying potassium channel Kir2.1 have been identified in about two-thirds of kindreds with ATS [117, 139]. Up to 20% of individuals carrying pathogenic mutations may not exhibit any phenotypic features [139, 140, 141]. De novo mutations are frequent [141].

Although Andersen's original case had marked physical abnormalities with low-set ears, hypertelorism, mandibular hypoplasia, scaphocephalic cranium, clinodactyly, single transverse palm crease, central defect of soft and hard palate, and cryptorchidism, many patients with ATS have only subtle physical changes. The most common features are mandibular hypoplasia, hypertelorism, broad-based nose, low-set ears, clinodactyly, and syndactyly [142] (Figure 21.4). Symptomatic onset with episodic weakness is typically in the first or second decade. The PP is most commonly hypokalemic but may also be hyper- or normokalemic [141]. Electrocardiography may show bi-directional or polymorphic ventricular tachycardia, prolonged corrected QT interval, bigeminy, frequent ventricular ectopy or may be normal (Figure 21.2). A particularly frequent finding is a prominent "U" wave even in the presence of a normal serum potassium [139]. ATS is also classified as long QT syndrome 7 (LQT7). In comparison to other long QT syndromes the arrhythmias in ATS are less malignant [139].

However sudden cardiac death does occur and patients require careful cardiac evaluation [139, 140, 141]. A more recent study of ECGs from a large cohort of ATS patients established a distinct T-U-wave pattern that reliably distinguished between *KCNJ2*-mutation-positive ATS patients and those where no mutation could be found [143]. In many ATS patients the QT interval is in fact within the normal limits [143].

Thyrotoxic periodic paralysis (TPP)

Thyrotoxic periodic paralysis is most common in Asia, particularly China, Korea and Japan where more than 10% of male thyrotoxic patients may be affected [144, 145, 146, 147]. The overall incidence in thyrotoxic patients from these populations is approximately 2% [145] compared to only 0.1%–0.2% in Caucasians [148]. The male to female predominance is much more marked in TPP (between 20:1 and 76:1) [145, 149] compared to hypoPP (3:1) [111].

Most cases of TPP are sporadic but a few familial cases have also been described [150, 151]. The onset of symptoms is frequently between the second and fourth decade when hyperthyroidism is most common. Importantly, many cases have only subtle clinical signs of hyperthyroidism [145, 148]. Autoimmune thyrotoxicosis (Graves disease) is the most common underlying disorder but TPP may be caused by any form of hyperthyroidism in susceptible patients, including excessive administration of thyroid hormone replacement.TPP bears phenotypic resemblance to familial hypoPP. It is associated with low serum potassium during attacks, may be triggered by glucose/insulin administration, and may also be triggered by rest following exercise. Focal weakness can develop in more strenuously exercised muscles and attacks typically occur at night or on wakening in the morning [145]. The respiratory and cranial musculature tend to be spared. Morbidity and mortality are low but significant arrhythmias associated with severe hypokalemia have been reported [145, 152].

Differential diagnosis

The difference between myasthenia and PP is often straightforward. Attacks of weakness are more distinct in PP versus a more long-term fluctuation of muscle strength in myasthenia. Gentle exercise helps to lessen or abort PP attacks but worsens symptoms in myasthenia. The distribution of muscles affected is different (bulbar and extraocular muscles are frequently affected in myasthenia and spared in PP). Investigations (neuromuscular junction transmission deficit on repetitive nerve stimulation and single-fiber EMG, acetylcholine receptor antibodies, genetic testing) should distinguish between these two disorders. However, diagnostic difficulty may sometimes arise when distinguishing between the limb-girdle presentation of myasthenia and PP [153]. Patients with both myotonia congenita and paramyotonia/hyperPP can experience intermittent weakness as described earlier. Most other disorders causing acute or subacute muscle weakness (e.g., McArdle disease, Guillain–Barré syndrome, acute intermittent porphyria) are normally straightforward to exclude by appropriate history, clinical examination, and investigations.

General examination and laboratory tests in periodic paralysis

General examination of patients between attacks is often normal. Muscle strength testing may reveal persistent proximal weakness. Patients with hyperPP may show signs of action and percussion myotonia. Lid-lag may be a sensitive indicator of myotonia but it can occur in healthy volunteers. Subtle dysmorphic features may indicate ATS.

Laboratory investigations should establish potassium levels during attacks (ideally soon after the onset of attack) and exclude secondary causes of PP. All patients with hypoPP should have their thyroid function checked to exclude TPP. Routine ECG should be undertaken in all PP cases since the cranioskeletal features of ATS may be subtle. Patients with suspected ATS should undergo thorough cardiological work-up including prolonged ECG recordings, echocardiography, and exercise testing. Previously patients were often subjected to a range of provocative tests, many of which have now been superseded by the availability of genetic analysis and specialized neurophysiological investigations.

Genetic testing in periodic paralysis

Deoxyribonucleic acid (DNA) testing is now a major diagnostic tool in familial PP. However, even with extensive DNA sequencing of the ion channel genes known to be involved in PP, mutations are not detected in one-third of patients with either hyperPP or hypoPP [113]. Both *CACNA1S* and *SCN4A* are large genes containing 44 and 25 exons respectively. The genetic testing generally available in DNA diagnostic-service laboratories often only encompasses gene regions containing common mutations. It is therefore important to note that a negative genetic result from such a laboratory reduces the likelihood of, but does not exclude, a diagnosis of familial PP. The potassium channel gene *KCNJ2* mutated in ATS is a small single-exon gene and direct sequencing analysis of the whole gene is more feasible in the diagnostic laboratory setting. In ATS more than 30 mutations have been identified but approximately 30% of kindreds do not harbor mutations in *KCNJ2*. This could be partly because there may be undetected mutations in the promoter or intronic regions of the *KCNJ2* gene [139].

In patients with clear evidence of hypoPP, analysis for the known mutations in *CACNA1S* should be undertaken first. Mutations have so far only been described at residues 528 (R528H and R528G) and 1239 (R1239G and R1239H) and testing is therefore relatively straightforward. The R528H or R1239H mutations are each found in 40%–50% of genotyped hypoPP patients, while the R1239G mutation is rare [111, 112, 113, 115, 116, 154]. The R528G mutation has only been reported in a single Chinese kindred [155]. Less commonly (<10%) changes are found in *SCN4A* in hypoPP and exon 12 appears to be a hotspot [113, 114, 115, 116]. Testing of *KCNJ2* may also be helpful even in the absence of cardiac or distinctive physical features as some patients only present with one of the three typical features of ATS.

The DNA of patients with definite hyperPP and/or with evidence of myotonia should be analyzed for mutations in *SCN4A*. The two most commonly occurring mutations are T704M and M1592V [131, 156], accounting for 30%–70% and 15%–30% respectively of all genotyped patients with hyperPP depending on the population [61, 113]. Patients with ATS may less commonly suffer from hyperPP (without myotonia) and testing of *KCNJ2* may be indicated in selected cases. In patients where the clinical data are insufficient to decide whether the patient is suffering from hypo- or hyperPP, testing for the common mutations in both *SCN4A* and *CACNA1S* is a reasonable strategy.

Molecular pathophysiology

The structure of $Na_V1.4$ channels is similar to that of other cation channels and consists of four domains, each comprising six transmembrane segments. The fourth segment of each domain (S4) acts as the voltage sensor. Upon activation, a conformational change leads to channel opening and an inward flux of sodium ions leading to depolarization. This is followed by a process of "fast inactivation" which prevents further action potential generation. *SCN4A* mutations cause differing effects on gating including delayed or incomplete inactivation and enhanced activation, but the net effect is to cause an increase in Na^+ flux. Generally mutations that cause PMC/PAM lead to prolonged duration of the action potential and persistent after-discharges (myotonia) as described above. Those associated with hyperPP lead to sustained depolarization, electrical inexcitability, and muscle weakness. The exception to this gain-of-function mechanism are the hypoPP sodium channel mutations in the voltage-sensing S_4 segment of domain II, which enhance channel inactivation.

Mutations in both hypoPP1 (CACNA1S mutations) and hypoPP2 (SCN4A mutations) involve the outermost positively charged arginine residues of the voltage-sensing segments of domains II and IV in Cav1.1 and of domain II in Nav1.4. A recent report [157] indicates that mutations in these residues that result in loss of positive charge may produce a "cation leak" through the channel pore when the channel is in the resting closed state. Similar key arginine residues can be found in the voltage-sensing segments of a number of muscle and brain channels. This proposed new mechanism requires further study. The confirmation of this proposed "cation leak" may enhance our ability to understand the therapeutic efficacy of drugs such as acetazolamide and allow development of new therapeutic options. The causal mutations in ATS have dominant negative loss-of-function effects.

Neurophysiological assessment

Routine nerve conduction studies between attacks are normal. EMG may show myopathic changes particularly in those patients who have developed fixed weakness. In patients with hyperPP evidence of sarcolemmal hyperexcitability in the form of myotonic discharges, increased insertional activity, and spontaneous fibrillation and positive sharp waves may be found. Myotonic discharges can be present even in the absence of clinical symptoms or signs of (para)myotonia but the degree of abnormality tends to correlate with the clinical picture. The presence of myotonic discharges is not seen in hypoPP regardless of the underlying genetic defect (*CACNA1S*, *SCN4A* or *KCNJ2*) [3]. The detection of myotonia is therefore helpful in directing gene analysis to SCN4A.

During an attack the compound motor action potential (CMAP) amplitude and area are reduced. Needle EMG shows fibrillation potentials and positive sharp waves, a decrease in insertional activity, and there is an increased proportion of polyphasic motor unit potentials [122]. With severe paralysis the muscle may become completely inexcitable.

More specific tests include the use of provocation such as exercise, rest and cold in combination with EMG or CMAP monitoring. These include the long exercise test and short exercise test protocols [158, 159]. Fournier and colleagues have provided evidence that electrophysiological studies, particularly the short exercise test with and without cooling, can be very helpful in predicting genotype and directing genetic analysis [3, 4].

Muscle histopathology

Muscle biopsy is not usually indicated in making the diagnosis of PP. Commonly observed changes in muscle biopsies include vacuolar changes and tubular aggregates. Histopathological features generally do not distinguish between the subtypes of PP. Occasionally, a biopsy with typical changes may be helpful in patients who are evaluated with prominent myopathy in the absence of paralytic attacks. The changes appear to be more closely related to the degree of fixed weakness rather than the number of attacks. Histopathological abnormalities including glycogen accumulation have been reported in the absence of paralytic attacks or clinical myopathy [160].

Treatment of periodic paralysis

General advice

Simple advice to avoid recognized triggering factors can be helpful. Excessive exertion particularly when followed by a long period of rest, such as sleep overnight, should be avoided. During an attack gentle physical activity can abort symptoms. Many patients benefit from "warming down" after exercise. Dietary advice includes regular meals (to prevent fasting) and avoidance of potassium-rich foods (banana, melon, and a number of other fruits) in hyperPP. Ingestion of carbohydrate-containing drinks or snacks may abort attacks in hyperPP. Patients with hypoPP should avoid large, late-evening carbohydrate-rich meals.

Medication options

Potassium chloride can be used for an acute attack in hypoPP. Oral preparations are preferable and safer than intravenous administration. Regular use may reduce the frequency of attacks. Agents that reduce urinary potassium loss such as spironolactone (100 mg/day) or triamterene (150 mg/day) can also improve symptoms in hypoPP.

Patients with hyperPP may benefit from treatment to prevent hyperkalemia including thiazide diuretics [161] and inhaled β-agonists [162, 163, 164].

Inhibitors of carbonic acid anhydrase (acetazolamide, dichlorphenamide) are helpful in all forms of PP [161, 165]. Studies in hypoPP suggest that interictal low-grade weakness may also improve [166, 167]. None of the treatments used in PP have been proven to prevent the progressive myopathy seen in both hypoPP and hyperPP. The exact mechanism underlying the beneficial effect of carbonic anhydrase inhibitors remains unclear. One possibility is acidification of the channel microenvironment. The channel defect may be alleviated by a reduction in the muscle pH as shown in expression studies for some mutations [168]. A similar mechanism may explain why gentle exercise (known to cause transient hyperkalemia) can improve symptoms during a mild attack. Acetazolamide should be started low, at 62.5 or 125 mg daily, and gradually increased until a satisfactory response is achieved but usually not higher than 1000 mg/day given in two to three divided doses. Distal paresthesiae, headaches, and occasionally mood disturbance including depression can be experienced. An important long-term complication is the development of renal calculi in 10%–20% of patients [169]. Therefore, all patients should undergo baseline and yearly follow-up renal imaging to enable early detection and treatment of nephrolithiasis. Regular intake of citrus drinks reduces the development of renal calculi.

The efficacy of dichlorphenamide (50–300 mg/day) was shown in a double-blind placebo-controlled crossover trial [170]. The effectiveness of dichlorphenamide to prevent or reduce the severity and frequency of attacks in both hyperPP and hypoPP was clearly shown. Side-effects and consequent precautions are similar to those for acetazolamide.

Some reports suggest that acetazolamide can exacerbate symptoms in patients with hypoPP due to sodium channel mutations [64, 116] but others report benefit [168, 171]. Treatment-induced worsening with carbonic anhydrase inhibitors can also occur with other mutations and the patient should be warned and monitored accordingly. Patients with hyperPP and myotonia may also benefit from antimyotonic agents such as mexiletine (200–600 mg/day in two to three divided doses). Due to its cardiac side-effects mexiletine should be monitored with baseline and follow-up ECGs.

Treatment of Andersen–Tawil syndrome

Muscle and cardiac symptoms often occur independently in ATS and treatment of one has the potential to exacerbate the other. Carbonic anhydrase inhibitors are helpful and are the first-line treatment for paralytic attacks. The management of cardiac arrhythmias can range between simple monitoring to necessity of pacemaker or implantable cardioverter defibrillator. Case reports exist on the successful use of amiodarone [172] and imipramine [173, 174]. Imipramine does not interact with Kir2.1 channels [175] but it has inhibitory effects on many other cardiac potassium, sodium, and calcium channels [176]. β-Blockers have been tried [177]. Verapamil has been found beneficial in one patient [178] but worsened muscle symptoms in another [177].

Treatment of thyrotoxic periodic paralysis

Effective treatment of TPP requires correction of the endocrine abnormality. Once the patient becomes euthyroid the paralytic attacks cease and neurophysiological abnormalities disappear [80, 179]. The underlying susceptibility however remains and excessive thyroid supplementation may induce recurrence of attacks.

In contrast to the familial periodic paralyses no convincing benefit from carbonic anhydrase inhibitors has been described in TPP [180, 181]. Most centers use potassium supplementation, a β-blocker, or a combination to treat acute attacks.

β-Blockers can be used in the acute attack as well as a preventive measure. It has been suggested that hyperadrenergism during thyrotoxicosis contributes to the muscle weakness.

Periodic paralysis and anesthesia

Case reports exist of patients with PP having episodes of malignant hyperthermia [182, 183, 184]. In one of these patients a mutation in the ryanodine receptor has been identified [185]. Whether another unidentified mutation in a voltage-gated channel is responsible for the PP in this particular case is uncertain. From a practical point of view it is advisable to avoid volatile anesthetics although there is no definite evidence of an increased risk of malignant hyperthermia in this patient group. The more frequent anesthetic complication is an attack of paralysis following an intervention [112]. This is not unexpected given the known trigger factors (stress, immobility, cold, exertion during labor) in addition to anesthetic drugs. The management plan should take these factors into account (avoidance or minimization of pain, carbohydrate loads in hypoPP, fasting and cold in hyperPP, sympathomimetics, prolonged labor, etc.). Nondepolarizing muscle relaxants, propofol, and regional anesthesia have been found to be relatively safe [186, 187, 188, 189].

Neuromyotonia and episodic ataxia type 1

Potassium channelopathy

The episodic ataxias are inherited ataxic syndromes characterized by intermittent cerebellar dysfunction separated by periods of normality. Episodic ataxia type 1 (EA-1) patients often exhibit neuromyotonia. EA-1 is caused by mutations in the voltage-gated-potassium channel gene, *KCNA1* [190].

Clinical features

Clinically, EA-1 usually declares itself in the first or second decade of life. Patients experience disabling attacks of midline cerebellar dysfunction, manifesting as truncal and limb ataxia, dysarthria, and visual symptoms such as oscillopsia and visual blurring. These symptoms are often accompanied by nausea and headache. A coarse tremor of the arms and head is clinically evident in certain kindreds. These attacks are triggered by physical and emotional stress, chemical stressors, startle and sudden postural changes and can last from seconds to minutes. The frequency of these ataxic spells can vary amongst individuals from recurrent daily ictal episodes to infrequent monthly attacks. The episodes terminate spontaneously. Interictally, patients are asymptomatic with a normal neurological examination. The disease is non-progressive with the attack frequency attenuating over time, although patients may be left with a subtle impairment of cerebellar function.

The second cardinal feature of EA-1 is the presence of continuous persistent interictal motor activity in the form of myokymia or neuromyotonia, which is a consequence of peripheral nerve hyperexcitability. The term myokymia denotes spontaneous skeletal muscle contractions which produces a "rippling" quality. These fine rippling movements of muscle can be observed in the limbs and around the eyes and are also evident as small-amplitude side-to-side movements of the fingers in the outstretched hands. Myokymia in these patients is often subclinical, although invariably evident on EMG studies.

With the discovery of novel genetic lesions responsible for EA-1, the phenotypic spectrum of the disorder has widened [190, 191, 192, 193]. In addition to the classical description, phenotypic variants include EA-1 with partial epilepsy, EA-1 without myokymia and also isolated severe neuromyotonia [192]. Eunson *et al.* [192] described a family with a *KCNA1* gene mutation in which the proband, a 3-year-old boy, presented with increased tone in the limbs, his fists partially clenched, and small semi-rhythmical lateral movements of his fingers and rippling movements of his calf and hamstrings. His EMG confirmed continuous generalized myokymic activity. His 39-year-old father had no history of episodic ataxia or muscle stiffness but displayed subtle myokymia of his dorsal interossei. Isolated neuromyotonia has been previously described in autoimmune Isaac syndrome or acquired neuromyotonia, in which antibodies against the voltage-gated potassium channel result in its dysfunction. However this family indicates that isolated neuromyotonia can be caused by a genetic mutation in the Kv1.1 channel. A number of different neuromuscular findings are recognized including distal wasting with contractures, shortening of the Achilles tendon in children, and transient postural abnormality in infants such as flexion of the fingers, wrists, elbow, and knees [193]. Kinali and colleagues reported a case in a family in which the same mutation of the *KCNA1* gene in the mother and son resulted in two different clinical phenotypes [194]. The son presented in infancy with generalized muscle stiffness and motor developmental delay. He was also found to have mildly dysmorphic features, short stature, and an abnormal gait. His increased muscle tone resulted in marked kyphoscoliosis, elbow contractures and shortening of the Achilles tendon. His EMG demonstrated marked generalized myokymia. The boy's mother presented some years later with typical features of EA-1. On examination she had myokymia and mild skeletal abnormalities. Recently, a 10-year-old girl with EA-1 was found to have distal weakness with paresis of the extensors of the feet and prolonged spells of limb stiffness lasting up to 12 h [195]. There is also heterogeneity in the response to treatment with some kindreds being particularly resistant to drugs. Furthermore phenocopies without Kv1.1 mutations have been identified in two families.

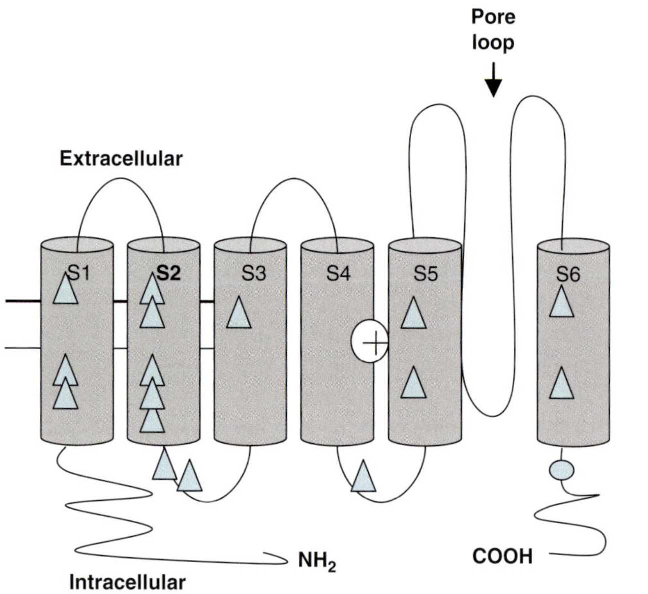

Figure 21.5. Structure of the Kvα1.1 channel subunit showing the six transmembrane segments (S1–S6), the voltage-sensing S4 segment and the pore-lining loop between S5 and S6. The triangles indicate the positions of known missense mutations; the circle represents the R147 stop which truncates most of the C-terminus. (Figure prepared by Dr. Stephanie Schorge.)

Molecular pathophysiology

Genetic linkage studies have mapped the EA-1 syndrome locus to chromosome 12p13 [190, 196] and to mutations in the *KCNA1* gene which encodes the voltage-gated potassium channel subunit Kvα1.1 (Figure 21.5) This is the mammalian ortholog of the *Shaker* channel, the first potassium channel to be identified in the fruit fly, *Drosophila melanogaster*. Over 16 missense mutations and one premature stop codon in the carboxyl terminus have been identified in EA-1 patients [190, 191, 192, 193, 197]. Several studies have demonstrated that mutant Kv1.1 subunits result in a significant reduction in peak potassium current amplitude relative to wild-type currents [193].

Treatment

Acetazolamide is a carbonic anhydrase inhibitor which may reduce the frequency of ataxic episodes in some individuals. Some loss of efficacy occurs with prolonged treatment. The precise mechanism of action in EA-1 is unknown, although it has been postulated to alter the pH in the vicinity of the ion channel, causing hyperpolarization of the cell membrane and thus reducing neuronal excitability [198]. Acetazolamide is commonly used as a diuretic and long-term use can result in the formation of renal calculi. Regular monitoring of kidney function is necessary to avoid renal complications. Some patients also respond to various anti-epileptic medications including carbamazepine, phenytoin, and phenobarbitone. Again the mechanisms of action remain to be elucidated although these observations may suggest that treatment may be specific to the mutations present as not all patients with EA-1 respond to these therapies.

Acknowledgments

Bertrand Fontaine thanks Emmanuel Fournier, Marianne Arzel-Hézode, Damien Sternberg, and Sophie Nicole for their generous contributions to the figures. Bertrand Fontaine acknowledges financial support from INSERM, AFM, and ANR-Maladies Rares as well as fruitful discussion with members of Resocanaux. Michael Hanna thanks Doreen Fialho, Susie Tomlinson, and Sanjeev Rajakulendran for generous help with the figures. Michael Hanna acknowledges financial support from the Medical Research Council, UK.

References

1. C. R. Heatwole, R. T. Moxley, 3rd, The nondystrophic myotonias. *Neurotherapeutics* **4** (2007), 238–251.
2. P. J. Lamont, R. L. Jacob, F. L. Mastaglia, N. G. Laing, An expansion in the ZNF9 gene causes PROMM in a previously described family with an incidental CLCN1 mutation. *J. Neurol. Neurosurg. Psychiatry* **75** (2004), 343.
3. E. Fournier, M. Arzel, D. Sternberg, *et al.*, Electromyography guides toward subgroups of mutations in muscle channelopathies. *Ann. Neurol.* **56** (2004), 650–661.
4. E. Fournier, K. Viala, H. Gervais, *et al.*, Cold extends electromyography distinction between ion channel mutations causing myotonia. *Ann. Neurol.* **60** (2006), 356–365.
5. P. Michel, D. Sternberg, P. Y. Jeannet, *et al.*, Comparative efficacy of repetitive nerve stimulation, exercise, and cold in differentiating myotonic disorders. *Muscle Nerve* **36** (2007), 643–650.
6. S. C. Cannon, Pathomechanisms in channelopathies of skeletal muscle and brain. *Annu. Rev. Neurosci.* **29** (2006), 387–415.
7. K. Jurkat-Rott, F. Lehmann-Horn, Muscle channelopathies and critical points in functional and genetic studies. *J. Clin. Invest.* **115** (2005), 2000–2009.
8. B. Fontaine, T. S. Khurana, E. P. Hoffman, *et al.*, Hyperkalemic periodic paralysis and the adult muscle sodium channel alphasubunit gene. *Science* **250** (1990), 1000–1002.
9. E. P. Hoffman, P. F. Lehmann-Horn, R. Rudel, Overexcited or inactive: ion channels in muscle disease. *Cell* **80** (1995), 681–686.
10. J. Thomsen, Töniche Krämpfe in willkürlich beweglichen Muskeln in Folge von ererbter psychisscher. *Arch. Psychiatrie Nervenkranheiten* **6** (1876), 702–718.
11. P. E. Becker, Zür frage der heterogenie der erblichen myotonien. *Nervenartz.* **28** (1957), 455–460.
12. F. Lehmann-Horn, V. Mailander, R. Heine, A. L. George, Myotonia levior is a chloride channel disorder. *Hum. Mol. Genet.* **4** (1995), 1397–1402.
13. S. Nagamitsu, T. Matsuura, M. Khajavi, *et al.*, A "dystrophic" variant of autosomal recessive myotonia congenita caused by novel mutations in the CLCN1 gene. *Neurology* **55** (2000), 1697–1703.
14. J. Rosenfeld, K. Sloan-Brown, A. L. George Jr., A novel muscle sodium channel mutation causes painful congenital myotonia. *Ann. Neurol.* **42** (1997), 811–814.
15. G. Drost, J. P. Van Dijk, D. F. Stegeman, B. G. Van Engelen, M. J. Zwarts, Maintaining constant voluntary force in generalized myotonia despite muscle membrane disturbances: insights from a high-density surface EMG study. *J. Clin. Neurophysiol.* **21** (2004), 114–123.
16. R. J. Lipicky, S. H. Bryant, Sodium, potassium, and chloride fluxes in intercostal muscle from normal goats and goats with hereditary myotonia. *J. Gen. Physiol.* **50** (1966), 89–111.
17. G. Mehrke, H. Brinkmeier, H. Jockusch, The myotonic mouse mutant ADR: electrophysiology of the muscle fiber. *Muscle Nerve* **11** (1988), 440–446.
18. K. Steinmeyer, C. Ortland, T. J. Jentsch, Primary structure and functional expression of a developmentally regulated skeletal muscle chloride channel. *Nature* **354** (1991), 301–304.
19. K. Steinmeyer, R. Klocke, C. Ortland, *et al.*, Inactivation of muscle chloride channel by transposon insertion in myotonic mice. *Nature* **354** (1991), 304–308.
20. J. A. Abdalla, W. L. Casley, H. K. Cousin, *et al.*, Linkage of Thomsen disease to the T cell receptor beta (TCRB) locus on chromosome 7q35. *Am. J. Hum. Genet.* **51** (1992), 579–584.
21. M. C. Koch, K. Steinmeyer, C. Lorenz, *et al.*, The skeletal muscle chloride channel in dominant and recessive human myotonia. *Science* **257** (1992), 797–800.
22. A. L. George Jr, M. A. Crackower, J. A. Abdalla, A. J. Hudson, G. C. Ebers, Molecular basis of Thomsen's disease (autosomal dominant myotonia congenita). *Nat. Genet.* **3** (1993), 305–310.
23. C. De Diego, J. Gamez, E. Plassart-Schiess, *et al.*, Novel mutations in the muscle chloride channel CLCN1 gene causing myotonia congenita in Spanish families. *J. Neurol.* **246** (1999), 825–829.
24. A. L. George Jr, K. Sloan-Brown, G. M. Fenichel, G. A. Mitchell, R. Spiegel, R. M. Pascuzzi, Nonsense and missense mutations of the muscle chloride channel gene in patients with myotonia congenita. *Hum. Mol. Genet.* **3** (1994), 2071–2072.
25. P. P. Koty, E. Pegoraro, G. Hobson, *et al.*, Myotonia and the muscle chloride channel: dominant mutations show variable penetrance and founder effect. *Neurology* **47** (1996), 963–968.
26. C. Lorenz, C. Meyer-Kleine, K. Steinmeyer, M. C. Koch, T. J. Jentsch, Genomic organization of the human muscle chloride channel CIC1 and analysis of novel mutations leading to Beckertype myotonia. *Hum. Mol. Genet.* **3** (1994), 941–946.
27. V. Mailander, R. Heine, F. Deymeer, F. Lehmann-Horn, Novel muscle chloride channel mutations and their effects on heterozygous carriers. *Am. J. Hum. Genet.* **58** (1996), 317–324.
28. C. Meyer-Kleine, K. Steinmeyer, K. Ricker, T. J. Jentsch, M. C. Koch, Spectrum of mutations in the major human skeletal

muscle chloride channel gene (CLCN1) leading to myotonia. *Am. J. Hum. Genet.* **57** (1995), 1325–1334.

29. H. Papponen, T. Toppinen, P. Baumann, *et al.*, Founder mutations and the high prevalence of myotonia congenita in northern Finland. *Neurology* **53** (1999), 297–302.
30. F. F. WuF, A. Ryan, J. Devaney, *et al.*, Novel CLCN1 mutations with unique clinical and electrophysiological consequences. *Brain* **125** (2002), 2392–2407.
31. J. Zhang, A. L. George Jr., R. C. Griggs, *et al.*, Mutations in the human skeletal muscle chloride channel gene (CLCN1) associated with dominant and recessive myotonia congenita. *Neurology* **47** (1996), 993–8.
32. C. Fahlke, T. Knittle, C. A. Gurnett, K. P. Campbell, A. L. George Jr., Subunit stoichiometry of human muscle chloride channels. *J. Gen. Physiol.* **109** (1997), 93–104.
33. C. Kubisch, T. Schmidt-Rose, B. Fontaine, A. H. Bretag, T. J. Jentsch, ClC1 chloride channel mutations in myotonia congenita: variable penetrance of mutations shifting the voltage dependence. *Hum. Mol. Genet.* **7** (1998), 1753–1760.
34. K. Steinmeyer, C. Lorenz, M. Pusch, M. C. Koch, T. J. Jentsch, Multimeric structure of ClC1 chloride channel revealed by mutations in dominant myotonia congenita (Thomsen). *EMBO J.* **13** (1994), 737–743.
35. C. Fahlke, E. Zachar, R. Rudel, Chloride channels with reduced single-channel conductance in recessive myotonia congenita. *Neuron* **10** (1993), 225–232.
36. R. Heine, A. L. George Jr., U. Pika, F. Deymeer, R. Rudel, F. Lehmann-Horn, Proof of a nonfunctional muscle chloride channel in recessive myotonia congenita (Becker) by detection of a 4 base pair deletion. *Hum. Mol. Genet.* **3** (1994), 1123–1128.
37. B. J. Simpson, T. A. Height, G. Y. Rychkov, *et al.*, Characterization of three myotonia-associated mutations of the CLCN1 chloride channel gene via heterologous expression. *Hum. Mutat.* **24** (2004), 185.
38. J. Zhang, M. C. Sanguinetti, H. Kwiecinski, L. J. Ptacek, Mechanism of inverted activation of ClC1 channels caused by a novel myotonia congenita mutation. *J. Biol. Chem.* **275** (2000), 2999–3005.
39. D. Fialho, S. Schorge, U. Pucovska, *et al.*, Chloride channel myotonia: exon 8 hotspot for dominant negative interactions. *Brain* **130**:Pt 12 (2007), 3265–3274.
40. F. Deymeer, F. Lehmann-Horn, P. Serdaroglu, *et al.*, Electrical myotonia in heterozygous carriers of recessive myotonia congenita. *Muscle Nerve* **22** (1999), 123–125.
41. E. Plassart-Schiess, A. Gervais, B. Eymard, *et al.*, Novel muscle chloride channel (CLCN1) mutations in myotonia congenita with various modes of inheritance including incomplete dominance and penetrance. *Neurology* **50** (1998a), 1176–1179.
42. M. Duno, E. Colding-Jorgensen, M. Grunnet, T. Jespersen, J. Vissing, M. Schwartz, Difference in allelic expression of the CLCN1 gene and the possible influence on the myotonia congenita phenotype. *Eur. J. Hum. Genet.* **12** (2004), 738–743.
43. D. C. Camerino, S. Pierno, A. de Luca, S. H. Bryant, Antimyotonic effects of tocainide enantiomers on skeletal muscle fibers of congenitally myotonic goats. *Neuromuscul. Disord.* **10** (2000), 160–164.
44. G. Meola, V. Sansone, Treatment in myotonia and periodic paralysis. *Rev. Neurol. (Paris).* **160** (2004), S55–S69.
45. J. Trip, G. Drost, B. G. Van Engelen, C. G. Faber, Drug treatment for myotonia. *Cochrane Database Syst. Rev.* (2006) CD004762.
46. C. S. Rogers, C. G. Vanoye, B. A. Sullenger, A. L. George Jr., Functional repair of a mutant chloride channel using a transsplicing ribozyme. *J. Clin. Invest.* **110** (2002), 1783–1789.
47. A. Von Eulenburg, Über eine familiäre durch 6 Generationen verfolgbare Form kongenitaler Paramyotonie. *Neurol. Zentralbl.* **5** (1886), 265–272.
48. Y. Pereon, G. Lande, S. Demolombe, *et al.*, Paramyotonia congenita with an SCN4A mutation affecting cardiac repolarization. *Neurology* **60** (2003), 340–342.
49. P. J. Blijham, G. Drost, D. F. Stegeman, M. J. Zwarts, Reduced muscle-fiber conduction but normal slowing after cold exposure in paramyotonia congenita. *Muscle Nerve* **37**:1 (2008), 23–26.
50. M. A. Weber, S. Nielles-Vallespin, H. B. Huttner, *et al.*, Evaluation of patients with paramyotonia at ^{23}Na MR imaging during cold-induced weakness. *Radiology* **240** (2006), 489–500.
51. G. C. Ebers, A. L. George, R. L. Barchi, *et al.*, Paramyotonia congenita and hyperkalemic periodic paralysis are linked to the adult muscle sodium channel gene. *Ann. Neurol.* **30** (1991), 810–816.
52. M. C. Koch, K. Ricker, M. Otto, *et al.*, Linkage data suggesting allelic heterogeneity for paramyotonia congenita and hyperkalemic periodic paralysis on chromosome 17. *Hum. Genet.* **88** (1991), 71–74.
53. L. J. Ptacekj, J. S. Trimmer, W. S. Agnew, J. W. Roberts, J. H. Petajan, M. Leppert, Paramyotonia congenita and hyperkalemic periodic paralysis map to the same sodium channel gene locus. *Am. J. Hum. Genet.* **49** (1991), 851–854.
54. A. I. McClatchey, D. Mckenna-Yasek, D. Cros, *et al.*, Novel mutations in families with unusual and variable disorders of the skeletal muscle sodium channel. *Nat. Genet.* **2** (1992), 148–152.
55. A. I. McClatchey, P. Van Den Bergh, M. A. Pericak-Vance, *et al.*, Temperature-sensitive mutations in the IIIIV cytoplasmic loop region of the skeletal muscle sodium channel gene in paramyotonia congenita. *Cell* **68** (1992), 769–774.
56. L. J. Ptacek, A. L. George Jr., R. L. Barchi, *et al.*, Mutations in an S4 segment of the adult skeletal muscle sodium channel cause paramyotonia congenita. *Neuron* **8** (1992), 891–897.
57. K. Borg, G. Ahlberg, M. Anvret, C4342Tmutation in the SCN4A gene on chromosome 17q in a Swedish family with paramyotonia congenita (Eulenburg) correlations with clinical, neurophysiological and muscle biopsy data. *Neuromuscul. Disord.* **7** (1997), 231–233.
58. H. Lerche, N. Mitrovic, V. Dubowitz, F. Lehmann-Horn, Paramyotonia congenita: the R1448P Na^+ channel mutation in adult human skeletal muscle. *Ann. Neurol.* **39** (1996), 599–608.
59. C. Meyer-Kleine, M. Otto, B. Zoll, M. C. Koch, Molecular and genetic characterisation of German families with paramyotonia congenita and demonstration of founder effect in the Ravensberg families. *Hum. Genet.* **93** (1994), 707–710.
60. E. Plassart, B. Eymard, L. Maurs, *et al.*, Paramyotonia congenita: genotype to phenotype correlations in two families and report of a new mutation in the sodium channel gene. *J. Neurol. Sci.* **142** (1996), 126–133.

61. E. Plassart, J. Reboul, C. S. Rime, *et al.*, Mutations in the muscle sodium channel gene (SCN4A) in 13 French families with hyperkalemic periodic paralysis and paramyotonia congenita: phenotype to genotype correlations and demonstration of the predominance of two mutations. *Eur. J. Hum. Genet.* **2** (1994), 110–124.

62. R. Rudel, F. Lehmann-Horn, Paramyotonia, potassium-aggravated myotonias and periodic paralyses. 37th ENMC International Workshop, Naarden, The Netherlands, 8–10 December 1995. *Neuromuscul. Disord.* **7** (1997), 127–132.

63. R. Sasaki, H. Takano, K. Kamakura, *et al.*, A novel mutation in the gene for the adult skeletal muscle sodium channel alpha-subunit (SCN4A) that causes paramyotonia congenita of von Eulenburg. *Arch. Neurol.* **56** (1999), 692–696.

64. S. Bendahhou, R. Cummins, N. Kwiecinski, G. Waxman, J. Ptacek, Characterization of a new sodium channel mutation at arginine 1448 associated with moderate paramyotonia congenita in humans. *J. Physiol (Lond.)* **518**:2 (1999), 337–344.

65. L. J. Ptacek, L. Gouw, H. Kwiecinski, *et al.*, Sodium channel mutations in paramyotonia congenita and hyperkalemic periodic paralysis. *Ann. Neurol.* **33** (1993), 300–307.

66. M. Bouhours, S. Luce, D. Sternberg, J. C. Willer, B. Fontaine, N. Tabti, A1152D mutation of the Na^+ channel causes paramyotonia congenita and emphasizes the role of DIII/S4S5 linker in fast inactivation. *J. Physiol. (Lond.)* **565** (2005), 415–427.

67. M. Bouhours, D. Sternberg, C. S. Davoine, *et al.*, Functional characterization and cold sensitivity of T1313a, a new mutation of the skeletal muscle sodium channel causing paramyotonia congenita in humans. *J. Physiol. (Lond.)* **554** (2004), 635–647.

68. S. C. Cannon, Spectrum of sodium channel disturbances in the nondystrophic myotonias and periodic paralyses. *Kidney Int.* **57** (2000), 772–779.

69. M. Chanine, A. L. George, Jr., M. Zhou, *et al.*, Sodium channel mutations in paramyotonia congenita uncouple inactivation from activation. *Neuron* **12** (1994), 281–294.

70. J. F. Desaphy, D. C. Camerino, V. Tortorella, A. De Luca, Effect of mexiletine on sea anemone toxin-induced non-inactivating sodium channels of rat skeletal muscle: a model of sodium channel myotonia. *Neuromuscul. Disord.* **9** (1999), 182–189.

71. H. Lerche, R. Heine, U. Pika, *et al.*, Human sodium channel myotonia: slowed channel inactivation due to substitutions for a glycine within the IIIIV linker. *J. Physiol. (Lond.)* **470** (1993), 13–22.

72. N. Mitrovic, A. L. George Jr., R. Rudel, F. Lehmann-Horn, H. Lerche, Mutant channels contribute <50% to Na^+ current in paramyotonia congenita muscle. *Brain* **122**:Pt 6 (1999), 1085–1092.

73. E. Plassart-Schiess, L. Lhuillier, A. L. George Jr., B. Fontaine, N. Tabti, Functional expression of the Ile693Thr Na^+ channel mutation associated with paramyotonia congenita in a human cell line. *J. Physiol. (Lond.)* **507**:Pt 3 (1998b), 721–727.

74. J. E. Richmond, D. E. Featherstone, P. C. Ruben, Human Na+ channel fast and slow inactivation in paramyotonia congenita mutants expressed in *Xenopus laevis* oocytes. *J. Physiol. (Lond.)* **499**:Pt 3 (1997), 589–600.

75. A. J. Tahmoush, K. L. Schaller, P. Zhang, T. Hyslop, T. Heiman-Patterson, J. H. Caldwell, Muscle sodium channel inactivation defect in paramyotonia congenita with the thr1313met mutation. *Neuromuscul. Disord.* **4** (1994), 447–454.

76. N. Yang, S. Ji, M. Zhou, *et al.*, Sodium channel mutations in paramyotonia congenita exhibit similar biophysical phenotypes in vitro. *Proc. Natl. Acad. Sci. U. S. A.* **91** (1994), 12785–12789.

77. A. De Luca, S. Pierno, A. Liantonio, *et al.*, New potent mexiletine and tocainide analogues evaluated in vivo and in vitro as antimyotonic agents on the myotonic ADR mouse. *Neuromuscul. Disord.* **14** (2004), 405–416.

78. J. F. Desaphy, A. De Luca, M. P. Didonna, A. L. George Jr., D. Camerino Conte, Different flecainide sensitivity of hNav1. 4 channels and myotonic mutants explained by state-dependent block. *J. Physiol. (Lond.)* **554** (2004), 321–334.

79. A. Duranti, C. Franchini, G. Lentini, *et al.*, Homologation of mexiletine alkyl chain and stereo-selective blockade of skeletal muscle sodium channels. *Eur. J. Med. Chem.* **35** (2000), 147–156.

80. C. E. Jackson, R. J. Barohn, L. J. Ptacek, Paramyotonia congenita: abnormal short exercise test, and improvement after mexiletine therapy. *Muscle Nerve* **17** (1994), 763–768.

81. B. Mohammadi, K. Jurkat-Rott, A. Alekov, R. Dengler, J. Bufler, F. Lehmann-Horn, Preferred mexiletine block of human sodium channels with IVS4 mutations and its pH dependence. *Pharmacogenet. Genomics* **15** (2005), 235–244.

82. M. P. Takahashi, S. C. Cannon, Mexiletine block of disease-associated mutations in S6 segments of the human skeletal muscle Na(+) channel. *J. Physiol. (Lond.)* **537** (2001), 701–714.

83. G. K. Wang, C. Russell, S. Y. Wang, Mexiletine block of wild-type and inactivation-deficient human skeletal muscle hNav1.4 Na+ channels. *J. Physiol. (Lond.)* **554** (2004), 621–633.

84. K. Ricker, R. T. Moxley, R. Heine 3rd, F. Lehmann-Horn, Myotonia fluctuans. A third type of muscle sodium channel disease. *Arch. Neurol.* **51** (1994), 1095–1102.

85. D. Ferriby, T. Stojkovic, D. Sternberg, J. F. Hurtevent, J. P. Hurtevent, P. Vermersch, A new case of autosomal dominant myotonia associated with the V1589M missense mutation in the muscle sodium channel gene and its phenotypic classification. *Neuromuscul. Disord.* **16** (2006), 321–324.

86. R. Heine, U. Pika, F. Lehmann-Horn, A novel SCN4A mutation causing myotonia aggravated by cold and potassium. *Hum. Mol. Genet.* **2**:9 (1993), 1349–1353.

87. M. C. Koch, K. Baumbach, A. L. George, K. Ricker, Paramyotonia congenita without paralysis on exposure to cold: a novel mutation in the SCN4A gene (Val1293Ile). *Neuroreport* **6** (1995), 2001–2004.

88. N. Mitrovic, A. L. George Jr., R. Heine, *et al.*, K(+)aggravated myotonia: destabilization of the inactivated state of the human muscle Na+ channel by the V1589M mutation. *J. Physiol. (Lond.)* **478**:Pt 3 (1994), 395–402.

89. R. W. Orrell, K. Jurkat-Rott, F. Lehmann-Horn, R. J. Lane, Familial cramp due to potassium-aggravated myotonia. *J. Neurol. Neurosurg. Psychiatry* **65** (1998), 569–572.

90. B. G. Schoser, J. M. Schroder, T. Grimm, D. Sternberg, W. Kress, A large German kindred with cold-aggravated myotonia and a heterozygous A1481D mutation in the SCN4A gene. *Muscle Nerve* **35** (2007), 599–606.

91. S. Vicart, D. Sternberg, B. Fontaine, G. Meola, Human skeletal muscle sodium channelopathies. *Neurol. Sci.* **26** (2005), 194–202.

92. F. F. Wu, E. Gordon, E. P. Hoffman, S. C. Cannon, A C-terminal skeletal muscle sodium channel mutation associated with myotonia disrupts fast inactivation. *J. Physiol. (Lond.)* **565** (2005), 371–380.

93. E. Colding-Jorgensen, M. Duno, J. Vissing, Autosomal dominant monosymptomatic myotonia permanens. *Neurology* **67** (2006), 153–155.

94. J. Trip, C. G. Faber, H. B. Ginjaar, B. G. Van Engelen, G. Drost, Warm-up phenomenon in myotonia associated with the V445M sodium channel mutation. *J. Neurol.* **254** (2007), 257–258.

95. G. M. Vita, A. Olckers, A. E. Jedlicka, *et al.*, Masseter muscle rigidity associated with glycine1306 to alanine mutation in the adult muscle sodium channel alpha-subunit gene. *Anesthesiology* **82** (1995), 1097–1103.

96. D. C. Aberfeld, L. P. Hinterbuchner, M. Schneider, Myotonia, dwarfism, diffuse bone disease and unusual ocular and facial abnormalities (a new syndrome). *Brain* **88** (1965), 313–322.

97. O. Schwartz, R. S. Jampel, Congenital blepharophimosis associated with a unique generalized myopathy. *Arch. Ophthalmol.* **68** (1962), 52–57.

98. D. Viljoen, P. Beighton, Schwartz-Jampel syndrome (chondrodystrophic myotonia). *J. Med. Genet.* **29** (1992), 58–62.

99. A. Giedion, Heterogeneity in Schwartz-Jampel chondrodystrophic myotonia. *Pediatr. Radiol.* **27** (1997), 454.

100. S. Nicole, H. Topaloglu, B. Fontaine, 102nd ENMC International Workshop on Schwartz-Jampel syndrome, 14–16 December, 2001, Naarden, The Netherlands. *Neuromuscul. Disord.* **13** (2003), 347–351.

101. S. Nicole, C. Ben Hamida, P. Beighton, *et al.*, Localization of the Schwartz-Jampel syndrome (SJS) locus to chromosome 1p34p36.1 by homozygosity mapping. *Hum. Mol. Genet.* **4** (1995), 1633–1636.

102. S. Nicole, C. S. Davoine, H. Topaloglu, *et al.*, Perlecan, the major proteoglycan of basement membranes, is altered in patients with Schwartz-Jampel syndrome (chondrodystrophic myotonia). *Nat. Genet.* **26** (2000), 480–483.

103. E. Arikawa-Hirasawa, A. H. Le, I. Nishino, *et al.*, Structural and functional mutations of the perlecan gene cause Schwartz-Jampel syndrome, with myotonic myopathy and chondrodysplasia. *Am. J. Hum. Genet.* **70** (2002a), 1368–1375.

104. M. Stum, C. S. Davoine, S. Vicart, *et al.*, Spectrum of HSPG2 (Perlecan) mutations in patients with Schwartz-Jampel syndrome. *Hum. Mutat.* **27** (2006), 1082–1091.

105. E. Arikawa-Hirasawa, S. G. Rossi, R. L. Rotundo, Y. Yamada, Absence of acetylcholinesterase at the neuromuscular junctions of perlecan-null mice. *Nat. Neurosci.* **5** (2002b), 119–123.

106. H. Topaloglu, A. Serdaroglu, M. Okan, K. Gucuyener, M. Topcu, Improvement of myotonia with carbamazepine in three cases with the Schwartz-Jampel syndrome. *Neuropediatrics* **24** (1993), 232–234.

107. T. P. Links, M. J. Zwarts, J. T. Wilmink, W. M. Molenaar, H. J. Oosterhuis, Permanent muscle weakness in familial hypokalaemic periodic paralysis. Clinical, radiological and pathological aspects. *Brain* **113**:Pt 6 (1990), 1873–1889.

108. I. M. Kantola, L. T. Tarssanen, Familial hypokalaemic periodic paralysis in Finland. *J. Neurol. Neurosurg. Psychiatry* **55** (1992), 322–324.

109. B. Fontaine, Primary periodic paralysis and muscle sodium channel. *Adv. Nephrol. Necker. Hosp.* **23** (1994), 191–197.

110. B. Fontaine, J. Vale-Santos, K. Jurkat-Rott, *et al.*, Mapping of the hypokalaemic periodic paralysis (HypoPP) locus to chromosome 1q31–32 in three European families. *Nat. Genet.* **6** (1994), 267–272.

111. A. Elbaz, J. Vale-Santos, K. Jurkat-Rott, *et al.*, Hypokalemic periodic paralysis and the dihydropyridine receptor (CACNL1A3): genotype/phenotype correlations for two predominant mutations and evidence for the absence of a founder effect in 16 Caucasian families. *Am. J. Hum. Genet.* **56** (1995), 374–380.

112. G. Fouad, M. Dalakas, S. Servidei, *et al.*, Genotype-phenotype correlations of DHP receptor alpha 1subunit gene mutations causing hypokalemic periodic paralysis. *Neuromuscul. Disord.* **7** (1997), 33–38.

113. T. M. Miller, M. R. Dias Da Silva, H. A. Miller, *et al.*, Correlating phenotype and genotype in the periodic paralyses. *Neurology* **63** (2004), 1647–1655.

114. D. E. Bulman, K. A. Scoggan, M. D. Van Oene, *et al.*, A novel sodium channel mutation in a family with hypokalemic periodic paralysis. *Neurology* **53** (1999), 1932–1936.

115. N. P. Davies, L. H. Eunson, M. Samuel, M. G. Hanna, Sodium channel gene mutations in hypokalemic periodic paralysis: An uncommon cause in the UK. *Neurology* **57** (2001), 1323–1325.

116. D. Sternberg, T. Maisonobe, K. Jurkat-Rott, *et al.*, Hypokalaemic periodic paralysis type 2 caused by mutations at codon 672 in the muscle sodium channel gene SCN4A. *Brain* **124** (2001), 1091–1099.

117. N. M. Plaster, R. Tawil, M. Tristani-Firouzi, *et al.*, Mutations in Kir2.1 cause the developmental and episodic electrical phenotypes of Andersen's syndrome. *Cell* **105** (2001), 511–519.

118. M. R. Ziegler, I. McQuarrie, Hereditary periodic paralysis. I. Effects of various induced changes in physiological state on paralytic attacks. *Metabolism* **1**:2 (1952), 116–128.

119. P. T. Rowley, B. Kliman, The effect of sodium loading and depletion on muscular strength and aldosterone excretion in familial periodic paralysis. *Am. J. Med.* **28** (1960), 376–385.

120. J. S. Resnick, W. K. Engel, Myotonic lid lag in hypokalaemic periodic paralysis. *J. Neurol. Neurosurg. Psychiatry* **30** (1967), 47–51.

121. A. Biemond, A. P. Daniels, Familial periodic paralysis and its transition into spinal muscular atrophy. *Brain* **57** (1934), 91–108.

122. A. G. Engel, E. H. Lambert, J. W. Rosevear, W. N. Tauxe, Clinical and electromyographic studies in a patient with primary hypokalaemic periodic paralysis. *Am. J. Med.* **38** (1965), 626–640.

123. J. A. Bender, Family periodic paralysis in a girl aged seventeen. *Arch. Neurol. Psychiatry* **35** (1936), 131–135.

124. T. P. Links, A. J. Smit, W. M. Molenaar, M. J. Zwarts, H. J. Oosterhuis, Familial hypokalemic periodic paralysis. Clinical, diagnostic and therapeutic aspects. *J. Neurol. Sci.* **122** (1994), 33–43.

125. J. De Keyser, J. Smitz, R. Malfait, G. Ebinger, Rhabdomyolysis in hypokalaemic periodic paralysis: a clue to the mechanism that terminates the paralytic attack? *J. Neurol.* **234** (1987), 119–121.

126. J. J. Schipperheyn, O. J. Buruma, P. J. Voogd, Hypokalaemic periodic paralysis and cardiomyopathy. *Acta Neurol. Scand.* **58** (1978), 374–378.

127. I. Gamstorp, Adynamia episodica hereditaria. *Acta Paediatr. Scand.* **45** (1956), 1–126.

128. R. B. Layzer, R. E. Lovelace, L. P. Rowland, Hyperkalemic periodic paralysis. *Arch. Neurol.* **16** (1967), 455–472.

129. M. Saunders, B. Ashworth, A. E. Emery, J. E. Benedikz, Familial myotonic periodic paralysis with muscle wasting. *Brain* **91** (1968), 295–304.

130. W. G. Bradley, R. Taylor, D. R. Rice, *et al.*, Progressive myopathy in hyperkalemic periodic paralysis. *Arch. Neurol.* **47** (1990), 1013–1017.

131. L. J. Ptacek, A. L. George Jr, R. C. Griggs, *et al.*, Identification of a mutation in the gene causing hyperkalemic periodic paralysis. *Cell* **67** (1991), 1021–1027.

132. D. C. Poskanzer, D. N. Kerr, A third type of periodic paralysis, with normokalemia and favourable response to sodium chloride. *Am. J. Med.* **31** (1961), 328–342.

133. K. R. Meyers, D. H. Gilden, C. F. Rinaldi, J. L. Hansen, Periodic muscle weakness, normokalemia, and tubular aggregates. *Neurology* **22** (1972), 269–279.

134. T. S. Danowski, E. R. Fisher, C. Vidalon, *et al.*, Clinical and ultrastructural observations in a kindred with normohyperkalaemic periodic paralysis. *J. Med. Genet.* **12** (1975), 20–28.

135. P. F. Chinnery, T. J. Walls, M. G. Hanna, D. Bates, P. R. Fawcett, Normokalemic periodic paralysis revisited: does it exist? *Ann. Neurol.* **52** (2002), 251–252.

136. S. M. De Silva, R. W. Kuncl, J. W. Griffin, D. R. Cornblath, S. Chavoustie, Paramyotonia congenita or hyperkalemic periodic paralysis? Clinical and electrophysiological features of each entity in one family. *Muscle Nerve* **13** (1990), 21–26.

137. J. Kim, Y. Hahn, E. H. Sohn, *et al.*, Phenotypic variation of a Thr704Met mutation in skeletal sodium channel gene in a family with paralysis periodica paramyotonica. *J. Neurol. Neurosurg. Psychiatry* **70** (2001), 618–623.

138. E. D. Andersen, P. A. Krasilnikoff, H. Overvad, Intermittent muscular weakness, extrasystoles, and multiple developmental anomalies. A new syndrome? *Acta Paediatr. Scand.* **60** (1971), 559–564.

139. M. Tristani-Firouzi, J. L. Jensen, M. R. Donaldson, *et al.*, Functional and clinical characterization of KCNJ2 mutations associated with LQT7 (Andersen syndrome). *J. Clin. Invest.* **110** (2002), 381–388.

140. G. Andelfinger, A. R. Tapper, R. C. Welch, C. G. Vanoye, A. L. George Jr., D. W. Benson, KCNJ2 mutation results in Andersen syndrome with sex-specific cardiac and skeletal muscle phenotypes. *Am. J. Hum. Genet.* **71** (2002), 663–668.

141. M. R. Donaldson, J. L. Jensen, M. Tristani-Firouzi, *et al.*, PIP2 binding residues of Kir2.1 are common targets of mutations causing Andersen syndrome. *Neurology* **60** (2003), 1811–1816.

142. S. Canun, N. Perez, L. G. Beirana, Andersen syndrome autosomal dominant in three generations. *Am. J. Med. Genet.* **85** (1999), 147–156.

143. L. Zhang, D. W. Benson, M. Tristani-Firouzi, *et al.*, Electrocardiographic features in Andersen-Tawil syndrome patients with KCNJ2 mutations: characteristic TU-wave patterns predict the KCNJ2 genotype. *Circulation* **111** (2005), 2720–2726.

144. K. M. Chen, T. P. Hung, T. Y. Lin, Periodic paralysis in Taiwan. Clinical study of 28 cases. *Arch. Neurol.* **12** (1965), 165–171.

145. A. J. McFadzean, R. Yeung, Periodic paralysis complicating thyrotoxicosis in Chinese. *Br. Med. J.* **1** (1967), 451–455.

146. K. P. Ober, Thyrotoxic periodic paralysis in the United States. Report of 7 cases and review of the literature. *Medicine (Baltimore)* **71** (1992), 109–120.

147. A. W. Kung, K. S. Lau, G. C. Fong, V. Chan, Association of novel single nucleotide polymorphisms in the calcium channel alpha 1 subunit gene (Ca(v)1.1) and thyrotoxic periodic paralysis. *J. Clin. Endocrinol. Metab.* **89** (2004), 1340–1345.

148. D. E. Kelley, H. Gharib, F. P. Kennedy, R. J. Duda Jr., P. G. Mcmanis, Thyrotoxic periodic paralysis. Report of 10 cases and review of electromyographic findings. *Arch. Intern. Med.* **149** (1989), 2597–2600.

149. S. Okinaka, K. Shizume, S. Iino, *et al.*, The association of periodic paralysis and hyperthyroidism in Japan. *J. Clin. Endocrinol. Metab.* **17** (1957), 1454–1459.

150. W. M. Kufs, M. Mcbiles, T. Jurney, Familial thyrotoxic periodic paralysis. *West. J. Med.* **150** (1989), 461–463.

151. M. R. Dias Da Silva, J. M. Cerutti, L. A. Arnaldi, R. M. Maciel, A mutation in the KCNE3 potassium channel gene is associated with susceptibility to thyrotoxic hypokalemic periodic paralysis. *J. Clin. Endocrinol. Metab.* **87** (2002), 4881–4884.

152. J. Fisher, Thyrotoxic periodic paralysis with ventricular fibrillation. *Arch. Intern. Med.* **142** (1982), 1362–1364.

153. A. Tsujino, C. Maertens, K. Ohno, *et al.*, Myasthenic syndrome caused by mutation of the SCN4A sodium channel. *Proc. Natl. Acad. Sci. U.S.A.* **100** (2003), 7377–7382.

154. L. J. Ptacek, R. Tawil, R. C. Griggs, *et al.*, Dihydropyridine receptor mutations cause hypokalemic periodic paralysis. *Cell* **77** (1994), 863–868.

155. Q. Wang, M. Liu, C. Xy, *et al.*, Novel CACNA1S mutation causes autosomal dominant hypokalemic periodic paralysis in a Chinese family. *J. Mol. Med.* **83**:3 (2005), 203–208.

156. C. V. Rojas, J. Z. Wang, L. S. Schwartz, *et al.*, A Met to Val mutation in the skeletal muscle Na+ channel alpha-subunit in hyperkalaemic periodic paralysis. *Nature* **354** (1991), 387–389.

157. S. Sokolov, T. Scheuer, W. A. Catterall, Gating pore current in an inherited ion channelopathy. *Nature* **446** (2007), 76–79.

158. P. G. McManis, E. H. Lambert, J. R. Daube, The exercise test in periodic paralysis. *Muscle Nerve* **9** (1986), 704–710.

159. E. W. Streib, S. F. Sun, M. Hanson, Paramyotonia congenita: clinical and electrophysiologic studies. *Electromyogr. Clin. Neurophysiol.* **23** (1983), 315–325.

160. O. J. Buruma, G. T. Bots, Myopathy in familial hypokalaemic periodic paralysis independent of paralytic attacks. *Acta Neurol. Scand.* **57** (1978), 171–179.

161. B. McArdle, Adynamia epdisodica hereditaria and its treatment. *Brain* **85** (1962), 121–148.

162. P. Wang, T. Clausen, Treatment of attacks in hyperkalaemic familial periodic paralysis by inhalation of salbutamol. *Lancet* **1** (1976), 221–223.

163. P. E. Bendheim, E. O. Reale, B. O. Berg, Beta-adrenergic treatment of hyperkalemic periodic paralysis. *Neurology* **35** (1985), 746–749.

164. M. G. Hanna, J. Stewart, A. H. Schapira, N. W. Wood, J. A. Morgan-Hughes, N. M. Murray, Salbutamol treatment in a patient with hyperkalaemic periodic paralysis due to a mutation in the skeletal muscle sodium channel gene (SCN4A). *J. Neurol. Neurosurg. Psychiatry* **65** (1998), 248–250.

165. J. S. Resnick, W. K. Engel, R. C. Griggs, A. C. Stam, Acetazolamide prophylaxis in hypokalemic periodic paralysis. *N. Engl. J. Med.* **278** (1968), 582–586.

166. R. C. Griggs, W. K. Engel, J. S. Resnick, Acetazolamide treatment of hypokalemic periodic paralysis. Prevention of attacks and improvement of persistent weakness. *Ann. Intern. Med.* **73** (1970), 39–48.

167. M. C. Dalakas, W. K. Engel, Treatment of "permanent" muscle weakness in familial hypokalemic periodic paralysis. *Muscle Nerve* **6** (1983), 182–186.

168. A. Kuzmenkin, V. Muncan, K. Jurkat-Rott, *et al.*, Enhanced inactivation and pH sensitivity of Na(+) channel mutations causing hypokalaemic periodic paralysis type II. *Brain* **125** (2002), 835–843.

169. R. Tawil, R. T. Moxley III, R. C. Griggs, Acetazolamide-induced nephrolithiasis: implications for treatment of neuromuscular disorders. *Neurology* **43** (1993), 1105–1106.

170. R. Tawil, M. P. McDermott, R. Brown Jr., *et al.*, Randomized trials of dichlorphenamide in the periodic paralyses. Working Group on Periodic Paralysis. *Ann. Neurol.* **47** (2000), 46–53.

171. M. K. Kim, S. H. Lee, M. S. Park, *et al.*, Mutation screening in Korean hypokalemic periodic paralysis patients: a novel SCN4A Arg672Cys mutation. *Neuromuscul. Disord.* **14** (2004), 727–731.

172. R. Junker, W. Haverkamp, E. Schulze-Bahr, L. Eckardt, W. Paulus, R. Kiefer, Amiodarone and acetazolamide for the treatment of genetically confirmed severe Andersen syndrome. *Neurology* **59**:3 (2002), 466.

173. R. J. Gould, C. N. Steeg, A. B. Eastwood, A. S. Penn, L. P. Rowland, D. C. De Vivo, Potentially fatal cardiac dysrhythmia and hyperkalemic periodic paralysis. *Neurology* **35** (1985), 1208–1212.

174. R. Tawil, L. J. Ptacek, S. G. Pavlakis, *et al.*, Andersen's syndrome: potassium-sensitive periodic paralysis, ventricular ectopy, and dysmorphic features. *Ann. Neurol.* **35** (1994), 326–330.

175. T. Kobayashi, K. Washiyama, K. Ikeda, Inhibition of G protein-activated inwardly rectifying K+ channels by various antidepressant drugs. *Neuropsychopharmacology* **29** (2004), 1841–1851.

176. R. E. Garcia-Ferreiro, D. Kerschensteiner, F. Major, F. Monje, W. Stuhmer, L. A. Pardo, Mechanism of block of hEag1 K+ channels by imipramine and astemizole. *J. Gen. Physiol.* **124** (2004), 301–317.

177. V. Sansone, R. C. Griggs, G. Meola, *et al.*, Andersen's syndrome: a distinct periodic paralysis. *Ann. Neurol.* **42** (1997), 305–312.

178. P. J. Kannankeril, D. M. Roden, F. A. Fish, Suppression of bidirectional ventricular tachycardia and unmasking of prolonged QT interval with verapamil in Andersen's syndrome. *J. Cardiovasc. Electrophysiol.* **15** (2004), 119.

179. C. E. Jackson, R. J. Barohn, Improvement of the exercise test after therapy in thyrotoxic periodic paralysis. *Muscle Nerve* **15** (1992), 1069–1071.

180. F. H. Norris, Jr., E. C. Clark, E. G. Biglieri, Studies in thyrotoxic periodic paralysis. *J. Neurol. Sci.* **13** (1971), 431–442.

181. R. T. Yeung, T. F. Tse, Thyrotoxic periodic paralysis. Effect of propranolol. *Am. J. Med.* **57** (1974), 584–590.

182. R. T. Paasuke, A. K. Brownell, Serum creatine kinase level as a screening test for susceptibility to malignant hyperthermia. *J. Am. Med. Assoc.* **255** (1986), 769–771.

183. C. Lambert, Y. Blanloeil, R. K. Horber, L. Berard, H. Reyford, M. Pinaud, Malignant hyperthermia in a patient with hypokalemic periodic paralysis. *Anesth. Analg.* **79** (1994), 1012–1014.

184. Y. A. Rajabally, M. El Lahawi, Hypokalemic periodic paralysis associated with malignant hyperthermia. *Muscle Nerve* **25** (2002), 453–455.

185. C. L. Marchant, F. R. Ellis, P. J. Halsall, P. M. Hopkins, R. L. Robinson, Mutation analysis of two patients with hypokalemic periodic paralysis and suspected malignant hyperthermia. *Muscle Nerve* **30** (2004), 114–117.

186. J. J. Aarons, R. E. Moon, E. M. Camporesi, General anesthesia and hyperkalemic periodic paralysis. *Anesthesiology* **71** (1989), 303–304.

187. E. M. Ashwood, W. J. Russell, D. D. Burrow, Hyperkalaemic periodic paralysis and anaesthesia. *Anaesthesia* **47** (1992), 579–584.

188. A. M. Cone, A. J. Sansome, Propofol in hyperkalaemic periodic paralysis. *Anaesthesia* **47** (1992), 1097.

189. J. F. Weller, R. A. Elliott, P. J. Pronovost, Spinal anesthesia for a patient with familial hyperkalemic periodic paralysis. *Anesthesiology* **97** (2002), 259–260.

190. D. L. Browne, S. T. Gancher, J. G. Nutt, *et al.*, Episodic ataxia/myokymia syndrome is associated with point mutations in the human potassium channel gene, KCNA1 *Nat. Genet.* **8**:2 (1994), 136–140.

191. S. Comu, M. Giuliani, V. Narayanan, Episodic ataxia and myokymia syndrome: a new mutation of potassium channel gene Kv1.1. *Ann. Neurol.* **40** (1996), 684–687.

192. L. H. Eunson, R. Rea, S. M. Zuberi, *et al.*, Clinical, genetic, and expression studies of mutations in the potassium channel gene KCNA1 reveal new phenotypic variability *Ann. Neurol.* **48** (2000), 647–656.

193. S. M. Zuberi, L. H. Eunson, A. Spauschus, *et al.*, A novel mutation in the human voltage-gated potassium channel gene (Kv1.1) associates with episodic ataxia type 1 and sometimes with partial epilepsy. *Brain* **122** (1999), 817–825.

194. M. Kinali, H. Jungbluth, L. H. Eunson, *et al.*, Expanding the phenotype of potassium channelopathy: severe neuromyotonia and skeletal deformities without prominent episodic ataxia. *Neuromuscul. Disord.* **14**:10 (2004), 689–693.

195. A. Kleinoltshauser, R. Een Jaloh, Episodic ataxia type 1 with distal weakness: a novel manifestation of a potassium channelopathy. *Neuropaediatrics* **35**:2 (2004), 147–149.

196. M. Litt, P. Kramer, D. Browne, *et al.*, A gene for episodic ataxia/myokymia maps to chromosome 12p13. *Am. J. Hum. Genet.* **55**:4 (1994), 702–709.

197. H. Lee, H. Wang, J. C. Jen, C. Sabatti, R. W. Baloh, S. F. Nelson, A novel mutation in KCNA1 causes episodic ataxia without myokymia. *Hum. Mutat.* **24**:6 (2004), 536.

198. E. R. Brunt, T. W. van Weerden, Familial paroxysmal kinesigenic ataxia and continuous myokymia. *Brain* **113** (1990), 1361–1382.

Chapter 22

Inflammatory myopathies

Marinos C. Dalakas and George Karpati

Introduction

Inflammatory myopathies (IM) constitute a heterogeneous group of subacute, chronic and, rarely, acute acquired diseases of skeletal muscle which have in common the presence of moderate to severe muscle weakness and inflammation on muscle biopsy. The diseases are clinically important because they represent the largest group of acquired and potentially treatable myopathies both in children and adults.

A practical classification of all the IM, based on etiology and pathogenesis, has four groups: (1) idiopathic IM (IIM), which together constitute the largest group and will be the main focus of this chapter; (2) secondary IM, occurring in association with other systemic or connective tissue diseases, or with bacterial, viral or parasitic infections; (3) infantile, childhood or congenital forms; and (4) miscellaneous forms.

Idiopathic inflammatory myopathies

Based on distinct clinical, immunopathological, histological, and prognostic criteria, as well as different responses to therapies, IIM can be separated into three major and distinct subsets: polymyositis (PM), dermatomyositis (DM), and inclusion body myositis (IBM). PM and DM would appear to have primarily an autoimmune pathogenesis, based on their association with other putative or definite autoimmune diseases or viral infections, the evidence for a T-cell-mediated myocytotoxicity (PM) or complement-mediated microangiopathy (DM) and their varying but generally favorable response to immunotherapies [1, 2, 3, 4, 5, 6, 7]. In IBM, the autoimmune features coexist with "degenerative" features including myonuclear abnormalities, a peculiar form of muscle fiber vacuolization, intrafiber deposition of amyloid as well as other "alien" molecules and mitochondrial abnormalities. This chapter will review the main clinical and microscopic features, the underlying immunopathology and the response to immunotherapeutic interventions.

Overall clinical features

The incidence of PM, DM, and IBM is approximately 1 in 100 000. DM affects both children and adults, and females more often than males, whereas PM is seen after the second decade of life and very rarely in childhood. IBM is three times more frequent in men than in women, is more common in Whites than in Blacks, and is most likely to affect people over the age of 50 years.

All three forms have in common a myopathy characterized by proximal and often symmetrical muscle weakness, which usually develops subacutely or chronically (weeks to months) or very insidiously, as in IBM. Patients usually report increasing difficulty with everyday tasks predominantly requiring the use of proximal muscles, such as getting up from a chair, climbing steps, stepping onto a curb, lifting objects or combing their hair. Fine motor movements that depend on the strength of distal muscles, such as buttoning a shirt, sewing, knitting or writing, are affected only late in the course of DM and PM but earlier in IBM, where distal weakness is common and may even predominate. Falling is common among patients with IBM because of early involvement of the quadriceps muscle and buckling of the knees. Ocular muscles remain normal, even in advanced, untreated disease, and if these muscles were affected, the diagnosis of IM would be in doubt. Facial muscles also remain normal except, rarely, in advanced disease. Mild facial muscle weakness, however, is seen in up to 60% of patients with sporadic IBM (s-IBM). The pharyngeal and neck flexor muscles are often involved, causing dysphagia or fatigue and difficulty in holding up the head. In advanced disease, and rarely in acute DM, respiratory muscles may also be affected. Severe weakness is almost always associated with muscular wasting. Sensation remains normal. The tendon reflexes are preserved but may be absent in severely weakened or atrophied muscles, especially in s-IBM, where atrophy of the quadriceps and the distal muscles is common. Exercise-induced myalgia and muscle tenderness may occur in some patients, usually early in the disease, particularly in DM but

Disorders of Voluntary Muscle, 8th edn., eds. George Karpati, David Hilton-Jones, Kate Bushby and Robert C. Griggs. Published by Cambridge University Press.

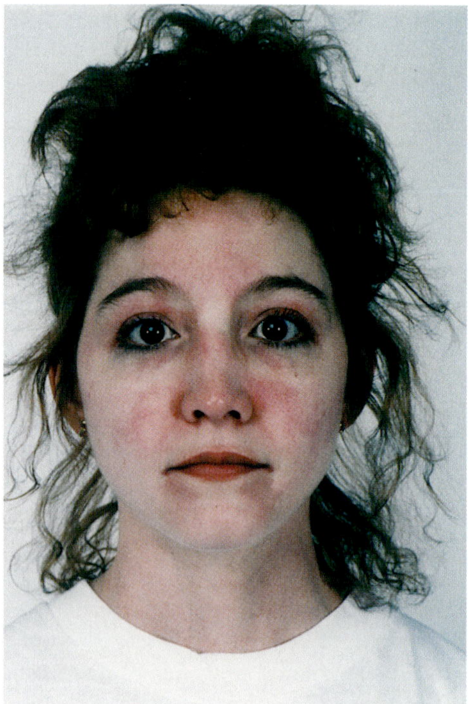

Figure 22.1. Typical skin changes in a young woman with dermatomyositis. The heliotrope rash is prominent around the eyelids, forehead, bridge of the nose, and cheeks. The "misery" is clear in her expression.

not in PM or s-IBM. Weakness in PM and DM progresses over a period of weeks or months, in contrast with the much slower progression of limb-girdle dystrophies, from which they sometimes need to be differentiated. However, IBM may progress very slowly for years, and its clinical features may simulate those of limb-girdle muscular dystrophy or peroneal muscular atrophy.

Specific features

Adult dermatomyositis

Dermatomyositis occurs in both children and adults. It is a distinct clinical entity identified by a characteristic rash accompanying or, more often, preceding the muscle weakness. The skin manifestations include a heliotrope rash (blue–purple discoloration) on the upper eyelids with edema (Figure 22.1), a flat red rash on the face and upper trunk, and erythema of the knuckles with a raised violaceous scaly eruption (Gottron rash) that later results in scaling of the skin. The erythematous rash can also occur on other body surfaces, including the knees, elbows, malleoli, neck, and anterior chest (often in a V sign), or back and shoulders (shawl sign), and is exacerbated by exposure to the sun. In some patients, the rash is pruritic especially in the scalp, chest, and back. Dilated capillary loops at the base of the fingernails are also characteristic of DM. The cuticles may be irregular, thickened, and distorted, and the lateral and palmar areas of the fingers may become rough and cracked, with irregular, "dirty" horizontal lines, resembling mechanics' hands. In racially pigmented skin the usual skin rash is difficult to ascertain. However, periorbital and/or pretibial edema may be detectable. The degree of weakness can be mild, moderate or severe leading to quadriparesis. At times, the muscle strength appears normal, hence the term "dermatomyositis sine myositis" [8]. When muscle biopsy is performed in such cases, however, significant perivascular and perimysial inflammation is often seen. DM in children resembles the adult disease except for more frequent extramuscular manifestations, as discussed below. A common early abnormality in children is "misery," defined as an irritable child that feels uncomfortable, has a red flush on the face, is fatigued, does not feel like socializing, and has a varying degree of proximal muscle weakness. A tiptoe gait caused by flexion contracture of the ankles is also common.

Dermatomyositis usually occurs alone but may overlap with systemic sclerosis and mixed connective tissue disease [2, 3]. Fasciitis and skin changes similar to those found in DM have occurred in patients with the eosinophilia-myalgia syndrome associated with ingestion of contaminated L-tryptophan [9, 10].

For the association of dermatomyositis with latent malignancy please refer to a later section ("Extramuscular manifestations").

Polymyositis

Patients with PM do not present with any distinctive clinical feature that would confirm the diagnosis. Unlike DM, in which the rash secures early recognition, the actual onset of PM is difficult to pinpoint. The patients present with subacute onset of proximal muscle weakness and very rarely myalgia, which may exist for several months before they seek medical advice. The diagnosis of PM is based on finding subacute inflammatory myopathy, which progresses steadily and occurs in adults who do not have a rash, involvement of the extraocular and facial muscles (mild facial weakness is seen in IBM but not in PM), family history of a neuromuscular disease, history of exposure to myotoxic drugs or toxins, endocrinopathy, neurogenic disease, dystrophy, biochemical muscle disorder or IBM, as determined by muscle pathology and histochemistry.

Polymyositis can be viewed as a syndrome from diverse causes that may occur separately or in association with systemic autoimmune or connective tissue diseases and certain known viral or bacterial infections. With the exception of d-penicillamine and zidovudine (AZT), in which there may be endomysial inflammatory infiltrates similar to those seen in PM, myotoxic drugs, such as emetine, chloroquine, steroids, cimetidine, ipecac, and statins, do not cause PM. Instead, they elicit a toxic noninflammatory myopathy that is histologically different from PM and does not require immunosuppressive therapy [2]. In a peculiar form of possible PM, an abnormally high prevalence of ragged red/blue fibers is present in addition to the usual myopathology of PM [11]. This myopathy shows less responsiveness to immunosuppressive therapy than the typical PM and most likely represents a form of IBM. In one of the author's experience (M.C.D.), repeated biopsies in some of these cases could reveal typical IBM.

Inclusion body myositis

Inclusion body myositis is the most common of the IM. It affects men more often than women and is more frequent above the age of 50 years. It is the most commonly acquired myopathy in men above 50 years of age. Although IBM may be suspected when a patient with presumed PM does not respond to therapy, involvement of distal muscles, especially foot extensors and deep finger flexors in almost all cases, should be a clue to an early clinical diagnosis [2, 4, 12, 13, 14, 15, 16, 17, 18, 19] to be confirmed by muscle biopsy. Some patients present with falls because their knees collapse owing to early weakness of the quadriceps muscles. Others present with weakness in the small muscles of the hands, especially the long finger flexors, and complain of inability to hold certain objects such as golf clubs, to play the guitar, to turn a key or tie a knot (Figure 22.2). The weakness and the accompanying atrophy can be asymmetrical, with preferential involvement of the quadriceps (Figure 22.3a), iliopsoas, triceps, biceps, and finger flexors in the forearm. This is in contrast to the hereditary or familial quadriceps-sparing IBM [20, 21, 22] in which the quadriceps remains strong in spite of the weakness in the other muscles (Figure 22.3b). The selective involvement of the flexor digitorum profundus has been confirmed with magnetic resonance imaging (MRI) [23]. Some dysphagia is common, occurring in up to 60% of the patients, especially late in the disease, but it rarely requires gastrostomy. Because of the distal and at times asymmetrical weakness and atrophy and the early loss of the patellar reflex, a lower motor neuron disease is often suspected, especially since serum creatine kinase (CK) activity is either not elevated or only moderately increased [2]. Sensory examination is generally normal except for a mildly diminished vibratory sensation at the ankles, presumably related to the patient's age. Contrary to early suggestions, the distal weakness does not represent neurogenic involvement but is part of the distal myopathic process, as confirmed with macro electromyography (EMG) [24]. However, an axonal neuropathy seems to occur in IBM patients more frequently than would be expected by chance alone [25]. In contrast to PM and DM in which facial muscles are spared, mild facial muscle weakness has been noted in 60% of IBM patients [13].

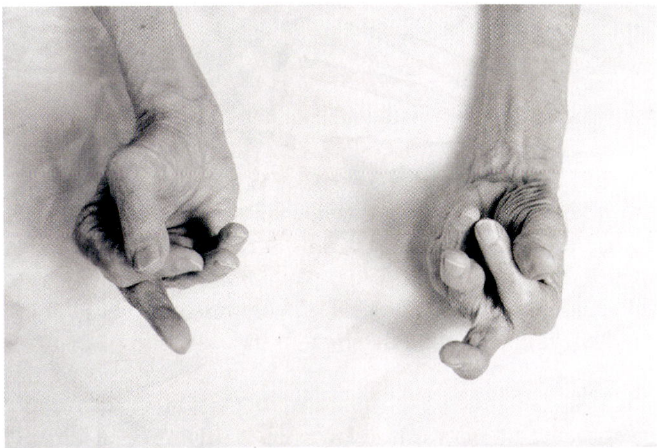

Figure 22.2. Severe preferential weakness in finger flexors in a patient with sporadic inclusion body myositis.

Sporadic IBM can be associated with systemic autoimmune or connective tissue diseases in up to 33% of affected patients [26, 27]. An increased frequency of DRb10301 and DQb10201 alleles associated with DR and DQ phenotypes has been documented in up to 75% of patients [28]. A frequent association with HLA-B8-DR3 haplotype has also been observed [27]. Familial aggregation of IBM with the typical clinical phenotype of s-IBM, and with histological and immunopathological features identical to the sporadic form, can also occur, as seen in other autoimmune disorders [29]; this has been designated as familial inflammatory IBM. Latent malignancy does not occur in sIBM.

Hereditary inclusion body myopathy (hIBM) does not really belong to the category of inflammatory myopathies as

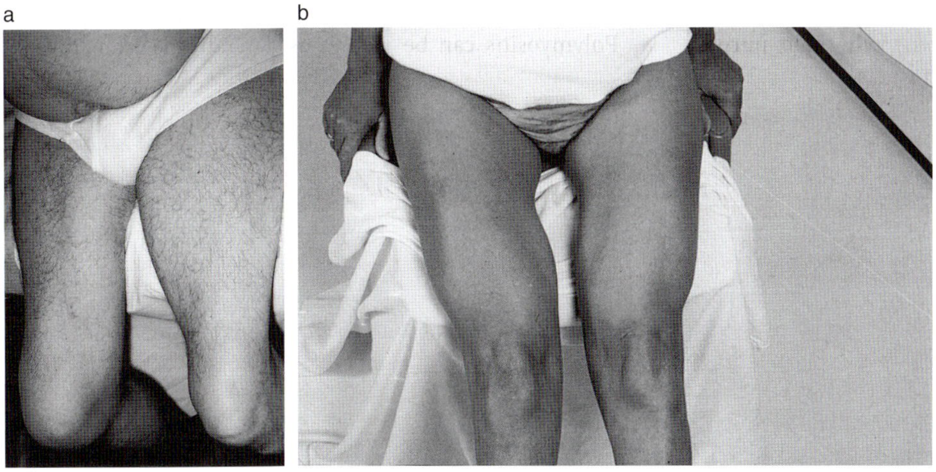

Figure 22.3a, b. Quadriceps changes in patients with inclusion body myositis (IBM). (a) Prominent muscle weakness and wasting in the quadriceps muscles of a patient with sporadic IBM. (b) A patient with hereditary sparing IBM, linked to chromosome 9p, showing the quadriceps-sparing phenotype in contrast to that seen in (a).

there is no inflammation in the biopsied muscle. However, other myopathological features are shared with sIBM and therefore a brief description is included here. hIBM is usually recessive but can, less frequently, be dominant, some with an associated leukoencephalopathy [30] and others with sparing of the quadriceps [14, 20 21, 22]. At present, HIBM includes various ill-defined vacuolar myopathies affecting distal more than proximal muscles and with clinical profiles that differ from the one described above for s-IBM [14, 22]. Hereditary IBM with sparing of the quadriceps occurs not only in Iranian Jews, as initially described [22, 31], but also in other ethnic groups [20, 22]. This disorder is linked to chromosome 9p1 and results from mutations in the UDP-*N*-acetylglucosamine 2-epimerase/*N*-acetylmannosamine kinase (*GNE*) gene [32]. IBM with Paget disease linked to mutations in the valosin-containing protein (VCP) has been also noted [33]. Further description and genetic data on hereditary IBM are not provided in this review because these diseases lack muscle inflammation and, therefore, do not represent a true inflammatory myopathy.

Progression of s-IBM is slow but steady. The degree of disability in relation to the duration of the disease has not been systematically studied. Review of the course of 14 randomly chosen patients with symptoms for more than 5 years revealed that 10 of them required a cane or other support for ambulation by the fifth year after onset of disease while three of five patients with symptoms for 10 years or more were using wheelchairs. Using quantitative muscle strength testing, a 10% drop in muscle strength over a 1- and 2-year period was noted [13]. Data from 86 consecutively studied patients revealed that progression is faster when the disease begins later in life. Patients whose disease began in their sixties required an assistive device many years later compared with those whose disease began in their seventies, presumably because of fewer reserves [34]. A long-term longitudinal study with evaluation of muscle strength every 6 months for 3 years has now been completed in 47 IBM patients; the results are currently being analyzed (Dalakas M. C., unpublished observations).

Extramuscular manifestations

In addition to the primary disturbance of the skeletal muscles of limbs, other manifestations may be prominent in patients with IIM. Dysphagia is most prominent in IBM and DM because of involvement of the oropharyngeal striated muscles and proximal esophagus. *Symptomatic* cardiac abnormalities in DM are rare and consist of atrioventricular conduction defects, tachyarrhythmias, low ejection fraction, and dilated cardiomyopathy, either from the disease itself or from hypertension associated with long-term steroid use. Cardiac involvement is not seen in IBM. Pulmonary involvement results from primary weakness of the thoracic muscles, drug-induced pneumonitis (e.g., from methotrexate) or interstitial lung disease. Interstitial lung disease may precede the myopathy or occur early in the disease, and develops in up to 10% of patients with

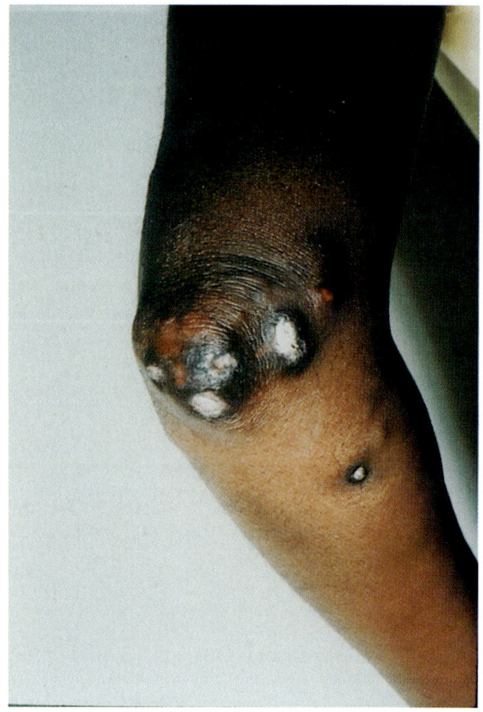

Figure 22.4. Prominent subcutaneous calcification extends to the surface, with ulcerations and infection in a 26-year-old woman with dermatomyositis.

PM or DM, the majority of whom have anti-Jo-1 antibodies (directed against histidyl-transfer RNA synthetase). Fatality related to adult respiratory distress syndrome has been noted in PM patients with anti-Jo-1 antibodies [35], emphasizing the diagnostic importance of these antibodies. Pulmonary capillary angiitis with varying degrees of diffuse alveolar hemorrhage has also been described [36]. Subcutaneous calcifications, sometimes extruding to the surface and causing ulcerations and infections (Figure 22.4), are found in patients with DM, mostly in children but also in some adults [37]. Intestinal infarcts are seen more often in childhood DM and result from vasculitis and infarction. Contractures of the joints are seen particularly in childhood DM. General systemic disturbances, such as fever, malaise, weight loss, arthralgia, and Raynaud phenomenon, can occur, particularly when the inflammatory myopathy is associated with a connective tissue disorder. Finally, there is an increased incidence of malignancies in patients with DM (particularly over 50 years of age), but not in PM or IBM. Because tumors are usually uncovered by abnormal findings in the medical history and physical examination rather than by a radiological blind search, it is our practice to recommend a complete physical examination, with focus on breast, pelvic, and rectal examinations, urinalysis, complete blood cell count, relevant blood chemistry tests (i.e., prostate-specific antigen or PSA) and carcinoembryonic antigen (CEA) and a chest X-ray film, to be repeated at 6-monthly intervals for at least 3 years. Some authorities recommend routine positron emission tomography (PET) scanning as a cost-effective screening method for malignancies in these patients. However, we have not followed this routine.

Diagnosis

The clinically suspected diagnosis of PM, DM or IBM is established or confirmed by elevated activity of the muscle-derived serum enzymes, electromyographic findings and, specifically, by the muscle biopsy.

Muscle-derived serum enzyme levels

The most sensitive indicator enzyme is CK, which, in the presence of active disease, can be elevated in serum by as much as 50 times the normal level, particularly in some cases of DM with muscle infarcts. Although serum CK usually parallels the disease activity, it can be normal in active DM and even, rarely, in active PM. In IBM, serum CK is not usually elevated more than tenfold, and in some patients may be normal even from the beginning of the illness. Serum CK may also be normal in patients with untreated, even active, childhood DM and in some patients with PM or DM associated with a connective tissue disease, reflecting the restriction of the pathological process to the intramuscular vessels and perimysium. Along with the serum CK, glutamate oxaloacetate transaminase (GOT), glutamate pyruvate transaminase (GPT), and lactate dehydrogenase (LDH) may be elevated, which sometimes is erroneously interpreted as a sign of liver disease. Serum aldolase activity may also be elevated.

Electromyography

Needle EMG shows myopathic motor unit potentials characterized by short-duration, low-amplitude polyphasic units on voluntary activation, and increased spontaneous activity with fibrillations, complex repetitive discharges, and positive sharp waves. This EMG pattern also occurs in a variety of acute, toxic and active myopathic processes and should not be considered diagnostic for the inflammatory myopathies. Mixed myopathic and neurogenic potentials (polyphasic units of short and long duration) are more often seen in IBM, but they can be seen in both PM and DM as a consequence of muscle fiber regeneration and chronicity of disease or the presence of an associated peripheral neuropathy. Contrary to previous reports, our findings using macro-EMG have failed to show a neurogenic pattern of involvement in patients with IBM [24] even though histological evidence of an axonal neuropathy may be present in some patients especially of older age. EMG studies, therefore, are generally useful for excluding primary neurogenic disorders in such patients [25].

Muscle biopsy

For definite diagnosis of an inflammatory myopathy, microscopic examination of a muscle biopsy is essential [4, 7, 38, 39]. For maximum diagnostic information, three major prerequisites are essential.

1. Proper choice of muscle. As a rule of thumb, a clinically moderately weak muscle offers the best chance for a positive biopsy. Imaging techniques such as computed tomography (CT) or MRI are rarely required to select an involved region of a muscle. Simultaneous biopsies from more than one site are to be discouraged, although a repeat biopsy from a different site occasionally becomes necessary. Open biopsy done by an expert is strongly recommended in preference to needle biopsy, since open biopsy offers a larger sample and is far better suited for ultrastructural study.
2. The biopsy specimens should be used for the preparation of cryostat sections, semi-thin plastic-embedded sections and, for selected patients, ultra-thin sections for ultrastructural scrutiny. Each of these preparations should be stained by appropriate techniques. Cryostat sections are to be used mainly for routine histological and histochemical stains and reactions and for class I major histocompatibility complex (MHC) immunocytochemistry. However, in selected patients, they are also used for immunocytochemical localization of various lymphocytic subsets, cytokines, adhesion molecules, and expression of "alien" molecules in muscle fibers in IBM, as well as immunoglobulins and complement components. Semi-thin plastic-embedded sections or laminin cytochemistry also offer reliable means to determine capillary density of muscle, which is essential information in the differential diagnosis of DM from PM and IBM [4, 40]. Electron microscopic examination is essential for the detection of tubuloreticular inclusions in endothelial cells of blood vessels in DM [41] or for the identification of the tubular filamentous inclusions in IBM [15, 16]. However, such studies are not always required for routine clinical diagnosis.
3. Interpretation of the biopsy requires special expertise in myopathology to avoid the several pitfalls that can lead to erroneous diagnosis (vide infra). The principal pathological features in the muscle biopsy are: changes affecting muscle fibers, alterations in blood vessels and the inflammatory cell profile, plus any special immunopathological features.

A constellation of these abnormalities is usually characteristic of DM, PM, IBM, or certain other forms of inflammatory myopathy. In some instances, the number of typical changes falls short of being pathognomonic for a given form of IM. In such cases, only a "probable" diagnosis is made. Table 22.1 summarizes these changes in adult DM, as well as in PM and IBM and Figures 22.5, 22.6, 22.7, 22.8, 22.9, 22.10, 22.11, 22.12, 22.13, 22.14, 22.15, 22.16 illustrate many of these changes.

A number of comments must be made about these changes. Several of these abnormalities are pathognomonic even in isolation. Muscle infarcts (Figure 22. 6.), perifascicular atrophy, A-band or focal myofibrillar loss (Figure 22.8), capillary necrosis (Figure 22.13a) [42, 43], membrane attack complex (MAC) deposition in vessel walls (Figure 22.13b) [44, 45],

Table 22.1. Pathological features in idiopathic inflammatory myopathies (IIM)

		Dermatomyositis	Polymyositis	Inclusion body myositis
Muscle fibers	Necrosis of muscle fibers			
	Scattered necrosis (Figure 22.5)	±	+	+
	Infarcts (Figure 22.6)	+	−	−
	Sluggish phagocytosis (Figure 22.6)	+	−	−
	Regeneration	±	+	+
	Atrophy			
	Grouped	−	−	−
	Scattered	+	+	+
	Perifascicular (Figure 22.7)	+	−	−
	Hypertrophy	−	−	+
	Z-disk streaming	+	+	+
	Zonal myofibrillar loss (Figure 22.8)	+	−	−
	A-band loss	+	−	−
	Intrinsic lysosomal activation with exocytosis	−	+	−
	Rimmed vacuoles and eosinophilic masses (Figure 22.9)	−	−	+
	Nuclear abnormalities (15-nm filaments) (Figure 22.10)	−	±	+
	Ragged-red fibers	−	−[a]	+
	Amyloid-staining inclusions (Figure 22.11)	−	−	+
	Ubiquitin-positive inclusions	−	−	+
	"Alien" molecules[b] (Figure 22.12)	−	−	+
	Adhesion molecules (ICAM-1)	+	−	−
Blood vessels	Increased capillarity	−	−	+
	Capillary necrosis ± loss (Figure 22.13a)	+	± (secondary)	−
	Undulating tubules and other endothelial abnormalities	+	−	−
	Arterial necrosis or thrombosis	+	−	−
	Immunoglobulin deposition	+	−	−
	Complement (5b-9) deposition (membrane attack complex) (Figure 22.13b)	+	−	−
	Adhesion molecules (VCAM-1)	+	−	−
Inflammatory and immunopathology	Lymphocytes			
	Endomysial (CD4+/CD8+ T-cells) (Figure 22.14)	+	+	+
	Septal (B-cells + CD4+ T-cells)	+	−	−
	Partial invasion (T cytotoxic CD8+ cells and activated macrophages) (Figure 22.15)	−	+	
	Plasma cells	−	±	−

Table 22.1. *(cont.)*

		Dermatomyositis	Polymyositis	Inclusion body myositis
	Expression of sarcolemmal MHC class I protein products (Figure 22.16)	+	+	+
Other	Marked regional variability in clinically affected muscles	+	–	–
	Interstitial fibrosis	+ (in severe cases)	+ (variable)	+ (focal)

Notes: +, Present; –, absent. Since microscopic scrutiny should be directed to muscle fibers, blood vessels and inflammatory cells changed in these domains are shown separately. Certain highly characteristic pathological changes are marked + and the presence of at least two of these changes in a given biopsy would provide a practically pathognomonic diagnosis for a given entity.

[a]Ragged-red fibers occur in rare cases of polymyositis that seem to constitute a treatment-resistant subgroup. [b]"Alien" molecules include α_1-chymotrypsin, apolipoprotein E, prion protein, β-amyloid precursor.

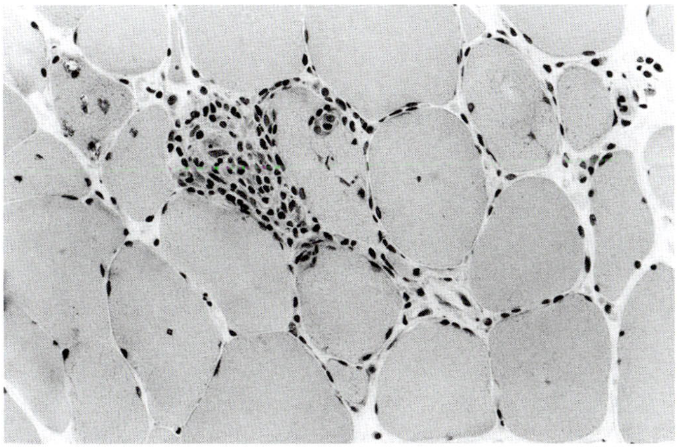

Figure 22.5. Adult polymyositis. A single necrotic fiber is undergoing phagocytosis by macrophages. (Hematoxylin and eosin, ×350.)

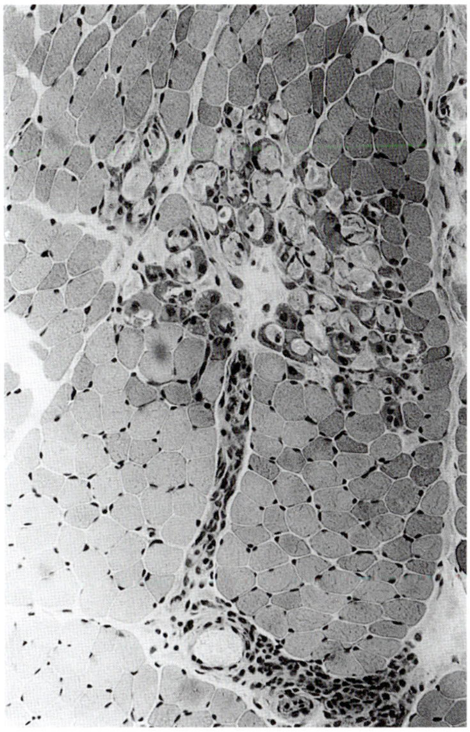

Figure 22.6. Childhood dermatomyositis. A triangular area contains necrotic fibers in which phagocytosis is sparse despite some activation of satellite cells, which appear as peripheral myoblasts. The entire area represents an infarct. An interfascicular septum leading downwards from the infarct is infiltrated by mononuclear cells. (Hematoxylin and eosin, ×350.)

arterial thrombosis and undulating tubules in endothelial cells are characteristic for DM. Partial invasion of non-necrotic muscle fibers by CD8+ cytotoxic lymphocytes and activated macrophages (Figure 22.15) is typical for either PM or IBM but does not occur in DM [46, 47]. Myopathology consisting of abundant necrotic fibers invaded by phagocytic macrophages but only with rare lymphocytic infiltrates needs to be differentiated from classical inflammatory myopathies. We have encountered such pictures of non-inflammatory necrotic myopathies in latent malignancy. The presence of multinucleated giant cells among elongated inflammatory ("epithelioid") cells, macrophages or lymphocytes is characteristic of granulomatous myopathy. The presence of encysted trichinella larvae in muscle fibers in the midst of a florid inflammatory reaction with abundant polymorphonuclear leukocytes is typical of *Trichinella* myositis.

In IBM, the presence of 15- to 18-nm tubular filamentous masses in nuclei or cytoplasm of muscle fibers (Figure 22.10) is helpful in confirming the diagnosis of IBM but its demonstration may require extensive ultrastructural scrutiny [48]. However, it has become clear that these filamentous masses are not disease-specific for s-IBM and neither are rimmed vacuoles (Figure 22.9) [31]. The blue granules that are located in or along the wall of the vacuoles correspond to whorls of cytomembranes or myelin figures, detectable by electron microscopy. On epon-embedded sections, the actual vacuolar space is much less conspicuous than on cryostat sections. The round or oval masses (2–4 mm by 6–8 mm) correspond to masses of irregularly stacked 14- to 18-mm-thick filaments, which, on suitable orientation, can be shown to be tubular. The contention of a group of investigators that these filaments are identical to the paired helical filaments found in neurons in Alzheimer disease [49] has not been confirmed. The nature of the tubular filaments is still obscure. They do not represent

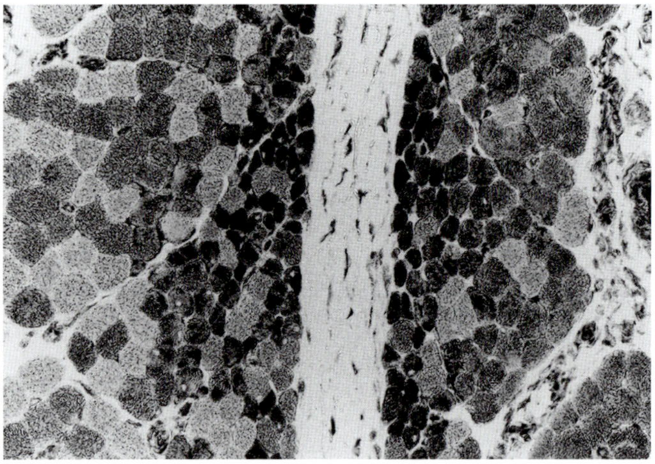

Figure 22.7. Adult dermatomyositis. A narrow mantle of the periphery of two adjacent fascicles separated by an interfascicular septum contains markedly atrophic fibers with excessive oxidative enzyme activity. The interior of the fascicle appears normal. (NADH-tetrazolium reductase stain, ×140.)

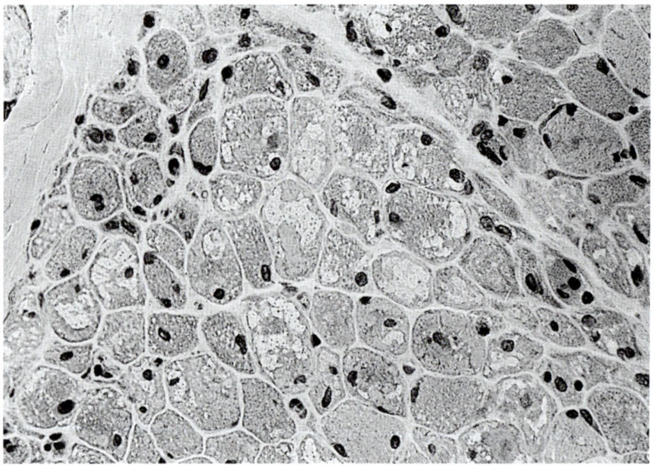

Figure 22.8. Adult dermatomyositis. Many muscle fibers contain irregular, optically empty areas, from where the myofibrils have been lost ("punched out" zones). Myonuclei are conspicuous by their large size and sometimes internal location. (Hematoxylin and eosin, ×350.)

viral particles. They may consist of altered myonuclear matrix material (vide infra).

Electron microscopy is necessary to show precisely the myonuclear abnormalities. These include abnormal heterochromatin distribution indicative of either a shut-off or activation ("dysregulation") of genomic activity, masses of the typical IBM tubular filaments, and actual nuclear disintegration. In rare instances, the nuclear IBM filaments can be caught in the process of being discharged to the cytoplasm as a result of myonuclear breakdown (Figure 22.10).

Congophilic material, best visualized by Texas-red fluorescence optics (Figure 22.11), can be found in a variable number of fibers usually in or near rimmed vacuoles [50, 51, 52]. However, this is by no means specific for IBM, as it has been found in other myopathies [53], or even in chronic neurogenic conditions such as the postpolio syndrome [54]. The same applies to a

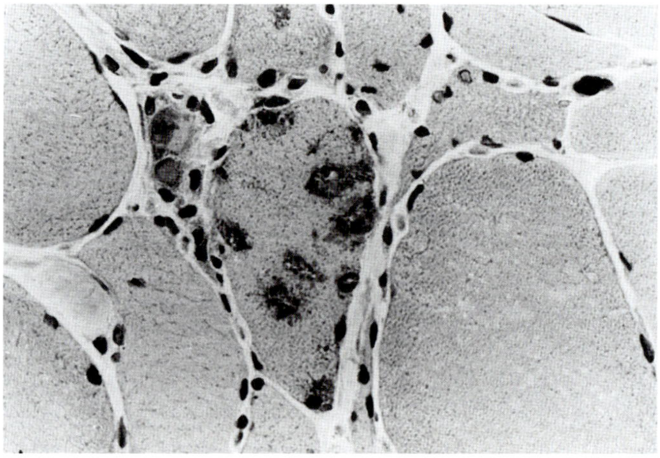

Figure 22.9. Sporadic inclusion body myositis. A muscle fiber contains several "rimmed" vacuoles. Most of these are at the periphery of the fiber. (Modified trichrome, ×520.)

variety of "alien" molecules (Figure 22.11), such as β-amyloid and its precursor protein, α-chymotrypsin, tau proteins, apolipoprotein E, prion protein, etc. [51, 55], which are found in a small percentage of fibers. In IBM, the β-amyloid appears targeted for lysosomal degradation via macroautophagy, as recent studies indicate [56]. Ubiquitin-positive masses are relatively frequent but are also nonspecific [51].

A single-stranded DNA-binding protein accumulates in up to 5% of muscle fibers. This is demonstrated by *in situ* hybridization using a variety of DNA probes [57]. The sites of these accumulations correspond to existing or disintegrated myonuclei (Figure 22.12). The identity of this protein is undetermined.

The rimmed vacuoles have been proposed to be a consequence of the myonuclear breakdown based partly on the observation that they express myonuclear molecules [58]. Ragged-red, cytochrome oxidase-negative muscle fibers with mitochondrial excess are common. Multiple mitochondrial DNA deletions have been demonstrated in most examined cases [59].

Uniform expression of class I MHC products at the surface of most muscle fibers is characteristic of PM and IBM (Figure 22.16), whereas in DM this phenomenon may be evident only in the perifascicular or other random regions [60, 61]. Ubiquitous expression of MHC class I does not occur in limb-girdle dystrophy, denervating diseases or metabolic myopathies (except in regenerating fibers or in fibers invaded by macrophages and lymphoid cells), which makes MHC immunostaining a very helpful diagnostic tool.

The most common cause of a clinical misdiagnosis of inflammatory myopathies is an erroneous pathological interpretation of the biopsy.

A relatively common erroneous practice is to consider PM and DM as the "DM–PM complex." Another source of confusion is the failure to distinguish IBM from PM. In the vast majority of patients, clear distinctions between these entities

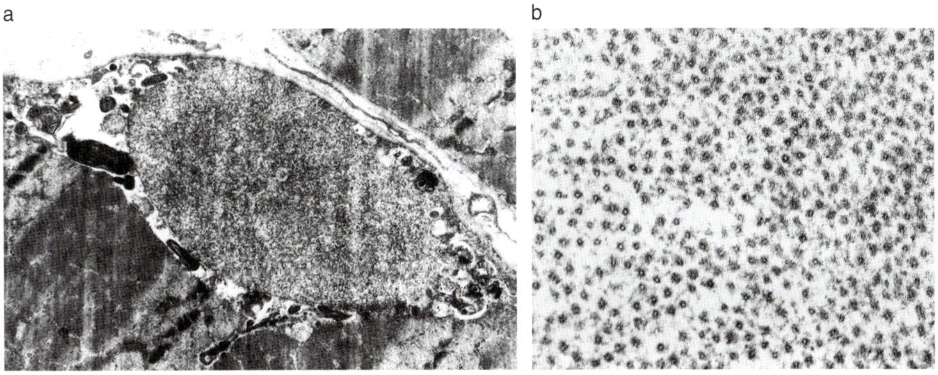

Figure 22.10a, b. Nuclear abnormalities. (a) A large collection of abnormal filaments is present on the surface of a muscle fiber. The filamentous mass is surrounded by whorls of cytomembrane, which on light microscopy would appear as a rimmed vacuole. The shape and size of the filamentous mass suggest that it used to fill a myonucleus, but the nuclear membrane has been fully dissolved. (b) High power shows the 18 nm diameter filaments, typical of inclusion body myositis, to be tubular.

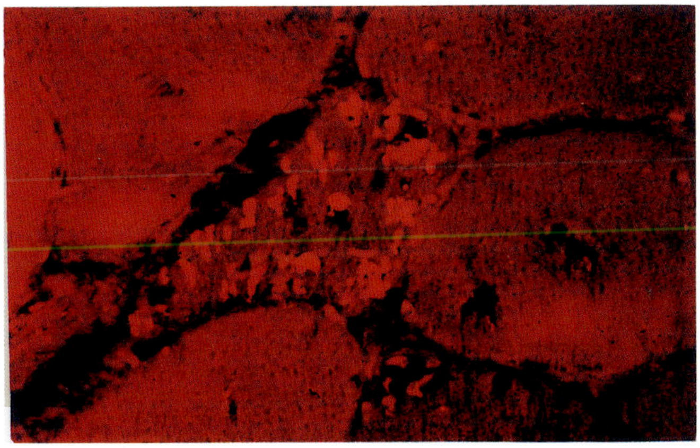

Figure 22.11. Sporadic inclusion body myositis. A muscle fiber contains numerous congophilic fluorescent masses positive with Texas and optics. (Congo red, ×520.)

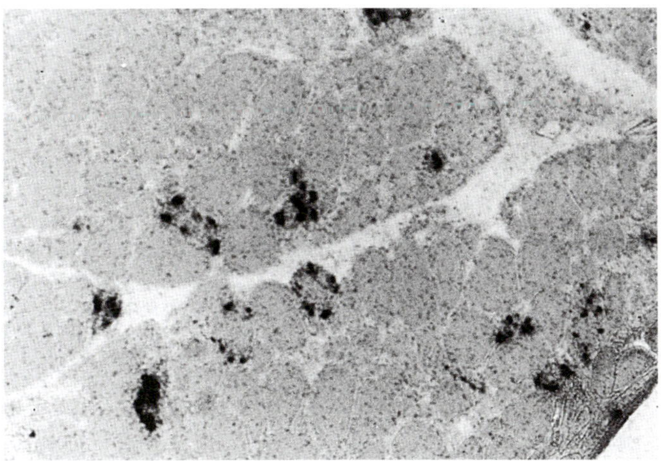

Figure 22.12. Sporadic inclusion body myositis. Radioautograph using a radiolabeled single-stranded M13 phage DNA shows discrete binding sites in scattered muscle fibers. The binding sites are in or near rimmed vacuoles or in myonuclei (×140).

can be made reliably, which is important for investigative, therapeutic, and prognostic reasons.

There are a number of pitfalls that could lead to erroneous interpretation of the muscle biopsy. Failure to assess blood vessel pathology may occur through lack of awareness of its importance or lack of appropriate preparations or stains to assess it. The failure to find IBM filaments is usually related to inadequate electron microscopy samples and an insufficient search. The failure to distinguish between muscle fiber necrosis and partial invasion of muscle fibers by cytotoxic lymphocytes and macrophages is usually related to the lack of awareness of this phenomenon. In DM, the pathological involvement may be spotty and a given biopsy may not contain convincing pathological changes ("skip areas") requiring repeat biopsy. In other instances, even if the biopsy contains changes typical of perifascicular atrophy, the lack of inflammatory cell infiltrates in the biopsy could lead to the conclusion of "nonspecific abnormalities." In some diseases other than inflammatory myopathies (i.e., Duchenne muscular dystrophy, myasthenia gravis, dysferlinopathy, calpainopathy, merosin-deficient muscular dystrophy), endomysial infiltration by lymphocytes may also occur [62, 63]. Regarding IBM, there are a number of cases with typical clinical features whose biopsies demonstrate inflammation, like the one seen in PM, but without the classic vacuoles. These patients were recently labeled has having a PM/IBM [64]. A careful view of these biopsies however shows a large number of Cox-negative fibers and signs of chronicity (large fibers, splitting, increased connective tissue) that denote probably IBM. Errors in the histological diagnosis of IBM when the typical vacuoles are not obvious occur in 15% of the cases [64] and can be avoided by a combined evaluation of the clinical with the histological and immunopathological findings.

In addition to muscle biopsy, skin biopsy may be indicated in DM, preferably from a clinically involved area; however, pathological alteration is often present in clinically uninvolved skin. The changes include a thinning of the epithelial cell layer with attenuation or absence of rete pegs, perivascular mononuclear inflammatory cell infiltrates, and edema of the superficial dermis.

Etiology and pathogenesis

Immune-mediated mechanisms

Immunopathology of dermatomyositis

The primary antigenic target in DM is the vascular endothelium of the endomysial capillaries and to a lesser extent of

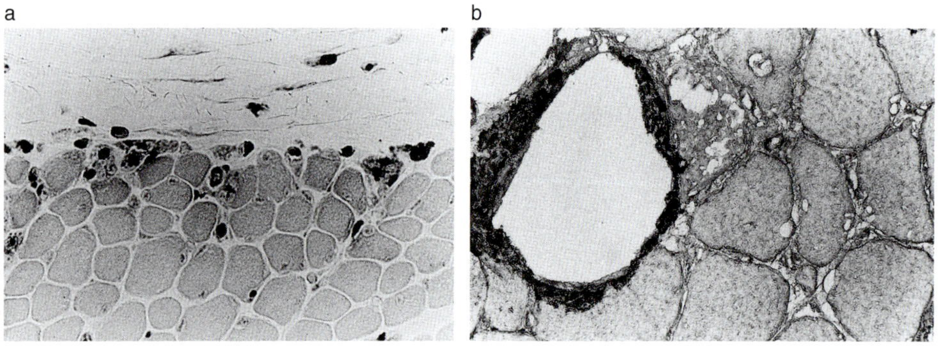

Figure 22.13a, b. Adult dermatomyositis. (a) Acid-phosphatase-positive macrophages mark the sites of endomysial capillaries. The macrophages are presumably engaged in phagocytosis of necrotic endothelial cells (×350). (b) A large vein shows immunoreactive membrane attack complex deposited in its wall (×520).

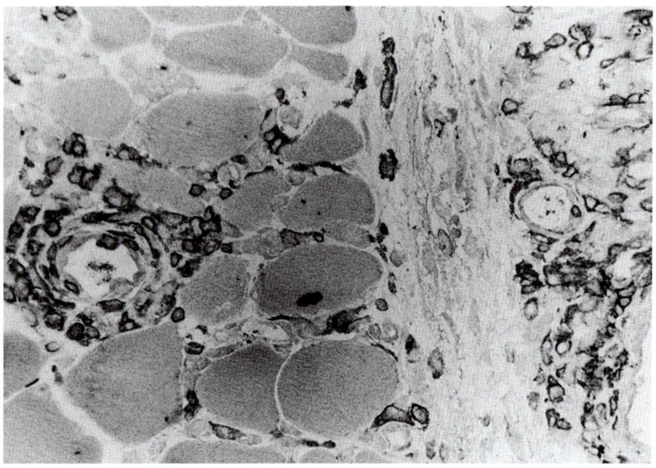

Figure 22.14. Adult dermatomyositis. Helper T-cells surround an endomysial arteriole on the right. On the left, an interfascicular septum contains mainly B-lymphocytes. (Immunoperoxidase with antibodies for CD4 and CD20 antigens, respectively; ×350.)

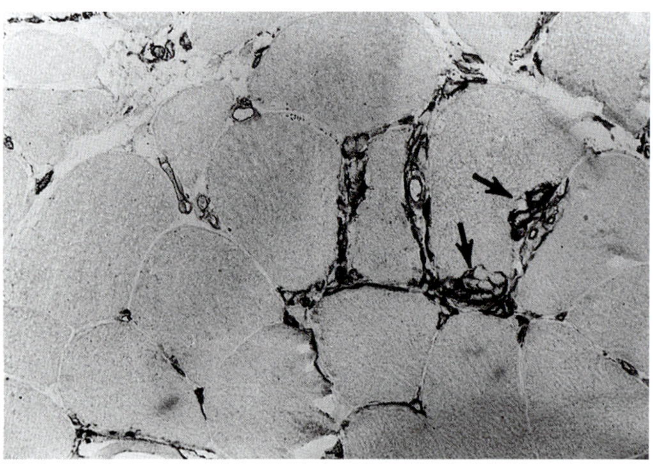

Figure 22.15. Adult polymyositis. CD8 antigen-bearing (cytotoxic) lymphocytes partially invade a non-necrotic muscle fiber (arrows) (×320).

larger blood vessels. The disease begins when putative antibodies directed against endothelial cells activate complement C3 which subsequently forms C3b and C4b fragments and leads to formation of C5b-9 (MAC), the lytic component of the complement pathway [44, 45, 65, 66]. MAC, C3b, and C4b are detected early in the patient's serum [67] and are deposited on capillaries before inflammatory or structural changes are seen in the muscle [44, 45, 65]. Sequentially, the complement-mediated alterations begin with swollen endothelial cells followed by vacuolization and necrosis of capillaries, perivascular inflammation, and ischemic muscle fiber damage [3, 43, 68]. The characteristic perifascicular atrophy is probably a reflection of the normally occurring relative hypoperfusion in the perifascicular zones. Finally, there is a marked reduction in the number of capillaries per muscle fiber with compensatory dilatation of the lumen of the remaining capillaries [3, 37, 69]. The release of cytokines and chemokines [70, 71, 72, 73, 74, 75] related to complement activation upregulate VCAM-I and ICAM-I on the endothelial cells. These molecules serve as ligands for the integrins VLA-4, LFA-I, and Mac-I expressed on T-cells and facilitate their exit through the blood vessel wall to the perimysial and endomysial spaces (Figure 22.17). Immunophenotypic analysis of the lymphocytic infiltrates demonstrates B-cells and CD4+ cells in the perimysial and perivascular regions and plasmacytoid dendritic cells in the perifascicular regions, supporting the view that a humoral-mediated mechanism plays the major role in the disease. Other molecules upregulated in DM, especially in the perifascicular regions where many regenerating and degenerating fibers are prominent, include TGF-β [76], MHC-I, NCAM, calpain, αB-crystallin, cathepsins, amyloid precursor protein, STAT-I probably triggered by interferon-γ, and MxA triggered by α/β interferon [77, 78, 79]. Using gene arrays, a number of adhesion molecules, cytokines, and chemokine genes have been found upregulated in the muscles of DM patients. A biologically relevant gene is the one for the KAL-1 adhesion molecule because it is significantly downregulated in patients who improved after therapy [80]. The KAL-I protein is upregulated in vitro by TGF-β and may have a role in inducing fibrosis [80]. Another interesting protein identified by gene arrays, with specificity for DM, is the myxovirus resistance MxA protein, which is induced by α-interferon and, like so many other proteins mentioned above, is predominantly immunolocalized in the perifascicular regions [79, 81]. The cellular source of the abundant α/β-interferon in DM is probably the large number of plasmacytoid dendritic cells found in these regions, suggesting that in DM the innate immune response is also involved in a pattern similar to systemic lupus erythematosus [79]. On this basis, this author has proposed that in DM the myofibers may be primarily injured by chronic overproduction of α/β-interferon-inducible proteins, challenging the long-lasting view of a primary microangiopathy. Such a proposed theory, however, does not explain the reduced number of capillaries found throughout the fascicle and not just the perifascicular regions. Further, α/β-interferon-inducible genes are also overexpressed in the patients' blood, not only in DM but also in PM [82], casting doubt on the specificity of this protein in DM patients. Another gene expression profiling study in the muscles of genetically susceptible children with childhood DM has also shown α/β- and γ-interferon-inducible genes implying a virus-driven autoimmune dysregulation [83]. However, no viruses have been amplified from the muscles of these patients [84, 85].

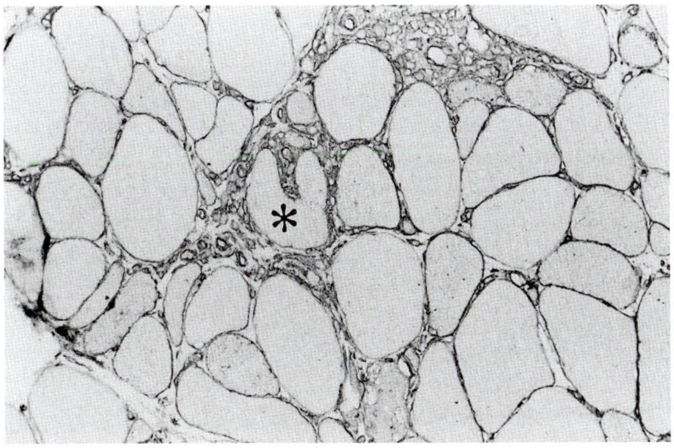

Figure 22.16. Adult polymyositis. Immunoreactive class I major histocompatibility complex protein is present at the surface of all muscle fibers as well as the surface of endomysial mononuclear inflammatory cells. The asterisk indicates a fiber that is partially invaded by inflammatory cells (×350).

Serum autoantibodies

Various autoantibodies against nuclear (antinuclear antibodies) and cytoplasmic antigens are found in up to 20% of patients with inflammatory myopathies [2, 86, 87, 88]. The antibodies to cytoplasmic antigens are directed against cytoplasmic ribonucleoproteins, which are involved in translation and protein synthesis. They include antibodies against various synthetases, translation factors, and proteins of the signal-recognition particles. The antibody anti-Jo-1 accounts for 75% of all the antisynthetases; it is clinically useful because up to 80% of patients with anti-Jo-1 antibodies have interstitial lung disease. In general, these antibodies may be nonmuscle-specific because they are directed against ubiquitous targets; and they are almost always associated with interstitial lung disease even in patients who do not have active myositis. In addition, they are seen in all three subtypes (PM, DM, and IBM), in spite of their clinical and immunopathological differences. Therefore, their pathogenic role in producing muscle damage is doubtful. In general, anti-Jo-1 antibodies may be useful markers of a co-existing interstitial lung disease, while anti-SRP (signal recognition particle) antibodies may be markers of a necrotizing myopathy [89, 90].

Immunopathology of polymyositis and s-IBM

Polymyositis and s-IBM are T-cell-mediated diseases in which CD8+ cells invade major histocompatibility complex (MHC) class-I-antigen-expressing muscle fibers [3, 43, 46, 47, 91]. The immune components associated with this process are identical

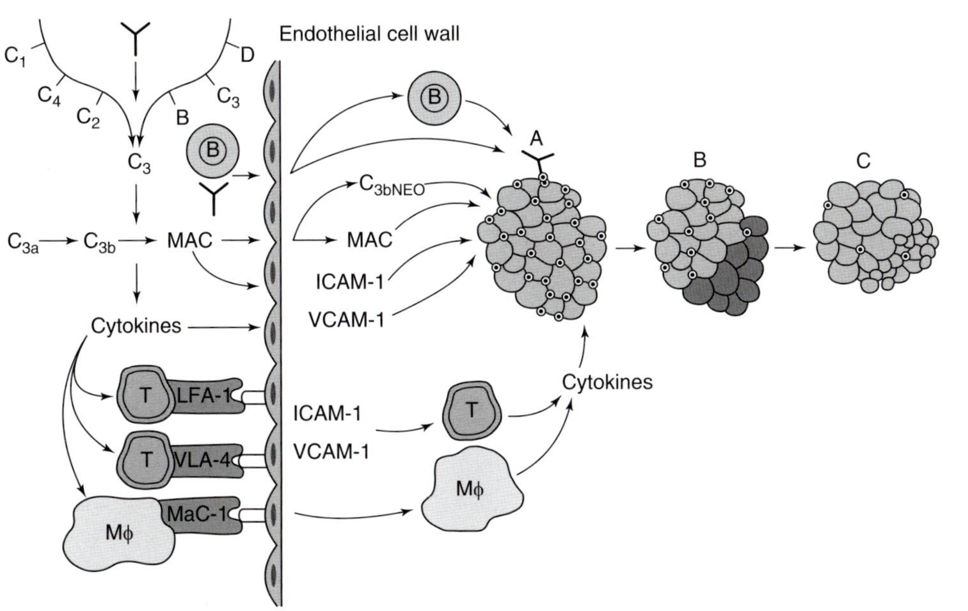

Figure 22.17. Diagrammatic illustration of the main immune factors connected with the pathogenesis of dermatomyositis from the initiation of the disease. MAC, membrane attack complex; ICAM-1, intercellular adhesion molecule 1, VCAM-1, vascular cell adhesion molecule 1; LFA-1, leukocyte function associated antigen; VLA-4, very late antigen 4; C, complement components, Mφ, macrophages. (See text for details.)

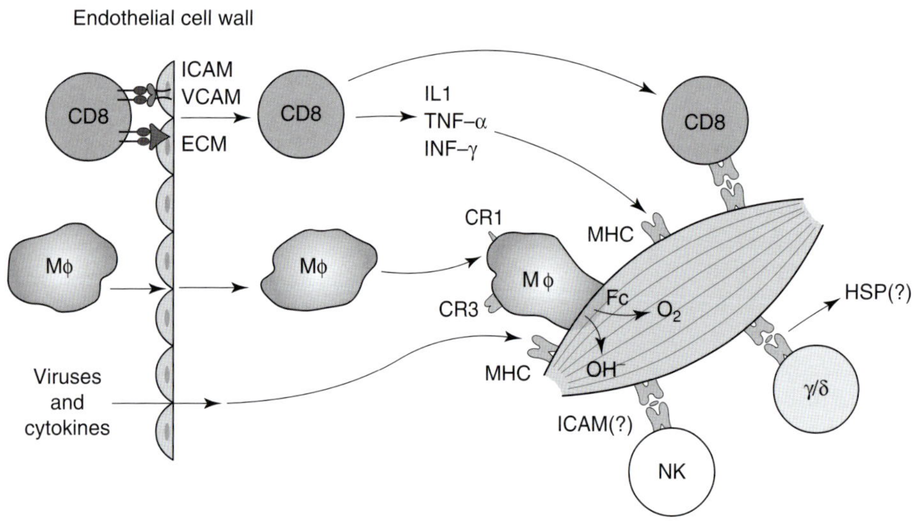

Figure 22.18. Diagrammatic illustration of the main immune factors associated with the immunopathogenesis of polymyositis and sporadic inclusion body myositis. ICAM, intercellular adhesion molecule; VCAM, vascular cell adhesion molecule, CD8, CD8+ T-cells; IL1, interleukin-1, TNF-α, tumor necrosis factor α; INF-γ, interferon γ; CR, cellular receptor; MHC, major histocompatibility complex; HSP, heat shock protein, NK, natural killer; Mφ, macrophages. (See text for details.)

in both PM and s-IBM, in spite of poor response to immunotherapies of the latter, and include the following (Figure 22.18).

Upregulation of MHC class I antigen on muscle fibers and formation of immunological synapses with the autoinvasive cytotoxic CD8+ T-cells –– In PM and s-IBM the CD8+ cells surround healthy non-necrotic muscle fibers, but which express MHC-class-I antigen, and which eventually invade [47]. Muscle fibers normally do not express detectable amount of MHC class I or II antigens. In PM and IBM however, widespread overexpression of MHC class I and occasionally class II is seen, even in areas remote from the inflammation [60, 61]. In other chronic myopathies or dystrophies, and in contrast to PM or s-IBM, the muscle fibers do not express the MHC class I antigen in a ubiquitous and consistent pattern [68], or the co-stimulatory molecules described below. Furthermore, in dystrophies the occasionally seen autoinvasive T-cells are not antigen-driven because they are clonally diverse, do not form the immunological synapses described below, and do not express the specific activation markers of cytotoxicity. The upregulation of MHC class I is probably related to overexpression of cytokines such as *IFN-γ*, *TNF-α* and *interleukins*, which in vitro can trigger MHC class I expression by human myotubes [92, 93, 94]. In transgenic mice, the MHC class I may act as an inciting event triggering an atypical, non-inflammatory myopathy with "myositis-specific" antibodies [95]. In human PM and IBM it is uncertain whether the upregulation of MHC class I alone is sufficient to drive T-cell activation and endomysial infiltration as proposed, because in several chronic cases of PM, MHC class I overexpression is not associated with endomysial inflammation [96]. Another MHC molecule, the nonpolymorphic, "non-classical" HLA-G, is upregulated in vitro by IFN-γ and is expressed on muscle fibers of patients with PM and IBM [97, 98]. Interestingly, HLA-G protects human muscle cells from immune-cell-mediated lysis in vitro, suggesting that it might (partially) protect muscle fibers in vivo [98].

Cytotoxic autoinvasive T-cells –– In PM and IBM the T-cells are activated, as evidenced by their expression of memory and activation markers CD45RO and ICAM-I, as well as MHC class I and inducible co-stimulator (ICOS) on their surface [3, 99]. A number of the activated autoinvasive CD8+ T cells are cytotoxic because they overexpress perforin and granzyme granules (both at the protein and mRNA levels). The perforin granules are vectorially directed toward the surface of the muscle fiber, inducing necrosis upon release [98, 100, 101]. These cells have also been shown to be cytotoxic in autologous myotubes in vitro [92]. Consequently, the perforin pathway seems to be the major cytotoxic effector mechanism in PM and IBM. In contrast, the Fas-Fas-L-dependent apoptotic process is not functionally involved despite expression of the Fas antigen on muscle fibers and of Fas-L on autoinvasive CD8+ cells [102, 103]. Whether the coexpression of the antiapoptotic molecules Bcl-2 [103], FLICE {Fas-associated death domain-like IL1-converting enzyme-inhibitory protein (FLIP); [104]}, and human IAP-like protein (hILP; Li and Dalakas [105]), confers resistance of muscle to Fas-mediated apoptosis remains speculative.

The autoinvasive T-cells are clonally expanded with rearrangement of the TCR genes –– The T-cells recognize an antigen via the T-cell receptor (TCR), a heterodimer of two α and β chains, encoded by multiple gene families in the V (variable), D (diversity), J (joining), and C (constant) regions of the TCR. The part of the TCR that recognizes an antigen is the CDR3 region, which is encoded by genes in the V-J and V-D-J segments of the TCR gene. If the endomysial T-cells are selectively recruited by a specific autoantigen, the use of the V and J genes of the TCR should be restricted and the amino acid sequence in their CDR3 region should be conserved. In patients with PM and IBM, but not in those with DM or dystrophies, only certain T-cells of specific TCRα and TCRβ families are recruited to the muscle from the circulation [93,

106, 107, 108, 109, 110]. Cloning and sequencing of the amplified endomysial TCR gene families has demonstrated a restricted use of the Jβ gene with conserved amino acid sequence in the CDR3 region indicating clonal selection and in situ expansion. The clonality of the autoinvasive T-cells has been confirmed with CDR3 spectratyping of the TCR Vβ chains in lymphocytes concurrently obtained from peripheral blood and muscles. This study has demonstrated a high degree of clonal restriction only in the endomysial T-cells, suggesting that T-cell clones expand within the muscle microenvironment after recognizing local antigens [111]. Combining spectratyping with molecular laser-assisted microdissection, and immunocytochemistry with sequencing of the most prominent TCR families has further shown that the clonally expanded T-cells are relevant to the muscle fiber injury because they are autoinvasive and express perforin [107, 111, 112, 113]. Sequential muscle biopsy specimens obtained during a 19- to 22-month period in several IBM patients have led to the conclusion that the clonally expanded Vβ families persist over time among the autoinvasive CD8+ cells even in different muscles [107, 110, 111, 112, 114, 115]. Collectively, in PM and s-IBM there is overwhelming evidence of clonal restriction of the autoinvasive endomysial T-cells, which are specifically recruited to the muscle and appear to expand in situ probably driven by local antigen(s). In an important case of PM, a single clone of γ/δ T-cells was the primary cytotoxic effector [116, 117, 118]. When the γ/δ TCR of the pathogenic T-cells was transfected into a TCR-deficient mouse hybridoma cell line [118], the transfectants could be stimulated with an as yet unknown autoantigen on human myoblasts [118]. This study provides the first indication that at least in γ/δ T-cell-mediated PM the autoaggressive T-cells recognize genuine muscle antigens.

Presence of co-stimulatory molecules, formation of immunological synapses, and presence of antigen presenting cells -- The clonally expanded autoinvasive CD8+ T-cells are primed to receive specific antigenic peptides presented by the MHC class I molecule to form an immunological synapse only in the presence of the B7 family of co-stimulatory molecules. Indeed, in PM and IBM the B7 family of molecules (B7-1, B7-2, BB1, ICOS-L, and CD40) are upregulated on MHC-I-positive muscle fibers, while their respective counter receptors (CD28, CTLA-4, ICOS, and CD40-L) are overexpressed on the autoinvasive CD8+ T-cells [98, 101, 119, 120]. Of relevance to the muscle fiber injury is the observation that the ICOS-positive T-cells at the synapses are cytotoxic, expressing perforin granules [101]. These findings, along with the intrinsic production of cytokines and chemokines directly by the muscle fiber as discussed later, imply that the muscle fiber can behave like an antigen presenting cell (APC) and it is not only the target of an attack but also an active participant in the immune response.

Myeloid dendritic cells (DC), the most potent cells in antigen presentation, are also abundantly found within the endomysial infiltrates of PM, DM, and IBM [81] and invade non-necrotic muscle fibers. These cells may present local antigens to T-cells and B-cells and contribute to muscle fiber injury. In PM and IBM as well as in DM, a large number of plasma cells and clonally expanded B-cells are found endomysially [121], suggesting that an antigen-specific humoral immune response, bypassing the lymphoid tissue, may also take place within the muscle. This observation is not unexpected, as ectopic germinal centers are frequently noted in targeted tissues in several autoimmune disorders, confirming that different effector mechanisms of T-cells and B-cells concurrently play an active role in the process of an autoimmune disease. The suggestion that in PM and IBM there is a humoral response associated with in situ production of autoantibodies [81] remains speculative.

Upregulation of cytokines, cytokine signaling, chemokines, and metalloproteinases -- Cytokines and chemokines are essential in enhancing the activation of T-cells and the induction of co-stimulatory molecules at the synapses as discussed earlier. Various cytokines including interleukins (IL-1, IL-2, IL-6 and IL-10), TNF-α, INF-γ, signal transducer and activation of transcription (STAT), transforming growth factor β (TGF-β), and granulocyte–macrophage colony-stimulating factor are variably overexpressed in the muscles of patients with PM and IBM [71, 77, 91, 122, 123, 124, 125]. Some of these molecules can also exert a direct cytotoxic effect on the muscle fibers.

Chemokines, such as MCP-1 and MIP-1a, Mig and IP-10, and the receptor for Mig, CXCR3, are strongly upregulated in all inflammatory myopathy muscles, at the protein and the mRNA level [74, 75, 125, 126]. Using gene array studies, the upregulated chemokine and cytokine genes were much higher in the muscles of patients with IBM compared to DM [80]. Various adhesion and extracellular matrix molecules such as VCAM and ICAM, thrombospondins and metalloproteinases are also upregulated in the tissues of patients with PM and IBM [127, 128] and may enhance the inflammatory response or promote tissue fibrosis in the late stages of the disease.

What has now become clear is that the human muscle, in vivo and in vitro, can also secrete proinflammatory cytokines upon cytokine stimulation in an auto-amplificatory mechanism, facilitating thereby the recruitment of activated T-cells to the muscle and contributing to the self-sustaining nature of endomysial inflammation [68, 75, 78, 98, 129].

Non-immune features in the muscles of inclusion body myositis reconciling the roles of inflammation and "degeneration" and the stress response -- In IBM, there is clear evidence of primary autoimmune and inflammatory features, as discussed above and summarized in Table 22.2. IBM is however a more complex disease as evidenced by the concomitant features of degeneration highlighted by the presence of rimmed vacuoles (almost always in fibers not invaded by T-cells), the intracellular deposition of Congo-red-positive amyloid, and the accumulation of β-amyloid-related molecules, β-APP, phosphorylated tau, presenilin-1, apolipoprotein, γ-tubulin, clusterin, α-synuclein,

Table 22.2. Factors supporting an immunopathogenic disease mechanism for sporadic inclusion body myositis

1. Immunogenetic association with DR*0301, DQ1*0201 alleles, and the B8-DR3-Dr52-DQ2 haplotype
2. DQ2 haplotype; the human leukocyte antigen (HLA)-A haplotype is associated with earlier disease onset
3. Occurrence of sporadic inclusion body myositis (s-IBM) in family members of the same generation (familial inflammatory IBM), as seen with other autoimmune disorders
4. Association with other autoimmune disorders and autoantibodies
5. Association with paraproteinemia at a significantly higher frequency than in age-matched controls (22.8% vs 2%)
6. Association with common variable immunodeficiency and natural killer cells
7. Association with HIV and human T-lymphotropic virus (HTLV) 1 infection (13 cases reported to date)
8. CD8+ autoinvasive T-cells surround major histocompatibility complex (MHC-) class-I-expressing fibers, express perforin and activation markers of cytotoxicity, and are clonally expanded
9. Ubiquitous upregulation of MHC class I antigen and co-stimulatory molecules on muscle fibers, even those not invaded by T-cells; the counter receptors of the co-stimulatory molecules are overexpressed on the autoinvasive T-cells
10. Strong upregulation of cytokines, chemokines, and their receptors at the protein, messenger RNA, and gene levels

gelsolin, and a number of oxidative stress or other cell stressor molecules. These accumulations are not however unique to s-IBM, because they are also observed to a similar extent in other vacuolar myopathies. What appears unique to IBM however, compared to other chronic vacuolar myopathies, is the strong presence of primary inflammation and the overexpression of MHC class I molecules on all the vacuolated fibers. The relationship between inflammation and degeneration is currently under intense study but there is evidence that the inflammatory mediators, such IL-1, can enhance the production and intracellular accumulation of amyloid and stressor proteins such as α-crystallin [78, 130]. Furthermore, the chronic upregulation of MHC class I appears to independently induce endoplasmic reticulum (ER) cell stress in the myofiber [131].

The assembly and folding of MHC class I occurs in the ER. It begins with the association of a heavy chain glycoprotein with β2-microglobulin, forming an unstable heterodimer complex that matures only when it binds to an antigenic peptide. The ER maintains quality control by processing, folding, and exporting MHC molecules loaded with antigen. If an MHC molecule does not bind to an appropriate antigen, the heavy chain glycoprotein is misfolded and removed from the ER and transported to the cytosol for degradation [68, 129]. In s-IBM, the muscle fibers are overloaded with MHC molecules, and the antigenic peptides may not undergo proper conformational change to bind to the MHC class I complex, leading to ER stress and further protein misfolding. This model is supported by the enhanced immunoproteasome activity noted [131, 132], enhanced MHC class I protein assembly [133], misfolding of accumulated glycoproteins and signs of a cell stress response [131, 134], with upstream upregulation of α-crystallin in intact and MHC-I-positive muscle fibers [78, 135]. Such stressor effects are also seen in transgenic mice that overexpress MHC class I, indicating that chronic overexpression of MHC class I alone might be sufficient to induce ER stress in the myofiber [131].

On the basis of the foregoing features we have suggested a complex pathogenic scenario as a hypothesis to explain the myopathological features of s-IBM.

Although the factors triggering immune and protein dysregulation or vacuolar formation remain unknown, one of the authors (M.C.D.) favors a primary inflammatory process that leads to degeneration [26, 28, 129, 136, 137], because: (1) IBM is frequently seen with autoimmune disorders and increasingly with HIV and HTLV-I infection; (2) T-cell invasion of non-necrotic fibers is found early and at a higher frequency than in the Congo-red-positive fibers [138]; (3) the cytotoxic T-cells at the immunological synapses do not recognize amyloid-related proteins as antigens (Dalakas and Raju unpublished observations); and (4) the cytokine-induced upregulation of MHC class I occurs early and is capable of triggering cell stress and degeneration [129, 131]. Most importantly, endomysial inflammation alone can cause muscle destruction and clinical weakness, as seen in PM; whether the tiny β-amyloid deposits alone are sufficient to trigger muscle degeneration in humans remains unclear especially since the same molecules accumulate in various vacuolar myopathies and muscular dystrophies caused by genetic mutations, while in other conditions these deposits appear innocuous [136]. Regardless of whether the primary event is a dysimmune or protein dysregulation process, there is now strong evidence that in IBM pro-inflammatory cytokines not only correlate with the intramuscular accumulation of amyloid, phosphorylated tau, ubiquitin, and αB-crystallin [78, 139] but also induce tau phosphorylation and amyloid aggregates. Cytokines also stimulate myofibers to produce inflammatory mediators in an autoamplificatory mechanism, enhancing further the chronicity of inflammation, amyloid formation, and cell stress.

The other author of this chapter (G.K.) however has hypothesized that the "degenerative" changes are the primary events while the inflammatory features are secondary. Furthermore, the initial events of the "degenerative" cascade take place in the myonuclei.

"Degenerative" events

1. The initial change is the accumulation of the intranuclear tubular filaments which may represent altered elements of

the myonuclear matrix. The cause of this seemingly critical change is not known but retroviral infections have been suspected (vide infra). In any event, the development of such changes likely occurs over a very long period of time in different muscle fibers giving rise to the "graying of the hair" phenomenon. The putative myonuclear matrix alterations could be responsible for altered myonuclear gene expression (dysregulation) with both upregulation and downregulation. The upregulated gene expression could be responsible for the appearance of the hitherto cited "alien" molecules, some of which may be toxic and also represent neoantigens.

2. Later stages of the myonuclear alterations lead to disintegration of myonuclei and the release of the nuclear contents into the cytoplasm. This would have two sets of immediate consequences. One is the appearance of cytoplasmic IBM filaments and the other is the development of the rimmed vacuoles as an effect of the highly basophilic nuclear content in the neutral pH cytoplasm. The finding of remnants of nuclear molecules supports this notion [58].
3. A more remote effect of myonuclear disintegration is myonuclear attrition, which brings about progressive shrinkage of muscle fibers. This occurs as the ratio of the myonuclear number to muscle fiber volume is a relatively steady quotient.

Inflammatory events

These may be related to the emergence of neoantigens as a result of transcriptional dysregulation of certain molecules. For example, the emergence of *intracellular* β-amyloid as a consequence of the overexpression of the β-amyloid precursor protein may be an example of a neoantigen that can trigger a cytotoxic lymphocytic attack on muscle fiber.

The mechanism of multiple deletions in the mitochondrial DNA and mitochondrial proliferation could also fit into the above scenario if the transcription of some of the nuclear-coded mitochondrial molecules are dysregulated. Some such molecules control mtDNA proliferation.

Regardless of what is the triggering event that leads to inflammation and protein dysregulation, the foregoing hypotheses would indicate that there are at least four mechanisms by which damage to muscle fibers in s-IBM can develop. These include myonuclear attrition-induced atrophy, toxic effects of some of the "alien" molecules, mitochondrial ox-phos deficiency, and autoimmune cytotoxic attack.

Viral infections

Several viruses, including coxsackievirus, influenza, paramyxoviruses, cytomegalovirus and Epstein-Barr virus, have been directly associated with chronic and acute myositis [69, 140, 141, 142]. A possible molecular mimicry phenomenon has been proposed with the coxsackieviruses because of structural homology between Jo-1 antibody and the genomic RNA of an animal picornavirus and the encephalomyocarditis virus [84, 86]. Very sensitive PCR studies, however, have repeatedly failed to confirm the presence of such viruses in these patients' muscle biopsies, suggesting that it is unlikely, although not impossible, for these viruses to replicate in the muscles of patients with PM, DM, and IBM [143].

The best evidence for possible viral connection in PM and IBM comes from the retroviruses. Monkeys infected with the simian immunodeficiency virus and humans infected with HIV and human T-cell lymphotropic virus (HTLV-1) develop PM or IBM. In humans infected with HIV or HTLV-1, an isolated inflammatory myopathy may occur as the initial manifestation of the retroviral infection, or myositis may develop later in the disease course [141, 144, 145, 146, 147, 148]. It is now becoming clear that the association of retroviruses with s-IBM is more than a coincidence because more than 30 cases of HIV/HTLV-1-positive patients with IBM have been reported or are known to us [129, 144, 149, 150, 151]. In these seropositive patients, the disease appears before the age of 50 but several years after the first manifestations of the retroviral infection, suggesting that in HIV-positive patients who live longer and harbor the virus for several years the disease is more frequently recognized. The clinical phenotype and muscle histology in HIV-IBM patients is identical to the retroviral-negative IBM. The predominant endomysial cells are CD8+ cytotoxic T cells which, along with macrophages, invade or surround MHC-class-I-antigen-expressing non-necrotic muscle fibers [152, 153]. Using in situ hybridization, polymerase chain reaction (PCR), immunocytochemistry, and electron microscopy, viral antigens could not be detected within the muscle fibers but only in occasional endomysial macrophages [129, 144, 152, 153, 154]. Molecular immunological studies using tetramers have shown that retrovirally specific cytotoxic T-cells, whose TCR contains amino acid residues for specific HLA/viral peptides, are recruited within the clonally expanded T-cells and invade muscle fibers [148, 149, 155]. We have interpreted these observations to suggest that in HIV-IBM and HTLV-1-IBM there is no evidence of persistent infection of the muscle fibers with the virus or viral replication within the muscle, but rather that the chronic retroviral infection, in genetically susceptible individuals, triggers a persistent inflammatory process that leads to s-IBM [148, 149].

The development of PM or IBM in HIV-positive patients should be distinguished from a toxic myopathy related to long-term therapy with zidovudine, which is characterized by fatigue, myalgia, mild muscle weakness, and mild elevation of serum CK activity [156, 157]. Zidovudine-induced myopathy, which generally improves when the drug is discontinued, is a mitochondrial disorder characterized histologically by the presence of "ragged-red/blue" fibers. Abnormal muscle mitochondria and depletion of the muscle mitochondrial DNA by zidovudine result from inhibition of γ-DNA polymerase, an enzyme found solely in the mitochondrial matrix.

Nonviral microbial myositis

Several animal parasites, such as protozoa (*Toxoplasma*, *Trypanosoma* spp.), cestodes (cysticerci), and nematodes (trichinae), may produce a focal of diffuse IM known as parasitic PM. *Staphylococcus aureus*, *Yersinia* spp., *Streptococcus* spp., and anaerobes may produce a suppurative myositis, known as tropical PM or pyomyositis. Pyomyositis, a previous rarity in western countries, can now be seen in rare patients with AIDS. Certain bacteria, such as *Borrelia burgdorferi* of Lyme disease and *Legionella pneumophila* of Legionnaires' disease, may infrequently be the cause of PM.

Hyperacute necrotizing fasciitis/myositis ("flesh-eating disease") [158]

In this very acute disease, there is galloping necrosis of large areas of fascia and muscle usually in the limb territory. It is usually caused by an exceptionally virulent strain of group A beta-hemolytic streptococcus behaving like a superantigen. The port of bacterial entry is usually a trivial cut or abrasion on the skin and the source is contact with carriers of the organism. It is not clear what predisposes people to this event but some type of immune system incompetence is probably a factor. Systemic varicella is a predisposing factor in children. Initial symptoms are swelling, pain, and redness of the involved area along with fever. The process of tissue necrosis develops rapidly at an estimated rate of 3 cm/h. Rapid diagnosis and prompt vigorous treatment with appropriate antibiotics are essential. One of the authors of this chapter (G.K.) has successfully used early intravenous immunoglobulins as well. Hyperbaric oxygen was also recommended. However, the disease is often diagnosed too late and generous amputation of the involved limb is the only means of avoiding a fatal outcome.

Inflammatory myopathies in collagen vascular diseases

Neuromuscular impairment may occur in any of the collagen vascular diseases from a variety of causes, such as muscle ischemia, cachexia, peripheral nerve involvement, musculoskeletal deformities, and therapeutic steroid-related side-effects. True IM is another possibility but occurs relatively infrequently. In a large series of patients with systemic sclerosis, a DM-like picture was found in about 12% of the patients, particularly in those with anti-PM-Scl antibodies [159]. Among the inflammatory myopathies, DM is the only form that truly overlaps with systemic sclerosis. In systemic lupus erythematosus, the true incidence in the form of PM has been estimated at 5%–8% [160]. In our experience, prominent MHC class I expression at the surface of muscle fibers appears to be a constant feature in these patients. In Sjögren syndrome, a DM and an IBM picture have both been observed; however, the overall incidence is low [161]. In rheumatoid arthritis and periarteritis nodosa, a clinically evident inflammatory muscle disease is very rare, although muscle biopsies may show focal interstitial or perivascular mononuclear inflammatory cell infiltrates and necrotic arteritis (Figure 22.13a), respectively, without major muscle fiber damage.

In practical terms, if a patient with any of the above collagenoses, as defined by rigorous diagnostic criteria, shows undue muscle weakness that cannot otherwise be explained, and particularly if serum CK activity is significantly elevated and if there is an EMG abnormality consistent with an IM, a muscle biopsy from a carefully selected site is justified.

It appears that DM or PM in association with collagen vascular diseases shows the same pathological features as the ones found in idiopathic DM and PM.

Miscellaneous forms of inflammatory myopathies

Granulomatous myopathy

Granulomatous myopathy can occur in a number of conditions [162]. While many patients with systemic sarcoidosis have asymptomatic microscopic granulomata in muscle, which can be helpful in the diagnosis, others manifest a clinical myopathy with a varying degree of severity. These patients present with an insidious limb-girdle syndrome that can also affect distal muscles [163]. The muscle biopsy shows non-caseating granulomas with giant cells. Muscle fiber damage is usually limited. In some patients, intranuclear filaments can be seen in myonuclei that are indistinguishable from those observed in IBM. In a special group of patients, usually post-menopausal women, a similar clinical and pathological picture in muscle is present without evidence of systemic sarcoidosis. In some of these patients myasthenia gravis may also develop. The relationship of this granulomatous myopathy to classical sarcoidosis is unclear.

A granulomatous myopathy may rarely develop into Crohn disease [164] and in association with thymoma. In some cases, no other associated conditions are found. Sarcoid myopathy can result in severe disability with poor response to steroids or anti-TNF-α agents; in contrast patients with idiopathic granulomatous myositis had a better prognosis [163].

Myopathy in hypersensitivity vasculitis

Vasculitis in muscle may be present in the many forms of IM including DM and the collagenoses. In addition, there are patients who present with a nonspecific vasculitis, which involves either skeletal muscles alone or their tissues as well. In many instances, the etiological factor remains obscure. In these patients, the pathology consists of mononuclear infiltration of vessel walls and their vicinity without necrosis or thrombosis of the vessels themselves. The clinical picture is variable but severe muscle weakness rarely develops.

Eosinophilic syndromes

Prominent presence of eosinophilic polymorphonuclear leukocytes in muscle (or fascia) can occur in isolation or with systemic eosinophilia, due to parasitic infection, vasculitis, hypereosinophilic syndrome or toxic factors.

In eosinophilic polymyositis [165], muscle involvement is part of a systemic hypereosinophilic syndrome. A marked systemic eosinophilia is present. Myocardium is often involved in the inflammatory process. Proximal limb muscles show stiffness, pain, and variable weakness. Serum CK activity is moderately elevated. The pathological picture is similar to that of idiopathic PM, except that there is a conspicuous presence of eosinophilic polymorphonuclear leukocytes in the inflammatory infiltrates. Recent evidence suggests that certain patients with genetically defined calpain gene mutations have eosinophilic infections in their muscle [63]. The frequency of this phenomenon and the role of eosinophils in myopathy remain unclear.

In eosinophilic fasciitis, the inflammatory reaction is restricted to the fascia and is best shown by a biopsy of the fascia lata [166]. Necrotizing fasciitis is a misnomer because the basic process is a hyperacute necrotizing myopathy caused usually by beta-hemolytic streptococci, presumably acting as a superantigen [167, 168]. It may follow a variety of wounds and surgical interventions. If early treatment with high-dose intravenous immunoglobulins and antistreptococcal antibiotics is missed, amputation of the affected limb may be necessary to avoid a fatal outcome [see Hyperacute necrotizing fasciitis/myositis ("flesh-eating disease") above].

The eosinophilia-myalgia syndrome was caused by the prolonged oral intake of large doses of a contaminated L-tryptophan preparation as a therapeutic agent, mainly for insomnia [9]. There was marked systemic eosinophilia with generalized myalgia and moderate muscle weakness [169]. Another important feature was thickening of the skin, mimicking scleroderma. In severe disease, myocarditis and other visceral involvements can supervene. The lymphocytic inflammatory infiltrates (CD81 cytotoxic cells) also included either abundant or few eosinophilic polymorphonuclear leukocytes, mainly in the perimysial region, but less often in the interstitial space of muscle as well [10, 170]. Muscle fiber necrosis was rare and serum CK activity did not rise significantly. Coexisting peripheral neuropathy may cause denervation atrophy. In some cases, the muscle biopsy showed no abnormality, despite clinical symptoms.

The pathogenic factor appears to be contamination of L-tryptophan with an acetaldehyde ditryptophan derivative, which seems to induce autosensitization. The disease usually subsides after cessation of exposure but resolution may be slow. Corticosteroid therapy may help to accelerate recovery.

Macrophagic myofasciitis

A distinctive inflammatory muscle disorder was recently identified in up to 80 French patients who presented with myalgias, fatigue, and mild muscle weakness [171]. Muscle biopsy revealed pronounced infiltration of the connective tissue around the muscle (epimysium, perimysium, and perifascicular endomysium) by sheets of periodic-acid-Schiff-base-positive macrophages and occasional CD81 T-cells. Serum CK or erythrocyte sedimentation rate may at times be elevated. Most patients respond to glucocorticoid therapy, and the overall prognosis is favorable. The pathology is almost always seen at the sites of previous vaccinations, even several months later, and has been linked to a type of aluminum component used as the substrate for preparation of the vaccines. Macrophagic myofasciitis has been reported exclusively from France.

Localized forms

Inflammatory myopathies, usually of the PM type, may be restricted to one muscle or to one group of muscles [172, 173]. These localized forms of IM may involve forearm muscles, quadriceps, sternomastoids, and masseter or shoulder-girdle muscles. The last is probably the best known variety, since it mimics facioscapulohumeral dystrophy [174]. It may be sporadic or familial (autosomal dominant). The response to corticosteroid therapy is poor.

Another form of localized muscle inflammation can occur in any large muscle presenting as a muscle mass [172]. Necrosis and regeneration of muscle fibers and focal inflammatory infiltrates are present. The etiology of this peculiar muscle reaction is unknown. It has to be differentiated from neoplasms or abscesses.

Inflammatory myopathy with "pipe-stem" capillaries

In three patients, a peculiar form of necrotizing myopathy and to a lesser extent IM with a microangiopathy has been described [175]. The hallmark of the pathology is so-called pipe-stem capillaries, which stand out because of their thickened wall. MAC was demonstrated in the walls of some of these vessels. The capillarization of the muscle is usually reduced. While there are similarities between this vascular pathology and that occurring in DM, the two entities are different. It should be noted that capillaries with thickened walls, presumably caused by a widening of the basal lamina, can occur in a variety of diseases including diabetes, collagen vascular disorders (such as systemic lupus erythematosus), as well as unspecified myopathies and neuropathies.

Drug-induced inflammatory myopathy

Recurrent intramuscular injection of pentazocine in habitual users of the analgesic drug produces a necrotic IM with a massive increase of endomysial and perimysial connective tissue, resulting in joint contractures. A peculiar effect of this process is the inability of arms to be fully lowered next to the trunk ("arm levitation phenomenon"). It is not known what chemical feature of pentazocine is responsible for this peculiar pathological reaction in muscle.

Systemic use of d-penicillamine [130], procainamide, and phenytoin may cause vasculitis involving skeletal muscles. Reduced muscle strength, however, is usually mild. d-Penicillamine, in fact, more often causes a myasthenia-like picture than vasculitis. Zidovudine, used in the treatment of AIDS, causes a mitochondrial myopathy that may coexist with endomysial inflammatory infiltrates related to HIV [156].

Graft-versus-host reaction

In the graft-versus-host reaction, interstitial infiltration of muscle with lymphocytes may occur, but clinical muscle weakness is mild or not discernible.

Combined inflammatory and mitochondrial myopathy

Combined inflammatory and mitochondrial myopathy occurs in middle-aged patients with a chronic limb-girdle syndrome and prominent quadriceps weakness [176, 177]. They have elevated serum CK activity with typical muscle pathological features of PM and mitochondrial myopathy. The response to corticosteroids is poor. Whether this entity is distinct from IBM remains unclear, but a number of cases appear to have IBM.

Special forms of myopathies in children

Benign acute childhood myositis

Benign acute childhood myositis (BACM) is also called myalgia cruris epidemica since the cardinal manifestations include acute pain and swelling of the muscles in the calves and anterior tibial compartment. The disease runs a self-limiting course of a few days up to 2 weeks [178]. Cases tend to cluster, which would be consistent with an infectious etiology. Influenza A and B virus have been found in patients with BACM [179]. Muscle biopsy may be normal or it may show intense lymphocytic infiltration and edema.

Childhood dermatomyositis

Childhood DM is the most common form of acquired muscle disease in childhood [65, 180]. Onset of symptoms may occur as early as 2 years of age. The peak incidence is 14–16 years of age. The female-to-male ratio of occurrence is about 3:2. In approximately 25% of children, an acute viral-like disease precedes the onset.

The course of the disease is usually subacute, but acute cases are not too infrequent. Symptoms include weakness of the shoulder and hip girdle muscles, as well as proximal limb muscles. Muscles are often tender to touch and may be swollen. Muscle pain and arthralgia are exaggerated by exercise. The skin rash is similar to that described in adult DM. Raynaud phenomenon does not occur and carcinoma is not associated with childhood DM.

Extramuscular manifestations, which are nowadays rare, may include ischemic necrosis of the intestinal wall with perforation. Subcutaneous calcinosis is not uncommon and causes skin ulceration and limb deformities. Interstitial pulmonary fibrosis is very rare. Childhood DM is self-limiting after a course of 2–4 years; however, if it is left untreated, severe residual muscle wasting and weakness may occur.

The serum CK activity is elevated and the EMG shows a characteristic pattern that is similar to that of adult DM.

The light and electron microscopy histological features on muscle biopsy are very similar to those of adult DM, but perifascicular atrophy and muscle infarcts are more common in childhood DM. The vascular changes include capillary necrosis, reduced capillary density of muscle, endothelial cell abnormalities and thrombosis of medium-sized arteries and veins.

Polymyositis in children

Chronic IM of the adult PM type is exceedingly rare in children [181]. Two peculiar types of chronic IM deserve comment. Although these entities are rare they are still important because they are potentially treatable and require differentiation from congenital muscular dystrophy and other congenital myopathies.

Infantile polymyositis with sick myonuclei

Infantile PM with sick myonuclei [182] develops during the first year. Early signs include an inability to stand, falling, weak arm elevation, and poor head control owing to weakness of neck muscles. The atrophy of arm muscles with relatively normal bulk of forearm musculature confers a "Popeye" type of arm contour. Craniobulbar deficits are lacking and there are no extramuscular manifestations. Tendon reflexes are usually lost early in the disease.

The EMG findings are similar to those described for adult idiopathic PM. Muscle biopsy abnormalities include interstitial infiltrates of lymphocytes but without partial invasion of muscle fibers of the type described in PM, marked smallness of most muscle fibers, scattered muscle fiber necrosis, and regeneration. Failed regeneration, however, is common and as a result numerous scattered foci of muscle fiber loss and fibrosis are common features. Sarcolemmal MHC class I expression in muscle fibers occurs, which tends to confirm the inflammatory nature of the disease.

A distinctive feature of the pathology consists of prominent myonuclear abnormalities (Figure 22.10) including abnormally large size, irregular or even bizarre shapes with cytoplasmic invaginations and various inclusions. Inclusions may take the form of 4-nm filaments resembling actin filaments, hexagonal arrays of 22-nm filaments and microtubules. Excess heterochromatin is present in many nuclei.

This disease appears to be self-limiting but even with corticosteroid therapy (which is somewhat helpful) major permanent muscle wasting and weakness remain.

Congenital inflammatory myopathy

In congenital IM [183, 184], fetal movements are reduced and muscular hypotonia is noted at birth. Motor milestones are considerably delayed. Muscle weakness involves the neck, limbs, face, and respiratory territories. Contractures are common in the limbs. Stretch reflexes are depressed or absent. Most patients have microencephaly and mental subnormality. The muscle biopsy reveals necrosis and regeneration, extensive muscle fiber loss and fibrosis, focal interstitial lymphocytic infiltration, and sarcolemmal MHC class I expression in large groups of nonregenerating muscle fibers. Dystrophin immunostaining of muscle fibers is normal.

Steroid responsiveness of this disease is variable but never dramatic and the central nervous system is not affected.

This syndrome must be differentiated from Fukuyama congenital dystrophy [185], as well as the Walker–Warburg syndrome and merosin-negative congenital dystrophy (see Chapter 13). In the last, the muscle biopsy may show prominent endomysial inflammatory infiltrates.

Treatment

Because the specific target antigens in DM, PM, and IBM are unknown, the presently employed immunosuppressive therapies do not selectively target either the autoreactive T cells or the complement-mediated process affecting intramuscular blood vessels. Instead, they induce a nonselective and largely nonspecific immunosuppression or immunomodulation. Furthermore, many of these therapies are empirical and are based mostly on uncontrolled experience.

The practical goal of therapy in IM is to improve the function in the activities of daily living and to improve muscle strength. In essence, the therapy is also designed to induce a remission of the dysimmune state or to minimize muscle fiber loss before a spontaneous remission occurs. Despite the fact that when the muscle strength improves the serum CK tends to fall concurrently, the reverse is not always true because most of the immunosuppressive therapies can result in a decrease of serum muscle enzymes without necessarily improving muscle strength. Unfortunately, this has been interpreted as "chemical improvement" and led to the erroneous practice of "chasing" or "treating" the serum CK level instead of the muscle weakness. This practice may lead to prolonged use of unnecessary immunosuppressive drugs and erroneous assessment of their efficacy [1, 2, 69, 186, 187].

Drugs of use in treating inflammatory myopathies

Corticosteroids

Prednisone is the first-line drug for treatment for DM or PM. Its action is unclear but it may exert a beneficial effect by inhibiting the recruitment and migration of lymphocytes to the areas of muscle inflammation and by interfering with the production of lymphokines. Its effect on IL-1 may be important because this lymphokine is myotoxic [188] and is secreted by the activated macrophages that invade the muscle fibers. Steroid-induced suppression of ICAM-1 may also be relevant because downregulation of ICAM-1 can prevent the passage of lymphocytes across the endothelial cell wall towards the muscle fibers.

Because the effectiveness and relative safety of prednisone therapy will determine the future need for stronger immunosuppressive drugs, our preference has been to start with a high-dose prednisone, 80–100 mg per day, early in the disease. After an initial period of 3–4 weeks, prednisone is tapered on alternate days over a 10-week period to 80–100 mg in a single daily dose by gradually reducing the alternate "off day" dose by 10 mg per week, or faster if necessitated by side-effects, though this carries a greater risk of breakthrough of disease. If there is evidence of efficacy, and no serious side-effects, the dosage is reduced gradually by 5–10 mg every 3–4 weeks until the lowest possible dose that controls the disease is reached. If, by the time the dosage has been reduced to 80–100 mg every other day (approximately 14 weeks after initiating therapy), there has been no objective benefit (defined as unimproved muscle strength) the patient may be considered unresponsive to prednisone and an accelerated tapering regimen is introduced while the next-in-line immunosuppressive drug is started [1, 69, 187]. An important alternative to high-dose oral steroids is high-dose intermittent intravenous methylprednisolone, at 500–1000 mg 2–3 times weekly, depending on disease severity and tolerance. In fact, this is the highly preferred first-line treatment of one of the authors (G.K.). This route of administration minimizes muscular (and extramuscular) side-effects, which are particularly prone to occur in the aged and those with malnutrition and disuse atrophy. In such cases, it is our preferred initial treatment. When the dose can be reduced, a switch to a much lower oral therapy can be made.

Although almost all the patients with bona fide PM or DM respond to steroids to some degree at least for some period of time, a number of them fail to respond or become steroid resistant. Many authorities recommend immunosuppressive drugs, such as azathioprine, along with corticosteroids at the outset, while others base the decision to start an immunosuppressive drug in patients with PM or DM on the following factors: (1) need for its "steroid-sparing" effect, when in spite of steroid responsiveness the patient has developed significant complications; (2) attempts to lower a high steroid dosage have repeatedly resulted in a new relapse; (3) an adequate dose of prednisone for at least a 2- to 3-month period has been ineffective; and (4) rapidly progressive disease with evolving severe weakness and respiratory failure. One author of this chapter (G.K.) prefers to use immunosuppressants at the outset, while the other author (M.D.) delays it for the above-cited special circumstances. The preference for selecting immunosuppressive therapy is, however, empirical. The choice is usually based on our own prejudices, our personal experience with each drug, and our own assessment of the relative efficacy and safety ratio. A number of immunosuppressive agents have been used.

Azathioprine

Azathioprine is a derivative of 6-mercatopurine; it is given orally. Although lower doses (1.5–2 mg/kg) are commonly used, we prefer higher doses, up to 3 mg/kg for effective immunosuppression. This drug is well tolerated, has relatively few side-effects and, empirically, it appears to be as effective for long-term therapy as the other drugs. If liver function tests become impaired, the drug should be stopped. Some degree of anemia however is tolerated.

Methotrexate

Methotrexate is an antagonist of folate metabolism. Although its superiority to azathioprine has not been established, it does have a faster action. It is often given orally starting at 7.5 mg weekly for the first 3 weeks (given in a total of three doses, 2.5 mg every 12 h), increasing gradually by 2.5 mg per week up to a total of 25 mg weekly. A relevant side-effect is methotrexate pneumonitis, which can be difficult to distinguish from the interstitial lung disease of the primary inflammatory myopathy, the latter often associated with Jo-1 antibodies.

Cyclophosphamide

Intravenous cyclophosphamide has not been effective in our hands [189].

Mycophenolate mofetil

This drug is very well tolerated at doses up to 2–3 g/day. It is helpful as a steroid-spring agent and it is preferable to azathioprine because it is better tolerated and has a faster action.

Ciclosporin

Although the toxicity of ciclosporin can now be monitored by measuring optimal trough serum levels (optimal levels are 100–250 mg/ml), its effectiveness in PM and DM needs confirmation [190]. The advantage of ciclosporin is that it acts faster than azathioprine or methotrexate and the results (positive or negative) may therefore become apparent early [191].

Plasmapheresis

A double-blind, placebo-controlled study did not show any advantage gained from plasmapheresis [192].

Total lymphoid irradiation

Total lymphoid irradiation has been helpful in rare patients and may have long-lasting benefit. The long-term side-effects of this treatment, however, should be seriously considered before deciding on this experimental and rather extreme approach. Total lymphoid irradiation has been ineffective in IBM [193].

Intravenous immunoglobulin

Intravenous immunoglobulin (IVIg) has been effective in DM and PM based on uncontrolled studies [194, 195, 196] and one controlled trial conducted for DM [197]. In DM, IVIg was effective not only in improving strength but also in the skin changes and the underlying immunopathology [197]. The improvements begin after the first IVIg infusion and are clearly evident by the second monthly infusion. Repeated infusions every 6–8 weeks may be required to maintain improvement.

Intravenous Ig may act in DM by inhibiting the deposition of activated complement fragment on the capillaries [67], by suppressing cytokines especially ICAM-1, or by saturating Fc receptors and interfering with the action of macrophages [198, 199, 200]. In PM the drug has been found to be effective in up to 80% of the patients based on uncontrolled studies [194].

Intravenous Ig has also exerted some benefit in up to 30% of IBM patients, although the changes were not statistically significant, based on our controlled double-blind study [198].

Rituximab, a B-cell-depleting monoclonal antibody, may be of benefit in some DM patients resistant to therapy [201]. A controlled study is underway.

Tacrolimus may also be of some benefit in difficult cases especially those associated with interstitial lung disease [202].

A treatment regimen

Until further controlled drug trials are completed, the following step-by-step empirical approach for the treatment of PM and DM is suggested:

Step 1: high-dose corticosteroid (oral or intermittent intravenous)

Step 2: initial and/or subsequent optional immunosuppressants, i.e., azathioprine, methotrexate, or mycophenolate

Step 3: if step 2 fails, try high-dose IVIg

Step 4: if step 3 fails, consider a trial, with guarded optimism, of one of the following agents, chosen according to the patient's age, degree of disability, tolerance, experience with the drug, and the patient's general health: rituximab, ciclosporin, cyclophosphamide or tacrolimus.

One team (G.K.) starts treatment in DM and PM with high-dose intermittent intravenous steroids (methylprednisolone, 1000–250 mg three times a week). This initial dose is gradually diminished according to clinical response. When the methylprednisolone is sufficiently reduced, for the sake of convenience there may be a switch to oral prednisone in patients younger than age 35 and not at a dose higher than 30 mg/day. In all patients careful attention is paid to bone density and appropriate preventative medication is used if indicated. Intravenous steroids produce substantially fewer side-effects than oral ones, particularly in patients older than 50 years and those with disuse atrophy and protein malnutrition.

In patients who do not have malignancy or pulmonary fibrosis, azathioprine 2–3 mg/kg per day is given at the very outset. If not tolerated, methotrexate up to 25 mg/week is used. Azathioprine or methotrexate is continued for at least 1 year.

In severe cases of DM, IvIg (40 g every 1–3 weeks) are given for a few months.

The ultimate aim of treatment is elimination of the etiological factor; this is rarely attainable at present. Short of that, the development of specific immunotherapies aimed at targeting precise pathogenic events operating in the particular inflammatory myopathy is the goal. This may include inhibition of antigen presentation, curtailment of inflammatory cell activation and mobility or inhibition of the production or action of specific pathogenic antibodies.

References

1. M. C. Dalakas, *Polymyositis and Dermatomyositis*. (Boston, MA: Butterworths, 1988.)
2. M. C. Dalakas, Polymyositis, dermatomyositis, and inclusion-body myositis. *N. Engl. J. Med.* **325** (1991), 1487–1498.
3. M. C. Dalakas, R. Hohlfeld, Polymyositis and dermatomyositis. *Lancet* **362**:9388 (2003), 971–982.
4. G. Karpati, S. Carpenter, Pathology of the inflammatory myopathies. *Baillière's Clin. Neurol.* **2** (1993), 527–556.
5. A. G. Engel, R. Hohlfeld, B. Q. Banker, The polymyositis and dermatomyositis syndrome. In *Myology*, eds. A. G. Engel, C. Franzini-Armstrong. (New York: McGraw-Hill, 2006), pp. 1335–1383.
6. G. Karpati, G. S. Currie, The inflammatory myopathies. In *Disorders of Voluntary Muscle*, eds. J. Walton, G. Karpati, D. Hilton-Jones. (Edinburgh: Churchill-Livingston, 1994), pp. 619–646.
7. F. L. Mastaglia, M. J. Garlepp, B. A. Phillips, P. J. Zilko, Inflammatory myopathies: clinical, diagnostic and therapeutic aspects. *Muscle Nerve* **27**:4 (2003), 407–425.
8. C. Otero, I. Illa, M. C. Dalakas, Is there dermatomyositis (DM) without myositis? *Neurology* **42** (1992), 388S.
9. P. A. Hertzmann, W. L. Blevins, J. Mayer, B. Greenfield, M. Ting, G. J. Gleich, Association of the eosinophilia-myalgia syndrome with the ingestion of tryptophan. *N. Engl. J. Med.* **322** (1990), 869–873.
10. I. Illa, S. Dinsmore, M. C. Dalakas, Immune-mediated mechanisms and immune activation of fibroblasts in the pathogenesis of eosinophilia-myalgia syndrome induced by l tryptophan. *Hum. Pathol.* **24** (1993), 702–709.
11. R. Temiz, C. C. Weihl, A. Pestronk, Inflammatory myopathies with mitochondrial pathology and protein aggregates. *J. Neurol. Sci.* **278**:1-2 (2009), 25–29.
12. G. Karpati, S. Carpenter, Evolving concepts about inclusion body myositis. In *Actualités Neuromusculaires: Acquisition Récentes*, eds. G. Serratrice, J. F. Pellesier, J. Pouget, *et al.* (Paris: Exp. Scient. Française, 1993), pp. 93–98.
13. E. A. Sekul, M. C. Dalakas, Inclusion body myositis: new concepts. *Semin. Neurol.* **13** (1993), 256–263.
14. R. C. Griggs, V. Askanas, S. DiMauro, *et al.*, Inclusion body myositis and myopathies. *Ann. Neurol.* **38** (1995), 705–713.
15. S. Carpenter, Inclusion body myositis, a review. *J. Neuropathol. Exp. Neurol.* **55** (1996), 1105–1114.
16. G. Karpati, Inclusion body myositis – Status 1997. *Neurologist* **3** (1997), 201–208.
17. M. C. Dalakas, Inflammatory, immune, and viral aspects of inclusion-body myositis. *Neurology* **66**:2 (Suppl 1) (2006), S33–S38.
18. M. Needham, F. L. Mastaglia, Inclusion body myositis: current pathogenetic concepts and diagnostic and therapeutic approaches. *Lancet Neurol.* **6**:7 (2007), 620–631.
19. M. Needham, F. L. Mastaglia, Sporadic inclusion body myositis: a continuing puzzle. *Neuromuscul. Disord.* **18**:1 (2008), 6–16.
20. K. Sivakumar, M. C. Dalakas, The spectrum of familial inclusion body myopathies in 13 families and description of a quadriceps sparing phenotype in non-Iranian Jews. *Neurology* **47** (1996), 977–984.
21. K. Sivakumar, M. C. Dalakas, Inclusion body myositis and myopathies. *Curr. Opin. Neurol.* **10** (1997), 413–420.
22. Z. Argov, R. Yarom, 'Rimmed vacuole myopathy' sparing the quadriceps: a unique disorder in Iranian Jews. *J. Neurol. Sci.* **64** (1984), 33–43.
23. E. A. Sekul, C. Chow, M. C. Dalakas, Magnetic resonance imaging of the forearm as a diagnostic aid in patients with inclusion body myositis. *Neurology* **48** (1997), 863–866.
24. C. A. Luciano, M. C. Dalakas, A macro-EMG study in inclusion-body myositis: no evidence for a neurogenic component. *Neurology* **48** (1997), 29–33.
25. J. M. Schroder, M. Molnar, Mitochondrial abnormalities and peripheral neuropathy in inflammatory myopathy, especially inclusion body myositis. *Mol. Cell. Biochem.* **174** (1997), 277–282.
26. B. M. Koffman, M. Rugiero, M. C. Dalakas, Autoimmune diseases and autoantibodies associated with sporadic inclusion body myositis. *Muscle Nerve* **21** (1998), 115–117.
27. U. A. Badrising, G. M. Schreuder, M. J. Giphart, *et al.*, Associations with autoimmune disorders and HLA class I and II antigens in inclusion body myositis. *Neurology* **63**:12 (2004), 2396–2398.
28. B. M. Koffman, K. Sivakumar, T. Simonis, D. Stroncek, M. C. Dalakas, HLA allele distribution distinguishes sporadic inclusion body myositis from hereditary inclusion body myopathies. *J. Neuroimmunol.* **84** (1998), 139–142.
29. K. Sivakumar, C. Semino-Mora, M. C. Dalakas, An inflammatory, familial, inclusion body myositis with autoimmune features and a phenotype identical to sporadic inclusion body myositis: studies in 3 families. *Brain* **120** (1997), 653–661.
30. A. J. Cole, R. Kuzniecky, G. Karpati, S. Carpenter, E. Andermann, F. Andermann, Familial myopathy with changes resembling inclusion body myositis and periventricular leucoencephalopathy. *Brain* **111** (1988), 1025–1037.
31. R. Massa, B. Weller, G. Karpati, E. Shoubridge, S. Carpenter, Familial inclusion body myositis among Kurdish-Iranian Jews. *Arch. Neurol.* **48** (1991), 519–522.
32. I. Eisenberg, N. Avidan, T. Potikha, *et al.*, The UDP-N-acetylglucosamine 2-epimerase/N-acetylmannosamine kinase gene is mutated in recessive hereditary inclusion body myopathy. *Nat. Genet.* **29**:1 (2001), 83–87.

33. G. D. Watts, J. Wymer, M. J. Kovach, *et al.*, Inclusion body myopathy associated with Paget disease of bone and frontotemporal dementia is caused by mutant valosin-containing protein. *Nat. Genet.* **36**:4 (2004), 377–381.

34. A. Peng, B. M. Koffman, J. D. Malley, M. C. Dalakas, Disease progression in sporadic inclusion body myositis (s-IBM): observations in 78 patients. *Neurology* **55** (2000), 296–298.

35. K. Clawson, C. V. Oddis, Adult respiratory distress syndrome in polymyositis patients with the anti-Jo-I antibody. *Arthritis Rheum.* **38** (1995), 1519–1523.

36. M. I. Schwarz, J. M. Sutarik, J. A. Nick, R. L. Leff, J. W. Emlen, R. M. Tuder, Pulmonary capillaritis and diffuse alveolar hemorrhage: a primary manifestation of polymyositis. *Am. J. Respir. Crit. Care Med.* **151** (1995), 2037–2040.

37. M. C. Dalakas, Calcifications in dermatomyositis. *N. Engl. J. Med.* **333** (1995), 978.

38. S. Carpenter, G. Karpati, The major inflammatory myopathies of unknown cause. *Pathol. Ann.* **16** (1981), 205–237.

39. A. G. Engel, B. Q. Banker, *Myology*. (New York: McGraw-Hill, 1986.)

40. S. Carpenter, G. Karpati, The pathological diagnosis of specific inflammatory myopathies. *Brain Pathol.* **2** (1992), 13–19.

41. F. Jerusalem, M. Rakusa, A. G. Engel, R. D. Macdonald, Morphometric analysis of skeletal muscle capillary ultrastructure in inflammatory myopathies. *J. Neurol. Sci.* **23** (1974), 391–401.

42. M. De Visser, A. M. Emslie-Smith, A. G. Engel, Early ultrastructural alterations in adult dermatomyositis. Capillary abnormalities precede other structural changes in muscle. *J. Neurol. Sci.* **94** (1989), 181–192.

43. A. M. Emslie-Smith, A. G. Engel, Microvascular changes in early and advanced dermatomyositis: a quantitative study. *Ann. Neurol.* **27** (1990), 343–356.

44. J. T. Kissel, J. R. Mendell, K. W. Rammohan, Microvascular deposition of complement membrane attack complex in dermatomyositis. *N. Engl. J. Med.* **314** (1986), 329.

45. J. T. Kissel, R. K. Halterman, K. W. Rammohan, J. R. Mendell, The relationship of complement-mediated microvasculopathy to the histologic features and clinical duration of disease in dermatomyositis. *Arch. Neurol.* **48** (1991), 26–30.

46. K. Arahata, A. G. Engel, Monoclonal antibody analysis of mononuclear cells in myopathies. I: Quantitation of subsets according to diagnosis and sites of accumulation and demonstration and counts of muscle fibres invaded by T cells. *Ann. Neurol.* **16** (1984), 193–208.

47. K. Arahata, A. G. Engel, Monoclonal antibody analysis of mononuclear cells in myopathies III. Immunoelectron microscopy aspects of cell-mediated muscle fibre injury. *Ann. Neurol.* **19** (1986), 112–125.

48. B. P. Lotz, A. G. Engel, H. Nishino, J. C. Stevens, W. J. Litchy, Inclusion body myositis. Observations in 40 patients. *Brain* **112** (1989), 727–747.

49. V. Askanas, W. K. Engel, M. Bilak, R. B. Alvarez, D. J. Selkoe, Twisted tubulofilaments of inclusion body myositis muscle resemble paired helical filaments of Alzheimer brain containing hyperphosphorylated tau. *Am. J. Pathol.* **144** (1994), 177–187.

50. V. Askanas, P. Serdaroglu, W. K. Engel, R. B. Alvarez, Immunocytochemical localization of ubiquitin in inclusion body myositis allows its light-microscopic distinction from polymyositis. *Neurology* **42** (1992), 460–461.

51. V. Askanas, W. K. Engel, R. B. Alvarez, G. G. Glenner, β-Amyloid protein immunoreactivity in muscle of patients with inclusion-body myositis. *Lancet* **339** (1992), 560–561.

52. V. Askanas, W. K. Engel, R. B. Alvarez, Enhanced detection of Congo-red-positive amyloid deposits in muscle fibers of inclusion body myositis and brain of Alzheimer disease using fluorescence technique. *Neurology* **43** (1993), 1265–1267.

53. J. L. De Bleecker, B. B. Ertl, A. G. Engel, Patterns of abnormal parotein expression in target formations and unstructured cores. *Neuromuscul. Disord.* **6** (1996), 339–349.

54. C. Semino-Mora, M. C. Dalakas, Rimmed vacuoles with β-amyloid and ubiquitinated filamentous deposits in the muscles of patients with long-standing denervation (post-poliomyelitis muscular atrophy): similarities with inclusion body myositis. *Hum. Pathol.* **29** (1998), 1128–1133.

55. J. R. Mendell, Z. Sahenk, T. Gales, L. Paul, Amyloid filaments in inclusion body myositis. *Arch. Neurol.* **48** (1991), 1229–1234.

56. J. D. Lünemann, J. Schmidt, D. Schmid, *et al.*, Beta-amyloid is a substrate of autophagy in sporadic inclusion body myositis. *Ann. Neurol.* **61**:5 (2007), 476–483.

57. J. Nalbantoglu, G. Karpati, S. Carpenter, Conspicuous accumulation of a single- stranded DNA binding protein in skeletal muscle fibres in inclusion body myositis. *Am. J. Pathol.* **144** (1994), 874–882.

58. S. A. Greenberg, J. L. Pinkus, A. A. Amato, Nuclear membrane proteins are present within rimmed vacuoles in inclusion body myositis. *Muscle Nerve* **34** (2006), 406–416.

59. R. Horvath, K. Fu, A. Genge, G. Karpati, E. A. Shoubridge, Characterization of the mitochondiral DNA abnormalities in the skeletal muscle of patients with inclusion body myositis. *J. Neuropathol. Exp. Neurol.* **57** (1998), 396–403.

60. G. Karpati, Y. Pouliot, S. Carpenter, Expression of immunoreactive major histocompatability complex products in human skeletal muscles. *Ann. Neurol.* **23** (1988), 64–72.

61. A. M. Emslie-Smith, K. Arahata, A. G. Engel, Major histocompatibility complex class I antigen expression, immunologicalization of interferon subtypes, and T cell-mediated cytotoxicity in myopathies. *Hum. Pathol.* **20** (1989), 224–231.

62. J. T. Kissel, K. L. Burrow, K. W. Rammohan for the CIDD Group, Mononuclear cell analysis of muscle biopsies in prednisone-treated and untreated Duchenne muscular dystrophy. *Neurology* **41** (1991), 667–672.

63. M. Krahn, A. Lopez de Munain, *et al.*, CAPN3 mutations in patients with idiopathic eosinophilic myositis. *Ann. Neurol.* **59**:6 (2006), 905–911.

64. N. Chahin, A. G. Engel, Correlation of muscle biopsy, clinical course, and outcome in PM and sporadic IBM. *Neurology* **70**:6 (2008), 418–424.

65. S. Carpenter, G. Karpati, S. Rothman, G. Walters, The childhood type of dermatomyositis. *Neurology* **26** (1976), 952–962.

66. J. N. Whitaker, W. K. Engel, Vascular deposits of immunoglobulin and complement in idiopathic inflammatory myopathy. *N. Engl. J. Med.* **286** (1972), 333–338.

67. M. Basta, M. C. Dalakas, High-dose intravenous immunoglobulin exerts its beneficial effect in patients with dermatomyositis by blocking endomysial deposition of activated complement fragments. *J. Clin. Invest.* **94** (1994), 1729–1735.

68. M. C. Dalakas, Mechanisms of disease: signaling pathways and immunobiology of inflammatory myopathies. *Nat. Clin. Pract. Rheumatol.* **4** (2006), 219–227.

69. M. C. Dalakas, Immunopathogenesis of inflammatory myopathies. *Ann. Neurol.* **37** (1995), 74–86.

70. D. P. Stein, M. C. Dalakas, Intercellular adhesion molecule-1 expression is upregulated in patients with dermatomyositis (DM). *Ann. Neurol.* **34** (1993), 268.

71. I. Lundberg, J. M. Brengman, A. G. Engel, Analysis of cytokine expression in muscle in inflammatory myopathies, Duchenne's dystrophy and non-weak controls. *J. Neuroimmunol.* **63** (1995), 9–16.

72. D. S. Tews, H. H. Goebel, Expression of cell adhesion molecules in inflammatory myopathies. *J. Neuroimmunol.* **59** (1995), 185–194.

73. D. S. Tews, H. H. Goebel, Cytokine expression profiles in idiopathic inflammatory myopathies. *J. Neuropathol. Exp. Neurol.* **55** (1996), 342–347.

74. J. L. De Paepe, B.De Bleecker, I. E. Vanwalleghem, J. M. Schröder, Differential expression of chemokines in inflammatory myopathies. *Neurology* **58**:12 (2002), 1779–1785.

75. R. Raju, O. Vasconcelos, R. Granger, M. C. Dalakas, Expression of IFN-gamma-inducible chemokines in inclusion body myositis. *J. Euroimmunol* **141**:1–2 (2003), 125–131.

76. K. Amemiya, C. Semino-Mora, R. P. Granger, M. C. Dalakas, Downregulation of TGF-beta1 mRNA and protein in the muscles of patients with inflammatory myopathies after treatment with high-dose intravenous immunoglobulin. *Clin. Immunol.* **94**:2 (2000), 99–104.

77. I. Illa, E. Gallardo, R. Gimeno, C. Serrano, I. Ferrer, C. Juárez, Signal transducer and activator of transcription 1 in human muscle: implications in inflammatory myopathies. *Am. J. Pathol.* **151**:1 (1997), 81–88.

78. J. Schmidt, *et al.*, Interplay between inflammatory and degeneration-associated molecules in sporadic IBM. *Brain* **131** (2008), 1228–1240.

79. S. A. Greenberg, J. L. Pinkus, G. S. Pinkus, *et al.*, Interferon-alpha/beta-mediated innate immune mechanisms in dermatomyositis. *Ann. Neurol.* **57**:5 (2005), 664–678.

80. R. Raju, M. C. Dalakas, Gene expression profile in the muscles of patients with inflammatory myopathies: effect of therapy with IVIg and biological validation of clinically relevant genes. *Brain* **128**:Pt 8 (2005), 1887–1896.

81. S. A. Greenberg, Proposed immunologic models of the inflammatory myopathies and potential therapeutic implications. *Neurology* **69**:21 (2007), 2008–2019.

82. R. J. Walsh, S. W. Kong, Y. Yao, *et al.*, Type I interferon-inducible gene expression in blood is present and reflects disease activity in dermatomyositis and polymyositis. *Arthritis Rheum.* **56**:11 (2007), 3784–3792.

83. Z. Tezak, E. P. Hoffman, J. L. Lutz, *et al.*, Gene expression profiling in DQA1*0501+ children with untreated dermatomyositis: a novel pathogenesis. *J. Immunol.* **168**:8 (2002), 4154–4163.

84. R. L. Leff, L. A. Love, F. W. Miller, *et al.*, Viruses in the idiopathic inflammatory myopathies: absence of candidate viral genomes in muscle. *Lancet* **339** (1992), 1192–1195.

85. M. Leon-Monzon, M. C. Dalakas, Absence of persistent infection with enteroviruses in muscles of patients with inflammatory myopathies. *Ann. Neurol.* **32** (1992), 219–222.

86. P. H. Plotz, M. Dalakas, R. L. Leff, L. A. Love, F. W. Miller, M. E. Cronin, Current concepts in the idiopathic inflammatory myopathies: polymyositis, dermatomyositis and related disorders. *Ann. Intern. Med.* **111** (1989), 143–157.

87. I. N. Targoff, Immune mechanisms of myositis. *Curr. Opin. Rheumatol.* **2** (1990), 882–888.

88. Q. Ge, D. S. Nilasena, C. A. O'Brien, M. B. Frank, I. N. Targoff, Molecular analysis of a major antigenic region of the 240 kD protein of Mi-2 autoantigen. *J. Clin. Invest.* **96** (1995), 1730–1737.

89. T. Miller, M. T. Al-Lozi, G. Lopate, A. Pestronk, Myopathy with antibodies to the signal recognition particle: clinical and pathological features. *J. Neurol. Neurosurg. Psychiatry* **73**:4 (2002), 420–428.

90. G. J. Hengstman, B. G. van Engelen, W. J. van Venrooij, Myositis specific autoantibodies: changing insights in pathophysiology and clinical associations. *Curr. Opin. Rheumatol.* **16**:6 (2004), 692–699.

91. M. C. Dalakas, Understanding the immunopathogenesis of inclusion-body myositis: present and future prospects. *Rev. Neurol. (Paris)* **158**:10 Pt 1 (2002), 948–958.

92. R. Hohlfeld, A. G. Engel, Coculture with autologous myotubes of cytotoxic T cells isolated from muscle in inflammatory myopathies. *Ann. Neurol.* **29** (1991), 498–507.

93. R. Mantegazza, F. Andreette, P. Bernasconi, *et al.*, Analysis of T cell receptor repertoire of muscle infiltrating T lymphocytes in polymyositis. *J. Clin. Invest.* **91** (1993), 2880–2886.

94. D. Michaelis, N. Goebels, R. Hohlfeld, Constitutive and cytokine-induced expression of human leukocyte antigens and cell adhesion molecules by human myotubes. *Am. J. Pathol.* **143**:4 (1993), 1142–1149.

95. K. Nagaraju, N. Raben, L. Loeffler, *et al.*, Conditional up-regulation of MHC class I in skeletal muscle leads to self-sustaining autoimmune myositis and myositis-specific autoantibodies. *Proc. Natl. Acad. Sci. U. S. A.* **97**:16 (2000), 9209–9214.

96. P. Englund, E. Lindroos, I. Nennesmo, L. Klareskog, I. E. Lundberg, Skeletal muscle fibers express major histocompatibility complex class II antigens independently of inflammatory infiltrates in inflammatory myopathies. *Am. J. Pathol.* **159**:4 (2001), 1263–1273.

97. H. Wiendl, M. Mitsdoerffer, D. Schneider, *et al.*, Muscle fibres and cultured muscle cells express the B7.1/2-related inducible co-stimulatory molecule, ICOSL: implications for the pathogenesis of inflammatory myopathies. *Brain* **126**:Pt 5 (2003) 1026–1035.

98. H. Wiendl, R. Hohlfeld, B. C. Kieseier, Immunobiology of muscle: advances in understanding an immunological microenvironment. *Trends Immunol.* **26**:7 (2005), 373–380.

99. J. L. De Bleecker, A. G. Engel, J. C. Winkelmann, Localization of dystrophin and beta-spectrin in vacuolar myopathies. *Am. J. Pathol.* **143**:4 (1993), 1200–1208.

100. N. Goebels, D. Michaelis, M. Engelhardt, *et al.*, Differential expression of perforin in muscle-inflammatory T cells in polymyositis and dermatomyositis. *J. Clin. Invest.* **97** (1996), 2905–2910.

101. J. Schmidt, G. Rakocevic, R. Raju, M. C. Dalakas, Upregulated inducible co-stimulator (ICOS) and ICOS-ligand in inclusion body myositis muscle: significance for CD8 + T cell cytotoxicity. *Brain* **127**:Pt 5 (2004), 1182–1190.

102. C. Schneider, R. Gold, M. C. Dalakas, *et al.*, MHC class I-mediated cytotoxicity does not induce apoptosis in muscle fibres nor in inflammatory T cells: studies in patients with polymyositis, dermatomyositis and inclusion body myositis. *J. Neuropathol. Exp. Neurol.* **55** (1996), 1205–1209.

103. L. Behrens, A. Bender, M. A. Johnson, R. Hohlfeld, Cytotoxic mechanisms in inflammatory myopathies. Co-expression of Fas and protective Bcl-2 in muscle fibres and inflammatory cells. *Brain* **120** (1997), 929–938.

104. K. Nagaraju, L. Casciola-Rosen, A. Rosen, *et al.*, The inhibition of apoptosis in myositis and in normal muscle cells. *J. Immunol.* **164**:10 (2000), 5459–5465.

105. M. Li, M. C. Dalakas, The muscle mitogen-activated protein kinase is altered in sporadic inclusion body myositis. *Neurology* **54**:8 (2000), 1665–1670.

106. T. P. O'Hanlon, M. C. Dalakas, P. H. Plotz, F. W. Miller, Predominant TCR-alpha-beta variable and joining gene expression by muscle-infiltrating lymphocytes in the idiopathic inflammatory myopathies. *J. Immunol.* **152** (1994), 2569–2576.

107. I. M. Fyhr, A. R. Moslemi, A. A. Mosavi, C. Lindberg, A. Tarkowski, A. Oldfors, Oligoclonal expansion of muscle infiltrating T cells in inclusion body myositis. *J. Neuroimmunol.* **79** (1997), 185–189.

108. A. Bender, N. Ernst, A. Iglesias, K. Dornmair, H. Wekerle, R. Hohlfeld, T cell receptor in polymyositis: clonal expansion of autoaggressive CD81 T cells. *J. Exp. Med.* **181** (1995), 1863–1868.

109. O. Benveniste, S. Herson, B. Salomon, *et al.*, Long-term persistence of clonally expanded T cells in patients with polymyositis. *Ann. Neurol.* **56**:6 (2004), 867–872.

110. D. Dimitri, O. Benveniste, O. Dubourg, *et al.*, Shared blood and muscle CD8 + T-cell expansions in inclusion body myositis. *Brain* **129**:Pt 4 (2006), 986–995.

111. M. Salajegheh, G. Rakocevic, R. Raju, A. Shatunov, L. G. Goldfarb, M. C. Dalakas, T cell receptor profiling in muscle and blood lymphocytes in sporadic inclusion body myositis. *Neurology* **69**:17 (2007), 1672–1679.

112. A. Bender, L. Behrens, A. G. Engel, R. Hohlfeld, T-cell heterogeneity in muscle lesions of inclusion body myositis. *J. Neuroimmunol.* **84** (1998), 86–91.

113. M. Hofbauer, S. Wiesener, H. Babbe, *et al.*, Clonal tracking of autoaggressive T cells in polymyositis by combining laser microdissection, single-cell PCR, and CDR3-spectratype analysis. *Proc. Natl. Acad. Sci. U. S. A.* **100**:7 (2003), 4090–4095.

114. K. Amemiya, R. P. Granger, M. C. Dalakas, Clonal restriction of T-cell receptor expression by infiltrating lymphocytes in inclusion body myositis persists over time. Studies in repeated muscle biopsies. *Brain* **123** (2000), 2030–2039.

115. K. Müntzing, C. Lindberg, A. R. Moslemi, A. Oldfors, Inclusion body myositis: clonal expansions of muscle-infiltrating T cells persist over time. *Scand. J. Immunol.* **2** (2003), 195–200.

116. R. Hohlfeld, A. G. Engel, L. I. Kunio, M. C. Harper, Polymyositis mediated by T lymphocytes that express the gamma/delta receptor. *N. Engl. J. Med.* 324 (1991), 877–881.

117. G. Puschke, D. Ruegg, R. Hohlfeld, A. G. Engel, Autoaggressive myocytotoxic T-lymphocytes expressing an unusual gamma delta T cell receptor. *J. Exp. Med.* **176** (1992), 1785–1789.

118. H. Wiendl, J. Malotka, B. Holzwarth, *et al.*, An autoreactive gamma delta TCR derived from a polymyositis lesion. *J. Immunol.* **169**:1 (2002), 515–521.

119. L. Behrens, M. Kerschensteimer, T. Misgeld, N. Goebels, H. Wekerle, R. Hohlfeld, Human muscle cells express a functional costimulatory molecule distinct from B7.1 (CD80) and B7.2 (CD86) in vitro and in inflammatory lesions. *J. Immunol.* **161**:11 (1998), 5943–5951.

120. K. Murata, M. C. Dalakas, Expression of the costimulatory molecule BB-1, the ligands CTLA-4 and CD28 and their mRNA in inflammatory myopathies. *Am. J. Pathol.* **155** (1999), 453–460.

121. E. M. Bradshaw, A. Orihuela, S. L. McArdel, *et al.*, A local antigen-driven humoral response is present in the inflammatory myopathies. *J. Immunol.* **178**:1 (2007), 547–556.

122. M. C. Dalakas, Molecular immunology and genetics of inflammatory muscle diseases. *Arch. Neurol.* **55** (1998), 1509–1512.

123. B. De Paepe, J. L. De Bleecker, Beta-chemokine receptor expression in idiopathic inflammatory myopathies. *Muscle Nerve* **31**:5 (2005), 621–627.

124. B. De Paepe, K. De Keyzer, J. J. Martin, J. L. De Bleecker, Alpha-chemokine receptors CXCR1-3 and their ligands in idiopathic inflammatory myopathies. *Acta Neuropathol.* **109**:6 (2005), 576–582.

125. D. Figarella-Branger, J. Pouget, R. Bernard, *et al.*, Limb-girdle muscular dystrophy in a 71-year-old woman with an R27Q mutation in the CAV3 gene. *Neurology* **61**:4 (2003), 562–564.

126. M. Civatte, C. Bartoli, N. Schleinitz, B. Chetaille, J. F. Pellissier, D. Figarella-Branger, Expression of the beta chemokines CCL3, CCL4, CCL5 and their receptors in idiopathic inflammatory myopathies. *Neuropathol. Appl. Neurobiol.* **31**:1 (2005), 70–79.

127. Y. C. Choi, M. C. Dalakas, Expression of matrix metalloproteinases in the muscle of patients with inflammatory myopathies. *Neurology* **54** (2000), 65–71.

128. M. Salajegheh, R. Raju, J. Schmidt, M. C. Dalakas, Upregulation of thrombospondin-1 (TSP-1) and its binding partners, CD36 and CD47, in sporadic inclusion body myositis. *J. Neuroimmunol.* **187**:1-2 (2007), 166–174.

129. M. C. Dalakas, Sporadic inclusion body myositis – diagnosis, pathogenesis and therapeutic strategies. *Nat. Clin. Pract. Neurol.* **2**:8 (2006b), 437–447.

130. M. C. Dalakas, Toxic and drug-induced myopathies. *J. Neurol. Neurosurg. Psychiatry* **80**:8 (2009), 832–838.

131. K. Nagaraju, L. Casciola-Rosen, I. Lundberg, *et al.*, Activation of the endoplasmic reticulum stress response in autoimmune

myositis: potential role in muscle fiber damage and dysfunction. *Arthritis Rheum.* **52**:6 (2005), 1824–1835.

132. I. Ferrer, B. Martín, J. G. Castaño, J. J. Lucas, D. Moreno, M. Olivé, Proteasomal expression, induction of immunoproteasome subunits, and local MHC class I presentation in myofibrillar myopathy and inclusion body myositis. *J. Neuropathol. Exp. Neurol.* **63**:5 (2004), 484–498.

133. G. Vattemi, W. K. Engel, J. McFerrin, V. Askanas, Endoplasmic reticulum stress and unfolded protein response in inclusion body myositis muscle. *Am J Pathol.* **164**:1 (2004), 1–7.

134. V. Askanas, W. K. Engel, Proposed pathogenetic cascade of inclusion-body myositis: importance of amyloid-beta, misfolded proteins, predisposing genes, and aging. *Curr. Opin. Rheumatol.* **15**:6 (2003), 737–744.

135. B. L. Banwell, A. G. Engel, AlphaB-crystallin immunolocalization yields new insights into inclusion body myositis. *Neurology* **54**:5 (2000), 1020–1021.

136. M. C. Dalakas, Interplay between inflammation and degeneration: using inclusion body myositis to study “neuroinflammation”. *Ann. Neurol.* **64**:1 (2008), 1–3.

137. M. C. Dalakas, I. Illa, Common variable immunodeficiency and inclusion body myositis: a distinct myopathy mediated by natural killer cells. *Ann. Neurol.* **37** (1995), 806–810.

138. J. N. Pruitt, 2nd, C. J. Showalter, A. G. Engel, Sporadic inclusion body myositis: counts of different types of abnormal fibers. *Ann. Neurol.* **39**:1 (1996), 139–143.

139. Murth *et al.*

140. S. M. Chou, Inclusion body myositis: a possible chronic persistent mumps myositis? *Hum. Pathol.* **17** (1986), 765–776.

141. M. C. Dalakas, G. H. Pezeshkpour, M. Gravell, J. L. Sever, Polymyositis in patients with AIDS. *J. Am. Med. Assoc.* **256** (1986), 2381–2383.

142. H. Nishino, A. G. Engel, B. K. Rima, Inclusion body myositis: the mumps virus hypothesis. *Ann. Neurol.* **25** (1989), 260–264.

143. M. C. Dalakas, Viral myopathies. In *Myology*, vol. II, eds. A. G. Engel, C. Franzini-Armstrong. (New York: McGraw-Hill, 2006), pp. 1419–1437.

144. E. J. Cupler, M. Leon-Monzon, J. Miller, C. Semino-Mora, T. L. Anderson, M. C. Dalakas Inclusion body myositis in HIV-I and HTLV-I infected patients. *Brain* **19** (1996), 1887–1893.

145. M. C. Dalakas, W. T. London, M. Gravell, J. L. Sever, Polymyositis in an immunodeficiency disease in monkeys induced by a type D retrovirus. *Neurology* **36** (1986), 569–572.

146. M. C. Dalakas, G. H. Pezeshkpour, Neuromuscular diseases associated with human immunodeficiency virus infection. *Ann. Neurol.* **23** Suppl. (1988), 38–48.

147. O. Morgan, C. P. St. Rodgers-Johnson, C. Mora, G. Char, HTLV-1 and polymyositis in Jamaica. *Lancet* **ii** (1989), 1184–1187.

148. M. C. Dalakas, G. Rakocevic, A. Shatunov, L. Goldfarb, R. Raju, M. Salajegheh, Inclusion body myositis with human immunodeficiency virus infection: four cases with clonal expansion of viral-specific T cells. *Ann. Neurol.* **61**:5 (2007), 466–475.

149. S. Ozden, M. Cochet, J. Mikol, A. Teixeira, A. Gessain, C. Pique, Direct evidence for a chronic CD8 + T-cell-mediated immune reaction to tax within the muscle of a human T-cell leukemia/lymphoma virus type 1-infected patient with sporadic inclusion body myositis. *J Virol.* **78**:19 (2004), 10320–10327.

150. M. C. Dalakas, Advances in the immunobiology and treatment of inflammatory myopathies. *Curr. Rheumatol. Rep.* **9**:4 (2007), 291–297.

151. K. Matsuura, K. Miura, M. Taki, *et al.*, Ocular following responses of monkeys to the competing motions of two sinusoidal gratings. *Neurosci. Res.* **61**:1 (2008), 56–69.

152. I. Illa, A. Nath, M. C. Dalakas, Immunocytochemical and virological characteristics of HIV-associated inflammatory myopathies: similarities with seronegative polymyositis. *Ann. Neurol.* **29** (1991), 474–481.

153. M. Leon-Monzon, I. Illa, M. C. Dalakas, Polymyositis in patients infected with HTLV-1 (the role of the virus in the cause of the disease. *Ann. Neurol.* **36** (1994), 643–649.

154. M. Leon-Monzon, L. Lamperth, M. C. Dalakas, Search for HIV proviral DNA and amplified sequences in the muscle biopsies of patients with HIV-polymyositis. *Muscle Nerve* **16** (1993), 408–413.

155. M. Saito, I. Higuchi, A. Saito, *et al.*, Molecular analysis of T cell clonotypes in muscle-infiltrating lymphocytes from patients with human T lymphotropic virus type 1 polymyositis. *J. Infect. Dis.* **186**:9 (2002), 1231–1241.

156. M. C. Dalakas, I. Illa, G. H. Pezeshkpour, *et al.*, Mitochondrial myopathy caused by long-term zidovudine therapy. *N. Engl. J. Med.* **332** (1995), 1098–1105.

157. W. Lewis, M. C. Dalakas, Mitochondrial toxicity of antiviral drugs. *Nat. Med.* **1**:5 (1995), 417–422.

158. H. D. Davies, Flesh-eating disease: a note on necrotizing fasciitis. *Can. J. Inf. Dis.* **12**:3 (2001), 136–140.

159. T. Mimori, Scleroderma-polymyositis overlap syndrome: clinical and seriologic aspects. *Int. J. Dermatol.* **26** (1987), 419–425.

160. R. A. Foote, S. M. Kimbrough, J. C. Stevens, Lupus myositis. *Muscle Nerve* **5** (1982), 65.

161. S. P. Ringel, J. Z. Forstot, E. M. Tan, C. Wehling, R. C. Griggs, D. Butcher, Sjögren’s syndrome and polymyositis or dermatomyositis. *Arch. Neurol.* **39** (1982), 157.

162. S. Carpenter, G. Karpati, Granulomatous myopathies. In: *Pathology of Skeletal Muscle*, eds. S. Carpenter, G. Karpati. (New York: Churchill-Livingstone, 1984), pp. 557–558.

163. K. Le Roux, N. Streichenberger, C. Vial, *et al.*, Granulomatous myositis: a clinical study of thirteen cases. *Muscle Nerve* **35**:2 (2007), 171–177.

164. D. B. Ménard, H. Haddad, J. G. Blain, R. Beaudry, G. Devroede, S. Masse, Granulomatous myositis and myopathy associated with Crohn’s disease. *N. Engl. J. Med.* **295** (1976), 818–819.

165. R. B. Layzer, M. A. Shearn, S. Satya-Murti, Eosinophilic polymyositis. *Ann. Neurol.* **1** (1977), 65–71.

166. D. B. Simon, S. F. Ringel, R. I. Sufit, Clinical spectrum of fascial inflammation. *Muscle Nerve* **5** (1982), 525.

167. T. M. File Jr., S. J. Tan, J. R. DiPersio, Group A streptococcal necrotizing fasciitis. Diagnosing and treating the ‘flesh-eating bacteria syndrome’. *Cleveland Clin. J. Med.* **65** (1998), 241–249.

168. M. A. Gardam, D. E. Low, R. Saginur, M. A. Miller, Group B streptococcal necrotizing fasciitis and streptococcal toxic shock-like syndrome in adults. *Arch. Int. Med.* **158** (1998), 1704–1708.

169. R. W. Martin, J. Duffy, A. G. Engel, *et al.*, The clinical spectrum of eosinophilia-myalgia syndrome associated with l tryptophan ingestion. *Ann. Int. Med.* **113** (1990), 124.

170. A. M. Emslie-Smith, A. G. Engel, J. Duffy, C. A. Bowles, Eosinophilia myalgia syndrome: I. Immunocytochemical evidence for a T-cell-mediated immune effector response. *Ann. Neurol.* **29** (1991), 524–528.

171. M. M. Gherardi, J. C. Ramirez, D. Rodríguez, *et al.*, IL-12 delivery from recombinant vaccinia virus attenuates the vector and enhances the cellular immune response against HIV-1 Env in a dose-dependent manner. *J. Immunol.* **162**:11 (1999), 6724–6733.

172. R. R. Heffner, V. W. Armbrustmacher, K. M. Earle, Focal myositis. *Cancer* **40** (1977), 301–306.

173. N. E. Bharucha, J. A. Morgan-Hughes, Chronic focal polymyositis in the adult. *J. Neurol. Neurosurg. Psychiatry* **44** (1981), 419–425.

174. T. L. Munsat, D. Piper, P. Cancilla, J. Mednick, Inflammatory myopathy with facioscapulohumeral distribution. *Neurology* **22** (1972), 335–347.

175. A. M. Emslie-Smith, A. G. Engel, Necrotizing myopathy with pipestem capillaries, microvascular deposition of the complement membrane attack complex (MAC), and minimal cellular infiltration. *Neurology* **41** (1991), 936–939.

176. S. Carpenter, G. Karpati, W. Johnston, E. Shoubridge, M. Gavel, Coexistence of polymyositis (PM) with mitochondrial myopathy (MM). *Neurology* **42**:Suppl. 3 (1992), 388.

177. G. Blume, A. Pestronk, B. Frank, D. R. Johns, Polymyositis with cytochrome oxidase negative muscle fibres. Early quadriceps weakness and poor response to immunosuppressive therapy. *Brain* **120** (1997), 39–45.

178. J. H. Anthony, P. G. Procopis, R. A. Ourvrier, Benign acute childhood myositis. *Neurology* **29** (1979), 1068–1071.

179. R. L. Ruff, D. Secrist, Viral studies in benign acute childhood myositis. *Arch. Neurol.* **39** (1982), 261.

180. B. Q. Banker, A. G. Engel, The polymyositis and dermatomyositis syndromes. In: *Myology*, eds. A. G. Engel, B. Q. Banker. (New York: McGraw Hill, 1986), pp. 1385–1422.

181. C. E. Thompson, Infantile myositis. *Dev. Med. Child Neurol.* **24** (1982), 307–313.

182. N. Sripathi, G. Karpati, S. Carpenter, A distinctive type of infantile inflammatory myopathy with abnormal myonuclei. *J. Neurol. Sci.* **136** (1996), 1–2.

183. S. M. Roddy, S. Ashwal, N. Peckham, S. Mortensen, Infantile myositis: a case diagnosed in the neonatal period. *Ped. Neurol.* **2** (1986), 241.

184. M. Shevell, B. Rosenblatt, C. M. Silver, S. Carpenter, G. Karpati, Congenital inflammatory myopathy. *Neurology* **40** (1990), 1111–1114.

185. R. K. Olney, R. K. Miller, Inflammatory infiltration in Fukuyama type congenital muscular dystrophy. *Muscle Nerve* **6** (1983), 75.

186. M. C. Dalakas, Current treatment of the inflammatory myopathies. *Curr. Opin. Rheumatol.* **6** (1994), 595–601.

187. M. C. Dalakas, Therapeutic approaches in patients with inflammatory myopathies. *Semin. Neurol.* **23**:2 (2003), 199–206.

188. M. Leon-Monzon, M. C. Dalakas, Interleukin-1 (IL-1) is toxic to human muscle. *Neurology* **44**: Suppl. (1994), A132.

189. M. E. Cronin, F. W. Miller, J. E. Hicks, M. Dalakas, P. H. Plotz, The failure of intravenous cyclophosphamide therapy in refractory idiopathic inflammatory myopathy. *J. Rheumatol.* **16** (1989), 1225–1228.

190. J. Heckmatt, N. Hasson, C. Saunders, *et al.*, Cyclosporin in juvenile dermatomyositis. *Lancet* **i** (1989), 1063–1066.

191. J. M. Grau, C. Herrero, J. Casademont, J. Fernandez-Sola, A. Urbano-Marquez, Cyclosporine A as first choice for dermatomyositis. *J. Rheumatol.* **21** (1994), 381–382.

192. F. W. Miller, S. F. Leitman, M. E. Cronin, *et al.*, Controlled trial of plasma exchange and leukopheresis in patients with polymyositis and dermatomyositis. *N. Engl. J. Med.* **326** (1992), 1380–1384.

193. J. J. Kelly Jr., H. Madoc-Jones, L. S. Adelman, P. L. Andres, T. L. Munsat, Total body irradiation is not effective in inclusion body myositis. *Neurology* **36** (1986), 1264–1266.

194. P. Cherin, S. Herson, B. Wechsler, *et al.*, Efficacy of intravenous immunoglobulin therapy in chronic refractory polymyositis and dermatomyositis. An open study with 20 adult patients. *Am. J. Med.* **91** (1991), 162–168.

195. B. Lang, R. M. Laxer, G. Murphy, E. D. Silverman, C. M. Roifman, Treatment of dermatomyositis with intravenous immunoglobulin. *Am. J. Med.* **91** (1991), 169–172.

196. S. Jan, S. Beretta, M. Moggio, L. Alobbati, G. Pellegrini, High-dose intravenous human immunoglobulin in polymyositis resistant to treatment. *J. Neurol. Neurosurg. Psychiatry* **55** (1992), 60–64.

197. M. C. Dalakas, I. Illa, J. M. Dambrosia, *et al.*, A controlled trial of high-dose intravenous immunoglobulin infusions as treatment for dermatomyositis. *N. Engl. J. Med.* **329** (1993), 1993–2000.

198. M. C. Dalakas, B. Sonies, B. Koffman, *et al.*, High-dose intravenous immunoglobulin (IVIg) combined with prednisone in the treatment of patients with inclusion-body myositis (IBM): a double blind, randomized controlled trial. *Neurology* **48** (1997), 332S.

199. M. C. Dalakas, E. A. Sekul, E. J. Cupler, K. Sivakumar, The efficacy of high dose intravenous immunoglobulin (IVIg) in patients with inclusion-body myositis (IBM). *Neurology* **48** (1997), 712–716.

200. M. C. Dalakas, Intravenous immunoglobulin therapy for neurological diseases. *Ann. Intern. Med.* **126** (1997), 721–730.

201. T. D. Levine, Rituximab in the treatment of dermatomyositis: an open-label pilot study. *Arthritis Rheum.* **52**:2 (2005), 601–607.

202. C. V. Oddis, F. C. Sciurba, K. A. Elmaqd, T. E. Starzl, Tacrolimus in refractory polymyositis with interstitial lung disease. *Lancet* **353**:9166 (1999), 1762–1763.

Chapter 23

Autoimmune and inherited disorders of neuromuscular transmission

Amelia Evoli, Hanns Lochmüller and Violeta Mihaylova

Introduction

The neuromuscular junction (NMJ) is a chemical synapse that converts motor nerve impulses into muscle contraction.

At normal NMJ (see Figure 23.1), the nerve terminal and muscle postsynaptic membrane are separated by a 50- to 100-nm-thick synaptic cleft, containing a basal lamina which anchors acetylcholinesterase and other synapse-specific proteins. The postsynaptic membrane has a characteristic folded architecture; the acetylcholine receptors (AChRs) are densely clustered at the top of the folds while voltage-gated sodium channels (VGSC) are concentrated at the bottom. AChRs co-aggregate with a complex network of proteins which participate in the formation and maintenance of the postsynaptic membrane. The nerve terminal contains ACh-loaded synaptic vesicles (each contains 5000–10 000 ACh molecules and corresponds to a quantum), which are packed at special sites of the presynaptic membrane (active zones) where voltage-gated calcium channels (VGCC) are located. When the action potential invades the nerve terminal, the opening of VGCC leads to a rapid increase in the local Ca^{2+} concentration, which triggers the exocytosis of synaptic vesicles and about 20–200 ACh quanta (depending on the species) are released in the synaptic cleft. Two ACh molecules bind each AChR and open the ion channel; the influx of cations (mainly Na^{+}) results in a local membrane depolarization, end-plate potential (EPP), which in turn activates the VGSC and a propagated muscle action potential ensues (the small depolarization caused by the release of a single ACh quantum is called a miniature end-plate potential – MEPP). In the motor nerve, VGSC close and voltage-gated potassium channels (VGKC) open, repolarizing the membrane to its resting level. EPP amplitude largely exceeds the threshold depolarization required for VGSC activation (safety factor of neuromuscular transmission). Diseases of the NMJ are characterized by an alteration, generally a reduction, of safety factor.

While the NMJ is vulnerable to a number of drugs and toxins, the main pathology is autoimmunity, as transmembrane proteins both at pre- and postsynaptic levels are exposed to circulating antibodies. In addition, mutations of genes encoding for different synaptic proteins are responsible for congenital myasthenic syndromes (CMS).

Since the late 1980s, a huge amount of research work has greatly expanded the understanding of these disorders and has markedly improved their clinical management.

Autoimmune diseases

Autoimmune diseases of the NMJ are caused by antibodies against membrane proteins at the motor end-plate. The target antigens are in most cases ion channels, the autoimmune attack resulting in a loss of function due to reduced number of these molecules. This disease group includes myasthenia gravis (MG), the Lambert–Eaton myasthenic syndrome (LEMS) and acquired neuromyotonia. Figure 23.1 shows a schematic view of the NMJ with the principal antigens involved.

Myasthenia gravis

Myasthenia gravis (MG) is the most common NMJ disease and one of the best understood autoimmune conditions. It is not a single entity, but rather a syndrome with different pathogenic scenarios.

Pathogenesis

Myasthenia gravis with antibodies to acetylcholine receptor (AChR-MG)

Myasthenia gravis is due to a postsynaptic defect of neuromuscular transmission, caused, in the great majority of patients, by antibodies against the AChR (AChR antibodies).

The AChR is a membrane glycoprotein consisting of five homologous subunits: $2\alpha1,\beta1,\varepsilon,\delta$ in normal adult muscle and $2\alpha1,\beta1,\gamma,\delta$ in embryonic/denervated muscle [1]. Serum AChR antibodies are detected by immunoprecipitation in 85%–90% of patients with generalized MG (GMG) and in 50% of cases with ocular MG (OMG). A large proportion of these polyclonal IgG, mainly IgG1 and IgG3, binds the so-called *main immunogenic region* (MIR) on the extracellular domain of each α-subunit. Anti-MIR antibodies are responsible for AChR cross-linking with increased internalization and degradation;

Disorders of Voluntary Muscle, 8th edn., eds. George Karpati, David Hilton-Jones, Kate Bushby and Robert C. Griggs. Published by Cambridge University Press. © Cambridge University Press 2010.

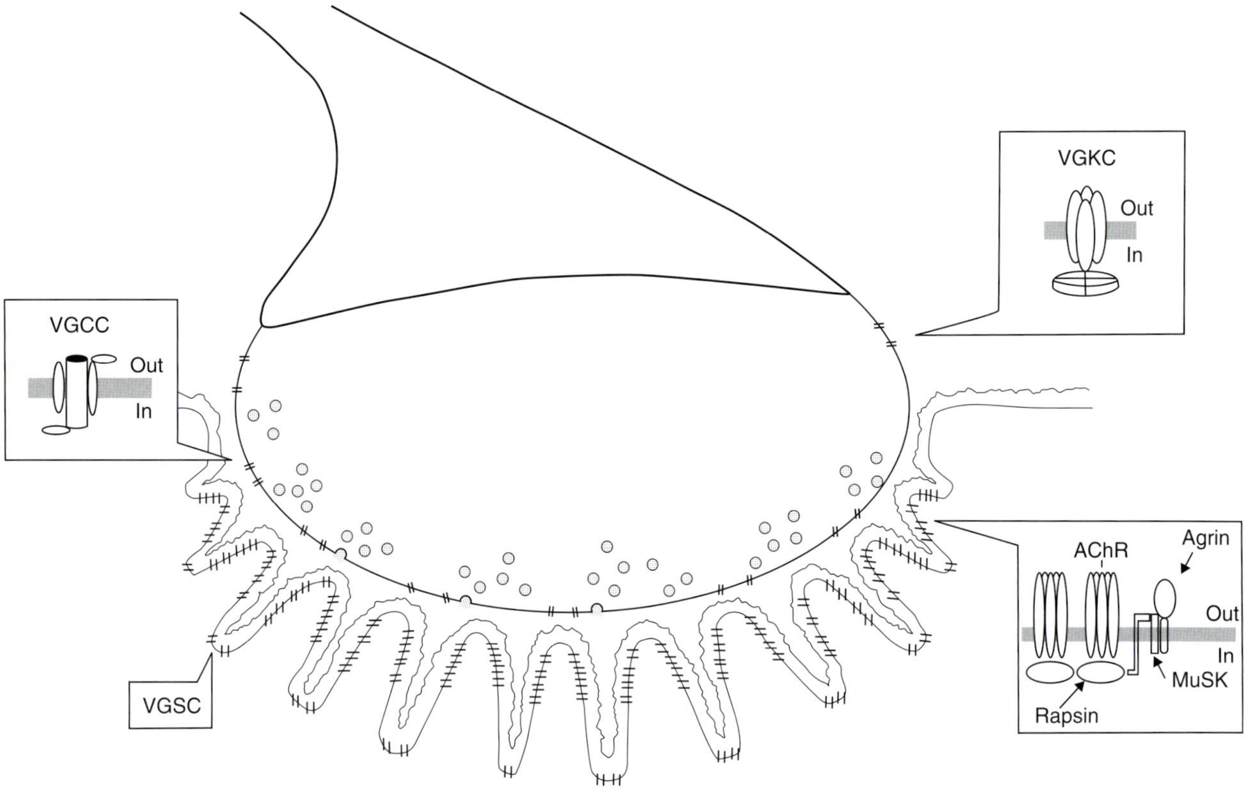

Figure 23.1. Schematic view of the neuromuscular junction with the principal antigens involved in autoimmune diseases. At the postsynaptic membrane the acetylcholine receptors (AChRs) are clustered at the top of the junctional folds while voltage-gated sodium channels (VGSC) are concentrated at the bottom. Muscle specific kinase (MuSK) and its ligands co-localize with the AChR. The motor nerve terminal contains voltage-gated potassium channels (VGKC) and voltage-gated calcium channels (VGCC). VGCC are concentrated at the sites of vesicle exocytosis.

complement-activating IgG cause lysis of the postsynaptic membrane, whereas functional block of the ACh-binding site is an uncommon effect [2]. The autoimmune attack results in AChR loss, simplification of the postsynaptic membrane, and widening of the synaptic cleft. These alterations reduce the response to ACh and, especially during sustained exercise when neurotransmitter release is physiologically reduced, the EPP may not reach the threshold to elicit a propagated muscle action potential. End-plate alterations together with clinical and electrophysiological MG features have been reproduced in animals immunized with AChR or injected with patients' IgG (experimental autoimmune MG, EAMG).

CD4+ T-cells have a pivotal role in MG and EAMG development: these cells recognize AChR epitopes in the context of major histocompatibility complex (MHC) class II molecules and have a helper function on B-cells, both Th1 and Th2 cytokines being relevant to antibody production [3]. As AChR-specific CD4+ T-cells are also present in healthy subjects, a defect in self-tolerance control can be hypothesized. Recently, a functional impairment of CD4+ CD25+ T regulatory (Treg) cells was reported in MG patients [4].

A pathogenic link between AChR-MG and the thymus has long been recognized. Patients with early-onset (<50 years) disease very frequently have a thymic hyperplasia, characterized by expanded perivascular spaces containing germinal centers. The hyperplastic thymus actively produces AChR antibodies and is regarded as the site of auto-sensitization against AChR [5]. Early-onset MG displays marked prevalence in women, high frequency of B8 DR3 DQ2 MHC alleles, and increased association with other autoimmune disorders [2]. In 10%–15% of patients, AChR-MG is associated with thymoma, a tumor of thymic epithelial cells. Thymoma does not produce AChR antibodies but appears to contribute to MG pathogenesis through export of mature CD4+ T-cells and decreased production of Treg cells [6]. MG with thymoma has a peak onset in the fifth and sixth decades; it shows neither sex prevalence nor MHC association. Late-onset MG is prevalent in men and is weakly associated with MHC B7 DR2 alleles; the thymus is generally atrophic (i.e., normal-for-age). Nearly 50% of late-onset patients and an even higher percentage of those with thymoma have serum IgG against the muscle proteins titin and ryanodine receptor. These antibodies are very uncommon in early-onset MG and their detection in young patients is predictive of an underlying thymoma [7].

Myasthenia gravis with antibodies to MuSK (MuSK-MG)

Serum antibodies to the muscle-specific kinase (MuSK) were first described in 2001 [8] and have proved fairly specific for AChR-negative MG.

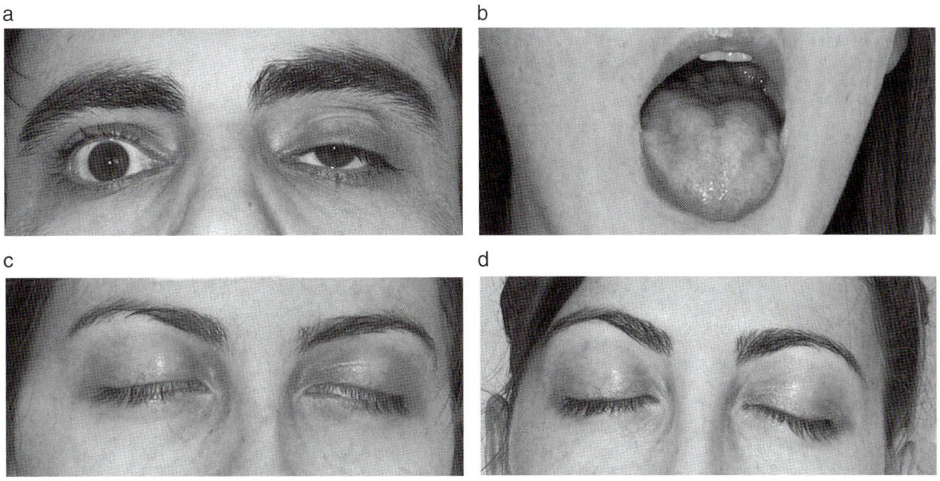

Figure 23.2a–d. Patterns of muscle weakness in patients with myasthenia gravis (MG). (a) Ptosis of the left eye. The palpebral fissure of the non-ptotic eye widens when the patient tries to open the ptotic eye. This phenomenon is quite common in MG and can be explained with Hearing's law. (b) Atrophy of the tongue with two lateral and one medial furrows (triple furrowed tongue). (c) Weakness of the orbicularis oculi muscle is responsible for incomplete eyelid closure and, when the patient attempts to close her eyes, the Bell phenomenon is evident. Improvement after treatment (d).

MuSK is a transmembrane polypeptide expressed selectively at NMJ [9]. It interacts through specific co-receptors with agrin, a nerve-derived protein, and with rapsyn, a cytoplasmic muscle protein. Although NMJ development involves many regulatory signals, the agrin/MuSK/rapsyn interaction is essential for AChR clustering. Moreover, the role of MuSK is required to maintain the postsynaptic apparatus throughout adult life [10].

MuSK antibodies are measured by radioimmunoassay using human recombinant ^{125}I-labeled MuSK as antigen; they bind to MuSK ectodomain and mainly belong to the IgG 4 subclass, which does not activate complement [11]. MuSK antibody effects have not been elucidated, as muscle biopsy studies from patients failed to show significant alterations of the postsynaptic membrane [12], whereas MuSK-immunized animals developed EAMG associated with AChR loss and reduction of the postsynaptic area [13]. Differences between muscle groups in susceptibility to MuSK immunization [14] may account for these discrepancies.

In this disease entity, the thymus generally lacks histological alterations [15] and does not seem to play a pathogenic role.

Different MuSK-associated phenotypes have been described, including a clinical picture indistinguishable from AChR-MG, a focal disease with involvement of neck, shoulder, and respiratory muscles [16] and a severe form with prevalent bulbar weakness and high frequency of respiratory crises [17].

Seronegative myasthenia gravis (SNMG)

This term currently applies to generalized MG with neither AChR nor MuSK antibodies [11]. The disease is clinically indistinguishable from AChR-MG, with an increased rate of mild forms.

In SNMG patients the thymus often shows hyperplastic changes [18] and muscle biopsy reveals postsynaptic alterations similar to those in AChR-MG [12]. These observations suggest that SNMG could belong to the same spectrum as early-onset MG [5] and that low-titer/low-affinity AChR antibodies could actually be present in these subjects. SNMG has not been described in association with thymoma.

About 50% of patients with OMG are seronegative (MuSK antibodies are rarely found in these cases). The high susceptibility of extrinsic ocular muscles (EOM) to MG could depend on intrinsic structural and molecular properties, which may increase NMJ vulnerability to the autoimmune attack [19]. AChR-positive and AChR-negative OMG do not differ on clinical grounds. The presence of a thymoma is uncommon and always associated with raised AChR antibody levels.

Neonatal myasthenia gravis (NMG)

This is a transient disease occurring in 10%–15% of newborns to MG women, due to antibody placental transfer. Symptoms (poor sucking, feeble cry, hypotonia and, in some cases, respiratory difficulty) are evident within the first 2 days of life and generally last 2–3 weeks. Treatment is symptomatic, with anticholinesterases together with tube feeding and assisted ventilation, when needed. There is no relationship between NMG and maternal clinical severity or antibody status, but treatment in the mother can prevent the occurrence of the disease in the child [20]. Arthrogryposis multiplex congenita is a severe complication of maternal MG, when antibodies are directed mainly against the AChR fetal isoform; in these cases, the mothers can be asymptomatic [2].

Clinical features

The hallmark of MG is fluctuating muscle weakness that increases with exercise and is relieved by rest. Although all voluntary muscles can be affected, some are more commonly involved, giving rise to a characteristic pattern of weakness in most cases. However, clinical presentation is notably variable, as both the extent and severity of symptoms differ from one patient to another.

The EOM are affected in the great majority of patients and ptosis and diplopia are the most common presenting symptoms. Ptosis is generally asymmetrical (see Figure 23.2a) and frequently alternating; diplopia is intermittent (especially in

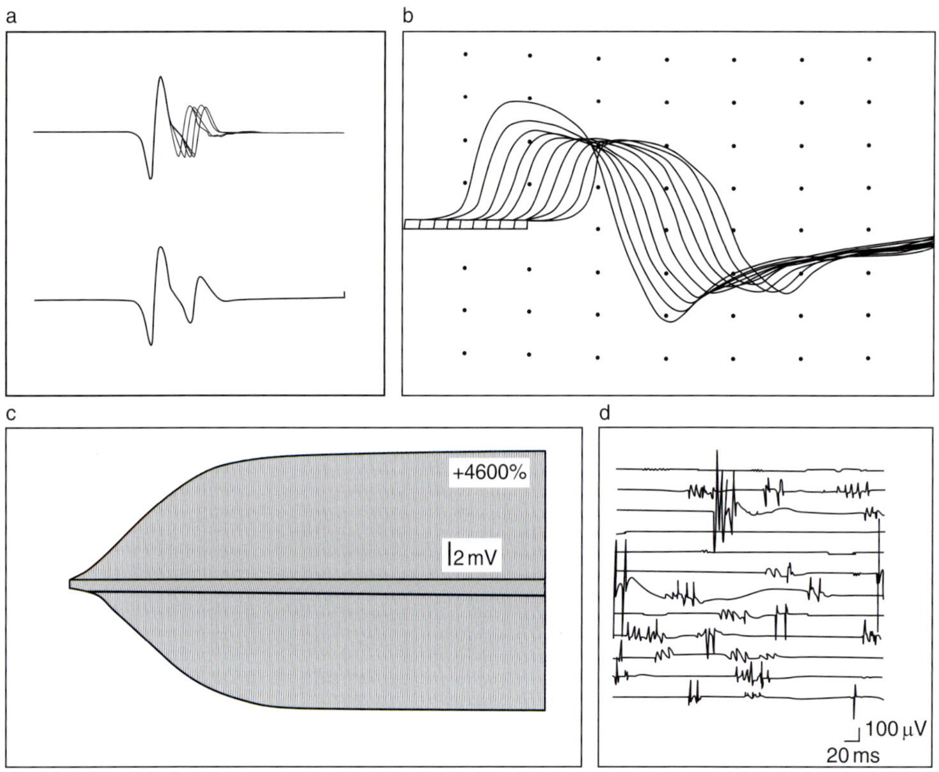

Figure 23.3a–d. EMG features. (a) Single-fiber electromyography in a patient with myasthenia gravis (orbicularis oculi muscle) showing an increased jitter as a second action potential wave group (upper panel), which is corrected by edrophonium injection (lower panel). (b) Low-rate (3/s) repetitive nerve stimulation in a patient with myasthenia gravis showing a 30% decrement in the compound muscle action potential (CMAP) amplitude. Supramaximal stimulation of brachial plexus at the Erb's point and CMAP recording from deltoid muscle. (c) High-rate (50/s) repetitive nerve stimulation in a patient with Lambert–Eaton myasthenic syndrome showing an abnormally low amplitude of the first CMAP with marked facilitation. Supramaximal stimulation of the ulnar nerve and CMAP recording from abductor digiti quinti muscle. (d) Myokymic discharges in a patient with acquired neuromyotonia. Spontaneous firing of single motor units as doublets, triplets, and multiplets. Needle EMG recording from gastrocnemius muscle.

the early stages) and variable, due to the involvement of different muscles at different times. These features are useful in differentiating myasthenia gravis from other causes of ophthalmoparesis, such as oculopharyngeal dystrophy, mitochondrial diseases and thyroid ophthalmopathy. In 12%–15% of cases, MG remains confined to ocular muscles; in the other patients the disease becomes generalized usually within 2 years from onset. Facial muscles are commonly affected with difficulty in closing the eyes tightly (Figure 23.2c, d), blowing out the cheeks, and the development of a vertical smile ("myasthenic snarl"). Limb weakness is almost invariably more marked in proximal muscles, but weakness of finger extension (sometimes with "dropping" of a single finger) is not rare. Among axial muscles, both neck flexors and extensors ("dropped head syndrome") are frequently involved. Weakness of the "bulbar" region (tongue, oropharyngeal, and laryngeal muscles) is responsible for eating problems, chewing difficulties, dysphagia, and dysarthria, while vocal cord paresis is an uncommon, life-threatening event. Lastly, although many patients with generalized MG have mild to moderate respiratory impairment, 20% suffer from respiratory crises, due to paralysis of the diaphragm and intercostal muscles.

Different score systems have been devised to assess the extent and severity of MG weakness. The Osserman scale [21] has been in use for more than 40 years; more recently, a new classification was proposed by the MG Foundation of America [22].

The disease affects all races, although clinical manifestations can vary between ethnic groups [23]. Recent studies have reported a steady increase in MG frequency, with an incidence of 4–11/million and a prevalence of 100–150/million. Interestingly, this finding appears to be due to an increased incidence of late-onset AChR-MG [24].

MuSK-MG frequency shows remarkable ethnic and geographical differences [11]. In clinical studies from Europe and North America, MuSK antibodies were found in around 40% of AChR-negative GMG patients (4%–6% of all GMG cases), with a striking prevalence in women.

Diagnosis

When MG is suspected on clinical grounds, the diagnosis is confirmed on the basis of serum antibody detection, electromyographic (EMG) evidence of a >10% compound muscle action potential (CMAP) decrement on low-rate repetitive nerve stimulation (RNS) or increased jitter on single-fiber electromyography (SF-EMG), and improvement with anticholinesterases.

AChR and MuSK antibodies are very specific and their detection in patients with congruent symptoms confirms the diagnosis unequivocally.

A decremental response on RNS can be obtained in most patients with GMG, when both distal and proximal limb muscles are tested [23] (see Figure 23.3b). SF-EMG is even more sensitive, being abnormal in more than 90% of patients, including those with mild or ocular disease (Figure 23.3a). However, the diagnostic yield of EMG depends on testing weak muscles. Accordingly, in MuSK-MG, which is often characterized by prevalent cranial weakness, neurophysiological studies may be abnormal in the facial muscles, but normal in limb muscles [25].

A clear improvement on anticholinesterase injection (edrophonium i.v./prostigmine i.m.) is observed in up to 90% of patients and strongly supports the diagnosis. However, a negative result does not exclude the possibility of MG. In particular, MuSK-positive patients can show lack of response and even worsening of symptoms [17].

Positive results on RNS or SF-EMG are not strictly specific for MG, as they can be observed in other neuromuscular disorders. "False" responses to edrophonium, mainly due to wrong interpretation of the response, have been reported in different diseases, including brain stem tumors. In practice, diagnostic difficulties mostly arise in SNMG, which must be differentiated from other NMJ disorders and various conditions that can mimic MG.

Once the diagnosis has been established, patients should undergo a radiological study of the thymus, together with a screening for other autoimmune diseases that may be associated and medical conditions that could complicate treatment.

Therapeutic modalities

Symptomatic therapy is based on anticholinesterases (mostly pyridostigmine), which increase the availability of ACh. These drugs are always first-line treatment, although normal muscle strength can be restored in only a minority of cases. Adverse effects mainly consist of gastric discomfort, diarrhea, salivation, and muscle cramps and can be reversed by reducing dosage, or by the addition of an antimuscarinic drug such as propantheline. Most MG patients benefit from anticholinesterases to a certain extent, with two exceptions: (1) ocular symptoms generally are scarcely improved; and (2) patients with MuSK antibodies can show an abnormal sensitivity to ACh, with increased weakness and various side-effects with low pyridostigmine doses [17].

Although the efficacy of thymectomy in MG has not been definitely established, retrospective studies showed higher remission rates in thymectomized patients [26]. Thymectomy is indicated for all thymoma cases and, when thymoma is excluded, should be considered for patients with GMG. An international multi-center trial is going on to determine whether thymectomy plus prednisone treatment in patients with generalized non-thymomatous AChR-MG confers additional benefits in comparison with prednisone alone [27]. Currently, in most centers, thymectomy is restricted to subjects with early-onset MG as this group appears to be the most likely to benefit from surgery. Patients with late-onset MG show a less satisfactory response, while the indication for thymectomy is controversial in the AChR-negative disease. Removal of a thymoma does not significantly improve the disease course; moreover, an invasive thymoma should be regarded as a potentially malignant tumor and – depending on surgical staging and tumor classification – postoperative radiotherapy and/or chemotherapy may be required.

Plasma-exchange and intravenous immunoglobulin (IVIg) induce a rapid, albeit short-term, improvement with comparable efficacy [28]. These treatments are mostly used in myasthenic emergencies, such as respiratory crises and severe bulbar weakness, and in preparation for thymectomy. On the other hand, they do not affect the long-term outcome [28, 29] and should always be used in association with immunosuppression.

Immunosuppressive therapy is indicated in patients with disabling MG and, although nonselective in mode of action, is highly effective in the majority of cases.

Owing to their short-latency effect, corticosteroids (mostly prednisone/prednisolone) are the first-line treatment in severely affected patients. In these cases, as symptoms can worsen in the first days of treatment, high-dose prednisone (100–120 mg on alternate days) should be started in hospital (some, but not all, specialists prefer gradual introduction over a couple of weeks in the hope of lessening the risk of initial deterioration); when symptoms are mild or purely ocular, treatment at lower doses can be undertaken in outpatients. Once stable improvement is achieved, prednisone is slowly tapered, to the minimum effective dose or to complete withdrawal. As MG often relapses during steroid tapering, prolonged treatment is generally needed with the risk of serious side-effects. In patients with unsatisfactory response or requiring high maintenance doses, other immunosuppressants must be considered [23]. These drugs can be administered from the beginning and can replace prednisone in long-term treatment, but owing to the delayed onset of clinical effect, they are generally used together with steroids in the initial phase of treatment. In general, combined therapy (steroids plus an immunosuppressant) appears to be more effective and safer than monotherapy [30]. Azathioprine is the antimetabolite most used in MG and, at an initial dose of 2.5–3 mg/kg body weight per day, is effective in most patients. Gastrointestinal hypersensitivity, leukopenia, and hepatotoxicity are the main adverse effects, which usually subside with dose reduction or withdrawal. Mycophenolate mofetil appears to be better tolerated due to its more selective effect on activated T and B cells [3, 31], but its efficacy remains uncertain. Of the calcineurin inhibitors, cyclosporine proved effective in a randomized trial [32] and has since been used mainly as an alternative to azathioprine. Tacrolimus is a promising agent, as shown by several uncontrolled studies [33]. The main problem with these drugs is nephrotoxicity, which requires careful monitoring. Cyclophosphamide is an alkylating agent whose use is currently confined to refractory MG. In selected cases, "immunoablative" therapy with high-dose cyclophosphamide has been described as effective and tolerably safe [34]. Biological drugs have recently been introduced in MG treatment. Rituximab, which transiently eliminates circulating B-cells, has been successfully used in refractory disease, while etanercept, a competitive blocker of tumor necrosis factor α, has been tried in small pilot studies [33]. Figure 23.4 shows a general treatment plan for MG.

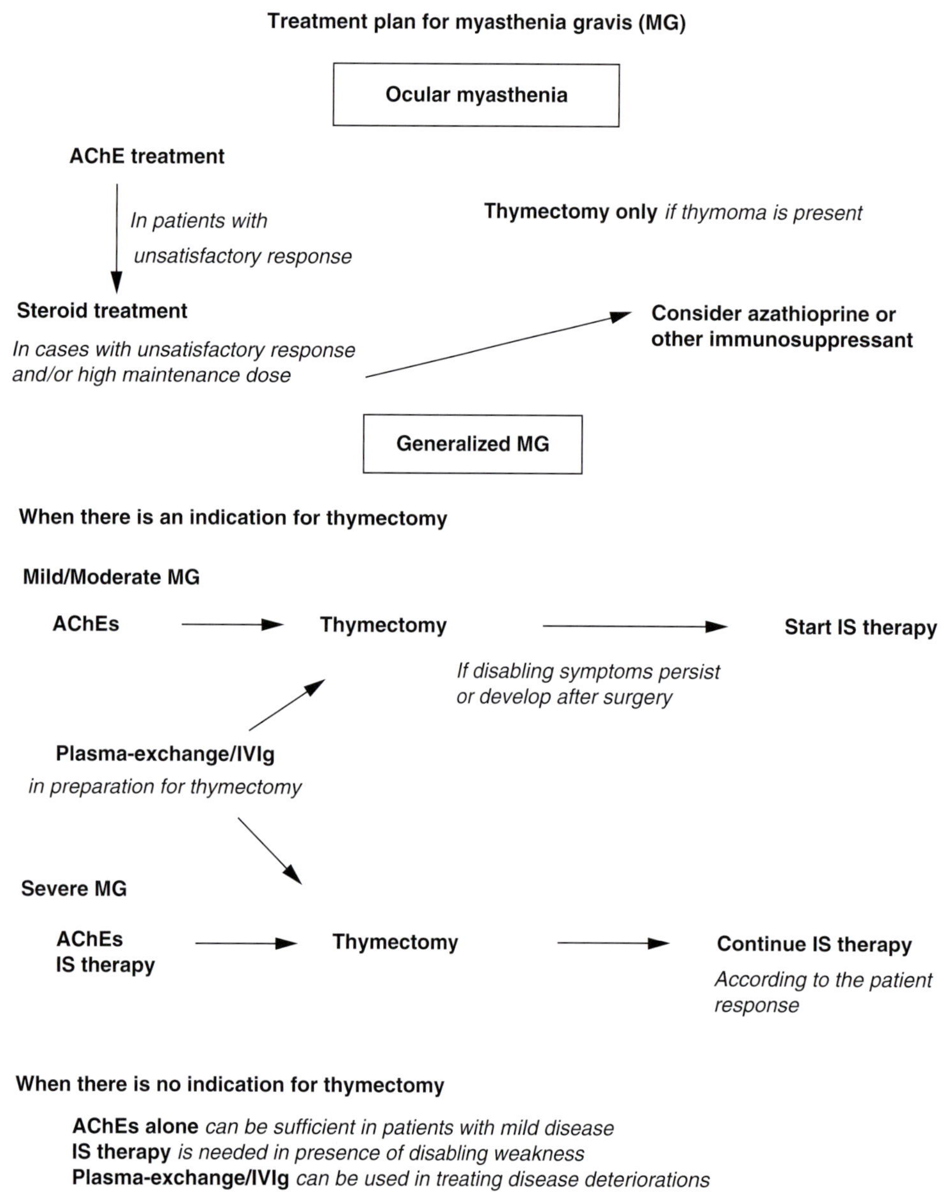

Figure 23.4. General treatment plan for myasthenia gravis. AChE, anticholinesterases; IS therapy, immunosuppressive therapy; IVIg, intravenous immunoglobulin.

The Lambert–Eaton myasthenic syndrome

Lambert–Eaton myasthenic syndrome (LEMS) is a presynaptic disorder of neuromuscular and autonomic transmission. It is paraneoplastic (P-LEMS) in 50%–60% of cases, generally related to small-cell lung carcinoma (SCLC). Nonparaneoplastic LEMS (NP-LEMS) is often associated with other autoimmune diseases.

Pathogenesis

The defect of neuromuscular transmission is a reduced quantal content, i.e., the number of ACh vesicles released by each nerve impulse. As a morphological correlate of this finding, there are both paucity and disorganization of active zone particles, which correspond to voltage-gated calcium channels (VGCC) on the nerve terminal membrane [35]. P/Q-type VGCC, which are responsible for neurotransmitter release at the mammalian NMJ, are the main antibody target in LEMS.

P/Q-VGCC are multimeric complexes formed from a pore-forming voltage-sensitive α1-subunit and auxiliary β, $\alpha 2\delta$ and γ subunits [36]. They are expressed in SCLC and antibodies induced against cancer cell determinants cross-react with the same antigen at the NMJ. The etiology of NP-LEMS is unknown. By a radioimmunoassay using ^{125}I-conotoxin-MVIIC, P/Q-type VGCC antibodies are detected in 90% of patients. They bind to the α1-subunit and cause channel loss through cross-linking and increased degradation [37]. The antibody pathogenic effect has been confirmed in passive transfer studies in mice [35]. P/Q-type VGCC antibodies are thought to be responsible for cerebellar degeneration which can occur in SCLC patients with or without concomitant LEMS [38].

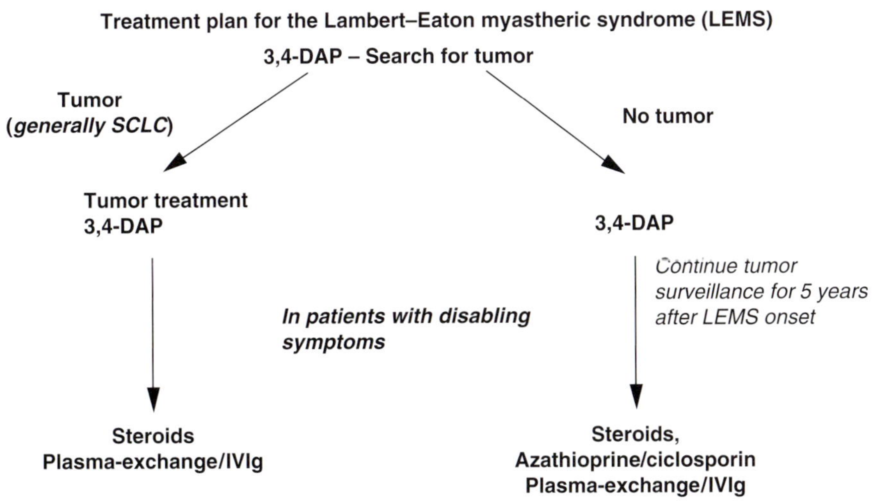

Figure 23.5. Treatment plan for the Lambert–Eaton myasthenic syndrome. 3,4 DAP, 3,4 diaminopyridine; SCLC, small-cell lung carcinoma; IVIg, intravenous immunoglobulin.

Some patients have serum antibodies against synaptogamin I, a synaptic vesicle protein that is exposed extracellularly during exocytosis; immunization with synthetic peptides corresponding to synaptogamin N-terminus induced LEMS features in rats [39].

Clinical features

Most patients complain of leg weakness with difficulty in walking; ocular and oropharyngeal symptoms are usually mild, and respiratory crises are uncommon. On examination, weakness is prevalent in proximal muscles of the legs and, less frequently, of the arms. The increase in muscle strength immediately after exercise (facilitation) and the elicitation of tendon reflexes after brief muscle contraction are characteristic signs. Autonomic symptoms, such as dry mouth, impotence, constipation, and postural hypotension, are reported in more than 80% of cases, with increased frequency in cancer patients.

Neurological symptoms usually precede the diagnosis of cancer. In rare instances, LEMS is associated with tumors other than SCLC, such as thymoma, breast cancer, and lymphomas.

The disease prevalence and annual incidence have been estimated at 2–2.5/million and 0.2–0.4/million, respectively [40]. P-LEMS patients are usually smokers, more frequently men, with a peak onset in the fifth to sixth decades. NP-LEMS can present at any age and shows an increased association with HLA-B8 DR3. P-LEMS does not differ on clinical grounds from NP-LEMS, other than having a more progressive course.

Diagnosis and therapeutic modalities

Clinical features, namely proximal muscle weakness and hypoactive tendon reflexes with facilitation, are strongly suggestive of LEMS. Diagnostic confirmation relies on P/Q-type VGCC antibody detection and EMG testing. Although in LEMS weakness is prevalent in proximal muscles, electrophysiological abnormalities are more easily detected in distal muscles. EMG typically shows abnormally small CMAP amplitudes at rest, a decremental response at low-rate RNS, and an incremental response (facilitation) during high-rate RNS or after brief contraction (see Figure 23.3c). Although a 100% CMAP increment is usually considered the gold standard for LEMS diagnosis, using a 60% increment as the cut-off has proven to be highly sensitive and specific [41].

Upon diagnosis of LEMS, a search for malignancy is imperative and, if the initial evaluation is negative, tumor surveillance should be continued for at least 5 years after the disease onset. P-LEMS responds to tumor treatment, while it can be quite refractory to other therapies.

Symptomatic treatment is with 3,4-diaminopyridine (DAP), a voltage-gated potassium channel (VGKC) blocker, which increases ACh release from the nerve terminal by prolonging nerve depolarization and so lengthening the VGCC open time. In most patients, DAP is effective in relieving both muscle and autonomic symptoms and is well tolerated at doses <100 mg/day [42]. Although anticholinesterases such as pyridostigmine are generally less effective than DAP they sometimes give a modest additional benefit when combined with DAP [29, 43]. Patients with disabling symptoms require pharmacological immunosuppression, which is performed mostly with prednisone and azathioprine, with the same strategy as in MG; the use of antimetabolites should perhaps be avoided in patients with SCLC (see Figure 23.5), although there is little direct evidence of complications. Plasma-exchange and IVIg induce significant, although temporary, improvement. The plasma-exchange takes longer to have an effect than in MG, probably reflecting a slower turnover of VGCC in comparison with AChR [44].

Acquired peripheral nerve hyperexcitability (PNH) syndromes

This disease group includes acquired neuromyotonia (Isaacs syndrome) and cramp-fasciculation syndrome (C–F). These disorders are thought to have the same pathogenesis, with clinical and EMG features reflecting quantitative rather than qualitative differences [45].

Pathogenesis

The association with other autoimmune diseases, namely MG, and the response to plasma-exchange suggested an autoimmune etiology, while the presence of myokymia in subjects with KCNA1 (Kv1.1) mutations implicates VGKC involvement. In line with these observations, immunization with patients' IgG induced a significant increase in quantal content in mice, mimicking the effect of 4-aminopyridine, a potassium channel blocker [46].

Peripheral nerve hyperexcitability syndromes are thought to be caused by antibodies against VGKC, which control neuronal excitability within the central and peripheral nervous systems. Kv1 (*Shaker*) VGKC consist of four transmembrane α-subunits and up to four cytoplasmic β-subunits [47]. These ion channels are characterized by a remarkable antigenic heterogeneity, as α-subunits coded by different genes (Kv1.1–Kv1.8) combine promiscuously and can associate with different β-subunits [48].

Using a radioimmunoassay with ^{125}I-labeled dendrotoxin, which binds to Kv1.1, Kv1.2, and Kv1.6, VGKC antibodies can be detected in 50% of patients with neuromyotonia [45], as well as in some patients with central nervous system (CNS) involvement (see below). The demonstration that patients' sera bind with different affinity to Kv1 α-subunits (which have different distribution in the peripheral and central nervous systems) can, at least in part, account for the diverse clinical phenotypes [49]. Antibodies cause channel loss through cross-linking and increased degradation, while complement activation does not seem to be relevant [50].

Clinical features

In neuromyotonia, the PNH manifests clinically with continuous muscle fiber activity. Symptoms can be focal or generalized. Patients complain of muscle twitching (myokymia), cramps, and fasciculations, more evident in trunk and limb muscles. Increased sweating is frequent, while pseudomyotonia, paresthesia, and muscle weakness are less common. Serum CK level can be increased and patients with long-standing disease develop muscle hypertrophy. C–F is regarded as a milder variant, being mainly characterized by post-exercise cramps.

VGKC antibodies can associate with CNS involvement. Morvan syndrome typically presents with a combination of PNH, insomnia, autonomic, and behavioral alterations. Some patients (mostly without peripheral signs) develop a limbic encephalitis (LE), with seizures, short-term memory loss, and brain MRI abnormalities consisting of increased T_2 signal in the mesial temporal areas [51]. PNH with and without CNS symptoms can be idiopathic or paraneoplastic, associated with thymoma, more rarely with SCLC [48].

Diagnosis and therapeutic modalities

In patients with neuromyotonia EMG typically shows spontaneous motor unit discharges as doublets, triplets or multiplets (myokymic discharges) with an intraburst frequency of 5–150 Hz. "Neuromyotonic discharges" consist of prolonged bursts at higher frequency (150–300 Hz), which begin and end abruptly [52]. Although characteristic, neuromyotonic discharges are not always detected and, in practice, evidence of myokymic discharges is diagnostic of a PNH condition (Figure 23.3d). Confirmation of acquired neuromyotonia requires the exclusion of other causes of myokymia. Whilst the detection of anti-potassium channel antibodies is essentially confirmatory of the diagnosis, in clinical practice they are often undetectable, at least by the standard assay. In C–F, EMG features are milder and mainly consist of after-discharges evoked by RNS [48].

Acquired PNH syndromes and related CNS disorders can be monophasic illnesses with spontaneous or treatment-induced remission. Symptomatic drugs, such as carbamazepine and phenytoin, which inhibit sodium channels are effective in relieving mild to moderate symptoms. When disability is severe, plasma-exchange and IVIg can induce marked, but only temporary, improvement; for longer-term benefit, immunosuppression with corticosteroids and azathioprine can be considered. Thymoma-associated PNH syndromes do not generally respond to tumor treatment while central disturbances can improve. Both Morvan syndrome and LE respond to plasma-exchange and in idiopathic LE early immunosuppressive treatment is highly effective.

Future perspectives

As in other autoimmune conditions, the main therapeutic objective is specific immunosuppression, which should eradicate the autoantibody production leaving the host defense unaltered. New therapeutic approaches have been investigated in EAMG. They comprise: T-cell tolerization, selective autoantibody removal, elimination of specific T- and B-cells, interference at different levels with antigen presentation, and dendritic cell-based immunotherapy [3, 53, 54]. Although effective in experimental settings, most of these strategies are still far from being applied to patients. However, increasing understanding both of disease mechanisms and immune system modulation raises hope for direct therapeutic interventions in the future.

Congenital myasthenic syndromes

Congenital myasthenic syndromes (CMS) are a genetically and phenotypically heterogeneous group of rare inherited disorders affecting neuromuscular transmission.

According to the localization of the impaired protein at the NMJ, CMS may be classified as presynaptic, synaptic basal-lamina-associated, and postsynaptic (Figure 23.6). Postsynaptic CMS are the most frequent, accounting for approximately 80% of all genetically diagnosed CMS, while presynaptic CMS are rare [55, 56, 57].

Clinically patients present with myasthenic signs and symptoms: exercise-induced muscle weakness and abnormal

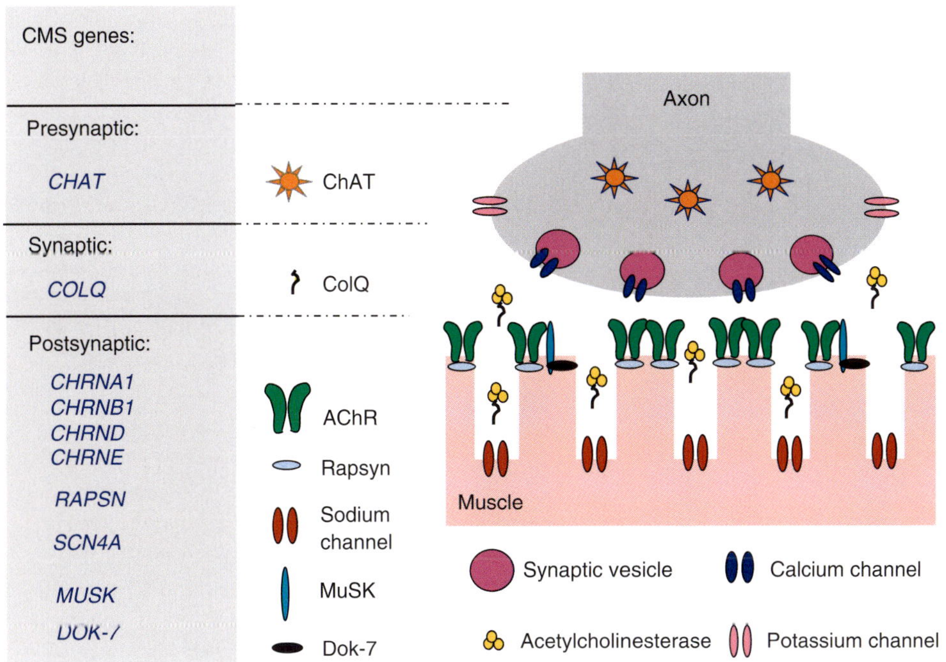

Figure 23.6. Known candidate genes for CMS and localization of their protein products at the neuromuscular junction.

fatigability, as well as ocular, bulbar, and respiratory disturbances. The symptoms usually present at birth or during infancy, though onset at a later age has been observed in some patients. Impaired neuromuscular transmission is evidenced by the decremental response on RNS and increased jitter and blocking on SF-EMG. There are no anti-AChR or anti-MuSK antibodies. Immunosuppressive therapy is ineffective.

Understanding of the molecular basis of the different types of CMS has rapidly evolved recently. To date, mutations in ten different genes, encoding post-, pre- or synaptic proteins, have been shown to cause CMS. The precise molecular diagnosis is of paramount importance not only for diagnosis and counseling but also for optimizing the treatment of each patient.

Presynaptic congenital myasthenic syndromes

Presynaptic CMS may be caused by either decreased synthesis, packaging in vesicles, or release of acetylcholine (ACh). So far, only mutations in the *CHAT* gene encoding choline acetyltransferase (ChAT) have been identified as causing presynaptic CMS [57].

Choline acetyltransferase catalyzes the reversible synthesis of ACh from acetyl CoA and choline at cholinergic synapses. Mutations in *CHAT* lead to reduced ChAT expression and impaired catalytic activity. CMS with underlying mutations in *CHAT* is associated with episodes of severe respiratory distress and bulbar weakness leading to apnea (CMS with episodic apnea) [58]. These bouts are precipitated by fever, infections, excitement, and overexertion. Some patients present with respiratory distress at birth, others are normal at birth and develop apneic attacks later during infancy or childhood [59]. Sometimes the apneic episodes are severe and assisted ventilation may be necessary for several months [60]. Between attacks the degree of muscle weakness varies: while some patients demonstrate ptosis and generalized weakness, others are free of symptoms (Figure 23.7f). However, weakness can be induced by exercise in the latter.

Between attacks, 2-Hz stimulation of rested muscles may not elicit a decremental response, but this can be induced by either exercise or a conditioning train of 10-Hz stimuli for 5–10 min [59].

CHAT mutations are recessive and mostly missense, the majority of them private, though there are exceptions. The missense mutation I336T has been identified in several independent kinships of Turkish origin, which implies a possible founder effect [61].

Congenital myasthenic syndrome patients with underlying mutations in *CHAT* are treated prophylactically with an oral acetylcholinesterase (AChE) inhibitor (e.g., pyridostigmine) to prevent respiratory crises, and with parenteral prostigmine methylsulfate during respiratory crises [55].

There are additional patients with a presumed presynaptic defect where the underlying genetic cause has not been determined yet [59, 62].

Synaptic basal-lamina-associated CMS: mutations in *COLQ*

The synaptic basal-lamina-associated CMS is caused by absence of the asymmetrical form of AChE from the synaptic space [63, 64]. The asymmetrical AChE at the endplate is composed of one, two, or three homotetramers of globular subunits ($AChE_T$) attached to a triple-stranded collagenic tail (ColQ) [55]. Recessive mutations in the *COLQ* gene encoding ColQ lead to endplate AChE deficiency.

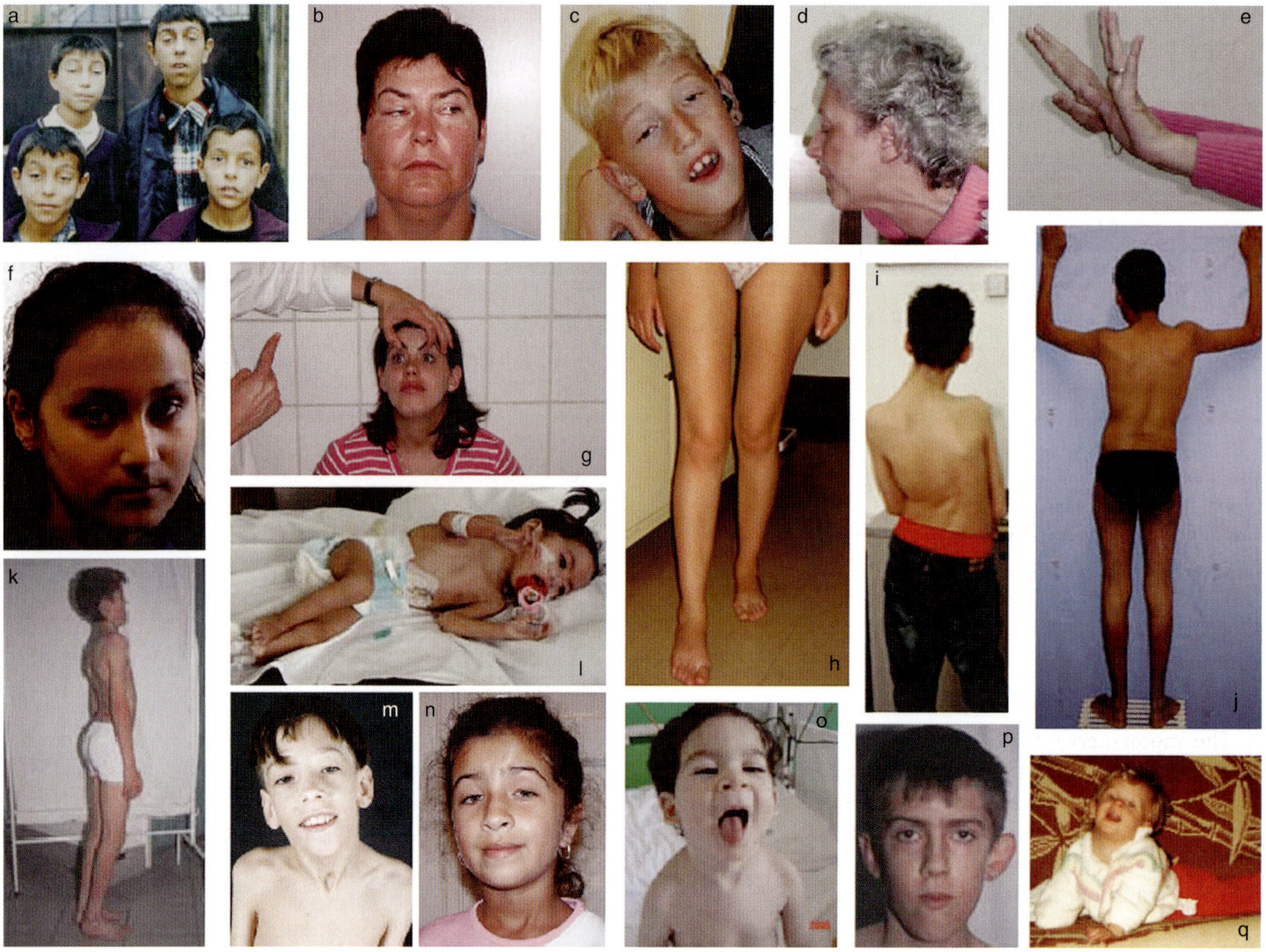

Figure 23.7a–q. Patients with congenital myasthenic syndromes (CMS). (a, g, n) Patients with CMS due to mutations of the ε-subunit gene. The patients have ptosis and ophthalmoparesis. (b) Patient with mutations of DOK7 gene. There is asymmetrical ptosis but eye movements are spared. (c) Patient with mutations of RAPSN. He presented with apnea and congenital contractures at birth. The patient has ptosis, facial weakness, elongated face, and episodic respiratory crises. (d, e) Patient with slow channel CMS (SCCMS) due to mutation of the β-subunit gene. Note weakness of neck and finger extensor muscles. (f) Patient with homozygous CHAT mutation. There is neither ptosis nor ophthalmoparesis. The patient experienced a sudden episode of cyanosis at age 1 year. (h) Patient with mutations of DOK7 gene. Note the inward rotation of the knees. (i) Patient with SCCMS due to kinetic mutation of ε-subunit gene. Note the severe scoliosis. (j) Patient with CMS due to homozygous mutation of COLQ gene. Note scoliosis, scapular winging, and muscle atrophy. (k, p) Patient with homozygous mutation in RAPSN. He presented with arthrogryposis multiplex and hypotonia at birth. Note the presence of moderate contractures at age 10 years (k), mild ptosis, elongated face, and protrusion of mandibule (p). (l) Patient with DOK7 mutations. She was hypotonic at birth, and needed assisted ventilation, and gastric tube feeding. (m) Patient with mutations of DOK7 gene. Note the scar from tracheostomy because of respiratory difficulties at birth, ptosis, and muscle atrophy. The patient became wheelchair-bound at the age of 9 years. (o) Patient with homozygous mutation of COLQ gene. He had hypotonia and respiratory distress at birth. Note ptosis and ophthalmoparesis. (q) Patient with mutations of COLQ gene. The patient presented with respiratory distress at birth and died at age 3½ years during respiratory crisis. Note neck and facial weakness.

The AChE is an enzyme responsible for the rapid hydrolysis of ACh released at the cholinergic synapses. The absence of the AChE prolongs the lifetime of ACh in the synaptic space, and this increases the duration of the endplate current so that it outlasts the refractory period of the muscle fiber and excites a second CMAP. There is overloading of the synaptic space with cations and evidence of endplate myopathy [55].

The patients present usually at birth or during the first year of life and motor developmental milestones are frequently delayed. Respiratory difficulties are common and may lead to death or need for assisted ventilation. Ptosis and ophthalmoparesis are frequently observed (Figure 23.7o). Delayed pupillary response to light is considered to be a clinical clue pointing to the diagnosis, however it is not a consistent finding [59, 65]. The muscle weakness affects predominantly proximal and axial muscles. The gait may be waddling and muscle atrophy may be observed. Some patients develop scoliosis during progression (Figure 23.7j). There is pronounced clinical heterogeneity: while some patients present at birth with severe weakness and progressive disease course (Figure 23.7q), others present at 6–7 years of age with mild weakness and slow or no progression. Interestingly, some *COLQ* mutant patients have a phenotype resembling CMS patients with *DOK7* mutations [65].

Electrophysiological studies demonstrate a decremental response on RNS. Double CMAP in response to a single nerve

stimulus is characteristic, but may be absent. Lack of objective long-term benefit from AChE inhibitors is the most consistent finding [65].

Recessive mutations in *COLQ* cause endplate AChE deficiency. More than 30 mutations have been identified to date [65, 66]. Q240X was found homozygously in six Palestinian Arab patients and in an Iraqi Jewish patient, indicating that this mutation could be a common cause of AChE deficiency in Near and Middle Eastern countries [67]. Similarly, four patients from three unrelated German families were found to be homozygous for the mutation T441A [65, 68]. The mutation Y430S was originally described in a consanguineous Spanish family and found later in other Spanish patients. The occurrence of the same mutation in seven unrelated Spanish families, four of them not being consanguineous, suggests a founder effect [63, 65, 69].

As yet, there is no established therapy for *COLQ* mutant CMS patients. However, patients gaining benefit from ephedrine treatment have been reported (see below).

Postsynaptic congenital myasthenic syndromes

A crucial step during NMJ formation is the concentration of densely packed AChR molecules at the postsynaptic membrane. The motor-nerve-derived proteoglycan agrin initiates AChR clustering via the muscle-specific receptor tyrosine kinase MuSK, the receptor-associated protein of the synapse rapsyn, and other as yet unidentified components. In addition to the AChR itself, mutations in several components of this signaling pathway were shown to cause CMS [57].

Mutations of the acetylcholine receptor genes

The muscle AChR is a pentamer existing in two isoforms, an adult form comprising $\alpha_2\beta\varepsilon\delta$ subunits and a fetal form comprising $\alpha_2\beta\delta\gamma$ subunits. Interestingly, recessive mutations of *CHRNG*, encoding the fetal γ-subunit, have been shown to cause Escobar syndrome, a congenital arthrogryposis syndrome with pterygia. Neuromuscular transmission in Escobar patients may be severely impaired in utero, but not after birth ("prenatal myasthenia") [70]. The AChR subunits are homologous, each consisting of a long N-terminal extracellular domain followed by three transmembrane domains (M1–M3), an intracellular cytoplasmic domain, a final transmembrane (M4) and an extracellular C-terminus [57].

Mutations involving subunits of AChR fall into two major classes: kinetic mutations with or without minor AChR deficiency, and low-expressor (AChR deficiency) mutations with or without minor kinetic effects. The kinetic mutations fall into two classes according to whether they cause slow-channel or fast-channel syndromes [56].

Slow-channel congenital myasthenic syndrome (SCCMS)

The name "slow-channel syndrome" originates from the abnormally slow decay of synaptic currents caused by abnormally prolonged opening events of the AChR channel. The prolonged end-plate potential (EPP) outlasts the refractory period of the muscle fiber action potential so that a single nerve stimulus evokes a characteristic repetitive CMAP. The prolonged, as well as spontaneous, channel openings overload the postsynaptic region with cations, including calcium, leading to end-plate myopathy [55].

The clinical phenotype may vary: in some SCCMS patients the disorder presents in early life and is considerably disabling, while others present later in life and have a slowly progressive disease course, resulting in little disability even in the sixth or seventh decade. Most patients show selective involvement of cervical and of wrist and finger extensor muscles (Figure 23.7d, e). Ptosis and ophthalmoparesis may also be observed. Progressive spinal deformities and respiratory restriction requiring ventilatory support are common complications during the evolution of the illness (Figure 23.7i) [55, 71, 72]. Repetitive stimulation reveals a decremental response at low stimulation frequency. The repetitive CMAP is of lower amplitude and has a faster decremental rate than the first CMAP [59]. However, repetitive CMAP may be absent.

Although the SCCMS is typically inherited in an autosomal dominant mode, variable penetrance and autosomal recessive inheritance have been reported in some patients [71].

To date, 22 slow-channel mutations have been published, most of them missense [57]. The different mutations frequently cause slow-channel closing, slow dissociation of ACh from the binding site or both [55].

The SCCMS are treated with quinidine sulfate or fluoxetine leading to progressive improvement of clinical symptoms, CMAP amplitudes, and decrement. A dramatic response 24 h after fluoxetine therapy was observed in a recently reported SCCMS patient [72, 73, 74].

Fast-channel syndrome

The fast-channel syndrome originates from abnormally fast decay of the synaptic response. Mutations in the AChR α-,δ-, and ε-subunits have been found to cause fast-channel syndrome by decreasing affinity for ACh, impairing gating efficiency or destabilizing the channel kinetics. The mutations cause loss of function and are typically recessive, but αF256L in the M2 domain of the α-subunit has a dominant negative effect. The patients present in the neonatal period with ocular, bulbar, or respiratory symptoms (even episodes of severe apnea), excessive fatigability, and delayed motor milestones. The clinical features are mild when the main effect of the mutation is on gating efficiency, or moderately severe when affinity for ACh or both affinity and gating efficiency are impaired. The fast-channel δE59K mutation also results in multiple joint contractures at birth because of reduced fetal movements [59, 75].

AChR mutations leading to receptor deficiency

Recessive mutations causing severe endplate AChR deficiency are the most common cause of CMS and concentrated in the ε-subunit. The likely reason for this is that the fetal γ-subunit can partially compensate for absence of the ε-subunit, whereas null mutations in the other subunit genes may not be compatible with postnatal survival [55].

Patients present usually at birth or during the first year of life with ptosis, poor cry, and feeding difficulties. The most characteristic symptom is ophthalmoparesis (Figure 23.7a, g, n). Frequently there is bulbar muscle weakness. Proximal muscle weakness is mild and respiratory crises are rarely observed. The disease course is usually benign with tendency towards improvement [56, 57].

Missense, frameshift, nonsense, splice site mutations as well as chromosomal microdeletions and mutations in the promoter region of *CHRNE* have been described. Though mutations in *CHRNE* have been described worldwide, they are a particularly common cause of CMS in Eastern Mediterranean countries [76].

The frameshift mutation ε1267delG of the ε-subunit disrupts the cytoplasmic loop and the M4 domain. ε1267delG is an old founder mutation causing CMS in patients with Gypsy ethnic origin dating back to ~800 years ago. CMS is one of the most common Mendelian disorders with ~4% heterozygous carrier rates in this population [77, 78]. Given the carrier frequency and the increased number of consanguineous marriages, pseudodominant inheritance is also possible [79]. Testing for ε1267delG mutation facilitates the genetic diagnosis in Gypsy CMS patients [80].

Other recurrent mutations in the *CHRNE* gene have been observed: the *CHRNE* 1293insG mutation was found with a rate of 20% in CMS patients originating from Maghreb. An ancient founder effect for this mutation was demonstrated by haplotyping with microsatellite markers and intragenic polymorphisms. Interestingly, 1293insG was repeatedly found in patients originating from Spain and Portugal too [56]. Another frequent *CHRNE* mutation in Spanish, Portuguese, and Brazilian patients is 70insG (unpublished observation).

Patients with AChR deficiency with underlying mutations in the *CHRNE* gene benefit from AChE inhibitors [57].

Mutations of the RAPSN gene

RAPSN gene encodes rapsyn (AChR-associated protein of the synapse), a 43-kDa postsynaptic peripheral membrane protein that interacts directly with AChRs and is essential for clustering the receptor molecules at the postsynaptic membrane of the neuromuscular junction [57]. The discovery of mutations in *RAPSN* came from CMS patients with demonstrated endplate AChR deficiency who carried no mutation in any subunit of the AChR [81].

Two distinct clinical phenotypes are associated with AChR deficiency due to *RAPSN* mutations: a rather severe early-onset (EO) phenotype and a mild late-onset (LO) phenotype. The EO phenotype is characterized by a disease onset at birth or in the first 2 years of life. In some cases, prenatal disease onset with reduced fetal movements in utero is noted. These children might be born with multiple flexion contractures in the upper and lower limbs and/or dysmorphic facial features, e.g., malformed low-set ears, elongated face, open mouth, high-arched palate, and prominent jaw (Figure 23.7c, k, p). Patients with EO phenotype have a history of muscle hypotonia, poor suck and cry, bilateral ptosis, episodes of severe generalized weakness, and respiratory distress, usually triggered by febrile infections. In contrast to patients with *CHRNE* mutations, eye movements are not restricted. One patient without any myasthenic symptoms between episodic crises has also been reported [57].

In contrast, patients with LO phenotype are asymptomatic during childhood. First disease symptoms occur in adolescence or early adulthood. Disease course is benign, usually with bilateral ptosis and mild muscle weakness. The LO phenotype is less frequent than the EO phenotype, but may be mistaken for seronegative myasthenia gravis. The lack of a clinical response to immunosuppressive treatments should alert the clinician to the possibility of LO CMS particularly with *RAPSN* mutations [57].

More than 30 different *RAPSN* mutations have been published so far. In contrast to patients with *CHRNE* or *COLQ* mutations, CMS patients with *RAPSN* null mutations on both alleles were not reported. Complete loss of rapsyn expression is probably not compatible with postnatal life, similar to the situation in rapsyn-deficient mice. Most patients with *RAPSN* mutations in the translated region of the gene carry one single missense mutation, N88K, on at least one allele. It has been suggested that most *RAPSN* N88K alleles detected worldwide derive from a single founder event that occurred in an ancient Indo-European population [57]. Therefore, screening for N88K should be an early consideration in the diagnostic work-up of CMS patients.

All *RAPSN* mutations described so far show a recessive inheritance pattern, although in the case of N88K – given its relatively high frequency – pseudodominant inheritance is possible [57]. *RAPSN* mutations are a frequent cause of CMS, accounting for around 10% of all CMS cases.

Patients with *RAPSN* mutations benefit from AChE inhibitors and some of them derive further benefit from a combination with 3,4-DAP [59].

Mutations of the DOK7 gene

Recently, it has been shown that overexpression of Dok-7, a member of the Dok-family of cytoplasmic molecules, can induce aneural activation of MuSK and subsequent clustering of AChR in cultured myotubes [82].

Dok-7 has a pleckstrin-homology (PH) domain and a phosphotyrosine-binding (PTB) domain in the N-terminal moiety and multiple tyrosine residues in the C-terminal region.

Mutations in the *DOK7* gene were found in patients with recessive CMS with predominant limb-girdle weakness.

Patients with *DOK7* mutations usually present during the second year of life with difficulties in walking or running. Typically, they achieve motor milestones at a normal age, though there are exceptions. Late onset of symptoms (in adolescence or even in the 20s) as well as onset at birth or in the first months of life are also possible (Figure 23.7l). The majority of the patients have ptosis, but no ophthalmoparesis (Figure 23.7b). Facial and bulbar weakness is frequent. Atrophy of the tongue has also been reported in some patients. Proximal weakness is greater than the distal weakness. The gait is often waddling and sometimes accompanied by inward rotation of knees ("sinuous gait") (Figure 23.7h). Prior to identification of the gene, these patients were classified as limb-girdle myasthenic syndrome (LG-CMS), although they show clear, clinical differences from another group of patients named LG-CMS, as outlined below. Most patients develop scoliosis and/or lordosis and muscle atrophy in the course of the disease (Figure 23.7m). The vital capacity is reduced in most of the adult patients and some require nocturnal ventilation. Respiratory crises may be observed. Patients with *DOK7* mutations often show fluctuations of symptoms over longer periods (good or bad weeks), not the typical daytime dependence as observed in other CMS or myasthenia gravis. The clinical course is variable: while in some patients the disease progresses leading to loss of ambulation, others demonstrate a stable clinical course with no or slight progression. RNS shows abnormal decremental response and single CMAP. Muscle biopsy results are unspecific and do not show tubular aggregates. There is no long-term benefit from esterase inhibitors, but an initial beneficial response and positive edrophonium test may be observed [83, 84].

So far, 18 different mutations of the *DOK7* gene have been reported and most of them are located in exon 7, facilitating genetic testing. The C-terminal domain frameshift mutation 1124_1127dupTGCC is of particular interest as it was found on at least 1 allele in all but 3 out of 12 kinships and in all but 4 of 24 kinships in 2 independent studies [83, 84].

Limb-girdle myasthenia with tubular aggregates

This is a rare autosomal recessive disorder with as yet unidentified genetic defect. Patients present usually during childhood or adolescence with proximal muscle weakness, but spared cranial muscles. There are no respiratory crises. Serum CK level may be increased. There are tubular aggregates on muscle biopsy. Unlike patients with *COLQ* and *DOK7* mutations, these patients have a long-term benefit from esterase inhibitors [85, 86, 87].

Mutations of the *MUSK* gene and the *SCN4A* gene have been observed in single patients only [82, 88, 89].

The salient clinical features of the most frequent CMS forms are summarized in Table 23.1.

Genotype–phenotype correlations

The genotype–phenotype correlations in CMS are complicated because of the limited number of patients with identical mutations and the phenotypic heterogeneity even within kinships. The poorly characterized signaling pathways downstream of MuSK and the as yet unidentified molecules acting at the NMJ provide a host of potential modifiers of the disease phenotype. However, there are some general conclusions that can be drawn from the published CMS observations.

Patients with AChR deficiency due to *CHRNE* mutations have no respiratory crises in contrast to patients with *RAPSN* and *CHAT* mutations. The eye movements are restricted in patients with *CHRNE* mutations while patients with *RAPSN* and *CHAT* mutations have no ophthalmoparesis. In contrast to patients with *COLQ* mutations, patients with *CHRNE* mutations have no respiratory difficulties and less frequently have delayed motor milestones. Unlike patients with SCCMS and *DOK7* and *COLQ* mutations, patients with *CHRNE* mutations usually have no progression and clear benefit from esterase inhibitors.

Diagnostic approaches

Most importantly, the threshold for suspecting a neuromuscular transmission defect should be rather low and may be based on clinical observations only. Muscle weakness starting in infancy or early childhood in the absence of sensory symptoms, together with normal CK and unspecific biopsy findings, showing fluctuation over time or upon activity are the most important clinical observations. Supportive technical results are helpful in establishing the diagnosis, but may not be obtainable in every patient.

Clinically, the various CMS forms share common features. The onset is most frequently early in life. The newborns present with poor cry and suck, respiratory distress, feeding difficulties, muscle hypotonia, and ptosis. The early motor development is frequently delayed. During childhood the patients cannot keep up with their peers in sports, and there is abnormal fatigability and exercise-induced weakness. Some patients develop spinal deformities and muscle atrophy. Ptosis and ophthalmoparesis are also frequently observed.

The electrophysiological studies frequently demonstrate impaired neuromuscular transmission: decremental response on RNS and increased jitter and blocking on SF-EMG. RNS should be carried out on two distal and two proximal muscles. Because myasthenia gravis is more frequent than CMS and both disorders share many symptoms, testing for antibodies against AChR and MuSK is necessary to differentiate CMS from autoimmune myasthenia gravis, especially in older children and young adults. A conventional muscle biopsy is usually not helpful in differentiating different CMS subtypes, but may be needed to exclude other neuromuscular disorders.

Molecular genetic testing is indispensable for CMS diagnosis. There are some clinical clues facilitating molecular diagnosis (Table 23.2).

Haplotype analysis is applicable to families with at least two affected siblings, leading to exclusion of loci and reducing the number of candidate genes to be sequenced [90].

Differential diagnosis

A variety of conditions need to be considered in the differential diagnosis of CMS (Table 23.3). However, detailed history and

Table 23.1. Comparison of key clinical features of the frequent CMS forms [57, 65]

	CHRNE (AChR deficiency)	RAPSN	DOK7	COLQ	CHAT	SCCMS
Onset	First year of life, no LO	Birth to first year of life EO; LO possible	Second year of life; LO possible	Birth to seventh year of life; no LO	Birth to first year of life; no LO	Birth to late twenties; LO possible
Presenting symptoms	Bilateral ptosis, feeding difficulties, poor suck and cry	Hypotonia, muscle weakness, ptosis, respiratory crises, arthrogryposis multiplex congenita; LO – ptosis, mild weakness	Walking difficulties; difficulties in running; waddling gait	Ptosis, hypotonia, poor suck and cry, respiratory insufficiency; poor head control	Hypotonia, apnea	Ptosis, muscle weakness
Congenital joint contractures, dysmorphic facial features	No	Frequent	No	No	No	No
Ptosis	Yes	Yes	Yes	Yes	Yes	Yes
Ophthalmoparesis	Yes	No	No	Yes (in more than 50%)	No	Possible
Facial and bulbar weakness	Yes	Yes	Yes	Yes	Yes	Yes
Extremities, axial weakness, scoliosis	Generalized fatigable weakness	Generalized fatigable weakness	Limb-girdle weakness, waddling or sinuous gait, axial weakness, scoliosis	Generalized weakness, sometimes predominant limb-girdle weakness, waddling gait, axial weakness, scoliosis	Generalized fatigable weakness	Severe weakness EO, mild weakness LO, axial weakness, scoliosis
Respiratory crises	Very rare	Yes, especially during infections	Progressive deterioration of respiratory function, crises also possible	Yes	Yes	Progressive deterioration of respiratory function, crises also possible
Fluctuation of weakness	Daytime dependent	Daytime dependent	Day-to-day fluctuations	Daytime dependent, day-to-day fluctuations also possible	No weakness or only mild weakness between crises	Daytime dependent
Progression	Usually benign course, no progression	Usually no progression, sometimes improvement in later childhood	Often slowly progressive	Often slowly progressive	Unknown	Often slowly progressive
Response to esterase inhibitors	Clearly positive in most	Clearly positive in most	No effect or only short-term benefit, sometimes worsening	No effect or worsening	Clearly positive in most	No effect or worsening

Notes: AChR, acetylcholine receptor; CMS, congenital myasthenic syndromes; EO, early onset; LO, late onset.

Table 23.2. Clinical clues facilitating genetic testing for CMS

Symptom/finding	CMS form, probable responsible gene/ mutations
Autosomal dominant inheritance	SCCMS
Origin (Southeastern Europe)	*CHRNE*
Origin (Central Europe)	*RAPSN* N88K or *DOK7* 1124_1127dupTGCC
Origin (Roma)	*CHRNE* 1267delG
No response (or worsening) to esterase inhibitors	*COLQ*, *DOK7*, SCCMS,
Repetitive CMAP	SCCMS, *COLQ*
Late onset	*RAPSN*, *DOK7*, SCCMS
Predominant involvement of proximal muscles, waddling gait and scapular winging	*DOK7*, *COLQ*
Selective involvement of neck, wrist and finger extensors	SCCMS
Episodes of respiratory distress	*CHAT*, *RAPSN*, *COLQ*

Notes: CMAP, compound muscle action potential; SCCMS, slow-channel congenital myasthenic syndrome.

Table 23.3. Differential diagnosis of CMS

Neonatal period, infancy	Childhood, adulthood
Birth trauma	Mitochondrial myopathy
SMA1	SMA 2 and 3
Congenital myopathies	Motor neuron disease
Congenital muscular dystrophies	Muscular dystrophies (FSHD, LGMD, OPMD)
Congenital myotonic dystrophy	Autoimmune MG (seronegative)
Möbius syndrome	
Infantile botulism	
Congenital fibrosis of external ocular muscles (CFEOM)	

Notes: FSHD, facioscapulohumeral dystrophy; LGMD, limb-girdle muscular dystrophy; MG, myasthenia gravis; OPMD, oculopharyngeal muscular dystrophy; SMA, spinal muscular atrophy.

clinical examination, electrophysiological studies, muscle biopsy findings, and molecular genetic testing would usually differentiate CMS from other disease entities.

Therapeutic and preventive modalities

The diverse underlying genetic defects in CMS result in different pathophysiology. Therefore, the administration of the best therapeutic agent depends on the precise molecular diagnosis. CMS that decrease the synaptic response to ACh are treated with drugs that augment cholinergic stimulation, namely AChE inhibitors and 3,4-diaminopyridine (3,4-DAP) [55]. Most patients show clear benefit from AChE inhibitors, namely patients with AChR deficiency due to *CHRNE* and *RAPSN* mutations. In contrast, AChE inhibitors show little benefit in CMS due to *DOK7* mutations or in the SCCMS, and may dramatically worsen symptoms in esterase deficiency due to *COLQ* mutations. 3,4-DAP is often used as an "add-on" medication when AChE inhibitors alone are not sufficient to obtain the desired therapeutic effect or side-effects prevent a higher, more effective dosing of AChE inhibitors.

Anticholinesterase medications benefit patients with presynaptic CMS caused by defects of *CHAT*. Oral prophylactic treatment with AChE inhibitors should be administered even in patients asymptomatic between crises as it may prevent or mitigate respiratory complications [54]. The parents should be instructed in using an inflatable rescue bag and a fitted mask during crisis and during transport to the hospital [59].

In end-plate AChE deficiency, AChE inhibitors should be avoided, since they are ineffective or even worsen symptoms. Moreover, AChE-deficient patients may be more prone to muscarinic side-effects [59].

Benefit from therapy with ephedrine was anecdotally reported in *COLQ*- and *DOK7*-mutant patients [65, 69, 83, 84]. However, more research is needed to give recommendations on ephedrine use for these conditions.

The SCCMS is treated with quinidine or fluoxetine, both acting as long-lived open-channel blockers of AChR [59]. These drugs should be avoided in other CMS.

Patients and parents should be advised that a number of drugs (such as simple antibiotics) and anesthetics may cause serious risks by negatively influencing neuromuscular transmission. They should therefore carry an emergency card and present it to any health care professional who prescribes or administers drugs.

Genetic counseling

Molecular diagnosis is pivotal for genetic counseling. Although recessive inheritance appears most common, some CMS (SCCMS) are inherited in dominant traits. When the exact molecular defect in the proband is identified, testing for carrier status should be performed in all siblings and prenatal diagnosis is feasible. Identification of presymptomatic *CHAT* or *RAPSN* mutation carriers among the siblings is important for early administration of esterase inhibitors. Molecular diagnosis is necessary for definitive establishment of the mode of inheritance even when pedigree analysis would suggest a certain pattern of inheritance (variable penetrance; de novo mutations; pseudodominant inheritance).

Future perspectives

Congenital myasthenic syndromes have proven to be suitable models to study the neuromuscular transmission. Although mutations in several genes have already been identified as causing CMS, in approximately half of CMS patients the underlying genetic defects still await identification. The discovery of new CMS genes and proteins and the investigation of their function will add more detail to the knowledge of the molecular processes at the NMJ. The generation of transgenic mice carrying particular mutations (e.g., *RAPSN* N88K or *DOK7* 1124_1127dupTGCC) would be very interesting for evaluation of the function of these proteins in vivo as well as for testing new therapeutic agents. Moreover, clinical studies are warranted to assess the long-term outcome and prognosis of CMS patients and to test new treatments.

Acknowledgment

A. Evoli thanks M. Stampanoni Bassi for his technical assistance. Hanns Lochmüller and Violeta Mihaylova are grateful to the patients and their referring physicians for their cooperation. Violeta Mihaylova received a Bayhost Fellowship from the Bavanian State.

References

1. J. M. Lindstrom, Nicotinic acetylcholine receptors of muscles and nerves: comparison of their structures, functional roles, and vulnerability to pathology. *Ann. N. Y. Acad. Sci.* **998** (2003), 41–52.
2. A. Vincent, Unravelling the pathogenesis of myasthenia gravis. *Nat. Rev. Immunol.* **2** (2002), 797–804.
3. B. M. Conti-Fine, M. Milani, H. Kaminski, Myasthenia gravis: past, present, and future. *J. Clin. Invest.* **116** (2006), 2843–2854.
4. A. Balandina, S. Lècart, P. Dartevelle, A. Saoudi, S. Berrih-Aknin, Functional defect of regulatory CD4+CD25+ T cells in the thymus of patients with autoimmune myasthenia gravis. *Blood* **105** (2005), 735–741.
5. M. I. Leite, M. Jones, P. Ströbel, *et al.*, Myasthenia gravis thymus: complement vulnerability of epithelial and myoid cells, complement attack on them, and correlations with autoantibody status. *Am. J. Pathol.* **171** (2007), 893–905.
6. P. Ströbel, A. Rosenwald, N. Beyersdorf, *et al.*, Selective loss of regulatory T cells in thymomas. *Ann. Neurol.* **56** (2004), 901–904.
7. F. Romi, G. O. Skeie, N. E. Gilhus, J. A. Aarli, Striational antibodies in myasthenia gravis: reactivity and possible clinical significance. *Arch. Neurol.* **62** (2005), 442–446.
8. W. Hoch, J. McConville, S. Helms, J. Newsom-Davis, A. Melms, A. Vincent, Auto-antibodies to the receptor tyrosine kinase MuSK in patients with myasthenia gravis without acetylcholine receptor antibodies. *Nat. Med.* **7** (2001), 365–368.
9. L. Strochlic, A. Cartaud, J. Cartaud, The synaptic muscle-specific kinase (MuSK) complex: new partners, new functions. *Bioessays* **27** (2005), 1129–1135.
10. V. Witzemann, Development of the neuromuscular junction. *Cell. Tissue Res.* **326** (2006), 263–271.
11. A. Vincent, M. I. Leite, Neuromuscular junction autoimmune disease: muscle specific kinase antibodies and treatments for myasthenia gravis. *Curr. Opin. Neurol.* **18** (2005), 519–525.
12. H. Shiraishi, M. Motomura, T. Yoshimura, *et al.*, Acetylcholine receptors loss and postsynaptic damage in MuSK antibody-positive myasthenia gravis. *Ann. Neurol.* **57** (2005), 289–293.
13. S. Jha, K. Xu, T. Maruta, *et al.*, Myasthenia gravis induced in mice by immunization with the recombinant extracellular domain of rat muscle-specific kinase (MuSK). *J. Neuroimmunol.*, **175** (2006), 107–117.
14. K. Xu, S. Jha, W. Hoch, S. E. Dryer, Delayed synapsing muscles are more severely affected in an experimental model of MuSK-induced myasthenia gravis. *Neuroscience.* **143** (2006), 655–659.
15. L. Lauriola, F. Ranelletti, N. Maggiano, *et al.*, Thymus changes in anti-MuSK-positive and -negative myasthenia gravis. *Neurology* **64** (2005), 536–538.
16. D. B. Sanders, K. El-Salem, J. M. Massey, J. McConville, A. Vincent, Clinical aspects of MuSK antibody positive seronegative MG. *Neurology* **60** (2003), 1978–1980.
17. A. Evoli, P. A. Tonali, L. Padua, *et al.*, Clinical correlates with anti-MuSK antibodies in generalized seronegative myasthenia gravis. *Brain* **126** (2003), 2304–2311.
18. M. I. Leite, P. Ströbel, M. Jones, *et al.*, Fewer thymic changes in MuSK antibody-positive than in MuSK antibody-negative MG. *Ann. Neurol.* **57** (2005), 444–448.
19. L. L. Kusner, A. Puwanant, H. J. Kaminski, Ocular myasthenia. Diagnosis, treatment and pathogenesis. *Neurologist* **12** (2006), 231–239.
20. A. P. Batocchi, L. Majolini, A. Evoli, M. M. Lino, C. Minisci, P. Tonali, Course and treatment of myasthenia gravis during pregnancy. *Neurology* **52** (1999), 447–452.
21. K. E. Osserman, G. Genkins, Studies in myasthenia gravis: review of a twenty-year experience in over 1200 patients. *Mt. Sinai J. Med.* **38** (1971), 497–537.
22. A. Jaretzski 3rd, R. J. Barohn, R. M. Ernstoff, *et al.*, Myasthenia gravis: recommendations for clinical research standards. Task Force of the Medical Scientific Advisory Board of the Myasthenia Gravis Foundation of America. *Neurology* **55** (2000), 16–23.
23. J. C. Keesey, Clinical evaluation and management of myasthenia gravis. *Muscle Nerve* **29** (2004), 484–505.
24. F. E. Somnier, Increasing incidence of late-onset anti-AChR antibody-seropositive myasthenia gravis. *Neurology* **65** (2005), 928–930.
25. M. E. Farrugia, R. P. Kennett, J. Newsom-Davis, D. Hilton-Jones, A. Vincent, Single-fiber electromyography in limb and facial muscles in muscle-specific kinase antibody and acetylcholine receptor antibody myasthenia gravis. *Muscle Nerve* **33** (2006), 568–570.
26. G. S. Gronseth, R. J. Barohn, Thymectomy for myasthenia gravis. *Curr. Treat. Options Neurol.* **4** (2002), 203–209.
27. J. Newsom-Davis, G. Cutter, G. I. Wolfe, *et al.*, Status of the thymectomy trial for nonthymomatous myasthenia gravis patients receiving prednisone. *Ann. N. Y. Acad. Sci.* **1132** (2008), 344–347.
28. P. Gajdos, S. Chevret, K. Toyka, Intravenous immunoglobulin for myasthenia gravis. *Cochrane Database Syst. Rev.* **2** (2006), CD002277.
29. G. O. Skeie, S. Apostolski, A. Evoli, *et al.*, Guidelines for the treatment of autoimmune neuromuscular transmission disorders. *Eur. J. Neurol.* **13** (2006), 691–699.

30. J. Palace, J. Newsom-Davis, B. Lecky, The Myasthenia Study Group, A randomized double-blind trial of prednisolone alone or with azathioprine in myasthenia gravis. *Neurology* **50** (1998), 1778–1783.

31. V. Chaudhry, D. R. Cornblath, J. W. Griffin, R. O'Brien, D. B. Drachman, Mycophenolate mofetil: a safe and promising immunosuppressant in neuromuscular diseases. *Neurology* **56** (2001), 94–96.

32. R. S. A. Tindall, T. J. Phillips, J. A. Jollins, L. Wells, K. Hall, A clinical therapeutic trial of cyclosporine in myasthenia gravis. *Ann. NY. Acad. Sci.* **681** (1993), 539–551.

33. J. Sieb, Myasthenia gravis: emerging new therapy options. *Curr. Opin. Pharmacol.* **5** (2005), 303–307.

34. D. B. Drachman, R. J. Jones, R. A. Brodsky, Treatment of refractory myasthenia: "rebooting" with high-dose cyclophosphamide. *Ann. Neurol.* **53** (2003), 29–34.

35. H. Fukunaga, A. G. Engel, B. Lang, J. Newsom-Davis, A. Vincent, Passive transfer of Lambert-Eaton myasthenic syndrome with IgG from man to mouse depletes the presynaptic membrane active zones. *Proc. Natl. Acad. Sci. U. S. A.* **80** (1983), 7636–7640.

36. W. A. Catterall, Structure and function of voltage-gated Ca^{2+} channels. *Annu. Rev. Cell. Dev. Biol.* **16** (2000), 521–555.

37. A. Nagel, A. G. Engel, B. Lang, J. Newsom-Davis, T. Fukuoka, Lambert-Eaton myasthenic syndrome IgG depletes presynaptic membrane active zone particles by antigenic modulation. *Ann. Neurol.* **24** (1988), 552–558.

38. T. Fukuda, M. Motomura, Y. Nakao, *et al.*, Reduction of P/Q-type calcium channels in the postmortem cerebellum of paraneoplastic cerebellar degeneration with Lambert-Eaton myasthenic syndrome. *Ann. Neurol.* **53** (2003), 21–28.

39. M. Takamori, Lambert-Eaton myasthenic syndrome as an autoimmune calcium channelopathy. *Biochem. Biophys. Res. Commun.* **322** (2004), 1347–1351.

40. P. W. Wirtz, J. G. van Dijk, P. A. van Doorn, *et al.*, The epidemiology of the Lambert-Eaton myasthenic syndrome in the Netherlands. *Neurology* **63** (2004), 397–398.

41. S. H. Oh, K. Kurokawa, G. C. Claussen, H. F. Ryan Jr., Electrophysiological diagnostic criteria in the Lambert-Eaton myasthenic syndrome. *Muscle Nerve* **32** (2005), 515–520.

42. D. B. Sanders, Lambert–Eaton myasthenic syndrome: diagnosis and treatment. *Ann. N. Y. Acad. Sci.* **998** (2003), 500–508.

43. J. Newsom-Davis, A treatment algorithm for Lambert-Eaton myasthenic syndrome. *Ann. N. Y. Acad. Sci.* **841** (1998), 827–831.

44. J. Newsom-Davis, J. N. M. Murray, Plasma-exchange and immunosuppressive treatment in the Lambert-Eaton myasthenic syndrome. *Neurology* **34** (1984), 480–485.

45. I. K. Hart, P. Maddison, J. Newsom-Davis, A. Vincent, K. R. Mills, Phenotypic variants of autoimmune peripheral nerve hyperexcitability. *Brain* **125** (2002), 1887–1895.

46. P. Shillito, P. C Molenaar, A. Vincent, *et al.*, Acquired neuromyotonia: evidence for autoantibodies directed against K^+ channels of peripheral nerves. *Ann. Neurol.* **38** (1995), 714–722.

47. G. Yellen, The voltage-gated potassium channels and their relatives. *Nature* **419** (2002), 35–42.

48. S. Vernino, Autoimmune and paraneoplastic channelopathies. *Neurotherapeutics* **4** (2007), 305–314.

49. K. A. Kleopa, L. B. Elman, B. Lang, A. Vincent, S. S. Scherer, Neuromyotonia and limbic encephalitis sera target mature Shaker-type K^+ channels: subunit specificity correlates with clinical manifestations. *Brain* **129** (2006), 1570–1584.

50. H. Tomimitsu, K. Arimura, T. Nagado, *et al.*, Mechanism of action of voltage-gated K^+ channel antibodies in acquired neuromyotonia. *Ann. Neurol.* **56** (2004), 440–444.

51. C. Buckley, A. Vincent, Autoimmune channelopathies. Nat. *Clin. Pract. Neurol.* **1** (2005), 22–33.

52. L. Gutmann, L. Gutmann, Myokymia and neuromyotonia. *J. Neurol.* **251** (2004), 138–142.

53. R. S. Duan, H. Link, B. G. Xiao, Long-term effects of IFN-gamma, IL-10, and TGF-beta-modulated dendritic cells on immune response in Lewis rats. *J. Clin. Immunol.* **25** (2005), 50–56.

54. K. Kostelidou, N. Trakas, S. J. Tzartos, Extracellular domains of the beta, gamma and epsilon subunits of the human acetylcholine receptor as immunoadsorbents for myasthenic autoantibodies: a combination of immunoadsorbents results in increased efficiency. *J. Neuroimmunol.* **190** (2007), 44–52.

55. A. Engel, S. Sine, Current understanding of congenital myasthenic syndromes. *Curr. Opin. Pharmacol.* **5** (2005), 308–321.

56. D. Beeson, D. Hantai, H. Lochmuller, A. Engel, 126th International Workshop: Congenital myasthenic syndromes 24–26 September 2004, Naarden, the Netherlands. *Neuromuscul. Disord.* **15** (2005), 498–512.

57. J. S. Müller, V. Mihaylova, A. Abicht, H. Lochmuller, Congenital myasthenic syndromes: spotlight on genetic defects of neuromuscular transmission. *Expert. Rev. Mol. Med.* **9**:22 (2007), 1–20.

58. K. Ohno, A. Tsujino, J. Brengman, *et al.*, Choline acetyltransferase mutations cause myasthenic syndrome associated with episodic apnea in humans. *Proc. Natl. Acad. Sci. U. S. A.* **98**:4 (2001), 2017–2022.

59. A. Engel, K. Ohno, S. Sine, Congenital myasthenic syndromes: progress over the past decade. *Muscle Nerve* **27** (2003), 4–25.

60. N. Barisic, J. Muller, E. Paucic-Kirincic, *et al.*, Clinical variability of CMS-EA (congenital myasthenic syndromes with episodic apnea) due to identical CHAT mutations in two infants. *Eur. J. Paediatr. Neurol.* **9** (2005), 7–12.

61. C. Schmidt, A. Abicht, K. Krampfl, *et al.*, Congenital myasthenic syndromes due to a novel missense mutation in the gene encoding choline acetyltransferase. *Neuromuscul. Disord.* **13** (2003), 245–251.

62. M. Milone, T. Fukuda, X. M. Shen, *et al.*, Novel congenital myasthenic syndromes associated with defects in quantal release. *Neurology* **66** (2006), 1223–1229.

63. C. Donger, E. Krejci, A. P. Serradell, *et al.*, Mutation in the human acetylcholinesterase-associated collagen gene, COLQ, is responsible for congenital myasthenic syndrome with end-plate acetylcholinesterase deficiency (type Ic). *Am. J. Hum. Genet.* **63** (1998), 967–975.

64. K. Ohno, J. Brengman, A. Tsujino, A. Engel, Human endplate acetylcholinesterase deficiency caused by mutations in the collagen-like tail subunit (ColQ) of the asymmetric enzyme. *Proc. Natl. Acad. Sci. U.S.A.* **95** (1998), 9654–9659.

65. V. Mihaylova, J. Muller J. Vilchez, *et al.*, Clinical and molecular genetic findings in 22 COLQ-mutant congenital myasthenic syndromes. *Brain* **131** (2008), 747–759.

66. K. Ohno, A. Engel, Congenital myasthenic syndromes: gene mutations. *Neuromuscul. Disord.* **14** (2004), 117–122.

67. Y. A. Shapira, M. E. Sadeh, M. P. Bergtraum, *et al.*, Three novel COLQ mutations and variation of phenotypic expressivity due to G240X: synaptic congenital myasthenic syndrome in three patients due to a novel missense mutation (T441A) of the COLQ gene. *Neurology* **58** (2002), 603–609.

68. J. S. Müller, S. Petrova, R. Kiefer, *et al.*, Congenital endplate acetylcholinesterase deficiency responsive to ephedrine. *Neuropediatrics* **35** (2004), 183–189.

69. M. Bestue-Cardiel, A. Saenz de Cabezon-Alvarez, J. L. Capablo-Liesa, *et al.*, Escobar syndrome is a prenatal myasthenia caused by disruption of the acetylcholine receptor fetal γ subunit. *Neurology* **65** (2005), 144–146.

70. K. Hoffmann, J. S. Müller, S. Stricker, *et al.*, Recessive inheritance and variable penetrance of slow-channel congenital myasthenic syndromes. *Am. J. Hum. Genet.* **79** (2006), 303–312.

71. R. Croxen, C. Hatton, C. Shelley, *et al.*, Long-term improvement of slow-channel congenital myasthenic syndrome with fluoxetine. *Neurology* **59** (2002), 162–168.

72. J. Colomer, J. S. Müller A. Vernet, *et al.*, Quinidine sulfate therapy for the slow-channel congenital myasthenic syndrome. *Neuromuscul. Disord.* **16** (2006), 329–333.

73. C. M. Harper, A. G. Engel, Treatment of slow-channel congenital myasthenic syndrome with fluoxetine. *Ann. Neurol.* **43** (1998), 480–484.

74. C. M. Harper, T. Fukodome, A. G. Engel, Acetylcholine receptor δ subunit mutations underlie a fast-channel myasthenic syndrome and arthrogryposis multiplex congenital. *Neurology* **60** (2003), 1710–1713.

75. S. Brownlow, R. Webster, R. Croxen, *et al.*, Chromosome 17p-linked myasthenias stem from defects in the acetylcholine receptor ε-subunit gene. *J. Clin. Invest.* **108** (2001), 125–130.

76. L. Middleton, K. Ohno, K. Christodoulou, *et al.*, A common mutation (ε1267delG) in congenital myasthenic patients of Gypsy ethnic origin. *Neurology* **53** (1999), 1076–1082.

77. A. Abicht, R. Stucka, V. Karcagi, *et al.*, Mutation history of the Roma/Gypsies. *Neurology* **53** (1999), 1564–1569.

78. B. Morar, D. Gresham, D. Angelicheva, *et al.*, Case report: congenital myasthenic syndrome in a Gypsy family showing a pseudodominant pattern of inheritance. *Am. J. Hum. Genet.* **75** (2004), 596–609.

79. A. Herczegfalvi, A. Abicht, V. Kargaci, H. Lochmüller, 125th ENMC International Workshop: Neuromuscular disorders in the Roma (Gypsy) population, 23–25 April 2004, Naarden, The Netherlands. *Acta Myologica* **19** (2000), 49–51.

80. L. Kalaydjieva, H. Lochmüller, I. Tournev, *et al.*, Rapsyn mutations in humans cause endplate acetylcholine receptor deficiency and myasthenic syndrome. *Neuromuscul. Disord.* **15** (2005), 65–71.

81. K. Ohno, A. G. Engel, X.-M. Shen, *et al.*, The muscle protein Dok-7 is essential for neuromuscular synaptogenesis. *Am. J. Hum. Genet.* **70** (2002), 875–885.

82. K. Okada, A. Inoue, M. Okada, *et al.*, Phenotypical spectrum of DOK7 mutations in congenital myasthenic syndromes. *Science* **312**:6 (2006), 1802–1805.

83. J. S. Müller, A. Herczegfalvi, J. Vilchez, *et al.*, Clinical features of the DOK7 neuromuscular junction synaptopathy. *Brain* **130**:6 (2007), 1497–1506.

84. J. Palace, D. Lashley, J. Newson-Davis, *et al.*, Familial myasthenia with "tubular aggregates" treated with prednisone. *Brain* **130**: Pt6 (2007), 1507–1515.

85. T. R. Johns, J. F. Campa, L. S. Adelman, Familial neuromuscular disease with type 1 fiber hypoplasia, tubular aggregates, cardiomyopathy, and myasthenic features. *Neurology* **73** (1973), 426.

86. B. H. Dobkin, M. A. Verity, Familial limb-girdle myasthenia with tubular aggregates. *Neurology* **28** (1978), 1135–1140.

87. E. Furui, K. Fukushima, T. Sakashita, *et al.*, MUSK, a new target for mutations causing congenital myasthenic syndrome. *Muscle Nerve* **20** (1997), 599–603.

88. F. Chevessier, B. Faraut, A. Ravel-Chapuis, *et al.*, Myasthenic syndrome caused by mutation of the SCN4A sodium channel. *Hum. Mol. Gen.* **13** (2004), 3229–3240.

89. A. Tsujino, C. Maertens, K. Ohno, *et al.*, Myasthenic syndrome caused by mutations of the SCN4A sodium channel. *Proc. Natl. Acad. Sci. U. S. A.* **100** (2003), 7377–82.

90. M. Von der Hagen, J. Schallner, A. M. Kaindl, *et al.*, Facing the genetic heterogeneity in neuromuscular disorders: linkage analysis as an economic diagnostic approach towards the molecular diagnosis. *Neuromuscul. Disord.* **16** (2006), 4–13.

Chapter 24

Endocrine and toxic myopathies

Zohar Argov and Frank L. Mastaglia

A number of endocrine disorders may cause neuromuscular complications which may sometimes be the presenting symptoms of the disorder and are usually reversible once the endocrine condition is corrected. Endocrine myopathies should be part of the differential diagnosis of myalgia, cramps, weakness, fatigability, muscular atrophy or hypertrophy, and of an unexpected deterioration or acceleration of a pre-existing neuromuscular disorder. Muscle involvement is most common in hyperthyroidism and hypothyroidism, and may also occur in patients with parathyroid and adrenal cortical disorders, acromegaly, diabetes mellitus, or hypogonadism [1].

Hypothyroid myopathy

Hypothyroidism can lead to a number of neuromuscular symptoms and signs, most commonly muscle pain, stiffness, cramping, and subclinical weakness [2]. Occasionally a more severe myopathy, with a proximal or diffuse pattern of weakness, elevated serum creatine kinase (CK), and myopathic electromyographic (EMG) findings with prominent spontaneous potentials occurs [3], and may resemble polymyositis [4]. Slowing in muscle contraction and relaxation ("pseudomyotonia"), and in the relaxation phase of the tendon reflexes (classically the ankle jerk) is a useful confirmatory sign of hypothyroidism, although rarely noticed. Myoedema (the mounding phenomenon) may be demonstrable by direct muscle percussion in some patients. Very rarely, adults with long-standing untreated hypothyroidism may develop diffuse muscular hypertrophy and painful muscle spasms on movement (Hoffman syndrome). A similar diffuse pattern of muscle hypertrophy may occur in some children with untreated congenital hypothyroidism (Kocher–Debre–Semelaigne syndrome). Patients with hypothyroidism may also present with rhabdomyolysis or asymptomatic elevation of the serum CK [5]. Hypothyroidism also predisposes to the development of a statin-induced myopathy and statins may unmask previously undiagnosed hypothyroid myopathy [5]. The muscular symptoms usually improve after commencement of thyroxine replacement therapy but recovery is often slow in cases of severe hypothyroid myopathy.

A muscle biopsy may be required in atypical cases or if the muscle symptoms do not improve after treatment with thyroxine. The biopsy findings are variable and include type I and II fiber atrophy or hypertrophy, reduced type II fiber numbers [6], and muscle fiber necrosis and regeneration in some cases [3, 7]. Other changes in long-standing cases include core-like areas devoid of enzyme activity and containing granulofilamentous material, and calcium deposits [3]. Experimental studies have shown that hypothyroidism causes a marked increase in the proportion of type I (slow-twitch) fibers in the limb and respiratory muscles, and conversion of fast- to slow-twitch myosin isoforms [8].

Hyperthyroid myopathy

A clinical myopathy occurs in only a small proportion of patients with hyperthyroidism. However, subclinical weakness and atrophy, particularly of proximal limb muscles, is commonly found especially in patients with long-standing hyperthyroidism [2], and quantitative EMG studies also show a high frequency of subclinical myopathy. The weakness is most prominent in proximal muscle groups, but may be more diffuse, including the bulbar and respiratory muscles in severe cases [1]. Myalgia and muscle cramps occur in some cases. Muscle fasciculations may occur but are uncommon, and when associated with brisk reflexes and bulbar symptoms the condition may resemble motor neuron disease [9]. The CK level is usually normal (and even below the range of normal) but may be elevated in rare cases of thyroid storm.

A muscle biopsy is only necessary in patients with atypical features, or if symptoms fail to improve after treatment of the hyperthyroidism when the possibility of an associated inflammatory or other myopathy should be considered. The biopsy findings in hyperthyroid myopathy are nonspecific, with variable degrees of atrophy of type I and II fibers [6] and small interstitial lymphocytic infiltrates in some cases. Experimental studies have shown reduced numbers of type I fibers [8] and a switch in expression from slow to fast myosin isoforms in hyperthyroid animals [10].

Disorders of Voluntary Muscle, 8th edn., eds. George Karpati, David Hilton-Jones, Kate Bushby and Robert C. Griggs. Published by Cambridge University Press.

Thyrotoxic periodic paralysis

A form of periodic paralysis closely resembling familial hypokalemic periodic paralysis can occur in patients with thyrotoxicosis and may sometimes be the presenting feature [11, 12]. It occurs mainly in people of Asian origin, but has also been increasingly reported from Western countries [11]. It is much more common in males than females, typically occurring in young adult males 20–40 years of age [11], and can be associated with any etiological form of thyrotoxicosis, including drug-induced varieties. Unlike primary forms of periodic paralysis, no specific genetic basis has been identified. The severity of the thyrotoxicosis is variable and its clinical signs at the time of presentation may be subtle or absent. The attacks of weakness are usually precipitated by meals with a high carbohydrate content or alcohol, or may occur following strenuous physical activity. They may also occur spontaneously, particularly early in the morning on waking and may last for several hours or even days. The weakness initially affects the limb and trunk muscles but may progress to flaccid quadriplegia in severe attacks. In some cases the weakness is asymmetrical and more severe in muscles that were strenuously exercised.

The attacks are usually associated with hypokalemia ($K^+ < 3$ mmol/l), which is thought to result from intracellular potassium shifts due to increased activity of the Na^+/K^+-ATPase pump [11]. A number of factors may be responsible for this, including the effects of excessive thyroid hormones, an enhanced β-adrenergic response, and an exaggerated insulin response to carbohydrate loading. Affected individuals may also have an underlying predisposition to excessive activation of the Na^+/K^+-ATPase pump by thyroid hormone or other factors [11]. An association with certain polymorphisms in the β-adrenergic receptor gene has been found in Chinese patients, as well as an association with certain HLA haplotypes [11, 12].

Treatment of the acute attacks requires cautious potassium replacement intravenously or orally, with careful monitoring of the serum K^+ level to avoid rebound hyperkalemia, and β-blockade with propranolol (3–4 mg/kg orally) [11]. Some patients with hypophosphatemia may also require phosphate infusions. Prevention of attacks involves avoiding known precipitating factors, administration of propranolol, and definitive treatment of the thyrotoxicosis [11, 12].

Thyroid ophthalmopathy

This is characterized by exophthalmos due to swelling of the orbital contents, diplopia and, in severe cases, extraocular muscle palsies and visual loss due to optic nerve compression. Enlargement of the extraocular muscles, which is usually symmetrical, can be demonstrated by computerized tomography (CT) or magnetic resonance imaging (MRI) of the orbits. The condition is associated with Graves disease in about 90% of cases, and less frequently with Hashimoto thyroiditis. It is thought to be due to a T-cell-mediated process against common antigen(s) shared by the orbital tissues and the thyroid gland [13] and the thyrotropin receptor and thyroglobulin have been implicated as possible target antigens. The orbital fibroblasts and adipocytes are thought to be the primary target of the immune response but there is also some evidence for an antibody-dependent, cell-mediated cytotoxic process involving extraocular muscle antigens [13].

Treatment involves administration of glucocorticoids intravenously or orally, and correction of the associated hyperthyroidism or hypothyroidism. Other options in resistant cases include intravenous immunoglobulin, immunosuppressive agents (ciclosporin), somatostatin analogs (octreotide), and orbital radiotherapy [13]. Orbital decompression may be necessary in some cases with optic nerve compression if vision is threatened.

Adrenal myopathies

A myopathy of variable severity may occur in patients with Cushing syndrome or ectopic adrenocorticotropic-hormone-(ACTH-) producing tumors. A proximal myopathy is common in patients with Cushing disease, being found in as many as 80% of patients in some series, and recovers slowly after hypophysectomy [14]. A myopathy associated with skin hyperpigmentation has also been described in patients with excessive ACTH secretion following adrenalectomy for Cushing disease (Nelson syndrome) and in patients with primary hyperaldosteronism (Conn syndrome) who may also develop hypokalemic periodic paralysis [1, 15]. The clinical and laboratory features of the steroid myopathies are discussed below.

Complaints of fatigue, muscle weakness, and cramping are common in patients with Addison disease. Occasional patients may develop a more severe generalized myopathy, which may also affect the respiratory muscles, and which is reversible after cortisone replacement therapy [16]. The CK level is not usually elevated and the EMG and muscle biopsy findings are nonspecific. Rarely, patients with adrenal insufficiency who have elevated serum potassium levels may develop a severe hyperkalemic myopathy or periodic paralysis.

Hyperparathyroidism

Patients with primary hyperparathyroidism may present with complaints of muscle weakness and fatigability on exertion, which recover after parathyroidectomy, but in the modern era when the diagnosis is often made purely on biochemical grounds, many patients are asymptomatic or develop a mild sensory peripheral neuropathy [17, 18]. Although there are well-documented reports in the older literature of patients with a severe proximal myopathy and muscular atrophy, and other neurological abnormalities such as hyperreflexia, fasciculations of the tongue, and gait abnormalities [18, 19], such patients are only rarely encountered in current clinical practice [20]. Patients with secondary hyperparathyroidism due to chronic renal failure may also develop a similar myopathy [1].

Investigations in patients with primary hyperparathyroidism have shown evidence of impaired muscle function, with reduced muscle twitch and tetanic tension [20], and mild impairment of neuromuscular transmission in some cases [17]. Muscle biopsy findings in patients with myopathy include type I and II fiber atrophy [19] and mild fiber type grouping, but the biopsy is often normal in less affected cases [20].

Osteomalacia

The occurrence of a painful proximal myopathy – often with disproportionate weakness of the gluteal muscles and a waddling gait, and with bone tenderness and pain on movement – is well recognized in adults with osteomalacia and may also occur in children with rickets [1]. The frequency of myopathy in osteomalacia has varied from 73% to 97% in different series, and in one series the myopathy was the initial presenting problem in 30% of cases [21]. It may be associated with vitamin D deficiency of dietary origin or due to malabsorption, or with abnormal vitamin D metabolism associated with renal tubular acidosis or anticonvulsant therapy [21, 22]. Secondary hyperparathyroidism is usually present, with low serum phosphate, normal or raised serum calcium, and a raised serum alkaline phosphatase level, which is a useful screening test. The serum CK level is usually normal. The bone pain and weakness usually improve gradually after vitamin D supplements are commenced.

Muscle biopsy studies have shown type II fiber atrophy (in rats it was mostly type IIB [23]), and other minor nonspecific changes [21, 22]. A physiological study of the effects of vitamin D deficiency in rabbits showed reduced calcium uptake by the sarcoplasmic reticulum and reduced troponin C levels [24].

Hypoparathyroidism

Patients with hypocalcemia due to hypoparathyroidism commonly suffer from tetany, with associated muscle cramps and paresthesiae, but do not usually develop a symptomatic myopathy. There are reports in the older literature of a myopathy with mild nonspecific muscle biopsy changes, and of asymptomatic elevation of the serum CK and lactate dehydrogenase (LDH) activity, with recovery after administration of calcium and vitamin D (see [25]. Prolonged hypocalcemia in rats has also been shown to lead to elevation of the serum CK activity [26]. However, there have not been any systematic studies in the modern era and doubt remains as to the existence of the entity of hypoparathyroid myopathy.

Pituitary disorders

Subjective complaints of weakness and fatigue are common in acromegalic patients and about half have a proximal myopathy with mild weakness and muscle strength out of proportion to the increased size of the muscles [27, 28]. The CK level may be mildly elevated and quantitative EMG demonstrates a reduction in motor unit potential duration [28]. Histological changes in muscle biopsies are nonspecific and include hypertrophy or atrophy of type I and type II fibers, glycogen accumulation, muscle fiber necrosis, and tubular aggregates in some cases [29]. The mechanism of the myopathy has not been investigated but may involve effects of excess growth hormone on carbohydrate metabolism and secondary downstream effects mediated through insulin growth factor-1 (IGF-1).

Deficiency of growth hormone in patients with hypopituitarism may contribute to the subjective complaints of muscular weakness and fatigue and to the impaired muscle development in children. However, the effects of growth hormone deficiency on skeletal muscle have not been systematically investigated.

Diabetes mellitus

A focal ischemic myopathy with infarction of the thigh muscles has been reported in poorly controlled diabetics [30]. The condition presents with acute onset of unilateral pain, swelling, and a palpable mass in the quadriceps or hamstring muscles and CT or MRI is helpful in confirming the diagnosis without resorting to muscle biopsy. Recovery usually occurs spontaneously and surgical intervention is not required, but the condition may recur in the same or the opposite leg.

Diabetes mellitus may occur in association with a mitochondrial myopathy [31] and cytopathy, particularly in patients with the A3243G $tRNA^{Leu}$ mutation [32]. It may also be associated with syndromes of partial or generalized lipodystrophy and myopathy [1]. The condition of diabetic amyotrophy, which causes painful proximal muscle weakness and atrophy in the lower limbs, is due to a proximal diabetic neuropathy or plexusradiculopathy and not a myopathy [33].

Drug-induced myopathies

Numerous drugs can cause weakness or muscle pain as a side-effect when used in therapeutic doses (the term "drug" in this chapter also includes drugs of addiction). Some medications have a direct myotoxic effect, others do so indirectly by inducing a metabolic or immunological disturbance, while a third group causes weakness by interfering with the function of the neuromuscular junction. The incidence of drug-induced neuromuscular disorders is difficult to establish, partly because many such side-effects are not recognized and because reactions to certain drugs are idiosyncratic and occur only rarely. There is therefore need for a high level of clinical awareness of this possibility to allow early withdrawal of the offending medication and prevent permanent or more severe muscle damage. Meticulous recording of drug history and early reporting to the medical community, so that other cases may not be missed, will increase recognition and awareness of these side-effects.

Experimental studies have provided a better understanding of the basic cellular mechanisms of action of drugs. However, the basic mechanism that underlies the therapeutic effect of a compound is not necessarily always responsible for the adverse myotoxic effects. Detailed discussion will be limited to the more important conditions and the reader is referred to other reviews for more specific information [34, 35, 36].

Table 24.1. Some of the drugs which can cause myalgia and muscle cramps

Statins	Ciclosporin
Fibrates	Nicotinic acid
Diuretics	Cimetidine
Antiarrhythmics	Lithium
β-adrenergic agonists	Salbutamol
Chemotherapeutic agents	D-Penicillamine
Calcium channel blockers (nifedipine)	Gold
Depolarizing muscle relaxants (suxamethonium)	

Table 24.2. Drugs causing painful myopathies

Myotoxic effect	Hypokalemia	Inflammatory myopathy
Statins (all)	Diuretics	D-Penicillamine
Fibrates	Purgatives	L-Tryptophan
EACA (ε-aminocaproic acid)	Liquorice	Procainamide
Emetine	Fluoroprednisolone	L-DOPA
Heroin	Carbenoxolone	Phenytoin
Amiodarone	Amphotericin	Cimetidine
Iopamidol		Statins
Zidovudine		Aluminum-containing vaccination
Proton pump inhibitors		

Clinical syndromes

Muscle damage can be induced by local injection of the drug into the muscle or by a more widespread effect on skeletal muscle tissue. The resulting clinical syndromes vary in their mode of onset and rate of progression, as well as the severity of myalgia and degree and extent of muscle weakness.

1. *Myalgia and asymptomatic CK elevation.* Muscle pain and cramps are common complaints in patients with various diseases, but the possibility that they may also be a side-effect of their medications should always be considered (Table 24.1). The drug-induced pain is not of a specific nature and weakness is not a feature. Modest elevation of serum CK may be found and asymptomatic CK elevation may itself be the only sign of myotoxicity in some patients. The EMG is almost always normal. These features are usually reversible once the drug is withdrawn, but muscle discomfort may persist in some cases (e.g., with statins). It should be recognized however that myalgia may also herald the onset of a more severe necrotizing myopathy and acute rhabdomyolysis.
2. *Focal myopathy.* Intramuscular injections cause local muscle damage as a consequence of the needle insertion and the toxic effect of the injected substance. The drugs reported to be associated with focal muscle damage include local anesthetics (lidocaine), diazepam, digoxin, chloroquine, opiates, chlorpromazine, paraldehyde, pentazocine, and other drugs of addiction (if injected repeatedly). Local pain may be the prominent symptom initially, but focal atrophy and replacement of muscle by fibrous tissue may occur at a later stage. Weakness of the affected muscle may be found but more commonly the only sign of muscle damage is an elevated serum CK level.
3. *Painful myopathy.* This is usually an acute or subacute syndrome with myalgia, muscle tenderness, and proximal weakness. Axial muscles may also be involved, but the cranial and respiratory muscles are not usually involved. The tendon reflexes are depressed when the weakness is severe in most of these myopathies; however, in hypokalemic myopathy loss of tendon reflexes may be an early finding. The serum CK is usually markedly elevated and myoglobin may be detected in the urine. The EMG shows typical findings of a myopathy, which may be associated with fibrillation potentials, mimicking the findings in acute myositis. Muscle biopsy shows features of a noninflammatory necrotizing myopathy. This syndrome is usually caused by drugs with direct myotoxic effects (Table 24.2) but may also be seen as a result of drug-induced hypokalemia or in some cases of drug-induced myositis in which the inflammatory changes in the biopsy are absent or inconspicuous.
4. *Acute rhabdomyolysis.* This is the most worrisome, life-threatening myopathic side-effect of medications and represents the most extreme form of acute necrotizing myopathy. It is characterized by an abrupt onset of severe and diffuse myalgia and rapidly evolving flaccid weakness. Muscle swelling, which may even require fasciotomy, is common. Myoglobinuria usually occurs, leading to dark-colored urine ("cola-like" urine) with a positive reaction for "blood" on bedside testing, but without the presence of red blood cells on microscopic examination. Direct measurements of myoglobin, when available, will confirm the finding. Myoglobinuria can lead to acute renal failure with various secondary metabolic impairments, the most alarming of which is a rapid rise in serum potassium level. Emergency dialysis is indicated in such cases, while for most other patients early treatment with fluids and bicarbonate infusions will suffice. The serum CK is markedly elevated and may reach levels of several hundred thousand. The EMG reveals a myopathic pattern with spontaneous activity. Muscle biopsy is not indicated when the offending medication is clearly identified, but when done will show widespread necrosis with, at times, a mild reactive inflammatory response. With prompt treatment recovery usually occurs over a period of weeks.

Table 24.3. Drugs inducing rhabdomyolysis

Statins	Heroin
Fibrates	Cocaine
ε-aminocaproic acid	Amphetamines
Isoniazid	Barbiturates
Amphotericin B	Ethanol abuse

Table 24.4. Malignant hyperthermia

Conditions which increase susceptibility	Ryanodine receptor mutations (dominant inheritance)
	Noonan-like syndrome
	Central core disease
	Myotonia congenital
	Osteogenesis imperfecta
	Duchenne muscular dystrophy(?)
	Myotonic dystrophy(?)
Precipitating drugs	Suxamethonium
	Halothane
	Cyclopropane
	Chloroform
	Methoxyflurane
	Ketamine
	Enflurane
	Ether

Most of the medications that can cause a necrotizing myopathy have the potential to induce acute rhabdomyolysis (see Table 24.3). A special situation exists with the use of drugs of addiction, when crush injury caused by prolonged periods of immobilization may result in rhabdomyolysis. Thus, ethanol abuse is probably the most common cause of nontraumatic rhabdomyolysis [37]. Drug-induced hyperkinetic syndromes (e.g., due to phenylcyclidine use) may also lead to rhabdomyolysis in extreme cases.

5. *Malignant hyperthermia (MH).* This condition is caused by a combination of genetic susceptibility and administration of specific medications, usually during anesthesia (Table 24.4). It is characterized by generalized muscular rigidity, severe hyperpyrexia, marked metabolic acidosis, myoglobinuria, and marked elevation of serum CK activity. If not recognized and treated immediately, MH has a high fatality rate. Malignant hyperthermia should be distinguished from the neuroleptic malignant syndrome, in which an acute extrapyramidal disorder is caused by antipsychotic medications. The latter is a central nervous system (CNS) disorder but many of its features, including rigidity, high fever, and elevated CK, resemble MH.

   Malignant hyperthermia is thought to result from the sudden, drug-induced release of calcium ions into the cytoplasm, leading to sustained activation of the myofibrillar apparatus. Thus the treatment is aimed at blocking calcium release from the sarcoplasmic reticulum, and the drug of choice is dantrolene sodium [38].

   Since this disorder is associated with a genetic tendency [most frequently ryanodine receptor (*RYR1*) mutations, which are also associated with core myopathies], functional testing of muscle samples is available in some laboratories for family members of patients with a history of MH. Muscle is exposed to halothane or to caffeine, and contractions induced by very low levels indicate MH susceptibility. For such persons, specialized protocols of anesthesia are available (see review by Halsall and Robinson [38]).
6. *Painless myopathy.* This is a chronic or subacute condition that may mimic a primary myopathy. In clinical practice it is seen mainly in patients taking glucocorticoids (especially 9α-fluorinated steroids) for prolonged periods, but other drugs such as chloroquine and colchicine may be the cause. Proximal muscles are symmetrically weakened, with the pelvic girdle muscles and the quadriceps being affected initially, and muscle atrophy may ensue. The tendon reflexes may also be depressed in those patients whose myopathy is the result of medications with an associated neuropathic side-effect. With some medications the serum CK levels may be elevated, but not with glucocorticoids.
7. *Myotonia.* While drug-induced myotonia is currently not seen with present-day medications, it was reported in the past with the cholesterol-lowering agent 20,25-diazacholesterol. A number of drugs can however aggravate myotonia in patients with a pre-existing myotonic syndrome or may unmask a subclinical myotonic disorder. The medications to be avoided in patients with myotonia are suxamethonium, propranolol (and other β-adrenergic blockers), furosemide, acetazolamide, and ritodrine.

Steroid myopathy

Muscle weakness and wasting are common complications of prolonged glucocorticoid administration [39], usually with other signs of chronic steroid usage. Weakness is insidious in onset affecting particularly the quadriceps and pelvic girdle musculature. Other proximal muscles may become involved later but the cranial and respiratory muscles are rarely affected. Dysphonia may occur as a result of a localized myopathy of the laryngeal muscles in patients using inhaled corticosteroids.

Serum CK and aldolase levels are normal or reduced. EMG findings are typically those of low-amplitude and short-duration motor unit potentials without spontaneous activity. Histological studies show selective atrophy of type II fibers, in particular type IIB, and increased glycogen in type IIA fibers.

Estimates of the incidence of steroid myopathy associated with daily treatment lasting more than 90 days vary from 2% to 21%. The dose and duration of steroid treatment leading to myopathy vary with the glucocorticoid preparation. Although any glucocorticoid can produce steroid myopathy, the fluorinated steroids (triamcinolone, betamethasone, and dexamethasone) are more likely to produce weakness. With prednisone or prednisolone myopathy is most likely to develop with doses over 40 mg per day but may also occur with prolonged administration of lower doses. Distinguishing between worsening of the condition for which steroids are prescribed, in particular inflammatory myopathies and inflammatory CNS disorders, and steroid myopathy may be difficult. Steroid myopathy takes time to develop; therefore, weakness developing within the first month of steroid treatment is more likely to be due to a flare of the basic condition. Steroid myopathy usually occurs with other stigmata of steroid usage; in their absence weakness is probably not steroid induced.

Corticosteroids cause myopathy by inhibiting mRNA transcription and the synthesis of muscle-specific proteins [40] and also increase protein degradation [41]. The resulting physiological and biochemical disturbances are numerous, affecting glycolytic activity, contractile properties, membrane excitability, and calcium metabolism.

The best way to treat steroid myopathy is to decrease the steroid dosage, but this may not always be possible. Conversion to a non-fluorinated preparation and to alternate-day dosing may reduce the overall side-effects of steroids including the myopathy. Even when steroids are stopped, recovery may be slow particularly in patients with severe weakness. Malnutrition and inactivity worsen steroid myopathy and an adequate protein intake and regular program of exercise are both important to prevent or delay the development of weakness.

Lipid-lowering agent myopathies

Probably all drugs that lower serum cholesterol have a potential for myotoxicity. Clofibrate was originally identified as a cause of necrotizing myopathy and the more modern fibrates also carry a myotoxic hazard as does nicotinic acid. However, the main risk of myotoxicity is with the statin group of drugs, which are now the most widely used lipid-lowering agents. These compounds inhibit the function of a key enzyme in cholesterol biosynthesis, 3-hydroxy-3-methylglutaryl coenzyme A (HMG-CoA) reductase, causing a reduction of not only serum lipid levels but also a number of important intermediaries including ubiquinone (coenzyme Q_{10}). The magnitude of the myotoxic risk, the exact syndromes, and the mechanisms of this side-effect are still controversial [42, 43, 44, 45]. In the early clinical trials of these agents, myotoxicity was reported in only ~0.1% of patients on monotherapy, but it now seems likely that this was an underestimate.

Statin myotoxicity may present in the following ways:

1. Asymptomatic rise of serum CK, which is usually mild to moderate and disappears after withdrawal of the medication. In a subgroup of patients there is an exaggerated CK elevation after exercise [44] and exercise-induced muscle damage. There is debate as to when to stop statins in asymptomatic patients with a recorded CK elevation (whether it is determined to be a change from a pretreatment level or not). It is not recommended to stop statins if the CK level is less than 3–5 times the normal upper limit [46, 47].
2. Myalgia or cramps, usually but not always associated with CK elevation. Most of these patients do not have overt weakness. It is recommended to stop statins in such patients and not to try another medication from this group; however the risk that such patients will develop a more serious complication on re-challenge remains unknown. Both asymptomatic CK elevations and myalgia may persist after withdrawal of statins in some patients [48].
3. Rhabdomyolysis, which may be severe and even fatal. More than 3500 cases have been recorded in which rhabdomyolysis occurred in patients on statins [49] with an estimated death rate of 7.8% [44]. Some statins are more hazardous, as was the case with cerivastatin, which was withdrawn from usage, but all statins have been reported to cause rhabdomyolysis.
4. Inflammatory myopathy (polymyositis or dermatomyositis) has been reported in at least 15 patients on statin treatment [48]. In some of these patients withdrawal of the offending medication led to resolution of the myopathy but most required immunotherapy. The onset of this complication was only after prolonged use of the statins (months or even years) and a possible coincidental disorder cannot be excluded. However, statins are known to possess autoimmune effects [42, 48, 50], including an association with myasthenia, and upregulation of major histocompatibility complex (MHC) class I expression on muscle fibers in patients with persistent myopathic symptoms [48].

Several factors may make the patient more susceptible to statin myotoxicity: high dose, the use of more than one cholesterol-lowering agent, renal insufficiency, obstructive liver disease, and co-administration of drugs that are metabolized by the CYP3A4 isoenzyme of the cytochrome P450 system (Table 24.5). Most currently used statins are metabolized by this system in the liver, and those which are not (e.g., pravastatin) are thought to carry a lower risk, although there is no proof that this is the case for humans.

It is not known whether a relatively high serum CK before commencement of statin therapy carries an increased risk of myotoxicity. Thus, there is a controversy about

Table 24.5. Drugs which Increase the risk of developing statin myotoxicity

Ciclosporin	Macrolide antibiotics
Gemfibrozil	Niacin
Fibrates (others)	Nefazodone
Nicotinic acid	Amiodarone
HIV protease inhibitors	Verapamil
Azole antifungals	

the routine monitoring of serum CK before and during the early statin prescription [42]. We recommend that this should be done in order to avoid unnecessary stoppage of the medication if myalgic complaints appear. Also there is no definite evidence that patients with a pre-existing myopathy are more at risk, despite the suggestion that some patients with statin-induced rhabdomyolysis have an underlying metabolic myopathy [51].

The exact mechanism by which statins produce muscle damage is unknown but several hypotheses have been suggested. The prevailing theory is that all drugs that interfere with cholesterol biosynthesis deplete muscle membranes of some essential lipid components, but there have been several other postulated mechanisms to explain the statin-induced myopathy: mitochondrial dysfunction due to reduced synthesis of ubiquinone, induction of apoptosis, alteration of ionic conduction in membranes, and increased protein catabolism. The use of supplementary ubiquinone (CoQ_{10}) was not proven to be protective [45, 52].

Critical illness myopathy (CIM)

This syndrome of severe skeletal muscle weakness may develop in patients treated in an intensive care unit (ICU), usually with respiratory support, for periods longer than 10 days. Numerous such cases have been reported [53] and the condition has also been referred to as “acute quadriplegic myopathy” (AQM) and “critical illness neuromuscular abnormalities” (CINMA). Its frequency is unknown but it has been suggested that up to 50% of ICU patients with respiratory support, sepsis, and multi-organ failure develop some form of neuromuscular disorder, and about 20% develop a myopathy [53].

The clinical picture is that of severe flaccid weakness of voluntary limb and neck muscles with paralysis of respiratory muscles (mainly the diaphragm), leading to difficulties in weaning patients off the respirator. Facial weakness may infrequently be found. The tendon reflexes are either lost or markedly diminished and typically there is no sensory impairment, although this is difficult to evaluate in sedated patients. A similar syndrome may develop as a result of peripheral nerve disorder (“critical illness neuropathy,” CIN) and both CIM and CIN may co-exist in the same patient.

One of the main controversial points is the contribution of drugs to the development of this condition, especially glucocorticoids and neuromuscular blocking agents of the curariform type, which were initially considered to be the cause. While most reported patients with CIM were being treated with respiratory assistance plus prolonged use of neuromuscular blockers and frequently also corticosteroids [54], in some cases only one or neither of these agents had been used.

The serum CK is usually elevated but not to extreme levels and some patients have normal levels. EMG findings are heterogeneous: a mix of myopathic potentials and “neurogenic features” can be found and even spontaneous activity was recorded. Nerve conduction studies are usually normal but the compound muscle action potentials may be attenuated. The electrophysiological hallmark of CIM is loss of membrane excitability, manifested by a reduced or absent response to direct muscle stimulation in vivo [55]. Muscle biopsy may show either nonspecific changes such as atrophy of both fiber types, angulated fibers, and fiber size variation, or myofiber necrosis and apoptotic changes, but the unique feature found in up to 80% of CIM patients is selective loss of thick (myosin) filaments with preservation of Z-bands [56] on electron microscopy.

The causes of CIM and its pathophysiology are still unclear. Several contributing/risk factors have been identified: older age (although the condition has also been reported in children), protracted ICU course with prolonged inactivity, protein malnutrition, and associated asthma, liver or heart transplantation, marked hyperglycemia, and sepsis. Observations in an animal model have shown that myosin loss only occurs if the muscle is denervated before the administration of corticosteroids [57]. Thus loss of neural activation rather than an effect of neuromuscular blocking agents may be the key factor in the development of this condition. Such animals also show reduced muscle membrane excitability which is due to impaired sodium channel activation [55, 58].

The prognosis of CIM is usually relatively good and most patients who survive the intensive care treatment make a gradual functional recovery over a period of several months, although there may be residual symptoms in some cases.

Mitochondrial myopathy

Several medications, including statins, can produce a myopathy by compromising mitochondrial function, but few cause a histologically confirmed mitochondrial myopathy. The best characterized is zidovudine (AZT), which causes a progressive, painful proximal myopathy, often exacerbated by exercise, which is thought to be dose-related [59]. Symptoms of weakness and fatigue may start within a few months of commencing the medication. The serum CK is normal or only mildly increased. Electromyography may show fibrillations and positive waves as well as myopathic changes in the proximal limb muscles. A clear distinction between AZT myopathy and HIV myositis is sometimes difficult to make. Ragged-red fibers are found, but inflammatory infiltrates are usually absent in AZT myopathy. The myopathy is due to inhibition of mtDNA replication resulting in its depletion.

Germanium, an antineoplastic agent and constituent of some health supplements, affects mitochondria in many organ systems, often leading to renal failure and anemia. It can also cause a myopathy with ragged-red fibers and vacuolization of muscle fibers. Mitochondria contain dense granules on electron microscopy.

Drug-induced autophagic myopathies

Several drugs that share amphiphilic cationic properties [60] impair lysosomal metabolism and can cause a myopathy with autophagic degeneration of muscle fibers. These include the antimalarials chloroquine and hydroxychloroquine as well as the less frequently used agents perhexiline and amiodarone [34]. Autophagic vacuoles are also found in the muscles of patients who develop myopathy with vincristine or colchicine treatment. Both these agents interfere with tubulin polymerization and more commonly cause a peripheral neuropathy. Perhexiline and amiodarone are also capable of causing a neuropathy which is demyelinating in nature, whereas chloroquine may cause a mild axonal neuropathy. Thus the clinical syndrome of neuromuscular toxicity with all these agents is that of neuromyopathy with painless muscle weakness and wasting, loss of tendon reflexes, and variable sensory findings. Serum CK levels are variable but may be elevated especially with colchicine. Electrophysiological studies demonstrate impaired nerve conduction in addition to mixed myopathic and neurogenic EMG changes. The number of vacuolated fibers may be prominent, especially with chloroquine, affecting both fiber types. The myopathy slowly reverses after discontinuation of the medications usually over a period of a few months.

Hypokalemic myopathies

Drugs that cause chronic hypokalemia may induce muscle damage [61]. The most common agents are diuretics and laxatives when used therapeutically or abused. The antifungal drug amphotericin B produces potassium depletion as part of its renal toxicity. Liquorice (licorice), which contains glycyrrhizic acid, and carbenoxolone, a drug for peptic ulcer disease that contains the related compound glycyrrhetinic acid (enoxolone), have an aldosterone-like effect that induces potassium loss. Toluene and lithium may also induce potassium depletion.

With all the above medications, the myopathy may be associated with loss of tendon reflexes, and in some cases myalgia and profound muscle weakness are observed. The serum CK is markedly elevated and even rhabdomyolysis episodes were reported. Histology shows a vacuolar myopathy sometimes associated with necrosis and regeneration [34].

Drug-induced inflammatory myopathies

There are four forms of inflammatory myopathy that have been attributed to medications: polymyositis, dermatomyositis, macrophagic myofasciitis, and the eosinophilia-myalgia syndrome. One of the major problems in evaluating the reported cases of these complications is that the term "myositis" is sometimes used loosely in patients with subacute muscle weakness and high CK levels, and is not always supported by the histological changes in muscle. This is especially noted with some cases of statin-induced myositis and polymyositis reported in association with proton pump inhibitors [47, 62]. Yet, several agents are recognized to cause inflammatory muscle disease that is very similar to idiopathic polymyositis Some such as D-penicillamine [63] and interferon [64] do so by inducing an immune response. In others, a toxic pathophysiology for the inflammatory response is likely: due to a chemical contaminant in the case of L-tryptophan-induced eosinophilic myositis [65]; and aluminum in the vaccination-related macrophagic myofasciitis [66]. Dermatomyositis is more clearly accepted as an aberrant immune-mediated disorder but it is probably the rarest form of drug-induced inflammatory myopathy [67].

In all the above conditions the subacute development of myalgia, muscle weakness, high CK, and markers of inflammation and autoimmunity can be found in association with inflammatory infiltrates in muscle and in the surrounding connective tissues. Treatment with glucocorticoids is sometimes necessary when the withdrawal of the offending medication does not lead to recovery.

Alcoholic myopathies

Acute and possibly chronic forms of alcoholic myopathy exist [37]. Excessive ingestion of alcohol may result in acute necrotizing myopathy characterized by rapid onset of severe muscle pain, cramps, weakness, swelling, and tenderness, which may be generalized or focal. The severity of the clinical picture is variable depending on the amounts of the binge drinking. Histological changes include myofiber necrosis, loss of oxidative enzyme activity, and mild mononuclear infiltrates. Recovery time depends on the severity of muscle destruction and may take several months [34].

The existence of an isolated chronic alcoholic myopathy is more controversial. The insidious onset of painless weakness and wasting affecting mainly the limb-girdle muscles is observed in chronic alcoholics, but may be attributed to peripheral neuropathy. The serum CK levels are usually normal and muscle histology shows mainly type II fiber atrophy. Abstinence may lead to gradual improvement of both the clinical symptoms and the histological changes.

Chronic alcoholism may also induce a hypokalemic myopathy [68], especially when there is associated hypomagnesemia. Weakness, hypotonia, and depressed deep tendon reflexes occur and this may progress rapidly to flaccid paralysis with

Table 24.6. Drug-induced myasthenia in humans: clinical presentations and mechanisms

Drug	Clinical presentations					Mechanism[a]
	Rapid myasthenia	Slow myasthenia	Unmasking of myasthenia	Aggravation of myasthenia	Postoperative respiratory depression	
Antibiotics and antimicrobials						
Neomycin	+				+	Combined
Kanamycin	+			+?	+	Presynaptic
Streptomycin	+	+		+	+	Combined
Gentamicin	+			+		Presynaptic
Tobramycin					+	Presynaptic
Amikacin					+	Presynaptic
Polymyxin B (polymixin B)	+				+	Combined
Colistin	+			+	+	Combined
Tetracyclines				+		Postsynaptic
Lincomycin					+	Combined
Clindamycin					+	Combined
Erythromycin				+		Presynaptic?
Ampicillin			+			Unknown
Imipenem				+		Unknown
Clarithromycin	+?					Unknown
Bretylium	+					Postsynaptic
Emetine	+					Unknown
Ciprofloxacin			+	+		Unknown
Cardiovascular drugs						
β-blockers	+		+			Combined
Quinidine			+	+	+	Presynaptic
Procainamide	+	+		+		Combined
Verapamil	+			+		Combined
Trimetaphan	+				+	Unknown
Statins		+		+		Immune
Central nervous system drugs						
Phenytoin (diphenylhydantoin)	+	+	+			Combined
Trimethadione		+				Immune?
Lithium			+		+	Presynaptic?
Chlorpromazine				+		Combined
Benzhexol (trihexyphenidyl)	+					Unknown
Gabapentin			+	+		Unknown

Table 24.6. *(cont.)*

Drug	Clinical presentations					Mechanism[a]
	Rapid myasthenia	Slow myasthenia	Unmasking of myasthenia	Aggravation of myasthenia	Postoperative respiratory depression	
Antirheumatic agents						
D-Penicillamine	+	+			+	Immune
Chloroquine	+	+			+	Combined
Prednisone				+		Postsynaptic
Other drugs						
Procaine/lignocaine (lidocaine)	+?					Presynaptic
D, L-Carnitine		+				Unknown
Lactate				+		Presynaptic
Methoxyflurane	+					Unknown
Magnesium	+			+		Presynaptic
Contrast agents				+		Unknown
Citrate anticoagulation				+		Presynaptic?
Aprotinin				+		Unknown
Ritonavir			+?			Unknown
Levonorgestrel			+			Unknown
Desferrioxamine (desferrioxamine)			+?			Unknown
Interferons-α and -β		+		+		Immune
Pyrantel pamoate			+	+		Unknown

Note: [a]Neuromuscular junction affected pre- or postsynaptically or as a combination of both. ? Indicates a clear mechanism has not been established.

elevation of the serum CK level. Strength improves with potassium and magnesium replacement.

Drug-induced myasthenic syndromes

A substantial number of drugs and other therapeutic agents may interfere with neuromuscular junction transmission (NMT), producing various clinical disorders. These agents may either augment a transmission defect in patients with a pre-existing myasthenic disorder or interact with other drugs to produce NMT block, and may even produce a myasthenic syndrome de novo.

Clinical presentations

1. *Rapid-onset drug-induced myasthenia.* The development, within days, of myasthenic features in an apparently normal person should always be suspected as being drug-related. When the symptoms and signs develop shortly after starting a new medication, correct diagnosis is relatively easy. Most commonly affected are the respiratory muscles, with the dramatic onset of respiratory failure, or the extraocular muscles, with the appearance of ptosis and double vision. Rapid resolution of these signs after drug withdrawal is considered proof that the myasthenia was drug-induced. A number of drugs have been implicated in causing such a syndrome (Table 24.6), usually through a combination of their strong NMT blocking effects and an underlying subclinical neuromuscular junction defect.
2. *Slow-onset drug-induced myasthenia.* The gradual evolution of myasthenia over a period of weeks to months has been linked to a number of drugs (Table 24.6). The clinical syndrome is very similar to idiopathic myasthenia gravis (MG) and may be accompanied by a similar immune response. The major difference is that upon withdrawal of

the offending medication gradual recovery is observed in the drug-induced disorder. Full recovery after drug withdrawal, however, does not occur in all patients and MG may persist, with a need for immunosuppressive therapy. The causal role of the drug in this situation can only be confirmed retrospectively when full recovery occurs and there is no recurrence during a prolonged period of follow-up.

3. *Unmasking myasthenia gravis.* Previously undeclared MG that first manifests after exposure to a drug and persists even after the medication is withdrawn is the feature of this group. Typically, a drug with NMT-blocking properties is administered to a "healthy" subject and a myasthenic syndrome appears within a short time (usually days but sometimes a few weeks). Withdrawal of the drug does not affect the overall clinical course, although transient improvement can be observed. In many of these patients, typical immunological features of MG are already present at diagnosis.
4. *Aggravated myasthenia gravis.* Aggravated MG is by now probably the most common presentation of drug-induced NMT impairment, and many drugs have been implicated (Table 24.6). When a patient with relatively mild or well-controlled MG is given a drug and worsening of symptoms occurs, recognition of the drug's contribution is straightforward. However, when the drug is given for a disease that itself is detrimental to MG (e.g., antibiotics for infection) its additional harmful effects may be overlooked. Knowledge of the possible harmful effects of a drug is essential for the management of patients with MG, but the use of such a drug is not necessarily an absolute contraindication if it is indicated and is the most appropriate drug to use.
5. *Postoperative respiratory depression.* Delayed recovery of muscle function, especially that of the respiratory muscles, after anesthesia can have many causes, such as erroneous overdosage, pseudocholinesterase deficiency with depolarizing muscle relaxant usage, and drug-induced impairment of NMT in patients with previously undetected MG or myasthenic syndrome. In many instances, the offending drug augments the function of NMT blockers traditionally used for muscle relaxation. In other cases, the patients may be unduly susceptible to the neuromuscular-blocking activity of a drug. Patients with other diseases that reduce the safety factor for NMT, such as poliomyelitis, rapidly progressive amyotrophic lateral sclerosis, polymyositis, and hypocalcemia, should be closely monitored for similar post-anesthetic complications.

Identification

Recognition of one of the above-mentioned clinical syndromes is the first and essential part in identifying a possible hazardous drug for myasthenic patients. In drugs with strong neuromuscular-blocking activity (e.g., the aminoglycoside antibiotics) and relatively frequent use in MG, the deleterious effects become easily apparent. Drugs with weaker effects or infrequent use in MG are identified through rare single case reports (Table 24.6). This poses a problem because it is not always clear from such reports that the drug is the sole causative factor. A possible method for determining that a certain drug is hazardous, especially one rarely used in MG, is to re-challenge with the medication. However, this is potentially dangerous and raises ethical considerations. The traditional step in identifying a hazardous drug was to perform in vitro testing. Such experiments are important in elucidating the mechanisms of neuromuscular blockade by a drug but cannot always be used as proof for the drug-induced myasthenic disorder. It is our belief that the experimental autoimmune MG (EAMG) animal model should be used to identify potentially hazardous drugs clearly when only single clinical observations are available. The major disadvantage of EAMG for drug testing is that it is available in only a few laboratories.

Mechanisms

Drug-induced myasthenia results from a direct pharmacological NMT-blocking property of the medication. The site of block may be presynaptic, postsynaptic, or a combination of both actions. NMT block may occur only when the safety factor of the neuromuscular junction is lowered either by another disorder or by the medication itself (e.g., hypocalcemia induced by citrate anticoagulants) or when serum levels of the drug are unduly high (e.g., in renal insufficiency). The mechanism is completely different in immune-mediated drug-induced myasthenia, when a drug induces a disorder similar to idiopathic MG through an effect on immunoregulatory mechanisms (Table 24.6). For detailed discussion of the mechanisms involved the reader is referred to our previous reviews [69, 70].

Management

As in any drug-induced disorder, recognition and withdrawal of the suspected agent are the most important steps in management. A few patients may develop a severe disease that will require immunosuppressive therapy. In acute severe myasthenia, maintenance of respiratory function is essential. Although the pharmacological block resolves within hours to days, shortening the respirator time is a goal. This can be achieved by agents that counteract the neuromuscular block induced by the offending drug. Positive response to edrophonium should be followed by neostigmine (1.0–2.5 mg intramuscular). It should be repeated every 4 h if the edrophonium test remains positive. As combined block is common in drug-induced myasthenia, calcium infusions (1 ampoule of calcium 10% given slowly) should be administered with the acetylcholinesterase inhibitors.

Avoidance of a possible drug complication in myasthenics requires special consideration in two clinical situations: infection and elective operations. Myasthenic patients are prone to infection, mainly respiratory, and it is essential to achieve early control of the infection as it can aggravate the myasthenic condition. However, numerous antibiotics are known to impair NMT. If an ambulatory myasthenic patient needs antibiotics, it is mandatory to choose a "safe" drug. Newer antibiotics that have not passed the time trial in myasthenia should not be regarded as safe even if no reports of drug-induced MG exist. Myasthenic patients may require surgery, and a safe choice of anesthetics is needed. Halothane may still be the best choice. Monitoring of the state of the neuromuscular junction by the "train of four" method has long been practiced by anesthesiologists and is recommended for every patient with MG during surgery and in the early postoperative period. Whenever possible, muscle relaxants should be avoided in myasthenia, especially the curariform agents.

References

1. R. W. Orrell, Endocrine myopathies. In *Handbook of Clinical Neurology*, eds. F. L. Mastaglia, D. Hilton-Jones. (UK: Elsevier, 2007), pp. 343–355.
2. R. F. Duyff, J. Van den Bosch, D. M. Laman, B. J. van Loon, W. H. Linssen, Neuromuscular findings in thyroid dysfunction: a prospective clinical and electrodiagnostic study. *J. Neurol. Neurosurg. Psychiatry* **68**:6 (2000), 750–755.
3. F. L. Mastaglia, V. J. Ojeda, H. B. Sarnat, B. A. Kakulas, Myopathies associated with hypothyroidism: a review based upon 13 cases. *Aust. N. Z. J. Med.* **18**:6 (1988), 799–806.
4. M. G. Madariaga, Polymyositis-like syndrome in hypothyroidism: review of cases reported over the past twenty-five years. *Thyroid* **12**:4 (2002), 331–336.
5. J. Rush, S. Danzi, I. Klein, Role of thyroid disease in the development of statin-induced myopathy. *Endocrinologist* **16** (2006), 279–285.
6. C. M. Wiles, A. Young, D. A. Jones, R. H. Edwards, Muscle relaxation rate, fibre-type composition and energy turnover in hyper- and hypo-thyroid patients. *Clin. Sci. Lond.* **57**:4 (1979), 375–384.
7. K. R. Scott, Z. Simmons, P. J. Boyer, Hypothyroid myopathy with a strikingly elevated serum creatine kinase level. *Muscle Nerve* **26**:1 (2002), 141–144.
8. M. A. Johnson, J. L. Olmo, F. L. Mastaglia, Changes in histochemical profile of rat respiratory muscles in hypo- and hyperthyroidism. *Q. J. Exp. Physiol.* **68**:1 (1983), 1–13.
9. P. J. Shaw, D. Bates, P. Kendall-Taylor, Hyperthyroidism presenting as pyramidal tract disease. *Br. Med. J.* **297**:6660 (1988), 1395–1396.
10. A. F. Dulhunty, The rate of tetanic relaxation is correlated with the density of calcium ATPase in the terminal cisternae of thyrotoxic skeletal muscle. *Pflügers Arch.* **415**:4 (1990), 433–439.
11. A. W. Kung, K. S. Lau, W. M. Cheung, V. Chan, Thyrotoxic periodic paralysis and polymorphisms of sodium-potassium ATPase genes. *Clin. Endocrinol. Oxf.* **64**:2 (2006), 158–161.
12. S. H. Lin, Thyrotoxic periodic paralysis. *Mayo Clin. Proc.* **80**:1 (2005), 99–105.
13. L. Bartalena, W. M. Wiersinga, A. Pinchera, Graves' ophthalmopathy: state of the art and perspectives. *J. Endocrinol. Invest.* **27**:3 (2004), 295–301.
14. A. A. Khaleeli, R. H. Edwards, K. Gohil, *et al.*, Corticosteroid myopathy: a clinical and pathological study. *Clin. Endocrinol. Oxf.* **18**:2 (1983), 155–166.
15. T. Atsumi, S. Ishikawa, T. Miyatake, M. Yoshida, Myopathy and primary aldosteronism: electron microscopic study. *Neurology* **29**:10 (1979), 1348–1353.
16. A. Mier, C. Laroche, J. Wass, M. Green, Respiratory muscle weakness in Addison's disease. *Br. Med. J.* **297**:6646 (1988), 457–458.
17. S. Ljunghall, G. Akerstrom, G. Johansson, Y. Olsson, E. Stalberg, Neuromuscular involvement in primary hyperparathyroidism. *J. Neurol.* **231**:5 (1984), 263–265.
18. S. A. Turken, M. Cafferty, S. J. Silverberg, *et al.*, Neuromuscular involvement in mild, asymptomatic primary hyperparathyroidism. *Am. J. Med.* **87**:5 (1989), 553–557.
19. B. M. Patten, J. P. Bilezikian, L. E. Mallette, A. Prince, W. K. Engel, G. D. Aurbach, Neuromuscular disease in primary hyperparathyroidism. *Ann. Intern. Med.* **80**:2 (1974), 182–193.
20. C. Joborn, J. Rastad, E. Stalberg, G. Akerstrom, S. Ljunghall, Muscle function in patients with primary hyperparathyroidism. *Muscle Nerve* **12**:2 (1989), 87–94.
21. J. A. Russell, Osteomalacic myopathy. *Muscle Nerve* **17**:6 (1994), 578–580.
22. L. E. Mallette, B. M. Patten, W. K. Engel, Neuromuscular disease in secondary hyperparathyroidism. *Ann. Intern. Med.* **82**:4 (1975), 474–483.
23. M. Swash, M. S. Schwartz, M. K. Sargeant, Osteomalacic myopathy: an experimental approach. *Neuropathol. Appl. Neurobiol.* **5**:4 (1979), 295–302.
24. J. J. Pointon, M. J. Francis, R. Smith, Effect of vitamin D deficiency on sarcoplasmic reticulum function and troponin C concentration of rabbit skeletal muscle. *Clin. Sci. Lond.* **57**:3 (1979), 257–263.
25. E. Shane, K. A. McClane, M. R. Olarte, J. P. Bilezikian, Hypoparathyroidism and elevated muscle enzymes. *Neurology* **30**:2 (1980), 192–195.
26. T. Ishikawa, M. Kanayama, T. Oba, T. Horie, Hypocalcemic induced increase in creatine kinase in rats. *Pediatr. Neurol.* **18**:4 (1998), 326–330.
27. A. A. Khaleeli, R. D. Levy, R. H. Edwards, *et al.*, The neuromuscular features of acromegaly: a clinical and pathological study. *J. Neurol. Neurosurg. Psychiatry* **47**:9 (1984), 1009–1015.
28. F. L. Mastaglia, D. D. Barwich, R. Hall, Myopathy in acromegaly. *Lancet* **2**:7679 (1970), 907–909.
29. F. L. Mastaglia, Pathological changes in skeletal muscle in acromegaly. *Acta Neuropathol. Berl.* **24**:4 (1973), 273–286.
30. L. Kiers, Diabetic muscle infarction: magnetic resonance imaging (MRI) avoids the need for biopsy. *Muscle Nerve* **18**:1 (1995), 129–130.
31. F. Mechler, P. R. Fawcett, F. L. Mastaglia, P. Hudgson, Mitochondrial myopathy. *J. Neurol. Sci.* **50**:2 (1981), 191–200.
32. J. Finsterer, Genetic, pathogenetic, and phenotypic implications of the mitochondrial A3243G tRNALeu(UUR) mutation. *Acta. Neurol. Scand.* **116**:1 (2007), 1–14.

33. G. Said, F. Elgrably, C. Lacroix, *et al.*, Painful proximal diabetic neuropathy: inflammatory nerve lesions and spontaneous favorable outcome. *Ann. Neurol.* **41**:6 (1997), 762–770.

34. F. L. Mastaglia, Z. Argov, Toxic and iatrogenic myopathies. In *Handbook of Clinical Neurology: Myopathies*, eds. F. L. Mastaglia, D. Hilton-Jones. (Amsterdam: Elsevier, 2007), pp. 321–341.

35. J. P. Sieb, T. Gillessen, Iatrogenic and toxic myopathies. *Muscle Nerve* **27**:2 (2003), 142–156.

36. R. J. Walsh, A. A. Amato, Toxic myopathies. *Neurol. Clin.* **23**:2 (2005), 397–428.

37. A. Urbano-Marquez, J. Fernandez-Sola, Effects of alcohol on skeletal and cardiac muscle. *Muscle Nerve* **30**:6 (2004), 689–707.

38. P. J. Halsall, R. L. Robinson, Malignant hyperthermia and associated conditions. In *Handbook of Clinical Neurology: Myopathies*, eds. F. L. Mastaglia, Z. Argov. (Amsterdam: Elsevier, 2007), pp. 107–124.

39. A. Anagnos, R. L. Ruff, H. J. Kaminski, Endocrine neuromyopathies. *Neurol. Clin.* **15**:3 (1997), 673–696.

40. S. R. Rannels, D E. Rannels, A E. Pegg, L. S. Jefferson, Glucocorticoid effects on peptide-chain initiation in skeletal muscle and heart. *Am. J. Physiol.* **235**:2 (1978), E134–E139.

41. A. F. Clark, G. N. DeMartino, K. Wildenthal, Effects of glucocorticoid treatment on cardiac protein synthesis and degradation. *Am. J. Physiol.* **250**:6 Pt 1 (1986), C821–C827.

42. L. Christopher-Stine, Statin myopathy: an update. *Curr. Opin. Rheumatol.* **18**:6 (2006), 647–653.

43. R. S. Rosenson, Current overview of statin-induced myopathy. *Am. J. Med* **116**:6 (2004), 408–416.

44. P. D. Thompson, P. Clarkson, R. H. Karas, Statin-associated myopathy. *J. Am. Med. Assoc.* **289**:13 (2003), 1681–1690.

45. M. Ucar, T. Mjorndal, R. Dahlqvist, HMG-CoA reductase inhibitors and myotoxicity. *Drug Saf.* **22**:6 (2000), 441–457.

46. Z. Argov, Drug-induced myopathies. *Curr. Opin. Neurol.* **13**:5 (2000), 541–545.

47. R. C. Pasternak, S. C Smith, Jr., C. N. Bairey-Merz, S. M. Grundy, J. I. Cleeman, C. Lenfant, ACC/AHA/NHLBI clinical advisory on the use and safety of statins. *J. Am. Coll. Cardiol.* **40**:3 (2002), 567–572.

48. M. Needham, V. Fabian, W. Knezevic, P. Panegyres, P. Zilko, F. L. Mastaglia, Progressive myopathy with up-regulation of MHC-I associated with statin therapy. *Neuromuscul. Disord.* **17**:2 (2007), 194–200.

49. M. A. Omar, J. P. Wilson, FDA adverse event reports on statin-associated rhabdomyolysis. *Ann. Pharmacother.* **36**:2 (2002), 288–295.

50. B. Noel, Autoimmune disease and other potential side-effects of statins. *Lancet* **363**:9425 (2004), 2000.

51. G. D. Vladutiu, Z. Simmons, P. J. Isackson, *et al.*, Genetic risk factors associated with lipid-lowering drug-induced myopathies. *Muscle Nerve* **34**:2 (2006), 153–162.

52. L. Marcoff, P. D. Thompson, The role of coenzyme Q10 in statin-associated myopathy: a systematic review. *J. Am. Coll. Cardiol.* **49**:23 (2007), 2231–2237.

53. R. D. Stevens, D. W. Dowdy, R. K. Michaels, P. A. Mendez-Tellez, P. J. Pronovost, D. M. Needham, Neuromuscular dysfunction acquired in critical illness: a systematic review. *Intensive Care Med.* **33**:11 (2007), 1876–1891.

54. D. Lacomis, M. J. Giuliani, A. Van Cott, D. J. Kramer, Acute myopathy of intensive care: clinical, electromyographic, and pathological aspects. *Ann. Neurol.* **40**:4 (1996), 645–654.

55. M. M. Rich, S. J. Bird, E. C. Raps, L. F. McCluskey, J. W. Teener, Direct muscle stimulation in acute quadriplegic myopathy. *Muscle Nerve* **20**:6 (1997), 665–673.

56. D. Lacomis, D. W. Zochodne, S. J. Bird, Critical illness myopathy. *Muscle Nerve* **23**:12 (2000), 1785–1788.

57. R. Massa, S. Carpenter, P. Holland, G. Karpati, Loss and renewal of thick myofilaments in glucocorticoid-treated rat soleus after denervation and reinnervation. *Muscle Nerve* **15**:11 (1992), 1290–1298.

58. M. M. Rich, M. J. Pinter, Sodium channel inactivation in an animal model of acute quadriplegic myopathy. *Ann. Neurol.* **50**:1 (2001), 26–33.

59. M. C. Dalakas, I. Illa, G. H. Pezeshkpour, J. P. Laukaitis, B. Cohen, J. L. Griffin, Mitochondrial myopathy caused by long-term zidovudine therapy. *N. Engl. J. Med.* **322**:16 (1990), 1098–1105.

60. D. Drenckhahn, R. Lullmann-Rauch, Experimental myopathy induced by amphiphilic cationic compounds including several psychotropic drugs. *Neuroscience* **4**:4 (1979), 549–562.

61. K. K. George, R. Pourmand, Toxic myopathies. *Neurol. Clin.* **15**:3 (1997), 711–730.

62. D. W. Clark, J. Strandell, Myopathy including polymyositis: a likely class adverse effect of proton pump inhibitors? *Eur J Clin Pharmacol* **62**:6 (2006), 473–479.

63. G. J. Carroll, R. K. Will, J. B. Peter, M. J. Garlepp, R. L. Dawkins, Penicillamine induced polymyositis and dermatomyositis. *J. Rheumatol.* **14**:5 (1987), 995–1001.

64. K. M. Kalkner, L. Ronnblom, A. K. Parra Karlsson, *et al.*, Antibodies against double-stranded DNA and development of polymyositis during treatment with interferon. *Q. J. Med.* **91**:6 (1998), 393–399.

65. L. D. Kaufman, Neuromuscular manifestations of the L-tryptophan-associated eosinophilia-myalgia syndrome. *Curr. Opin. Rheumatol.* **2**:6 (1990), 896–900.

66. R. K. Gherardi, M. Coquet, P. Cherin, *et al.*, Macrophagic myofasciitis lesions assess long-term persistence of vaccine-derived aluminium hydroxide in muscle. *Brain* **124**:Pt 9 (2001), 1821–1831.

67. C. M. Magro, J. T. Schaefer, J. Waldman, D. Knight, K. Seilstad, D. Hearne, Terbinafine-induced dermatomyositis: a case report and literature review of drug-induced dermatomyositis. *J. Cutan. Pathol.* (2007), DOI: 101111/j.600–0560.

68. J. Finsterer, B. Hess, C. Jarius, C. Stollberger, H. Budka, B. Mamoli, Malnutrition-induced hypokalemic myopathy in chronic alcoholism. *J. Toxicol. Clin. Toxicol.* **36**:4 (1998), 369–373.

69. Z. Argov, F. L. Mastaglia, Drug therapy: disorders of neuromuscular transmission caused by drugs. *N. Engl. J. Med.* **301**:8 (1979), 409–413.

70. Z. Argov, F. L. Mastaglia, Drug-induced neuromuscular disorders in man. In *Disorders of Voluntary Muscle*, eds. J. Walton, G. Karpati, D. Hilton-Jones. (Avon: Churchill-Livingstone, 1994), pp. 989–1029.

Chapter 25

Myofibrillar myopathies

Duygu Selcen

Definition of myofibrillar myopathies

The term myofibrillar myopathies (MFM) was proposed in 1996 as a descriptive term for a group of chronic neuromuscular diseases associated with a common morphological phenotype but diverse molecular etiology [1, 2]. MFM are characterized by a distinct pathological pattern of myofibrillar dissolution associated with accumulation of myofibrillar degradation products and ectopic expression of multiple proteins that include desmin, αB-crystallin, dystrophin, and congophilic amyloid material.

Salient microscopic diagnostic criteria

Routine histochemical studies reveal abnormal fiber regions of irregular shape and size that harbor amorphous, granular or hyaline structures best recognized in trichromatically stained frozen sections, vacuolated muscle fibers with membranous material within or lining the vacuoles, and sharply decreased oxidative enzyme activity in many abnormal fiber regions. The abnormal fibers sometimes contain large and often multiple congophilic inclusions. Immunohistochemical studies indicate ectopic accumulation of multiple proteins in the abnormal fiber regions. Electron microscopy demonstrates disintegration of myofibrils that begins at the Z-disk, accumulation of degraded filamentous material in various patterns, aggregation of membranous organelles and glycogen in spaces vacated by myofibrils, and degradation of dislocated membranous organelles in autophagic vacuoles.

Genotype–phenotype correlations

There is no consistent genotype–phenotype correlation that has been established in MFM patients, except that cataracts were present in affected members of one of the three reported kinships with αB-crystallinopathy [3].

Salient clinical phenotypical features

Although the clinical phenotypes vary, in most MFM patients the disease begins in adult life, evolves slowly, and affects distal as well as proximal muscles. Cardiomyopathy and peripheral neuropathy are present in a subset of MFM patients.

Symptoms elicited at the time of diagnosis consist of slowly progressive weakness, paresthesias, muscle wasting, stiffness, aching or cramps of skeletal muscle, dyspnea, dysphagia, dysarthria, nasal voice, joint contractures, head drop, and palpitations.

In clinically affected patients, the distribution of weakness can be only proximal, only distal, or both proximal and distal. Mild facial weakness can also be present. Conspicuous muscle atrophy, elbow, wrist and hip contractures, and profound distal sensory deficits can accompany the muscle weakness.

Clinical features in the desminopathy subset of myofibrillar myopathy

Mutations in desmin causing MFM were first reported in 1998 by Goldfarb and coworkers [4] and Munoz-Marmol and coworkers [5]. The desminopathy patients reported to date are similar to other MFM patients in terms of distribution of weakness, serum creatine kinase (CK) level, and electromyography (EMG) findings. The age of onset is usually between the second and fourth decades of life, with a wide range between 10 and 61 years of age. The distribution of weakness is distal or both proximal and distal. Muscle atrophy, mild facial weakness, dysphagia, dysarthria, and respiratory insufficiency can occur. The serum CK level is normal or mildly elevated. EMG studies usually show abnormal irritability and myopathic motor unit potentials (MUPs). Cardiomyopathy is a common manifestation. The family history is consistent with dominant inheritance, and rarely with recessive inheritance. Some cases are sporadic [6, 7].

Recently, an autosomal dominant mutation in desmin was identified in a large kinship previously diagnosed as scapuloperoneal syndrome of the Kaeser type [8].

Clinical features in the αB-crystallinopathy subset of myofibrillar myopathy

A mutation in αB-crystallin was detected in 1998 in a previously reported French kinship [3], and in 2 of the 63 MFM

Disorders of Voluntary Muscle, 8th edn., eds. George Karpati, David Hilton-Jones, Kate Bushby and Robert C. Griggs. Published by Cambridge University Press.

patients observed at the Mayo Clinic in 2003 [9]. Affected members of the French family presented in early adult life, had symmetrical proximal and distal muscle weakness and atrophy, respiratory involvement, hypertrophic cardiomyopathy, palato-pharyngeal weakness, and cataracts. The CK was moderately elevated and the EMG showed myopathic MUPs. The two Mayo patients had adult-onset and slowly progressive myopathy and neuropathy. One patient presented with respiratory failure but he also suffered from scleroderma which may have accounted for the restrictive ventilatory defect, but his affected brother who did not have scleroderma also had respiratory muscle involvement. The second patient presented with slowly progressive weakness and occasional muscle cramps in the fifth decade. He later developed mild biatrial enlargement. The serum CK level was normal in one and sixfold higher than the upper limit of normal in the other. EMG studies showed abnormal irritability and myopathic MUPs in both as well as neurogenic changes in the first patient. Both had muscle atrophy and histological evidence of peripheral neuropathy, but did not have cataracts on direct ophthalmoscopy.

Clinical features in the myotilinopathy subset of myofibrillar myopathy

In 2000, a missense mutation in myotilin was detected in a large kinship that had previously been linked to the myotilin locus at 5q31 [10]. In this kinship, proximal leg and arm muscle weakness appeared in the third decade of life. Distal muscle weakness became apparent later in the course of the disease. Tight heel cords and a nasal dysarthric speech were frequently observed. The serum CK level was normal to 15-fold elevated. Some patients had hypoactive tendon reflexes. Two years later, a second kinship with a similar phenotype was found to have a missense mutation in myotilin [11].

Myofibrillar myopathies are characterized by distinct morphological alterations that typically begin at the Z-disk. Because myotilin is a Z-disk component, we searched for mutations in myotilin in the Mayo cohort of patients whose muscle specimens showed MFM pathology. In 2004, we identified four mutations in six unrelated patients with MFM pathology [12], followed later by detection of three other patients with myotilin mutations. The mean age of onset was 60 years. In three patients the weakness was more prominent distally than proximally. Cardiac involvement without signs of coronary artery disease was evident in three. Evidence for peripheral nerve involvement reflected by clinical, EMG, and histological findings, or a combination of these, was apparent in all. Subsequent studies by other investigators identified additional patients with mutations in myotilin. All had progressive weakness of proximal and/or distal limb muscles, and some had dysarthric, nasal speech, hypoactive tendon reflexes, respiratory failure, or cardiomyopathy. Intrafamily phenotypic variability was present in some kinships [13, 14, 15, 16].

Clinical features in the zaspopathy subset of myofibrillar myopathy

Zaspopathy was first described in 2005 by Selcen and Engel [17] in 11 MFM patients who carried heterozygous missense mutations in *ZASP*. The mean age of onset was in the sixth decade. Most patients presented with muscle weakness but one patient whose father had muscle weakness presented with palpitations and mild hyperCKemia. Seven of 11 patients had family histories consistent with autosomal dominant inheritance. The weakness was more prominent distally than proximally in five, and distal only in one. Two patients had only proximal muscle weakness. The three remaining patients had both proximal and distal muscle weakness.

Cardiac involvement without signs of coronary artery disease was present in three patients. In one of these, cardiac symptoms antedated the muscle weakness by 10 years. Peripheral nerve involvement by clinical, EMG, or histologic criteria was present in five patients.

Subsequently, a large kinship, originally described by Markesbery *et al.* [18] as well as five other kinships with distal myopathy and MFM pathology were found to carry one of the previously described mutations in *ZASP* [19].

Clinical features in the filaminopathy subset of myofibrillar myopathy

In 2005, a nonsense mutation in the last exon of filamin C was reported in 17 affected individuals of a large German kinship by Vorgerd and coworkers [20]. Eight examined patients presented between 37 and 57 years of age with slowly progressive weakness of the distal leg muscles. The serum CK level was elevated up to eightfold. Four patients had signs of respiratory insufficiency, one had an incomplete right bundle branch block, and three had a peripheral neuropathy. Three MFM kinships carrying the same mutation were identified in the Mayo MFM cohort (unpublished observations by D. Selcen). The age of onset and the clinical presentation were similar to those reported by Vorgerd and coworkers [20]. In 2007, Kley and coworkers [21] observed two additional families with the same nonsense mutation and with similar clinical and pathological findings.

Diagnostic approaches

The diagnosis of MFM should be considered in any slowly progressive myopathy associated with proximal and distal weakness, mild or no CK elevation, neuropathy, cardiomyopathy, abnormal electrical irritability on EMG (which can include myotonic discharges), and dominant inheritance. However, not all these features are present in all patients, and other disorders can mimic some or all features of MFM.

Muscle pathology

The diagnosis of MFM in a generic sense is established by muscle biopsy. In trichrome-stained sections, the abnormal fibers harbor an admixture of amorphous, granular, and hyaline deposits that vary in shape and size, and are dark blue or blue red in color (Figure 25.1a, d, and g). Many abnormal fiber regions, and especially the hyaline structures, are devoid of oxidative enzyme activity (Figure 25.1h). Some hyaline structures are intensely congophilic (Figure 25.1k). Some muscle fibers harbor small vacuoles containing membranous material.

Signs of denervation, consisting of groups of atrophic fibers composed of fibers of either histochemical type and increased reactivity of atrophic fibers for nonspecific esterase (Figure 25.1l), are observed in some patients. Abnormal and ectopic accumulation of multiple proteins including myotilin (Figure 25.1b), αB-crystallin (Figure 25.1f), dystrophin (Figure 25.1j), sarcoglycans, neural cell adhesion molecule (NCAM), desmin (Figure 25.1e), plectin, gelsolin (Figure 25.1i), ubiquitin (Figure 25.1c), and filamin C are present [7, 12, 13, 17, 20]. In addition, abnormal accumulation of phospho-tau, actin, amyloid βA4, clusterin [13], a mutant nonfunctional ubiquitin, p62, a multimeric signal protein [22] as well as glycoxidation and lipoxidation markers and neuronal, inducible, and endothelial nitric oxide synthases, and superoxide dismutase have been observed in myotilinopathy and desminopathy muscle specimens [23]. Recently, the aberrant increase of neuron-related proteins such as ubiquitin C-terminal hydrolase L1, synaptosomal-associated protein 25, synaptophysin, and α-internexin were observed in myotilinopathy muscle specimens. This was attributed to decreased activity of the neuron-restrictive silencer factor (NRSF)/RE1 silencing transcription factor (REST) [24].

The muscle biopsy findings in MFM patients are generally similar with the following exceptions. With mutations in desmin or αB-crystallin, the pathological alterations tend to be less severe and more monotonous, the congophilic deposits are less numerous and less intensely fluorescent, and ubiquitin expression is not enhanced, but the ectopic expression of dystrophin is more intense than in other types of MFM.

Electron microscopy reveals that the earliest pathological alterations in MFM characteristically occur at the Z-disk (Figure 25.2). These changes consist of streaks of dense material emanating from the Z-disks (arrows in Figure 25.3b) or of less-dense material dappled with spots of denser material (asterisks in Figure 25.3a and b). In fiber regions in which the Z-disks have disintegrated, the sarcomeres and myofibrils are no longer recognizable, and dislocated membranous organelles and glycogen accumulate in clusters in spaces vacated by disintegrating myofibrils (Figure 25.4). At a still more advanced stage, large fiber regions harbor fragmented filaments and Z-disk remnants that aggregate into pleomorphic inclusions. In other fiber regions, the degraded and fragmented filaments accumulate in hyaline structures composed of compacted fragmented filaments of variable electron density and entrained glycogen granules (Figure 25.5a and b). The dislocated membranous organelles are trapped and degraded in autophagic vacuoles that can undergo exocytosis (Figure 25.6).

Mutation analysis

Mutations in desmin, αB-crystallin, myotilin, Zasp, and filamin C are currently recognized causes of MFM.

Desmin is encoded by a single gene, *DES*, located at 2q35. Since 1998, no fewer than 25 mutations have been identified in desmin [6]. Most mutations are autosomal dominant or sporadic heterozygous missense amino acid changes, but small in-frame amino acid deletions, splice donor- or acceptor-site mutations, and one frameshift mutation have also been reported [4, 6]. A homozygous in-frame deletion of seven amino acids caused a severe phenotype with inability to form desmin filaments in vitro [5].

In 1998, Vicart and coworkers [3] identified a heterozygous missense mutation (R120G) in αB-crystallin, encoded by *CRYAB* on chromosome 11q22.3, in the kinship described in 1978 by Fardeau and associates [25]. Subsequently, Selcen and Engel [9] found two truncation mutations in *CRYAB* in two patients. The first mutation was 464delCT that generates eight missense codons followed by a stop codon and predicts a C-terminal-truncated protein consisting of 162 instead of 175 residues. The second mutation was a C-to-T transition at position 451 (451C > T) that generates a stop codon (Q151X) and predicts a protein consisting of 150 residues. Thus both mutations remove a significant segment of the flexible C-terminal extension of αB-crystallin essential for the solubilization and chaperone function of the protein [26, 27].

In 2000, a Thr57Ile mutation in myotilin was detected in a large kinship [10]. Two years later, a second kinship with a similar phenotype was found to have a Ser55Phe mutation in myotilin [11]. In 2004, four myotilin mutations were found in six unrelated patients in the Mayo MFM cohort [12] followed by detection of two other patients with previously identified myotilin mutations. Subsequently, other investigators identified additional MFM patients with mutations in myotilin, including members of a kinship originally described under the rubric of "spheroid body myopathy" [13, 14, 15, 16]. All myotilin mutations reported to date are heterozygous missense amino acid changes, and all but one mutation fall in *MYOT* exon 2 [10, 11, 12, 13, 14, 15, 28].

Zaspopathy resulting in MFM was first described in 11 MFM patients who carried heterozygous missense mutations in *ZASP* [17]: Ala147Thr and Ala165Val in exon 6, and Arg268Cys in exon 9. The Ala165Val mutation is within, and the A147Thr mutation is immediately before, the ZM motif needed for interaction with α-actinin [29]. Subsequently, a large kinship, originally described by Markesbery *et al.* [18], as well as five other kinships with distal myopathy and MFM pathology were found to carry the same Ala165Val mutation in *ZASP*. These six kinships and three of the zaspopathy kinships observed at the Mayo Clinic may have a common founder [19].

In 2005, a dominant Trp2710X mutation was detected in the last exon of filamin C in a large German kinship [20]. Recently, two additional families with the same nonsense

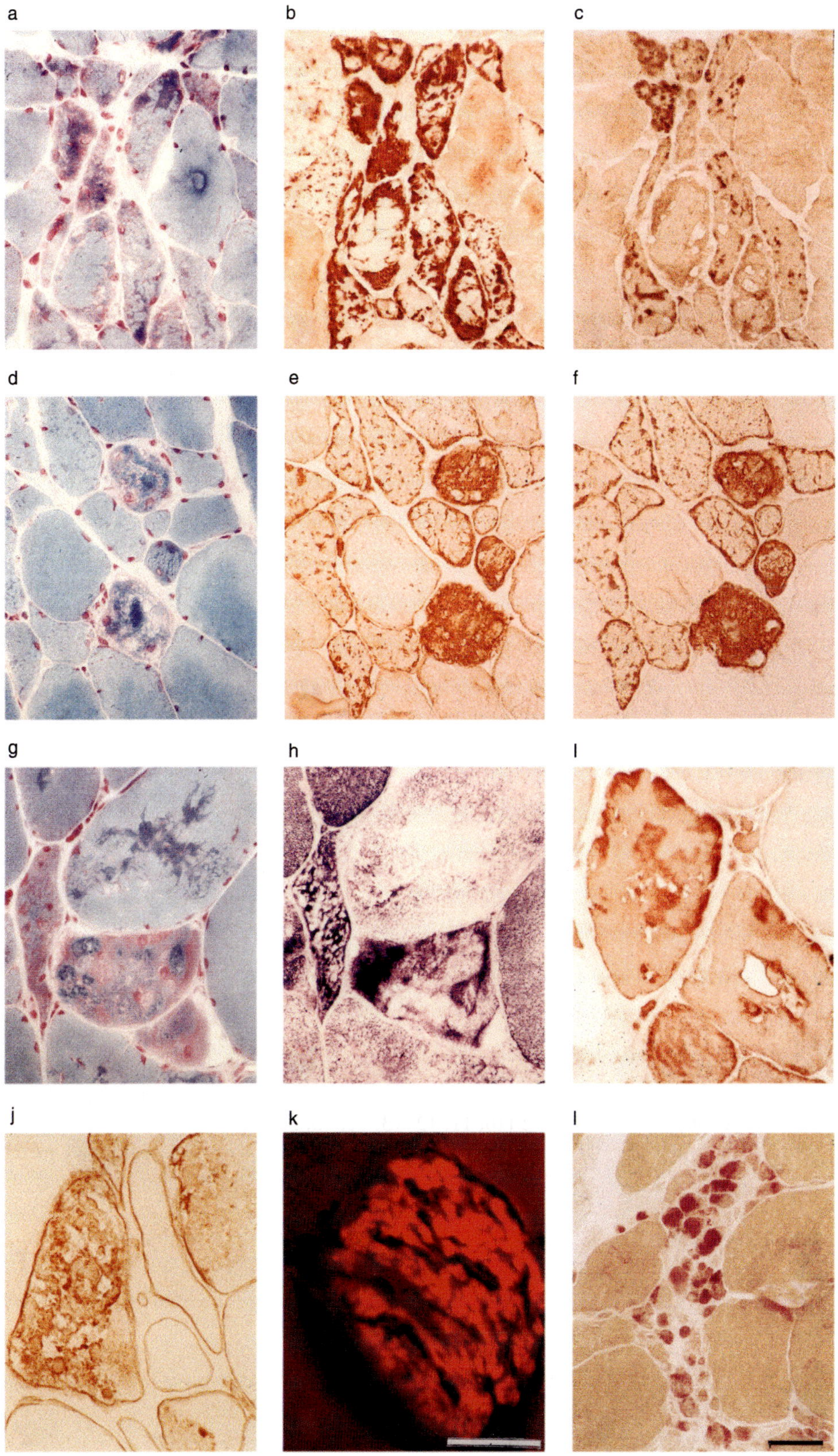

Figure 25.1a–l. Histochemical and immunocytochemical features of a myotilinopathy specimen. Note accumulation of myotilin (b), ubiquitin (c), desmin (e), αB-crystallin (f), gelsolin (i), and dystrophin (j), and sharply circumscribed decreases of NADH dehydrogenase enzyme activity (h) in fiber regions that appear abnormal in serial trichrome sections (a, d, and g). Serial sections for gelsolin (i) and dystrophin (j) are not shown. Intensely fluorescent congophilic deposits are associated with many hyaline deposits (k). Grouped atrophic fibers have increased reactivity for nonspecific esterase (l). Bar in l (also applies to a–j) and in k = 50 μm. (From [12], with permission.)

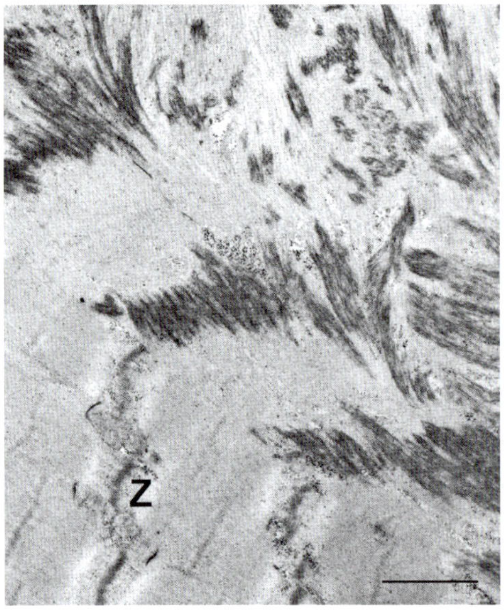

Figure 25.2. Normal Z-disks are replaced by stripes of dense material. The myofibrils are out of register. Z, Z-disk. Bar = 1 µm. (From [6], with permission.)

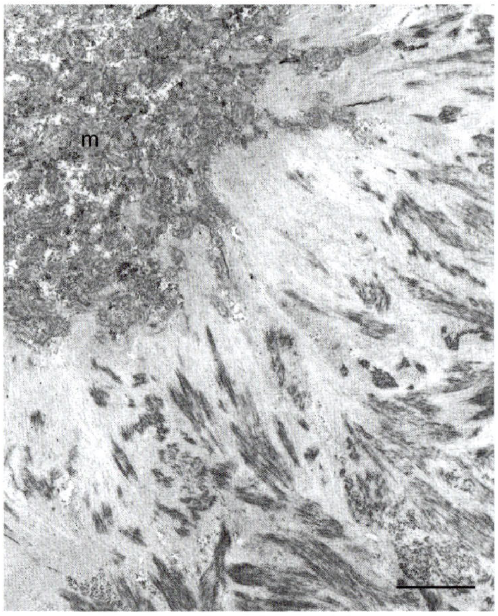

Figure 25.4. Abnormal fiber region harbors material that had emanated from Z-disks and a cluster of dislocated mitochondria (m). Bar = 1 µm. (From [17], with permission.)

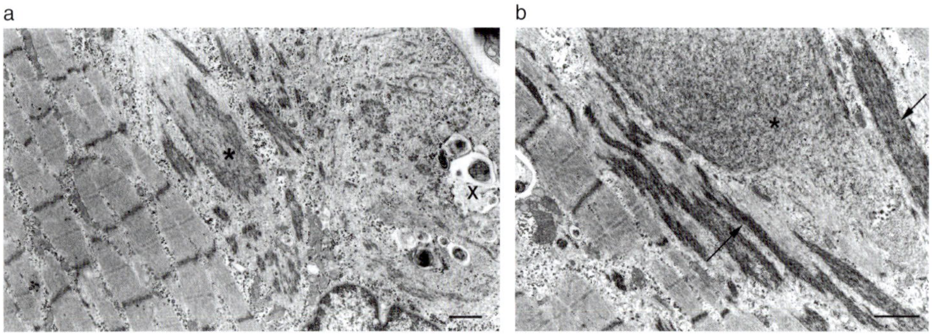

Figure 25.3a, b. Streaks of dense material (arrows in b) and less-dense material are interspersed with dappled small spots of dense material (asterisks in a and b) of Z-disk origin. Degraded material is accumulating in small autophagic vacuoles (X in a). Bars = 1 µm. (From [12], with permission.)

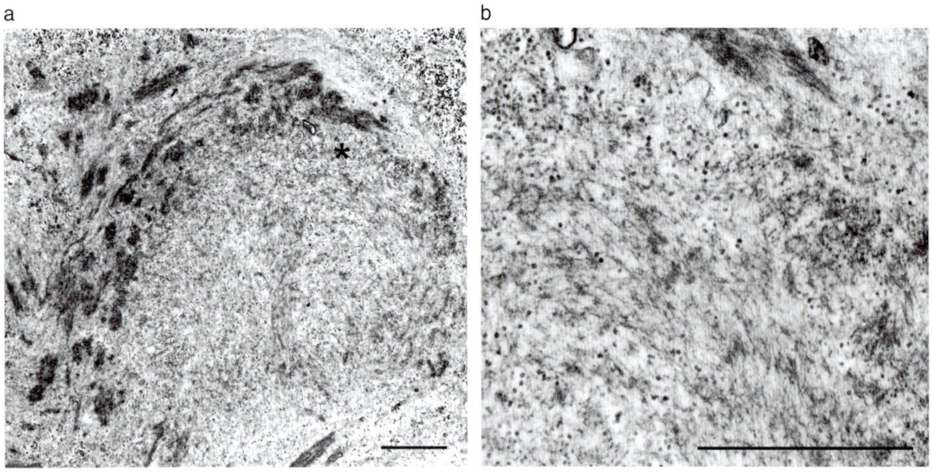

Figure 25.5a, b. (a) Large hyaline structures observed by light microscopy consist of compacted and fragmented filaments of variable electron density. (b) A higher magnification of region marked by asterisk in (a) resolves filamentous profiles. Bar = 1 µm. (From [12], with permission.)

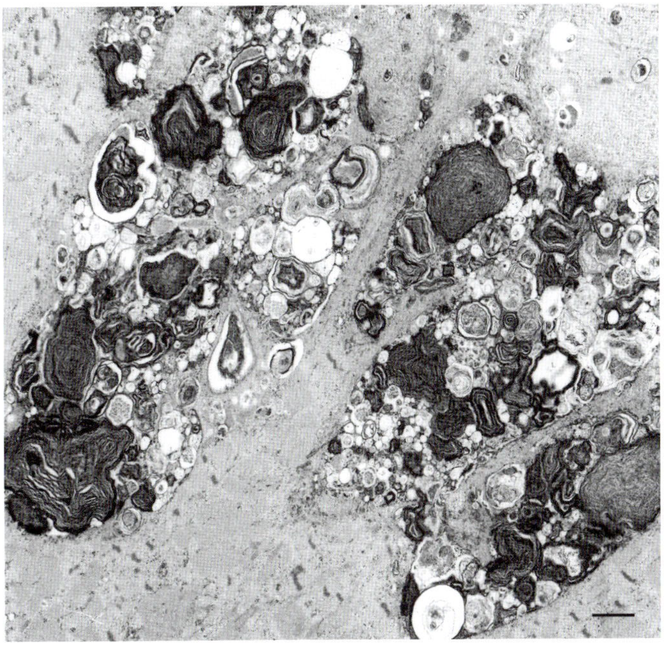

Figure 25.6. Large autophagic vacuoles harbor myeloid structures and debris. Bar = 1 μm. (From [6], with permission.)

mutation in filamin C were reported. These three German families may have a common founder [21].

Muscle imaging

Recently, several investigators performed muscle imaging studies in MFM patients (see Table 25.1) [8, 13, 14, 16, 19, 30, 31, 32]. There is a significant overlap between the magnetic resonance imaging (MRI) findings in the different diseases. Moreover, the MRI findings are a snapshot in time and depend on the stage of the disease. In a recent report by Fischer and coworkers [32] patients with desminopathy and the single patient with an αB-crystallin mutation had no MRI evidence for quadriceps involvement but our four desminopathy and two αB-crystallinopathy patients exhibited mild to moderate quadriceps muscle weakness and atrophy on clinical examination. Hence, we should be cautious in using MRI to diagnose MFM, or a specific type of MFM, unless data accumulate on many more patients in different stages of their disease as well as in disease controls

Therapeutic and preventative approaches

No known measures mitigate the slow but relentless progression of MFM. Corticosteroids have not been shown to be of benefit. Physical therapy, consisting of passive exercises, orthoses, and other supporting devices, is helpful in the more advanced cases. Respiratory support consisting of continuous (CPAP)

Table 25.1. Muscle imaging in myofibrillar myopathy (MFM)

Muscles	Desminopathy [8, 30, 32]	αB-Crystallinopathy [32]	Myotilinopathy [13, 14, 16, 31, 32]	Zaspopathy [19, 32]	Filaminopathy [32]
Gluteus maximus	+	+	+	+	
Sartorius	+	+	+		
Gracilis	+	+			
Iliopsoas	+				
Rectus femoris					
Vastus intermedius			+	+	+
Vastus medialis			+	+	+
Vastus lateralis			+	+	
Adductor magnus	+		+	+	+
Semimembranosus	+		+	+	+
Semitendinosus	+	+	+		
Biceps femoris	+		+	+	+
Soleus	+		+	+	+
Peroneal	+	+		+	
Medial gastrocnemius	+		+	+	+
Tibialis anterior	+		+	+	

or bilevel (BIPAP) positive airway pressure ventilation, initially at night and later in the daytime, are indicated in patients with respiratory failure and signs of hypercapnia.

Periodic monitoring for the appearance of cardiomyopathy should be done in all patients and pacemaker and an implantable cardioverter defibrillator (ICD) should be considered in individuals with arrhythmia and/or cardiac conduction defects. Patients with progressive or life-threatening cardiomyopathy are candidates for cardiac transplantation.

Genetic counseling

Most MFM cases are sporadic; when a reliable family history can be obtained, it is usually of dominant inheritance. Rare cases have been reported to have autosomal recessive or X-linked inheritance. Obtaining a reliable family history is difficult because of the late onset of the disease, death of the parent before the onset of the symptoms, or failure to recognize the disorder in family members.

Future directions

We must better understand the pathophysiology of this emerging group of dominant diseases. We need to identify the signaling mechanisms between the Z-disk and the nucleus, and investigate the abnormal nuclear transcription of multiple proteins when the Z-disk begins to fail. We should also continue to search for mutations in other genes, because identifying the underlying gene defect is the first step toward developing an effective therapy.

References

1. S. Nakano, A. G. Engel, A. J. Waclawik, A. M. Emslie-Smith, N. A. Busis, Myofibrillar myopathy with abnormal foci of desmin positivity. I. Light and electron microscopy analysis of 10 cases. *J. Neuropathol. Exp. Neurol.* **55** (1996), 549–562.
2. J. L. De Bleecker, A. G. Engel, B. B. Ertl, Myofibrillar myopathy with abnormal foci of desmin positivity. II. Immunocytochemical analysis reveals accumulation of multiple other proteins. *J. Neuropathol. Exp. Neurol.* **55** (1996), 563–577.
3. P. Vicart, A. Caron, P. Guicheney, *et al.*, A missense mutation in the alphaB-crystallin chaperone gene causes a desmin-related myopathy. *Nat. Genet.* **20** (1998), 92–95.
4. L. G. Goldfarb, K. Y. Park, L. Cervenakova, *et al.*, Missense mutations in desmin associated with familial cardiac and skeletal myopathy. *Nat. Genet.* **19** (1998), 402–403.
5. A. M. Munoz-Marmol, G. Strasser, M. Isamat, *et al.*, A dysfunctional desmin mutation in a patient with severe generalized myopathy. *Proc. Natl. Acad. Sci. U. S. A.* **95** (1998), 11312–11317.
6. L. G. Goldfarb, P. Vicart, H. H. Goebel, M. C. Dalakas, Desmin myopathy. *Brain* **127** (2004), 723–734.
7. D. Selcen, K. Ohno, A. G. Engel, Myofibrillar myopathy: clinical, morphological and genetic studies in 63 patients. *Brain* **127** (2004), 439–451.
8. M. C. Walter, P. Reilich, A. Huebner, *et al.*, Scapuloperoneal syndrome type Kaeser and a wide phenotypic spectrum of adult-onset, dominant myopathies are associated with the desmin mutation R350P. *Brain* **130**:Pt 6 (2007), 1485–1496.
9. D. Selcen, A. G. Engel, Myofibrillar myopathy caused by novel dominant negative alpha B-crystallin mutations. *Ann. Neurol.* **54** (2003), 804–810.
10. M. A. Hauser, S. K. Horrigan, P. Salmikangas, *et al.*, Myotilin is mutated in limb girdle muscular dystrophy 1A. *Hum. Mol. Genet.* **9** (2000), 2141–2147.
11. M. A. Hauser, C. B. Conde, V. Kowaljow, *et al.*, Myotilin mutation found in second pedigree with LGMD1A. *Am. J. Hum. Genet.* **71** (2002), 1428–1432.
12. D. Selcen, A. G. Engel, Mutations in myotilin cause myofibrillar myopathy. *Neurology* **62** (2004), 1363–1371.
13. M. Olive, L. G. Goldfarb, A. Shatunov, D. Fischer, I. Ferrer, Myotilinopathy: refining the clinical and myopathological phenotype. *Brain* **128** (2005), 2315–2326.
14. I. Penisson-Besnier, K. Talvinen, C. Dumez, *et al.*, Myotilinopathy in a family with late onset myopathy. *Neuromuscul. Disord.* **16** (2006), 427–431.
15. T. Foroud, N. Pankratz, A. P. Batchman, *et al.* A mutation in myotilin causes spheroid body myopathy. *Neurology* **65** (2005), 1936–1940.
16. J. Berciano, E. Gallardo, R. Dominguez-Perles, *et al.*, Autosomal-dominant distal myopathy with a myotilin S55F mutation: sorting out the phenotype. *J. Neurol. Neurosurg. Psychiatry* **79**:2 (2008), 205–208.
17. D. Selcen, A. G. Engel, Mutations in ZASP define a novel form of muscular dystrophy in humans. *Ann. Neurol.* **57** (2005), 269–276.
18. W. R. Markesbery, R. C. Griggs, R. P. Leach, L. W. Lapham, Late onset hereditary distal myopathy. *Neurology* **24** (1974), 127–134.
19. R. Griggs, A. Vihola, P. Hackman, *et al.*, Zaspopathy in a large classic late-onset distal myopathy family. *Brain* **130** (2007), 1477–1484.
20. M. Vorgerd, P. F. van der Ven, V. Bruchertseifer, *et al.*, A mutation in the dimerization domain of filamin C causes a novel type of autosomal dominant myofibrillar myopathy. *Am. J. Hum. Genet.* **77** (2005), 297–304.
21. R. A. Kley, Y. Hellenbroich, P. F. M. van der Ven, *et al.*, Clinical and morphological phenotype of the filamin myopathy: a study of 31 German patients. *Brain* **130** (2007), 3250–3264.
22. M. Olivé, F. W. van Leeuwen, A. Janue, D. Moreno, B. Torrejon-Escribano, I. Ferrer, Expression of mutant ubiquitin (UBB + 1) and p62 in myotilinopathies and desminopathies. *Neuropathol. Appl. Neurobiol.* **34**:1 (2008), 76–87.
23. A. Janue, M. Olivé, I. Ferrer, Oxidative stress in desminopathies and myotilinopathies: a link between oxidative damage and abnormal protein aggregation. *Brain Pathol.* **17** (2007), 377–388.
24. M. Barrachina, J. Moreno, S. Juves, D. Moreno, M. Olivé, I. Ferrer, Target genes of neuron-restrictive silencer factor are abnormally up-regulated in human myotilinopathy. *Am. J. Pathol.* **171** (2007), 1312–1323.
25. M. Fardeau, J. Godet-Guillain, F. M. Tome, *et al.*, A new familial muscular disorder demonstrated by the intra-sarcoplasmic accumulation of a granulo-filamentous material which is dense on electron microscopy. *Rev. Neurol. (Paris)* **134** (1978), 411–425.

26. R. H. P. H. Smulders, J. A. Carver, R. A. Lindner, M. A. M. van Boekel, H. Bloemendal, W. W. de Jong, Immobilization of the C-terminal extension of bovine alpha A-crystallin reduces chaperone-like activity. *J. Biol. Chem.* **271** (1996), 29060–29066.

27. U. P. Andley, S. Mathur, T. A. Griest, J. M. Petrash, Cloning, expression, and chaperone-like activity of human alpha A-crystallin. *J. Biol. Chem.* **271** (1996), 31973–31980.

28. S. Shalaby, Y. Hayashi, K. Goto, I. Nonaka, S. Noguchi, I. Nishino, A novel myotilin mutation in exon 9: The first LGMD1A identified in Japan. *Neuromuscul. Disord.* **17** (2007), 880.

29. T. Klaavuniemi, A. Kelloniemi, J. Ylanne, The ZASP-like motif in actinin-associated LIM protein is required for interaction with the alpha-actinin rod and for targeting to the muscle Z-line. *J. Biol. Chem.* **279** (2004), 26402–26410.

30. M. Sugawara, K. Kato, M. Komatsu, *et al.*, A novel de novo mutation in the desmin gene causes desmin myopathy with toxic aggregates. *Neurology* **55**:7 (2000), 986–990.

31. D. Fischer, C. S. Clemen, M. Olivé, *et al.*, Different early pathogenesis in myotilinopathy compared to primary desminopathy. *Neuromuscul. Disord.* **16** (2006), 361–367.

32. D. Fischer, R. A. Kley, K. Strach, *et al.*, Muscle imaging differentiates primary desminopathies from myofibrillar myopathies. *Neuromuscul. Disord.* **17** (2007), 879.

Chapter 26

Hereditary inclusion body myopathies

Zohar Argov and Stella Mitrani-Rosenbaum

Entity definition

The hereditary inclusion body myopathies are a group of adult-onset neuromuscular disorders that share the histological and ultrastructural features of cytoplasmic autophagic ("rimmed") vacuoles (Figure 26.1) and inclusions composed of clusters of tubular filaments [1, 2, 3, 4]. They differ from sporadic inclusion body myositis by their Mendelian mode of inheritance and the lack of inflammation (although inflammatory infiltrates have been described in occasional patients, see below), as well as their phenotypic presentation. Several hereditary myopathies with similar histological features are also classified as "distal myopathies," because of their mode of presentation. Thus, the chapter on distal myopathies (Chapter 16) describes conditions that could also be termed hereditary inclusion body myopathies. However, the identification of the gene defect involved in a distinctive and common form of this group, the *GNE*-related myopathy [5], has set the stage for a more useful classification of these conditions. We use the term hereditary inclusion body myopathy (HIBM, in the singular form) only for the worldwide *GNE*-related recessive disorder (IBM2 in the McKusick classification) and will focus on this myopathy. The chapter will, however, summarize other rare hereditary myopathies with rimmed vacuoles.

Diagnostic criteria

Table 26.1 lists the current diagnostic features of HIBM; however, histology is not mandatory in all patients, since with a typical clinical pattern, molecular diagnosis suffices and biopsy can be avoided. Some patients may, however, present with phenotypic variations that require diagnostic biopsy. We do not include the electron microscopy (EM) finding of inclusions as a required diagnostic criterion since muscle EM is infrequently performed, and it is often difficult to detect these inclusions as they are not present in most fibers.

Molecular genetics and pathogenesis

UDP-*N*-acetylglucosamine 2-epimerase/*N*-acetylmannosamine kinase (*GNE*) was first identified as the disease-causing gene in the large Persian Jewish cluster of HIBM, all sharing a single homozygous missense mutation, a T-to-C transition converting methionine to threonine at codon 712 (M712T) [5]. Later, this single homozygous *GNE* mutation was identified in Jewish and non Jewish patients from other Middle Eastern communities [6, 7, 8]. This founder Middle Eastern mutation was also identified in countries outside the Middle East but in a compound heterozygote genotype [9, 10].

Several other mutations in *GNE* were detected in Japanese patients with the disorder first described by Nonaka as distal myopathy with rimmed vacuoles (DMRV) [11, 12, 13, 14, 15, 16, 17], providing final evidence that HIBM and DMRV are the same disease. Interestingly, in most Japanese patients the disease results from the presence of two different *GNE* mutations (compound heterozygosity) and only one or two mutations (V572L, D176V) appear commonly in homozygosity and are thought to be founders [12, 13].

It is now recognized that HIBM is a worldwide disorder and about 50 different *GNE* mutations have been found in families of diverse origins other than Middle Eastern and Japanese, such as Italian, Spanish, Greek, German, Irish, Mexican, Caucasian, and Afro-Americans from the USA, and various Asian countries, mostly with compound heterozygosity genotypes ([5, 7, 9, 18, 19, 20, 21, 22, 23, 24, 25, 26, 27] and unpublished families tested in our laboratory). The majority of the mutations are missense but five mutations resulting in a premature stop codon have been identified [5, 10, 20, 22], but never in a homozygous form.

The product of the *GNE* gene is a 722-amino-acid protein, UDP-*N*-acetylglucosamine 2-epimerase/*N*-acetylmannosamine kinase, which is a bifunctional enzyme: the epimerase domain is located at the N-terminal part of GNE (up to amino acid 378) and the kinase domain at the C-terminus, from amino acid 410 [28, 29]. The mutations related to HIBM are dispersed throughout the gene-coding exons, both in the epimerase- and in the kinase-coding sequences, and several such mutations from both domains are often combined in the compound heterozygous patients (Figure 26.2).

Disorders of Voluntary Muscle, 8th edn., eds. George Karpati, David Hilton-Jones, Kate Bushby and Robert C. Griggs. Published by Cambridge University Press.

Pathogenesis

UDP-*N*-acetylglucosamine 2-epimerase/*N*-acetylmannosamine kinase (GNE) is the key enzyme in the metabolic pathway leading to the synthesis of sialic acid [30]. Sialic acids, the most abundant terminal monosaccharides on glycoconjugates in eukaryotic cells, comprise a family of more than 50 naturally occurring carboxylated amino sugars with a scaffold of nine carbon atoms, which are components of complex *N*-glycans and many *O*-glycans glycoconjugates [31].

The first two steps of this cytosolic pathway are catalyzed by the two distinct functional domains of GNE (Figure 26.3). First, the UDP-GlcNAc 2-epimerase domain synthesizes ManNAc from UDP-GlcNAc, then the ManNAc kinase phosphorylates ManNAc to generate ManNAc 6-phosphate [28, 29]. Three subsequent steps lead to the synthesis of the active form of sialic acid, CMP-sialic acid, which is the donor of sialic acid to the terminal sugar in a glycan chain.

Several different mechanisms regulate GNE, most importantly feedback inhibition of epimerase activity by CMP-sialic acid [32]. Point mutations in the CMP-sialic acid binding site of GNE in humans (at codons 263–266, Figure 26.2) result in disabled feedback inhibition, and lead to the very rare metabolic disease sialuria, characterized by highly abundant production and secretion of sialic acid by the patients [33].

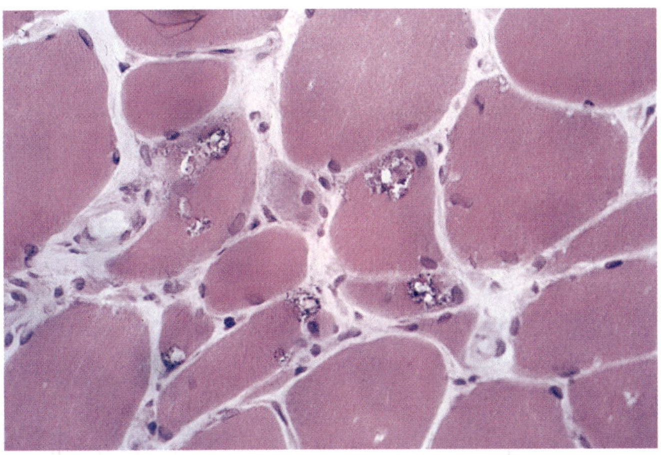

Figure 26.1. The typical vacuoles in an early biopsy of tibialis anterior in hereditary body inclusion myopathies. (H&E stain, D. Soffer with permission.)

To date, in HIBM, no mutation has been detected in these specific codons responding to feedback inhibition but it has not yet been determined if these four codons represent the full extent of this regulatory mechanism in GNE.

GNE is essential for embryonic development: specific knockout inactivation of the gene in mice results in drastic reduction of sialylation of embryonal cells and in embryonal lethality at day E8.5 [34]. These findings could explain why the combination of two nonsense mutations has not been detected in vivo in any HIBM patient, since it leads to total absence of the GNE protein. Marked GNE deficiency has not been observed in HIBM patients; in fact, GNE protein is expressed at equal levels in HIBM patients and normal control subjects [35]. Furthermore, no mislocalization of GNE in skeletal muscle could be documented [35, 36]: the GNE protein is located at the Golgi compartment in a variety of human cells including muscle. This subcellular localization is in good agreement with the established role of GNE as the key enzyme of sialic acid biosynthesis, since the sialylation of glycoconjugates takes place in the Golgi complex.

The first hypothesis considered in HIBM pathogenesis is a change in the sialylation pattern potentially caused by defective GNE activity. However, investigations of the GNE enzymatic functions showed that the extent of the activity reduction in lymphocytes, myoblasts, and myotubes of HIBM patients varied only between 30% and 60% [16, 37, 38], making it difficult to explain how such partial enzymatic activity reduction

Table 26.1. Salient diagnostic criteria of hereditary inclusion body myopathy (HIBM)

1. Isolated skeletal muscle disease
2. Onset in adulthood
3. Distal leg muscle weakness at presentation
4. Quadriceps sparing during progression
5. Presence of "rimmed" vacuoles with few other pathological changes
6. Mild elevation of serum creatine kinase
7. Autosomal recessive inheritance with mutations in the *GNE* gene

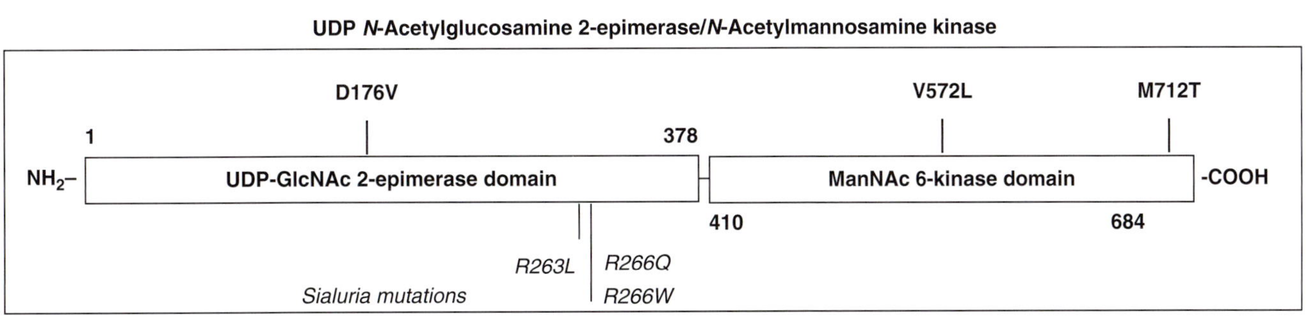

Figure 26.2. Schematic representation of the *GNE* gene and of the currently identified main founder mutations in the Middle East (M712T) and in Japan (D176V and V572L). The site of the sialuria mutations is indicated. The positions of the amino acids defining both enzymatic domains of GNE are indicated.

could lead to markedly reduced sialic acid production. This difficulty arises from the following considerations: firstly, in normal tissue GNE activity exploits only 5% of its potential [39] and theoretically this could be augmented in HIBM by compensatory activation; second, the existence of the feedback process, which enhances sialic acid synthesis when CMP-sialic acid is low, should have operated through the remaining activity of GNE; third, the presence of additional kinases in the cell, such as *N*-acetylglucosamine kinase (NAGK), which are able to use *N*-acetyl mannosamine as a substrate and therefore compensate for the partial defective function of the kinase activity of GNE, at least in HIBM cells carrying the homozygous M712T mutation (the common Middle Eastern mutation).

Analysis of patients' cells [16, 17, 37, 38] revealed a broad range of bound sialic acid levels, overlapping with those of normal controls. These results indicate that, since in most HIBM patients significant reduction in sialylation was not found, this by itself cannot fully explain the cellular impairment. It should be noted that in a few patients, a modest to marked decrease in membrane sialylation did occur. Reports on changes in the α-dystroglycan and NCAM sialylation patterns, as proficient markers of glycosylation defects, are even more controversial as they again show normal results in some HIBM patients and very abnormal findings in others [16, 17, 38, 40, 41]. Furthermore, even when low α-dystroglycan sialylation was reported, it did not seem to have functional consequences for the affected cells, at least in structural terms, since the α-laminin–α-dystroglycan bonds were maintained and sarcolemma integrity preserved. This is in contrast with the scenario observed in alpha dystroglycanopathies where α-dystroglycan hyposialylation results in the loss of α-laminin binding and the disintegration of the sarcolemma [42].

Interestingly, an overall reduction of 25% in membrane-bound sialic acid was observed in various organs of heterozygous GNE knockout mice including abdominal muscle (the only muscle tissue analyzed in these experiments). However, the extent of GNE expression and activity in those mice and tissues was not documented [43]. In spite of these biochemical findings those heterozygous mice appeared healthy and did not develop myopathy, even after 2 years. These findings raise a general question about the regulation of the feedback mechanism which, if working as proposed, should not allow sialic acid to decrease when supposedly 50% of GNE activity remains. Moreover, how a decrease in sialic acid, assuming it takes place in HIBM patients, can account for the disease pathogenesis remains unknown.

Recently a transgenic mouse overexpressing the human GNE D176V mutation, which is one of the most prevalent mutations among Japanese DMRV patients, was crossed with a heterozygous GNE knockout mouse (Gne+/–) to obtain Gne (–/–) transgenic hGNED176V animals [44]. These Gne(–/–) hGNED176V-Tg mice showed hyposialylation in muscle and other organs, similar to the heterozygous GNE knockout mice [43], but in contrast to the latter, which stayed healthy, they exhibited a reduction in muscle performance from 32 weeks of age and HIBM-like muscle pathology after 42 weeks of age. To date, this is the only animal model likely to be useful for future therapeutic trials, although the role of hyposialylation in the pathomechanism of HIBM is not yet resolved.

Various directions have been undertaken to explore other hypotheses, and to try to unravel novel potential functions for GNE, which could lead to better insights into the pathogenesis of HIBM. Among those, satellite cell dysfunction [45], modulatory effects on other biochemical pathways [39], and an undetermined nuclear activity [36] are to be noted. Still, at present there is no consensus explanation for HIBM pathogenesis.

Clinical phenotypic features

The age of onset is typically in the third decade, and although onset before age 20 and after age 45 can occur, this is rare [46, 47, 48, 49, 50]. Weakness at onset is typically in the anterior compartment of the leg leading to bilateral footdrop, but rarely weakness onset may be proximal in the leg without distal weakness [6]. Usually, the iliopsoas is the first and the most affected of the hip muscles with a lesser degree of weakness in the glutei, hamstrings, and adductors as the disorder evolves. The quadriceps muscle remains strong (normal power or minimal reduction) despite the continuous weakening of all other proximal lower limb muscles and this feature is found even in wheelchair-bound or bedridden patients. This unique pattern of quadriceps sparing myopathy (QSM) [46] is observed in the majority of patients with *GNE* defects reported worldwide and facilitates the clinical recognition of this condition. However, in a minority of patients (less than 5%) the quadriceps may also become very weak [47, 51, 52].

The disease progresses slowly to affect the upper limbs, mainly the scapular musculature, but weakening of the distal muscles of the arm and the hand at later stages occurs. Neck flexors may also become affected and mild facial weakness occur [53]. Ankle tendon reflexes may be lost and sensory subjective complaints are sometimes reported, but there are no objective signs of neuropathy. The heart, brain, and other organs are not involved in HIBM.

The rate of progression of HIBM is variable and many patients remain ambulatory even 15 years or more after disease onset. Complete loss of ambulation occurs early however in those rare patients with marked quadriceps involvement. Those patients who reached the seventh and even eighth decade of life were markedly incapacitated, without major respiratory difficulties (and most still had evidence of quadriceps sparing).

Genotype–phenotype correlation

Variable modes of onset and severity as described above and variation in the histological features (e.g., presence of inflammation, see below) are all observed in the Middle Eastern

Jewish cluster of HIBM, and sometimes even in the same large family. They all share not only the same homozygous M712T mutation but a similar founder haplotype of about 700 kb flanking the *GNE* region. Thus, at this stage it is hard to see how potential "modifiers'" could be genetically linked to the *GNE* region. The clinical–histological spectrum is shared by other patients worldwide and no mutational changes have been identified to cause a different disorder. Since currently no homozygous nonsense mutation genotype has been found in any patient we suspect that either this is a lethal situation (as in the animal knockout model) or that it causes a very different condition yet to be identified. It should be noted that in the few patients with mutations in the central part of the *GNE* gene resulting in sialuria no specific myopathy has been described.

Diagnostic approaches

Routine laboratory tests of muscle disease are nondiagnostic. Serum creatine kinase (CK) activity is usually modestly elevated (up to 4 times the upper maximal normal value) but normal levels may be observed initially. Conventional concentric needle electromyography (EMG) frequently shows spontaneous activity in the tibialis anterior, but not in other muscles. The motor units are small and polyphasic in most muscles, but reduced recruitment with prolonged, large and even polyphasic units were also recorded in some affected muscles [46, 48]. Nerve conductions are normal even in those patients with sensory complaints and reduced tendon reflexes.

The typical histopathological features of HIBM are vacuolated myofibers associated with variable (usually mild) neurogenic and myopathic changes [2] (Figure 26.1). The number of vacuolated fibers is extremely variable in affected muscles, and no correlation between either disease severity or progression rate and their number has been reported. The vacuoles may appear to be surrounded by granular eosinophilic material on hematoxylin and eosin staining (hence the term "rimmed" vacuoles) but they are not truly membrane bound and are classified as "autophagic" vacuoles [54]. The "classical" diagnostic feature of HIBM may be found only on EM: the presence of collections of 15- to 21-nm cytoplasmic tubofilamentous inclusions, usually near the vacuoles. Inflammation is not a feature of HIBM and its absence was considered a diagnostic criterion; however, recently patients with genetically confirmed HIBM have been observed to have inflammatory infiltrates in a muscle sample [6, 15, 21]. As mentioned above, the expression level of the GNE protein is not informative, because it is unchanged in patients. Testing for *GNE* mutations is the main diagnostic approach since direct biochemical evaluation and interpretation of GNE activity in muscle (or another tissue) are too complicated. In regions with a high prevalence of a single founder mutation, its direct evaluation will suffice, but in all other circumstances it is necessary to sequence the entire gene.

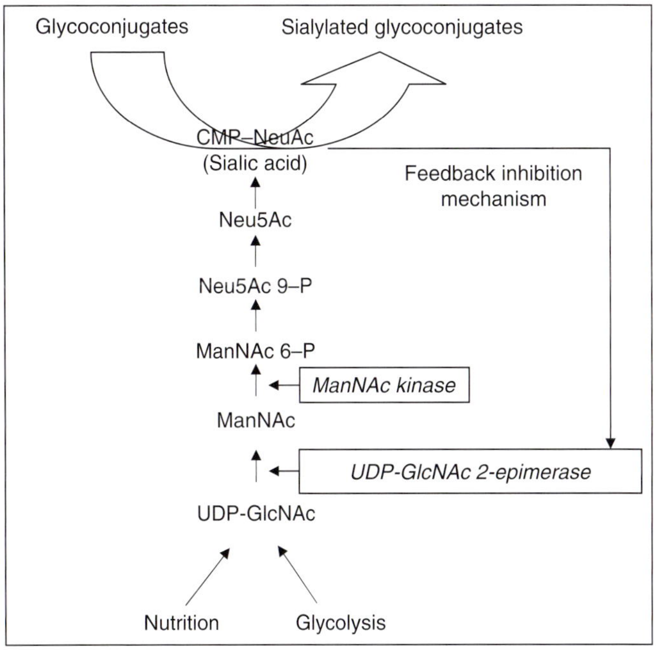

Figure 26.3. The sialic acid biosynthetic pathway.

Therapy

The assumption that reduced sialylation is part of the pathogenesis of HIBM led to a small trial of intravenous immunoglobulin (IVIg) in a small number of patients. IVIg contains high sialic acid levels and it was hypothesized that some form of transfer will occur to the defective muscle cell. This short trial showed mainly a subjective improvement [55]. Another therapeutic hypothesis is that increased supply of ManNAc, a natural precursor of sialic acid (Figure 26.3) will further drive the sialic acid synthesis pathway to compensate for presumed reduction in metabolism. This is based on the finding that sialylation could be restored in cells from a GNE knockout mouse by feeding them with ManNAc [34]. Sialylation in an animal model with *GNE* mutation was also improved by ManNAc [56]. However, this latter model yielded only renal disease and the relevance of this finding to human HIBM disease is unclear. ManNAc has not been tried yet in the recently described transgenic Gne (–/–)hGNED176V-Tg myopathic animal model [44]. Some patients have taken high doses of ManNAc but there is no helpful information on the risks/benefits of this therapy.

Addendum – ManNAC has now been shown to improve function in the transgenic animal model and a human study is planned.

Genetic counseling

Counseling in HIBM is similar to that for other recessively inherited disorders. One should however be aware of the variable severity of the disease even in the same family while trying to predict the outcome of a homozygous or compound heterozygous person. Furthermore, currently there are two known subjects belonging to genetically confirmed HIBM families who are homozygous for *GNE* mutations but show no signs of myopathy at their late 60 s [6, 13].

Future perspectives

Although the cellular biochemistry of GNE as a key enzyme in the biosynthesis of sialic acid has been thoroughly investigated, its role in normal muscle as well as in muscle with presumed defective GNE activity remains to be determined. The process by which *GNE* mutations lead to myopathy is certainly not well understood and controversy exists as to whether abnormal sialylation is a major part of the pathogenesis. Elucidating the metabolic basis may help in designing potential metabolic therapy before gene therapy becomes available. To elucidate the pathophysiology of HIBM it will be essential to unravel potential new pathways which involve GNE. A recent report by Krause *et al.* [36] localizes the GNE protein not only in the cytosolic part of the Golgi apparatus but also in the nucleus, thus revealing a new perspective on the function of this molecule. In another study, using a yeast two-hybrid assay with a human brain library, the collapsin response mediator protein 1 (CRMP-1) was found to bind to GNE [57], but the biological significance of this finding is not yet clear. A more comprehensive approach to identifying possible alternative GNE functions is the analysis of HIBM muscle tissue at the transcriptome and at the proteomic levels. Those ongoing studies could open new avenues for understanding HIBM pathogenesis.

Quadriceps sparing to the degree it occurs in HIBM is a distinctive characteristic. To date, no explanation exists for this phenotype, related to either embryogenesis and development [58], or GNE activity, which is similar to that in other affected muscles in HIBM [38]. Understanding this phenomenon may facilitate understanding of the pathomechanisms of HIBM, and have implications for therapy.

Other hereditary inclusion body myopathies

The feature of "rimmed" vacuolar myopathy is found in other hereditary neuromuscular conditions and few have a defined gene defect or a linkage site. We will briefly mention those conditions with clear genotypic and phenotypic characteristics that are not discussed elsewhere in this book.

Inclusion body myopathy, Paget disease, and frontotemporal dementia (IBMPFD)

This is an adult-onset syndrome presenting as proximal rimmed vacuolar myopathy and bone thickening [59]. Dementia appears about a decade later in more than one-third of the patients. This dominantly inherited disorder was found to be associated with several missense mutations in valosin-containing protein [60].

Proximal myopathy with ophthalmoplegia and congenital contractures

This dominantly inherited disorder, reported in only a single Swedish family [61], presents as newborn joint contractures which may resolve with time. Ophthalmoplegia is detected in the first decade of life and proximal weakness is observed later in adulthood. A histological diagnostic feature, in addition to the rimmed vacuoles, is lack of type 2A muscle fibers. A missense mutation in the myosin heavy chain IIA gene is responsible for this disorder [62].

Other conditions

The following hereditary inclusion body myopathies were reported in single families and have no known genotypic identification: scapuloperoneal syndrome [63]; dominantly inherited progressive proximal weakness [64]; myopathy and brain white matter abnormality [65]; and facioscapulohumeral syndrome [66)].

Acknowledgments

HIBM research in our Institute has been supported over the years by large donations from patients' support groups, Hadassah Chapters, Advancement of Research in Myopathies (ARM), and Neuromuscular Disease Foundation (NDF), for which we are thankful for both past and future support. Research grants were endowed by the Chief Scientist, Israeli Ministry of Health, U.S. Israel Binational Science Foundation (BSF), Hadasit-Applied Research Fund, Fritz Thyssen Foundation, Mizutani Foundation for Glycoscience, Association Française contre les Myopathies (AFM), German Israel Fund (GIF), and Israel Science Foundation (ISF).

References

1. R. C. Griggs, V. Askanas, S. DiMauro, *et al.*, Inclusion body myositis and myopathies. *Ann. Neurol.* **38** (1995), 705–715.
2. Z. Argov, D. Soffer, Hereditary inclusion body myopathies. In *Structural and Molecular Basis of Skeletal Muscle Disease*, ed. G. Karpati. (Basel: ISN Neuropath Press, 2002), pp. 274–276.
3. V. Askanas, W. K. Engel New advances in inclusion-body myositis. *Curr. Opin. Rheumatol.* **5** (1993), 732–741.
4. V. Askanas, W. K. Engel, Newest approaches to diagnosis of sporadic inclusion-body myositis and hereditary inclusion-body myopathies, including molecular-pathologic similarities to Alzheimer disease. In *Inclusion-Body Myositis and Myopathies*, eds. V. Askanas, G. Serratrice, W. K. Engel. (Cambridge: Cambridge University Press, 1998), pp. 3–78.
5. I. Eisenberg, N. Avidan, T. Potikha, *et al.*, The UDP-*N*-acetylglucosamine 2-epimerase/*N*-acetylemannosamine kinase is mutated in recessive hereditary inclusion body myopathy. *Nat. Genet.* **29** (2001), 83–87.
6. Z. Argov, I. Eisenberg, G. Grabov-Nardini, *et al.*, Hereditary inclusion body myopathy: the Middle Eastern genetic cluster. *Neurology* **60** (2003), 1519–1523.
7. I. Eisenberg, G. Grabov-Nardini, H. Hochner, *et al.*, Mutation spectrum of the GNE gene in hereditary inclusion body myopathy sparing the quadriceps. *Hum. Mutat.* **21** (2003), 99.
8. R. Amouri, A. Driss, K. Muruyama, M. Kefi, I. Nishino, F. Hentati, Allelic heterogeneity of GNE gene mutation in two Tunisian families with autosomal recessive inclusion body myopathy. *Neuromuscul. Disord.* **15** (2005), 361–363.

9. A. Broccolini, M. Pescatori, A. D'Amico, *et al.*, An Italian family with autosomal recessive inclusion-body myopathy and mutations in the GNE gene. *Neurology* **59** (2002), 1808–1809.

10. H. Tomimitsu, J. Shimizu, K. Ishikawa, N. Ohkoshi, I. Kanazawa, H. Mizusawa, Distal myopathy with rimmed vacuoles (DMRV). New GNE mutations and splice variant. *Neurology* **62** (2004), 1607–1610.

11. T. Kayashima, H. Matsuo, A. Satoh, *et al.*, Nonaka myopathy is caused by mutations in the UDP-*N*-acetylglucosamine-2-epimerase/*N*-acetylmannosamine kinase gene (GNE). *J. Hum. Genet.* **47** (2002), 77–79.

12. A. Arai, K. Tanaka, T. Ikeuchi, *et al.*, A novel mutation in the GNE gene and a linkage disequilibrium in Japanese pedigrees. *Ann. Neurol.* **52** (2002), 516–519.

13. I. Nishino, S. Noguchi, K. Murayama, *et al.*, Distal myopathy with rimmed vacuoles is allelic to hereditary inclusion body myopathy. *Neurology* **59** (2002), 1689–1693.

14. H. Tomimitsu, K. Ishikawa, J. Shimizu, N. Ohkoshi, I. Kanazawa, H. Mizusawa, Distal myopathy with rimmed vacuoles: novel mutations in the GNE gene. *Neurology* **59** (2002), 451–454.

15. I. Yabe, T. Higashi, S. Kikuchi, *et al.*, GNE mutations causing distal myopathy with rimmed vacuoles with inflammation. *Neurology* **61** (2003), 384–386.

16. S. Noguchi, Y. Keira, K. Murayama, *et al.*, Reduction of UDP-*N* acetylglucosamine 2-epimerase/*N*-acetylmannosamine kinase activity and sialylation in distal myopathy with rimmed vacuoles. *J. Biol. Chem.* **279** (2004), 11402–11407.

17. F. Saito, H. Tomimitsu, K. Arai, *et al.*, A Japanese patient with distal myopathy with rimmed vacuoles: missense mutations in the epimerase domain of the UDP-*N*-acetylglucosamine 2-epimerase *N*-acetylmannosaminekinase (GNE) gene accompanied by hyposialylation of skeletal muscle glycoproteins. *Neuromuscul. Disord.* **14** (2004), 158–161.

18. D. Darvish, P. Vahedifar, Y. Huo, Four novel mutations associated with autosomal recessive inclusion body myopathy (MIM: 600737). *Mol. Gen. Metab.* **77** (2002), 252–256.

19. O. M. Vasconcelos, R. Raju, M. C. Dalakas, GNE mutations in an American family with quadriceps-sparing IBM and lack of mutations in s-IBM. *Neurology* **59** (2002), 1776–1779.

20. R. Del Bo, P. Baron, A. Prelle, *et al.*, Novel missense mutation and large deletion of GNE gene in autosomal-recessive inclusion-body myopathy. *Muscle Nerve* **28** (2003), 113–117.

21. S. Krause, B. Schlotter-Weigel, M. C. Walter, *et al.*, A novel homozygous missense mutation in the GNE gene in a patient with quadriceps-sparing hereditary inclusion body myopathy associated with muscle inflammation. *Neuromuscul. Dis.* **13** (2003), 830–834.

22. A. Broccolini, E. Ricci, D. Cassandrini, *et al.*, Novel GNE mutations in Italian families with autosomal recessive hereditary inclusion-body myopathy. *Hum. Mutat.* **23** (2004), 632.

23. M. Huizing, G. Rakocevic, S. E. Sparks, *et al.*, Hypoglycosylation of alpha-dystroglycan in patients with hereditary IBM due to GNE mutations. *Mol. Genet. Metab.* **81** (2004), 196–202.

24. L. S. Ro, G. J. Lee-Chen, Y. R. Wu, M. Lee, P. Y. Hsu, C. M. Chen, Phenotypic variability in a Chinese family with rimmed vacuolar distal myopathy. *J. Neurol. Neurosurg. Psychiatry* **76** (2005), 752–755.

25. B. J. Kim, C. S. Ki, J. W. Kim, D. H. Sung, Y. C. Choi, S. H. Kim, Mutation analysis of the GNE gene in Korean patients with distal myopathy with rimmed vacuoles. *J. Hum. Genet.* **51** (2006), 137–140.

26. T. Liewluck, T. Pho-Iam, C. Limwongse, *et al.*, Mutation analysis of the GNE gene in distal myopathy with rimmed vacuoles (DMRV) patients in Thailand. *Muscle Nerve* **34** (2006), 775–778.

27. C. Chu, H. Kuo, T. Yeh, L. Ro, S. Chen, C. Huang, Heterozygous mutations affecting the epimerase domain of the GNE gene causing distal myopathy with rimmed vacuoles in a Taiwanese family. *Clin. Neurol. Neurosurg.* **109** (2007), 250–256.

28. S. Hinderlich, R. Stasche, R. Zeitler, W. Reutter, A bifunctional enzyme catalyzes the first two steps in *N*-acetylneuraminic acid biosynthesis of rat liver. Purification and characterization of UDP-*N*-acetylglucosamine 2 epimerase/*N*-acetylmannosamine kinase. *J. Biol. Chem.* **272** (1997), 24313–24318.

29. K. Effertz, S. Hinderlich, W. Reutter, Selective loss of either the epimerase or kinase activity of UDP-*N*-acetylglucosamine 2 epimerase/*N*-acetylmannosamine kinase due to site-directed mutagenesis based on sequence alignments. *J. Biol. Chem.* **274** (1999), 28771–28778.

30. T. Keppler, S. Hinderlich, J. Langner, R. Schwartz-Albiez, W. Reutter, M. Pawlita, UDP-GlcNAc 2-epimerase: a regulator of cell surface sialylation. *Science* **284** (1999), 1372–1376.

31. S. Kelm, R. Schauer, Sialic acids in molecular and cellular interactions. *Int. Rev. Cytol.* **175** (1997), 137–240.

32. S. Kornfeld, R. Kornfeld, E. Neufeld, P. J. O'Brien, The feedback control of sugar nucleotide biosynthesis in liver. *Proc. Natl. Acad. Sci. U.S.A.* **52** (1964), 371–379.

33. R. Seppala., V. P. Lehto, W. A. Gahl, Mutations in the human UDP-*N*-acetylglucosamine 2-epimerase gene define the disease sialuria and the allosteric site of the enzyme. *Am. J. Hum. Genet.* **64** (1999), 1563–1569.

34. M. Schwarzkopf, K. P. Knobeloch, E. Rohde, *et al.*, Sialylation is essential for early development in mice. *Proc. Natl. Acad. Sci. U.S.A.* **99** (2002), 5267–5270.

35. S. Krause, A. Aleo, S. Hinderlich, *et al.*, GNE protein expression and subcellular distribution are unaltered in HIBM. *Neurology* **69** (2007), 655–659.

36. S. Krause, S. Hinderlich, S. Amsili, *et al.*, Localization of UDP-GlcNAc 2-epimerase/ManAc kinase (GNE) in the Golgi complex and the nucleus of mammalian cells. *Exp. Cell Res.* **304** (2005), 365–379.

37. S. Hinderlich, I. Salama, I. Eisenberg, *et al.*, The homozygous M712T mutation of UDP-*N*-acetylglucosamine 2-epimerase/*N*-acetylmannosamine kinase results in reduced enzyme activities but not in altered cellular sialylation in hereditary inclusion body myopathy. *FEBS Lett.* **566** (2004), 105–109.

38. I. Salama, S. Hinderlich, Z. Shlomai, *et al.*, No overall hyposialylation in hereditary inclusion body myopathy myoblasts carrying the homozygous M712T GNE mutation. *Biochem. Biophys. Res. Commun.* **328** (2005), 221–226.

39. Z. Wang, Z. Sun, A. V. Li, K. J. Yarema, Roles for UDP-GlcNAc 2-epimerase/ManNAc 6-kinase outside of sialic acid biosynthesis: modulation of sialyltransferase and BiP expression, GM3 and GD3 biosynthesis, proliferation, and apoptosis, and ERK1/2 phosphorylation. *J. Biol. Chem.* **28137** (2006), 27016–27028.

40. A. Broccolini, C. Gliubizzi, E. Pavoni, *et al.*, α-Dystroglycan does not play a major pathogenic role in autosomal recessive hereditary inclusion-body myopathy. *Neuromuscul. Disord.* **15** (2005), 177–184.

41. E. Ricci, A. Broccolini, T. Gidaro, *et al.*, NCAM is hyposialylated in hereditary inclusion body myopathy due to GNE mutations. *Neurology* **66** (2006), 755–758.

42. M. Brockington, D. J. Blake, P. Prandini, *et al.*, Mutations in the fukutin-related protein gene (FKRP) cause a form of congenital muscular dystrophy with secondary laminin α2 deficiency and abnormal glycosylation of α-dystroglycan. *Am. J. Hum. Genet.* **69** (2001), 1198–1209.

43. D. Gagiannis, A. Orthmann, I. Danssmann, M. Schwarzkopf, W. Weidemann, R. Horstkorte, Reduced sialylation status in UDP-*N*-acetylglucosamine-2-epimerase/*N*-acetylmannosamine kinase (GNE)-deficient mice. *Glycoconj. J.* **24** (2007), 125–130.

44. M. C. Malicdan, S. Noguchi, I. Nonaka, Y. K. Hayashi, I. Nishino, A Gne knockout mouse expressing human GNE D176V mutation develops features similar to distal myopathy with rimmed vacuoles or hereditary inclusion body myopathy. *Hum. Mol. Genet.* **16** (2007), 2669–2682.

45. S. Amsili, Z. Shlomai, R. Levitzki, *et al.*, Characterization of hereditary inclusion body myopathy myoblasts: possible primary impairment of apoptotic events. *Cell Death Differ.* **14** (2007), 1916–1924.

46. Z. Argov, R. Yarom, "Rimmed vacuole myopathy" sparing the quadriceps: a unique disorder in Iranian Jews. *J. Neurol. Sci.* **64** (1984), 33–43.

47. N. Sunohara, I. Nonaka, N. Kamei, E. Satayoshi, Distal myopathy with rimmed vacuoles formation: a follow up study. *Brain* **112** (1989), 65–83.

48. M. Sadeh, M. Gadoth, H. Hadar, E. Ben David, Vacuolar myopathy sparing the quadriceps. *Brain* **116** (1993), 217–232.

49. K. Sivakumar, M. C. Dalakas, The spectrum of familial inclusion body myopathies in 13 families and a description of a quadriceps-sparing phenotype in non-Iranian Jews. *Neurology* **47** (1996), 977–984.

50. E. Satayoshi, N. Sunohara, I. Nonaka, Distal myopathy with rimmed vacuoles, inclusion-body myositis, and related disorders in Japan. In *Inclusion-Body Myositis and Myopathies*, eds. V. Askanas, G. Serratrice, W. K. Engel. (Cambridge: Cambridge University Press, 1998), pp. 244–251.

51. M. Y. Neufeld, M. Sadeh, B. Assa, M. Kushnir, A. D. Korczyn, Phenotypic heterogeneity in familial inclusion body myopathy. *Muscle Nerve* **18** (1995), 546–548.

52. M. Sadeh, Z. Argov, Hereditary inclusion body myopathy in Jews of Persian origin: clinical and laboratory data. In *Inclusion-Body Myositis and Myopathies*, eds. V. Askanas, G. Serratrice, W. K. Engel. (Cambridge: Cambridge University Press, 1998), pp. 191–199.

53. Z. Argov, M. Sadeh, I. Eisenberg, G. Karpati, S. Mitrani-Rosenbaum, Facial involvement in hereditary inclusion body myositis. *Neurology* **50** (1998), 1925–1926.

54. A. M. Cuervo, Autophagy: many paths to the same end. *Mol. Cell. Biochem.* **263** (2004), 55–72.

55. S. Sparks, G. Rakocevic, G. Joe, *et al.*, Intravenous immune globulin in hereditary inclusion body myopathy: a pilot study. *BMC Neurol.* **7** (2007), 3.

56. B. Galeano, R. Klootwijk, I. Manoli, *et al.*, Mutation in the key enzyme of sialic acid biosynthesis causes severe glomerular proteinuria and is rescued by *N*-acetylmannosamine. *J. Clin. Invest.* **117** (2007), 1585–1594.

57. W. Weidemann, U. Stelzl, U. Lisewski, *et al.*, The collapsin response mediator protein 1 (CRMP-1) and the promyelocytic leukemia zinc finger protein (PLZF) bind to UDP-*N*-acetylglucosamine 2-epimerase/*N*-acetylmannosamine kinase (GNE), the key enzyme of sialic acid biosynthesis. *FEBS Lett.* **580** (2006), 6649–6654.

58. I. R. Konigsberg, The embryonic origin of muscle. In *Myology*, Vol. 1, First Edition, eds. A. G. Engel, B. Q. Banker. (New York: McGraw-Hill, 1986), pp. 39–71.

59. G. D. J. Watts, M. Thorne, M. J. Kovach, A. Pestronk, V. E. Kimonis, Clinical and genetic heterogeneity in chromosome 9p associated hereditary inclusion body myopathy: exclusion of GNE and three other candidate genes. *Neuromuscul. Disord.* **13** (2003), 559–567.

60. G. D. Watts, J. Wymer, M. J. Kovach, *et al.*, Inclusion body myopathy associated with Paget disease of bone and frontotemporal dementia is caused by mutant valosin-containing protein. *Nat. Genet.* **36** (2004), 377–381.

61. N. Darin, M. Kyllerman, J. Wahlstrom, T. Martinsson, Autosomal dominant myopathy with congenital joint contractures, ophthalmoplegia, and rimmed vacuoles. *Ann. Neurol.* **44** (1998), 242–248.

62. T. Martinsson, A. Oldfors, N. Darin, *et al.*, Autosomal dominant myopathy: missense mutation (Glu-706-Lys) in the myosin heavy chain IIa gene. *Proc. Natl. Acad. Sci. U.S.A.* **97** (2000), 14614–14619.

63. K. C. Wilhelmsen, D. M. Blake, T. Lynch, *et al.*, Chromosome12-linked autosomal dominant scapuloperoneal muscular dystrophy. *Ann. Neurol.* **39** (1996), 507–520.

64. H. E. Neville, L. L. Baumbach, S. P. Ringel, *et al.*, Familial inclusion body myositis: evidence for autosomal dominant inheritance. *Neurology* **42** (1992), 897–902.

65. A. J. Cole, R. Kuzniecky, G. Karpati, S. Carpenter, E. Andermann, F. Andermann, Familial myopathy with changes resembling inclusion body myositis and periventricular leucoencephalopathy. *Brain* **111** (1988), 1025–1037.

66. D. McKee, G. Karpati, S. Carpenter, W. Johnson, Familial inclusion body myositis (IBM) mimics facioscapulohumeral dystrophy (FSHD) (abstr). *Neurology* **42** (Suppl 3) (1992), 302.

Chapter 27

Other myopathies

Giovanni Meola and Michael Swash

Introduction

Myopathies are often associated with skeletal wasting and muscle weakness, but muscle wasting can occur as a consequence of diseases such as malignant cancers (cachexia), connective tissue disease, vitamin and nutritional deficiencies, chronic illness or disuse.

Similarly, aging is associated with a progressive loss of muscle bulk associated with increasing frailty, weakness, and loss of functional independence. Wasting of skeletal muscle occurs for different reasons in different disorders. For example, loss of muscle mass may have a neurogenic origin, due to denervation, or can result from cytokine upregulation causing activation of protein degradative pathways, as in cancer-associated cachexia.

Muscles maintain their mass and function through a balance between protein synthesis and protein degradation, a concept that implies equal rates of anabolic and catabolic activity. Thus muscle bulk increases – hypertrophy – when protein synthesis exceeds protein degradation. These processes of muscle hypertrophy [1] and atrophy [2] depend on alterations in intracellular signaling. There are several major pathways leading to muscle breakdown, including the ubiquitin-proteasome pathway [3, 4], the calpain-calpastatin pathway [5], the lysosomal pathway [6] and apoptosis, also known as programmed cell death [7], and most clinical examples of muscle wasting can be explained by activation of one or more of these pathways. However, not all these pathways are activated in every condition.

In this chapter we will identify a number of different muscle wasting conditions not due to commonly defined conditions. We shall describe the mechanisms responsible for the loss of muscle mass and associated weakness in each instance.

Muscle wasting conditions

We have not attempted a description of every condition in which muscle wasting occurs. For example we have not described the muscle wasting associated with conditions such as sepsis, chronic obstructive pulmonary disease (COPD), chronic heart failure, chronic kidney disease or HIV-AIDS [8, 9]. Instead, we have focused on common muscle wasting conditions or circumstances, such as aging, disuse atrophy, malignant disease, and other conditions (nutritional deficiencies, amyloid myopathy, Marinesco–Sjögren myopathy, and connective tissue diseases).

Aging

Most serious consequences of aging relate to its effects on skeletal muscle. *Sarcopenia* is a term that has been widely used to describe the slow, progressive loss of muscle mass with advancing age. Sarcopenia is characterized not only by loss of skeletal muscle mass, but also by the gradual decline of functional properties of muscle, including a decrease in force capacity, reduction in maximum velocity of muscle fiber shortening, and a general slowing of contraction and relaxation.

This age-related decline in muscle function is considered to be related to a decrease in both muscle quantity (mass) and muscle quality. The latter term encompasses many factors including strength per muscle sectional area, age-dependent changes in fiber type proportions, and metabolic characteristics. Loss of muscle "mass" occurs through a decrease in contractile protein content due to loss of individual muscle fibers and a decrease in the size of the remaining fibers. This age-related loss of contractile tissue can also be described in terms of changes in rates of protein degradation and protein synthesis [10]. Thus it has been suggested that although increased muscle protein synthesis may occur in an attempt to maintain muscle mass, it is ineffective and so increased protein degradation is the main determinant of sarcopenia [11]. Various age-related changes in gene expression have been reported in age-related sarcopenia. These include impaired activity of mitochondrial proteins, abnormal differential expression of gene-regulating energy metabolism, decreased capacity to maintain DNA repair with aging, increased stress responses, the effects of altered immune/inflammatory responses, changes in RNA binding and splicing, and alterations of proteasome degradation [12].

Disorders of Voluntary Muscle, 8th edn., eds. George Karpati, David Hilton-Jones, Kate Bushby and Robert C. Griggs. Published by Cambridge University Press.

Another well-documented effect of aging in muscle is a decline in the size and number of muscle fibers. These changes affect the different muscle fiber types selectively, a process termed "age-related motor-unit remodeling," that involves muscle fiber denervation and consequent reinnervation [13]. This age-related change is thus primarily dependent on changes in motor neurons, associated with loss of the functional capacity to maintain the terminal innervation ratio. This remodeling of aged muscle fiber type distribution tends towards a slower phenotype. The muscle cross-sectional area is significantly reduced, especially in type II fibers (type II atrophy), whereas type I fibers remain relatively unaffected [14]. This process results in predominant loss of type II fibers with aging, leaving a higher proportion of type I fibers [15]. It is possible, also, that changes in post-translational modification of myosin play a role in the age-related changes to skeletal muscle [16].

Neurogenic muscle atrophy with aging

Although elderly people do not usually complain of muscle weakness the capacity to develop isometric force decreases with aging, such that it is about 30% reduced after the age of 60 years [17, 18]. Burke *et al.* [19] found that grip strength decreased by almost 50% between the ages of 25 and 79 years. These changes have been ascribed to loss of motor units found in histological studies of anterior horn cell numbers in aged persons during the twentieth century [20, 21]. There is little understanding of the cause of the increase in fibrous connective tissue found in aged muscle, but it has been suggested that this may correlate with age-related neurogenic change.

Muscle disuse, immobilization

A prolonged decrease in muscle contractile activity, such as occurs following the adoption of a sedentary lifestyle, during periods of prolonged bed rest, inactivity as a consequence of congestive heart failure, limb casting, and muscle unloading in tendon or joint injury, is associated with metabolic and structural changes in contractile proteins in skeletal muscle [22].

These disuse-induced changes result in a decreased muscle fiber cross-sectional area principally affecting type II fibers, with consequent decreased muscle mass, reduced force capacity, and a general shift toward a fast muscle phenotype [23].

The loss of muscle mass associated with disuse is believed to be mediated by a decrease in muscle protein synthesis and an increase in protein degradation. Evidence for inhibition of protein synthesis pathways includes a decrease in the levels of Akt and decreased Akt phosphorylation [24, 25]. On the other hand, increased protein degradation has been attributed to the activation of three distinct proteolytic pathways: the Ca^{2+}-dependent calpain pathway, the lysosomal cathepsin pathway, and the ubiquitin-proteasome system [26]. Experimental studies in animals suggest that whilst the ubiquitin-proteasome system may be responsible for the majority of the proteolysis associated with disuse, lysosomal proteases play an important role during prolonged periods of disuse. Only relatively small changes in the mRNA levels of Ca^{2+}-dependent proteases were observed during disease atrophy [23].

Eccentric exercise

Cachexia

Some muscle wasting disorders are characterized by a slow but progressive loss of muscle mass, such as occurs in sarcopenia, whereas other clinical conditions such as cachexia are associated with a more rapid loss of muscle structure and function.

Loss of muscle mass is sometimes complicated and hastened by other medical conditions, e.g., cardiovascular disease, and by medications, such as β-blockers, that can reduce the capacity to perform physical activity.

In cachexia, muscle wasting is associated with reduced protein synthesis, increased protein breakdown (increased catabolism) and increased oxidative damage. In cancer-associated cachexia, intervention with nutritional supplementation may improve the outcome in some patients [27]. Although increased protein catabolism is the main mechanism underlying muscle wasting in cachexia, the question has arisen whether abnormal trophism or a hypertrophism response might also have a pathogenic role. An impaired anabolic response might be the consequence of cancer-dependent reduced expression of positive regulators (e.g., MyoD) or over-expression of negative regulators, such as myostatin, of skeletal muscle growth.

Guttridge *et al.* [28] have recently suggested that impaired regeneration may be a key pathogenic factor for loss of muscle mass in cachexia. MyoD is a member of a skeletal muscle-specific family of transcription factors, also known as myogenic regulatory factors, that play a determinant role in myogenesis in cooperation with other regulators of muscle mass. In addition, a negative relation between myostatin mRNA expression and disease-related muscle wasting has been described [29]. The possible role of myostatin in the pathogenesis of cachexia remains to be elucidated.

Malignant disease

Carcinomatous myopathy

A nonspecific cachexia associated with muscle wasting and weakness is a common, non-specific, feature of advanced carcinomatous disease. *Carcinomatous neuromyopathy* is a term used to describe a heterogeneous group of conditions involving abnormalities of peripheral nerve, neuromuscular junction, and muscle, which are associated with, and may precede diagnosis of, a number of neoplasms. Paraneoplastic neurological syndromes are remote effects of cancer that, by definition, are not caused by direct tumor invasion or metastases, by infection, ischemia, metabolic and nutritional deficits, or by surgery or other cancer treatments. Immunological factors are believed to be important in the pathogenesis of paraneoplastic syndromes because antibodies and T-cell responses against nervous system antigens have been defined for many of these disorders. It is assumed that the immunological response is elicited by the ectopic expression of neuronal antigens by the tumor. Expression of these "onconeural" antigens is limited to the tumor and the nervous system. In most cases, at the time of presentation of the neurological symptoms, most patients presenting to the neurologist have not yet been diagnosed with cancer, and the diagnosis therefore depends initially on the recognition of the likely cause from the semiology of the clinical syndrome itself. In many other instances, however, the paraneoplastic syndrome develops in the context of diagnosed cancer or lymphoma, and complicates the clinical picture.

Detection of paraneoplastic antibodies can help diagnose the neurological syndrome as paraneoplastic and, in neurological practice, may direct the search for an underlying neoplasm. Often, it is appropriate to involve the oncologist or hematologist in the tumor work-up. On the other hand, in patients known to have cancer, the development of a paraneoplastic syndrome may herald recurrence of the tumor. In these patients, however, it is especially important to rule out metastatic complications of the known cancer first. Despite the presumed autoimmune etiology of paraneoplastic syndromes, treatment with various forms of immunotherapy have been disappointing, with a few exceptions. Rapid detection and immediate treatment of the underlying tumor appears to offer the best chance of stabilizing the patient and preventing further neurological deterioration.

Lambert–Eaton myasthenic syndrome (LEMS) associated with neoplasia often presents with clinical features "suggestive" of a "myopathy" and can represent an example of carcinomatous myopathy although, in many cases of LEMS, an idiopathic, autoimmune-based causation is evident without an underlying cancer (see below).

Lambert–Eaton myasthenic syndrome (LEMS)

Patients with LEMS present with proximal weakness of the lower extremities and fatigability. Bulbar symptoms may also occur, perhaps more frequently than reported in the literature, but bulbar features are generally milder than in myasthenia gravis. Respiratory weakness can occur. Deep tendon reflexes, especially those in the legs, are diminished or absent but may reappear after exercise. Autonomic features, especially dryness of the mouth, impotence, reduced sweating in a segmental or limb-based distribution, and mild/moderate ptosis, ultimately develop in 95% of patients. Approximately 70% of patients have cancer, almost always a small cell lung cancer (SCLC). Other tumors may cause LEMS, including small cell carcinomas of the prostate and cervix, lymphomas, and other adenocarcinomas. The incidence of LEMS in patients with SCLC is estimated to be around 3%. Clinically and serologically, the 30% without identifiable tumors are indistinguishable from paraneoplastic LEMS patients, although LEMS may have a more progressive course in patients with SCLC.

The typical pattern of electromyographic abnormalities is the hallmark of LEMS. This includes a low compound muscle action potential (CMAP) at rest with a decreased response at low rates of repetitive stimulation (3 Hz) and an incremental response at high rates of repetitive stimulation (50 Hz) or following 15–30 s of maximal voluntary contraction.

Most patients with LEMS have antibodies against P/Q-type calcium channels that are located presynaptically in the neuromuscular junction [30]. About 20% have anti-MysB antibodies reactive with the β-subunit of neuronal calcium channels [31].

In patients with paraneoplastic LEMS, effective management of the tumor frequently leads to neurological improvement, associated with reduced antibody levels. Symptomatic treatment with drugs that facilitate the release of acetylcholine from motor nerve terminals, such as 3,4-diaminopyridine (DAP), may be helpful. In a placebo-controlled randomized trial, DAP in a dose of 5–20 mg three to four times daily was effective as long-term treatment, alone or in combination with other treatments. The maximum recommended daily dose of DAP is 80 mg; at higher doses, seizures may occur. Cholinesterase inhibitors, such as pyridostigmine (30–60 mg, every 6 h), may improve dryness of the mouth and sometimes partially relieve fatigue and weakness. Removal of the pathogenic anti-P/Q-type calcium channel antibodies by plasma exchange or intravenous immunoglobulin (IVIg) can give quick but transient relief. In general, LEMS responds less favorably to immunotherapy than does myasthenia gravis.

Nutritional myopathy

Vitamin D deficiency

Muscle weakness is common in disorders of calcium and phosphorus homeostasis, including primary and secondary hyperparathyroidism, hypoparathyroidism, and other abnormalities of bone metabolism. In contrast to hyperparathyroidism and osteomalacia, hypoparathyroidism has only rarely been associated with overt myopathy.

Primary hyperparathyroidism and osteomalacia

The myopathy associated with primary hyperparathyroidism or osteomalacia is characterized by the gradual onset of symmetrical proximal weakness with atrophy. Significant lower-extremity weakness leads to a waddling gait or even to the inability to walk in some patients.

Besides proximal weakness and atrophy, examination of patients with hyperparathyroidism often reveals brisk muscle stretch reflexes with flexor plantar responses, and there are rare reports of spasticity and extensor plantar responses. In addition, 29%–57% of patients experience stocking and glove impairment of pain or vibratory sensation and decreased muscle stretch reflexes suggestive of an underlying peripheral neuropathy. Finally, neurobehavioral abnormalities, including memory loss, poor concentration, personality changes, inappropriate behavior, anxiety, and hallucinations, can also occur. *Secondary hyperparathyroidism* can occur in patients with chronic renal failure, who may develop weakness similar to that observed in primary hyperparathyroidism and osteomalacia. Lower-extremity weakness predominates early on with eventual progression to involvement of all four limbs.

The *myopathy of vitamin D deficiency* may present with a limb-girdle pattern of weakness that may be painful [32]. This syndrome is important to recognize and occurs, for example, in vegans living in developed western societies when sunlight exposure is reduced by wearing occlusive culturally important clothing. Vitamin D deficiency may also occur with reduced absorption in steatorrhea, or when certain drugs that interfere with Vitamin D metabolism are used, for example phenytoin.

Myopathy secondary to hypoparathyroidism is unusual, although paresthesias and tetany secondary to hypocalcemia are characteristic. There are only a few reports of mild proximal weakness in patients with hypoparathyroidism. Syriou *et al.* [33] described ten patients with myopathy and raised creatine kinase associated with hypocalcemia and hypoparathyroidism.

Primary hyperparathyroidism is most often caused by a single overactive parathyroid gland, usually an adenoma or, uncommonly, a carcinoma. In 15% of cases, diffuse hyperplasia of all the parathyroid glands is the cause. Secondary hyperparathyroidism can result from resistance to the metabolic action of parathyroid hormone leading to hypocalcemia, hyperphosphatemia, and osteomalacia. Chronic renal failure is not infrequently associated with secondary hyperparathyroidism. In chronic renal failure, reduction of 1,25-dihydroxy vitamin D conversion causes decreased intestinal absorption of calcium and decreased renal phosphorus clearance, which leads to secondary hyperparathyroidism and osteomalacia.

Hypoparathyroidism is seen in a number of conditions, including complications of thyroid or parathyroid surgery, thyroid radiation therapy, drugs, sepsis, infiltrative diseases of the parathyroid, and autoimmune, hereditary, or developmental disorders.

The mechanism of weakness in hyperparathyroidism and osteomalacia is not known. Some authors have suggested a neurogenic basis, but others have suspected a myopathic process. Muscle biopsies usually demonstrate nonspecific myopathic features such as type 2 fiber atrophy. Elevated levels of parathyroid hormone are associated with impaired energy production, transfer, and utilization, and enhanced muscle proteolysis.

In addition, parathyroid hormone may diminish the sensitivity of contractile myofibrillary proteins to calcium and activate a cytoplasmic protease, thus impairing the bioenergetics of muscle [34].

In hyperparathyroidism, serum calcium levels are usually elevated and serum phosphate levels are low, whereas urinary excretion of calcium is low and excretion of phosphate is high. In patients with concurrent hypoalbuminemia, serum calcium levels may be normal, and in these cases ionized calcium should be measured and is typically elevated. Increased urinary excretion of cyclic adenosine monophosphate in the presence of hypercalcemia is indicative of hyperparathyroidism.

In osteomalacia, serum calcium levels are low or normal and serum phosphate is variably low depending on the degree of secondary hyperparathyroidism. Serum vitamin D levels are also usually low. Urinary excretion of calcium is low (except in cases secondary to renal tubular acidosis), whereas excretion of phosphate is high.

Electromyography can be normal or show small polyphasic motor unit potentials with early recruitment of units during minimal effort, suggestive of a myopathic process.

Muscle biopsies usually demonstrate nonspecific myopathic features with atrophy predominantly of type 2 fibers but occasionally also of type 1 fibers.

Parathyroidectomy is the treatment of choice for symptomatic patients with primary hyperparathyroidism. Patients with secondary hyperparathyroidism usually improve with vitamin D and calcium replacement or, if they are in end-stage renal failure, with renal transplantation.

Likewise, the myopathy associated with osteomalacia responds well to vitamin D and calcium replacement and to treatment of the underlying condition responsible. The rare myopathy associated with hypoparathyroidism improves following correction of hypocalcemia and hyperphosphatemia with vitamin D and calcium.

Vitamin E deficiency myopathy

Vitamin E deficiency may be associated with a primary myopathy in humans [35], in addition to other neurological features, especially a painful sensory neuropathy. There are also a number of hereditary conditions which cause this deficiency [36]. Vitamin E deficiency is rare in humans, requiring a chronic deficiency, but may be seen in malabsorption syndromes such as short gut syndrome, chronic cholestasis, cystic fibrosis, and abetalipoproteinemia.

Vitamin E deficiency myopathy has been described in a 7-year-old boy with a complex syndrome characterized by severe malabsorption from birth, who developed progressive external ophthalmoplegia, proximal muscle weakness, peripheral neuropathy, hyporeflexia, and bilateral Babinski signs. Abnormalities on neurological examination included elevated creatine phosphokinase and aldolase, slowed distal sensory latencies, type 2 muscle fiber atrophy, and a plasma vitamin E level of only 8 μg/dl (normal, 550–1500 μg/dl). Treatment with oral water-solubilized vitamin E 400 IU daily, representing more than 50 times the normal daily intake, was begun, with repeat laboratory studies at 3-month intervals. Over a 16-month period, plasma vitamin E content gradually increased to 350 μg/dl, associated with clinical improvement and a reduction in creatine kinase level in the blood.

Alcoholic myopathy

Alcoholic myopathy has been described as occurring in two forms. Acute alcoholic myopathy is a rare condition affecting approximately 1% of alcoholics and is characterized by acute myalgias, weakness, very high creatine kinase levels, and often by renal impairment with associated myoglobinuria and rhabdomyolysis implicating morbidity and mortality. Muscle biopsy reveals acute muscle necrosis, and varying degrees of inflammatory infiltrate affecting both types of muscle fibers [37]. However, it is worth noting that these severe symptoms usually normalize after alcohol withdrawal and under general medical support.

In contrast, chronic ingestion of more than 100g/day alcohol for more than 10 years may lead to progressive proximal weakness and muscle atrophy involving legs and arms. This syndrome is characterized by decreased muscle strength, but a normal or only slightly elevated creatine kinase level. This chronic alcoholic myopathy is not associated with extensive muscle necrosis. Moreover, it is worth noting that, in contrast to acute alcoholic myopathy, type 2b fibers (anaerobic, glycolytic, fast-twitch) are mainly affected, whereas type I fibers – aerobic, slow-twitch fibers – are relatively resistant.

The etiology of the alcoholic myopathy is probably multifactorial, including protein malnutrition, metabolic effects related to the possible role of acetaldehyde, decreased amino acid availability, and reduced insulin-like growth factor (IGF-I) activity, as well as free-radical-induced membrane damage. Ethanol-induced protein metabolism disturbances have been suggested as mediated by reduced IGF-I factor activity. Insulin is itself a potent anabolic hormone, capable of stimulating protein synthesis in striated muscles. Thus, IGF-I, as a mediator of the synthesis of *muscle* proteins, modulates striated muscle metabolism. Moreover, IGF-1 is believed to play an antiapoptotic role in myocytes as well as a trophic role during differentiation of myoblasts into myotubes. Impairment of protein synthesis, resulting from acute and chronic ethanol intoxication, is also thought to be associated with upregulated IGF-binding protein activity. These proteins, whether phosphorylated or non-phosphorylated, inhibit IGF-I-induced protein synthesis, through IGF-I receptor effects, and prevent IGF-I-stimulated glucose uptake in myoblasts.

Another possible pathogenetic pathway implicated in alcohol intoxication involves free-radical-mediated muscle damage. Reactive oxygen species (ROS) have been considered to be associated with the decrease in cardiac creatine kinase activity in acute ethanol intoxication.

Alcohol-exposed muscle fiber membranes have shown impaired calcium uptake and release, and also decreased Na^{+}/K^{+}-ATPase activity. Another important factor in the pathogenesis of myopathic change in alcoholism is Ca^{2+}-mediated signaling. It has been suggested that increased Ca^{2+}-ATPase (SERCA1) activity associated with chronic, excessive ethanol ingestion may result from a specific process of tolerance and adaptation in alcoholics. Similarly this would explain the absence of leakage of muscle creatine kinase related to chronic ethanol intoxication in contrast to the acute myopathy [38].

Amyloid myopathy

Amyloid myopathy is a rare disorder of adults and diagnosis is often difficult or not suspected [39]. Myopathy results from the deposition of insoluble amyloid fibrils in skeletal muscle, in most cases as a consequence of the secretion of immunoglobulin light chains associated with plasma cell dyscrasia (primary or AL amyloidosis). Cases associated with inherited forms of amyloidosis due to transthyretin or gelsolin mutations have also been described. In primary amyloidosis, amyloid myopathy may be present in the context of multi-organ impairment, but rarely it constitutes the only clinical manifestation. It is characterized by progressive proximal weakness with increased creatine kinase level, mimicking polymyositis or limb-girdle muscular dystrophy; other typical features are muscle pseudohypertrophy, which has a characteristic "hard" feel, and macroglossia. Atypical syndromes with unusual presentation including rhabdomyolysis have been reported [40].

Amyloid myopathy is probably an underdiagnosed condition and it should be considered in the differential diagnosis of any adult with progressive myopathy. The presence of a monoclonal protein in serum or urine is an important diagnostic clue in this myopathy and we recommend immune electrophoresis of serum and urine as part of the routine investigation for all chronic progressive myopathies of uncertain origin, even including isolated hyperCKemia and rhabdomyolysis.

Several mechanisms have been proposed to explain the clinical features associated with deposition of amyloid in skeletal muscle, such as impairment of microvascular circulation due to infiltration of small vessels in muscle and peripheral nerves, inducing ischemic myopathy or denervation atrophy. Another proposed mechanism is mechanical interference caused by amyloid deposits in muscle. Immune-mediated mechanisms have been postulated in two patients with amyloid myopathy and rhabdomyolysis. Autoantibody binding to muscle proteins, or light chain deposition in the membrane of muscle fibers has also been proposed. Sundblad *et al.* [41] reported a 54-year-old man who, in the context of multi-organ impairment with acute renal failure, developed an episode of rhabdomyolysis with proximal muscular weakness. Immunoblot studies revealed serum antiskeletal muscle antibody reactivity, with binding to several muscular proteins. A putative antibody-mediated component was therefore postulated in the pathogenesis of rhabdomyolysis in this case.

Marinesco–Sjögren myopathy

Marinesco–Sjögren syndrome (MSS, MIM 248800) is a multi-organ disorder with autosomal recessive inheritance [42]. It is characterized by cerebellar ataxia, mental retardation, congenital cataracts, short stature, and frequently hypogonadism. Muscle involvement in MSS patients was reported many years ago, but the importance and progressive nature of this feature in MSS has been underestimated, probably because of the complex central nervous system (CNS) symptoms and signs. However, muscle atrophy has been reported in half of the patients and most muscle biopsy reports have described myopathic changes [43]. Ultrastructurally, the muscle pathology in MSS is rather distinctive with autophagic rimmed vacuolar changes and a peculiar dense membrane surrounding occasional nuclei [44, 45]. Other nuclear changes and apoptosis have also been reported [46].

Muscle weakness in MSS was originally considered to be a consequence of CNS-mediated hypotonia and a myopathic component was not fully documented until the report by Sewry *et al.* [44]. Mahjneh *et al.* [47] also found a rimmed vacuolar myopathy in a muscle biopsy study of nine Finnish patients. Muscle computed tomography (CT) showed that the distal muscles of the extremities were affected first, with predominant involvement of interossei, thenar, and peroneus muscles, and with pes planovalgus. Proximal muscles became involved later. Gracilis and sartorius muscles were also affected although, curiously, these muscles are rarely involved in other muscular dystrophies [48]. Neuropathy was neither clinically nor pathologically evident in the muscles studied.

In conclusion, myopathy is an early feature of MSS, and irreversible replacement of muscle tissue with fat and connective tissue is more extensive than expected from previous studies.

Connective tissue disease

Systemic sclerosis (SSc)

Skeletal muscle involvement is a common feature in systemic sclerosis (SSc). Muscle weakness is found in up to 90% of SSc patients when systematically assessed. Clinical, biological, and electromyographic features are similar to those of polymyositis or dermatomyositis, except for a very high proportion of patients with mild symptoms. SSc-associated myopathy is more prevalent in diffuse SSc and may be associated with cardiomyopathy. The pathophysiological process leading to SSc-associated myopathy is likely to be complex, given the heterogeneity of the muscle pathology, including signs of microangiopathy, with inflammatory infiltrates in about half of the cases, and prominent interstitial fibrosis. Conflicting results have been reported regarding the correlation between the clinical presentation and the pathological muscle features. Nevertheless there is general agreement that histologically proven inflammatory myopathies usually regress with high-dose corticosteroid therapy, or even low-dose steroids when there are detectable anti-PM/Scl antibodies. In contrast, non-inflammatory myopathies often result in milder clinical expression but do not respond to immunosuppressive treatment [49].

Systemic lupus erythematosus (SLE)

Myopathy occurs in up to 50% of SLE patients and is associated with elevated serum creatine kinase, proximal muscle weakness, and ribonucleoprotein antibodies [50]. Muscle biopsy in patients with SLE may show inflammation, vasculitic changes of small vessels, type 2 fiber atrophy, vessel wall thickening, neurogenic muscular atrophy and, rarely, inclusion bodies. These highly variable histopathological findings suggest different pathological mechanisms due to SLE itself, SLE-related conditions and treatment, and independent disorders.

Myopathy in SLE most commonly results from vasculitis of the small vessels in muscle, with pathology reminiscent of dermatomyositis, although on rare occasions the pathophysiology more closely resembles polymyositis with inflammatory involvement of muscle fibers themselves. These findings should be distinguished pathologically from medication-associated myopathy resulting from steroids or hydroxychloroquine sulfate therapy.

Rheumatoid disease

Myositis can occur as part of an overlap syndrome, in which either polymyositis or dermatomyositis is associated with another connective tissue disorder such as scleroderma, mixed connective tissue disease, Sjögren syndrome, systemic lupus erythematosus, and rheumatoid arthritis [51]. Effects on the skin, joints, kidneys, eyes, and salivary glands are identical to those seen for each of these disorders in isolation, and the serological abnormalities are also similar. Weakness in patients with these connective tissue diseases is actually relatively common and is usually related to disuse secondary to pain as well as type 2 fiber atrophy from chronic steroid use. Nevertheless, true myositis does occur and it is important to document the nature of the muscle involvement with serological and electromyographic studies and (often) muscle biopsy. The prognosis is often related to the underlying disorder; treatment may have to be modified based on the associated condition.

Sarcoid myopathy and granulomatous myopathy

Sarcoidosis is a systemic inflammatory disorder of unknown cause that is characterized by noncaseating epithelioid granulomas on microscopy. Neurological presentation is rare, affecting only about 5% of all cases and involving the meninges, hypothalamus, pituitary gland, spinal cord, and cranial and peripheral nerves. Cranial neuropathies, particularly Bell's palsy, are the most frequent manifestation of neurosarcoidosis, but myopathy occurs in 7%–12% of neurosarcoidosis patients alongside other neurological signs and symptoms. However, muscle involvement in sarcoidosis usually remains asymptomatic. As most patients with a neurological manifestation of sarcoidosis (97%) also have signs of systemic involvement, isolated muscle manifestations of sarcoidosis seem to be a rarity.

Table 27.1. Granulomatous myopathy

Primary granulomatous myopathy (sarcoid myopathy), without granuloma manifestation in other organs
Secondary granulomatous myopathy
Sarcoidosis
Vasculitis (Churg–Strauss syndrome, Wegener granulomatosis)
Connective tissue disease (progressive systemic sclerosis, rheumatoid arthritis)
Inflammatory bowel disease (Crohn disease, primary biliary cirrhosis)
Infectious myopathy (fungus infections, leprosy, syphilis, tuberculosis)
Autoimmune overlap syndrome with myasthenia gravis, myocarditis, thyroiditis, and thymoma
Inorganic agents (aluminum, beryllium, titanium)

In one case a muscle biopsy taken from the left brachial biceps muscle disclosed noncaseating epithelioid granulomas, multinuclear giant cells, and lymphoplasmacellular infiltration. Immunohistochemistry demonstrated abundant lymphocyte immunoreactivity for the T-cell-associated antigens CD3 and CD45R0, and a few scattered CD20-positive B-cells. Incubation with an antibody against the CD68 antigen disclosed several macrophages.

The serum angiotensin converting enzyme (ACE) level may not be specific as a diagnostic test, but its sensitivity has been established at least for pulmonary sarcoidosis. The presence of noncaseating muscle granulomas is the diagnostic hallmark for sarcoid myopathy. However, incidental noncaseating granulomas have been found in "blind," and asymptomatic muscle biopsy specimens in as many as 50% of sarcoid patients without clinical evidence of muscle disease.

Sarcoid myopathy can present in three distinct forms:

1. Subacute myositis with proximal weakness, myalgias, and fever
2. Chronic myopathy with diffuse atrophy or occasional pseudohypertrophy and progressive, symmetrical weakness, usually with normal serum creatine kinase, and granulomatous inflammation on muscle biopsy
3. Nodular sarcoid myopathy with palpable nodes, which rarely lead to muscle pain or impaired muscular function

Chronic myopathy is the most common form associated with systemic sarcoidosis. Although granulomatous myopathy is commonly associated with sarcoidosis, other granulomatous myopathies have to be considered in the differential diagnosis and must be excluded (Table 27.1).

Granulomatous myopathy without evidence of sarcoidosis was associated with milder, predominantly distal weakness that responded poorly to steroids. Whether an isolated granulomatous myopathy represents a disease entity in its own right or an isolated manifestation of sarcoidosis remains controversial.

The etiology of sarcoidosis and the reason for selective organ involvement are not known. Steroids remain the mainstay of therapy for progressive or persistent sarcoidosis. Most patients with sarcoid myopathy respond to steroid treatment, but the response and course of the disease are unpredictable and often require an extended course of treatment [52]. In cases with insufficient response to steroid therapy, methotrexate (7.5–15 mg per week) may provide benefit, if only to reduce the steroid dose.

References

1. S. C. Kandarian, R. W. Jackman, Intracellular signalling during skeletal muscle atrophy. *Muscle Nerve* **33** (2006), 155–165.
2. R. Bassel-Duby, E. N. Olson, Signaling pathways in skeletal muscle remodeling. *Ann. Rev. Biochem* **75** (2006), 19–37.
3. P. R. Cao, H. J. Kim, S. H. Lecker, Ubiquitin-protein ligases in muscle wasting. *Int. J. Biochem. Cell. Biol.* **37** (2005), 2088–2097.
4. M. J. Tisdale, The ubiquitin-proteasome pathway as a therapeutic target for muscle wasting. *J. Support. Oncol.* **3** (2005), 209–217.
5. M. Bartoli, I. Richard, Calpains in muscle wasting. *Int. J. Biochem. Cell. Biol.* **37** (2005), 2115–2133.
6. S. Busquets, C. Garcia-Martinez, M. Olivan, *et al.*, Overexpression of UCP3 in both murine and human myotubes in linked with the activation of proteolytic systems: a role in muscle wasting? *Biochim. Biophys. Acta* **1760** (2006), 253–258.
7. P. M. Siu, S. E. Always, Deficiency of the Bax gene attenuates denervation-induced apoptosis. *Apoptosis* **11** (2006), 967–981.
8. G. Mantovani, S. Anker, A. Inui, *et al.*, *Cachexia and Wasting: A Modern Approach.* (New York, NY: Springer, 2006.)
9. W. E. Mitch, Proteolytic mechanisms, not malnutrition, cause loss of muscle mass in kidney failure. *J. Renal Nutr.* **16** (2006), 208–211.
10. K. E. Yarasheski, Exercise, aging, and muscle protein metabolism. *J. Gerontol.* **58A** (2003), M918–M922.
11. S. R. Kimball, J. P. O'Malley, J. C. Anthony, *et al.*, Assessment of biomarkers of protein anabolism in skeletal muscle during the life span of the rat: sarcopenia despite elevated protein synthesis. *Am. J. Physiol. Endocrinol. Metab.* **287** (2004), 772–780.
12. P. G. Giresi, E. J. Stevenson, J. Theilhaber, *et al.*, Identification of a molecular signature of sarcopenia. *Physiol. Genomics* **21** (2005), 255–263.
13. A. A. Vandervoort, Aging of the human neuromuscular system. *Muscle Nerve* **25** (2002), 17–25.
14. E. I. Dedkov, A. B. Borisov, B. M. Carlson, Dynamic of post-denervation atrophy of young and old skeletal muscles: differential responses of fiber types and muscle types. *J. Gerontol. A. Biol. Sci. Med. Sci.* **58** (2003), 984–991.
15. K. M. Chan, T. J. Doherty, W. F. Brown, Contractile properties of human motor units in health, aging and disease. *Muscle Nerve* **24** (2001), 1113–1133.

16. P. Höök, V. Sriramoju, L. Larsson, Effects of aging on actin sliding speed on myosin from single skeletal muscle cells of mice, rats and humans. *Am. J. Physiol. Cell. Physiol.* **280** (2001), C782–C788.

17. M. J. Campbell, A. J. McComas, F. Petito, Physiological basis of ageing in muscles. *J. Neurol. Neurosurg. Psychiatry* **36** (1973), 174–182.

18. C. Bosco, P. V. Komi, Influence of ageing on the mechanical behaviour of leg extensor muscles. *Eur. J. Appl. Physiol.* **45** (1980), 209–219.

19. R. E. Burke, W. W. Tuttle, C. W. Thompson, *et al.*, The relation of grip strength and grip strength endurance to age. *J. Appl. Physiol.* **5** (1953), 618–630.

20. D. Duncan, A determination of the number of nerve fibers in the eighth thoracic and largest lumbar ventral roots of the albino rat. *J. Comp. Neurol.* **59** (1934), 47–60.

21. E. Gardner, Decrease in human neurones with age. *Anat. Rec.* **77** (1940), 529–536.

22. B. J. Krawiec, R. A. Frost, T. C. Vary, *et al.*, Hindlimb casting decreases muscle mass in part by proteasome-dependent proteolysis but independent of protein synthesis. *Am. J. Physiol. Endocrinol. Metab.* **289** (2005), E969–E980.

23. E. J. Stevenson, P. G. Giresi, A. Koncarevic, *et al.*, Global analysis of gene expression patterns during disuse atrophy in rat skeletal muscle. *J. Physiol. (Lond.)* **551** (2003), 33–48.

24. S. C. Bodine, E. Latres, S. Baumhueter, *et al.*, Identification of ubiquitin ligases required for skeletal muscle atrophy. *Science* **294** (2001), 1704–1708.

25. S. C. Bodine, T. N. Stitt, M. Gonzales, *et al.*, Akt/mTOR pathway is a crucial regulator of skeletal muscle hypertrophy and can prevent muscle atrophy in vivo. *Nat. Cell. Biol.* **3** (2001), 1014–1019.

26. M. B. Reid, Response of the ubiquitin-proteasome pathway to changes in muscle activity. *Am. J. Physiol. Regul. Integr. Comp. Physiol.* **288** (2005), R1423–R1431.

27. M. A. Van Bokhorst-de van der Schueren, Nutritional support strategies for malnourished cancer patients. *Eur. J. Oncol. Nurs.* **9**:2 (2005), 74–83.

28. D. C. Guttridge, M. V. Mayo, L. W. Madrid, *et al.*, NF-kappaB-induced loss of MyoD messenger RNA possible role in muscle decay and cachexia. *Science* **289** (2000), 2363–2366.

29. K. A. Readon, J. Davis, R. M. Kapsa, *et al.*, Myostatin, insulin-like growth factor-1, and leukaemia inhibitory factor mRNAs are upregulated in chronic human disuse muscle atrophy. *Muscle Nerve* **24** (2001), 893–899.

30. M. Motomura, I. Johnston, B. Lang, *et al.*, An improved diagnostic assay for Lambert-Eaton myasthenic syndrome. *J. Neurol. Neurosurg. Psychiatry* **58** (1995), 85–87.

31. M. R. Rosenfeld, E. Wong, J. Dalmau, *et al.*, Cloning and characterization of a Lambert-Eaton myasthenic syndrome antigen. *Ann. Neurol.* **33** (1993), 113–120.

32. J. J. van der Heyden, A. Verrips, H. J. ter Laak, *et al.*, Hypovitaminosis D-related myopathy in immigrant teenagers. *Neuropediatrics* **35** (2004), 290–292.

33. V. Syriou, A. Kolitsa, L. Pantazi, *et al.*, Hypoparathyroidism in a patient presenting with severe myopathy and skin rash. Case report and review of the literature. *Hormones* **4** (2005), 161–164.

34. E. E. Ubogu, R. L. Ruff, H. J. Kaminski, Endocrine myopathies (hyper- and hypofunctioning of adrenal, thyroid, pituitary, and parathyroid glands and iatrogenic steroid myopathy). In *Myology*, Third Edition, eds. A. G. Engel, C. Franzini-Armstrong. (New York: McGraw-Hill Inc., 2004), pp. 1713–1738.

35. L. G. Tomasi, Reversibility of human myopathy caused by vitamin E deficiency. *Neurology* **29** (1979), 1182–1186.

36. N. Gordon, Hereditary vitamin-E deficiency. *Dev. Med. Child Neurol.* **43** (2001), 133–135.

37. C. H. Lang, S. R. Kimball, R. A. Frost, *et al.*, Alcohol myopathy: impairment of protein synthesis and translation initiation. *Int. J. Biochem. Cell. Biol.* **33** (2001), 457–473.

38. K. Ohlendieck, S. Harmon, M. Koll, *et al.*, An essential role for Rho, Rac, and Cdc42 GTPases in cell cycle progression through G1. *Metabolism* **52** (2003), 1102–1112.

39. J. E. Chapin, M. Kornfeld, A. Harris, Amyloid myopathy: characteristic features of a still underdiagnosed disease. *Muscle Nerve* **31** (2005), 266–272.

40. C. Rodolico, A. Mazzeo, A. Toscano, *et al.*, Amyloid myopathy presenting with rhabdomyolysis: evidence of complement activation. *Neuromuscul. Disord.* **16** (2006), 514–517.

41. A. Sundblad, A. Porwit, M. Ostad, *et al.*, Antibody reactivities to skeletal muscle proteins in a patient with k light chain secreting multiple myeloma, generalised amyloidosis and rhabdomyolysis. *Eur. J. Haematol.* **67** (2001), 189–193.

42. C. Lagier-Tourenne, L. Tranebaerg, D. Chaigne, *et al.*, Homozygosity mapping of Marinesco-Sjogren syndrome to 5q31. *Eur. J. Hum. Genet.* **11** (2003), 770–778.

43. D. W. Superneau, W. Wertelecki, H. Zellweger, *et al.*, Myopathy in Marinesco-Sjogren syndrome. *Eur. Neurol.* **26** (1987), 8–16.

44. C. A. Sewry, T. Voit, V. Dubowitz, Myopathy with unique ultrastructural feature in Marinesco-Sjögren syndrome. *Ann. Neurol.* **24** (1988), 576–580.

45. A. Komiyama, I. Nonaka, K. Hirayama, Muscle pathology in Marinesco-Sjögren syndrome. *J. Neurol. Sci.* **89** (1989), 103–113.

46. K. Sasaki, K. Suga, S. Tsugawa, *et al.*, Muscle pathology in Marinesco-Sjögren syndrome: a unique ultrastructural feature. *Brain Dev.* **18** (1996), 64–67.

47. I. Mahjneh, A. K. Anttonen, M. Somer, *et al.*, Myopathy is a prominent feature in Marinesco-Sjögren syndrome. A muscle computed tomography study. *J. Neurol.* **253** (2006), 301–306.

48. M. Swash, M. M. Brown, C. Thakkar, CT muscle imaging and the clinical assessment of neuromuscular disease. *Muscle Nerve* **18** (1995), 708–714.

49. B. Ranque, F. J. Authier, A. Berenze, *et al.*, Systemic sclerosis-associated myopathy. *Ann. N. Y. Acad. Sci.* **1108** (2007), 268–282.

50. M. J. Garton, D. A. Isenberg, Clinical features of lupus myositis versus idiopathic myositis: a review of 30 cases. *Br. J. Rheumatol.* **36** (2000), 1067–1074.

51. F. L. Mastaglia, M. J. Garlepp, B. A. Phillips, *et al.*, Inflammatory myopathies: clinical, diagnostic and therapeutic aspects. *Muscle Nerve* **27** (2003), 407–425.

52. C. Berger, C. Sommer, H. M. Meinck, Isolated sarcoid myopathy. *Muscle Nerve* **26** (2002), 553–556.

Index